Instructional Course Lectures

Volume 46 1997

American Academy
of Orthopaedic Surgeons

Instructional Course Lectures

Volume 46 1997

Edited by
Dempsey S. Springfield, MD
Professor and Chairman
Leni & Peter W. May Department of Orthopaedics
Mount Sinai Medical Center
New York, New York

American Academy
of Orthopaedic Surgeons
6300 North River Road
Rosemont, IL 60018

American Academy of Orthopaedic Surgeons

Instructional Course Lectures
Volume 46

Vice President, Educational Programs: Mark W. Wieting
Director, Department of Publications: Marilyn L. Fox, PhD
Senior Editor: Bruce Davis
Associate Senior Editors: Joan Abern, Lisa Moore
Production Manager: Loraine Edwalds
Production Coordinators: David M. Stanley, Sophie Tosta
Production Assistant: Jana Ronayne
Layout and Design: Geraldine Dubberke
Publications Secretary: Tom Pender

ISBN 0-89203-161-1

Contributors

Robert S. Adelaar, MD, Professor of Surgery, Vice Chairman, Department of Orthopedics, Medical College of Virginia, Richmond, Virginia

Gina B. Aharonoff, MPH, Assistant Director, Geriatric Hip Fracture Research Group, Hospital for Joint Diseases, New York, New York

David W. Altchek, MD, Assistant Attending Orthopaedic Surgeon, Sports Medicine and Shoulder Service, The Hospital for Special Surgery, New York, New York

David Amiel, PhD, Professor of Orthopaedics, University of California San Diego, Department of Orthopaedics, La Jolla, California

Howard S. An, MD, Director of Spine Surgery, Associate Professor of Orthopedic Surgery, Medical College of Wisconsin, Milwaukee, Wisconsin

David C. Ayers, MD, Associate Professor of Orthopaedic Surgery, Director of Joint Replacement Surgery, SUNY Department of Orthopaedic Surgery, SUNY Health Science Center, Syracuse, New York

Bernard R. Bach, Jr, MD, Associate Professor, Department of Orthopaedic Surgery, Director, Sports Medicine Section, Rush Medical College, Rush Presbyterian-St. Luke's Medical Center, Chicago, Illinois

Richard A. Balderston, MD, Chief, Scoliosis Service, Rothman Institute, Thomas Jefferson University, Philadelphia, Pennsylvania

Timothy C. Beals, MD, Assistant Professor, Department of Orthopedics, University of Utah School of Medicine, Salt Lake City, Utah

Randal R. Betz, MD, Medical Director of Spinal Cord Injury Unit, Shriners Hospitals, Philadelphia Unit, Philadelphia, Pennsylvania

R. Dale Blasier, MD, FRCS(C), Associate Professor of Orthopaedic Surgery, Division of Pediatric Orthopaedics, Arkansas Children's Hospital, University of Arkansas for Medical Sciences, Little Rock, Arkansas

Lawrence B. Bone, MD, Associate Professor, Department of Orthopaedic Surgery, SUNY Buffalo, Buffalo, New York

Kenneth Brummel-Smith, MD, Medical Director, Long Term Care Division, Providence Health Systems, Oregon, Portland, Oregon

Robert Bucholz, MD, Professor and Chairman, Department of Orthopaedic Surgery, University of Texas Southwestern, Dallas, Texas

Joseph A. Buckwalter, MD, MS Professor of Orthopaedics, University of Iowa, Iowa City, Iowa

T. Jeff Chandler, EdD, Director of Research and Education, Sports Medicine, Lexington Clinic, Lexington, Kentucky

Robert H. Cofield, MD, Frank R. and Shari Caywood Professor of Orthopaedics, Mayo Medical School, Vice-Chair, Department of Orthopedics, Mayo Clinic/ Mayo Foundation, Rochester, Minnesota

William Cole, PhD, FRACS, FRCSC, Professor and Head, Division of Orthopaedic Surgery, Hospital for Sick Children, Toronto, Ontario, Canada

Patrick M. Connor, MD, The Shoulder and Elbow Center, Miller Orthopaedic Clinic, Charlotte, North Carolina

Jerome M. Cotler, MD, The Everett J. and Marian Gordon Professor of Orthopaedic Surgery, Department of Orthopaedic Surgery, Jefferson Medical College of Thomas Jefferson University, Philadelphia, Pennsylvania

Michael J. Coughlin, MD, Department of Orthopaedic Surgery, St. Alphonsus Regional Medical Center, Boise, Idaho

Richard D. Coutts, MD, Adjunct Professor of Orthopaedics, University of California San Diego, Department of Orthopaedics, La Jolla, California

Frances Cuomo, MD, Associate Chief, Shoulder Service, Orthopaedic Department, Hospital for Joint Diseases, New York, New York

Douglas A. Dennis, MD, Professor, Colorado School of

Mines, Director, Rose Musculoskeletal Laboratory, Rose Institute for Joint Replacement, Denver, Colorado

Thomas A. Einhorn, MD, Professor of Orthopaedics, Department of Orthopaedics, Mount Sinai School of Medicine, New York, New York

Gerard A. Engh, MD, President, Anderson Orthopaedic Research Institute, Arlington, Virginia

A. Louise Fincher, EdD, ATC, Coordinator of Research and Education, Joe W. King Orthopedic Institute, Houston, Texas

Evan L. Flatow, MD, Herbert Irving Associate Professor of Orthopaedic Surgery, Associate Chief, The Shoulder Service, New York Orthopaedic Hospital, Columbia-Presbyterian Medical Center, New York, New York

William E. Garrett, Jr, MD, PhD, Associate Professor of Orthopedics, Department of Orthopedics, Duke University, Durham, North Carolina

Victor M. Goldberg, MD, Charles H. Herndon Professor and Chairman, Department of Orthopaedics, Case Western Reserve University, University Hospitals of Cleveland, Cleveland, Ohio

James A. Goulet, MD, Associate Professor, Orthopaedic Surgery, University of Michigan, Ann Arbor, Michigan

Stuart A. Green, MD, Clinical Professor, Department of Orthopaedic Surgery, University of California, Irvine, Irvine, California

Sigvard T. Hansen, Jr, MD, Professor of Orthopaedics, University of Washington, Harborview Medical Center, Seattle, Washington

Arlen D. Hanssen, MD, Associate Professor, Orthopedic Surgery, Mayo Medical School, Rochester, Minnesota

Wilson C. Hayes, PhD, Maurice E. Mueller Professor of Biomechanics, Harvard Medical School, Orthopedic Surgery, Beth Israel Deaconess Medical Center, Boston, Massachusetts

John Jacquemin, MD, Orthopaedic Resident, University of Cincinnati, Department of Orthopaedic Surgery, Cincinnati, Ohio

Norman A. Johanson, MD, Associate Professor of Orthopaedic Surgery, Department of Orthopaedics, Temple University School of Medicine, Philadelphia, Pennsylvania

Lanny L. Johnson, MD, Clinical Professor of Orthopaedic Surgery, Michigan State University, Okemos, Michigan

Parviz Kambin, MD, Professor of Orthopaedic Surgery, Director, Spinal Center, Allegheny University Hospitals, MCP Division, Allegheny University of the Health Sciences, MCP Hahnemann School of Medicine, Philadelphia, Pennsyslvania

Steven E. Kann, MD, Mary S. Stern Hand Surgery Fellowship, Cincinnati, Ohio

Bryan T. Kelly, MD, Resident, Department of Orthopaedics, Hospital for Special Surgery, New York, New York

W. Ben Kibler, MD, Medical Director, Lexington Clinic Sports Medicine Center, Lexington, Kentucky

Donald T. Kirkendall, PhD, Clinical Assistant Professor, Department of Physical and Occupational Therapy, Duke University Medical Center, Durham, North Carolina

Kenneth J. Koval, MD, Chief, Fracture Service, Hospital for Joint Diseases, New York, New York

Joseph M. Lane, MD, Director, Metabolic Bone Disease Service, Chief Laboratory of Orthopaedic Applied Clinical Research, Department of Orthopaedics, Hospital for Special Surgery, New York, New York

Moo-Hyung Lee, MD, Orthopaedic Surgeon, Clinical Fellow, Sports Medicine, Markham Stouffville Hospital, Markham, Ontario, Canada

Andrew S. Levy, MD, Assistant Clinical Professor, Orthopaedic Surgery, University of Medicine and Dentistry of New Jersey, Newark, New Jersey

Thomas N. Lindenfeld, MD, Associate Director, Cincinnati Sportsmedicine and Orthopaedic Center, Cincinnati, Ohio

Beven Livingston, PT, ATC, Clinical Specialist, Sportsmedicine, Lexington Clinic, Lexington, Kentucky

E. Antero Mäkelä, MD, Associate Professor and Surgeon-in-Chief, Department of Orthopaedics and Traumatology, Kuopio University Hospital, Kuopio, Finland

Roger A. Mann, MD, Associate Clinical Professor, University of California, San Francisco School of Medicine, Department of Orthopaedic Surgery, San Francisco, California

Arthur Manoli II, MD, Professor and Chairman, Chief, Foot and Ankle Surgery, Department of Orthopedic Surgery, University of South Alabama, Mobile, Alabama

Paul R. Manske, MD, Department of Orthopaedic Surgery, Washington University, St. Louis, Missouri

Geoffrey McCullen, MD, Clinical Instructor of Orthopedic Surgery, Department of Orthopedic Surgery, Naval Medical Center San Diego, University of California San Diego, San Diego, California

Roy A. Meals, MD, Associate Clinical Professor, Department of Orthopaedic Surgery, University of California, Los Angeles, Los Angeles, California

James D. Michelson, MD, Associate Professor, Associate Director and Vice Chairman, Johns Hopkins School of Medicine, Baltimore, Maryland

Anthony Miniaci, MD, FRCSC, Head, Sports Medicine, Associate Professor, Orthopaedic Surgery, The Toronto Hospital, Western Division, University of Toronto, Toronto, Ontario, Canada

Michael P. Muldoon, MD, Lieutenant Commander, Medical Corps United States Navy, Director, Adult Reconstructive Service, Department of Orthopedics, Naval Medical Center, San Diego, California

Gregory R. Mundy, MD, Professor and Head, Division of Endocrinology and Metabolism, Department of Medicine, University of Texas Health Science Center at San Antonio, San Antonio, Texas

Paraic Murray, MSc, MCh (Orth), FRCS Ed (Orth), Consultant Orthopaedic Surgeon, Royal College of Surgeons in Ireland, Beaumont Hospital, Dublin, Ireland

Elizabeth R. Myers, PhD, Assistant Professor of Orthopedic Surgery, Harvard Medical School, Department of Orthopedic Surgery, Beth Israel Deaconess Medical Center, Boston, Massachusetts

Mark S. Myerson, MD, Director, Foot and Ankle Services, The Union Memorial Hospital, Baltimore, Maryland

Carl L. Nelson, MD, Professor and Chairman, Department of Orthopaedic Surgery, Director, Center for Hip and Knee Surgery, University of Arkansas for Medical Sciences, Little Rock, Arkansas

Barry Oakes, MD, Department of Anatomy, Monash University, Melbourne, Australia

Steven A. Olson, MD, Assistant Profesor, Co-Director of Orthopaedic Trauma, Department of Orthopaedic Surgery, University of California–Davis Medical Center, Sacramento, California

Douglas R. Osmon, MD, Assistant Professor of Medicine, Infectious Diseases, Mayo Clinic, Rochester, Minnesota

Wesley Parke, PhD, Professor and Chairman, Emeritus, Department of Anatomy and Structural Biology, University of South Dakota School of Medicine, Vermillion, South Dakota

Nancy L. Parks, MS, Senior Project Director, Anderson Orthopaedic Research Institute, Arlington, Virginia

Vincent D. Pellegrini, Jr, MD, Michael and Myrtle Baker Professor, Chairman, Department of Orthopaedics and Rehabilitation, Pennsylvania State University, Milton S. Hershey Medical Center, Hershey, Pennsylvania

Michael S. Pinzur, MD, Professor of Orthopaedic Surgery, Department of Orthopaedic Surgery, Loyola University, Stritch School of Medicine, Maywood, Illinois

Hollis G. Potter, MD, Chief, MRI Section, Assistant Professor of Radiology, Department of Radiology, Hospital for Special Surgery–Cornell University Medical College, New York, New York

John J. Regan, MD, Associate Clinical Professor, University of Texas Southwestern Medical Center, Dallas, Texas

Edward H. Riley, MD, Chief Resident, Department of Orthopaedics, UCLA, Los Angeles, California

Cecil H. Rorabeck MD, FRCSC, Professor and Chairman, Division of Orthopaedic Surgery, London Health Sciences Centre, University Hospital, London, Ontario, Canada

Ron G. Rosenfeld, MD, Professor and Chairman, Department of Pediatrics, Oregon Health Services University, Portland, Oregon

Jeffrey A. Russell, MS, ATC, Director, Joe W. King Orthopedic Institute, Houston, Texas

Robert L. Sah, MD, ScD, Assistant Professor of Bioengineering, University of California San Diego, Department of Bioengineering, La Jolla, California

Bruce J. Sangeorzan, MD, Professor of Orthopedic Surgery, University of Washington, Seattle, Washington

Jonathan L. Schaffer, MD, Instructor, Department of Orthopedic Surgery, Brigham and Women's Hospital, Harvard Medical School, Boston, Massachusetts

Mark E. Schweitzer, MD, Associate Professor of Radiology and Orthopedic Surgery, Department of Radiology, Thomas Jefferson University Hospital, Philadelphia, Pennsylvania

Mary Louise Skovron, DrPH, Assistant Professor and Director, Musculoskeletal Epidemiology, Hospital for Joint Diseases, New York University Medical Center, New York, New York

Kevin P. Speer, MD, Assistant Professor, Division of

Orthopedic Surgery, Duke University Medical Center, Durham, North Carolina

Peter J. Stern, MD, Professor and Chairman, University of Cincinnati College of Medicine, Department of Orthopaedic Surgery, Cincinnati, Ohio

Carol C. Teitz, MD, Associate Professor, Orthopaedic Surgery, University of Washington, Seattle, Washington

David Templeman, MD, Assistant Professor, Department of Orthopaedic Surgery, University of Minnesota, Minneapolis, Minnesota

Paul Tornetta III, MD, Director of Orthopaedic Trauma, Kings County Hospital Center, SUNY Health Science Center at Brooklyn, Brooklyn, New York

Stephen B. Trippel, MD, Associate Professor of Orthopaedics, Massachusetts General Hospital, Harvard Medical School, Boston, Massachusetts

Alexander R. Vaccaro, MD, Assistant Professor, Thomas Jefferson University and the Rothman Institute, Department of Orthopaedic Surgery, Philadelphia, Pennsylvania

Robert Vander Griend, MD, Associate Professor, Department of Orthopaedics, University of Florida, Gainesville, Florida

Hugh G. Watts, MD, Shriners Hospital for Crippled Children, Los Angeles Unit, Clinical Professor, University of California, Los Angeles, Los Angeles, California

Leo A. Whiteside, MD, Director, Biomechanical Research Laboratory, Orthopaedic Surgeon, Barnes West County Hospital, Research Assistant Professor of Surgery, Orthopaedic Surgery, Washington University, St. Louis, Missouri

Philip Z. Wirganowicz, MD, Acting Instructor in Musculoskeletal Oncology, Department of Orthopaedics, University of Washington, Seattle, Washington

Edward M. Wojtys, MD, Associate Professor, Department of Surgery, University of Michigan, Ann Arbor, Michigan

G. William Woods, MD, Chief, Sports Medicine and Surgery of the Knee, Texas Orthopedic Hospital, Houston, Texas

Hansen Yuan, MD, Professor, Orthopaedic and Neurological Surgery, State University of New York Health Science Center at Syracuse, Syracuse, New York

Joseph D. Zuckerman, MD, Chief, Shoulder Service, Chairman, Department of Orthopaedic Surgery, Hospital for Joint Diseases, New York, New York

Preface

The Committee on Instructional Courses works throughout the year to select and help refine the instructional courses for the upcoming annual Academy meeting. After the annual meeting, the Committee is charged with selecting those courses that are to be published in the next year's *Instructional Course Lectures* volume. The Committee must select material which is of interest to you and which has not been recently published. This may seem like an impossible task, but each year a new and exciting publication is produced. This year's committee hopes our efforts will be equal to those of past years.

That the Academy can continue to produce an annual volume of such high quality may be attributed to the hard work of numerous people. In volume 46, there are 96 authors who voluntarily gave of their intellect and time to put to paper what they teach during their Instructional Course. This is no easy task, as any of you who have tried to write a scholarly paper can attest. This volume's authors have done a wonderful job of writing, and we are sure you will learn from their efforts. We must thank the other instructional course lecturers as well. Their diligent efforts mean that each year there is more material than there is room to include.

The second group who are vital to this publication are the members of the Academy's Department of Publications under the direction of Marilyn L. Fox, PhD. Bruce Davis and Sophie Tosta are the two staff most responsible for this volume. The editor selected the instructional courses to be included in the volume and invited the authors to submit their manuscripts. Then Bruce and Sophie sent each author instructions and a timetable. They also followed up with the authors, reminding them of their responsibilities. Geraldine Dubberke, in addition to updating manuscripts as they were processed, put in many hours at the computer to create the final page layout for the entire volume. In addition, because some of the manuscripts are selected for publication in the *Journal of Bone and Joint Surgery*, staff worked with the *Journal* and especially with James D. Heckman, MD, to assure that those manuscripts chosen were finished in time for publication. Dr. Heckman edited those manuscripts published in the *Journal*, which took some of the burden off the Editor of the *Instructional Course Lectures* volume. The committee thanks all of the publications staff for their efforts. Without them the volume you are holding would not exist. The committee thanks Dr. Heckman for his superb editing.

The committee decided to include five symposia in this year's volume. These symposia were chosen because of their unique quality. This presented a special challenge to the authors and Department of Publications but they did a wonderful job and these symposia are an excellent addition.

The Committee knows you will enjoy this ICL and learn from it. It has been educational and fun putting it together.

Dempsey S. Springfield, MD
New York, New York
Editor

Richard H. Gelberman, MD
St. Louis, Missouri
Chairman, Committee on Instructional Courses

W. Dilworth Cannon, MD
San Francisco, California

Douglas W. Jackson, MD
Long Beach, California

Douglas J. Pritchard, MD
Rochester, Minnesota

Joseph D. Zuckerman, MD
New York, New York

Contents

SECTION IV

SECTION V

Shoulder

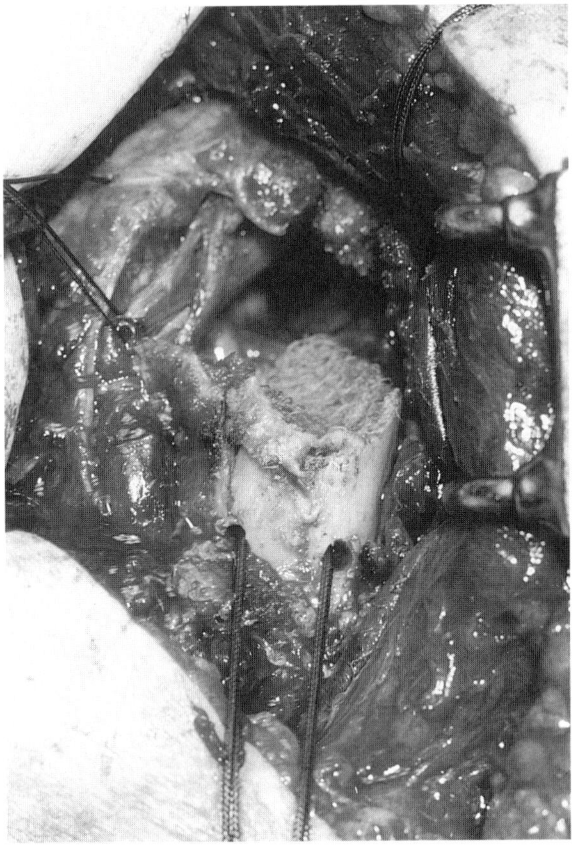

CHAPTER 1

Pathophysiologic Alterations in Shoulder Injury

W. Ben Kibler, MD
William E. Garrett, Jr, MD, PhD

Shoulder pathology results from acute macrotrauma or chronic repetitive microtrauma (Outline 1). Acute macrotrauma implies an event—a one-time incident that instantly converts a normal anatomic structure to an abnormal, clinically symptomatic structure. Examples of this process include traumatic anterior dislocation or an acute acromioclavicular joint sprain.

Repetitive microtrauma, the more common causative factor in shoulder pathology, represents a process—a chronic series of events in which normal tissues are converted to abnormal but asymptomatic tissues. Under continued athletic stress, these tissues become increasingly abnormal and eventually develop clinical symptoms.[1] This process results in a failure of homeostasis of cellular activities in the face of continued athletic demand. This homeostatic failure includes changes in size and shape of mitochondria, changes in mitochondrial enzyme levels,[2] alterations in calcium release and uptake,[3] and alterations in fiber formation, kinking, and cross links.[2] The eventual result of this degenerative process is the absence of normal cell matrix, whether it be ligament, tendon, muscle, or bone. Investigations of shoulder pathology and pathogenesis indicate that this process is present in rotator cuff injury, and the degeneration here is similar to that seen in specimens from other areas of tendinous injury, such as the elbow or foot.[4,5,6] This abnormal cellular matrix produces poorly organized tissues that cannot respond to normal biologic signals for repair and recovery, collagen orientation, or maturation.[7]

Outline 1
Acute macrotrauma and chronic microtrauma

Acute Macrotrauma
One-Time Event

Normal tissues → Abnormal tissues with clinical symptoms
- Fractures of clavicle
- Acute traumatic shoulder dislocation
- Acromioclavicular joint sprain

Chronic Microtrauma
Process

Normal tissues → Abnormal but asymptomatic tissues → Abnormal clinically symptomatic tissues
- Rotator cuff tendinitis
- Nontraumatic capsuloligamentous instability
- Attritional labral tears

It appears that initiation of these degenerative changes is due to the cumulative result of mechanical strain on the cell by multiple repetitive tensile loads and that these changes represent a materials failure caused by these loads.[8,9] Vascular and hormonal changes also play a role, but their roles appear to be secondary in the model studied.[8]

These cellular changes create alterations in tissue function. Scar formation occurs as a result of tensile load, occurring at the muscle-tendon junction, in the supportive connective tissue, and in the capsule, creating stiffness in the muscle and inflexibility of the joints. Muscle strength weakness results from tissue injury, pain, or muscle fiber abnormality, and this loss of muscle strength causes problems due to individual muscle weakness, strength or force couple imbalance, and inability to absorb loads due to weakness in eccentric muscle contraction.[10]

These alterations can be objectively measured as decreases in joint range of motion, muscle flexibility, strength production, strength balance, or work output. Although they can be present without producing overt clinical symptoms, they do impose biomechanical inefficiencies on the athlete. These inefficiencies include increased humeral translation due to lack of glenohumeral internal rotation,[11] superior humeral translation due to rotator cuff weakness in the face of normal deltoid strength,[12] and abnormal scapular position, motion, and rotation due to trapezius and serratus anterior muscle weakness.[13] They have been implicated as risk factors in producing injuries in various anatomic areas including the shoulder,[14] plantar fascia,[6] and the lower extremity.[15]

These alterations may be considered intrinsic risk factors that the athlete brings to the functional demands of the sport.[16] These create a predisposed athlete, who may then interact with the extrinsic risk factors (sport-specific motions, forces or loads, surfaces, or equipment) in such a way that the tissues become injured to the point of clinical symptoms. Therefore, the onset of clinical symptoms can occur long after the initiation of the pathologic process, and the clinical symptoms may reflect only a small part of all of the tissue alterations that may be present. Examples of this pathologic mechanism around the shoulder include chronic rotator cuff tendinosis, attritional labral tears, and nontraumatic capsuloligamentous instability.

In either the macrotrauma or microtrauma situation, the pathologic process alters the normal bony, ligamentous, or muscular constraint systems so that the normal path of the instant center of rotation is not constrained. Pathology may involve only one of the constraint systems, but because the constraint systems interact to allow mobility while conferring stability, there is usually some involvement of several constraints. The constraint systems may fail individually (one system only), concurrently (two or three at the same time), or consecutively (failure of one followed by failure of others) (Outline 2). The initiating factor in the pathology is commonly local, but alterations in other parts of the kinematic chain may produce loads or stresses that have clinical expression at the shoulder, due to the shoulder's role as a funnel for developed forces.

From a rehabilitation standpoint, alterations in the muscular constraint system are the most important, because they can be modified and improved by appropriate protocols and because of the important role the muscular system plays in complementing and increasing the efficiency of the other constraint systems. Alterations in muscle may be either anatomic or neurologic.

Anatomic alterations may be caused by direct blow trauma and muscle damage, but such injuries are rare, and their effect on shoulder function is small. Disuse or altered use is the most common factor in anatomic alterations. The muscle requires a certain level of activation and feedback to maintain normal size and physiologic function. Immobilization and disuse cause severe loss of muscle size over short periods of time.[17] Because muscle strength is proportional to muscle mass, ability to generate torque or absorb a load is similarly diminished.

A most visible response by skeletal muscle to decreased use or disuse is the loss of mass. This loss of mass reflects a loss of muscular protein, indicating that protein degradation exceeds protein synthesis during the period of decreased use. About 70% of the protein of a muscle fiber is as myofibrils.[18] Therefore, loss of mass is reflective of a loss of myofibrillar proteins of the individual muscle fibers. In muscle disuse, protein synthesis decreases in the first day by as much as 50%, and then remains fairly constant.[19] Therefore, a balance of degradation and synthesis is achieved after about 30 days.

If a muscle is immobilized in a shortened position or is not used in ways that allow full range of motion, or if the muscle is shortened due to inflexibility, the normal length/tension relationship is shifted, resulting in decreased maximum tension and strength-generating capacity.[17] Booth immobilized rat hindlimbs for varying intervals and determined the rate of atrophy.[20] This research showed that the half time to atrophy from immobilization was 5 to 6 days, which reaches a steady state after about 21 days. These types of findings indicate that the major fraction of loss of muscle mass occurs very early.

While the overall muscle mass declines with decreased use, protein losses differ between and within muscles. To determine if immobilization affects fast- or slow-twitch muscle differently, areas of the specific muscle fiber types are measured from samples of muscle. Fiber area is a reasonable variable to use because it should be sensitive to changes in myofibrillar protein. Both slow- and fast-twitch muscles lose cross-sectional area. However, the slow-twitch fibers show a greater relative change than the fast-twitch fibers.

Neurologic alterations affect the muscular constraint system by altering local strength development, and by altering the organization of the motor firing patterns necessary for force-dependent kinematic chain activity. Most of the muscle weakness seen in the postoperative or post-injury period is due to decreased neural drive,[17] which is the activation and coordination of muscle firing patterns. Neurologic and psychological research in recent years have called attention to the fact that central nervous system control of motor function is based, in part, on stored specific patterns of sequential muscle activation that guide a complex motor task. This motor pattern is learned through repetition and practice. The stored motor pattern can be recalled easily with little thought. Even a skilled player with excellent knowledge of a tennis serve would be inefficient serving with the non-dominant arm. The lack of practice with the nondominant side does not allow the creation of a reproducible hard-wired motor control program, even with the same knowledge base and sensory feedback mechanisms. Many factors, including joint effusions, pain from any source, disuse, and different abnormalities, such as altered proprioception, decrease the neural drive stimulus. It appears that for months after an injury maximum strength output is closely related to available neural drive.

The force-dependent motor patterns responsible for smooth generation and transfer of force through a coordinated succession of joint positions and movements are highly dependent on the neurologic integrity of

Outline 2
Methods of constraint system failure

Individual
- Fractured clavicle (bony)
- Acute Bankhart lesion (ligamentous)

Concurrently
- Rotator cuff tear (muscular) with anterior dislocation (ligamentous)
- Bony Bankhart lesion (bony) and capsular stretch (ligamentous)

Consecutively
- Rotator cuff weakness (muscular) → decreased capsular stiffness and laxity (ligamentous)
- Posterior cuff weakness and inflexibility (muscular) → anterior humeral translation and labral tear (ligamentous)

each of the joints. If the length-dependent patterns that operate around individual joints are not working right because of weakness, inhibition, or other problems with neural drive, then the force-dependent patterns break down and are altered, thereby decreasing the efficiency and maximal force production from those patterns.[21]

Both anatomic and neurologic alterations in muscle are present at the same time during the pathologic process. Their clinical effect is to decrease the amount and effectiveness of muscle strength production. These alterations are widespread in a muscle-dependent joint like the shoulder and should be checked for closely.

Scapular muscle failure, which is commonly seen in shoulder pathology,[13,22,23] appears to be a nonspecific response to glenohumeral pain, injury, or pathology. It appears in 68% to 100% of cases.[23] Disruption of the force couples has deleterious effects on the four purposes of the scapula in overhead activities. Lack of acromial elevation, due to upper trapezius weakness, increases impingement with shoulder abduction. Trapezius, rhomboid, and serratus anterior weakness impairs the scapula's ability to position itself as a congruent socket for the moving humerus; to stabilize itself as an anchor for origins of the rotator cuff, deltoid, biceps, and triceps; and to move smoothly from retraction to protraction during the throwing motion.[13] Finally, this weakness, by interrupting the kinetic chain, disrupts funneling of velocity and force, and does not allow a stable base for the arm to work.

Rotator cuff injury, caused either by impingement or by partial- or full-thickness tears, results in failure of energy and force production, but its most deleterious effects are on the force couples that position and stabilize the glenohumeral joint. Supraspinatus weakness decreases capsular stiffness[24] and and also decreases concavity/compression.[25] Infraspinatus/teres minor weakness alters the deltoid force couple for abduction, leading to excessive superior translation.[26] Subscapularis weakness can lead to overstretching of the anterior capsular structures and cause excessive anterior translation.[27] Internal/external rotation force couple imbalance, with relatively strong internal rotators and relatively weak external rotators, is another common problem.[28] This imbalance decreases concavity/compression and, in concert with restricted glenohumeral internal rotation, increases anterior translation.

Pathology in other links of the kinematic chain may affect the muscular constraints. Biomechanical flaws or anatomic injuries, such as ankle sprains, knee pathology, or back inflexibility or weakness, create a catch-up situation if the distal kinematic links have to increase their energy or force production to maintain normal force production at the hand. The arm muscles, with their smaller cross-sectional area, cannot initiate or maintain this higher level of activity well and are put at risk of fatigue and injury. Our studies have shown that, in a mathematical model, a decrease of 10% of trunk/leg kinetic energy requires an 18.5% increase in shoulder velocity or a 40% increase in shoulder mass to achieve the same resultant energy at the hand.[29]

Sensory feedback and knowledge of outcome can positively influence motor performance. However, these feedback mechanisms can also have a negative influence on the motor pattern. Sensations of pain, stiffness, or instability can disrupt a previously acquired motor control program. These disruptions may persist even when the pain resolves, due possibly to continued anticipation of pain or harm, or a more permanent alteration in motor pattern.

Implications for Rehabilitation

Pathology around the shoulder, caused by either macrotrauma or microtrauma, creates associated alterations in the tissue flexibility, strength, or strength balance, alterations that add to tissue injury and disrupt the constraint systems around the shoulder. The muscular constraint system plays a key role in all of the constraint systems and is affected by both anatomic and neurologic alterations. Rehabilitation strategies must therefore address these muscle-specific changes and the central nervous system alterations. Even the recovery of strength, motion, and endurance does not always allow normal return to function. The motor patterns must be recalled or recreated and practiced. Also, because the shoulder is an important link in the kinematic chain of throwing activities, biomechanical flaws or injuries in other links may have major or minor effects on shoulder pathology and function.

Any evaluation framework set up to initiate the rehabilitation process must take all of these factors into account. It must start with the complete and accurate diagnosis, which includes not only the clinical symptoms and signs such as pain, swelling, catching, or instability, but must also include anatomic alterations—inflexibility, strength deficit, or strength imbalance; biomechanical alterations—scapular instability and decreased internal rotation with increased anterior translations; and subclinical performance adaptations—3/4 arm positioning, and leading with the body, which occur as a result of the pathologic process.[30] These alterations affect and magnify the clinical symptoms, alter athletic performance, and affect the completeness and efficacy of rehabilitation. They may be local or distant in the kinematic chain.

For macrotrauma pathology, the evaluation may be relatively simple, because there may be few associated alterations. However, for chronic repetitive microtrauma pathology, which accounts for the great majority of shoulder problems, these alterations are common and may be widespread.

The complete and accurate diagnosis can provide a comprehensive view of the entire spectrum of anatomic and biomechanical abnormalities the athlete has, abnormalities that must be normalized in treatment. This diagnosis is then used as the basis for the exercise prescription for functional treatment and rehabilitation.

References

1. Leadbetter WB: An introduction to sports-induced inflammation, in Leadbetter WB, Buckwalter JA, Gordon SL (eds): *Sports-Induced Inflammation: Clinical and Basic Science Concepts.* Park Ridge, IL, American Academy of Orthopaedic Surgeons, 1990, pp 3–23.
2. Kannus P, Jozsa L: Histopathological changes preceding spontaneous rupture of a tendon: A controlled study of 891 patients. *J Bone Joint Surg* 1991;73A:1507–1525.
3. Armstrong RB: Initial events in exercise-induced muscular injury. *Med Sci Sports Exerc* 1990;22:429–435.
4. Iannotti JP: Lesions of the rotator cuff: Pathology and pathogenesis, in Matsen FA III, Fu FH, Hawkins RJ (eds): *The Shoulder: A Balance of Mobility and Stability.* Rosemont, IL, American Academy of Orthopaedic Surgeons, 1993, pp 239–251.
5. Kibler WB: Pathophysiology of overload injuries around the elbow. *Clin Sports Med* 1995;14:447–457.
6. Kibler WB, Goldberg C, Chandler TJ: Functional biomechanical deficits in running athletes with plantar fasciitis. *Am J Sports Med* 1991;19:66–71.
7. Leadbetter WB, Mooar PA, Lane GJ, et al: The surgical treatment of tendinitis: Clinical rationale and biologic basis. *Clin Sports Med* 1992;11:679–712.
8. Warren GL, Hayes DA, Lowe DA, et al: Materials fatigue initiates eccentric contraction–induced injury in rat soleus muscle. *J Physiol* 1993;464:477–489.
9. Garrett WE Jr, Tidball J: Myotendinous junction: Structure, function, and failure, in Woo SL-Y, Buckwalter JA (eds): *Injury and Repair of the Musculoskeletal Soft Tissues.* Park Ridge, IL, American Academy of Orthopaedic Surgeons, 1988, pp 171–207.
10. Mair SD, Seaber AV, Glisson RR, et al: The role of fatigue in susceptibility to acute muscle strain injury. *Am J Sports Med* 1996;24:137–143.
11. Harryman DT II, Sidles JA, Clark JM, et al: Translation of the humeral head on the glenoid with passive glenohumeral motion. *J Bone Joint Surg* 1990;72A:1334–1343.
12. Speer KP, Garrett WE Jr: Muscular control of motion and stability about the pectoral girdle, in Matsen FA III, Fu FH, Hawkins RJ (eds): *The Shoulder: A Balance of Mobility and Stability.* Rosemont, IL, American Academy of Orthopaedic Surgeons, 1993, pp 159–172.
13. Kibler WB: Role of the scapula in the overhead throwing motion. *Contemp Orthop* 1991;22:525–532.
14. Silliman JF, Hawkins RJ: Current concepts and recent advances in the athlete's shoulder. *Clin Sports Med* 1991;10:693–705.
15. Knapik JJ, Bauman CL, Jones BH, et al: Preseason strength and flexibility imbalances associated with athletic injuries in female collegiate athletes. *Am J Sports Med* 1991;19:76–81.
16. Meeuwisse WH: Assessing causation in sport injury: A multifactorial model. *Clin J Sports Med* 1994;4:166–170.
17. Garrett WE Jr, Best TM: Anatomy, physiology and mechanics of skeletal muscle, in Simon SR (ed): *Orthopaedic Basic Science.* Rosemont, IL, American Academy of Orthopaedic Surgeons, 1994, pp 89–125.
18. Lieber RL (ed): *Skeletal Muscle Structure and Function: Implications for Rehabilitation and Sports Medicine.* Baltimore, MD, Williams & Wilkins, 1992.
19. Thomason DB, Biggs RB, Booth FW: Protein metabolism and beta-myosin heavy-chain mRNA in unweighted soleus muscle. *Am J Physiol* 1989;257:R300–R305.
20. Booth FW: Time course of muscular atrophy during immobilization of hindlimbs in rats. *J Appl Physiol* 1977;43:656–661.
21. Nichols TR: A biomechanical perspective on spinal mechanisms of coordinated muscular action: An architecture principle. *Acta Anat* 1994;151:1–13.
22. Paine RM, Voight M: The role of the scapula. *J Orthop Sports Phys Ther* 1993;18:386–391.
23. Warner JJ, Micheli LJ, Arslanian LE, et al: Scapulothoracic motion in normal shoulders and shoulders with glenohumeral instability and impingement syndrome: A study using Moire topographic analysis. *Clin Orthop* 1992;285:191–199.
24. Cain PR, Mutschler TA, Fu FH, et al: Anterior stability of the glenohumeral joint: A dynamic model. *Am J Sports Med* 1987;15:144–148.
25. Matsen FA III, Harryman DT II, Sidles JA: Mechanics of glenohumeral instability. *Clin Sports Med* 1991;10:783–788.
26. Inman VT, Saunders JB, Abbott LC: Observations on the function of the shoulder joint. *J Bone Joint Surg* 1944;26:1–30.
27. Jobe FW, Moynes DR: Delineation of diagnostic criteria and a rehabilitation program for rotator cuff injuries. *Am J Sports Med* 1982;10:336–449.
28. Warner JJ, Micheli LJ, Arslanian LE, et al: Patterns of flexibility, laxity, and strength in normal shoulders and shoulders with instability and impingement. *Am J Sports Med* 1990;18:366–375.
29. Kibler WB: Current concepts of shoulder biomechanics: Pathology and treatment. *J South Orthop Assoc* 1994;3:254–271.
30. Kibler WB, Chandler TJ, Pace BK: Principles of rehabilitation after chronic tendon injuries. *Clin Sports Med* 1992;11:661–671.

CHAPTER 2

Proximal Humeral Replacement for Complex Fractures: Indications and Surgical Technique

Joseph D. Zuckerman, MD
Frances Cuomo, MD
Kenneth J. Koval, MD

Introduction

The treatment of complex proximal humeral fractures presents a challenge to orthopaedic surgeons. First, these fractures are osteoporotic fractures, which by definition represent metaphyseal fractures that occur primarily in women over the age of 50. The osteoporosis results in compromised bone quality, which limits the potential to achieve secure internal fixation. Second, the muscular attachments of the proximal humerus and the associated deforming forces make it difficult to obtain and maintain an acceptable closed reduction. Third, radiographic evaluation of the fractures can also be challenging because of the displacement patterns and the overlapping bony structures. And fourth, fractures that result in displacement of the articular segment and the tuberosities are at significant risk for the development of osteonecrosis.

These were important factors in the development of humeral head replacement as a treatment option for complex proximal humeral fractures. The decision to proceed with proximal humeral replacement and tuberosity/rotator cuff reconstruction for the treatment of acute proximal humeral fractures should be based on a careful evaluation of injury factors and patient factors. The degree of displacement is an important injury factor because it indicates the degree of soft-tissue injury and the risk of osteonecrosis. Nondisplaced comminution and compromised bone quality are also important factors that limit the ability to obtain secure internal fixation that allows for an early range of motion program. Fractures that significantly compromise the integrity of the articular surface of the humeral head may also be more appropriately treated by primary prosthetic replacement.

Important patient factors include the age and functional needs of the patient. Elderly patients with lower functional demands are probably more suitable candidates for proximal humeral replacement than younger patients who will subject the shoulder to more strenuous activities. The presence of pre-existing functional deficits in the involved extremity must also be considered before deciding to proceed with a reconstructive procedure. Patients must also be able to participate in a structured postoperative rehabilitative program, which is essential for a successful outcome. The decision to proceed with a proximal humeral replacement should reflect a careful consideration of these injury factors to formulate a treatment plan individualized for each patient.

Although the indications for prosthetic replacement following acute proximal humeral fractures are not absolute, there are specific injuries for which it is preferred. These include: (1) Four-part fractures and fracture-dislocations, probably the most common indication for proximal humeral replacement (Fig. 1). (2) Three-part fractures and fracture-dislocations in elderly patients with osteoporotic bone, particularly in the presence of nondisplaced comminution. (3) Chronic anterior or posterior humeral head dislocations with impression fractures that involve more than 40% of the articular surface. (4) Head-splitting fractures that cannot be adequately reduced and internally fixed. (5) Anatomic neck fractures in which internal fixation is not possible.

The nonmodular proximal humeral replacement developed by Neer has been used more extensively than any of the more recently developed modular and nonmodular prostheses.[1-3] Today, there are a variety of implants available that provide different design options, including modularity with a wide range of head sizes, both Morse taper and reverse Morse taper articulations, smooth or coated surfaces, and cobalt chromium or titanium implants.[4] Although many variations in prosthetic design are available, the most important aspect of this procedure is the surgical technique. Proper technique is required for a successful outcome. Conversely, improper surgical technique will result in unsatisfactory outcome regardless of the prosthesis used.

The surgical technique described will be based on treatment of an acute four-part fracture, which is the most common fracture indication for proximal humeral replacement. The basic principles of this procedure include: (1) utilization of a deltopectoral approach that preserves the origin and insertion of the deltoid muscle; (2) insertion of the proximal humeral prosthesis to restore humeral length and proper retroversion; and (3) fixation of the tuberosities to the prosthesis, to the humeral shaft, and to each other that is secure enough to optimize postoperative function.

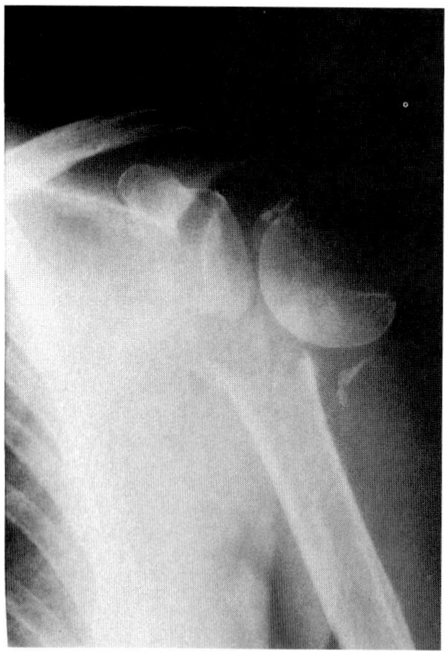

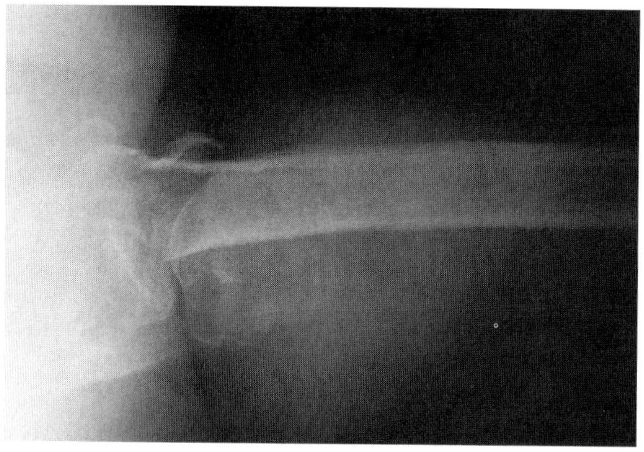

Fig. 1 Radiographs show a four-part fracture of the proximal humerus. The anteroposterior view, **left,** shows displacement of the articular segment and shaft fragments. The displacement of the lesser tuberosity is evident on the axillary view, **right,** while displacement of the greater tuberosity can be visualized on both views.

The success of this procedure depends, in large part, on close attention to the technical details of the procedure and the utilization of meticulous surgical technique.

Positioning

The patient should be placed on the operating table in a supine position. The head of the operating table should be elevated approximately 30° in a modified beach chair position. A small bolster should be placed behind the involved shoulder. The patient should be moved to the side of the table so that the upper extremity can be placed into maximum extension without obstruction by the operating table (Fig. 2). The patient should be secured to the operating table to minimize any changes in position intraoperatively. The entire upper extremity should be prepped and draped to allow full mobility during the procedure.

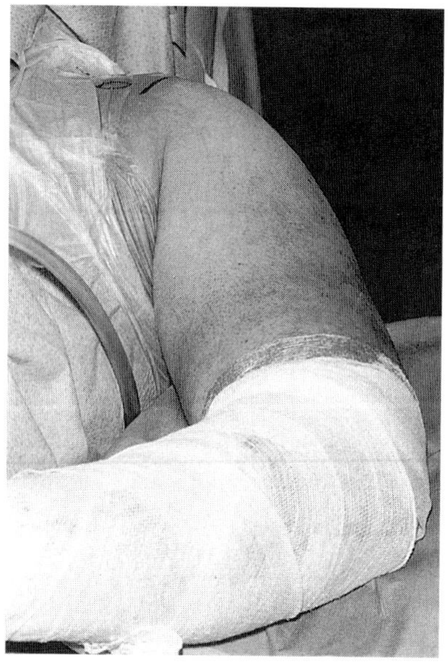

Fig. 2 Proper patient positioning is essential. The operating table should be elevated 30°, with the patient moved off the side of the table to allow complete mobility of the upper extremity. Support of the upper extremity on a Mayo stand adjacent to the operating table can be helpful during the procedure.

Surgical Approach

A straight deltopectoral incision is used that begins just lateral to the tip of the coracoid process and extends distally and laterally to the insertion of the deltoid (Fig. 3). The subcutaneous tissues are divided and medial and lateral flaps are elevated to expose the deeper muscular layers. The deltopectoral interval is identified by localization of the cephalic vein. The cephalic vein is usually retracted laterally with the deltoid muscle. In some instances, the cephalic vein is more easily retracted medially with the pectoralis major. In either case, care should be taken to preserve the cephalic vein throughout the procedure. The subdeltoid space is mobilized, as is the pectoralis major. The conjoined tendon muscles are identified and the clavipectoral fascia is divided at the medial edge of the conjoined tendon muscles. The fracture hematoma is usually evident after dividing the clavipectoral fascia. The conjoined tendon muscles and the pectoralis major are retracted medially and the deltoid is

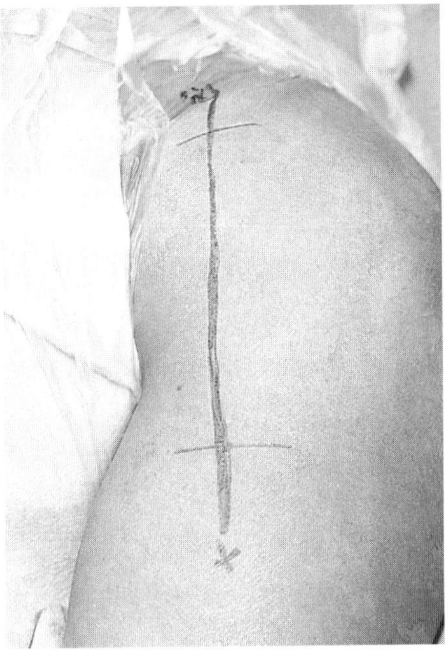

Fig. 3 A deltopectoral incision is used that extends from the area just lateral to the coracoid to the deltoid insertion.

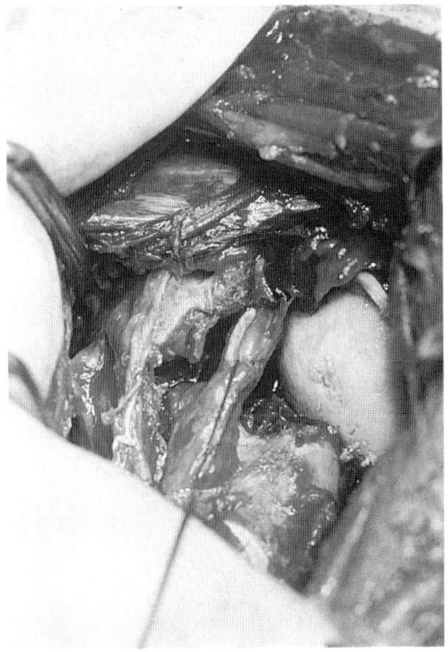

Fig. 4 The initial exposure should identify the biceps tendon. This assists in localizing the lesser tuberosity and greater tuberosity. In this intraoperative photograph, the articular segment is visualized lateral to the biceps tendon and the displaced lesser tuberosity is located medially.

retracted laterally. This can be most easily accomplished with the use of a self-retaining type of retractor. After the fracture hematoma has been evacuated, the deeper structures can be visualized. The biceps tendon should be identified and tagged with a suture (Fig. 4). The biceps tendon provides an orientation to the greater and lesser tuberosities. The lesser tuberosity is located medial to the biceps tendon and the greater tuberosity is located superiorly and laterally. Each tuberosity should be tagged with a #2 suture for easier mobilization. These sutures should be placed at the tendon insertion site because this is generally the most secure area; placement of the sutures through the tuberosity itself can result in fragmentation. The lesser tuberosity is mobilized and retracted medially while the greater tuberosity is retracted laterally and superiorly. This will allow visualization of the articular segment. In four-part fractures this segment is generally devoid of soft-tissue attachments and is easily removed. The coracoacromial ligament should be identified at its coracoid attachment and followed to its acromial attachment. Although in the past we have preferred to resect the ligament to decrease postoperative adhesions in this area, more recently our efforts have been to preserve the ligament because of its potential contribution to anterosuperior stability.

With the articular segment removed and the tuberosities retracted, the glenoid articular surface should be inspected. In the vast majority of situations, the articular surface of the glenoid is intact. It should be visualized to confirm the absence of pre-existing degenerative changes or acute injury. The axillary nerve can usually be easily palpated at the anteroinferior aspect of the glenoid. Continuity of the axillary nerve can be confirmed by the "tug test" which consists of palpation of the nerve as it comes around the humeral neck on the underside of the deltoid and as it passes inferior to the glenoid. A gentle back and forth "tugging" motion confirms its continuity. At this point the humerus should be placed in extension to expose the proximal portion of the humeral shaft.

Humeral Shaft Preparation

After the humerus has been placed in extension, the proximal humeral shaft can be accessed easily. A series of intramedullary broaches should be used to prepare the canal. Broaching should be continued until there is good cortical contact. At this point a trial component of appropriate size can be inserted. Because of the degree of proximal bone loss, it is necessary to place the prosthesis in a "proud" position. However, it is usually difficult to maintain the prosthesis in this position and to control rotation during trial reductions. To overcome this problem we have found it helpful to use a surgical sponge wrapped around the prosthesis (Fig. 5). This fills the canal and maintains the prosthesis in proper position. The desired position of retroversion is 20° to 35°. This can be modified if there is a pre-existing chronic dislocation or fracture-dislocation.

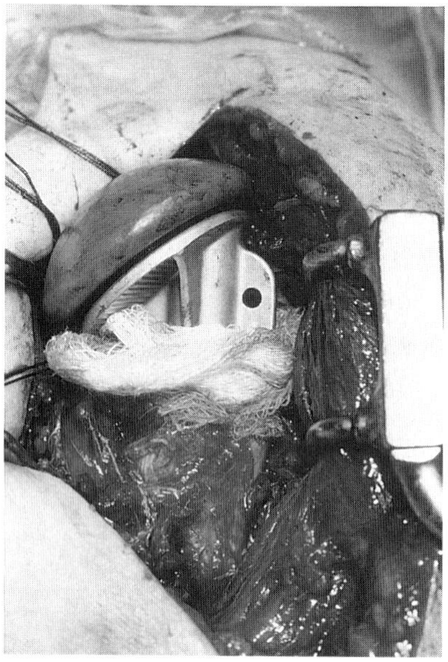

Fig. 5 Because of the degree of proximal bone loss, proper positioning of the trial prosthesis can be enhanced by use of a surgical sponge wrapped around the implant. This allows the prosthesis to be maintained in a "proud" position and maintains the proper position of retroversion.

The position of retroversion should be confirmed by comparing the position of the prosthesis with the transepicondylar axis. In addition, the position of the lateral or anterior flange of the prosthesis in relation to the adjacent humeral cortex should be marked and used to confirm proper position during cementing. The choice of head size should be based on the size of the removed humeral head regardless of whether the system used is modular or nonmodular. With the implant in place, the trial reduction can be performed.

The trial reduction is a critical part of the procedure because it defines the parameters needed to obtain a stable construct. After the humeral head is reduced onto the glenoid, the greater and lesser tuberosities are pulled into position. The biceps tendon is allowed to fall between the tuberosities. Traction on the tuberosity sutures not only maintains the tuberosities in position but also provides a more realistic assessment of stability. The self-retaining retractor should be relaxed for an accurate assessment of soft-tissue tension. Assessment of posterior, inferior, and anterior stability should be assessed by translating the humeral head in these directions. Up to 50% of posterior translation of the humeral head on the glenoid is acceptable; up to 50% of inferior translation is also acceptable. However, anterior translation should not exceed 25%. If these parameters are exceeded, the position of the component should be reevaluated to confirm that it has not subsided or rotated in the canal. If soft-tissue laxity is excessive, a larger humeral head should be used. Conversely, if soft-tissue tension is excessive, a smaller humeral head may be necessary. In either situation, repeat assessment of stability is required to confirm that the proper components and position have been chosen. When the proper position and component size are confirmed, the trial prosthesis should be removed.

At this point two drill holes should be placed through the humeral cortex into the medullary canal. These holes should be placed approximately 1.5 to 2 cm distal to the level of the surgical neck component in proximity to the bicipital groove. Two #5 nonabsorbable sutures are passed through one drill hole into the medullary canal and then out through the second drill hole (Fig. 6). These sutures will be used for tuberosity fixation. The medullary canal should be irrigated copiously and any loose cancellous bone removed. The use of the cement restrictor is based upon personal preference. We generally use a cement restrictor to enhance cement distribution. However, we avoid any formal pressurization of the cement to decrease the possibility of humeral shaft fracture. The canal should be packed with a sponge to obtain adequate drying before cementing.

The cement is mixed and poured into a vented 60 cc Toomey-type syringe approximately one minute after mixing (Fig. 7). This syringe should be vented by preparing a hole at the 20 to 30 cc level. This hole allows air to escape during insertion of the plunger so that a continuous column of cement is formed. The cement is then injected into the canal. During insertion of the prosthesis it is essential to maintain the prosthesis in the proper "proud" position as well as in the desired position of retroversion. The prosthesis should be held in position until the cement is completely set to avoid inadvertent subsidence or rotation into an unacceptable position. When the cementing is complete, the position should be confirmed. When a modular component is used, the modular head should be impacted into place, making certain that the taper is dry and free of any debris.

Tuberosity Fixation

Fixation of the tuberosities to the prosthesis and the shaft is a critical component of this procedure. Proper reattachment and secure fixation will enhance the probability of a successful outcome in terms of range of motion and overall function. However, careful attention must be given to the technical aspects of this portion of the procedure. Heavy (#5) nonabsorbable sutures should be used. These sutures are generally passed through the rotator cuff tendons just at their insertion into the tuberosities. The biceps tendon is allowed to fall between the tuberosities and is incorporated into the fixation. This results in a "functional

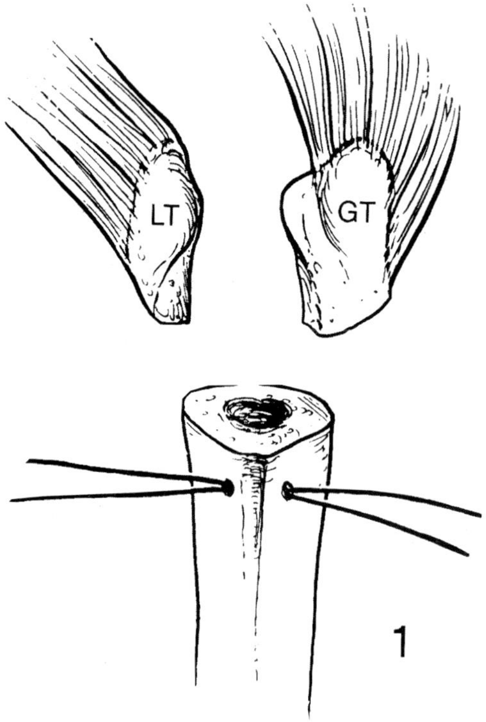

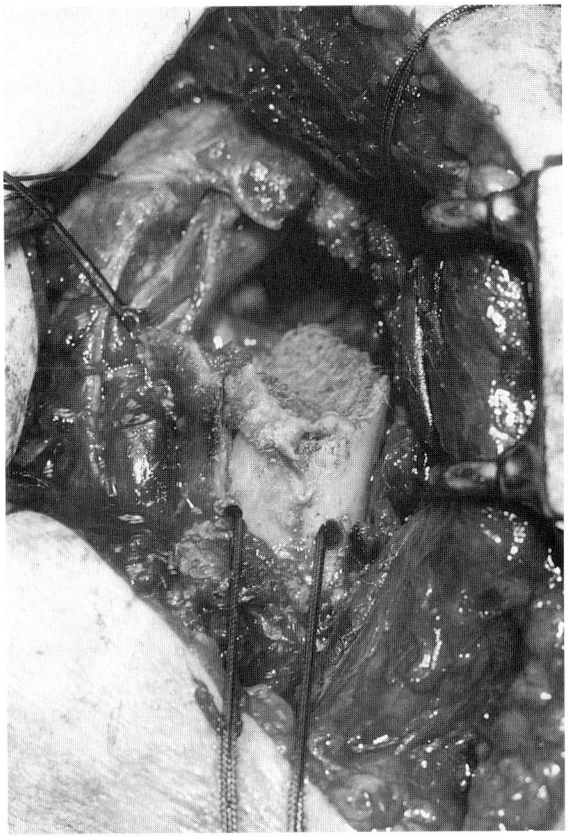

Fig. 6 After preparation of the humeral shaft, two drill holes are placed through the humeral cortex, one medial and one lateral to the bicipital groove. Heavy nonabsorable sutures are passed through the drill holes. The sutures will be used for tuberosity reattachment. This step is shown both graphically, **left,** and intraoperatively, **right.**

tenodesis" but probably preserves at least a portion of its humeral head depressor function.

The principles of tuberosity fixation include: (1) placement of longitudinal sutures to bring the tuberosities into a position below the prosthetic articular surface and into contact with the humeral shaft; and (2) transverse suture fixation, which brings the tuberosities into contact with each other and maintains the tuberosities in the distal position obtained with the longitudinal sutures. This is analogous to the principles of fixation of the greater trochanter in hip surgery, in which longitudinal wires are used to advance the trochanter distally into the proper position and transverse wires are used to secure the trochanter in this position.

At this point the two longitudinal sutures, which have already been passed through the humeral cortex, are used. The first longitudinal suture should be placed in a figure-of-eight fashion through the supraspinatus tendon as it inserts into the greater tuberosity and then through the upper portion of the subscapularis tendon as it inserts into the lesser tuberosity (Fig. 8, *top*). The second longitudinal suture should be passed in similar fashion through the infraspinatus tendon as it inserts into the greater tuberosity and through the lower portion of the subscapularis tendon as it inserts into the lesser tuberosity (Fig. 8, *top*). These sutures are passed but not tied. The first transverse suture is then passed through the supraspinatus tendon as it inserts into the greater tuberosity, through the upper hole of the lateral keel of the prosthesis and then through the upper portion of the subscapularis tendon as it inserts into the lesser tuberosity. The second transverse suture is passed, in similar fashion, through the infraspinatus tendon through the lower hole in the lateral keel and through the lower portion of the subscapularis tendon (Fig. 8, *top*). The suture tying sequence is important. The first longitudinal suture should be tied first. This will advance the tuberosities distally below the articular surface of the prosthesis and into contact with the humeral cortex, which is essential to obtain bone to bone healing. The second longitudinal suture should then be tied for enhanced fixation (Fig. 8, *bottom left*). When the tuberosities are confirmed to be in proper position, the superior transverse suture is tied followed by the inferior transverse suture. Transverse fixation

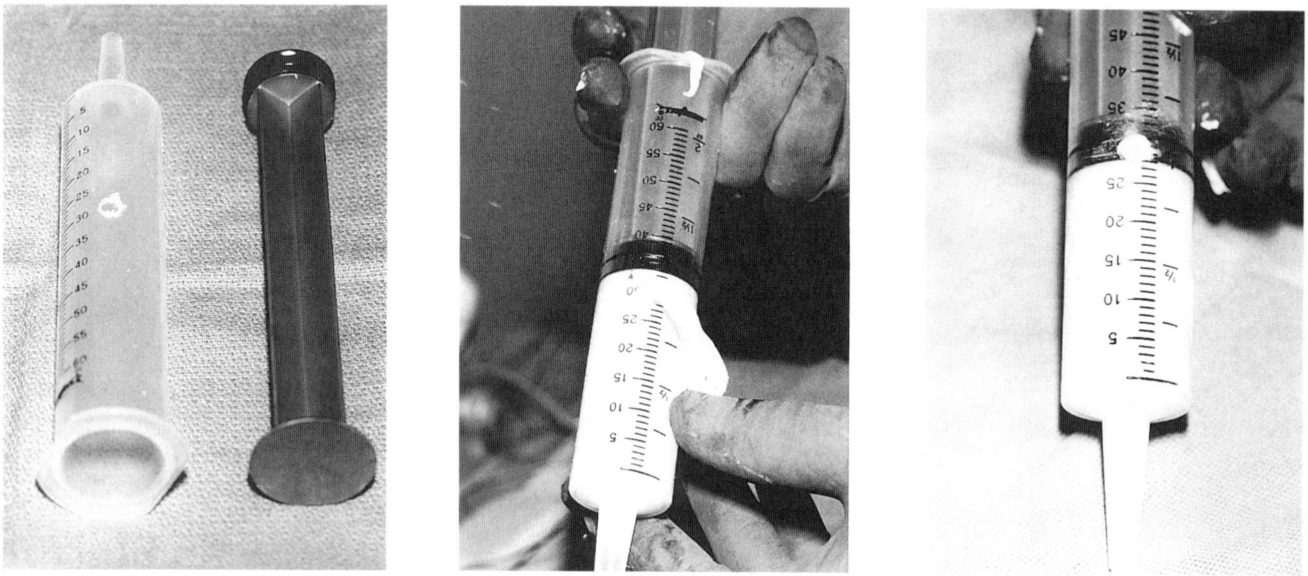

Fig. 7 Insertion of cement into the humeral canal can be enhanced by use of a vented syringe. A 60 cc Toomey-type syringe, **left,** is prepared by placing a hole through the wall of the syringe at the 30 cc level. Cement in its liquid stage is then poured into the syringe. The plunger is then inserted. Air and excess cement is then released through the vent hole, **center.** With this technique, a column of cement can be obtained for continuous injection into the humeral canal, **right.**

brings the tuberosities into contact with each other and maintains the position, obtained by the longitudinal sutures (Fig. 8, *bottom center*). Tuberosity reattachment should be performed with the arm in approximately 20° of abduction, neutral flexion, and 10° to 20° external rotation. When the tuberosity fixation is completed, the stability of the fixation should be carefully assessed (Fig. 8, *bottom right*). Range of motion in forward elevation, external rotation, internal rotation, and abduction should be performed to determine the specific limits of motion that will be allowed in the postoperative rehabilitation program. In addition, we have found that bone grafting the tuberosities can enhance the healing potential. Cancellous bone from the humeral head should be placed in the area of contact between the shaft and the tuberosities as well as between the tuberosities.

Closure includes repair of the rotator interval with #1 or #2 nonabsorbable sutures (Fig. 8, *bottom center*). This repair should be performed with the humerus in external rotation to decrease the possibility that rotator interval closure will restrict rotation. A closed suction drain is usually placed deep to the deltopectoral interval and brought out through the skin distally and laterally. The deltopectoral interval is repaired with absorbable suture, as is the subcutaneous tissue. This skin closure is performed with either sutures or staples. A sterile dressing is applied and the upper extremity is placed in a sling.

We feel it is very important to obtain a complete set of radiographs in the operating room. These should include an AP view of the shoulder with the humerus in internal rotation (on the chest) and maximum external rotation as defined by the intraoperative assessment. An axillary view should also be obtained (Fig. 9). These radiographs provide excellent visualization of the position of the prosthesis as well as the position of the tuberosities.

Postoperative Rehabilitation

On the first postoperative day, the patient is started on a rehabilitation program that consists of active range of motion of the elbow, wrist, and hand and passive range of motion of the shoulder. External rotation should be limited based upon the intraoperative evaluation. This is important to avoid any excess stress on the tuberosity repair that could compromise healing. Internal rotation is allowed to the chest. These exercises are continued for the first 6 to 8 weeks. Radiographs are obtained approximately 2 weeks following surgery to confirm the position of the tuberosities. Additional radiographs are obtained at 6 to 8 weeks following surgery to assess the degree of tuberosity healing. If tuberosity healing is sufficient, the sling is discontinued and an active range-of-motion program is begun. The patient is encouraged to use the involved upper

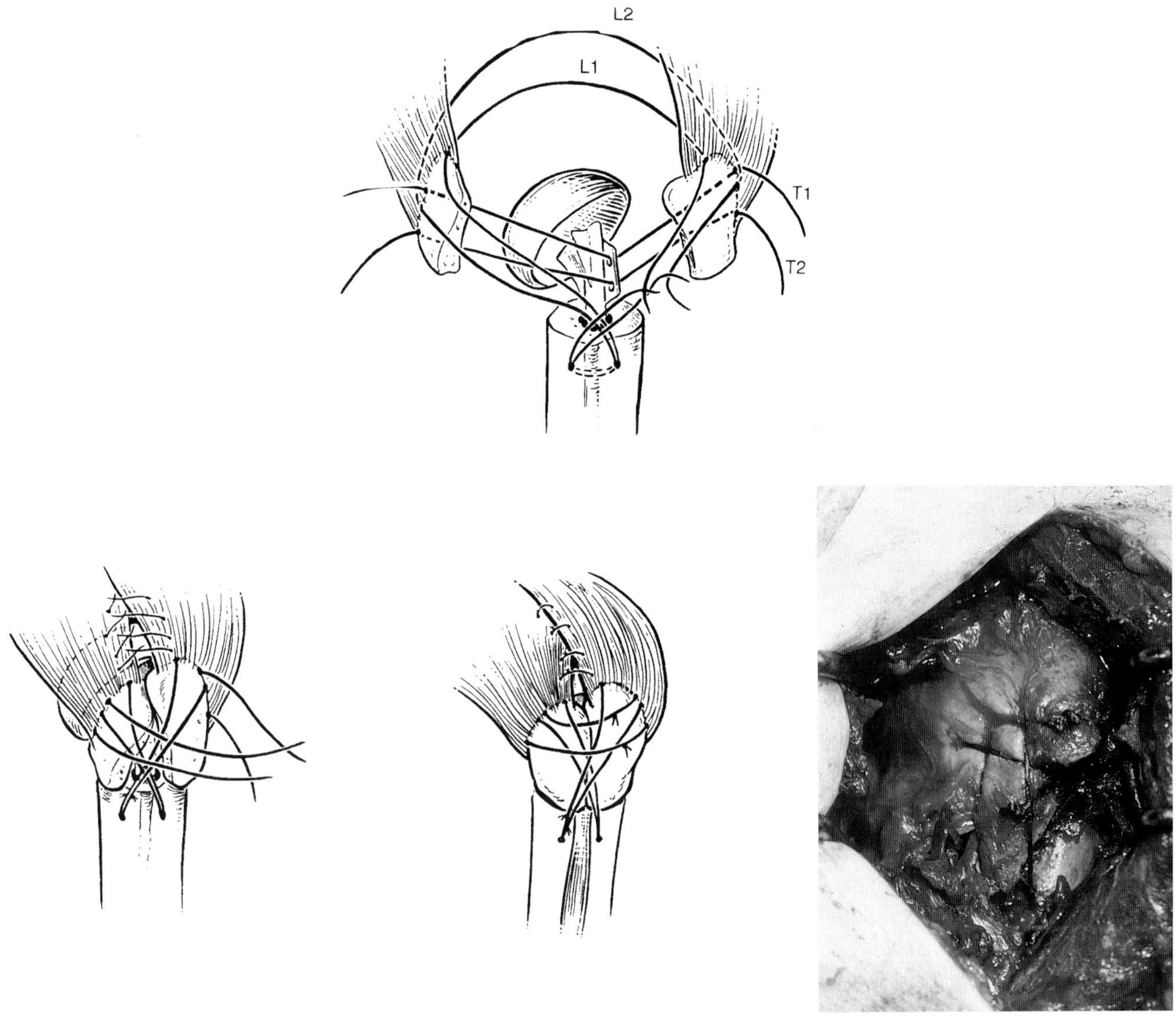

Fig. 8 Fixation of the tuberosities is achieved by placement of two longitudinal sutures (L1 and L2) from the humeral canal to the tuberosities as well as two transverse sutures (T1 and T2) through the tuberosities and through the lateral keel of the implant, **top.** The longitudinal sutures are tied first followed by the transverse sutures, **bottom left.** The rotator interval sutures are passed prior to completion of tuberosity attachment but are not tied until the tuberosity repair is completed. After all the sutures have been tied, **bottom center** and **bottom right,** the security of the fixation should be assessed by range of motion testing.

extremity for activities of daily living. Passive range of motion is continued with gentle stretching to increase the overall range. At 8 weeks following surgery, isometric deltoid and internal and external rotator strengthening exercises are begun. Vigorous strengthening exercises are not begun until active forward elevation of at least 90° is obtained. Our experience has shown that patients can expect continued recovery during the first year following surgery, although most recovery will occur during the first 6 months.

Results

Since the introduction of proximal humeral replacement for treatment of acute proximal humeral fractures there have been many reports in the orthopaedic literature documenting the outcomes of this procedure.[5-8] In general, the reported results have been quite variable. Some series have reported more than 90% satisfactory results, while other series have reported less than 50%.[1-4,6,9] The variability is difficult to explain but is probably related to both patient selection and

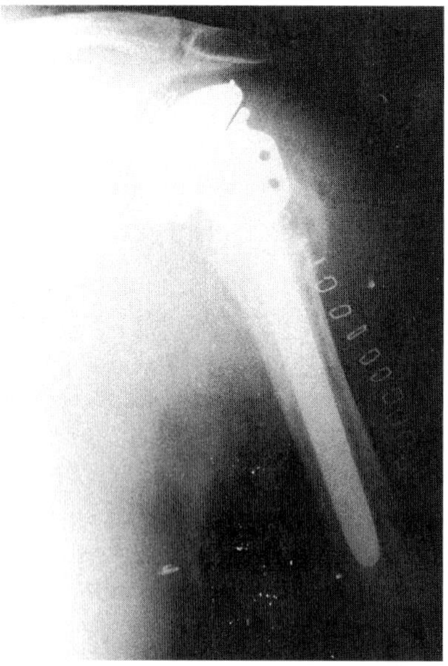

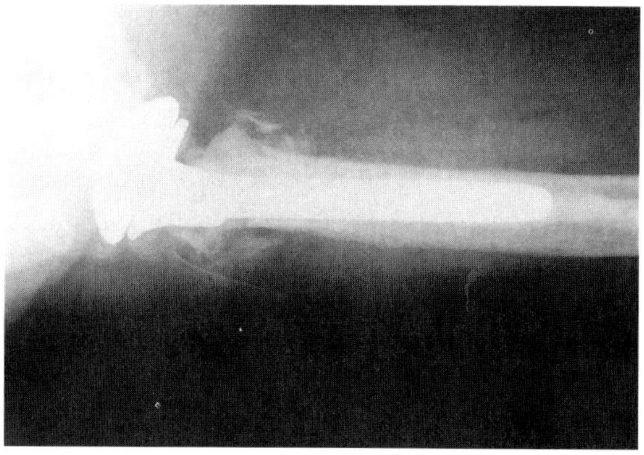

Fig. 9 Radiographs should be obtained in the operating room and should include an AP view with internal and external rotation, **left,** as well as an axillary view, **right.** These radiographs will confirm the proper position of the prosthesis as well as the position of the tuberosities adjacent to the prosthesis and in contact with the humeral shaft.

the outcome criteria used.[2,10] Surgical technique and postoperative rehabilitation are also important factors that can have a direct impact on the outcome. In general, the cumulative experience reported in the literature has shown that when this procedure is followed, patients are generally comfortable and pain is not a significant problem. However, functional recovery, ie, range of motion and the ability to use the upper extremities for activities of daily living, is inconsistent and somewhat unpredictable, particularly for use of the involved extremity at the shoulder level and above. This important information should be provided to patients before they undergo this procedure.

In summary, proximal humeral replacement has an important place in the treatment of complex proximal humeral fractures and fracture-dislocations, particularly for those fractures in which bone quality or comminution preclude the ability to obtain secure internal fixation and those at risk for the development of osteonecrosis. A successful outcome depends on many factors, including meticulous surgical technique with careful attention to restoration of soft-tissue tension and secure tuberosity fixation. Use of a structured and directed postoperative rehabilitation program is also an important component of the overall treatment plan.

References

1. Fischer RA, Nicholson GP, McIlveen SJ, et al: Primary humeral head replacement for severely displaced proximal humerus fractures. *Orthop Trans* 1992;16:779.
2. Hawkins RJ, Switlyk P: Acute prosthetic replacement for severe fractures of the proximal humerus. *Clin Orthop* 1993;289:156–160.
3. Moeckel BH, Dines DM, Warren RF, et al: Modular hemiarthroplasty for fractures of the proximal part of the humerus. *J Bone Joint Surg* 1992;74A:884–889.
4. Schai P, Imhoff A, Preiss S: Comminuted humeral head fractures: A multicenter analysis. *J Shoulder Elbow Surg* 1995;4:319–330.
5. Frich LH, Sojbjerg JO, Sneppen O: Shoulder arthroplasty in complex acute and chronic proximal humeral fractures. *Orthopedics* 1991;14:949–954.
6. Goldman RT, Koval KJ, Cuomo F, et al: Functional outcome after humeral head replacement for acute three-and-four-part proximal humeral fractures. *J Shoulder Elbow Surg* 1995;4:81–86.
7. Green A, Limbird RS, Barnard L: Humeral head replacement for acute four part fractures. *Orthop Trans* 1992;16:335.
8. Kraulis J, Hunter G: The results of prosthetic replacement in fracture-dislocations of the upper end of the humerus. *Injury* 1976;8:129–131.
9. Willems WJ, Lim TE: Neer arthroplasty for humeral fracture. *Acta Orthop Scand* 1985;56:394–395.
10. Tanner MW, Cofield RH: Prosthetic arthroplasty for fractures and fracture-dislocations of the proximal humerus. *Clin Orthop* 1983;179:116–128.

Complications of Humeral Head Replacement for Proximal Humeral Fractures

Michael P. Muldoon, MD
Robert H. Cofield, MD

Introduction

Prosthetic replacement of the humeral head is one treatment option for certain complex proximal humeral fractures, but a simpler treatment method should always be used when possible. Because complications can arise related to the misapplication of this form of treatment, great care must be taken in arriving at the specific diagnosis within this fracture category. Diagnosis may be possible by the use of standard, plain radiographs, or additional images, such as computed tomographic (CT) scans, may be necessary.[1-6]

The fracture classification system developed by Neer[7] is the one most commonly used, because it is based on anatomy, is easy to remember, and has direct implications for treatment decisions. It is recommended that humeral head replacement be considered for four-part fractures (which are almost always fracture-dislocations), humeral head splitting or crushing fractures, and a few three-part fractures in older patients with extensive osteopenia or comminution.[1,3,4,8-12] As experience with the applications of this classification system and treatment selection evolved, certain subgroups of fractures within these categories, such as valgus-impacted four-part fractures, might be more amenable to reduction and fixation than previously anticipated.[13-21] In addition, there are delayed complications of certain proximal humeral fractures that might also be most readily treated by prosthetic humeral head arthroplasty, such as osteonecrosis of the head segment, malunion involving the head segment,[22] nonunion of a proximal humeral fracture that includes a small osteopenic head fragment, or traumatic arthritis of the glenohumeral joint with a relatively preserved glenoid surface.

Several authors have reported patient series in which prosthetic humeral head replacement was used for the above indications. In 1970, Neer[11] reported on 43 shoulders with three- and four-part proximal humeral fractures; 38 achieved a satisfactory outcome. Subsequently, other authors[23-27] have also reported on the use of humeral head replacement in acute fractures, and this group of authors achieved 43 satisfactory results in 68 shoulders. Most patients achieved pain relief; several had persistent weakness and some stiffness. More recently, other authors have stressed the importance of restoring anatomic joint alignment with emphasis on management of the soft tissues and humeral tuberosities.[2,28-33] The frequency of satisfactory results may be improving.

Information on the outcome of humeral head replacement for chronic fractures is more limited.[34] Tanner and Cofield[26] reported on a group of patients who were treated for chronic fractures. Many of the patients had pain relief, but restoration of shoulder function was less consistent. Others have found measurably poorer results in those patients treated for chronic fractures versus those treated with a prosthesis in the acute setting and have suggested using humeral head replacement acutely when possible.[35] It is also said that complication rates are higher when applying this treatment method to chronic fractures.[35,36]

It is apparent that the indications for humeral head replacement secondary to proximal humeral fractures, whether acute or chronic, are reasonably well outlined, and a number of clinical reports indicate the type of results that can be achieved. A variety of complications have been recognized as a result of this form of treatment, but their frequency and significance are not defined. This chapter will review the available literature addressing complications, outline our experience, suggest preventive measures, and detail treatment options.

Literature

The complications that have been associated with humeral head replacement for proximal humeral fractures are listed in Outline 1. These complications may occur acutely or develop over time. They also can occur singly, or in combination, as when rotator cuff tearing is associated with instability.

Table 1 outlines the recognized complications following humeral head replacement for acute trauma in nine patient series. Overall, 71 complications developed in 203 shoulders (35%). Infection was uncommon, but more common than typically described for elective treatment of shoulder disorders using humeral head prostheses. Nerve injuries do occur; however, it may be difficult to determine if the nerve injury was present preoperatively, or present preoperatively to a mild degree and exacerbated by the procedure. Intraoperative fractures are very uncommon. The most common complication is shoulder instability, which

Outline 1
Complications of humeral head replacement for proximal humeral fractures

Problems with wound healing
Infection, early or delayed
Nerve injury, contusion/stretch or laceration
Humeral fracture
Component malposition
Instability
Problems with tuberosity healing: nonunion, malunion, resorption
Rotator cuff tearing
Reflex dystrophy
Periarticular fibrosis
Heterotopic ossification
Component loosening
Glenoid arthritis

may occur in the presence of tuberosity and rotator cuff problems or may exist without those additional complications. Tuberosity nonunion or malunion are also frequent complications, about which more will be mentioned later. Reflex dystrophy is surprisingly frequent. Heterotopic bone is uncommon, except in one patient series. The same can be said of glenoid arthritis in these patient series.

Complications related to delayed treatment of chronic fractures are outlined in Table 2. Overall, there were 41 complications in 100 shoulders, which is not substantially different than the frequency of complications seen in acute fractures. The distribution of complications is also remarkably similar.

There is only one article, that of Compito and associates[2] in 1994 on arthroplasty in acute shoulder trauma, that has organized information about the complications seen in failed prosthetic replacement for diplaced proximal humeral fractures. There were 30 failures in this series. The most common complication associated with failure was detachment of the greater tuberosity. Loosening of the humeral prosthesis occurred in 13 shoulders, 11 of which were uncemened. Two of the loosened prostheses were also infected. Other factors associated with failure included noncompliance with rehabilitation, nerve injury, glenoid erosion with arthritis, malposition of the humeral prosthesis, instability, and ectopic bone formation. Many of these complications are under the surgeon's control and are technical in nature. However, there are a number of complications that can occur despite technically adequate surgery, including failure of tuberosity healing, infection, nerve injury associated with the original trauma, subsequent development of glenoid arthritis, instability related to capsular disruption, and ectopic bone formation.

It is apparent that the frequency of complications is rather high and that complications are quite varied. Apparently, special care must be taken to prevent infection and to avoid new or additional nerve injury. Careful attention must be directed to the tuberosity repair and security of the rotator cuff and shoulder capsule. Although seldom emphasized in these reports, it seems clear that attention to component size and position, and security of component fixation are paramount to success.[37] It is clear that some patients with trauma may not always participate in cautious but persistent postoperative rehabilitation,[2] although this issue is not usually addressed in the literature. This behavior may, in fact, be associated with problems with tuberosity healing, rotator cuff tearing or instability, or alternatively it may be associated with periarticular stiffness, which seems to be underrepresented in these reports on complications.[9,31,38,39]

Mayo Clinic Experience

Patients and Methods

The Department of Orthopedics at the Mayo Clinic maintains a total joint registry such that all patients with arthroplasty are identified and periodically contacted for ongoing follow-up assessment. The registry was used to identify all humeral head replacements

Table 1
Complications in acutely treated cases

Reference	No. Shoulders	Wound Healing, Infection	Nerve Injury	Intra-operative Fracture	Instability	Tuberosity Nonunion or Malunion	Rotator Cuff Tear	Reflex Dystrophy	Heterotopic Bone	Glenoid Arthritis
Neer[11]	43	1	1			2			1	
Kraulis and Hunter[23]	11			1	4		1	2		
Tanner and Cofield[26]	16	1	1		4	4		1	1	1
Des Marchais et al[25]	8		1		1				1	
Stableforth[27]	16	2				4				
Neumann et al[30]	22		1							
Pietu et al[32]	35		2		9			2		
Moeckel et al[28]	22	1				1			9	
Hawkins and Switlyk[33]	20	1	1					2		7
Totals	203	6	7	1	18	11	1	7	12	8

Table 2
Complications in patients with delayed treatment (chronic fracture-related problems)

Reference	No. Shoulders	Infection	Nerve Injury	Intra-operative Fracture	Instability	Tuberosity Nonunion or Malunion	Rotator Cuff Tear	Reflex Dystrophy	Hetero-topic Ossification	Component Malposition
Tanner et al[26]	28	1	1		2	2	7	1	1	
Huten and Duparc[34]	18			2	2	3			7	1
Frich et al[35]	27	2			4					
Neumann et al[30]	7					1				
Dines et al[36]	20		1		2	1				
Totals	100	3	2	2	10	7	7	1	8	1

performed for acute proximal humeral fractures and for chronic proximal humeral fractures from 1979 to 1995. Twenty-six patients with 28 proximal humeral fractures who were treated with humeral head replacement for an acute injury were identified. Surgery was performed within 2 months following injury, with 23 of the 28 shoulders operated on within 2 weeks of injury. This group included 15 women and 11 men; the average age was 65 years (range, 25 to 89 years). The fractures were classified as four-part fractures or fracture-dislocations in 19 shoulders, three-part fractures or fracture-dislocations in six, and head-splitting fractures in three. At the time of surgery, 21 of the humeral head implants were cemented within the humerus, and seven were press-fitted. All patients were included to assure that all complications were recognized within the time constraints of the follow-up period. Three patients were followed less than 1 year, seven between 1 and 2 years, and the remainder for more than 2 years. Average follow-up was 56 months (range, 2 to 184 months).

Fifty-five patients with 55 involved shoulders were treated for problems that arose subsequent to initial treatment for a proximal humeral fracture or fracture-dislocation. Fifty-three patients had humeral head implants alone. In two shoulders, a glenoid component was also placed because of wear identified at the time of surgery.[40] The problems that led to surgery included nonunion in 17 shoulders, osteonecrosis of the humeral head in nine, traumatic glenohumeral arthritis in nine, proximal humeral malunion in eight, a poor result of a previously placed humeral head replacement (aching pain and stiffness) in eight, chronic dislocation in two, a flail shoulder related to excessive bone resection in one, and heterotopic ossification in one. In this group with chronic fractures, there were 30 women and 25 men. The average age was 56 years (range, 19 to 80 years). Forty-one had undergone a previous surgical procedure in treatment of their fracture. In this patient subgroup, seven were followed for less than 1 year, one for 1 to 2 years, and the remainder for greater than 2 years. The average length of follow-up was 57 months and ranged from 5 to 156 months. At surgery, 38 of the implants were cemented to the humerus, and 17 were press-fitted.

Results

The purpose of this chapter is to analyze complications. However, the results are reported to illustrate the rather typical nature of this patient group. In those treated with humeral head replacement within 2 months of injury, all but two patients had either no or mild shoulder pain. Average active elevation was 112°. In those treated surgically within 2 weeks of their injury, average active elevation was 126°. Active elevation was below 90° in 11 shoulders. Of these patients, seven had complications, and three others had radiographic evidence of tuberosity resorption. Four shoulders developed some radiolucency surrounding the implant; in three, this was incomplete. One noncemented implant was considered to be loose. A small amount of osteolysis was present around the proximal portion of one implant. There were no instances of tuberosity malunion. There was tuberosity nonunion in two shoulders and resorption of the greater tuberosity in six shoulders. In six shoulders, there was a variable degree of glenoid arthritis; it was mild in four. There was more than a mild amount of prosthetic humeral head translation on the glenoid in 13 shoulders; in eight the translation was superior, in two it was anterior, in two it was inferior, and in one it was posterior.

In the group of 55 shoulders with chronic fracture problems treated with a humeral head replacement, 14 had more than mild residual pain. Eleven of these patients classified their pain as moderate and three as severe. Active elevation averaged 61° preoperatively and 97° postoperatively (range, 20° to 170°). Patients who had a failed humeral head replacement had noticeably worse results than others in this grouping. Pain relief was less consistent, and average active elevation was 42°. On radiographic assessment, six implants were surrounded by some degree of radiolucency; in two noncemented components, these lucencies were complete. Tuberosity nonunion and tuberosity malunion were each present in two shoulders. Tuberosity resorption was present in seven shoulders. Twenty-one shoulders had some degree of glenoid arthritis. There was more than a mild amount of prosthetic humeral head translation on the glenoid in 20 shoulders. In ten cases of subluxation that might be considered more than mild, the subluxation was superior in six and anterior in four. With moderate to severe subluxation, the direction of instability was superior in five, posterior in three, and anterior in two.

Complications

In the six cases with infection, three were in the acute fracture group and three in the chronic fracture group (Table 3). In one of the patients with acute fracture, early closed fracture reduction failed; 10 days later the patient was treated with an endoprosthesis. Two weeks later, infection was suspected, and an aspirate grew *Staphylococcus epidermidis*. Antibiotics were administered intravenously, and 5 years later the patient was infection-free. In the other two patients treated for acute fractures, infections developed 21 and 24 months following surgery (Fig. 1); one patient had diabetes mellitus. An aspirate from one shoulder grew *S epidermidis*; the other grew *S aureus*. Both patients were subsequently treated with resection arthroplasty. Of the three patients with chronic fracture problems with infections, superficial infection (*S aureus*) developed in one patient 3 weeks following surgery. Surgical debridement was required, but the wound healed satisfactorily, and at follow-up the patient was infection-free. The other two patients presented at 4 and 6 months following surgery. In one, the culture was negative; in the other, *S aureus* was cultured. Both were treated with resection arthroplasty. Thus, in these limited numbers of patients, those with acute problems were treated successfully with either debridement and antibiotics or antibiotics alone. Those with chronic problems required resection arthroplasty because of the combination of septic arthritis and osteomyelitis surrounding the implant.

Table 3
Complications of humeral head replacement for proximal humeral fractures (Mayo Clinic Series)

	Acute	Chronic	Totals
No. shoulders	28	55	83
Infection	3	3	6
Nerve injury	0	0	0
Fracture	0	3	3
Instability	2	10	12
Tuberosity nonunion	2	2	4
Tuberosity malunion	0	2	2
Rotator cuff tear	2	4	6
Reflex dystrophy	1	0	1
Implant malposition	0	3	3
Glenoid arthritis	2	7	9
Implant loosening	1	2	3
Totals	13	36	49

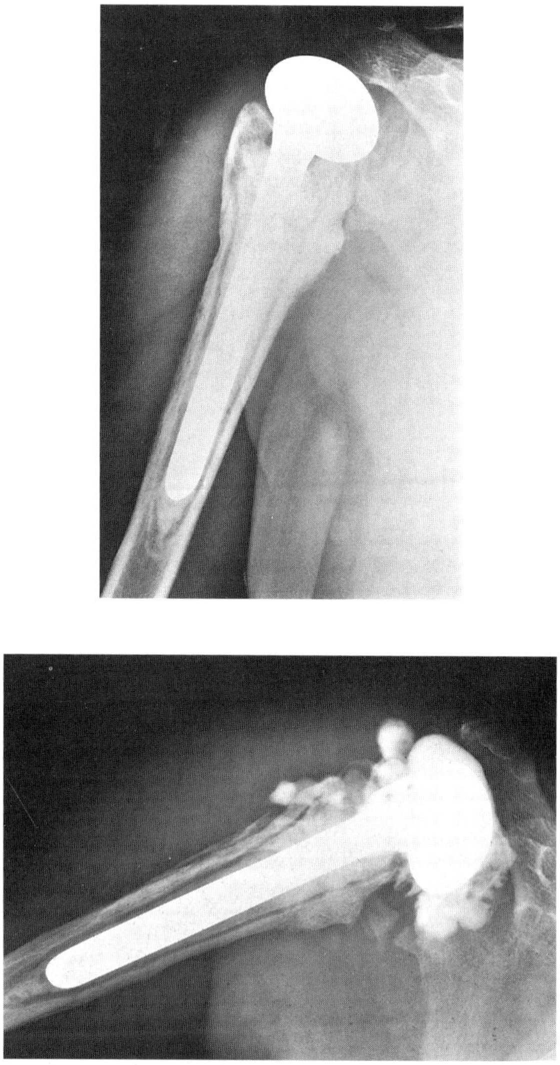

Fig. 1 **Top,** Radiograph of a 27-year-old man 2 years following placement of a humeral head prosthesis for a four-part proximal humeral fracture. At this time he presented with moderate to severe pain. A large complete lucent zone can be seen between the cement and bone surrounding the stem of the humeral head prosthesis, and there is some resorption of the humeral metaphyseal bone. **Bottom,** Aspiration and shoulder arthrography were performed. The aspirate grew *Staphylococcus aureus*. The arthrogram shows multiple synovial diverticula indicative of fistula formation. A resection arthroplasty was performed.

Three patients had humeral shaft fractures; two of these fractures occurred intraoperatively. One of the fractures healed following management with a long-stemmed prosthesis and cerclage cables. Another fracture was treated with circling bands. Unfortunately, infection developed and resection arthroplasty was necessary; the fracture healed. The third fracture occurred in a patient who subsequently developed multiple myeloma with a lesion at the tip of the prosthesis. This fracture was managed nonsurgically, but the patient soon died.

Two patients with acute fractures had moderate to severe instability. Inferior subluxation developed in one, but it resolved over a matter of weeks, with excellent results. Anterior-inferior subluxation associated with proximal humeral bone loss and component malposition (with poor results) developed in the other patient, who was elderly and declined reoperation. In those shoulders treated for chronic fracture problems, instability developed in ten. In four of these, the instability was clearly associated with rotator cuff tearing and was superior in direction. Posterior subluxation recurred in two patients who had been treated for chronic posterior dislocations. One of these patients experienced improvement with external support and exercise. Degenerative arthritis developed in the second patient, and revision total shoulder arthroplasty was performed (Fig. 2). At surgery, excessive retrotorsion of the implant was identified, and component malposition was believed to have played an important role in this patient's condition. Anterior instability developed in two patients. In one of the patients, the instability was associated with increased antetorsion of the prosthesis (malposition) and rotator cuff tearing; in the other patient, the condition was related to stretching of the anterior repair in combination with a generalized stiffness occurring in the early postoperative period. Two other patients with superior subluxation had severely compromised results. One had greater tuberosity nonunion but refused further treatment. The other developed degenerative joint disease and revision total shoulder arthroplasty was performed. Thus, instability is recognized as the most common complication; it can occur after treatment for acute or chronic fractures, in any direction and in any degree. Superior instability is usually associated with injury to the rotator cuff or tuberosity. Anterior instability is usually associated with failure of healing or stretching of the anterior structures. Posterior instability often precedes prosthetic treatment. In our patients, three of the ten in whom moderate or severe instability developed had associated component malposition.

Tuberosity nonunion developed in two shoulders following treatment for an acute fracture and in two shoulders following treatment for a chronic fracture. In the acute fractures, one involved the lesser tuberosity and was minimally symptomatic. The second involved the greater tuberosity. In this patient, infection developed and resection arthroplasty was performed at 24 months following surgery. In the shoulders with chronic fractures, both involved the greater tuberosity and one, in addition, involved the lesser tuberosity. One of these patients was minimally symptomatic relative to pain but had only 45° of active abduction (Fig. 3). This

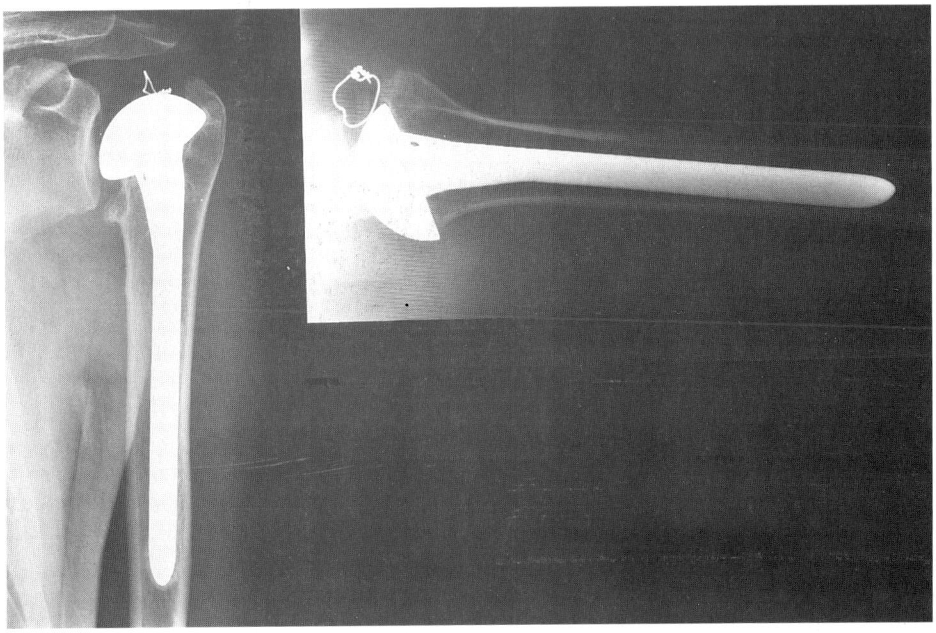

Fig. 2 Radiographs of a 32-year-old man in whom a humeral head prosthesis was placed 7 years earlier for treatment of a comminuted proximal humeral fracture. He now has moderate to severe pain. Anteroposterior and axillary radiographs show tuberosity malunion and nonunion, probable undersizing of the humeral head implant, posterior glenohumeral subluxation, and traumatic arthritis. Revision total shoulder arthroplasty was performed, and 11 years later he has only occasional moderate pain, 115° of active abduction, and 30° of external rotation.

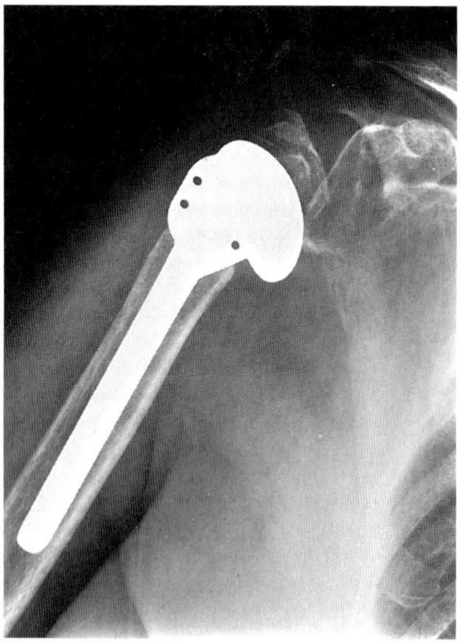

Fig. 3 Radiograph of a 72-year-old woman who had humeral head replacement for a four-part proximal humeral fracture. She has inferior glenohumeral subluxation, probable component loosening, and greater tuberosity nonunion. Despite these findings, she has only mild pain, but active abduction of only 10° with passive abduction of 90° and external rotation of 50°. She elected not to undergo revision surgery.

80-year-old woman elected not to have further surgery. A second patient had only mild pain, surprisingly good strength, and a satisfactory result at 8 months of follow-up. Thus, interestingly, in this patient group, tuberosity nonunion was not particularly associated with pain. When the lesser tuberosity alone was involved, the patient was minimally symptomatic. When the greater tuberosity was affected, active abduction and strength were somewhat compromised, but to a variable degree.

In two patients with chronic fractures, tuberosity malunion occurred after humeral head replacement. Both patients had required greater tuberosity osteotomy as part of their reconstructive procedure, and one required additional bone grafting to replace proximal humeral bone deficiency. In one patient, the tuberosity resorbed somewhat. There was 110° of active elevation, and the patient was satisfied. In the second patient, the patient with bone grafting, moderate pain continued. The patient had only 80° of active elevation and was dissatisfied with the result.

Rotator cuff tearing developed in two patients treated for acute fractures and in four treated for chronic fracture problems. In the acute fracture group, one tear developed 6 months after surgery following a fall. The subscapularis and supraspinatus were rerepaired. Unfortunately, this patient subsequently had a seizure and retore the repair. A second surgery resulted in only 50° of active abduction at follow-up. In the second patient, rotator cuff tearing was seen 14 months after surgery, and was associated with superior subluxation. The patient was noncompliant for self-protection and rehabilitation, was 71 years old, and no further treatment was entertained. In those four patients treated for chronic fracture, two rotator cuff tears were seen 6 months after surgery. One of the tears was associated with a seizure and anterior dislocation. The subscapularis was surgically repaired. With the second tear, surgical repair of the supraspinatus was performed and the infraspinatus was reinforced with fascia lata graft. In the third patient, a diagnosis was made 2 years after surgery. The patient had dystonia, and no further treatment was elected. In the fourth patient, a diagnosis was made at 10 years. This condition occurred in association with degenerative arthritis, and the humeral head implant was converted to a total shoulder arthroplasty. Thus, rotator cuff tearing can occur with both acute and chronic fractures. Tearing often occurs subsequent to a second injury, but can occur without history of injury. Those tears that did occur following injury were all surgically repaired, and chronic tears were evaluated for elective surgery based on the number of symptoms and the patient's needs and limitations.

Reflex dystrophy developed in only one patient, following treatment for an acute fracture. The dystrophy included shoulder stiffness. The patient was helped by nerve blocks, but at 6 months had only 90° of elevation. At 6-year follow-up, she remained dissatisfied with her fracture treatment.

As noted earlier, implant malposition occurred in three patients with instability. These were the only patients believed to have component malposition. In the shoulder of one patient, the implant was seated too inferiorly in the humerus. In the second, the implant was placed in too much retroversion, and in the third, it was placed in too much anteversion. All three patients had a poor result. One required conversion to a total shoulder arthroplasty because of associated degenerative arthritis.

Severe glenoid arthritis developed in two patients in the acute fracture group. One had minimal symptoms at a 7-year follow-up. In the second patient, the arthritis developed in association with prosthetic loosening; revision to a total shoulder arthroplasty was required after 11 years. Glenoid arthritis developed in seven shoulders treated for chronic fracture problems (Fig. 4). In two, an initial total shoulder arthroplasty was placed because of glenoid wear at surgery. Five had glenoid wear over time and were converted to total shoulder arthroplasty 2 to 12 years following their humeral head replacement. An eighth patient would have been converted to a total shoulder arthroplasty but was treated with glenoid reshaping because of significant glenoid bone loss.

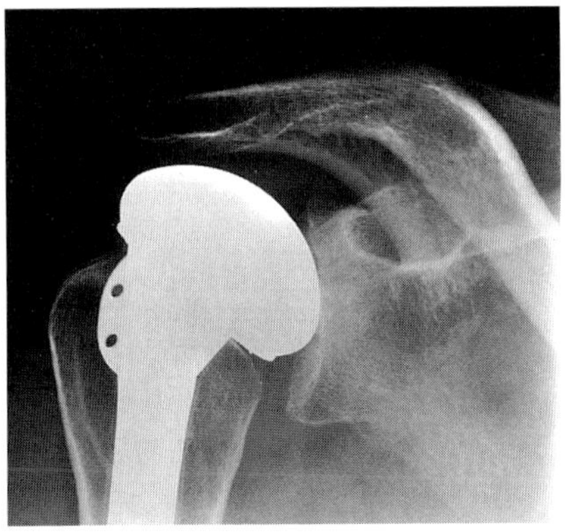

Fig. 4 A 41-year-old man underwent humeral head replacement for a fixed posterior fracture-dislocation of the shoulder. Six years later he has occasional moderate pain, 120° of active abduction, and -10° of external rotation. The radiograph shows loss of cartilage on the glenoid articular surface indicative of glenoid arthritis.

Humeral component loosening has been quite uncommon. One patient in the acute fracture group developed loosening of a press-fitted humeral component at 11 years. In the chronic fracture group, a second shoulder with press-fitting was revised at 10 years to a cemented total shoulder arthroplasty. A second patient with chronic fracture had been treated with a cemented humeral head replacement; at 3 years this patient had a complete lucent line 1.5 mm in diameter and the component was considered loose, but not symptomatic enough to require revision surgery. Of the humeral head replacements, 59 were fixed with cement at the time of surgery, and 24 were press-fitted. It appears that either method is satisfactory if secure fixation is obtained at the time of surgery.

In summary, in the patients treated with a humeral head replacement for acute fractures, there were seven different types of complications. Infections were somewhat more common than one might expect. Tuberosity nonunion or malunion and rotator cuff tearing was less common than the literature has suggested. Glenoid arthritis occasionally developed, as did implant loosening. Overall, there were 11 patients who developed 13 complications in the group of 28 shoulders (46%). In the patients with chronic fractures, there were nine different types of complications. Again, infection was slightly more common than is seen in elective shoulder surgery. Instability, which was much more common in the acute fracture patients, may be associated with problems such as tuberosity healing or rotator cuff tearing or may occur in the absence of these associated complications. Implant malposition occasionally occurred, as did implant loosening. The late development of glenoid arthritis is possible, but it was not of such frequency that routine total shoulder arthroplasty would be advocated in lieu of humeral head replacement alone—when the cartilage is normal or near normal. Overall, there were 29 patients who developed 36 complications in the group of 55 shoulders (65%).

Table 4
Reoperations (Mayo Clinic Series)

	Acute	Chronic	Totals
Debridement for infection	0	1	1
Resection for infection	2	2	4
Rotator cuff repair	2	2	4
Glenoid recontouring	0	1	1
TSA for glenoid wear	1	7	8
Totals	5	13	18 (22%)

Reoperations

In those patients treated for acute fracture problems, two underwent resection arthroplasty in treatment for infection. One patient had two rotator cuff rerepairs, and a glenoid component was later placed in one shoulder because of glenoid arthritis. In those with chronic fractures, debridement for infection was performed in one shoulder, resection arthroplasty for infection in two, rotator cuff repairs in two, and glenoid arthritis symptomatic enough to require treatment developed in eight; in seven of these, a glenoid component was placed. It can be seen that the need for reoperation is about equally frequent in acute fractures and in chronic fracture conditions, and, overall, 18 reoperations were necessary (22%). This reinforces the high rate of complications for this form of treatment in these patient groups (Table 4).

Preventive Measures

Without question, the concomitant damage to the soft tissues is an important contributing factor to the slightly higher incidence of infection in acute fractures. Before elective prosthetic shoulder arthroplasty is performed for acute fractures, the axilla should be washed, powdered, and padded before surgery to prevent maceration, the skin carefully cleansed, and prophylactic antibiotics administered.

Exposure must be ample during surgery. The deltopectoral approach is usually adequate for acute fracture surgery. With chronic fractures, it may be necessary to enlarge exposure, performing an anteromedial approach that uses the deltopectoral interval and by releasing the deltoid from the clavicle and anterior acromion. This procedure will allow more careful dissection of the tissue planes, avoiding injury to the nerves, and also lessening forces on the humerus, the latter being necessary to prevent the occasional intraoperative humeral fracture.

It is important to place the implant in correct position and to fix it securely. Rotational position can be ascertained by use of a combined intramedullary and extramedullary humeral resection guide. Correct height can be determined by traction on the limb and also by careful study of the fracture pattern. If an implant with tissue-ingrowth capabilities is used, there must be security of fixation, both in the humeral canal and in the humeral metaphysis. If both areas are not intact to allow secure fixation, methylmethacrylate cement should be used to secure the implant to the humerus. Currently, there are many sizes of humeral heads available in the multiple modular systems, and use of the proper size will help in adjusting tension across the tuberosity and promoting rotator cuff repair, and hopefully will lessen any tendency for instability.

The tuberosities should be secured with both horizontal and vertical suturing. The horizontal sutures may be lateral only, encompassing the tuberosities and the holes in the lateral fin of the implant, or they may be lateral and medial, encircling the implant beneath the humeral head component and continuing laterally much as the pattern for lateral suturing alone. The vertical suturing will be box-shaped, figure-of-8-shaped, or both. We prefer to use at least two, perhaps three, horizontal sutures and two vertical sutures, one of which is in the figure-of-8 style. Wire tends to fragment and probably should not be used. The fate of cables in this situation is uncertain. The preferred nonabsorbable suture material, or nonabsorbable tape, is preferred.

In chronic fracture problems, the concomitant use of a glenoid component should be considered. If there is moderate cartilage wear, it may well be efficacious to place a glenoid component at the time of humeral head replacement. However, please recall that of the 55 shoulders treated for chronic fracture problems in the Mayo Clinic series, to date only seven have required revision for glenoid arthritis.

Early passive motion within the limits of the security of the tuberosity and rotator cuff repair, determined at the time of surgery, will help prevent adhesions and stiffness. It will also prevent subacute stretching of the tuberosity and rotator cuff repair and, hopefully, retard the potential for the development of dystrophic changes within the limb.

Because many of the patients with these fractures and requiring treatment are elderly, planning for postoperative social arrangements is very important. These patients will not be able to live alone for at least the first month following surgery, and they will need assistance with their physical therapy for at least this long, if not longer.

Treatment Options

Prompt diagnosis of a postoperative infection is paramount. Aspiration is usually required, often done in association with arthrography to determine the presence or absence of sinus tracts. In the acute infection, occasionally antibiotics alone will suffice in the presence of a very susceptible and low-virulence organism. Otherwise, debridement is in order in addition to the intravenous antibiotic treatment. Certain individuals develop delayed acute infections that often mimic septic arthritis. Again, debridement might be a consideration for a low-grade infection with an organism of lesser virulence. Typically, however, either a one-stage or two-stage implant exchange must be considered. We prefer to delay a two-stage exchange for at least 6 to 8 weeks. Chronic infections often present not only as septic arthritis but have a significant element of osteomyelitis. Resection arthroplasty has been the standard treatment of choice. The success of delayed reimplantation in the shoulder is unknown. Following infections, there is often substantial involvement of the shoulder capsule and rotator cuff, making delayed reimplantation less desirable than it might be, for instance, in the hip.

Nerve injuries are not that uncommon. The nerve injury may occur at the time of an acute fracture or after surgical treatment. It is important to define the nerve injury as accurately as possible. Nerve recovery almost always begins before 6 weeks after surgery. If it does not occur by that time or there is no significant improvement, electrodiagnostic studies are useful. Patients can then be followed for continued assessment of their recovery. Exploration might well be considered in certain local nerve injuries, particularly musculocutaneous or axillary nerve injuries, depending on the level of the surgeon's confidence relative to the nerve not being injured by a laceration or incorporation in a suture repair. If recovery from a local nerve injury is not seen either clinically or with electrical testing by 6 months, exploration should be considered.

A few patients have postoperative humeral fractures at the level of the tip of the prosthesis or slightly proximal or distal to this. Typically, if the fracture is reducible, external support will suffice. If the fracture is nonreducible or remains mobile after 3 months of external support, cerclage or plate fixation, depending upon the pattern of the fracture, should be considered. If, as a part of fracturing, the implant becomes loose, consideration should be given to revising the implant and fixing the fracture. Typically, this is done with a long-stem implant, with or without cerclage, again depending on the fracture pattern.

In patients with a mild to moderate degree of subluxation, the instability often requires no treatment.

This is particularly true for early inferior subluxation, which often resolves over time and with isometric exercises for the biceps, triceps, and deltoid muscles. Subluxation in a superior direction is almost always combined with rotator cuff stretching or tearing or tuberosity nonunion or malunion. Whether or not revision surgery is considered depends on the patient's symptom level and physical demands. There is a tendency toward repair if subluxation occurs following an acute injury, and conservative treatment methods are more likely to be used when subluxation occurs over time. Subluxation or dislocation in the anterior direction will almost always occur in combination with disruption of the subscapularis or displacement of the lesser tuberosity. In this setting, there is a strong tendency for surgical repair of the anterior structures with or without a reinforcing graft. For subluxations in the posterior direction, or for dislocations for that matter, capsular plication or repair posteriorly are possible if the joint is otherwise well-balanced and the anterior structures are supple; however, the anterior structures are often contracted. These structures need to be lengthened and the humeral component revised, adjusting its torsion and also adjusting the size of the humeral head. If there is posterior glenoid wear associated with the posterior humeral subluxation, total shoulder arthroplasty is quite likely the treatment of choice.

A variety of tuberosity and rotator cuff problems occur. There is a tendency to repair acute disruptions, especially when these are associated with instability. When these problems develop over time, surgery is often elective, depending on pain, functional limitations, and patient demands.

Finally, there are a number of situations in which implant revision surgery will be the only treatment choice. This is particularly true if a patient develops severe pain in association with glenoid arthritis, and also, if there is component malposition with poor function and subluxation or dislocation. Also, implant revision surgery would be indicated when there is component loosening associated with significant symptoms.

Summary

The indications for humeral head replacement in acute fractures and in chronic fracture problems have been studied over many decades and are reasonably well defined. Complications have probably been understudied. Many different complications occur, and their frequency and the need for reoperation is quite high. Because of the variety of complications that occur, familiarity with preventive measures and treatment options is important, not only to deal with complications arising from endoprostheses, but also to treat musculoskeletal infections, nerve injuries, fractures, instability, nonunion of tuberosities, malunion, and rotator cuff or capsule contracture or tearing. Physicians also must be able to integrate reparative/reconstructive surgery with a program of postoperative rehabilitation. The challenges are many. Treatment often provides considerable improvement for the patient, but often the extent of the improvement is somewhat less than optimal.

References

1. Cofield RH: Comminuted fractures of the proximal humerus. *Clin Orthop* 1988;230:49–57.
2. Compito CA, Self EB, Bigliani LU: Arthroplasty and acute shoulder trauma: Reasons for success and failure. *Clin Orthop* 1994;307:27–36.
3. Connor PM, D'Alessandro DF: Role of hemiarthroplasty for proximal humeral fractures. *J South Orthop Assoc* 1995;4:9–23.
4. Schai P, Von Flüe M, Staubli AE, et al: Functional results of Neer II type hemi-arthroplasty joint replacement of multifragment humerus head fractures. *Helv Chir Acta* 1991; 57:799–804.
5. Sidor ML, Zuckerman JD, Lyon T, et al: The Neer classification system for proximal humerus fractures: An assessment of interobserver reliability and intraobserver reproductibility. *J Bone Joint Surg* 1993;75A:1745–1750.
6. Siebenrock KA, Gerber C: The reproducibility of classification of fractures of the proximal end of the humerus. *J Bone Joint Surg* 1993;75A:1751–1755.
7. Neer CS II: Displaced proximal humeral fractures: I. Classification and evaluation. *J Bone Joint Surg* 1970;52A: 1077–1089.
8. Dines DM, Altchek DW: Hemiarthroplasty techniques for proximal humerus fractures. *Complic Orthop* 1991;6:25–31.
9. Kristiansen B, Christensen SW: Proximal humeral fractures: Late results in relation to classification and treatment. *Acta Orthop Scand* 1987;58:124–127.
10. Mills KL: Severe injuries of the upper end of the humerus. *Injury* 1974;6:13–21.
11. Neer CS II: Displaced proximal humeral fractures: II. Treatment of three-part and four-part displacement. *J Bone Joint Surg* 1970;52A:1090–1103.
12. Schlegel TF, Hawkins RJ: Displaced proximal humeral fractures: Evaluation and treatment. *J Am Acad Orthop Surg* 1994;2:54–66.
13. Cuomo F, Flatow EL, Maday MG, et al: Open reduction and internal fixation of two- and three-part displaced surgical neck fractures of the proximal humerus. *J Shoulder Elbow Surg* 1992;1:287–295.
14. Darder A, Darder A Jr, Sanchis V, et al: Four-part displaced proximal humeral fractures: Operative treatment using Kirschner wires and a tension band. *J Orthop Trauma* 1993;7:497–505.
15. Esser RD: Open reduction and internal fixation of three- and four-part fractures of the proximal humerus. *Clin Orthop* 1994;299:244–251.
16. Hawkins RJ, Bell RH, Gurr K: The three-part fracture of the proximal part of the humerus: Operative treatment. *J Bone Joint Surg* 1986;68A:1410–1414.
17. Jakob RP, Miniaci A, Anson PS, et al: Four-part valgus impacted fractures of the proximal humerus. *J Bone Joint Surg* 1991; 73B:295–298.
18. Kristiansen B, Christensen SW: Plate fixation of proximal humeral fractures. *Acta Orthop Scand* 1986;57:320–323.
19. Paavolainen P, Björkenheim JM, Slätis P, et al: Operative treatment of severe proximal humeral fractures. *Acta Orthop Scand* 1983;54:374–379.

20. Sturzenegger M, Fornaro E, Jakob RP: Results of surgical treatment of multifragmented fractures of the humeral head. *Arch Orthop Trauma Surg* 1982;100:249–259.
21. Towfigh H, Buhl W, Obertacke U: Results of treatment after conservative and surgical management of proximal humerus fractures. *Aktuelle Traumatol* 1993;23:354–360.
22. Fourrier P, Martini M: Post-traumatic avascular necrosis of the humeral head. *Int Orthop* 1997;1:187–190.
23. Kraulis J, Hunter G: The results of prosthetic replacement in fracture-dislocations of the upper end of the humerus. *Injury* 1976;8:129–131.
24. Marotte JH, Lord G, Bancel P: Neer arthroplasty in complex fractures and fracture-dislocations of the shoulder: 12 cases. *Chirurgie* 1978;104:816–821.
25. Des Marchais JE, Benazet JP: Evaluation de l'hémi-arthroplastie de Neer dans le traitement des fractures de l'humerus. *Can J Surg* 1983;26:469–471.
26. Tanner MW, Cofield RH: Prosthetic arthroplasty for fractures and fracture-dislocations of the proximal humerus. *Clin Orthop* 1983;179:116–128.
27. Stableforth PG: Four-part fractures of the neck of the humerus. *J Bone Joint Surg* 1984;66B:104–108.
28. Moeckel BH, Dines DM, Warren RF, et al: Modular hemiarthroplasty for fractures of the proximal part of the humerus. *J Bone Joint Surg* 1992;74A:884–889.
29. Neer CS II, McIlveen SJ: Humeral head replacement with reconstruction of the tuberosities and the cuff in 4-fragment displaced fractures: Current results and technics. *Rev Chir Orthop Reparatrice Appar Mot* 1988;74(suppl 2):31–40.
30. Neumann K, Muhr G, Breitfuss H: Primary humerus head replacement in dislocated proximal humeral fracture: Indications, technique, results. *Orthopade* 1992;21:140–147.
31. Rietveld AB, Daanen HA, Rozing PM, et al: The lever arm in glenohumeral abduction after hemiarthroplasty. *J Bone Joint Surg* 1988;70B:561–565.
32. Pietu G, Deluzarches P, Gouin F, et al: Complex injuries of the proximal humerus treated with humeral head prosthesis: Apropos of 21 cases reviewed after a median 4-year follow-up. *Acta Orthop Belg* 1992;58:159–169.
33. Hawkins RJ, Switlyk P: Acute prosthetic replacement for severe fractures of the proximal humerus. *Clin Orthop* 1993;289: 156–160.
34. Huten D, Duparc J: Prosthetic arthroplasty in recent and old complex injuries of the shoulder. *Rev Chir Orthop Reparatrice Appar Mot* 1986;72:517–529.
35. Frich LH, Sojbjerg JO, Sneppen O: Shoulder arthroplasty in complex acute and chronic proximal humeral fractures. *Orthopedics* 1991;14:949–954.
36. Dines DM, Warren RF, Altchek DW, et al: Posttraumatic changes of the proximal humerus: Malunion, nonunion, and osteonecrosis. Treatment with modular hemiarthroplasty or total shoulder arthroplasty. *J Shoulder Elbow Surg* 1993;2:11–21.
37. Dines DM, Warren RF: Modular shoulder hemiarthroplasty for acute fractures: Surgical considerations. *Clin Orthop* 1994;307: 18–26.
38. Siebler G, Kuner EH: Late results following the surgical treatment of proximal humerus fractures in adults. *Unfallchirurgie* 1985;11:119–127.
39. Willems WJ, Lim TE: Neer arthroplasty for humeral fracture. *Acta Orthop Scand* 1985;56:394–395.
40. Neer CS II, Watson KC, Stanton FJ: Recent experience in total shoulder replacement. *J Bone Joint Surg* 1982;64A:319–337.

CHAPTER 4

Complications of Internal Fixation of Proximal Humeral Fractures

Patrick M. Connor, MD
Evan L. Flatow, MD

Introduction

The majority of proximal humeral fractures can be managed successfully with nonsurgical treatment. However, approximately 20% of displaced fractures and fracture-dislocations of the proximal humerus do poorly with closed management[1-10] and require surgery. Open reduction and internal fixation (ORIF) of displaced two- and three-part proximal humerus fractures and fracture-dislocations have generally provided satisfactory clinical results.[1,2,7,11-18] In addition, some authors have advocated ORIF of select four-part fractures in young patients with good bone stock.[17,19-31] Techniques of internal fixation have included various combinations of pins, screws, plates, intramedullary rods, wires, and/or sutures. Regardless of the type of fixation used, intraoperative or postoperative complications can and do occur, often leading to a worse clinical outcome than that obtained following nonsurgical management.[32]

The clinical decision-making process in the management of proximal humeral fractures is often predicated on the avoidance of complications. Thus, it is important for surgeons who treat these injuries with internal fixation to be familiar with potential complications, their relative risks, and how to avoid them. This is especially true given epidemiologic data, which projects an increased incidence of proximal humeral fractures in the ensuing years as the population ages.[33-35] This chapter reviews complications associated with internal fixation of proximal humeral fractures, provides recommendations for the surgeon on how to avoid these complications, and outlines surgical and nonsurgical treatment options when complications are encountered.

Nonunion

Nonunions of proximal humeral fractures, whether treated initially with nonsurgical management or internal fixation, most commonly occur at the level of the surgical neck (Fig. 1).[7,12,16,36-42] There is some evidence that internal fixation per se is a risk factor for the development of proximal humeral nonunions,[37,43] presumably through interruption of blood supply associated with the soft-tissue dissection. Additional factors associated with nonunion include inadequate reduction and/or poor initial fixation, comminution at the fracture site, soft-tissue interposition (eg, biceps tendon, capsule, deltoid muscle), osteopenia, systemic disease (eg, diabetes, rheumatoid arthritis), polytrauma, and excessive mobilization of the limb during the rehabilitation process.[7,16,36,38,39,41,42,44-47]

This latter risk factor often presents a difficult clinical situation, especially in the treatment of surgical neck fractures. "Too aggressive" or "too early" postoperative rehabilitation will risk nonunion at the fracture site, while "too little" or "too late" motion predisposes to postoperative stiffness and a poor clinical outcome. To circumvent this problem, the initial fixation must provide sufficient stability to enable early, passive postoperative motion within precise ranges as determined at the time of surgery. Passive motion within these ranges should then continue for 6 to 8 weeks postoperatively. As radiographic healing often occurs later than clinical healing, it is important to determine if the humeral shaft and head move together as a unit with rotation of the arm at the side. If there is clinical evidence of union at the fracture site after 6 to 8 weeks, motion can then gently be advanced. Stretching to the extremes of motion and active strengthening exercises should be avoided until radiographic evidence of healing is present.

As hardware fixation in soft, osteoporotic bone is often less than optimal, the use of polymethylmethacrylate reinforcement has been proposed.[48] Although this technique can be useful in the proximal humerus, care must be taken to place the cement only at the site of fixation and to keep it away from the healing fracture surfaces. If used improperly, the cement can impede healing and predispose to nonunion (Fig. 2).

The pathophysiology of surgical neck nonunions has been described by Neer[12,45] and others.[36,41,46] The proximal (head) fragment is often fixed by capsular contractures, and motion of the distal (shaft) fragment is primarily due to the pull of the pectoralis major and deltoid muscles. A true synovial-lined pseudarthrosis may occur as joint fluid communicates with the fracture site and retards union.[12,45] When this occurs, the head fragment becomes characteristically osteopenic and progressive resorption of cancellous bone

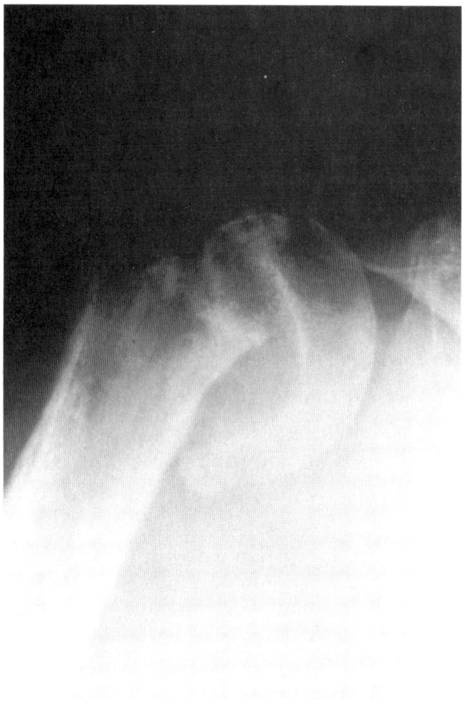

Fig. 1 Nonunions of the proximal humerus, whether treated initially with internal fixation or nonsurgical management, most commonly occur at the level of the surgical neck.

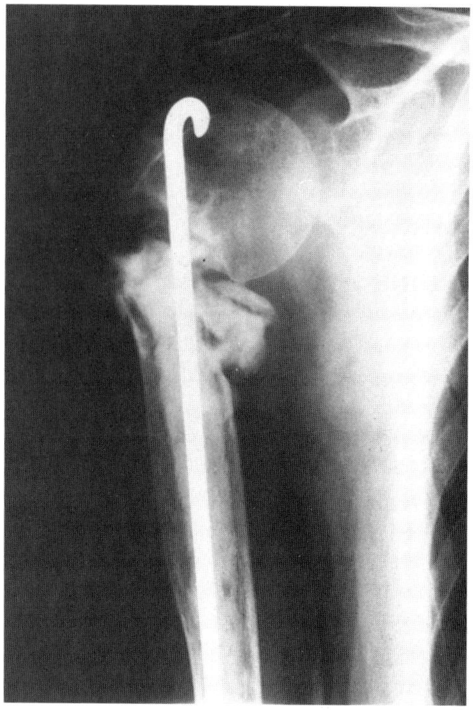

Fig. 2 Surgical neck fracture treated with intramedullary rod fixation and polymethylmethacrylate augmentation; no bone graft was used. Cement, inappropriately placed at the fracture site, predisposed to nonunion.

results in cavitation of the humeral head, making treatment with plate and screw fixation difficult or impossible.[12,36,38,39,41,45,46]

The treatment of surgical neck nonunions is fraught with difficulty, as shown in Neer's series, in which 35 of 50 patients had failed previous attempts of fixation.[45] Neer advocated using flexible intramedullary nails with tension band sutures, iliac crest bone graft, and a postoperative spica cast. Reoperation for removal of fixation and release of adhesions is the planned second stage of treatment. Neer[45] and others[36,38,46] have reported satisfactory results using this technique. Patients who have had previous surgery, however, have been shown to have inferior results using this technique as compared to those who were initially treated nonsurgically.[36] If the bone stock of the proximal head fragment is of sufficient quality, ORIF with a plate (T-plate, semitubular blade-plate, or custom proximal humerus blade-plate) and iliac crest bone graft has provided encouraging results in several reports.[37,39,44,47,49,50]

When a surgical neck nonunion is associated with posttraumatic arthritis or severe cavitation of the humeral head, prosthetic replacement is indicated (Fig. 3).[7,12,16,36,38,39,41,45,46] Although complications are not uncommon and improvements in shoulder function unpredictable, both ORIF and hemiarthroplasty of surgical neck nonunions provide relatively consistent pain relief.

Nonunions of tuberosities after internal fixation are much less common than those of the surgical neck, but can be equally disabling. More commonly, tuberosities are displaced along the pull of their attached muscle(s) and heal in a malunited position. Usual causes are inadequate initial reduction or fixation, inappropriately early active postoperative rehabilitation, or repeat trauma. Greater tuberosity nonunions may be associated with painful subacromial impingement, loss of external rotation due to abutment of the greater tuberosity on the posterior glenoid rim, and weakness due to the associated rotator cuff tear. Proper diagnosis is essential, and a complete radiographic trauma series is often supplemented with computed tomography (CT). Nonsurgical treatment of symptomatic greater tuberosity nonunions is generally unsuccessful. Surgical treatment through a superior deltoid-splitting approach consists of subacromial decompression (if indicated), mobilization of the greater tuberosity and attached rotator cuff tendon(s), debridement of fibrous tissue on the cancellous surfaces of both the tuberosity and the proximal humerus, and fixation with nonabsorbable sutures or tension band wires. If the tuberosity fragment is large and has a lateral cortical spike of bone, fixation with a cancellous screw and a

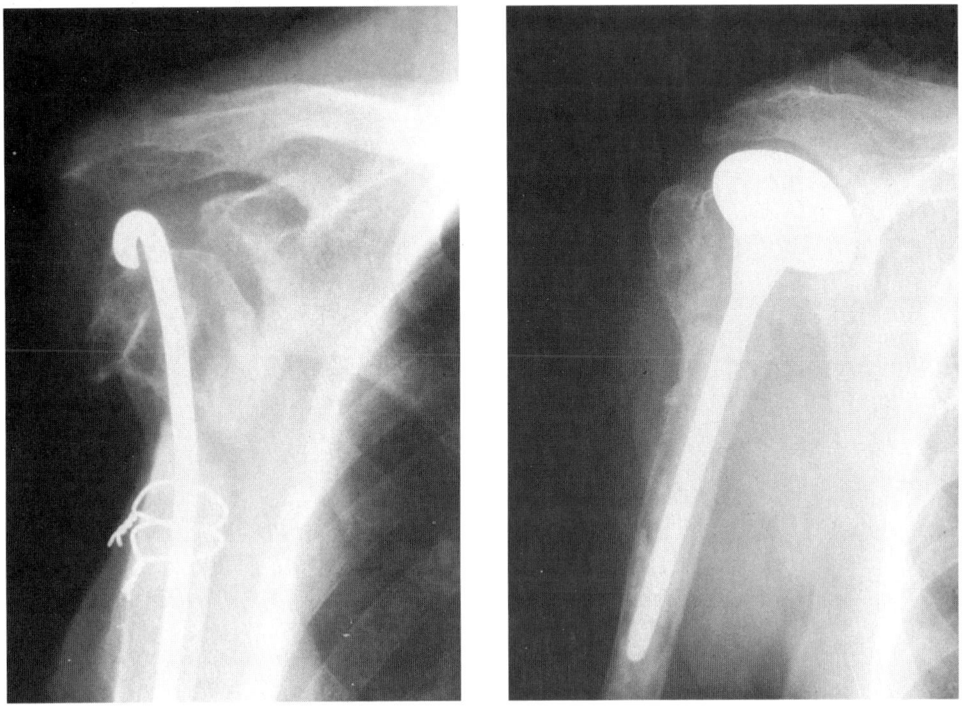

Fig. 3 Surgical neck nonunion after internal fixation with associated posttraumatic arthritis which required prosthetic replacement.

supplemental tension band can be done.[51] Postoperative management should consist of passive motion only for 6 to 8 weeks until healing.

Postoperative lesser tuberosity nonunions are rare and usually involve displacement of the lesser tuberosity/subscapularis unit after hemiarthroplasty for four-part fractures. If associated with pain and disability, exploration through a deltopectoral approach, mobilization, and revision fixation can be performed. Postoperative management should be similar to that after repair of subscapularis avulsions.[52]

Malunion

Although the importance of accuracy of closed reduction of proximal humeral fractures has been questioned,[53-56] failure to restore proximal humeral anatomy with internal fixation has repeatedly been associated with unsatisfactory results.[4,7,11,12,17,19,22,25,50,57-62] Most often, malunions result from technical errors in reduction and/or fixation (Fig. 4). In a review of 20 proximal humeral fractures treated with internal fixation, Hägg and Lundberg[59] showed a relation between malunion and restricted function as four of five shoulders with malunions had unsatisfactory results. Paavolainen and associates[17] failed to achieve anatomic reduction in five of 41 shoulders with internal fixation, leading to subacromial impingement by hardware, reoperations, and poor results.

Varus malunion of the surgical neck can lead to a decrease of abduction as well as subacromial impingement of the greater tuberosity and/or hardware (Fig. 5).[50,58,61,62] Apex anterior angulation of the surgical neck greater than 20° to 30° can result in limitations of elevation as well as subacromial impingement with flexion.[58] Superior or posterior malunion of the greater tuberosity of more than 1.0 cm leads to pain and disability with stiffness, subacromial impingement, and/or posterior glenoid abutment. Greater tuberosity malunions of 5 mm to 10 mm can also cause significant symptoms, especially in the young active patient.[1,2,12,14,63] Lesser tuberosity malunions, although uncommon, can be associated with subcoracoid impingement and weakness of internal rotation.

Because such serious disability is associated with proximal humerus malunion after internal fixation, avoidance of this complication becomes paramount.[1,2,7,12-15,38,64] Regardless of the method of initial fixation, stable anatomic reduction must be achieved. Intraoperative fluoroscopy can be used to assess reduction, stability, and the position of hardware (if applicable). An intraoperative assessment of the stable ranges of motion is required for the physician to direct postoperative passive rehabilitation. Active motion should be avoided until clinical healing has occurred.

Not only is the bony malalignment problematic, but soft-tissue contractures and scarring after internal fixation also complicate treatment of proximal humeral

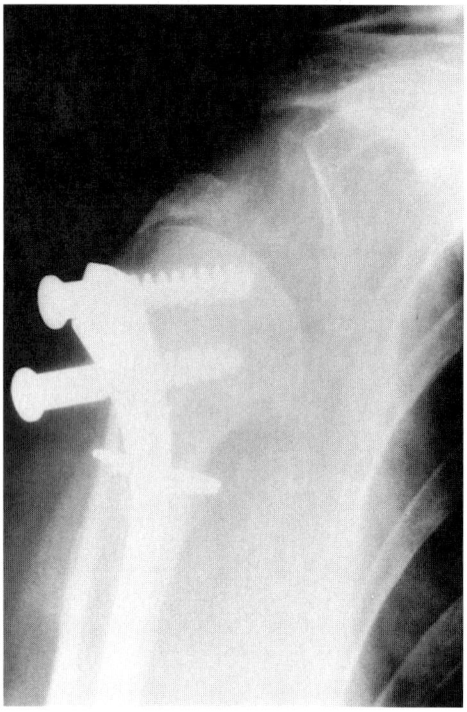

Fig. 4 This three-part proximal humeral fracture treated with internal fixation[28] resulted in malunion of the greater tuberosity fragment and prominent hardware.

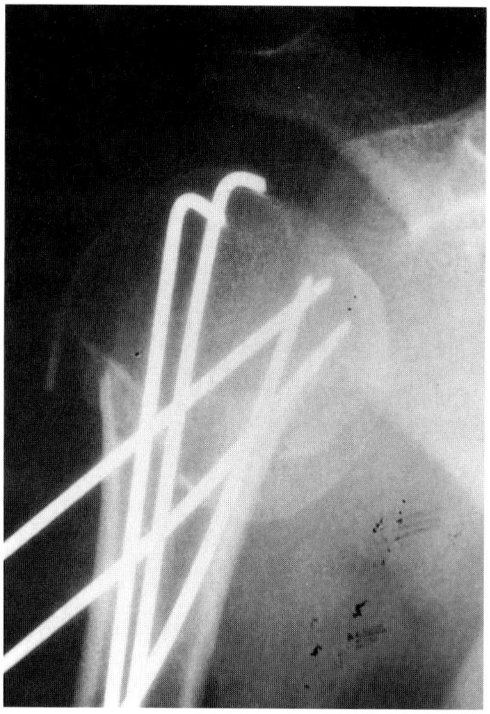

Fig. 5 Varus malunion of a surgical neck fracture after open reduction and internal fixation with percutaneous pins. This type of alignment predisposes to subacromial impingement of the greater tuberosity with elevation.

malunions.[12] Most shoulders with symptomatic malunions have concomitant stiffness. If the patient has failed an extensive course of physical therapy and rehabilitation, surgical treatment often can be limited to a release of adhesions, obtaining clearance by an anterior acromioplasty, and performing a greater tuberosity exostectomy (if applicable).[12] Severe malunions (eg, two-plane malunions of the surgical neck, greater tuberosity malunions with significant posterior and/or superior displacement), which require osteotomy, reduction, and internal fixation, are difficult management problems (Fig. 6).[65] Surgical attention must be directed to soft-tissue scarring and contractures as well as the bony pathology. Proximal humeral replacement is considered if the nonunion is associated with posttraumatic arthritis or osteonecrosis.[12,57,66-70] This alternative usually provides adequate pain relief but somewhat unpredictable improvements of function.

Hardware Complications

Pins, screws, plates, intramedullary rods, wires, and custom implants have all been used for fixation of proximal humeral fractures. Hardware, however, has been associated with many complications after proximal humeral fixation, including nonunion, malunion, osteonecrosis (ON), subacromial impingement, joint destruction, heterotopic ossification, and infection. Moreover, several studies have reported a high reoperation rate for hardware removal.[13,17-21,23,25,28,50,62,71,72] Preoperatively, the surgeon should be familiar not only with the "personality" of the fracture, but also with any patient characteristics that may influence fixation. Also, it is obviously important to be familiar with the relative risks of hardware complications and their implications.

Because the shoulder requires early postoperative motion to prevent stiffness, the hardware/bone fixation interface is necessarily stressed prior to bony union. In young patients with good bone stock, this issue usually has little clinical significance. However, in older patients with osteoporotic bone, this interface is at risk for failure. Hardware loosening is much more common than breaking, because stresses are concentrated at the hardware/bone interface(s) rather than within the plate and/or the screw(s) (Fig. 7). Szyszkowitz and associates[30] reported an approximate 10% incidence of plate and screw loosening after ORIF of proximal humeral fractures and found that loosening of K-wires was almost universal. A review of 349 proximal humeral fractures treated with internal fixation from the literature reveals a 12.6% incidence of loss of fixation.[7,15,17,18,20,21,23,25,28,30,71,73]

The foremost consideration is that the soft, osteoporotic bone of the proximal humerus in elderly

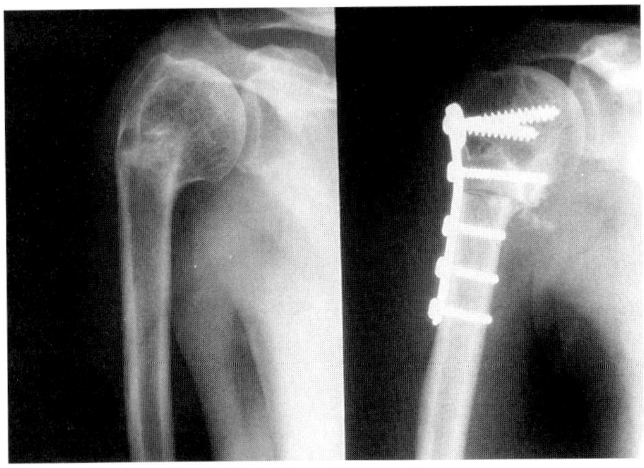

Fig. 6 Surgical neck malunion associated with a decrease in active elevation as well as painful subacromial impingement. Osteotomy, bone graft, internal fixation, and releases of extensive glenohumeral adhesions were performed.

patients predisposes hardware that relies on bone-to-bone fixation (eg, screws, plates) to fail.[1,2,12,13-15,25,62,74] As the bone/tendon junction of the tuberosities is often stronger than the poor quality bone of the proximal humerus, many surgeons prefer techniques of ORIF using suture or wire fixation that incorporate this bone/tendon junction.[1,2,7,12-15,72,75] These techniques have the further advantage of avoiding the higher incidence of subacromial impingement and ON seen with plates and screws.[1,2,7,16,25,30,38,62,72,73,76,77]

Although considered by some as a benign technique, percutaneous pin fixation of unstable proximal humeral fractures has been associated with a relatively high incidence of complications.[23,71,78] In a study of 48 cases in which this technique was used, there were 10 cases of humeral head ON (two complete, eight incomplete), nine malunions, five infections, four failures of fixation, and four reoperations.[23] Stoller and Gerber[78] noted displacement of pins in ten of 28 cases (36%), and there were two postoperative proximal humeral shaft fractures that occurred at the lateral cortical perforations.[78] Kocialkowski and Wallace[71] reported a 41% incidence of pin displacement as well as a postoperative radial nerve palsy. This technique has fewer complications when performed on young patients with good quality bone, especially those with displaced, noncomminuted surgical neck fractures amenable to closed reduction. In addition, it is important for the patient to be reliable and compliant with postoperative care and rehabilitation.

Although inconsistently reported, reoperation for hardware removal to correct hardware complications is relatively common. In a review of 13 recent studies, reoperation was required in 81 of 429 cases (18.9%).[13,17-21,23,25,28,50,62,71,72] If hardware failure occurs in the early postoperative period, redisplacement of the fracture fragments is common, and surgery is indicated for removal of hardware and revision ORIF. If fixation failure occurs after bony healing (eg, smooth pins[71,79] or tension band wire[1,2,7,12,51,77]), reoperation may be necessary to preclude migration of hardware into the

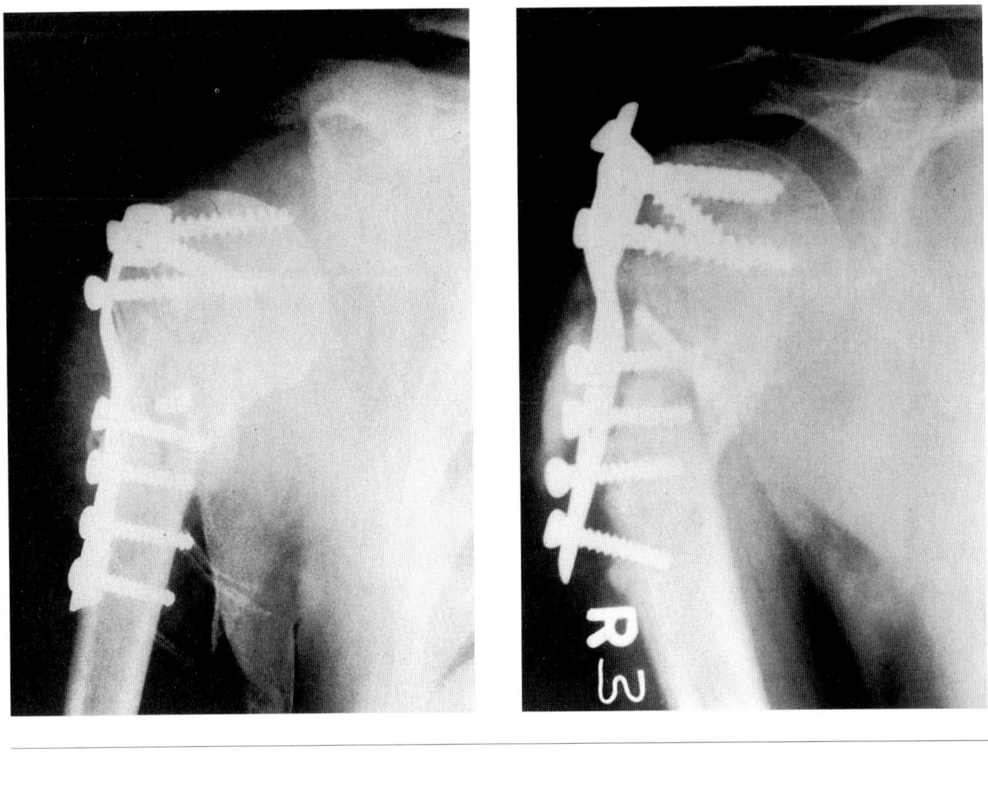

Fig. 7 Surgical neck fracture with comminution treated with ORIF using plate and screws. Although the initial postoperative radiograph, **left,** shows an anatomic reduction, loss of fixation resulted, **right.**

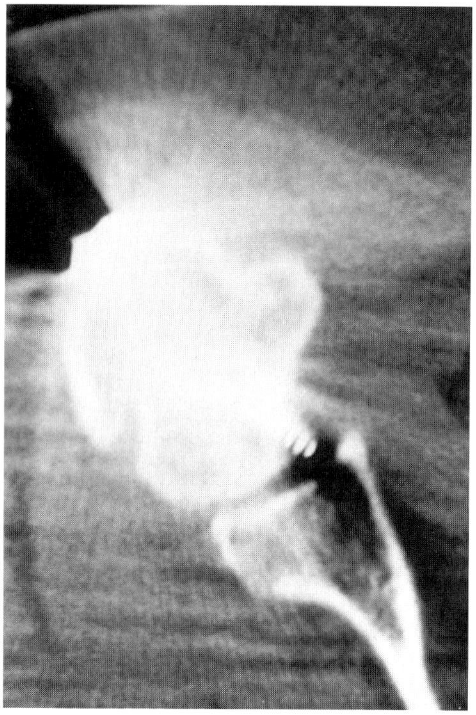

Fig. 8 Joint penetration of a screw through the humeral head subchondral bone. If humeral head screw or blade-plate fixation is chosen, intraoperative fluoroscopy should be used to assure that hardware does not penetrate into the joint.

subacromial space, the glenohumeral joint, or beyond. Another common cause of reoperation is for removal of prominent hardware in the subacromial space, which causes painful subacromial impingement.

Joint penetration from screw or blade-plate fixation is an avoidable and potentially disastrous complication (Fig. 8). As the highest quality bone of the humeral head is often subchondral,[74] efforts are often made to approach this bone with hardware to obtain good initial fixation. If screw or blade-plate fixation is chosen, intraoperative fluoroscopy is necessary to assure that the hardware does not penetrate through the subchondral bone. If joint penetration occurs, immediate recognition and hardware removal is necessary to prevent glenohumeral joint destruction.

Osteonecrosis

The blood supply to the proximal humerus is an important consideration in the understanding and treatment of complex proximal humeral fractures, as osteonecrosis (ON) is not an uncommon complication following these injuries. The major blood supply to the humeral head is from the anterior humeral circumflex artery.[80-82] Laing[82] first described the arcuate artery, which is a continuation of the ascending branch of the anterior humeral circumflex artery as it penetrates the bone at the proximal aspect of the bicipital groove. This tortuous artery supplies blood to a large portion of the humeral head, and provides branches to the greater and lesser tuberosities. Also, a smaller contribution to humeral head blood supply comes from branches of the posterior humeral circumflex and from the vascular rotator cuff through tendinous osseous anastomoses. Gerber and associates[81] demonstrated a rich extraosseous anastomosis between the anterior humeral circumflex, posterior humeral circumflex, thoracoacromial, and suprascapular arteries. They concluded that the anterior circumflex artery was the final common pathway for blood supply to the humeral head, and that almost the entire articular surface of the humeral head was supplied by its intraosseous continuation, the arcuate artery. They found that when the ascending branch of this artery is injured, the closer the injury is to its bony insertion, the greater the chance of significant disruption of the blood supply to the humeral head.[81] The findings of Brooks and associates[80] supported previous studies, and also highlighted the importance of the posteromedial arteries in the collateral circulation to the humeral head. Their findings support the possibility of maintained humeral head perfusion if the head fragment includes a significant portion of the posteromedial aspect of the proximal surgical neck.

The incidence of ON after internal fixation of displaced proximal humerus fractures has ranged from 0% to 90%,[4,5,7,9,15,17-19,23-28,30,31,59,62,76,83-87] in part highlighting the difficulty in diagnosis. Although ON of the humeral head can occur after nonsurgical treatment of high-energy fractures with large degrees of displacement, the likelihood of ON is greatly enhanced after ORIF.[59,62] This increased rate of ON after surgical fixation may be due to the deleterious effect of surgical trauma and/or the fact that the more severe injuries are usually treated with internal fixation.[59] Initial fixation of a proximal humeral fracture with a plate, which requires extensive exposure and soft-tissue dissection, increases the incidence of ON.[1,2,7,12,14,23,24,30,51,62,71,76,83,85]

The overall rate of ON can be reduced with "minimal fixation techniques," including tension band sutures or wires and/or narrow intramedullary fixation (eg, Ender rods). These techniques emphasize maintenance of vascularity, periosteum, and soft tissues while at the same time achieving stable fixation.[1,2,7,12-14,23,24,30,51,62,71,76]

Osteonecrosis may result in a stiff, painful shoulder with partial or total articular collapse, followed by loss of articular congruency, functional impairment, and, eventually, osteoarthrosis of the glenohumeral joint (Fig. 9).[22,62] Often, however, symptoms and radiographic evidence of ON may be delayed up to 2 years or more postoperatively.[4,19,59,87] Thus, the importance of long follow-up after internal fixation of proximal humeral

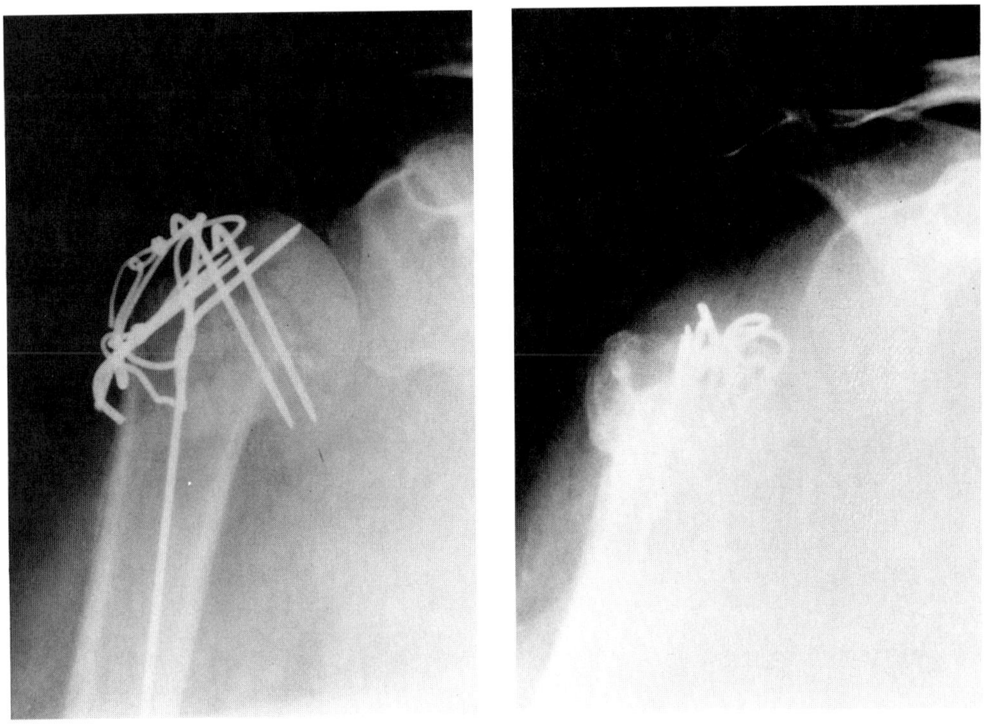

Fig. 9 **Left,** K-wire and cerclage wire fixation of a four-part proximal humerus fracture resulted in osteonecrosis and complete collapse of the articular surface, **right.** Hardware removal and hemiarthroplasty was required. (Reproduced with permission from Bigliani LU, Flatow EL, Pollock RG: Fractures of the proximal humerus, in Rockwood CA, Green DP, Bucholz RW, et al (eds): *Fractures in Adults*, ed 4. Philadelphia, PA, JB Lippincott, 1996, p 1095.)

fractures is stressed. Several authors have shown significantly worse results with complete humeral head ON compared to those without.[4,26,57,62,67,70,83,88,89] Others have stated that the presence of humeral head ON after internal fixation doesn't necessarily lead to unsatisfactory outcomes, especially if the tuberosities have been anatomically reduced and if articular congruency is maintained to some degree.[18,19,22,23,28,58,85,87] However, even if the initial reduction and fixation entirely restore normal anatomy, a satisfactory outcome is not assured if ON develops. On the contrary, articular collapse, prominent hardware, subacromial pain, stiffness, articular incongruity, and glenohumeral arthrosis often follow.

Symptomatic humeral head ON with articular incongruity and prominent hardware requires surgery. Removal of hardware, lysis of adhesions, capsular releases, and hemiarthroplasty are generally required. If surgery is performed relatively early after the development of articular collapse, reconstructive difficulties of more advanced disease (eg, severe soft-tissue contractures, glenoid arthrosis) may be avoided.[16]

Neurovascular Injury

The close vicinity of the brachial plexus, the axillary artery, and their branches to the proximal humerus place these structures at substantial risk. Although neurovascular injuries associated with proximal humeral fractures occur most commonly from the injury itself,[7,11,12,32,90-96] they also have been reported as complications from internal fixation. The most commonly injured nerve at the time of surgery is the axillary nerve, and the result is usually a transient neurapraxia.[11,14,16,28,62] It is important to be familiar not only with the normal anatomy of the axillary nerve,[97,98] but also with its potential deviations, given the associated fracture pattern. For example, the proximal shaft fragment of displaced surgical neck fractures is commonly draped medially over the axillary nerve and brachial plexus because of the pull of the pectoralis major muscle (Fig. 10). Also, with posterior fracture-dislocations, the axillary nerve is often very taut and is pulled in a more proximal direction than usual across the anterior aspect of the shoulder at the inferior border of the subscapularis. Diffuse brachial plexopathy as well as isolated injuries to the musculocutaneous, radial, and suprascapular nerves are also potential complications of internal fixation. Thus, it is important to avoid both direct and indirect (eg, traction) injury to the nerves during the surgical exposure and procedure.

Vascular injury at the time of internal fixation is a rare but potentially devastating complication. As with nerve injuries, vascular injuries also occur most often at the time of the injury. The injury, which occurs most commonly at the junction of the anterior humeral circumflex and axillary arteries,[11] can be caused by the sharp bone edges from the fracture site by vigorous manipulation of the fracture during exposure or reduction, or during mobilization of the lesser tuberosity/

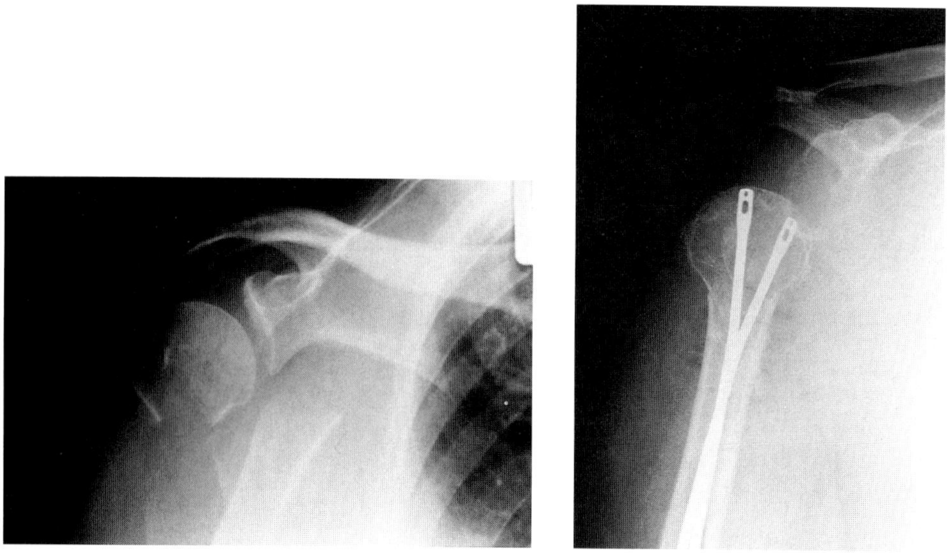

Fig. 10 **Left,** Severe displacement of a surgical neck fracture with the humeral shaft pulled medially by the pectoralis major. **Right,** Care was taken during open reduction and internal fixation of this fracture as the brachial plexus and axillary artery were draped over the proximal shaft.

subscaspularis unit. Care should be taken during medial dissection under the coracoid process and conjoined tendon, especially in older patients with fragile, atherosclerotic vessels. Also, if surgery is performed in a subacute or chronic setting, the chance of sustaining an intraoperative vascular injury is increased due to concomitant scarring and adhesions. If a significant vascular injury does occur at the time of surgery, exposure should be maximized and vascular surgery consultation obtained if necessary.

Subacromial Impingement

Subacromial impingement after internal fixation of proximal humeral fractures most commonly occurs with malunions and/or prominent hardware. As previously outlined, greater tuberosity fractures that heal in as little as 5 mm of superior or posterior displacement can cause painful subacromial impingement, with shoulder elevation or external rotation and secondary stiffness.[1,2,12,14,63,64] In addition, surgical neck fractures that heal in varus and/or apex anterior alignment cause deviation of the position of the greater tuberosity with elevation, also contributing to subacromial impingement.[50,58,61,62] Treatment of symptomatic subacromial impingement associated with malunions should initially be conservative, emphasizing stretching and rotator cuff strengthening. Surgical management of malunions has been outlined above.

Subacromial pain from prominent hardware is not an uncommon complication of internal fixation. Plates placed inappropriately high on the lateral aspect of the proximal humerus will impinge on the undersurface of the acromion with elevation and abduction (Fig. 11, *left*). Several studies have shown this complication to occur in as many as 10% to 15% of cases,[17,20,21,25] the majority of which require a second procedure for hardware removal. Intramedullary rods have also been reported to migrate proximally postoperatively, causing subacromial impingement (Fig. 11, *right*).[13,72,99]

All efforts should be made to avoid technical errors in hardware placement and fixation. If a plate is used, provisional fixation should be obtained initially and its position verified with intraoperative fluoroscopy or radiographs. If intramedullary fixation is chosen, Ender nails are favored over straight nails, as they afford three-point fixation for rotational control. In addition, the use of modified 3.3-mm Ender rods with an added hole above the eyelet[13,17] allows sutures to stabilize the rod with only 2 or 3 mm of metal projecting above the cortex. This is generally only a fraction of the thickness of the rotator cuff tendon, and the chance of symptomatic impingement is lessened. A similar custom hole for suture or wire incorporation has been reported with Rush rods as well.[100]

If prominent hardware requires removal, anterior acromioplasty and appropriate soft-tissue releases should be performed to allow generous subacromial clearance. An aggressive postoperative rehabilitation protocol should follow.

Frozen Shoulder

The reestablishment of shoulder motion after internal fixation of proximal humeral fractures is a challenging responsibility. Satisfactory radiographic evidence of healing may accompany a poor functional outcome if soft-tissue considerations are not met.[16] Although it has been stated that "a painless glenohumeral joint, even if movement is limited, is more

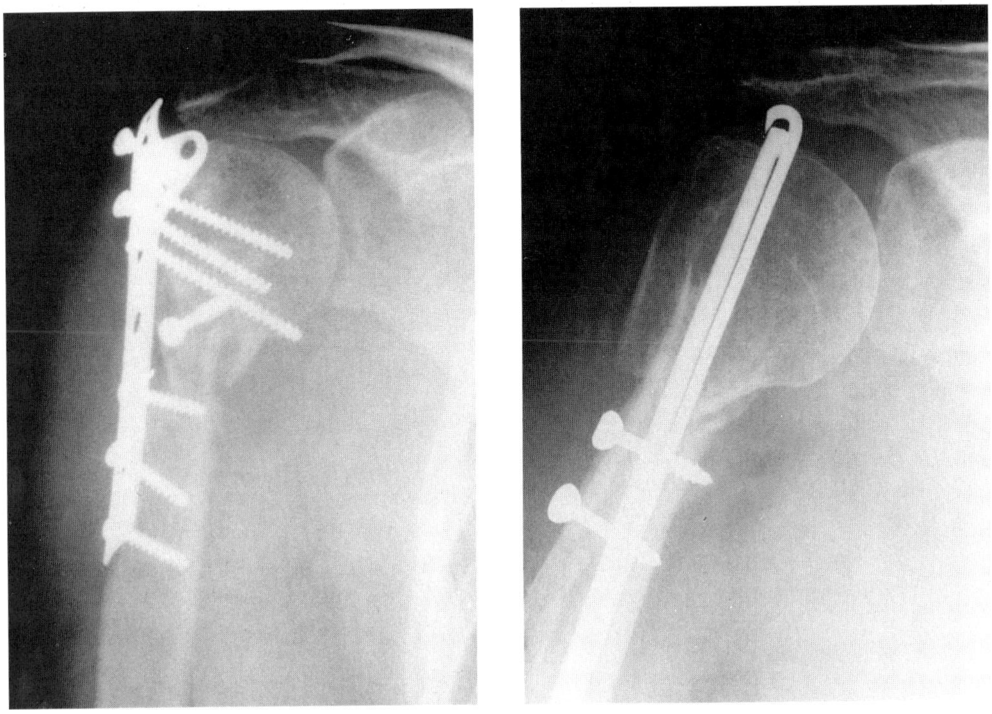

Fig. 11 Left, This plate, placed too high on the lateral aspect of the proximal humerus, caused subacromial impingement and required removal. **Right,** These intramedullary rods migrated proximally following open reduction and internal fixation. This caused impingement and also required removal.

important than full range of motion,"[17] a satisfactory postoperative outcome is unlikely if a functional arc of shoulder motion is not restored.

It is difficult to determine the incidence of clinically significant motion loss after proximal humeral fracture fixation. Variations in range of motion achieved postoperatively depend on many factors, including the age of the patient, type of fracture and associated soft-tissue disruption, associated injuries, delay in surgery, postoperative therapy regimen, and comorbid conditions.

At the time of surgery, the importance of achieving fixation stable enough to allow early postoperative motion cannot be overemphasized. Merely reapproximating fracture fragments together with internal fixation and immobilizing the shoulder in a sling for several weeks while awaiting "early healing" predisposes the shoulder to soft-tissue adhesions and capsular contractures, which often cannot be overcome with late rehabilitation. If stable fixation cannot be achieved at the time of surgery, a different method of fixation or conversion to hemiarthroplasty should be performed.

The patient's role in rehabilitation and the expected postoperative course should be discussed with the patient prior to surgery. In this way, when postoperative motion is initiated, the patient will have a better appreciation of the long-term objectives of the rehabilitation process. Patient motivation is important after fracture fixation, and the surgeon and therapist should provide encouragement throughout the entire course of rehabilitation, which may take up to 18 months for full benefit to be achieved.[1,2,4,12,38,101]

If postoperative motion limitations are recalcitrant to all conservative rehabilitation efforts and are clinically symptomatic, open release of adhesions and contractures is indicated. Hardware removal should be considered if applicable. Forceful manipulation under anesthesia, which can fracture the weakened and osteoporotic bone, is to be avoided.[1,2,12,16,41,62,77,102] It is, of course, imperative that an aggressive postoperative rehabilitation regimen follows.

Infection

The shoulder is uniquely protected from postoperative infections by its excellent soft-tissue and muscle coverage, collateral blood supply, and the fact that the majority of proximal humeral fractures are closed injuries. However, when infections do occur following fracture fixation, the problem can be devastating. Septic arthritis of the glenohumeral joint leads to cartilage destruction and secondary arthrosis, and osteomyelitis of the proximal humerus is not uncommon.

Several studies have reported deep infections following proximal humeral fixation,[7,17,23,25,26,30,59,72,103] but this complication is rare. More commonly, superficial infections (eg, cellulitis) have been reported, particularly after percutaneous pin fixation.[23,59,71,72] If a pin track infection occurs, it is advisable to remove the offending pin(s) and administer antibiotics. Due to the hematoma, which is universally present after internal fixation of these injuries, the risk for seeding the infection deep into the glenohumeral joint is present.[102] For this reason, cellulitis should be carefully monitored for resolution.

If a deep infection occurs after proximal humeral fracture fixation, aggressive irrigation, debridement, and appropriate parenteral antibiotics are indicated. Borrowing from experiences following infection of hip and knee arthroplasty infections, we have used an antibiotic-impregnated spacer in the shape of a shoulder prosthesis for local antibiotic delivery as well as to maintain soft-tissue spacing. Exchange arthroplasty after eradication of the infection has provided encouraging results.[104]

Heterotopic Ossification

Heterotopic ossification (HO) after proximal humeral fracture fixation may occur in up to 10% of cases, but it rarely affects clinical outcome.[1,2,7,12,16,62] Predisposing factors for development of postoperative HO include excessive soft-tissue injury (eg, fracture-dislocations), repeated closed manipulations, delayed treatment, and concomitant traumatic brain injury (Fig. 12).[7,12,105,106] Other patients who may be at increased risk of developing HO include those with active spondylitis, hypertrophic pulmonary osteoarthropathy, hypertrophic arthritis, and a history of previous HO.[107] Although prophylactic indomethacin or radiation treatment has been considered in these high-risk patients,[107] the role of prophylaxis remains unclear.

Management of HO about the shoulder is similar to that of other joints. In no case should an attempt be made to remove the extra bone before it has reached maturity. Serial radiographs, bone scans, and serum alkaline phosphatase levels may be followed to help determine the activity of bone remodeling, and observation should take place for at least a year after the injury. If the bone is mature and the limitation of motion disabling, reexploration for removal of HO is performed, sometimes requiring both anterior and posterior approaches. Postoperative treatment with indomethacin or radiation is suggested to help prevent recurrence.

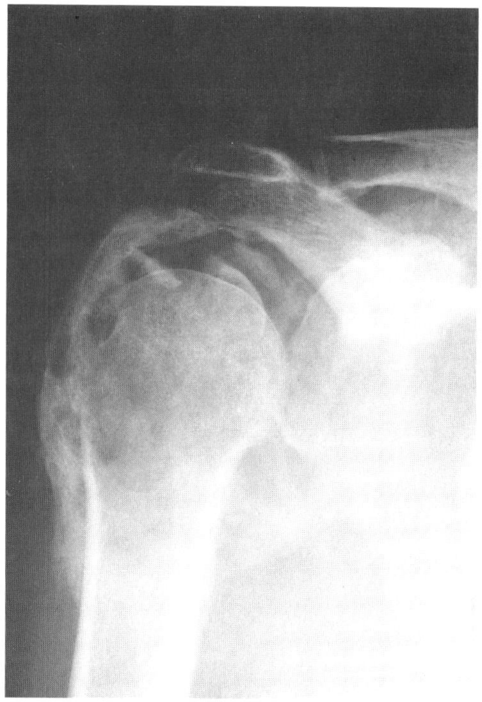

Fig. 12 This patient with an anterior fracture-dislocation of the greater tuberosity also had a closed head injury. Closed reduction failed to reduce the greater tuberosity fragment. Open reduction and internal fixation was performed and severe heterotopic ossification developed within 3 months.

Other Complications

Inferior Subluxation

Postoperative anterior and posterior instability is rare after internal fixation of proximal humeral fractures, but inferior subluxation is common.[7,12,16,102,108-110] Cotton[111] first described this phenomenon in 1921, and attributed it to decreased tone of the shoulder girdle muscles. In addition, loss of the stabilizing effect of negative intra-articular pressure may play a role.[112] These theories of etiology have been reinforced through clinical observations of complete resolution in most patients by 6 to 12 weeks.[7,12,16,102,108-110] Management includes adequate sling support of the extremity and isometric exercises of the shoulder girdle muscles. If resolution does not occur by 3 months, the more problematic causes of failure to restore full humeral length at the time of internal fixation or axillary nerve injury should be considered.

Iatrogenic Fracture Displacement

Seven cases of iatrogenic displacement of an undisplaced surgical neck fracture at the time of either closed or open reduction of a concomitant anterior fracture-dislocation have been reported by Hersche and Gerber.[113] In each case, there was a displaced greater tuberosity fracture, and all cases with anatomic neck fractures progressed to humeral head ON. This potential complication emphasizes the importance of obtaining adequate radiographs before reduction of a fracture-dislocation is attempted. When faced with this clinical situation, these authors advocate provisional fixation of the surgical or anatomic neck fracture prior to reduction of the dislocation.[113]

Conclusion

Complications from internal fixation of proximal humeral fractures are most often associated with errors in diagnosis, technique, or rehabilitation. The principles of reestablishing normal anatomy with stable fixation that allows early postoperative rehabilitation are integral in avoiding complications. Emphasis should be placed on maximizing results from the index procedure, because the results of revision surgery are inferior.[1,2,69,70,114]

References

1. Bigliani LU: Fractures of the shoulder: Part I. Fractures of the proximal humerus, in Rockwood CA Jr, Green DP, Bucholz RW (eds): *Fractures in Adults*, ed 3. Philadelphia, PA, JB Lippincott, 1991, pp 871–927.
2. Bigliani LU: Fractures of the proximal humerus, in Rockwood CA Jr, Matsen FA III (eds): *The Shoulder.* Philadelphia, PA, WB Saunders, 1990, pp 278–334.
3. Clifford PC: Fractures of the neck of the humerus: A review of late results. *Injury* 1980;12:91–95.
4. Knight RA, Mayne JA: Comminuted fractures and fracture-dislocations involving the articular surface of the humeral head. *J Bone Joint Surg* 1957;39A:1343–1355.
5. Leyshon RL: Closed treatment of fractures of the proximal humerus. *Acta Orthop Scand* 1984;55:48–51.
6. Neer CS II: Displaced proximal humeral fractures: Part I. Classification and evaluation. *J Bone Joint Surg* 1970;52A:1077–1089.
7. Neer CS II: Displaced proximal humeral fractures: Part II. Treatment of three-part and four-part displacement. *J Bone Joint Surg* 1970;52A:1090–1103.
8. Stableforth PG: Four-part fractures of the neck of the humerus. *J Bone Joint Surg* 1984;66B:104–108.
9. Svend-Hansen H: Displaced proximal humeral fractures: A review of 49 patients. *Acta Orthop Scand* 1974;45:359–364.
10. Zyto K, Kronberg M, Brostrom LA: Shoulder function after displaced fractures of the proximal humerus. *J Shoulder Elbow Surg* 1995;4:331–336.
11. Bigliani LU: Treatment of two- and three-part fractures of the proximal humerus, in Barr JS Jr (ed): *Instructional Course Lectures XXXVIII.* Park Ridge, IL, American Academy of Orthopaedic Surgeons, 1989, pp 231–244.
12. Neer CS II: Fractures, in Neer CS II (ed): *Shoulder Reconstruction.* Philadelphia, PA, WB Saunders, 1990, pp 363–420.
13. Cuomo F, Flatow EL, Maday MG, et al: Open reduction and internal fixation of two- and three-part displaced surgical neck fractures of the proximal humerus. *J Shoulder Elbow Surg* 1992;1:287–295.
14. Flatow EL, Cuomo F, Maday MG, et al: Open reduction and internal fixation of two-part displaced fractures of the greater tuberosity of the proximal part of the humerus. *J Bone Joint Surg* 1991;73A:1213–1218.
15. Hawkins RJ, Bell RH, Gurr K: The three-part fracture of the proximal part of the humerus: Operative treatment. *J Bone Joint Surg* 1986;68A:1410–1414.
16. Norris TR: Fractures of the proximal humerus and dislocations of the shoulder, in Browner BD, Jupiter JB, Levine AM, et al (eds): *Skeletal Trauma: Fractures, Dislocations, Ligamentous Injuries.* Philadelphia, PA, WB Saunders, 1992, pp 1201–1290.
17. Paavolainen P, Björkenheim JM, Slätis P: Operative treatment of severe proximal humeral fractures. *Acta Orthop Scand* 1983;54:374–379.
18. Savoie FH, Geissler WB, Vander Griend RA: Open reduction and internal fixation of three-part fractures of the proximal humerus. *Orthopedics* 1989;12:65–70.
19. Darder A, Darder A Jr, Sanchis V, et al: Four-part displaced proximal humeral fractures: Operative treatment using Kirschner wires and a tension band. *J Orthop Trauma* 1993;7:497–505.
20. Esser RD: Treatment of three- and four-part fractures of the proximal humerus with a modified cloverleaf plate. *J Orthop Trauma* 1994;8:15–22.
21. Esser RD: Open reduction and internal fixation of three- and four-part fractures of the proximal humerus. *Clin Orthop* 1994;299:244–251.
22. Gerber C: Indications and techniques for open reduction internal fixation of three and four part proximal humerus fractures. Proceedings of the American Academy of Orthopaedic Surgeons 63rd Annual Meeting, Atlanta, GA. Rosemont, IL, American Academy of Orthopaedic Surgeons, 1996, p 311.
23. Jaberg H, Warner JJ, Jakob RP: Percutaneous stabilization of unstable fractures of the humerus. *J Bone Joint Surg* 1992;74A:508–515.
24. Jakob RP, Miniaci A, Anson PS, et al: Four-part valgus impacted fractures of the proximal humerus. *J Bone Joint Surg* 1991;73B:295–298.
25. Kristiansen B, Christensen SW: Plate fixation of proximal humeral fractures. *Acta Orthop Scand* 1986;57:320–323.
26. Kristiansen B, Christensen SW: Proximal humeral fractures: Late results in relation to classification and treatment. *Acta Orthop Scand* 1987;58:124–127.
27. Lim TE, Ochsner PE, Marti RK, et al: The results of treatment of comminuted fractures and fracture-dislocations of the proximal humerus. *Neth J Surg* 1983;35:139–143.
28. Mouradian WH: Displaced proximal humeral fractures: Seven years' experience with a modified Zickel supracondylar device. *Clin Orthop* 1986;212:209–218.
29. Resch H, Beck E, Bayley I: Reconstruction of the valgus-impacted humeral head fracture. *J Shoulder Elbow Surg* 1995;4:73–80.
30. Szyszkowitz R, Seggl W, Schleifer P, et al: Proximal humeral fractures: Management techniques and expected results. *Clin Orthop* 1993;292:13–25.
31. Yamano Y: Comminuted fractures of the proximal humerus treated with hook plate. *Arch Orthop Traumat Surg* 1986;105:359–363.
32. Stableforth PG: Abstract: Surgical or non-surgical management of displaced proximal humeral fractures. *J Bone Joint Surg* 1993;75B(suppl 2):194.
33. Hall MC, Rosser M: The structure of the upper end of the humerus with reference to osteoporotic changes in senescence leading to fractures. *Can Med Assoc J* 1963;88:290–294.
34. Kelsey JL, Browner WS, Seeley DG, et al: Risk factors for fractures of the distal forearm and proximal humerus: The study of osteoporotic fractures research group. *Am J Epidemiol* 1992;135:477–489.
35. Lind T, Kroner F, Jensen J: The epidemiology of fractures of the proximal humerus. *Arch Orthop Trauma Surg* 1989;108:285–287.
36. Bigliani LU, Nicholson GP, Pollock RG, et al: Operative treatment of non-unions of the surgical neck of the humerus. *J Shoulder Elbow Surg* 1994;3(suppl):S8.
37. Coventry MB, Laurnen EL: Ununited fractures of the middle and upper humerus: Special problems in treatment. *Clin Orthop* 1970;69:192–198.
38. Hawkins RJ, Angelo RL: Displaced proximal humeral fractures: Selecting treatment, avoiding pitfalls. *Orthop Clin North Am* 1987;18:421–431.
39. Healy WL, Jupiter JB, Kristiansen TK, et al: Nonunion of the proximal humerus: A review of 25 cases. *J Orthop Trauma* 1990;4:424–431.

40. Leach RE, Premer RF: Nonunion of the surgical neck of the humerus: Method of internal fixation. *Minn Med* 1965; 48:318–322.
41. Norris TR, Turner JA, Bovill D: Nonunion of the upper humerus: An analysis of the etiology and treatment in 28 cases, in Post M, Morrey BF, Hawkins RJ (eds): *Surgery of the Shoulder.* St. Louis, MO, Mosby-Year Book, 1990, pp 63–67.
42. Sorensen KH: Pseudarthrosis of the surgical neck of the humerus: Two cases, one bilateral. *Acta Orthop Scand* 1964; 34:132–138.
43. Johansson O: Complications and failures of surgery in various fractures of the humerus. *Acta Chir Scand* 1961;120:469–478.
44. Jupiter JB, Mullaji AB: Blade plate fixation of proximal humeral non-unions. *Injury* 1994;25:301–303.
45. Neer CS II: Nonunion of the surgical neck of the humerus. *Orthop Trans* 1983;7:389.
46. Norris TR, Turner JA: Surgical treatment of nonunion of the upper humerus shaft fracture in the elderly. *Orthop Trans* 1985;9:44.
47. Scheck M: Surgical treatment of nonunions of the surgical neck of the humerus. *Clin Orthop* 1982;167:255–259.
48. Rosen H: Nonunion and malunion, in Browner BD, Jupiter JB, Levine AM, et al (eds): *Skeletal Trauma: Fractures, Dislocations, Ligamentous Injuries.* Philadelphia, PA, WB Saunders, 1992, pp 501–541.
49. Bosworth DM: Blade plate fixation: Techniques suitable for fractures of the surgical neck of the humerus and similar lesions. *JAMA* 1949;141:1111–1113.
50. Sehr JR, Szabo RM: Semitubular blade plate for fixation in the proximal humerus. *J Orthop Trauma* 1988;2:327–332.
51. Cornell CN, Levine D, Pagnani MJ: Internal fixation of proximal humerus fractures using the screw-tension band technique. *J Orthop Trauma* 1994;8:23–27.
52. Gerber C, Krushell RJ: Isolated rupture of the tendon of the subscapularis muscle: Clinical features in 16 cases. *J Bone Joint Surg* 1991;73B:389–394.
53. DePalma AF, Cautilli RA: Fractures of the upper end of the humerus. *Clin Orthop* 1961;20:73–93.
54. Mills KL: Severe injuries of the upper end of the humerus. *Injury* 1974;6:13–21.
55. Moriber LA, Patterson RL Jr: Abstract: Fractures of the proximal end of the humerus. *J Bone Joint Surg* 1967;49A:1018.
56. Young TB, Wallace WA: Conservative treatment of fractures and fracture-dislocations of the upper end of the humerus. *J Bone Joint Surg* 1985;67B:373–377.
57. Bigliani LU: Malunion of four-part anterior fracture-dislocation following open reduction internal fixation. *Tech Orthop* 1994; 9:99–101.
58. Gristina AG, Bigliani LU, Neviaser RJ, et al: Symposium: Management of displaced fractures of the proximal humerus. *Contemp Orthop* 1987;15:61–93.
59. Hägg O, Lundberg B: Aspects of prognostic factors in comminuted and dislocated proximal humeral fractures, in Bateman JE, Welsh RP (eds): *Surgery of the Shoulder.* Philadelphia, PA, BC Decker, 1984, pp 51–59.
60. Keene JS, Huizenga RE, Engber WD, et al: Proximal humeral fractures: A correlation of residual deformity with long-term function. *Orthopedics* 1983;6:173–178.
61. Solonen KA, Vastamäki M: Osteotomy of the neck of the humerus for traumatic varus deformity. *Acta Orthop Scand* 1985;56:79–80.
62. Sturzenegger M, Fornaro E, Jakob RP: Results of surgical treatment of multifragmented fractures of the humeral head. *Arch Orthop Traumat Surg* 1982;100:249–259.
63. McLaughlin HL: Dislocation of the shoulder with tuberosity fracture. *Surg Clin North Am* 1963;43:1615–1620.
64. Duralde XA, Rodosky MW, Pollock RG, et al: Abstract: Operative treatment of malunions of proximal humerus fractures. *J Shoulder Elbow Surg* 1995;4(suppl):S11.
65. Gerber C: Reconstructive surgery following malunion of fractures of the proximal humerus in adults. *Orthopade* 1990; 19:316–323.
66. Dines DM, Warren RF, Altchek DW, et al: Posttraumatic changes of the proximal humerus: Malunion, nonunion, and osteonecrosis. Treatment with modular hemiarthroplasty or total shoulder arthroplasty. *J Shoulder Elbow Surg* 1993;2:11–21.
67. Frich LH, Sojbjerg JO, Sneppen O: Shoulder arthroplasty in complex acute and chronic proximal humeral fractures. *Orthopedics* 1991;14:949–954.
68. Neer CS II, Watson KC, Stanton FJ: Recent experience in total shoulder replacement. *J Bone Joint Surg* 1982;64A:319–337.
69. Norris TR, Green A, McGuigan FX: Late prosthetic shoulder arthroplasty for displaced proximal humerus fractures. *J Shoulder Elbow Surg* 1995;4:271–280.
70. Tanner MW, Cofield RH: Prosthetic arthroplasty for fractures and fracture-dislocations of the proximal humerus. *Clin Orthop* 1983;179:116–128.
71. Kocialkowski A, Wallace WA: Closed percutaneous K-wire stabilization for displaced fractures of the surgical neck of the humerus. *Injury* 1990;21:209–212.
72. Robinson CM, Christie J: The two-part proximal humeral fracture: A review of operative treatment using two techniques. *Injury* 1993;24:123–125.
73. Koval KJ, Sanders R, Zuckerman JD, et al: Modified-tension band wiring of displaced surgical neck fractures of the humerus. *J Shoulder Elbow Surg* 1993;2:85–92.
74. Saitoh S, Milne E, Latta L: Abstract: Osteoporosis of the proximal humerus. *Orthop Trans* 1990;14:372.
75. Muller B, Bonnaire F, Kuner EH: Biological osteosynthesis for fractures of the proximal humerus. *J Bone Joint Surg* 1993; 75B(supp 2):194.
76. Müller ME, Allgöwer M, Schneider R, et al (eds): *Manual of Internal Fixation: Techniques Recommended by the AO-ASIF Group,* ed 3. Berlin, Germany, Springer-Verlag, 1991.
77. Watson KC: Complications of internal fixation of proximal humeral fractures, in Bigliani LU (ed): *Complications of Shoulder Surgery.* Baltimore, MD, Williams & Wilkins, 1993, pp 190–201.
78. Stoller C, Gerber C: Secondary fracture of the humerus after closed reduction and percutaneous stabilization of a subcapital fracture. *J Shoulder Elbow Surg* 1994;3:100–106.
79. Lyons FA, Rockwood CA Jr: Migration of pins used in operations on the shoulder. *J Bone Joint Surg* 1990;72A:1262–1267.
80. Brooks CH, Revell WJ, Heatley FW: Vascularity of the humeral head after proximal humeral fractures: An anatomical cadaver study. *J Bone Joint Surg* 1993;75B:132–136.
81. Gerber C, Schneeberger AG, Vinh TS: The arterial vascularization of the humeral head: An anatomical study. *J Bone Joint Surg* 1990;72A:1486–1494.
82. Laing PG: The arterial supply of the adult humerus. *J Bone Joint Surg* 1956;38A:1105–1116.
83. Cofield RH: Comminuted fractures of the proximal humerus. *Clin Orthop* 1988;230:49–57.
84. Fourrier P, Martini M: Post-traumatic avascular necrosis of the humeral head. *Int Orthop* 1977;1:187–190.
85. Kofoed H: Revascularization of the humeral head: A report of two cases of fracture-dislocation of the shoulder. *Clin Orthop* 1983;179:175–178.
86. Kuner EH, Siebler G: Dislocation fractures of the proximal humerus: Results following surgical treatment. A follow-up study of 167 cases. *Unfallchirurgie* 1987;13:64–71.
87. Lee CK, Hansen HR: Post-traumatic avascular necrosis of the humeral head in displaced proximal humeral fractures. *J Trauma* 1981;21:788–791.

88. Schai P, Imhoff A, Preiss S: Comminuted humeral head fractures: A multicenter analysis. *J Shoulder Elbow Surg* 1995; 4:319–330.
89. Stewart MJ, Hundley JM: Fractures of the humerus: A comparative study in methods of treatment. *J Bone Joint Surg* 1955; 37A:681–692.
90. Henson GF: Vascular complications of shoulder injuries: A report of two cases. *J Bone Joint Surg* 1956;38B:528–531.
91. Johnson JR, Bayley JI: Early complications of acute anterior dislocation of the shoulder in the middle-aged and elderly patient. *Injury* 1982;13:431–434.
92. Leffert RD, Seddon H: Infraclavicular brachial plexus injuries. *J Bone Joint Surg* 1965;47B:9–22.
93. Linson MA: Axillary artery thrombosis after fracture of the humerus: A case report. *J Bone Joint Surg* 1980;62A:1214–1215.
94. McLaughlin HL (ed): *Trauma.* Philadelphia, PA, WB Saunders, 1959, pp 233–296.
95. Theodorides T, de Keizer C: Injuries of the axillary artery caused by fractures of the neck of the humerus. *Injury* 1976;8:120–123.
96. Zuckerman JD, Flugstad DL, Teitz CC, et al: Axillary artery injury as a complication of proximal humeral fractures: Two case reports and a review of the literature. *Clin Orthop* 1984;189:234–237.
97. Burkhead WZ Jr, Scheinberg RR, Box G: Surgical anatomy of the axillary nerve. *J Shoulder Elbow Surg* 1992;1:31–36.
98. Flatow EL, Bigliani LU: Tips of the trade: Locating and protecting the axillary nerve in shoulder surgery. The tug test. *Orthop Rev* 1992;21:503–505.
99. Weseley MS, Barenfeld PA, Eisenstein AL: Rush pin intramedullary fixation for fractures of the proximal humerus. *J Trauma* 1977;17:29–37.
100. Weise K, Meeder PJ, Wentzensen A: Indications and technique of osteosynthesis in dislocated fractures of the humeral head in adults. *Langenbecks Arch Chir* 1980;351:91–98.
101. Neer CS II: Four-segment classification of displaced proximal humeral fractures, in Evans EB (ed): American Academy of Orthopaedic Surgeons *Instructional Course Lectures XXIV.* St. Louis, MO, CV Mosby, 1975, pp 160–168.
102. Dameron TB Jr: Complications of treatment of injuries to the shoulder, in Epps CH (ed): *Complications in Orthopaedic Surgery,* ed 2. Philadelphia, PA, JB Lippincott, 1986, pp 247–276.
103. Moda SK, Chadha NS, Sangwan SS, et al: Open reduction and fixation of proximal humeral fractures and fracture-dislocations. *J Bone Joint Surg* 1990;72B:1050–1052.
104. Codd TP, Yamaguchi K, Pollock RG: Infected shoulder arthroplasties: Treatment with staged reimplantations versus resection arthroplasty. Proceedings of the American Academy of Orthopaedic Surgeons 62nd Annual Meeting, Orlando, FL. Rosemont, IL, American Academy of Orthopaedic Surgeons, 1995, p 343.
105. Garland DE: Clinical observations on fractures and heterotopic ossification in the spinal cord and traumatic brain injured populations. *Clin Orthop* 1988;233:86–101.
106. Wenner SM: Heterotopic ossification of the shoulder following head injury: A case report. *Clin Orthop* 1986;212:231–236.
107. Berg EE, Ciullo JV: Heterotopic ossification after acromioplasty and distal clavicle resection. *J Shoulder Elbow Surg* 1995;4: 188–193.
108. Fairbank TJ: Fracture-subluxations of the shoulder. *J Bone Joint Surg* 1948;30B:454–460.
109. Thompson FR, Winant EM: Comminuted fracture of the humeral head with subluxation. *Clin Orthop* 1961;20:94–97.
110. Yosipovitch Z, Goldberg I: Inferior subluxation of the humeral head after injury to the shoulder: A brief note. *J Bone Joint Surg* 1989;71A:751–753.
111. Cotton FJ: Subluxation of the shoulder: Downward. *Boston Med Surg J* 1921;185:405–407.
112. Gibb TD, Sidles JA, Harryman DT II, et al: The effect of capsular venting on glenohumeral laxity. *Clin Orthop* 1991;268: 120–127.
113. Hersche O, Gerber C: Iatrogenic displacement of fracture-dislocations of the shoulder: A report of seven cases. *J Bone Joint Surg* 1994;76B:30–33.
114. Connor PM, D'Alessandro DF: Role of hemiarthroplasty for proximal humeral fractures. *J South Orthop Assoc* 1995;4:9–23.

CHAPTER 5

Normal Shoulder Mechanics and Function

W. Ben Kibler, MD

Introduction

Knowledge of normal shoulder function is essential for implementing efficacious shoulder rehabilitation. Protocols that emphasize restoration of normal motions, force couples, and biomechanics will allow the quickest return to activity. This chapter reviews the current knowledge of the biomechanics and physiology of the shoulder. This knowledge can then provide a base for the clinical application of specific rehabilitation activities.

Mobility Versus Stability

The shoulder functions most effectively in a relatively limited set of anatomic conditions that create a balance between the mobility necessary to achieve the wide ranges of joint motion, the disparate joint and bone positions that are necessary for athletic activity (Table 1),[1-3] and the stability necessary to allow a normal path of the instant center of joint motion in the face of large forces and translatory and distraction loads that occur in normal throwing or serving (Table 2).[2,4]

Mobility is possible because of the "large ball/small socket" bony arrangement and the voluminous glenohumeral joint capsule, which does not restrict motion except at the extremes of motion.[5] The scapula is also highly mobile due to the limited bony constraint of the clavicle. The scapula can therefore retract and protract on the thoracic wall to follow the moving humerus and can rotate and elevate to avoid humeral impingement.

Stability is conferred by the interaction of bony, ligamentous, and muscular constraint systems that control the movement of the instant center of motion of the glenohumeral joint. Studies of this movement have shown that in the mid-ranges of motion, very little translation of the humerus occurs on the glenoid, but at the extremes of motion in flexion, abduction, or rotation, translation occurs within certain limits.[6-10] This means that despite the anatomic "small socket/large ball" discrepancy, the glenohumeral joint does function as a ball and socket joint in most positions during throwing or serving, being stabilized by the ligaments mainly at the extremes of motion.

Constraint Systems

The bony constraints do contribute to stability. The geometry of the joint surfaces allows smooth conformity of the two articular surfaces. The glenoid is enlarged and deepened by the labrum, which increases the conformity. The greater conformity increases the "concavity-compression" effect[11,12] to control translation. The conformity is maximized by a proper positioning of the scapula, with the glenoid, in relation to the moving arm.[6,13] This positioning will depend on proper scapular muscle activity. The glenohumeral joint has been statically compared to a "golf ball on a tee" in terms of its size relationships. A more appropriate description of the dynamic situation would be Rowe's comparison to a "ball on the seal's nose." As the ball (humerus) moves, the seal (scapula and glenoid) moves to maintain the balanced relationship.

Table 1
Normal joint motions and bony positions around the shoulder joint

Scapula	
Rotation through arc of 65° with shoulder abduction	
Translation on thorax up to 15 cm	
Glenohumeral	
Abduction	140°
Internal/external rotation	90°/90°
Translation	
Anterior/posterior	5 to 10 mm
Inferior/superior	4 to 5 mm
Total rotations	
Baseball	185°
Tennis	165°

Table 2
Forces and loads on the shoulder in normal athletic activity

Rotational velocities	
Baseball	7,000°/sec
Tennis serve	1,500°/sec
Tennis forehand	245°/sec
Tennis backhand	870°/sec
Angular velocities	
Baseball	1,150°/sec
Acceleration forces	
Internal rotation	60 N·m
Horizontal adduction	70 N·m
Anterior shear	400 N·m
Deceleration forces	
Horizontal abduction	80 N·m
Posterior shear	500 N·m
Compression	70 N·m

The ligamentous constraints are the primary stabilizers at extremes of motion in rotation, abduction, or flexion. They control both anterior/posterior and superior/inferior translation,[14-17] and also control coupled translation, or translation that occurs at the limit of normal rotation. Different parts of the ligamentous structures are the main restraints at different glenohumeral positions.[18,19] The ligaments work in a static fashion to limit translation and rotation,[20] but their stiffness and torsional rigidity are increased with concomitant muscle activity. Both rotator cuff activity[21] and biceps activity [22,23] have been shown to stiffen the capsule and decrease glenohumeral translation.

The muscular constraints work in several ways to allow stability. First, as has already been mentioned, they contribute to the other constraint systems by dynamic positioning of the scapula and by increasing capsuloligamentous stiffness. Second, they act as dynamic ligaments when their passive elements are used to limit joint excursion when the muscles are put on stretch.[24] Third, and most importantly, they act as parts of force couples around the joint, either by controlling the joint motion, by controlling the position of the bones and joint, or by controlling and directing the force through the joint.[25] Two types of force couples work around the shoulder joint (Outline 1).[25-27] The first is coactivation, or coordinated simultaneous activation of agonist and antagonist muscles about a joint. Coactivation creates low net torque around the joint but creates increased control of motion.[25] These activations are confined to muscles near the joint, involve a small number of muscles, and are controlled by and respond to length changes in the muscles.[26] Their major function is to control pertubations of the joint. Examples of this type would be the upper trapezius/levator scapulae working with the lower trapezius/serratus anterior to control scapular rotation,[27] the deltoid working with the subscapularis/infraspinatus/teres minor to control glenohumeral rotation,[28] and the subscapularis working with the infraspinatus/teres minor to control glenohumeral movement in the transverse plane.[27]

Outline 1
Force couples around the shoulder

Coordinated coactivation
- Low net torque
- Increased joint control
- Small number of muscles, close to joint
- Dependent on length changes in muscles

Examples of coordinated coactivation
- Upper trapezius/levator scapulae: Lower trapezius/serratus anterior to control scapular rotation
- Deltoid: Subscapularis/infraspinatus/teres minor to control glenohumeral rotation
- Subscapularis: Infraspinatus/teres minor to control glenohumeral movement

Agonist/Antagonist
- Increased joint torque and motion
- Larger number of muscles, distant and local to joint
- Coordinated sequencing
- Dependent on force changes of the activity

Examples of agonist/antagonist
- Trapezius/rhomboids: Serratus to control scapular retraction and protraction
- Pectoralis/latissimus dorsi: Posterior deltoid/infraspinatus/teres minor to control upper arm internal rotation

The second force couple is an agonist/antagonist activity, with coordinated activation of the agonist and inhibition of the antagonist muscles. This force couple increases joint torque and motion,[25] increases forces through the joint, and allows transfer of forces through the joint.[26] These activations are usually part of a sequence of activations involving many, often distant, muscles, and are controlled by and respond to force demands of the activity.[26] Examples would include the trapezius/rhomboids working with the serratus anterior to control scapular retraction and protraction,[27] and the pectoralis/latissimus dorsi working with the posterior deltoid/infraspinatus/teres minor to control upper arm internal rotation.[1,3]

Sequential coordinated muscle activation is necessary to produce the torques and accelerations necessary for throwing or serving. The intrinsic shoulder musculature does not have the capability to generate the recorded velocities. The cross-sectional area of the muscles is not large enough to generate the torques,[29] optimum arm velocity is not related to shoulder muscle strength,[30] peak torques and maximal velocities of the shoulder or of thrown objects decrease by about 50% as body parts are eliminated from the normal sequencing,[29,31,32] and peak velocity in female tennis players is more highly correlated with leg strength than arm strength.[33] Mathematical analysis, based on measured velocities throughout the tennis serve in elite players, shows that the shoulder link contributes about 13% of the total kinetic energy of the service motion[34] and is contributing 10% of the total forward arm velocity at the moment of ball impact.[35]

The sequential activation that occurs in the shoulder in most throwing or serving activities is a proximal-to-distal activation of the links in a kinematic chain.[36-38] The simplest representation of this chain is a kinetic chain,[36] in which each link is isolated and stops its function before the next link works. In actuality, the activation is more complex, with link activity overlapping.[37] However, from a standpoint of performance and rehabilitation, it is correct to say that this proximal-to-distal sequencing allows generation, summation, and transfer of velocities, energy, and accelerations from the proximal segments of the legs and back through the shoulder, to be added to the contributions of the distal segments of the arm. The shoulder not only functions as a small energy generator in this sequence, but also as a funnel for the transfer and concentration of the forces generated from the proximal links. The efficiency with which this is accomplished depends on the stability of the joint.

It appears that the primary force couple activation pattern of local muscles around the shoulder joint is the length-dependent, coordinated coactivation, stabilization pattern. This pattern regulates the transferred forces, allows humeral head compression, allows ball and socket motion in the mid-ranges of motion, and helps stiffen the capsule at the extremes of motion.

Conclusion

The normal shoulder experiences large motions and high forces that are generated rapidly and frequently. The shoulder functions locally as a constrained ball and socket joint with a predictable path of the instant center of joint motion. The shoulder functions in a proximal-to-distal kinematic chain sequence of force generation, funneling forces from the legs and back to the hand. The primary function of the local muscle firing patterns is as a coordinated coactivation force couple to control motion of the joint. Activities of the muscular constraint system enhance the effectiveness of the bony and ligamentous constraint systems.

Implications for Rehabilitation

From a rehabilitation perspective, the shoulder is a joint that is highly dependent on muscular activity, and it is dependent on both local and distant input for normal function. Once the clinical pathology has been treated, rehabilitation should be designed from these two perspectives to allow normal function.

Pain must be kept to a minimum, because it has a marked inhibitory effect on muscle peak torque and muscle coactivation. Modalities, medications, and judicious injections may be used to control pain.

Deficits in range of motion restrict normal shoulder function in several ways. Restricted glenohumeral internal rotation alters coupled translation, allowing anterior translation in the mid-ranges of motion;[6] changes the activation of the length-dependent force couple patterns;[26] and interferes with upper arm internal rotation, the most significant contributor to forward arm velocity in both the serve[35] and the forehand.[39] To get a true measure of glenohumeral range of motion, these deficits must be identified and objectively measured by goniometric evaluation.

The only way that muscles can be organized to function well repetitively and with precision through such rapid speeds and high loads is through learned motor patterns. These patterns position the body links in certain predetermined ways and activate muscles in precise agonist/antagonist force-dependent patterns and coordinated coactivation length-dependent patterns depending on the demands of the activity.[25,26,40] These motor patterns are more efficient, in terms of shorter duration, higher amplitude, and smoother coordination, in more skilled athletes.[41] Rehabilitation will be more effective if it focuses on reestablishing these patterns early. Cocontraction patterns for the scapula and shoulder[42] should be employed, as these are directly related to the demands the shoulder faces. Finally, functional progressions of throwing or serving,[42] employing the same motions as are present in the sport, complete the rehabilitation for normal shoulder function.

In addition to local treatment, evaluation and possible rehabilitation of the distant contributors to shoulder function should be done. Deficits in strength, strength balance, and flexibility in the legs, hips, and trunk should be sought. Restrictions of hip and back motion are common in throwing athletes[1,42,43] and should be included in the rehabilitation protocols. Maintenance of fitness of all other links of the kinematic chain can be done while early shoulder healing is progressing.[44,45] They can then be integrated into the shoulder rehabilitation program to allow normal force generation and transfer.[42]

References

1. Kibler WB: Evaluation of sports demands as a diagnostic tool in shoulder disorders, in Matsen FA III, Fu FH, Hawkins RJ (eds): *The Shoulder: A Balance of Mobility and Stability*. Rosemont, IL, American Academy of Orthopaedic Surgeons, 1993, pp 379–395.
2. Kibler WB, Chandler TJ: Racquet sports, in Fu FH, Stone DA (eds): *Sports Injuries: Mechanisms, Prevention, and Treatment*. Baltimore, MD, Williams & Wilkins, 1994, pp 531–550.
3. Fleisig GS, Dillman CJ, Andrews JR: Biomechanics of the shoulder during throwing, in Andrews JR, Wilk KE (eds): *The Athlete's Shoulder*. New York, NY, Churchill Livingstone, 1994, pp 355–368.
4. Pappas AM, Zawacki RM, Sullivan TJ: Biomechanics of baseball pitching: A preliminary report. *Am J Sports Med* 1985;13:216–222.
5. Perry J: Normal upper extremity kinesiology. *Phys Ther* 1978;58:265–278.
6. Harryman DT II, Sidles JA, Clark JM, et al: Translation of the humeral head on the glenoid with passive glenohumeral motion. *J Bone Joint Surg* 1990;72A:1334–1343.
7. Dempster WT: Mechanisms of shoulder movement. *Arch Phys Med Rehabil* 1965;46:49–70.
8. Cain PR, Mutschler TA, Fu FH, et al: Anterior stability of the glenohumeral joint: A dynamic model. *Am J Sports Med* 1987;15:144–148.
9. Howell SM, Galinat BJ, Renzi AJ, et al: Normal and abnormal mechanics of the glenohumeral joint in the horizontal plane. *J Bone Joint Surg* 1988;70A:227–232.
10. Bowen MK, Warren RF: Ligamentous control of shoulder stability based on selective cutting and static translation experiments. *Clin Sports Med* 1991;10:757–782.
11. Howell SM, Galinat BJ: The glenoid–labral socket: A constrained articular surface. *Clin Orthop* 1989;243:122–125.

12. Matsen FA III, Harryman DT II, Sidles JA: Mechanics of glenohumeral instability. *Clin Sports Med* 1991;10:783–788.
13. Moseley JB Jr, Jobe FW, Pink M, et al: EMG analysis of the scapular muscles during a shoulder rehabilitation program. *Am J Sports Med* 1992;20:128–134.
14. O'Connell PW, Nuber GW, Mileski RA, et al: The contribution of the glenohumeral ligaments to anterior stability of the shoulder joint. *Am J Sports Med* 1990;18:579–584.
15. Terry GC, Hammon D, France P, et al: The stabilizing function of passive shoulder restraints. *Am J Sports Med* 1991;19:26–34.
16. Warner JJ, Deng XH, Warren RF, et al: Static capsuloligamentous restraints to superior-inferior translation of the glenohumeral joint. *Am J Sports Med* 1992;20:675–685.
17. O'Brien SJ, Neves MC, Arnoczky SP, et al: The anatomy and histology of the inferior glenohumeral ligament complex of the shoulder. *Am J Sports Med* 1990;18:449–456.
18. Warren RF, Kornblatt IB, Marchand R: Static factors affecting posterior shoulder stability. *Orthop Trans* 1984;8:89.
19. Itoi E, Newman SR, Kuechle DK, et al: Dynamic anterior stabilisers of the shoulder with the arm in abduction. *J Bone Joint Surg* 1994;76B:834–836.
20. Warner JJP, Schulte KR, Imhoff AB: Current concepts in shoulder instability, in *Advances in Operative Orthopedics.* St. Louis, MO, CV Mosby, 1995, vol 3, pp 217–248.
21. Warner JJP, Caborn DNM, Berger R, et al: Dynamic capsuloligamentous anatomy of the glenohumeral joint. *J Shoulder Elbow Surg* 1993;2:115–133.
22. Rodosky MW, Harner CD, Fu FH: The role of the long head of the biceps muscle and superior glenoid labrum in anterior stability of the shoulder. *Am J Sports Med* 1994;22:121–130.
23. Itoi E, Kuechle DK, Newman SR, et al: Stabilising function of the biceps in stable and unstable shoulders. *J Bone Joint Surg* 1993;75B:546–550.
24. Hill AV: The mechanics of voluntary muscle. *Lancet* 1951;2:947–951.
25. Speer KP, Garrett WE Jr: Muscular control of motion and stability about the pectoral girdle, in Matsen FA III, Fu FH, Hawkins RJ (eds): *The Shoulder: A Balance of Mobility and Stability.* Rosemont, IL, American Academy of Orthopaedic Surgeons, 1993, pp 159–172.
26. Nichols TR: A biomechanical perspective on spinal mechanisms of coordinated muscular action: An architecture principle. *Acta Anat* 1994;151:1–13.
27. Inman VT, Saunders JB, Abbott LC: Observations on the function of the shoulder joint. *J Bone Joint Surg* 1944;26:1–30.
28. Perry J, Glousman R: Biomechanics of throwing, in Nicholas JA, Hershman EB (eds): *The Upper Extremity In Sports Medicine.* St. Louis, MO, CV Mosby, 1990, pp 725–748.
29. Alexander RM: Optimum timing of muscle activation for simple models of throwing. *J Theor Biol* 1991;150:349–372.
30. Bartlet LR, Storey MD, Simons BD: Measurements of upper extremity torque production and its relationship to throwing speed in the competitive athlete. *Am J Sports Med* 1989;17:89–91.
31. Toyoshima S, Hoshikawa T, Miyashita M: Contribution of body parts to throwing performance, in Nelson RC, Morehouse CA (eds): *Biomechanics of Sport.* Baltimore, MD, University Park Press, 1974, pp 169–174.
32. Whiting WC, Puffer JC, Finerman GA, et al: Three-dimensional cinematographic analysis of water polo throwing in elite performers. *Am J Sports Med* 1985;13:95–98.
33. Kraemer WJ, Triplett NT, Fry AC: An in-depth sports medicine profile of women college tennis players. *J Sports Rehab* 1995;4:79–98.
34. Kibler WB: Biomechanical analysis of the shoulder during tennis activities. *Clin Sports Med* 1995;14:79–85.
35. Elliott BC, Marshall R, Noffal G: Contributions of upper limb segment rotations during the power serve in tennis. *J Appl Biomech* 1995;11:433–442.
36. Kibler WB: Current concepts of shoulder biomechanics: Pathology and treatment. *J South Orthop Assoc* 1994;3:254–271.
37. Elliott BC: Tennis strokes and equipment, in Vaughan CL (ed): *Biomechanics of Sport.* Boca Raton, FL, CRC Press, 1989, pp 263–288.
38. Hong O, Roberts EM: A three dimensional six segment chain analysis of forceful overarm throwing. *Proceedings of the Second North American Congress on Biomechanics,* Chicago, IL, 1992, pp 55–56.
39. Elliott BC, Takahashi K, Noffal GC: The influence of holding the racket on the contribution of upper limb segment rotations in tennis forehand ground strokes. *Int J Appl Biomech,* in press.
40. Perry J: Anatomy and biomechanics of the shoulder in throwing, swimming, gymnastics, and tennis. *Clin Sports Med* 1983;2:247–270.
41. Gowan ID, Jobe FW, Tibone JE, et al: A comparative electromyographic analysis of the shoulder during pitching: Professional versus amateur pitchers. *Am J Sports Med* 1987;15:586–590.
42. Kibler WB, Livingston B, Bruce R: Current concepts in shoulder rehabilitation, in *Advances in Operative Orthopedics.* St. Louis, MO, CV Mosby, 1995, vol 3, pp 249–291.
43. Wilk KE, Arrigo C, Andrews JR: Current concepts in rehabilitation of the athlete's shoulder. *J South Orthop Assoc* 1994;3:216–231.
44. Fyfe I, Stanish WD: The use of eccentric training and stretching in the treatment and prevention of tendon injuries. *Clin Sports Med* 1992;11:601–624.
45. Herring SA: Rehabilitation of muscle injuries. *Med Sci Sports Exerc* 1990;22:453–456.

CHAPTER 6

Shoulder Rehabilitation: Clinical Application, Evaluation, and Rehabilitation Protocols

W. Ben Kibler, MD
Beven Livingston, PT, ATC
T. Jeff Chandler, EdD

Implementation of specific rehabilitation protocols for the shoulder must be based on basic science knowledge, and must be used in a logical, diagnosis- or activity-specific progression to achieve maximum efficiency. The goal of the rehabilitation program, functional restoration, is the same for each condition, but the starting point is widely variable, depending on the pathologic process (macrotrauma, microtrauma), type of treatment (rest, immobilization, surgery), and associated alterations (other injuries, inflexibility, strength deficit). This point reinforces the need for a complete and accurate diagnosis as a starting point for rehabilitation.

Evaluation Before Rehabilitation

Evaluation of the shoulder should include evaluation of the kinematic chain as well. The hips and knees should be assessed for any incompletely resolved injury. Special attention should be focused on hip rotation and flexion, especially on the non-dominant side, because these areas have been shown to be tight (Fig. 1).[1] Lumbar flexibility, both in flexion and lateral bending, should be measured, lumbar lordosis should be checked, and trunk musculature strength should be evaluated. Finally, the thoracic spine should be evaluated for scoliosis or kyphosis. Either of these conditions not only can alter spine motion in throwing, but also may disrupt normal scapulothoracic motion.

Evaluation of the scapula should be done from the back. Abnormalities of the scapular position, such as winging or excessive prominence, should be noted (Fig. 2). Scapular motion should be observed in both arm flexion and arm abduction (Fig. 3). Smooth symmetrical motion both in the ascending phase and in the descending phase should be observed. Asymmetry, which is usually noted in the descending phase, suggests weakness in the scapula force couple. Scapular stabilizer strength may be assessed by wall push-ups or by the "lateral slide" measurement (Fig. 4).[2] Both of these tests measure the ability of the scapular muscles to stabilize the scapula on the thoracic wall in response to an imposed load.

The acromioclavicular joint is important as a stabilizing strut and as a loadbearing joint when the arm is in the overhead position. Palpation for tenderness,

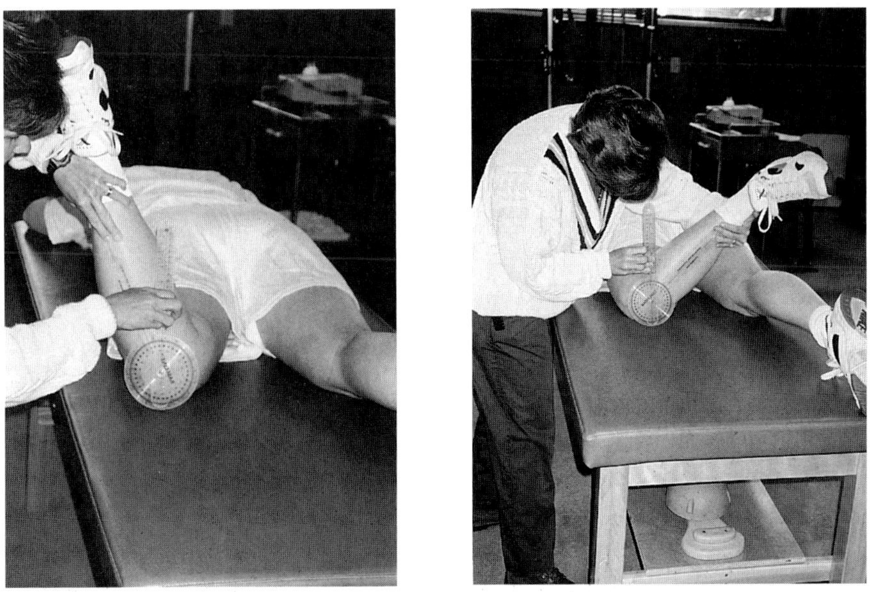

Fig. 1 Measurement of hip rotation. **Left,** internal rotation, and **right,** external rotation.

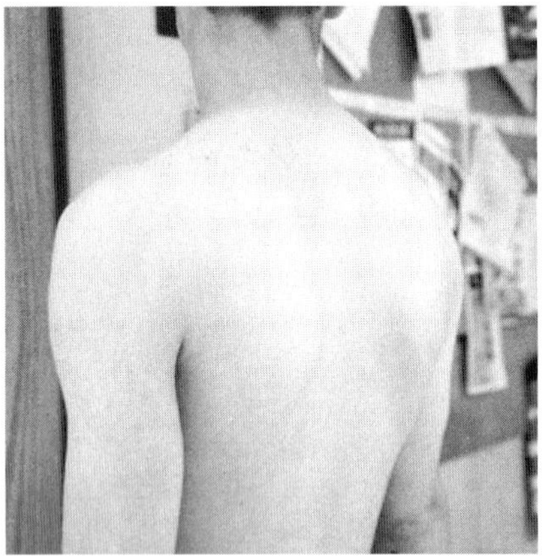

Fig. 2 Scapular prominence with arm at rest.

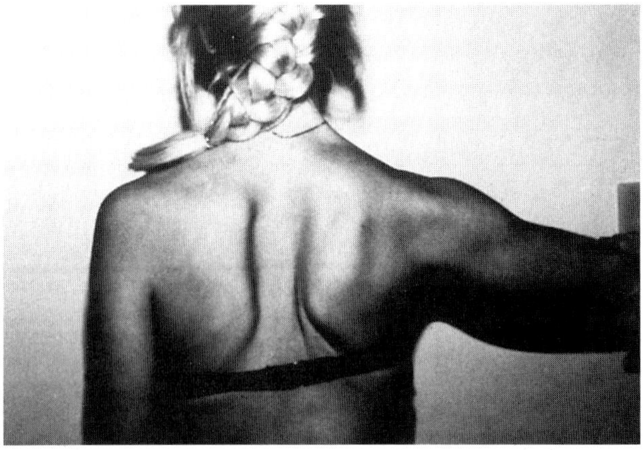

Fig. 3 Scapular winging with resisted abduction.

swelling, or crepitus should be done, and motion of the joint in both anterior/posterior and superior/inferior directions may be evaluated by stabilizing the scapula and using direct pressure to move the clavicle (Fig. 5).

Evaluation of the glenohumeral joint should include range of motion, strength, and provocative testing. Glenohumeral motion is a sensitive measure of shoulder pathology, and should be measured accurately by a goniometer, rather than by estimating spinous process levels.[3] The shoulder should be placed in the scapular plane, with the goniometer centered along the axis of rotation (Fig. 6). Abduction and horizontal abduction/adduction can be measured in the same fashion (Fig. 7).

Glenohumeral strength can be estimated by manual muscle testing, or it can be objectively described by isokinetic testing. Manual muscle testing is much better for evaluation of the individual components of the rotator cuff, which cannot be accurately evaluated by isokinetics.

Provocative tests for glenohumeral stability should be done after either treatment or surgery to assess the competence of the ligamentous constraints, to determine if full range-of-motion exercises and muscular loading can be done safely.

Phases of Rehabilitation

Our functional rehabilitation program is divided into three phases. Each phase is intended to resolve certain aspects of the tissue injuries or alterations that make up the shoulder problem (Outline 1).[4] There are specific goals, activity progressions, and criteria for movement to the next phase. Since this is a function-based program, all of the protocols tend to progress to some common end points in the later phases, regardless of the starting point.

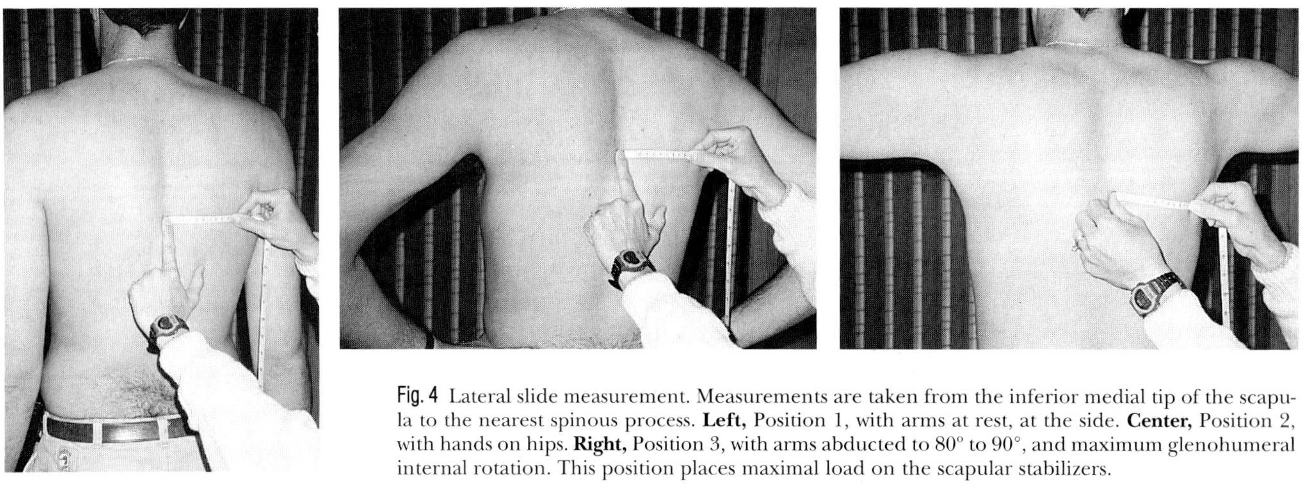

Fig. 4 Lateral slide measurement. Measurements are taken from the inferior medial tip of the scapula to the nearest spinous process. **Left,** Position 1, with arms at rest, at the side. **Center,** Position 2, with hands on hips. **Right,** Position 3, with arms abducted to 80° to 90°, and maximum glenohumeral internal rotation. This position places maximal load on the scapular stabilizers.

Acute Phase

The acute phase begins with the onset of clinical symptoms of injury or when the patient is seen for rehabilitation. Patient injuries vary widely, from acute fracture or dislocation, to a postoperative rotator cuff repair, to an overload tendinitis. In each instance, the focus is on resolving the clinical symptoms and the tissue injuries. This phase is the most diverse because of the wide spectrum of clinical symptoms and tissue injuries and the variety of treatments that are necessary. The objective of this phase is to create stable, healing tissues and improve joint health to allow more advanced rehabilitation.

Recovery Phase

The recovery phase continues rehabilitation of the tissue injury complex and, at the same time, addresses the tissue overloads and functional biomechanical deficits. Entry into this phase assumes that the injured tissues may be loaded in tension and compression so that normal strength and flexibility may now be reached. This phase is frequently the longest and most complex because of the large amount of work required to restore all of the alterations, both locally and distantly. Force couple restoration, full range of motion, scapular stability, and kinematic chain restoration are addressed in this phase. By the end of this phase, most of the protocols will be merging toward the common goals of gaining full motion and muscular balance.

Functional Phase

The functional phase addresses any remaining functional biomechanical deficits, corrects any subclinical adaptations that may have developed, and uses functional progressions to return to play. This is the final common pathway of all of the protocols. The athlete

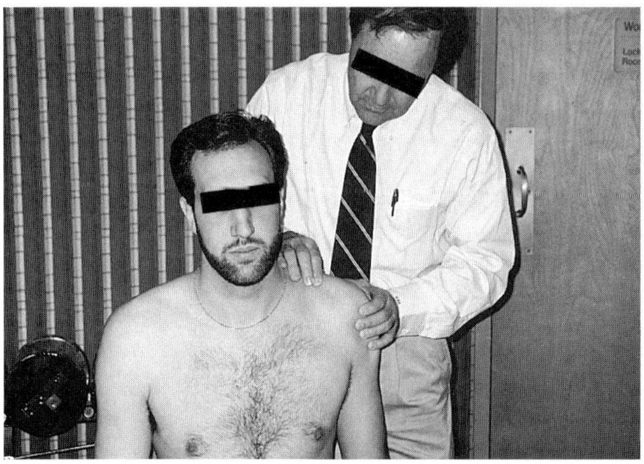

Fig. 5 Palpation for abnormal movement of the acromioclavicular joint.

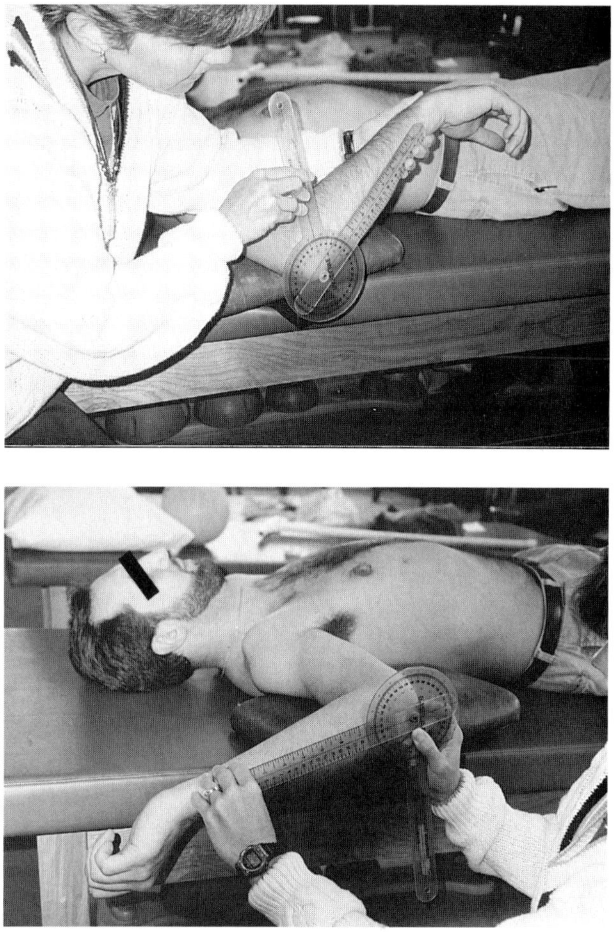

Fig. 6 Goniometric measurement of glenohumeral rotation. The humerus is placed in the scapular plane. **Top,** internal rotation, and **bottom,** external rotation.

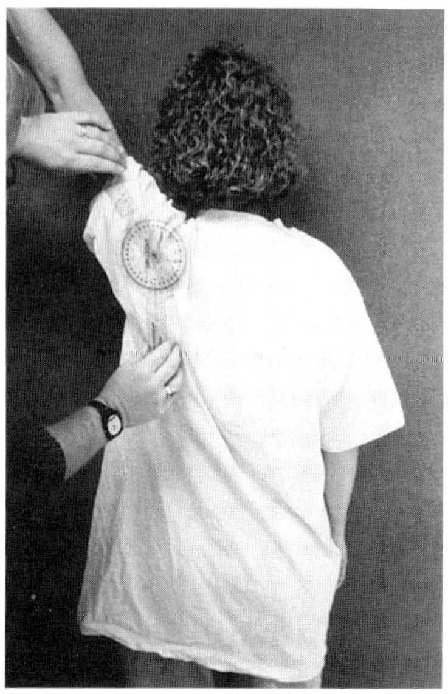

Fig. 7 Goniometric measurement of glenohumeral abduction.

Outline 1
Phases of rehabilitation and complexes addressed in each phase

Acute phase
- Clinical symptom complex
- Tissue injury complex

Recovery phase
- Tissue injury complex
- Tissue overload complex
- Functional biomechanical deficit complex

Functional phase
- Functional biomechanical deficit complex
- Subclinical adaptations complex

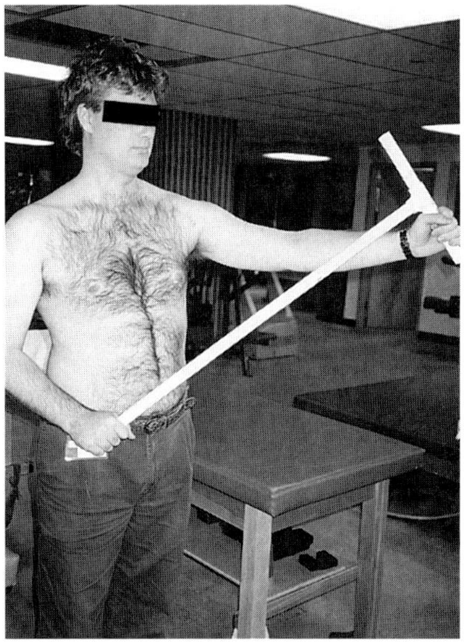

Fig. 8 Acute phase active assisted range of motion below 90°.

may start some modified athletic activity, such as hitting ground strokes only or throwing a limited number of pitches, but functional progressions of throwing, hitting, or serving need to be completed before full competition is allowed. These progressions test all of the mechanical parts of the normal overhead throwing or serving motion. Very few deviations from normal mechanics should be allowed, because these deviations will create extra stress when the athlete has to meet the normal demands inherent in the sport.

The functional phase should also be used to instruct the athlete in preventive activities, or "prehabilitation." The athlete who is injured as a result of participating in a sport will usually return to that sport and its demands after the injury is rehabilitated. A maintenance program of stretching, muscle balance exercises, power exercises, and kinematic chain exercise, all designed to improve the athlete's ability to withstand sports demands, is the best method of conditioning to prevent the overload injuries that are common around the shoulder.[5]

Specific Rehabilitation Protocols

Postoperative Rehabilitation Protocol

This general protocol will illustrate principles for rehabilitation of any postoperative problem. It assumes stable repair of the labrum, capsule, or rotator cuff, and ability to achieve 90° of abduction without impingement or excessive capsular stretch at the time of the operation. We try to get patients with labral repairs, shoulder reconstructions, and acromioplasties to 90° of passive or active assisted abduction by 3 weeks, and we try to get those with rotator cuff repairs to 90° passive or active assisted abduction by 4 to 6 weeks.

Acute Phase Goals during the acute phase are to heal tissue, to reduce pain and inflammation, to reestablish nonpainful range of motion below 90° of abduction, to retard muscle atrophy, to regain scapular control, and to maintain the fitness of the other components of the kinematic chain.

Tissue healing is accomplished by a combination of rest, short-term immobilization, nonsurgical modalities, and, if necessary, surgery.

Pain and inflammation are addressed by aggressive treatment to control pain in order to decrease inhibition-based muscle atrophy and decrease scapular instability due to serratus and/or trapezius inhibition. This is done with medication, either nonsteroidal drugs or the judicious use of steroids, orally or by injection; use of ultrasound, twice weekly for 2 weeks; cold compression devices; and joint protection, usually by sling or swathe, with gradual progression out of sling.

Range of motion should be started in pain-free arcs, kept below 90° abduction, and may be passive or active assisted. Modalities used include Codman's or other pendulum exercise equipment, manual capsular stretching and cross fiber massage, and T-bar or ropes and pulleys (Fig. 8).

Muscle atrophy is prevented by isometric exercises, with the arm below 90° abduction and 90° flexion. These exercises should be done following labral or capsular repair, but not following rotator cuff repair.

Scapular control is maintained by isometric scapular pinches and scapular elevation; closed chain weight shifts, with hands on table, shoulder flexed less than 60° and abducted less than 45° (Fig. 9); and tilt board or circular board weight shifts with same limitations.

The fitness of the rest of the kinematic chain is maintained by aerobic exercises, such as running, bicycling, or stepping; anaerobic agility drills; lower extremity strengthening, by machines, squat exercises, or open chain leg lifts; elbow and wrist strengthening by isometrics or rubber tubing; flexibility exercises, especially in areas that are shown to be tight on the

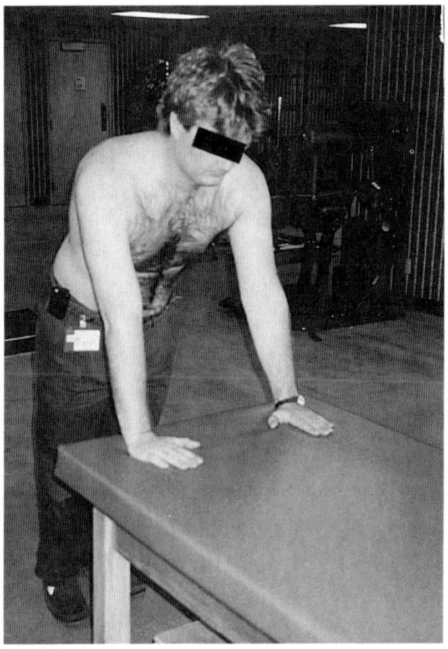

Fig. 9 Acute phase closed chain weight shifts. Arms are kept below 60° abduction.

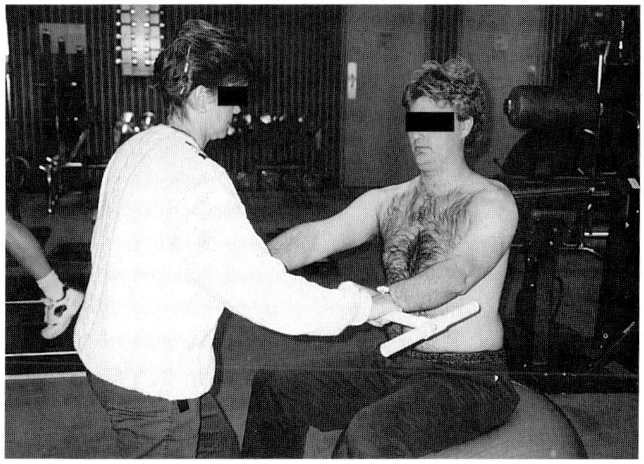

Fig. 10 Acute phase ball exercises. These exercises start the integration of the trunk into shoulder rehabilitation.

evaluation; and integration of the kinematic chain by leg and trunk stabilization on a ball, employing rotational and oblique patterns of contraction (Fig. 10).

The criteria for movement out of the acute phase are progression of tissue healing (healed or sufficiently stabilized for active motion and tissue loading); passive range of motion that is 66% to 75% of the opposite side; minimal pain; manual muscle strength of 4+ to 5 in nonpathologic areas; scapular control, with dominant side/nondominant side scapular asymmetry of less than 1.5 cm;[2] and kinematic chain function and integration.

Recovery Phase Goals during the recovery phase are a return to normal active and passive shoulder and glenohumeral motion; improvement of scapular control; normal upper extremity strength and strength balance; normal shoulder arthrokinematics in single, then multiple planes of motion; and normal kinematic chain and force generation patterns.

For range of motion, the goals are active assisted motion above 90° of abduction with wand (Fig. 11) and active assisted, then active, motion, both internal and external, with the scapula stabilized (Fig. 12). In this manner, glenohumeral rotation is normalized without substitution movements from the scapula.

Scapular control is improved by the use of scapular proprioceptive neuromuscular facilitation patterns, in diagonals; closed chain exercises at 90° of flexion and 90° of abduction, with scapular retraction and protraction and scapular elevation and depression (Fig. 13); modified push-ups; regular push-ups; medicine ball catch and push; and dips.

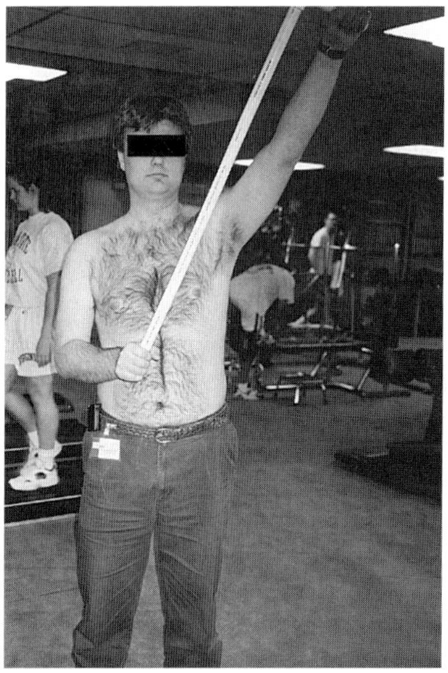

Fig. 11 Recovery phase active assisted range of motion in rotation.

Upper extremity strength and strength balance are regained by the use of glenohumeral proprioceptive neuromuscular facilitation patterns (Fig. 14); closed chain exercises at 90° of flexion and then at 90° of abduction (glenohumeral depressors and glenohumeral internal/external rotators); forearm curls; isolated rotator cuff exercises; and machines or weights for light bench press, military press, and pull downs. The resistance, which should initially be light, progresses as strength improves. Emphasis is placed on proper mechanics, proper technique, and joint stabilization.

The following three activities aid the recovery of

normal shoulder arthrokinematics. First is range of motion with arm at 90° of abduction, which is the position where most throwing and serving activities occur. The periarticular soft tissues must be completely loose and balanced at this position. Second is muscle activity at 90° of abduction. Normal muscle firing patterns must be reestablished at this position, both in organization of force generation and force regulation patterns and in proprioceptive sensory feedback. Closed chain patterns are an excellent method to reestablish the normal neurologic patterns for joint stabilization. Third are open chain exercises, including mild plyometric exercises. These exercises may be built upon the base of the closed chain stabilization to allow normal control of joint mobility.

Normal kinematic chain and force generation are achieved through normalization of all inflexibilities throughout the chain; normal agonist/antagonist force couples in legs by squats, plyometric depth jumps, lunges, and hip extensions; trunk rotation exercises, with medicine ball or tubing; integrated exercises with leg and trunk stabilization, including rotations (Fig. 15), diagonal patterns from hip to shoulder (Fig. 16), and medicine ball throws; and normal throwing or serving motion without resistance.

The criteria for moving out of the recovery phase are full nonpainful scapulothoracic motion; at least 90% of normal glenohumeral motion; lateral slide asymmetry less than 0.75 cm; normal back motion; rotator cuff strength of 4+ to 5 or higher; and normal kinematic chain function.

Functional Phase Goals during this phase are to increase power and endurance in the upper extremity; to increase normal multiple-plane neuromuscular control, locally, regionally, and in the entire kinematic chain; to instruct the patient in prehabilitation activities; and to resume sports-specific activity.

Development of increased power and endurance in the upper extremity is the first goal. Power is the rate of doing work. Work may be done to move the joint and the extremity, or it may be done to absorb a load and stabilize the joint or extremity. Power has a time component, and for shoulder activity, quick movements and quick reactions are the dominant ways of doing work. These exercises should, therefore, be done with relatively rapid movements in planes that approximate normal shoulder function (ie, 90° of abduction of the shoulder, trunk rotation and diagonal arm motions, and rapid external and internal rotation). Exercises include diagonal and multiplanar motions with tubing, light weights, small medicine balls, and isokinetic machines; and plyometrics, which include wall push-ups, corner push-ups, weighted ball throws, and tubing. Tubing exercises may be used to mimic any of the needed motions in throwing or serving. Medicine balls are very effective plyometric devices (Fig. 17). The weight of the ball creates a prestretch and an eccen-

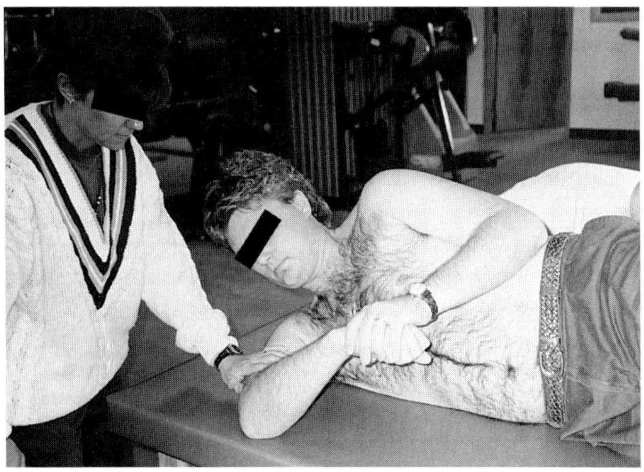

Fig. 12 Recovery phase glenohumeral rotation with scapula stabilized to stretch posterior shoulder capsule.

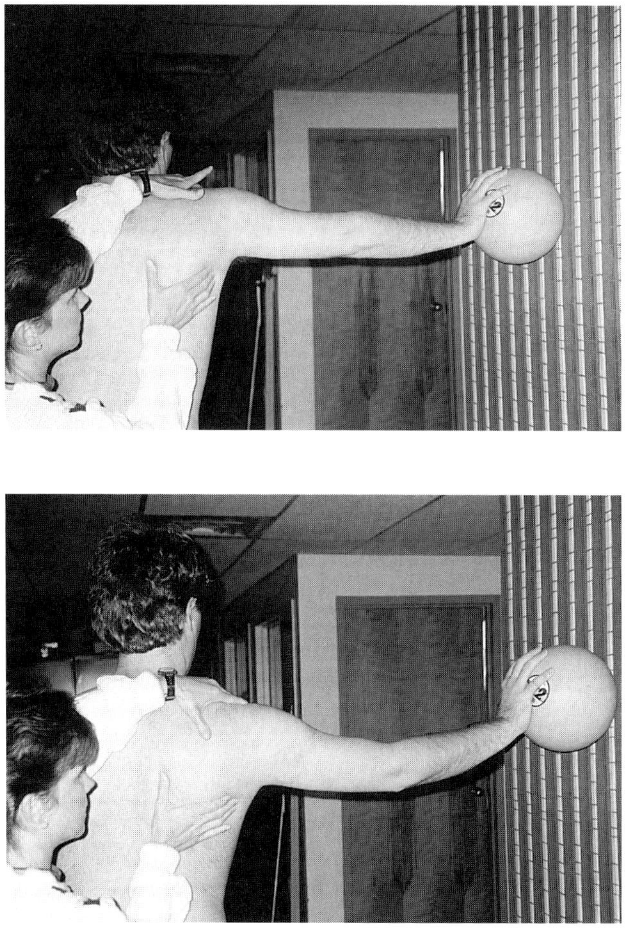

Fig. 13 Recovery phase closed chain exercises for scapular control. **Top,** scapular elevation, and **bottom,** scapular depression.

tric load when it is caught, creates a resistance, and demands a powerful agonist contraction to propel it forward again.

In order to increase multiple-plane neuromuscular control, the force dependent motor firing patterns should be reestablished. No subclinical adaptations, such as "opening up" (trunk rotation too far in front of shoulder rotation), 3/4 arm positioning on throwing, or excessive wrist snap, should be allowed. Help in this area can be obtained by watching preinjury videos or by using a knowledgeable coach in the particular sport.

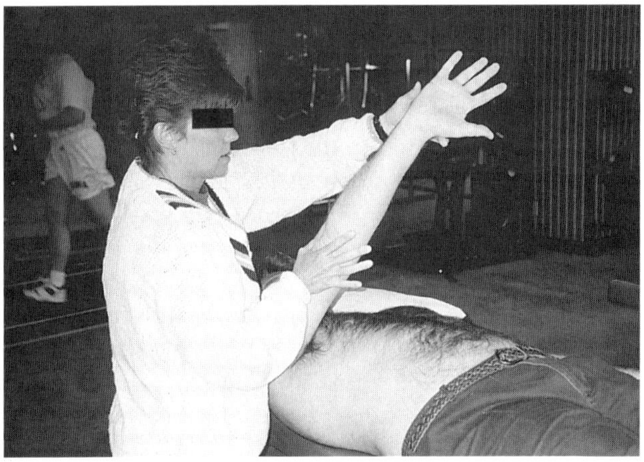

Fig. 14 Recovery phase glenohumeral proprioceptive neuromuscular facilitation patterns. The joint is rotated into internal and external rotation, and resisted in diagonal patterns.

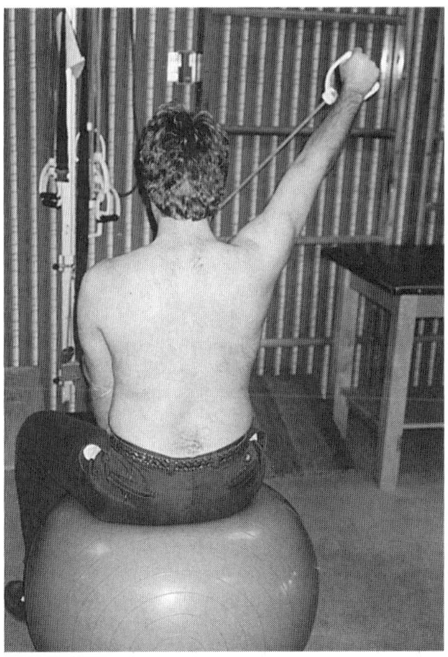

Fig. 15 Recovery phase trunk rotations. These may be done on the ball or while standing. The emphasis is to stabilize the pelvis and develop rotational strength.

Special care must be taken to completely integrate all of the components of the kinematic chain to generate and funnel the proper forces to and through the shoulder.

In setting up prehabilitation activities, it is important to remember that the athlete who is injured while playing a sport will most likely be going back to the same

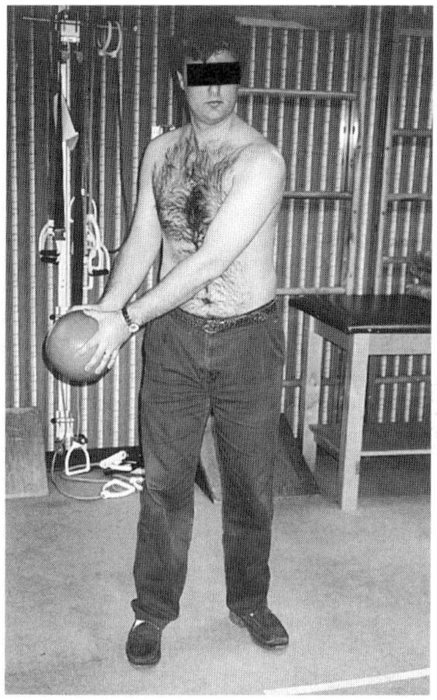

Fig. 16 Recovery phase diagonal patterns. Most throwing activities involve diagonal force generation and force regulation, starting from the legs, through the trunk, to the arm.

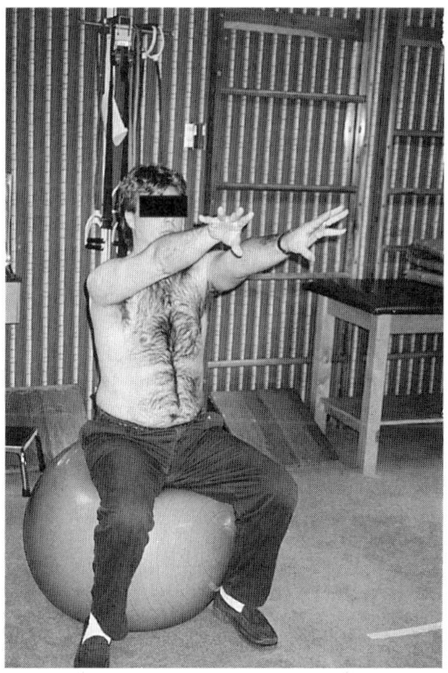

Fig. 17 Functional phase medicine ball plyometrics. Power should be emphasized, catching the ball, then pushing it back with a powerful thrust. Using the ball allows integration of the kinetic chain.

Outline 2
Return to play progression for throwing

45 ft: Warm up; throws with normal motion (25 × 2), (25 × 3)

60 ft: Warm up; throws with normal motion (25 × 2), (25 × 3)

90 ft: Warm up; throws with normal motion (25 × 2), (25 × 3)

120 ft: Warm up; throws with normal motion (25 × 2), (25 × 3)

60 ft off mound: 50% of normal velocity — fastball (15→30→45)

60 ft off mound: Batting practice at 50% — fastball (30→45→60)

60 ft off mound: Batting practice at 75% — fastball (15→30→45)

60 ft off mound: Batting practice at 75% — fastball, 50% breaking ball (45→60→75)

60 ft off mound: Batting practice at 75% both (60→90)

Simulated game: (75→90→105 pitches)

Outline 3
Return to play progression for serving

Arm movement in serve motion — no racquet
Upward ball toss and arm movement — racquet in hand
Hitting ball with arm movement, at net
Hitting ball across net standing at service line
Hitting ball across net standing at base line
Hitting ball with flat serve motion
Aiming serve into proper court
Full activity

sport and will be facing the same sports demands. The body should not only be healed from the symptomatic standpoint, but should be prepared for resuming the stresses inherent in playing the sport. In order to avoid overload injuries and further problems in sport,[5] a maintenance program is the best way to condition. This program emphasizes flexibility, including general body flexibility, with emphasis on sport-specific problems (shoulder internal rotation and elbow extension in the arm, low back, hip rotation and hamstrings in the legs); strengthening to regain the appropriate amount of strength in proper locations for sport-specific activities (quadriceps/hamstring strength for force generation, trunk rotation strength, strength balance for the shoulder); power to allow rapid movements in appropriate planes with light weights; and endurance, gained mainly through anaerobic exercises due to short duration, explosive, and ballistic activities seen in throwing and serving. These exercises should be based on the periodization principle of conditioning.[6]

In resumption of sport-specific activity, functional progressions of throwing or serving must be completed before full competition is allowed. These progressions will gradually test all of the mechanical parts of the throwing or serving motion. Very few deviations from normal parameters of arm motion, arm position, force generation, smoothness of all of the kinematic chain, and from preinjury form should be allowed, because most of these adaptations will be biomechanically inefficient. The athlete may move through the progressions as rapidly as possible. Progressions for throwing[7] and serving[8] are shown in Outlines 2 and 3.

The four criteria for return to play are normal clinical examination, normal shoulder arthrokinematics, normal kinematic chain integration, and completed progressions.

Other Shoulder Protocols

Protocols for nonoperative problems, such as impingement or rotator cuff tendinitis/tendinosis, vary from the detailed postoperative protocol mainly in the methods used in the acute phase. More emphasis is placed on resolving the symptoms of pain, swelling, or mechanical derangement. Medications, injections, ultrasound or other modalities, and relative rest are commonly used in the acute phase. We direct most of our attention to resolving pain because of its major effect on all shoulder functions. We try to implement the other aspects of the acute care protocol as soon as symptoms and tissue integrity allow. After the acute symptoms have been resolved, entry into the recovery phase will be implemented. The protocols are basically the same from this point on, differing only by whatever tissue overloads or biomechanical deficits are discovered on the prerehabilitation evaluation.

Summary

This chapter has discussed and illustrated a shoulder rehabilitation protocol based on restoration of the anatomy, biomechanics, physiology, and motor firing organization that is responsible for normal shoulder function. Many protocols exist in the literature, most of which appear to achieve good results.[4,7-11] There are no outcomes data to suggest the most efficacious protocols. Adherence to the basic principles outlined in these chapters appears to allow the best framework for constructing a good program.

References

1. Kibler WB: Evaluation of sports demands as a diagnostic tool in shoulder disorders, in Matsen FA III, Fu FH, Hawkins RJ (eds): *The Shoulder: A Balance of Mobility and Stability.* Rosemont IL, American Academy of Orthopaedic Surgeons, 1993, pp 379–395.
2. Kibler WB: Role of the scapula in the overhead throwing motion. *Contemp Orthop* 1991;22:525–532.
3. Kibler WB, Chandler TJ: The effect of age and tournament play on shoulder range of motion in elite tennis players. *Am J Sports Med* 1996;24:279–285.

4. Kibler WB, Chandler TJ, Pace BK: Principles of rehabilitation after chronic tendon injuries. *Clin Sports Med* 1992;11:661–671.
5. Chandler TJ, Kibler WB: Muscle training in injury prevention, in Renstrom P (ed): *Sports Injuries: Basic Principles of Prevention and Care.* Oxford, England, Blackwell Scientific, 1993, pp 252–261.
6. Kibler WB, Chandler TJ: Sport-specific conditioning. *Am J Sports Med* 1994;22:424–432.
7. Wilk KE: *Preventative and Rehabilitative Exercises for the Shoulder and Elbow.* Birmingham, AL, Alabama Sports Medicine Institute, 1991.
8. Kibler WB, Livingston BK, Bruce R: Current concepts in shoulder rehabilitation. *Adv Oper Orthop* 1996;3:249–300.
9. Wilk KE, Arrigo C, Andrews JR: Current concepts in the rehabilitation of the athlete's shoulder. *J South Orthop Assoc* 1994; 3:216–231.
10. Sobel J: Shoulder rehabilitation: Rotator cuff disease, in Pettrone FA (ed): *Athletic Injuries of the Shoulder.* New York, NY, McGraw-Hill, 1995, pp 245–270.
11. Pink MM, Screnar PM, Tollefson KD, et al: Injury prevention and rehabilitation in the upper extremity, in Jobe FW, Pink MM, Glousman RE, et al (eds): *Operative Techniques in Upper Extremity Sports Injuries.* St. Louis, MO, Mosby-Year Book, 1996, pp 3–14.

CHAPTER 7

Current Research on Muscle Activity About the Shoulder

Bryan T. Kelly, MD
Donald T. Kirkendall, PhD
Andrew S. Levy, MD
Kevin P. Speer, MD

Introduction

Electromyography (EMG) is a valuable tool for assessing muscle function and activity. Its fundamental utility is based on the close correlation of changes in a muscle's electrical activity with changes in force production from that muscle.[1,2] The electromyographic analysis of the shoulder has gained widespread acceptance since the pioneering work of Inman and associates[3] in 1944. Since that time, numerous questions regarding shoulder physiology have been addressed through this research modality. Electromyography research on the shoulder has ranged from the analysis of normal function[4-8] to the examination of muscle activation during shoulder rehabilitation protocols.[9-11] In addition, EMG has been used to compare the muscle activation of normal shoulders with abnormal shoulders[12] as well as to analyze shoulder muscle activation and coordination during sports activity.[13-17]

EMG offers an enticing opportunity to address clinically relevant questions regarding dynamic muscle activity. However, a major limitation of kinesiologic EMG research is the difficulty in making comparisons between EMG values obtained from identical muscles in different subjects, different muscles from the same subject, or even the same muscle from the same subject on different days. This difficulty is caused by subtle differences in muscle architecture, electrode placement, and electrode construction.[18-20] Because of such limitations, it is extremely important to standardize all aspects of shoulder EMG research. Through the development of strict instrumentation and normalization standards, our laboratory has been able to minimize many of the possible sources of technical error. Use of these standards should lead to results that have greater clinical utility and validity.

The chapter reviews three major areas of current research on muscle activity about the shoulder: technical considerations for shoulder EMG, with special attention to the standardization of recording and normalization procedures; clinically relevant questions regarding rotator cuff and shoulder synergist activity; and EMG analysis of muscle activity during therapeutic rehabilitation exercises.

Technical Considerations

Electrode Placement

Intramuscular fine-wire electrodes have been used for the examination of the deep muscles about the shoulder region since the classic work of Inman in 1944.[3] The use of bipolar indwelling electrodes was popularized with the development of the insertion technique described by Basmajian and Stecko[21] in 1962, in which two wires are introduced into the muscle via a single hypodermic needle and secured into the belly of the muscle by means of small hooks in the distal ends of the wires. This technique has gained widespread acceptance and has been used in a variety of different electromyography kinesiology studies analyzing the electrical signal from deep muscles in the body not amenable to evaluation with surface electrodes.[7-9,12,22-24]

The use of indwelling wire electrodes in electromyography studies provides many advantages. Wire electrodes can record muscles too deep to be detected by surface electrodes, they are less painful than needle electrodes, they have low sensitivity to movement artifact,[25] and they can easily be inserted and withdrawn.[26] Because they are relatively innocuous and less painful than needle electrodes, wire electrodes rarely interfere with activity and can thus be used in dynamic electromyography studies as well as during maximal voluntary contractions.[11,17] However, wire electrodes do have some drawbacks. A significant problem is the poor reproducibility of measurements demonstrated by imprecisely fabricated wire electrodes. Electromyography signals can range from clear maximal signals, to signals with submaximal voltage, to minimal or even short-circuited readings.[19]

Numerous studies have shown that indwelling electrodes have significantly less reliability than surface electrodes in test-retest situations.[18-20,27,28] Jonsson and Komi[19] have suggested some technical sources of error that are likely contributors to this reproducibility problem. These include variations in the starting positions of the two wires, as well as shifts in their relative positions as the needle is driven through the muscle. A further confounding factor is migration of the electrode tips with muscular contraction after placement. Wire migration commonly occurs with the first muscular contraction, but stability generally follows after several contractions. Hence, all intramuscular electrodes need some preliminary muscle motion to fix the wire hooks.[26,29,30] Because of these factors, the ultimate position of the electrode tip within the muscle is in large part left to chance. Unsystematic variation in the relative positions of the two leads can create significant inconsistency in the magnitude of the electrical signal obtained. A clear maximal signal can be obtained if the two wire tips end up 180° from each other and have completely independent pickup areas. The signal can be completely lost if the tips migrate toward each other and short circuit as a result of the tips touching. Some intermediate, submaximal signals can be obtained if the wire tips are located within overlapping pickup areas such that the common signals are subtracted when they pass through the differential amplifier (Fig. 1). Despite attempts to separate electrode tips by staggering their bared ends, migration of the electrodes after placement into the muscle will potentially lead to changes in the interelectrode distance and possibly even lead to short circuiting as described above. This phenomenon is especially problematic when the initial interelectrode distance is small, as is the case in the traditional, Basmajian single needle insertion technique. The migration can also be especially problematic when there is excessive movement of the electrode with muscular contraction. Electrodes placed in the subscapularis are subjected to large position changes due to significant scapular motion with normal shoulder function.

Despite the fact that optimal interdetection spacing for surface electrodes has been examined,[26,31,32] very little effort has been spent to determine optimal placement for indwelling electrodes. In an attempt to standardize indwelling wire electrode placement about the shoulder, the differences in the signal obtained from a bipolar electrode introduced into the muscle via a single hypodermic needle were compared with the signal obtained from an electrode with the two leads inserted separately at a distance of 1 cm (Fig. 2). We found that separated bipolar electrodes produced EMG signals with greater voltage, less variation, and higher partial correlation coefficients for the integrated EMG area versus force relationship. An electrical signal of greater amplitude has a greater ability to detect subtleties in the differential measurement of EMG values. An electrical signal with less intersubject variation represents a more reliable and reproducible recording method. An electrical signal that has a higher partial correlation coefficient with force measurement suggests an improved ability to reflect changes in the force generated by the subject.

We recommend the use of the separated bipolar electrode insertion technique, because it results in more accurate findings due to improved signal characteristics and the elimination of signal loss secondary to lead crossover. If investigators choose to continue to use the single needle bipolar construction technique, then extreme care should be taken during electrode fabrication. All attempts should be made to minimize electrode crossover by creating a significant difference in the hook length (suggested 2 to 3 mm) so that the bared ends cannot touch. Because of the learning curve associated with the placement and construction of bipolar leads, we recommend the separated bipolar insertion technique for investigators who are not practiced in the single needle insertion technique.

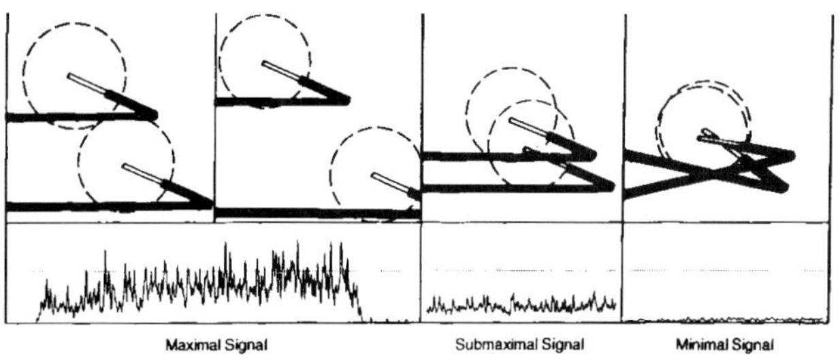

Fig. 1 Effects of interdetection spacing on the EMG signal. Separation of the two electrodes in a bipolar configuration to different pickup areas maximizes the EMG signal obtained. As the electrodes are moved closer together, there is increased overlap of the pickup areas, with an attendant decrease in the resultant EMG signal.

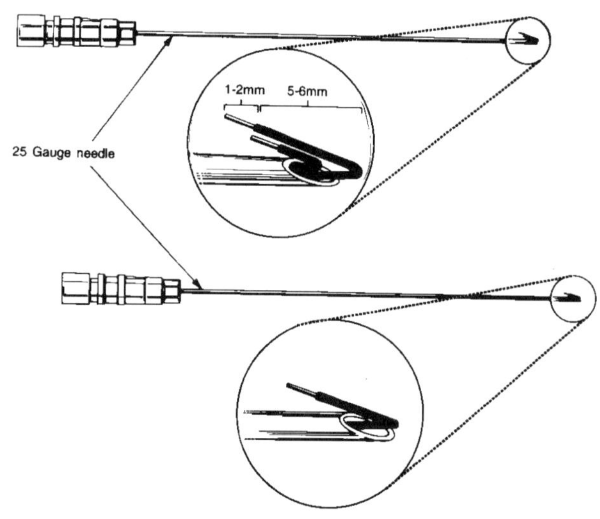

Fig. 2 Insertion technique for wire electrodes. The single needle insertion technique requires the placement of two wire electrodes in a single 25-gauge hypodermic needle. Both electrodes are driven into the muscle with one needle stick. To separate the two electrodes it is necessary to insert each wire individually using two separate hypodermic needles. This technique allows for improved control over the interdetection spacing.

Based on the findings in our laboratory and in conjunction with the results of earlier studies, we recommend a number of standardized procedures for the use of indwelling electrodes in shoulder electromyography studies addressing the rotator cuff muscles. Placement of each lead of the bipolar electrode into the muscle should be performed by using two separate hypodermic needles with a surface interdetection spacing of 1 cm. Positioning of the leads should place the center of the interdetection spacing at the appropriate locations defined for needle electromyography examination. (Ideal needle electrode locations are defined by Perotto and Delagi[33]). In order to control the depth of the needle placement by inserting the needle tip to the fossa of the scapula, 3.5-in, 25 gauge hypodermic needles should be used. The two leads of the electrode should be placed in longitudinal alignment with the muscle fibers for maximal electromyography signal generation.[26,34] Two millimeters of bared electrode tips should be left on the distal ends of the detecting surface.[26] If investigators choose to continue with the traditional single needle bipolar construction, strict attention must be paid to electrode fabrication. A minimum difference of 2 to 3 mm in hook length will reduce the likelihood of bare tip contact.

An optimal electromyographic signal is critical to accurate interpretation of muscle function. These technical considerations for the placement of indwelling wire electrodes about the shoulder are reviewed with the objective of standardizing a recording technique that will help improve signal characteristics and acquisition. Such standardization should lead to greater reproducibility of results and ultimately lead to results that have greater clinical utility and validity.

Normalization

As mentioned previously, a major limitation of kinesiologic EMG research is the difficulty in making comparisons between EMG values obtained from identical muscles in different subjects, different muscles from the same subject, or even the same muscle from the same subject on different days, due to subtle differences in muscle architecture, electrode placement, and electrode construction.[18-20]

Normalization of the EMG signal has been used to circumvent these comparison problems. All normalization techniques used have in common the conversion of absolute EMG values to relative values based on reference electrical activity. The activity of a given muscle during a specified task is compared to a reference value from that muscle and expressed as a percentage of that reference value.[35] The most common normalization technique is the use of the maximal voluntary contraction of a predetermined isometric movement as the reference EMG signal.[36-39] The normalization of EMG data is essential for the accurate comparison of signals between subjects, between muscles, or between test sessions.

Although the maximal voluntary contraction is the most commonly used normalization technique, the literature on identification of specific predefined positions that reproducibly elicit maximal electrical activity from muscles is sparse. Some researchers have made general recommendations to perform the normalization test in a position corresponding to the middle of the range of movement.[37,40] However, they have not identified any specific positions for the performance of a maximal isometric contraction. With regard to the shoulder, there are no accepted standard procedures for the production of maximal activity involving the shoulder girdle muscles.

If a maximal voluntary contraction is to be used as a reference value for normalization of EMG data, it is important that the neural activation being recorded truly reflects the maximal activation that the muscle can generate. In an attempt to further standardize shoulder EMG analysis, the optimal exercises for maximal neural activation of eight shoulder muscles (supraspinatus, infraspinatus, subscapularis, pectoralis major, latissimus dorsi, anterior, middle, and posterior deltoids) were identified. The 27 different isometric contraction positions we tested included the basic exercises of elevation, external rotation, and internal rotation at three degrees of initial humeral rotation (IR, NR, and ER), and three degrees of initial scapular elevation (0°, 45°, and 90°). Four tests were identified that resulted in the maximal neural activation of all eight shoulder muscles (Fig. 3): (1) 90° scapular elevation with -45° humeral rotation (IR) maximally activated the supraspinatus, anterior deltoid, and middle deltoid (Fig. 3, *top left*); (2) external rotation at 90° scapular elevation and -45° humeral rotation (IR) maximally activated the infraspinatus and posterior deltoid (Fig. 3, *top right*); (3) internal rotation at 90° scapular elevation and neutral humeral rotation maximally activated the subscapularis and latissimus dorsi (Fig. 3, *bottom left*); and (4) internal rotation at 0° elevation and neutral rotation maximally activated the pectoralis major (Fig. 3, *bottom right*).

Our results identify four standard testing positions that will provide maximal voluntary contraction normalization reference values for the eight muscles of the shoulder examined. Minimizing the number of tests required for normalization is desirable not only to lessen discomfort for the subject, but also to decrease the possibility of muscle fatigue that can lead to significant changes in the EMG signal obtained. A large battery of tests can be avoided if a small series of optimal tests can be identified that result in the consistent and reliable maximal activation of the entire muscle group being examined.

When using a maximal voluntary contraction as a

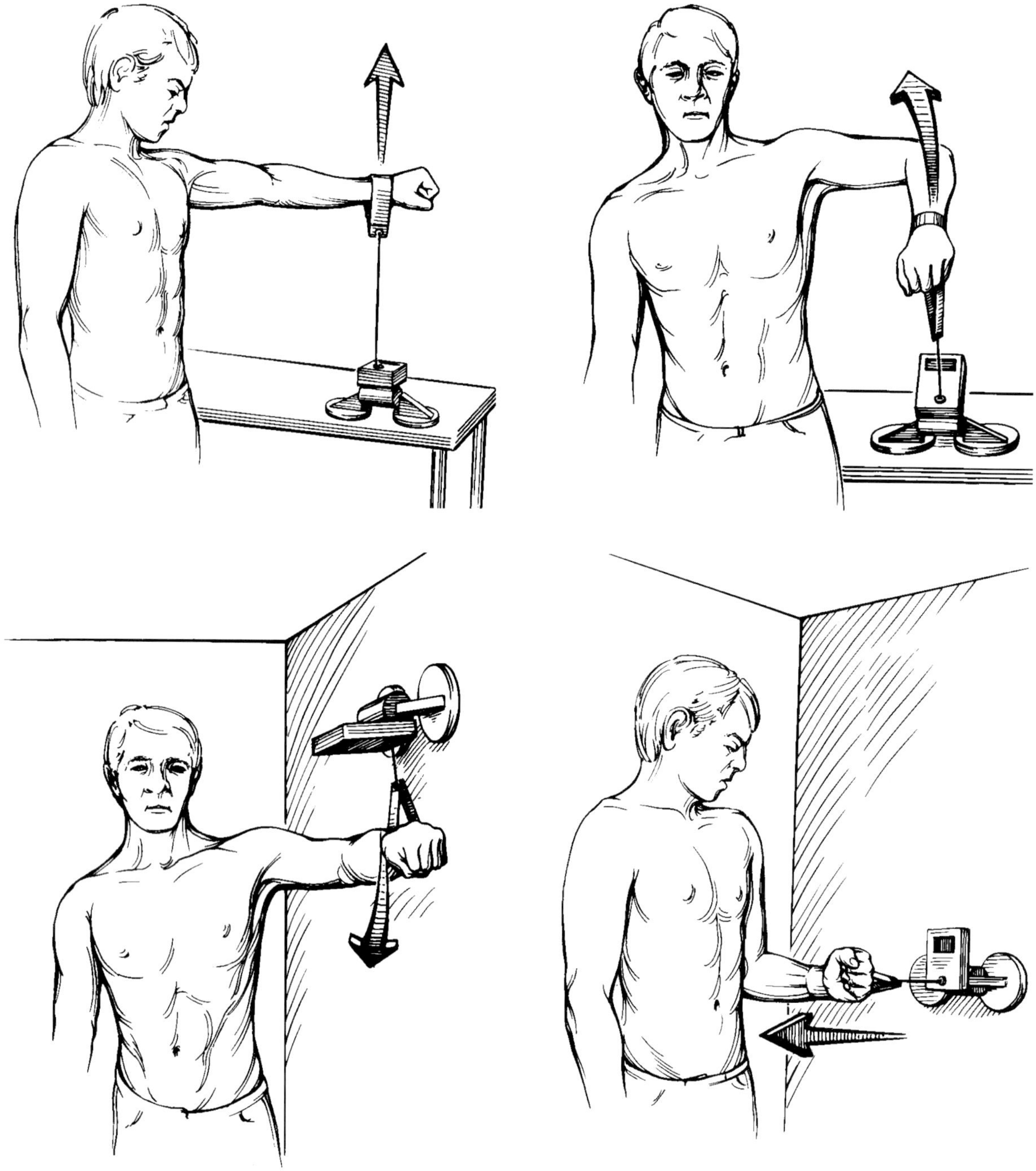

Fig. 3 Four optimal normalization test positions. **Top left,** Elevation at 90° scapular elevation and -45° humeral rotation resulted in maximal neural activation of the supraspinatus, anterior deltoid, and middle deltoid. **Top right,** External rotation at 90° scapular elevation and -45° humeral rotation resulted in maximal neural activation of the infraspinatus and posterior deltoid. **Bottom left,** Internal rotation at 90° scapular elevation and neutral humeral rotation resulted in maximal neural activation of the subscapularis and latissimus dorsi. **Bottom right,** Internal rotation at 0° scapular elevation and neutral humeral rotation resulted in maximal neural activation of the pectoralis major.

reference value for normalization, the test position must not only result in maximal neural activation of the muscle of interest, but it should reproducibly result in similar integrated EMG values. We found that the standardized optimal tests identified above are associated with increased test-retest reliability. Thus, through the standardization of the normalization test positions, we have identified not only the positions that correspond to a muscle's maximal neural activation, but also the positions that result in the greatest test-retest reliability. As a result, the strength and reliability of the maximal voluntary contraction normalization procedure is enhanced, and its usefulness as a reference value is optimized.

If the maximal voluntary contraction is to be used as the standard unit of neuromuscular system behavior, it must represent at least near-maximum force capacity of muscle. In the twitch interpolation test, a single electrical stimulus is superimposed on a muscle during a maximal voluntary contraction to ascertain whether or not additional electrical activity can be elicited. Based on this test, many investigators have concluded that the maximal voluntary contraction does result in at least 99% maximal muscle force.[41-43] However, other investigators have shown that neural supplementation can be achieved through the use of cutaneous stimulation[44] and a brief stretch.[45] These investigators conclude that, under certain conditions, maximal voluntary contractions do not represent the limit of a muscle's ability to elicit force; they suggest that there are complex neuromuscular and sensory interactions that result in modifications of muscle activation.[46] Such a conclusion, however, does not imply that the maximal voluntary contraction should not be used as a standard measure of muscle activation. Even if neural supplementation can produce neuromuscular activity greater than the maximal voluntary contraction activity, its utility as a reference value for EMG analysis is not lost. If such neural supplementation did occur during dynamic EMG studies, the "supramaximal" signals would merely be identified as greater than 100% of the maximal voluntary contraction.

The maximal voluntary contraction is an extremely useful normalization method, which allows for accurate interpretation of EMG data obtained from different muscles, different subjects, and different days. Our laboratory has identified four exercises that optimize shoulder muscle activation. These tests should lead to improved normalization procedures for dynamic shoulder EMG studies. They result in significantly larger EMG signals and improved test-retest reliability. In addition, because only four exercises are used, the potential effects of muscle fatigue, EMG signal changes, and subject discomfort are minimized. The standardization of maximal voluntary contraction normalization tests for the shoulder is one additional step toward the elimination of the many experimental variables inherent in EMG investigations. With the use of the normalization test positions proposed in our laboratory, the results of future dynamic EMG studies on the shoulder can be interpreted with greater confidence, accuracy, and validity.

Clinical Considerations

EMG Analysis of Manual Muscle Testing for Rotator Cuff Strength

Manual muscle testing (MMT) is an integral part of the physical examination of the shoulder.[47-54] When performed properly, this examination technique provides useful information about a muscle's capability to function in movement and its ability to provide stability and support.[55] However, without careful attention to detail and standardization of technique, the results may correlate poorly with accurate functional assessment.[56,57] Because seemingly minor changes in the positioning of the body can substantially affect the results of strength testing,[57] significant efforts have been made to standardize the MMT positions used for the assessment of the rotator cuff muscles. Recommendations for traditional testing positions for the shoulder have been based upon biomechanical studies examining the effects of joint position on force production,[56,58,59] cadaveric dissections of the involved musculature,[60] and clinical experience.[61-63] Unfortunately, the manual muscle examination of the rotator cuff has continued to challenge clinicians because of such factors as positional pain provocation in the injured shoulder, and the complex interactions of shoulder synergists with cuff physiology.[57,64,65]

Electromyography offers an ideal method for standardizing manual muscle examination techniques. Although some EMG studies have examined the neural activation of the supraspinatus muscle during different isometric testing positions,[63,66] a complete EMG examination of rotator cuff muscle activation during manual muscle testing positions has not been performed. Given the complexities of shoulder muscle physiology, and the subsequent challenge associated with isolated strength testing of the rotator cuff, EMG is a useful experimental tool for the refinement of this important clinical examination skill.

Our laboratory used EMG to identify the optimal MMT maneuvers for the assessment of rotator cuff strength based on the neural activation of three cuff muscles (supraspinatus, infraspinatus, and subscapularis) and five shoulder muscle synergists (pectoralis major, latissimus dorsi, anterior, middle, and posterior deltoid). A total of 29 manual muscle testing positions were examined. The 27 core test positions included the basic exercises of elevation, external rotation, and internal rotation at three degrees of initial humeral rotation (IR, NR, and ER), and three degrees of initial scapular elevation (0°, 45°, and 90°). The two additional tests were the Gerber push-off and the Gerber push-with-force (full, combined internal rotation with force). In order to most accurately assess the strength of a specific rotator cuff muscle, an optimal test should maximize the neural activation of the desired cuff muscle, simultaneously minimize the activation from involved synergist muscles, have good test-retest reliability, and minimize positional pain so that maximal effort can be exerted.

The optimal test for the supraspinatus was elevation at 90° of scapular elevation with +45° humeral rotation

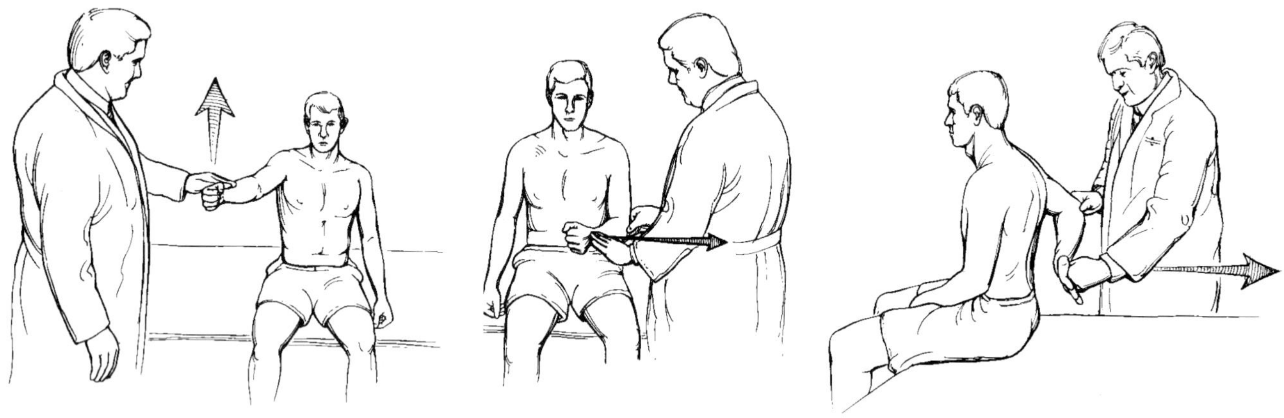

Fig. 4 Optimal manual muscle tests for the isolation of the rotator cuff muscles. **Left,** For the supraspinatus, elevation at 90° scapular elevation and +45° humeral rotation ("full can" position). **Center,** For the infraspinatus, external rotation at 0° scapular elevation and -45° humeral rotation. **Right,** For the subscapularis, the Gerber push-with-force. (Reproduced with permission from Kelly BT, Kadimas WR, Speer KP: The manual muscle examination for rotator cuff strength. *Am J Sports Med* 1996;24:581–588.)

(ER) ("full can") (Fig. 4, *left*). This test position differs from the traditional test position identified by Jobe and Moynes,[63] elevation at 90° of scapular elevation with -45° humeral rotation (IR) ("empty can"). Our findings indicate that there is no significant difference in supraspinatus activation with variation in humeral rotation. Furthermore, when the humerus is rotated externally (the "full can" position), there is slightly less relative activation from the infraspinatus, indicating better isolation of the supraspinatus. Perhaps most significant, however, is the decreased positional pain provocation associated with an externally rotated humerus. Internal rotation of the humerus at 90° of elevation results in the classic impingement position, in which the greater tuberosity is rotated under the acromial arch.[53] Such positional pain may decrease the reliability and accuracy of the manual muscle test of the supraspinatus.

The optimal test for the infraspinatus was external rotation at 0° elevation with -45° humeral rotation (Fig. 4, *center*). This position resulted in maximal activation of the infraspinatus and minimal activation of the supraspinatus and posterior deltoid. There is minimal pain provocation associated with this position. Kuhlman and associates[56] looked at the effect of joint angles on isometric and isokinetic strength measurements associated with external rotation. Their findings suggest that isometric strength of external rotation should be measured in 45° of scapular elevation with the shoulder in 45° of internal rotation.[56] However, isometric testing after block of the supraspinatus and infraspinatus was greatest at 0° to 30° of external rotation.[56] Iannotti reports that external rotation strength is most reliably tested with the arm in 0° of abduction and slight external rotation.[50] Our EMG analysis indicates that isolation of the infraspinatus is best performed at -45° (45° of internal rotation). Furthermore, our study demonstrated poor test-retest reliability of infraspinatus EMG activity when external rotation was performed at 45° of external rotation.

The optimal test for the subscapularis was the Gerber push-with-force[61] (Fig. 4, *right*). This test maximizes subscapularis activation and minimizes the activation from the pectoralis and the latissimus. Of the tests with significant reliability coefficients, the Gerber push-with-force resulted in the largest integrated EMG value for the subscapularis. In addition, this test avoids the impingement position associated with internal rotation at 90° of scapular elevation. The results from this EMG analysis corroborate the clinical findings observed by Gerber during his examination of patients with isolated rupture of the tendon of the subscapularis muscle.[61]

Through the use of an electromyographic analysis of the shoulder musculature, a methodologic analysis of the manual muscle examination of the rotator cuff was performed. By applying strict criteria for the identification of optimal manual muscle testing positions, we have addressed some of the confounding elements of this important clinical examination skill. By systematically identifying test positions that result in maximal activation of each of the three cuff muscles, minimal activation of involved shoulder synergists, good test-retest reliability, and decreased positional pain provocation, we have attempted to provide guidelines for a more accurate and reliable assessment of the strength and integrity of the rotator cuff.

EMG Analysis of the Long Head of the Biceps Tendon

The long head of the biceps tendon takes an intricate route to travel the distance from the upper arm to its insertion point on the supraglenoid tubercle and superior labrum. It enters the glenohumeral joint under a complex roof composed of fibers of the subscapularis tendon, the superior glenohumeral ligament, and the coracohumeral ligament. It is intra-articular but extrasynovial, and the humeral head rides up and down it, not unlike a pulley hanging from a rope.[67,68] Arthroscopic evaluation often shows capillary dilatation and erythema even when the shoulder is clinically asymptomatic. Despite all we know concerning its anatomy, the complete function of the long head of the biceps tendon remains unclear. Compounding this question is the theory that the majority of bicipital symptoms occur secondary to other shoulder pathologies.[69] Conditions such as bursitis, impingement, instability, and labral pathology often include bicipital tenderness to direct digital palpation.

The biceps brachi is one of several muscles that cross two joints. Its functional role at the elbow joint is relatively well-accepted; here, the biceps functions primarily as a forearm supinator and secondarily as an elbow flexor.[70] Recently, it has also been shown to function primarily as an elbow decelerator during the throwing motion. At the shoulder joint, however, the function of this muscle is less clear. Some authors have treated the tendon of the long head of the biceps as a vestigial structure, easily excised and tenodesed when symptomatic.[71,72] Others have attributed a vast number of functions to the long head of the biceps.[26,73-80] Previously, the long head of the biceps has been studied by cadaveric dissection with applied loads on the biceps and by direct observation during arthroscopy with applied loads on the biceps.[73,77-80] These studies have demonstrated bicipital function at the shoulder to be a head depressor, an anterior stabilizer, a posterior stabilizer, a limiter of external rotation, a lifter of the glenoid labrum, a head compressor, and a shunt muscle of the shoulder. The problem with many of these studies is the assumption that there is bicipital activity associated with shoulder activity to produce the desired function. However, although a muscle may be in a good position for a specific function, it may not be active when that function is performed.[81] Electromyography is a perfectly suited research modality for addressing the question of the functional role of the biceps tendon. Numerous EMG studies have been performed on the biceps in the last 50 years, producing a number of conflicting conclusions of bicipital function at the shoulder. Electromyographic studies have shown the role of the long head of the biceps to include shoulder flexion, shoulder abduction, shoulder internal rotation, shoulder external rotation, shoulder extension, anterior stabilization, and abduction only with resistance.[26,74-76,82] The majority of these studies, however, failed to adequately control the influence of EMG activity from elbow and forearm motion on the shoulder data. In a 1993 study with the elbow locked at 100° of flexion and neutral forearm rotation, Yamaguchi and associates found insignificant bicipital activity in all ranges of active shoulder motion (Yamaguchi K, Riew RD, Galatz LM, et al, personal communication, 1993).

We attempted to delineate the function of the long head of the biceps at the shoulder through EMG analysis. Efforts were made to rigorously control the influence of elbow activity on biceps analysis at the shoulder and to account for possible variation associated with elbow position, forearm position, speed of movement, and motion against resistance. The data from our laboratory demonstrate that when the elbow and forearm motion are strictly controlled (0° elbow flexion and neutral rotation), virtually no activity occurs in the long head of the biceps in response to a variety of shoulder motions (flexion, scapular abduction, external rotation at 90° glenohumeral abduction, internal rotation at 90° glenohumeral abduction, and extension), at varying speeds (170°/sec and 36°/sec), or in the presence of resistance (5 lb weight). Low-level EMG activity occasionally seen at the onset of fast flexion with a 5-lb weight was always accompanied by more substantial brachialis activity. This suggests that this minimal activity was in response to elbow function—either an isometric contracture or motion within the brace allowing small amounts of elbow flexion while initiating the movement of the weight at high speeds.

The vast array of conflicting EMG studies is better understood when the techniques are reviewed. In our laboratory, we placed a great deal of emphasis on rigidly controlling elbow and forearm position in order to prevent bicipital function at the elbow from influencing the data being recorded. Previous studies have failed to control this activity, and thus have not recorded isolated shoulder-related activity. The exception is the work of Yamaguchi and associates, who braced the elbow at 100°. Our data substantiated their findings of no isolated bicipital activity with shoulder motion. The measurements of no isolated bicipital activity in weighted and rapid motions adds to the magnitude of this finding.

Additional concerns regarding EMG methodology arise with the use of surface electrode monitoring of the brachioradialis as the elbow control in all of the previous studies. In our laboratory, thin wire leads were placed in the brachialis as the elbow control. Because the brachialis is the primary elbow flexor, the activity of this muscle (which parallels the distal biceps) should be a better indicator of elbow activity. This concept is ratified by the comparison of brachialis and brachioradialis activity. In several of the test conditions, the brachialis leads demonstrated low and moderate signal in response to elbow activity, while the brachioradialis surface leads remained silent. Based on this observation, the brachialis—not the brachioradialis—should be monitored to evaluate elbow activity.

The biceps brachi muscle crosses both the shoulder and elbow joints. We evaluated only the situation in which elbow and forearm activity are excluded. These data demonstrate that the long head of the biceps is not active in isolated shoulder motion when the elbow and forearm are controlled. This is supported by investigations in throwing athletes that demonstrated that bicipital function correlated with motion at the elbow, not at the shoulder.[76,83] Most recently, a radiographic study on patients' status post biceps tenodesis suggested that the biceps functions to prevent superior migration of the humeral head. Our laboratory results indicate that this or any other function attributed to the long head of the biceps is achieved by either a passive role (ie, proprioception) of the tendon, or an active role that achieves tension in association with elbow and forearm activity.

Rehabilitation

EMG of Aquatic Physical Therapy

Early active range of motion in the shoulder following injury or surgery is important to the restoration of normal shoulder kinematics and early return of shoulder function. Lack of motion about the pectoral girdle during the rehabilitative process will compromise the ability to attain the normal kinematic balance between the glenohumeral and scapulothoracic joints and may ultimately lead to rotator cuff or impingement-like symptoms.[84] The role of aquatic physical therapy is to allow active shoulder motion in an environment in which the injured or surgically repaired tissues are not adversely stressed (Fig. 5). Aquatic physical therapy has been used effectively for a wide variety of patient populations.[84-89] This rehabilitation approach is designed for the improvement of neuromuscular skeletal function in the postinjury or postoperative patient.[84,87] It is ideally suited for any patient with limited musculoskeletal function, as it offers the opportunity for purposeful movement that may not be possible within traditional land-based exercise programs.[84,85] The essential benefit of aquatic therapy for the rehabilitation of the injured shoulder is the buoyancy that the water provides to the upper extremity; studies have shown that in water, the arm can weigh as little as one eighth its original weight at 90° of abduction or forward flexion.[90]

Performing shoulder motion exercises in water allows an interim transition to more advanced dynamic strengthening or conditioning exercises on dry land. This active motion in water is both comforting to the patient and appropriate when antigravity motion would not be safe on dry land. Our clinical experience with over 500 patients in aquatic physical therapy has confirmed both its efficacy and safety in the immediate postsurgical or postinjury setting. Nonetheless, a substantial scientific basis for the effectiveness of this therapeutic modality has not been well elucidated.

We studied the neural activation of rotator cuff and shoulder synergist muscles (supraspinatus, infraspinatus, subscapularis, pectoralis major, anterior and middle deltoids) during standard aquatic therapy rehabilitation exercises and compared it with the same muscle activation during identical shoulder movements on dry land. Subjects performed the task of elevation from 0° to 90° with neutral rotation (Fig. 5). The exercise was performed on land and in water at three different speeds of elevation (3 s, 2 s, and 1 s). For all six muscles tested, neural activation during both the 3 s and 2 s test speeds was significantly less ($p < 0.05$) when performed in water versus on land. During the 1 s test, there was a consistent trend toward greater activation for all muscles when the exercise was performed in water. These EMG results confirm the lessened tissue tension resulting from shoulder movement during the slower aquatic rehabilitation movements as evidenced by the significantly decreased muscle neural activation in water versus on dry land.

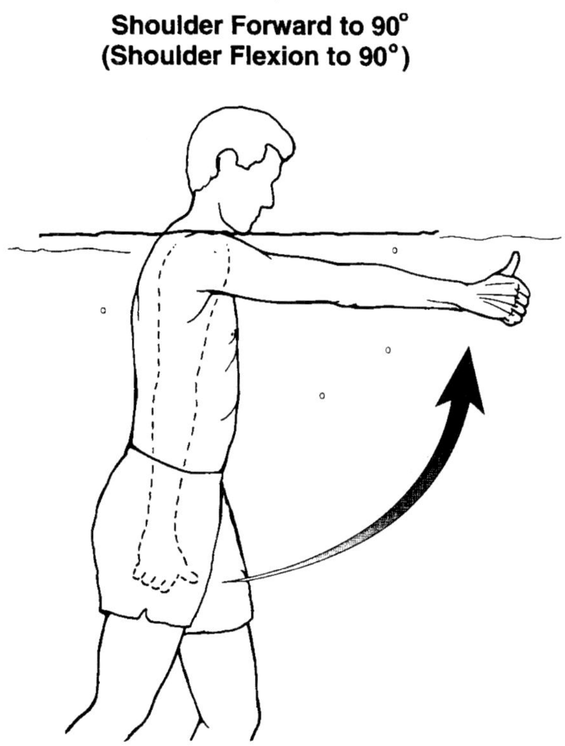

Fig. 5 Movement of the arm from 0° to 90° in aquatic physical therapy motion. The arm remains underwater throughout the entire movement, and the humerus remains in neutral rotation. This same movement was performed on dry land. The shoulder muscle activation at each of the two locations was compared.

Current aquatic physical therapy is based upon several important bioengineering principles. The basic forces acting on the patient while in the water consist of buoyancy, drag forces, and inertial forces. Additional factors affecting the patient include hydrostatic pressure and specific heat.[85,91] Through the integration and application of these principles, individualized programs can be developed that emphasize different aspects of rehabilitation that span from early active range of motion to progressive strength conditioning.

The concept of joint rehabilitation following injury and surgery has long been the subject of much debate. The development of an accelerated rehabilitation protocol after anterior cruciate ligament (ACL) reconstruction was spurred by the observations of Shelbourne and Nitz in the mid 1980s.[92,93] Prior to this time, postsurgical rehabilitation of the knee emphasized early limited range of motion and nonweightbearing on crutches for the first 6 weeks.[94] The essential features of the accelerated program included early restoration of full active range of motion, immediate full weightbearing, the use of closed-chain exercises, and the return to full sports participation within 4 to 6 months.[95,96] Shelbourne and Nitz clearly demonstrated that the accelerated rehabilitation program resulted in earlier restoration of motion, strength, and function without compromising stability.[95,96] Furthermore, the incidence of postsurgical complications, including loss of motion and subsequent gait abnormalities, quadriceps weakness, and/or patellofemoral pain, was markedly reduced in patients involved in the accelerated program.[92] Based on these findings, it is now well accepted that early active motion of the knee through the use of closed-chain exercises is imperative for successful rehabilitation of the ACL reconstruction patient.

The most appropriate rehabilitation process for the postsurgical shoulder has not been as clearly demonstrated. Although the trend in rehabilitation is toward earlier protected motion in conjunction with stabilizing exercises for the rotator cuff,[65] postoperative management still incorporates joint immobilization or delayed active motion. As in the knee, rehabilitative treatment that does not emphasize early active motion may result in postsurgical complications.[65] Strict immobilization may predispose the patient to functional instability secondary to rotator cuff inhibition, muscular atrophy, and poor neuromuscular control.[97] Although the use of passive dry land movement does limit subsequent joint stiffness, motion loss, and contracture, active motion is required for the return of normal motor patterns with normal kinematic balance between the glenohumeral and scapulothoracic complexes. Without early active motion, clinical symptoms suggestive of impingement and rotator cuff abnormality oftentimes ensue.[84]

Aquatic physical therapy can facilitate early active motion of the postsurgical or injured shoulder. Just as closed-chain exercises allow for early active motion of the knee, aquatic therapy allows for early active range of motion of the shoulder. Both are essential for a successful rehabilitation process that maximizes return of normal function and stability while also minimizing postsurgical complications. Incorporating this strategy into the shoulder rehabilitation regimen offers a new choice to many patients who cannot tolerate traditional dry land therapy. For the very painful and guarded shoulder, exercise and active motion in water may be the only effective method for shoulder rehabilitation. Postsurgical patients are able to initiate normal active shoulder movement within days of surgery, compared to a lag time of weeks for traditional active motion on land. Performing the exercises in water allows an interim step or transition before performing the exercises on dry land and against the full weight of gravity. The buoyancy effects of water allow less load on the repaired tissues so the active motion can be done earlier and more safely.[84]

The largest group of postoperative patients that we have treated with aquatic therapy is the rotator cuff repair group. This group seems to be most ideal for aquatic therapy because surgery for the repair of the rotator cuff and deltoid generally results in a globally dyskinetic shoulder. Other general indications that we use for aquatic intervention with shoulder rehabilitation include the painful shoulder that cannot tolerate conventional physical therapy, frozen shoulder (limited shoulder movement), patient need for restoration of biomechanically correct movement patterns, shoulder muscular endurance training, and the initiation of strength training as a precursor to land antigravity strengthening. The general principle for all of these indications is an early restoration of active movement in a safe and comfortable environment so that normal motor patterns can be restored. The renewed confidence that results from this environment enhances patient cooperation and benefits every area of rehabilitation.

Our EMG investigation of aquatic physical therapy provides clear scientific evidence that supports its use in the rehabilitation of the upper extremity. Our results clarify the neuromuscular basis for the positive effects that we have observed clinically. Decreased neural activation of a muscle is a direct indication of decreased force generation by that muscle.[1,46,98] Furthermore, decreased force production corresponds to decreased tissue tension. By demonstrating significantly decreased neural activation of the shoulder musculature during slow movement (3 s and 2 s elevation) in water compared to on land, we have confirmed the presence of lessened tissue tension. These findings underscore the relative safety of aquatic therapy in the

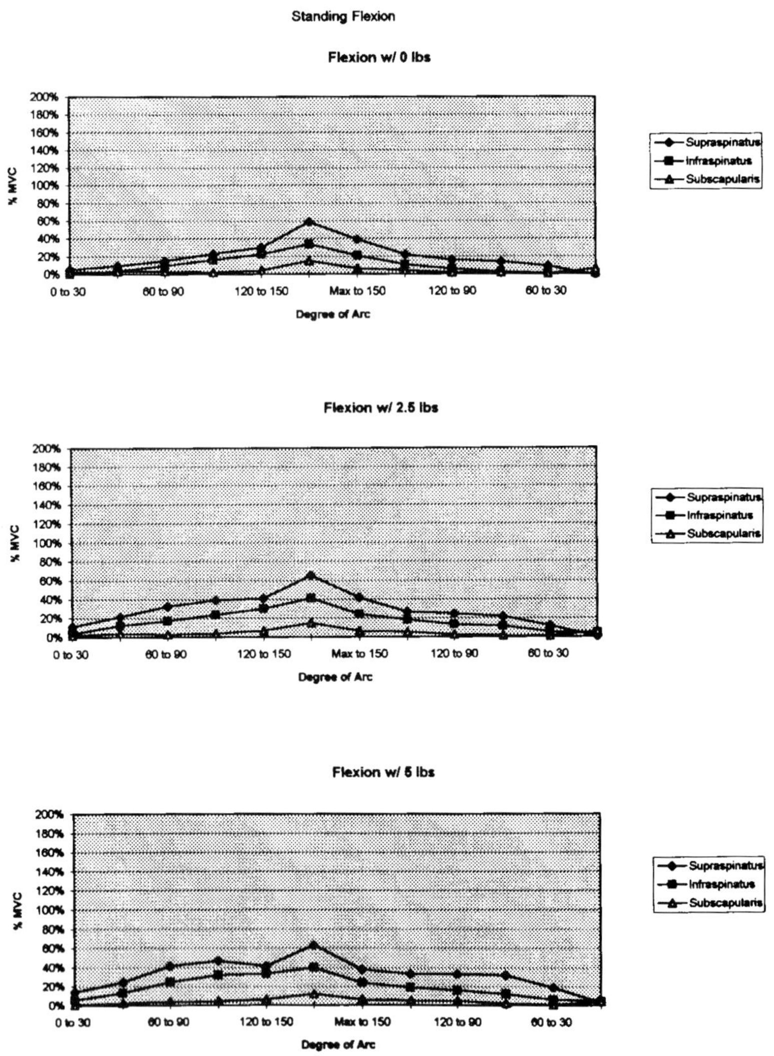

Fig. 6 Sample graphs demonstrating % MVC of the rotator cuff muscles throughout the movement of standing flexion with three different weights (0 lbs, 2.5 lbs, and 5 lbs). The % MVC of each of the muscles was determined at 30° arc intervals from 0° to maximum flexion (approximately 180°).

immediate postoperative or postinjury period and demonstrate that early active joint motion may be initiated without apparent compromise of the integrity of the repaired or injured tissue. This has been consistent with our clinical observations. As closed-chain kinematic exercises may allow safe, early active motion of the knee, we believe that aquatic physical therapy allows safe, early active motion of the shoulder.

EMG of Dynamic Shoulder Motion During Therapeutic Rotator Cuff Exercise

The research reviewed to this point used EMG analysis of the shoulder during either isometric movement or slow movements not requiring precise measurements of the arm in space. Through the integration of EMG analysis with digitized motion analysis, it is possible to determine more precisely the activation patterns of muscles throughout a range of dynamic movement.

Our current research is focusing on this integration of EMG and motion analyses. We researched the shoulder muscle activation of seven healthy males during seven different dynamic shoulder therapeutic rehabilitation exercises. The exercises used were ones designed for patients with rotator cuff tendinopathy and subacromial impingement syndrome. Each exercise was performed with weights of 0 lbs, 2.5 lbs, and 5 lbs. The EMG activity was synchronized with motion analysis equipment so that precise measurement of EMG activation throughout 30° arcs of movement could be examined.

The first four exercises studied were standing motions involving the movement of the arm from 0° (at the side) to 180° in three different planes (flexion, elevation with external rotation or "full can," elevation with internal rotation or "empty can," and abduction). The fifth exercise was horizontal abduction or abduction of the arm from 0° to 90° while lying in the prone position. The final two exercises involved internal and external rotation while lying in the supine position. Subjects were videotaped with reflective tracking balls on their arms and the motions were video time matched with the electromyographic data collected from eight shoulder muscles (supraspinatus, infraspinatus, subscapularis, pectoralis major, latissimus dorsi, anterior, middle and posterior deltoids). The analog video data were digitized and integrated with the EMG data. Precise angle data were calculated (every 30° of motion arc) and correlated to the muscle activation throughout the range of motion. A summary of our findings is presented below.

Standing Elevation Exercises (Flexion, Full Can, Empty Can, and Abduction) Of the three rotator cuff muscles studied, the supraspinatus demonstrated the greatest activation (% of maximum voluntary contraction, or MVC) (supraspinatus > infraspinatus > subscapularis) (Fig. 6). We identified two distinct patterns of muscle activation that we defined as phasic and tonic. Phasic activity was characterized by activation patterns beginning at ≤ 20% MVC and increasing to a peak that was at least 40% MVC or greater. This activation pattern was seen in the supraspinatus muscles of three of the seven subjects tested. Tonic activity was characterized by activation patterns beginning at ≥ 20% MVC and remaining within 40% MVC throughout the range of motion. This pattern of activity was seen in four of the seven subjects tested. If there was a difference, activation was greater during concentric motion than eccentric motion. With increasing weight, the supraspinatus was more involved in the initiation of movement. Muscle activation occurred earlier in the range of movement with more resistance, but the peak MVC remained nearly the same. If there was a difference, the supraspinatus was more active as the arm motion moved from the sagittal to scapular to coronal plane. The major synergist muscles involved during these standing exercises were the anterior and middle deltoids.

Of the three rotator cuff muscles studied, the infraspinatus demonstrated the second greatest activation (% MVC) (supraspinatus > infraspinatus > subscapularis). All subjects demonstrated a tonic activation pattern (beginning at ≥ 20% MVC and remaining within 40% MVC throughout the range of motion). As with the supraspinatus, activation was greater during concentric motion than eccentric motion. Also similar to the supraspinatus, with increasing weight the infraspinatus was more involved in the initiation of movement. Muscle activation occurred earlier with more resistance but the peak MVC remained nearly the same. There was no significant difference in infraspinatus activation with the change in plane of motion.

The subscapularis demonstrated the least amount of activation of the muscles studied. Subscapularis activity demonstrated a tonic pattern of activation in all subjects. Activation was consistently ≤ 20% MVC. If there was a peak in activation, it occurred at the maximum arc of motion. Similar to both the supraspinatus and infraspinatus, if there was a change in activation with increasing weight, then the subscapularis was activated earlier and more involved with the initiation of movement. If there was a change in activation with plane of motion, the activation was larger as subjects moved from the sagittal to scapular to coronal plane.

In comparing the activation patterns of the supraspinatus during elevation with external rotation ("full can") and elevation with internal rotation ("empty can"), we found no significant differences. Three of the seven subjects demonstrated greater activation during the full can exercise, while another three of the seven subjects demonstrated greater activation during the empty can exercise. The remaining subject had identical supraspinatus activation during the two elevation exercises. Since there was no difference in activation between these two exercises, we feel that the full can exercise should be used for rehabilitation given the decreased pain provocation with an externally rotated humerus.

Prone Horizontal Abduction Exercise As with the standing exercises, the supraspinatus demonstrated the greatest level of activation (% MVC) (supraspinatus > infraspinatus > subscapularis). All subjects tested demonstrated a phasic activation pattern. As with the standing exercises, activation was greater during concentric motion than during eccentric motion. With increasing weight, the supraspinatus was more involved in the initiation of movement. As with the standing exercises, muscle activation occurred earlier with more resistance, but the peak MVC remained essentially unchanged. The major synergist muscle involved in this movement arc was the posterior deltoid.

The infraspinatus demonstrated the second greatest level of activation (% MVC) (supraspinatus > infraspinatus > subscapularis). Four of the seven subjects tested demonstrated a phasic activation pattern and three of the seven subjects demonstrated a tonic activation pattern. As with the supraspinatus, activation was greater during concentric motion than eccentric motion. With increasing weight, the infraspinatus was more involved in the initiation of movement and muscle activation occurred earlier, but the peak MVC remained essentially unchanged.

All of the findings for the subscapularis were identical to those for the supraspinatus and infraspinatus with regard to differences in concentric and eccentric motion and changes in activation pattern with increasing weight. However, the subscapularis was the least active of the three rotator cuff muscles, and all seven subjects demonstrated tonic activation patterns.

Supine Rotational Exercises Of the three rotator cuff muscles tested, the infraspinatus demonstrated the greatest level of activation (% MVC) during supine ER (infraspinatus > supraspinatus > subscapularis). All subjects demonstrated tonic, low-level activity in all three rotator cuff muscles. There were no cases of phasic activity for any of the muscles. Maximum activity occurred variably throughout the motion of external rotation. There was not a predictable peak at the extreme of motion. As with the other exercises, with increasing weight, the muscles were more involved in the initiation of movement and there was a shift of the peak activation to the left (earlier in the range of motion). The major synergist muscle involved in the motion of supine external rotation was the posterior deltoid. The posterior deltoid paralleled the activity of the infraspinatus in a phasically synergistic manner. However, in six out of seven subjects, the infraspinatus signal (% MVC) was greater than the posterior deltoid.

For all subjects tested in supine IR, there was tonic, low-level activity with no incidence of phasic activity. There was no differential cuff activity. Curiously, the subscapularis did not demonstrate the greatest level of activation. Unlike the other exercises studied, there was no change in rotator cuff activity with the addition of weight. The level of activity remained low for all weights tested. The major synergist muscles involved in supine internal rotation were the pectoralis and latissimus (pectoralis > latissimus). The involvement of the pectoralis and latissimus were increased with increasing resistance and their maximum activity occurred variably throughout the motion of internal rotation.

The results from this study provide an objective quantification of the actions and interactions of the rotator cuff and shoulder synergists during a full range of dynamic movement. Such a methodologic analysis offers a more comprehensive understanding of the intricacies of the complex muscle physiology around the shoulder.

Conclusion

Electromyography can be a valuable tool for the assessment of muscle function. However, in order to obtain results with the optimal clinical validity and utility, it is imperative to strictly control for as many of the potentially confounding variables as is possible. We have attempted to do so and also develop guidelines for the standardization of shoulder EMG testing procedures. We feel that such standardizing procedures will aid in the elimination of at least some of the variables that plague this research area. We have applied these standard testing procedures to the clinical arena, and have only just begun to look at a variety of clinically relevant questions regarding shoulder muscle physiology. With the continued application of strict testing procedures, and the appropriate implementation of the EMG analysis of shoulder muscle function, we are confident that an improved understanding of the complexities of the shoulder joint will result.

References

1. Perry J, Bekey GA: EMG-force relationships in skeletal muscle. *Crit Rev Biomed Eng* 1981;7:1–22.
2. Solomonow M, Baratta R, Zhou BH, et al: Historical update and new developments on the EMG-force relationships of skeletal muscles. *Orthopedics* 1986;9:1541–1543.
3. Inman VT, Saunders JB, Abbott LC: Observations on the function of the shoulder joint. *J Bone Joint Surg* 1944;26:1–30.
4. Bradley JP, Tibone JE: Electromyographic analysis of muscle action about the shoulder. *Clin Sports Med* 1991;10:789–805.
5. Hirschberg GG, Dacso MM: The use of electromyography in the study of clinical kinesiology of the upper extremity. *Am J Phys Med* 1953;32:13–21.
6. Järvholm U, Palmerud G, Herberts P, et al: Intramuscular pressure and electromyography in the supraspinatus muscle at shoulder abduction. *Clin Orthop* 1989;245:102–109.
7. Kronberg M, Nemeth G, Broström LA: Muscle activity and coordination in the normal shoulder: An electromyographic study. *Clin Orthop* 1990;257:76–85.
8. Pearl ML, Perry J, Torburn L, et al: An electromyographic analysis of the shoulder during cones and planes of arm motion. *Clin Orthop* 1992;284:116–127.
9. Ballantyne BT, O'Hare SJ, Paschall JL, et al: Electromyographic activity of selected shoulder muscles in commonly used therapeutic exercises. *Phys Ther* 1993;73:668–682.
10. McCann PD, Wootten ME, Kadaba MP, et al: A kinematic and electromyographic study of shoulder rehabilitation exercises. *Clin Orthop* 1993;288:179–188.
11. Townsend H, Jobe FW, Pink M, et al: Electromyographic analysis of the glenohumeral muscles during a baseball rehabilitation program. *Am J Sports Med* 1991;19:264–272.
12. Kronberg M, Brostrom LA, Nemeth G: Differences in shoulder muscle activity between patients with generalized joint laxity and normal controls. *Clin Orthop* 1991;269:181–192.
13. Clarys JP, Cabri J: Electromyography and the study of sports movements: A review. *J Sports Sci* 1993;11:379–448.
14. Glousman R: Electromyographic analysis and its role in the athletic shoulder. *Clin Orthop* 1993;288:27–34.
15. Gowan ID, Jobe FW, Tibone JE, et al: A comparative electromyographic analysis of the shoulder during pitching: Professional versus amateur pitchers. *Am J Sports Med* 1987;15:586–590.
16. Morris M, Jobe FW, Perry J, et al: Electromyographic analysis of elbow function in tennis players. *Am J Sports Med* 1989;17:241–247.
17. Pink M, Perry J, Browne A, et al: The normal shoulder during freestyle swimming: An electromyographic and cinematographic analysis of twelve muscles. *Am J Sports Med* 1991;19:569–576.
18. Giroux B, Lamontagne M: Comparisons between surface electrodes and intramuscular wire electrodes in isometric and dynamic conditions. *Electromyogr Clin Neurophysiol* 1990;30:397–405.
19. Jonsson B, Komi PV: Reproducibility problems when using wire electrodes in electromyographic kinesiology, in Desmedt JE (eds): *New Developments in Electromyography and Clinical Neurophysiology*. Basel, Switzerland, S Karger, 1973, pp 540–546.

20. Kadaba MP, Wootten ME, Gainey J, et al: Repeatability of phasic muscle activity: Performance of surface and intramuscular wire electrodes in gait analysis. *J Orthop Res* 1985;3:201–211.
21. Basmajian JV, Stecko G: A new bipolar electrode for electromyography. *J Appl Physiol* 1962;17:849.
22. Gartlan MG, Peterson KL, Luschei ES, et al: Bipolar hooked-wire electromyographic technique in the evaluation of pediatric vocal cord paralysis. *Ann Otol Rhinol Laryngol* 1993;102:695–700.
23. Nemeth G, Kronberg M, Broström LA: Electromyogram (EMG) recordings from the subscapularis muscle: Description of a technique. *J Orthop Res* 1990;8:151–153.
24. Wolf LB, Segal RL, Wolf SL, et al: Quantitative analysis of surface and percutaneous electromyographic activity in lumbar erector spinae of normal young women. *Spine* 1991;16:155–161.
25. Notermans SLH, Goor C (eds): *Current Practice of Clinical Electromyography*. Amsterdam, Holland, Elsevier, 1984.
26. Basmajian JV, De Luca CJ (eds): *Muscles Alive: Their Functions Revealed by Electromyography*, ed 5. Baltimore, MD, Williams & Wilkins, 1985.
27. Komi PV, Buskirk ER: Reproducibility of electromyographic measurements with inserted wire electrodes and surface electrodes. *Electromyography* 1970;10:357–367.
28. Viitasalo JH, Komi PV: Signal characteristics of EMG with special reference to reproducibility of measurements. *Acta Physiol Scand* 1975;93:531–539.
29. Jonsson B, Bagge UE: Displacement, deformation and fracture of wire electrodes for electromyography. *Electromyography* 1968;8:329–347.
30. Jonsson B, Reichmann S: Displacement and deformation of wire electrodes in electromyography: A roentgenologic study. *Electromyography* 1969;9:201–211.
31. Jensen C, Vasseljen O, Westgaard RH: The influence of electrode position on bipolar surface electromyogram recordings of the upper trapezius muscle. *Eur J Appl Physiol* 1993;67:266–273.
32. Lynn PA, Bettles ND, Hughes AD, et al: Influences of electrode geometry on bipolar recordings of the surface electromyogram. *Med Biol Eng Comput* 1978;16:651–660.
33. Perotto A, Delagi EF (eds): *Anatomical Guide for the Electromyographer: The Limbs and Trunk*, ed 3. Springfield, IL, Charles C Thomas, 1994.
34. Long C, Brown ME: Electromyographic kinesiology of the hand: Muscles moving the long finger. *J Bone Joint Surg* 1964;46A:1683–1706.
35. Mirka GA: The quantification of EMG normalization error. *Ergonomics* 1991;34:343–352.
36. Hagberg M, Sundelin G: Discomfort and load on the upper trapezius muscle when operating a wordprocessor. *Ergonomics* 1986;29:1637–1645.
37. Westgaard RH: Measurement and evaluation of postural load in occupational work situations. *Eur J Appl Physiol* 1988;57:291–304.
38. Yang JF, Winter DA: Electromyographic amplitude normalization methods: Improving their sensitivity as diagnostic tools in gait analysis. *Arch Phys Med Rehabil* 1984;65:517–521.
39. Zuniga EN, Simons EG: Nonlinear relationship between averaged electromyogram potential and muscle tension in normal subjects. *Arch Phys Med Rehabil* 1969;50:613–620.
40. Nieminen H, Takala EP, Viikari-Juntura E: Normalization of electromyogram in the neck–shoulder region. *Eur J Appl Physiol* 1993;67:199–207.
41. Belanger AY, McComas AJ: Extent of motor unit activation during effort. *J Appl Physiol* 1981;51:1131–1135.
42. Bellemare F, Woods JJ, Johansson R, et al: Motor-unit discharge rates in maximal voluntary contractions of three human muscles. *J Neurophysiol* 1983;50:1380–1392.
43. Hales JP, Gandevia SC: Assessment of maximal voluntary contraction with twitch interpolation: An instrument to measure twitch responses. *J Neurosci Methods* 1988;25:97–102.
44. Howard JD, Enoka RM: Enhancement of maximum force by contralateral-limb stimulation. *J Biomech* 1987;20:980.
45. Lagasse PP: Muscle strength: Ipsilateral and contralateral effects of superimposed stretch. *Arch Phys Med Rehabil* 1974;55:305–310.
46. Enoka RM, Fuglevand AJ: Neuromuscular basis of the maximum voluntary force capacity of muscle, in Grabiner MD (ed): *Current Issues in Biomechanics*. Champaign, IL, Human Kinetics, 1993, pp 215–236.
47. Boublik M, Hawkins RJ: Clinical examination of the shoulder complex. *J Orthop Sports Phys Ther* 1993;18:379–385.
48. Cofield RH: Physical examination of the shoulder: Effectiveness in assessing shoulder stability, in Matsen FA III, Fu FH, Hawkins RJ (eds): *The Shoulder: A Balance of Mobility and Stability*. Rosemont, IL, American Academy of Orthopaedic Surgeons, 1993, pp 331–343.
49. Hawkins RJ, Bokor DJ: Clinical evaluation of shoulder problems, in Rockwood CA Jr, Matsen FA III (eds): *The Shoulder*. Philadelphia, PA, WB Saunders, 1990, vol 1, pp 149–177.
50. Iannotti JP: Evaluation of the painful shoulder. *J Hand Ther* 1994;7:77–83.
51. Jackins S, Matsen FA III: Management of shoulder instability. *J Hand Ther* 1994;7:99–106.
52. Kvitne RS, Jobe FW: The diagnosis and treatment of anterior instability in the throwing athlete. *Clin Orthop* 1993;291:107–123.
53. Rowe CR: Examination of the shoulder, in Rowe CR (ed): *The Shoulder*. New York, NY, Churchill Livingstone, 1988, pp 53–63.
54. Silliman JF, Hawkins RJ: Clinical examination of the shoulder complex, in Andrews JR, Wilk KE (eds): *The Athlete's Shoulder*. New York, NY, Churchill Livingstone, 1994, pp 45–58.
55. Kendall FP, McCreary EK, Provance P (eds): *Muscles, Testing and Function: With Posture and Pain*, ed 4. Baltimore, MD, Williams & Wilkins, 1993.
56. Kuhlman JR, Iannotti JP, Kelly MJ, et al: Isokinetic and isometric measurement of strength of external rotation and abduction of the shoulder. *J Bone Joint Surg* 1992;74A:1320–1333.
57. Sapega AA: Muscle performance evaluation in orthopaedic practice. *J Bone Joint Surg* 1990;72A:1562–1574.
58. Maddux REC, Kibler WB, Uhl T: Isokinetic peak torque and work values for the shoulder. *J Orthop Sports Phys Ther* 1989;10:264–269.
59. Howell SM, Imobersteg AM, Seger DH, et al: Clarification of the role of the supraspinatus muscle in shoulder function. *J Bone Joint Surg* 1986;68A:398–404.
60. Kolts I: A note on the anatomy of the supraspinatus muscle. *Arch Orthop Trauma Surg* 1992;111:247–249.
61. Gerber C, Krushell RJ: Isolated rupture of the tendon of the subscapularis muscle: Clinical features in 16 cases. *J Bone Joint Surg* 1991;73A:389–394.
62. Jobe FW, Jobe CM: Painful athletic injuries of the shoulder. *Clin Orthop* 1983;173:117–124.
63. Jobe FW, Moynes DR: Delineation of diagnostic criteria and a rehabilitation program for rotator cuff injuries. *Am J Sports Med* 1982;10:336–339.
64. Rabin SI, Post M: A comparative study of clinical muscle testing and Cybex evaluation after shoulder operations. *Clin Orthop* 1990;258:147–156.
65. Wilk KE, Arrigo C: Current concepts in the rehabilitation of the athletic shoulder. *J Orthop Sports Phys Ther* 1993;18:365–378.
66. Worrell TW, Corey BJ, York SL, et al: An analysis of supraspinatus EMG activity and shoulder isometric force development. *Med Sci Sports Exerc* 1992;24:744–748.
67. Burkhead WZ Jr: The biceps tendon, in Rockwood CA Jr, Matsen FA III (eds): *The Shoulder*. Philadelphia, PA, WB Saunders, 1990, vol 2, pp 791–836.

68. DePalma AF, Callery GE: Bicipital tenosynovitis. *Clin Orthop* 1954;3:69–85.
69. Neer CS II: Anterior acromioplasty for the chronic impingement syndrome in the shoulder: A preliminary report. *J Bone Joint Surg* 1972;54A:41–50.
70. Hollinshead WH (ed): *The Back and Limbs.* London, England, Cassell, 1958.
71. Kessel L, Watson M: The painful arc syndrome: Clinical classification as a guide to management. *J Bone Joint Surg* 1977; 59B:166–172.
72. Neviaser TJ, Neviaser RJ, Neviaser JS, et al: The four-in-one arthroplasty for the painful arc syndrome. *Clin Orthop* 1982; 163:107–112.
73. Andrews JR, Carson WG Jr, McLeod WD: Glenoid labrum tears related to the long head of the biceps. *Am J Sports Med* 1985; 13:337–341.
74. Basmajian JV, Latif A: Integrated actions and functions of the chief flexors of the elbow: A detailed electromyographic analysis. *J Bone Joint Surg* 1957;39A:1106–1118.
75. Bierman W, Yamshon LJ: Electromyography in kinesiologic evaluations. *Arch Phys Med Rehabil* 1948;29:206–211.
76. Glousman R, Jobe F, Tibone J, et al: Dynamic electromyographic analysis of the throwing shoulder with glenohumeral instability. *J Bone Joint Surg* 1988;70A:220–226.
77. Itoi E, Kuechle DK, Newman SR, et al: Stabilizing function of the biceps in stable and unstable shoulders. *J Bone Joint Surg* 1993;75B:546–550.
78. Kumar VP, Satku K, Balasubramaniam P: The role of the long head of biceps brachii in the stabilization of the head of the humerus. *Clin Orthop* 1989;244:172–175.
79. Neer CS II: Impingement lesions. *Clin Orthop* 1983;173:70–77.
80. Rodosky MW, Harner CD, Fu FH: The role of the long head of the biceps muscle and superior glenoid labrum in anterior stability of the shoulder. *Am J Sports Med* 1994;22:121–130.
81. Brunnstrom S: Muscle testing around the shoulder girdle: A study of the function of shoulder-blade fixators in seventeen cases of shoulder paralysis. *J Bone Joint Surg* 1941;23: 263–272.
82. Ting A, Jobe FW, Barto P, et al: An EMG analysis of the lateral biceps in shoulders with rotator cuff tears: Annual meeting of the third open meeting of the Society of American Shoulder and Elbow Surgeons, San Francisco, CA, 1987. *Orthop Trans* 1987;11:237.
83. Jobe FW, Tibone JE, Perry J, et al: An EMG analysis of the shoulder in throwing and pitching: A preliminary report. *Am J Sports Med* 1983;11:3–5.
84. Speer KP, Cavanaugh JT, Warren RF, et al: A role for hydrotherapy in shoulder rehabilitation. *Am J Sports Med* 1993;21: 850–853.
85. Campion MR (ed): *Adult Hydrotherapy: A Practical Approach.* Oxford, England, Heinemann Medical Books, 1990.
86. Gehlsen GM, Grigsby AS, Winant DM: Effects of an aquatic fitness program on the muscular strength and endurance of patients with multiple sclerosis. *Phys Ther* 1984;64:653–657.
87. Goldby LJ, Scott DL: Editorial: The way forward for hydrotherapy. *Br J Rheumatol* 1993;32:771–773.
88. Golland A: Basic hydrotherapy. *Physiotherapy* 1981;67:258–262.
89. Tovin BJ, Wolf SL, Greenfield BH, et al: Comparison of the effects of exercise in water and on land on the rehabilitation of patients with intra-articular anterior cruciate ligament reconstructions. *Phys Ther* 1994;74:710–719.
90. Morrey BF, An KN: Biomechanics of the shoulder, in Rockwood CA Jr, Matsen FA III (eds): *The Shoulder.* Philadelphia, PA, WB Saunders, 1990, vol 1, pp 208–245.
91. Edlich RF, Towler MA, Goitz RJ, et al: Bioengineering principles of hydrotherapy. *J Burn Care Rehabil* 1987;8:580–584.
92. Fu FH, Woo SLY, Irrgang JJ: Current concepts for rehabilitation following anterior cruciate ligament reconstruction. *J Orthop Sports Phys Ther* 1992;15:270–278.
93. Shelbourne KD, Klootwyk TE, DeCarlo MS: Update on accelerated rehabilitation after anterior cruciate ligament reconstruction. *J Orthop Sports Phys Ther* 1992;15:303–308.
94. Paulos L, Noyes FR, Grood E, et al: Knee rehabilitation after anterior cruciate ligament reconstruction and repair. *Am J Sports Med* 1981;9:140–149.
95. Shelbourne KD, Wilckens JH: Current concepts in anterior cruciate ligament rehabilitation. *Orthop Rev* 1990;19:957–964.
96. Shelbourne KD, Nitz P: Accelerated rehabilitation after anterior cruciate ligament reconstruction. *Am J Sports Med* 1990; 18:292–299.
97. Wilk KE, Andrews JR: Rehabilitation following arthroscopic subacromial decompression. *Orthopedics* 1993;16:349–358.
98. Milner-Brown HS, Stein RB: The relation between the surface electromyogram and muscular force. *J Physiol* 1975;246: 549–569.

Hand

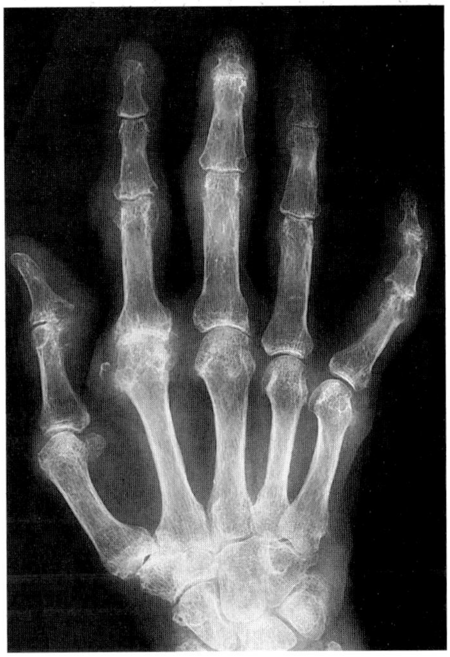

CHAPTER 8

Simulators of Hand Infections

Steven E. Kann, MD
John Jacquemin, MD
Peter J. Stern, MD

Inappropriate treatment of pathologic processes that mimic infection can have catastrophic consequences. Prompt recognition may prevent unnecessary surgical intervention and permit appropriate therapy. The purpose of this chapter is to acquaint the physician with infection simulators, to demonstrate how they can be confused with infection, and to give guidelines for treatment.

Acute Calcific Tendinitis

Acute calcific tendinitis may involve the hand and wrist as well as the shoulder, elbow, hip, or knee. Cohen,[1] in 1924, was the first to describe calcium deposition in the hands and extremities. The condition may be confused with infection because of the acute onset of symptoms; subtle radiographic findings; and physical findings of erythema, edema, severe pain, and, occasionally, fever.[2-8]

In the hand and wrist, the condition most commonly presents during middle age, with a slight preponderance in women.[8,9] Two cases in children have been reported.[9,10] The etiology is unknown, but it has been theorized that a focal area of tissue necrosis caused by trauma or disease in conjunction with an alkaline environment permits calcium salts to precipitate.[9] The calcium deposits usually occur in or adjacent to ligaments and tendons.[3,5,9]

The onset of symptoms is acute, with severe pain that is well localized over the tendon or ligament that contains the calcium deposit. The entire hand and wrist may be erythematous and swollen, with the specific region of the calcium deposit demonstrating point tenderness. The erythema and edema may extend proximally, mimicking cellulitis or lymphangitis, but there is no accompanying lymphadenopathy. The pain is often severe and is aggravated by both active and passive motion.[11,12] There are no accompanying abnormalities in laboratory values, and the condition can be associated with a febrile response.[9,13] Because the calcium deposits may be small and difficult to identify radiographically, it is important that radiographs be made centered on the region of maximum tenderness and in multiple projections to maximize visualization of the deposit. By region, the calcific deposits tend to be found in the ligaments of the phalanges, the intrinsic muscles of the palm, and the extensor or flexor tendons of the wrist. The most common site affected is the flexor carpi ulnaris tendon[5,9,14] near its insertion into the pisiform. In this location, the calcific deposit may be very small and easily overlooked on radiographs. A special radiographic view, made with the forearm in mid-supination, throws the pisiform into relief and demonstrates even a very small calcium deposit (Fig. 1).[12] There is no relationship between the size of the calcium deposit and the magnitude of the pain, erythema, or swelling. The radiographic finding of a dense, amorphous, well-circumscribed soft-tissue calcification confirms the diagnosis.[9]

Calcific tendinitis is a self-limited condition that resolves with or without treatment. Carroll and associates[9] noted that the symptoms subsided in about 3 weeks without treatment. However, there are reports in the literature of earlier resolution of the symptoms with intervention. With simple splinting, the time until relief of the symptoms was decreased to an average of 9 days, and relief was obtained in an average of 6 days with injection of 1% procainamide.[4,5] Dilley and Tonkin[3] found that relief occurred in an average of 7 or 8 days with the use of splints and anti-inflammatory medication. The symptomatic relief obtained from an

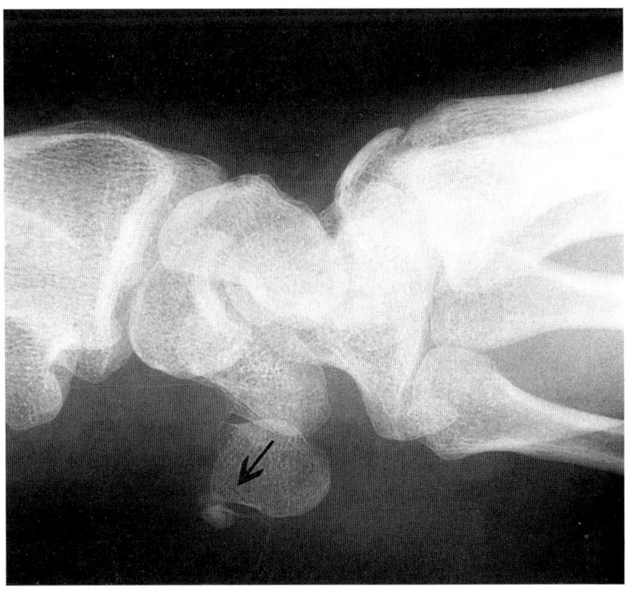

Fig. 1 Radiograph of a hand with calcific tendinitis of the flexor carpi ulnaris. The calcific deposit (arrow) where the flexor carpi ulnaris inserts into the pisiform is best visualized on the oblique radiograph.

injection of procainamide is the result of the release of tension within the deposit and the dissemination and absorption of the calcium salts.[12] The addition of a corticosteroid to the local anesthetic does not appear to enhance the efficacy of the injection.[9,12] Of note, radiographic evidence of resolution lags behind clinical resolution of the symptoms by several weeks.

If the deposit is unusually large, then aspiration of the calcium salts may be performed. In rare cases in which the symptoms have been present for more than a month and the calcification appears very dense radiographically, an injection is not likely to be effective. In this situation, surgical excision should be considered, and complete resolution of the symptoms can be anticipated within 24 to 48 hours.[9] Recurrence of the calcific tendinitis after resolution has occasionally been reported.[3,5,8-10]

Bites of the Brown Recluse Spider (Loxoscelism)

The brown recluse spider, which at one time was indigenous to Central and South America, can now be found in all 50 United States. Most reported bites, however, occur in the southern and midwestern states. The local and systemic manifestations of the bite are variable, which complicates treatment.

This spider is able to live in a variety of conditions. It can tolerate extreme ranges in temperature, needs little food over extended periods, and can live inside or outside but prefers a dark, secluded habitat.[15,16] It is approximately 0.5 to 2 in (1 to 5 cm) in length, and it can be identified by a violin-shaped mark on its cephalothorax and by six eyes in three pairs as opposed to eight eyes, as are found in most spiders.[16]

In a classic bite scenario, the spider is living in clothing, bed sheets, or blankets that have been stored in a dark place and often bites when the victim is putting on clothes or rolling over in bed. The bite is perceived as a sharp sting or may go unnoticed. The spider often escapes, and diagnosis is based solely on the history and the physical findings. The local reaction produces an urticarial rash that may progress to full-thickness skin necrosis.[15] The magnitude of tissue injury depends on the amount of venom injected and on the patient's immune status.[15] After several hours, a small hemorrhagic or erythematous blister develops that may be surrounded by a halo of ischemia. The erythema may spread rapidly and progress to a violaceous color. Snyder and Leonard[17] stated: "A non-healing ulcer with red, white, and blue phenomenon (erythema, ischemia, and cyanosis) is pathognomonic of a brown recluse spider bite." Over a 24- to 48-hour period, the affected area can expand, resulting in full-thickness skin loss in an area up to 30 cm in diameter (Fig. 2).[18] If left untreated, the lesion forms an eschar, followed by ulceration in approximately 14 days. Depending on its severity and size, the lesion can take weeks or months to heal. Systemic reactions to the venom have also been reported and range from nausea, vomiting, fever, chills, and arthralgia to disseminated intravascular coagulation, convulsions, and massive hemolysis leading to renal failure and death.[19,20]

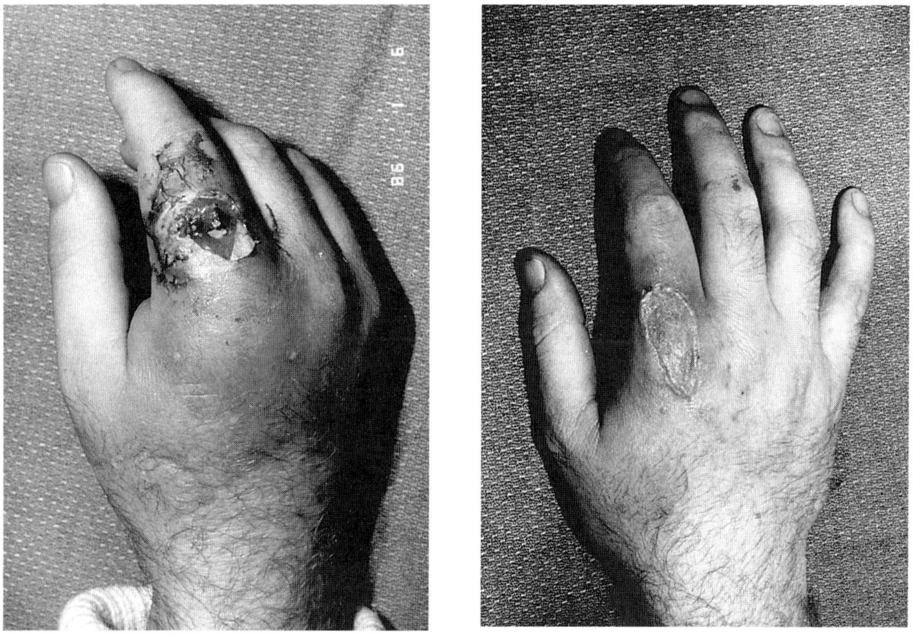

Fig. 2 Photographs of a hand that was bitten by a brown recluse spider. **Left,** Approximately 2 days after the bite, there was epidermolysis and a halo of erythema. **Right,** Ultimately, there was full-thickness skin necrosis that necessitated debridement and skin-grafting.

The overall approach to the treatment of loxoscelism is directed at three areas. First, the symptoms must be treated with antipyretics, sedatives, analgesics, and antipruritics. The second area of concern is the local wound. Treatment options include antihistamines, antibiotics, vasodilators, steroids (applied locally or systemically), operative excision, antivenin, hyperbaric oxygen, and oral administration of dapsone.[21-26] Unfortunately, there have been few prospective evaluations of these therapies in animals or humans.[26,27] The literature indicates that corticosteroids and early surgical excision are not consistently beneficial, and early surgical excision may be followed by delayed wound-healing and the formation of an abscess and scar.[16,24,27] Rees and associates,[27] in a prospective study of humans, demonstrated that treatment with dapsone and antibiotics reduced the prevalence of secondary infections as well as the need for surgical intervention. When an operation is necessary, it should be delayed until a mature eschar has formed and there is a need for skin grafting. Dapsone should be used with caution; it has not been approved by the Food and Drug Administration for this application and, in rare instances, can cause hemolysis and agranulocytosis.

The treatment of the systemic symptoms and signs is supportive. All patients should have a baseline complete blood-cell count and urinalysis. Patients who have any systemic signs should be managed intensively with supportive therapy (intravenous administration of fluids and continuous monitoring of hemoglobin, renal electrolytes, platelet count, and coagulation factors) on an inpatient basis.

In conclusion, despite the variability in presentation and outcome associated with loxoscelism, close observation and treatment should be initiated to decrease the possibility of substantial local and systemic morbidity and, in rare circumstances, death.

Pyogenic Granuloma

The cause of pyogenic granuloma remains obscure. Its name is a misnomer, as it is not primarily a true infection. Many authors have thought that it is caused by chronic or repetitive irritation or trauma, with subsequent infection resulting in a proliferative, vascular response to an infectious organism of low virulence.[28,29] However, other authors have believed that, because of the histologic findings and the absence of trauma or irritation in some patients, it is an acquired vascular lesion, possibly with secondary infection. It has a strong association with pregnancy and the use of oral contraceptives. These lesions are found primarily in the oral mucosa, but they have been seen in the hand.[28] Clinically, pyogenic granuloma must be differentiated from melanoma, particularly amelanotic melanoma. The primary and secondary small lesions may spread and can confuse the diagnosis.[28] The lesion has also been described in two case reports as an intravenous pyogenic granuloma of the hand.[30,31]

Grossly, the lesion is raised, red, and friable. On the hand, it is a papular lesion that bleeds easily and is usually found on the volar surface of the palm or digits (Fig. 3). Histologic examination demonstrates both granulation tissue and inflammatory cells. The lesions range from 1 mm to 1 cm in diameter. They may develop spontaneously or follow an untreated laceration. There is an initial period of rapid growth, which may be alarming and may lead to suspicion of a cutaneous malignant tumor.

There are numerous methods of treatment, including radiation, cauterization with silver nitrate, electrocautery, laser therapy, curettage, tangential removal, and surgical excision performed with or without a wide margin.[29,32-35] All of these approaches may be followed by recurrence.[36-39]

We recommend application of silver nitrate once or twice daily for ten days for the treatment of small lesions (less than 0.5 cm in diameter). For those that do not respond or for larger lesions, surgical excision with use of magnification, removal of a small cuff of normal tissue, and meticulous hemostasis is effective. Treatment with antibiotics is usually unnecessary.

In the rare case of a pyogenic granuloma occurring on the hand during pregnancy or with the use of oral contraceptives, it is advisable to wait until the

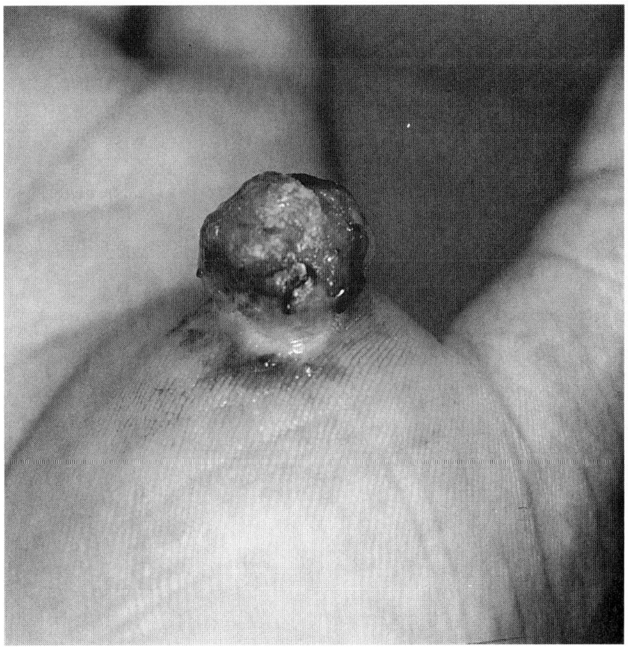

Fig. 3 Photograph of a pyogenic granuloma. The lesion developed following a laceration that was not surgically closed. It was excised, and the skin edges were approximated. It did not recur.

pregnancy is completed or for the patient to abstain from the use of the contraceptives for 4 to 8 weeks. Any source of irritation, such as a ring, should be removed. Most lesions resolve spontaneously without surgical intervention. In the event that the lesion is large or that a pregnant patient requests an excision, curettage or limited excision will suffice. Recurrence is uncommon.[28]

Pyoderma Gangrenosum

Pyoderma gangrenosum is a rare, destructive, cutaneous lesion that presents as a painful, rapidly enlarging ulcer.[40-43] It was first described by Brunsting and associates,[44] in 1930, and its etiology remains unclear. It is thought to be caused by a deficiency in the host immune system, and 80% of patients who have pyoderma gangrenosum have a coexisting systemic disease,[45] most commonly ulcerative colitis. Fifty percent of patients who have pyoderma gangrenosum have ulcerative colitis, but only 5% of patients who have ulcerative colitis have pyoderma gangrenosum.[43] Other associated diseases include Crohn disease, chronic active hepatitis, a carcinoid, diverticulosis, a myeloproliferative disorder, rheumatoid arthritis, diabetes mellitus, iron-deficiency anemia, and polyarteritis nodosa.[40-43,46] However, 10% to 20% of patients who have pyoderma gangrenosum have no evidence of systemic disease.[42,47-49] The differential diagnosis includes erythema multiforme, necrotizing vasculitis, Sweet syndrome, bacterial pyoderma, blastomycosis, brown recluse spider bite, and necrobiosis lipoidica diabeticorum.[49]

The lesions begin as red or black papules that arise acutely and are very painful. The lesion may also be associated with a fever. Within hours, pustules develop, spread rapidly, and undergo central necrosis (Fig. 4). The border, which is irregular, raised, and violaceous, advances centrifugally at a rate of 1 to 2 cm a day. The lesion is surrounded by an erythematous halo. In the initial stage, it is virtually indistinguishable from a pyogenic wound infection.[49,50] If they are left untreated, most lesions eventually cease advancing and become indolent. Histologic findings include a mixture of neutrophils and lymphocytes in small abscesses within the dermis.

The treatment of pyoderma gangrenosum should consist of local wound care (including changes of the dressing, application of topical sulfone compounds, and the use of a whirlpool), systemic treatment of the skin lesion, and the search for an associated systemic disease.[50] Incision and drainage are contraindicated. Surgical excision and closure of the wound can exacerbate the disease and leave a larger defect. Laurencin and Shoen[51] described the excision of what was thought to be an infected ulcer. The lesion recurred at the resection margin within 24 hours, and this rapid reappearance of the lesion at the clear margins is one of the hallmarks of the disease.[52] Occasionally, the lesion may result in substantial necrosis, necessitating amputation.

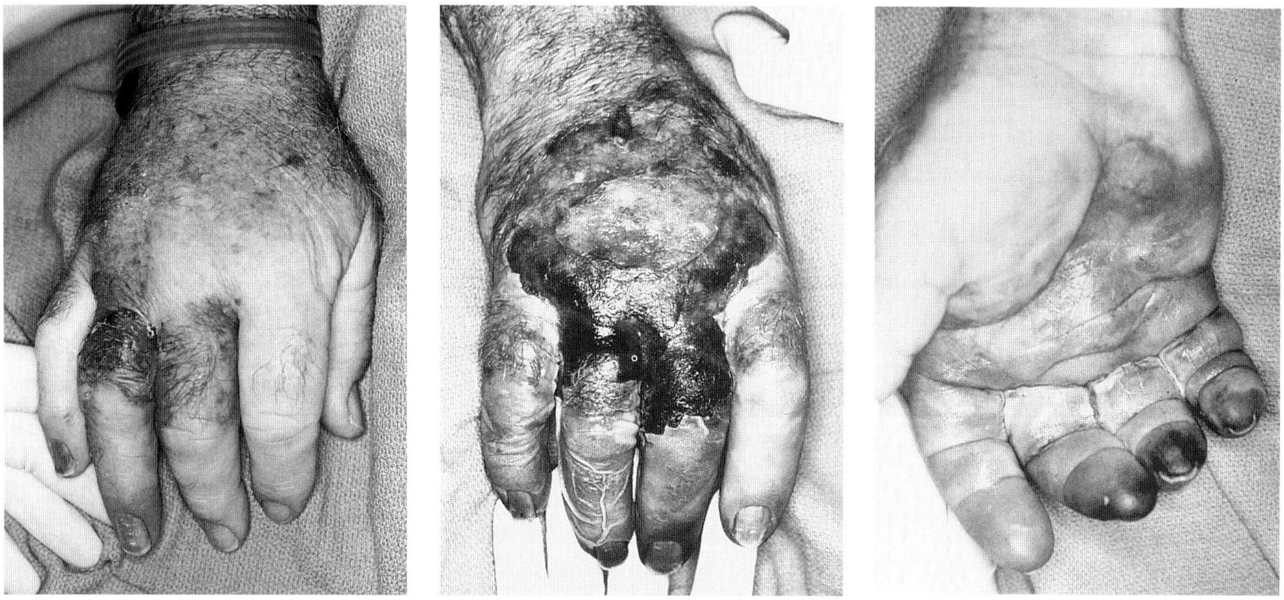

Fig. 4 Photographs of pyoderma gangrenosum of the hand in a patient who had ulcerative colitis. (Courtesy of John D. Wyrick, MD) **Left,** Hemorrhagic blisters had been present for 3 days. **Center** and **right,** Dorsal and palmar photographs, made at 10 days, revealed progression to digital necrosis. The patient died as a result of complications of the ulcerative colitis.

Systemic use of steroids (60 to 80 mg of prednisone a day) has been very successful in decreasing pain and resulting in the resolution of the lesion.[40,43,46,47,53] If the use of corticosteroids is contraindicated because of the underlying disease (as with diabetes), then a sulfone such as orally administered dapsone[54] or cyclosporin can be substituted.[55]

Metastatic Lesions of the Hand

Metastatic lesions distal to the elbow are distinctively rare and nearly always occur in bone. Metastasis to soft tissue is extremely rare. A review of the world literature by Kerin,[56] in 1983, identified only 156 metastatic tumors in the hand. Wu and Guise[57] reported three metastatic lesions in the hand in 41,000 patients who had cancer. Despite the rarity of the lesion, awareness of its possibility is important to prevent a misdiagnosis of infection and, hence, a delay in proper treatment.[58] During a 43-year period, Amadio and Lombardi[59] identified 18 patients who had 22 metastatic lesions of the hand. The distal phalanx was the most common location, and the lung was the most common primary site. This is consistent with the literature, in which it was reported that more than 40% of metastases to the hand (55 of 129 in four series) arose from a primary lung tumor.[56,60-62] The other sites of primary lesions are the breast, kidney, colon, thyroid, head and neck, and prostate.

The most common presenting symptom is continuous aching. The signs include erythema and swelling, with swelling in the phalanx presenting within 6 to 8 weeks[2] and metacarpal swelling, which presents later because of the thicker soft-tissue envelope. If it is left untreated, the tumor may fungate, leading the unwary physician to suspect infection (Fig. 5, *left*). Radiographs typically reveal osteolysis within an associated soft-tissue mass (Fig. 5, *right*). A biopsy specimen should be taken for histologic study and a culture specimen should be obtained to check for infection when any process destroys bone.

Most patients who have a metastatic lesion of the hand do not live for more than 6 months.[2] In one large review, the median duration of survival was less than 5 months.[59] Because of the poor prognosis, palliation is the primary goal for these patients. If the lesion is distal, conservative amputation provides the most rapid resolution of pain, obviates drainage from chronic wounds, and preserves maximum function of the hand. For more proximal lesions, local resection, with or without adjuvant radiation therapy, is effective in the short term and, again, preserves maximum function of the hand. Of the common primary tumors, carcinoma of the breast is most sensitive to radiation therapy. Despite such a dismal prognosis, there have been cases

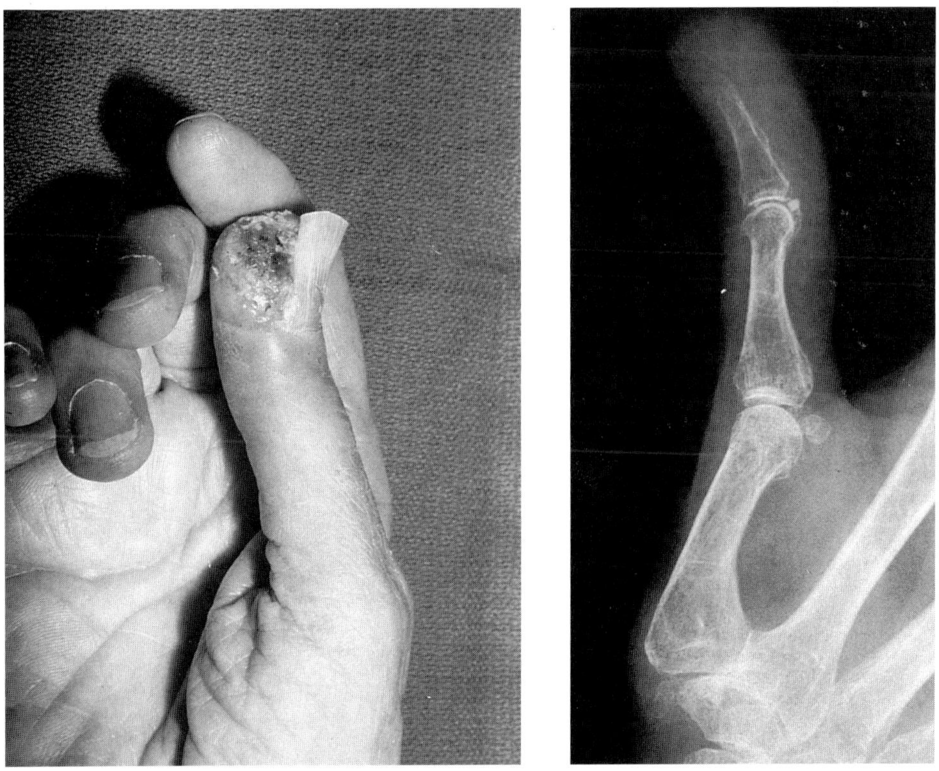

Fig. 5 Metastatic carcinoma of the distal phalanx in a patient who was seen with what was thought to be a chronic paronychia. **Left,** Photograph of the hand, showing an ulcerating lesion of the thumb pulp. **Right,** Radiograph showing osteolysis of the tuft. Biopsy of a specimen showed metastatic squamous-cell carcinoma from the lung.

in which wide excision of an isolated metastatic lesion resulted in a long-term disease-free interval.[59]

Foreign-Body Reaction

Injuries of the hand involving a foreign body are common. Usually the foreign body is removed; however, sometimes the patient is unaware of the penetration or the foreign body is not retrievable. Retained foreign bodies generate both acute and chronic inflammatory reactions, with the intensity of the reaction dependent on the type of material and the presence of any natural or synthetic toxins.[63-67] Chronic inflammation leads to isolation of the foreign body by granulomatous tissue.[63,66]

Most patients recall acute pain at the time of the initial injury. This may be followed by an asymptomatic period of weeks or months. There are several reports of previously asymptomatic patients being seen for an acute inflammatory reaction in the hand resulting from a foreign body that was deposited weeks or months earlier.[68-70]

The symptoms of a foreign-body reaction are those of acute or chronic inflammation. When a foreign body is deposited in or near a joint, the symptoms include the acute onset of pain, effusion of the joint, erythema, and a decreased range of motion. These findings simulate septic arthritis.[70-73] A foreign body may also puncture or lie in proximity to tendon sheaths, causing aseptic inflammation, pain, and swelling.[70,74,75] Erosion of bone in the hand following an initial diagnosis of osteomyelitis and failed treatment with antibiotics has often led to a biopsy or resection during which a sterile foreign body surrounded by a granuloma has been identified.[68,75,76]

The diagnosis of a retained foreign body depends on clinical suspicion and imaging studies. Plain radiographs made in multiple projections are the first step. Russell and associates[77] showed that adequate radiographs can demonstrate most foreign bodies. However, wood and plastic are difficult to demonstrate on plain radiographs,[77] and computed tomography and magnetic resonance imaging may prove useful for the identification of such material.[77,78] In the last several years, the use of ultrasound in the diagnosis of foreign bodies in the hand has gained popularity.[79-82] This technique, while labor-intensive and operator-dependent, may supplant other techniques because it is less costly.

Treatment consists of surgical removal. If there is secondary infection, culture of specimens and a short course of appropriate antibiotics are indicated. The complications of secondary infection, migration of the foreign body, and continued inflammation with damage to surrounding structures all militate against nonsurgical treatment.[69,70,78,83]

Factitious Diseases

Factitious disease of the hand presenting as an infection is unusual. Causes include factitious disorder and malingering.[84] Factitious conditions may occur alone or in conjunction with another psychiatric illness, such as conversion reaction.[84] Regardless, factitious disorders are characterized by the patient controlling the signs and symptoms of the illness without being aware of his or her motive.[84] In contrast, malingering is not strictly considered a mental illness, because the patient consciously attempts to deceive others.[84] The motive for secondary gain can be monetary or legal.

Grunert and associates[85] classified factitious disease of the hand into three categories on the basis of physical presentation: self-mutilation and manipulation of a wound (Fig. 6), edema, and contractures. Some of the more common examples of self-mutilation include debridement, excoriation, and extension of wounds or surgical incisions. In addition, new lesions or symptoms may develop along atypical paths of lymphatic drainage or in previously uninvolved areas.[85-88] Patients who have factitious edema may have sharp demarcations or even ligature marks.[89,90] Contractures of the hand may be simple or bizarre and cannot be explained on an anatomic basis. Frequently, these contractures involve muscles, nerves, or tendons that are unrelated to the described injury.

The diagnosis of factitious disease of the hand can be frustrating, time-consuming, and expensive. A high index of suspicion and thorough, nonconfrontational evaluations are necessary. Several studies have stressed the importance of serial examinations to record the appearance of new wounds or a decrease in findings after the application of an occlusive dressing or a cast.[86,89] Phelps and associates[88] applied fluorescein to the wound of one patient and then applied an occlusive dressing. Subsequent examination with a Wood lamp detected fluorescence under the nails of the uninjured hand, which confirmed manipulation of the wound. Phelps and associates[88] recommended this procedure for detection of factitious disease. In our experience, culture of specimens from self-inflicted wounds often reveals several different types of organisms, including bacteria such as *Enterobacter cloacae* and *Escherichia coli* that are not usually associated with infections in the hand.

After the physician has determined that an injury of the hand is factitious, the patient may be managed nonsurgically. A nonconfrontational explanation of the facts is recommended, because many authors have described severe emotional and psychiatric consequences of doctor-patient confrontations.[91,92] Referral to a psychiatric professional is necessary to diagnose and treat underlying disorders. The prognosis for patients diagnosed with factitious disease is mixed. Grunert and associates[85] found that angry or hostile

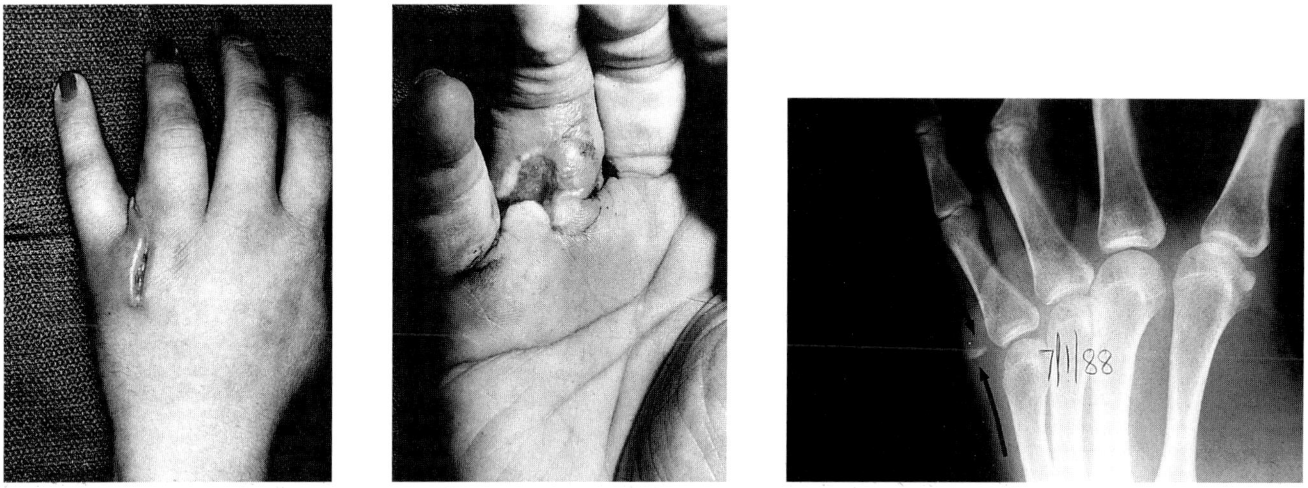

Fig. 6. A health-care professional who was referred for treatment of what she called spontaneously acquired nonhealing wounds. **Left** and **center,** Dorsal and palmar photographs of the hand. **Right,** A radiograph of the hand revealed a piece of glass (arrows). The patient subsequently admitted to self-inflicted manipulation of the wounds.

patients who manipulated their wounds were especially prone to have a poor result.

Gout

Gout, in our experience, is among the most common simulators of hand infection. Any man who is older than 40 years of age and is seen for the acute onset of soft-tissue, tenosynovial, or synovial swelling should be carefully questioned regarding a history of hyperuricemia.

Gout is the most common of the crystalline deposition diseases, with descriptions that date back to Hippocrates.[93] Its pathogenesis begins with hyperuricemia and the saturation of a joint space, tendon sheath, or bursa with monosodium urate crystals.[94,95] In some individuals, urate crystallizes out of solution and causes an inflammatory reaction in the involved tissue. While the exact triggering mechanism is unknown, many factors, such as temperature, age, previous damage to the tissue, and heredity, may play a role.[95,96]

History aids in the diagnosis of gout, with most patients (1,802 of 1,900 in one study[97]) being middle-aged or elderly men.[98] Women who are affected are almost exclusively postmenopausal, as estrogen promotes the excretion of urate.[94,95,99] Indeed, the onset in premenopausal women necessitates additional investigation to check for enzyme defects or renal disease. Obesity and a high alcohol intake are also frequently associated with gout.[94,95] Medications, such as thiazide diuretics or antimetabolites, can cause hyperuricemia and may precipitate an acute flare-up of gout.[94,100,101]

Questioning about a history of joint pain or a family history of gout is warranted. Any previous episodes of monarthritis, particularly in the metatarsophalangeal joint of the great toe, the midtarsal joint, or the knee, that developed quickly and subsided should raise suspicion of gout.[94] A history of chronic or severe gout in the lower extremity increases the likelihood of involvement of an upper extremity.[94] A family history of gout may be found in as many as 40% of patients.[94,97,102]

Gout is often confused with an infectious process as gout attacks may occur after an operation, infection, trauma, or illness.[96,101,103-110] A recent study of hospitalized patients who had crystal synovitis found that symptoms had developed in 75% after they were admitted for nonmusculoskeletal health problems.[105] Gouty arthritis may be precipitated even after minor trauma.[101,109,111] Postoperative attacks of gout mimicking infection of the treated hand have been reported in patients who have had a carpal tunnel release.[96,104]

Physical examination of the wrist and hand yields similar findings in gout and in infectious arthritis or tenosynovitis.[94,96,101,104] Gout presents with erythema, acute swelling, and pain that is exacerbated by active or passive motion. Patients with these symptoms may also be febrile.[107,112] Tophi are not present in new-onset attacks, but they should be sought elsewhere as evidence of chronic disease (Fig. 7).[113,114] Aspiration with crystalline analysis is helpful for establishing a diagnosis and thereby avoiding surgical intervention.

Laboratory studies are nonspecific. Both gout and infection may yield elevated erythrocyte-sedimentation rates and leukocyte counts.[94,115,116] Serum levels of uric acid, while helpful, are not diagnostic and are normal in 23% to 46% of patients.[94,117,118]

Analysis of the synovial fluid is the primary means of diagnosing gout.[94,113,116] Even a few milliliters of synovial

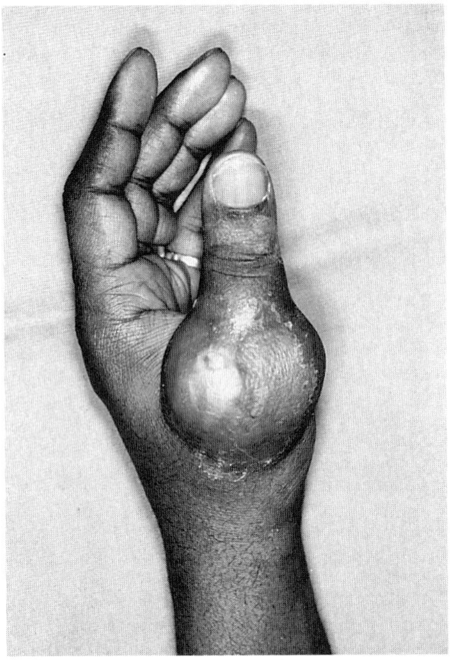

Fig. 7 Photograph showing a tophus of the metacarpophalangeal joint of the thumb, which had begun to drain. The patient had been referred for incision and drainage of a chronic infection of the joint.

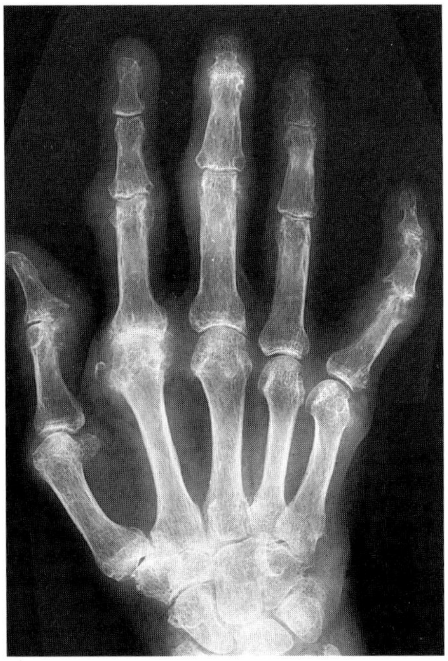

Fig. 8. Radiograph of the hand of a patient who had chronic gout. There are typical findings of asymmetrical joint involvement, periarticular erosions, and multiple soft-tissue tophi. The interphalangeal joint of the thumb demonstrates a classic periarticular erosion with an overhanging margin of bone.

fluid can be analyzed for urate crystals.[94] Detection of negatively birefringent crystals with a polarizing microscope confirms the diagnosis.[94,116] Determination of glucose, leukocyte, and protein levels in the synovial fluid may be helpful but is frequently nonspecific in the differentiation of infection from gout.[94,108,116] Gram stains and cultures should be performed for all patients, as gout and infection may occur together.[119,120]

Radiographs are useful in the diagnosis of chronic, but not acute, gout. Radiographic examination of patients with new acute-onset gout reveals only soft-tissue swelling or effusion of the joint. In chronic gout, tophaceous deposits (which appear as soft-tissue masses) may be detected. Additionally, well-marginated erosions of bone may occur. These are typically round or oval, are oriented along the long axis of the bone, and may be intra-articular, periarticular, or at a distance from the joint. They may be large (more than 5 mm in diameter) and can be surrounded by a sclerotic border. In many patients, the erosion is partially surrounded by an overhanging margin of bone. In the hand and wrist, any joint may be involved. Preservation of the joint space (until late in the disease) and asymmetrical joint involvement help to distinguish gout from rheumatoid arthritis (Fig. 8).[121]

Medical treatment of inflammation and pain is the first priority in the management of patients who have acute gout.[122,123] Colchicine and high-dose nonsteroidal anti-inflammatory drugs are the first line of treatment.[94,109] The recommended dosage of colchicine for acute attacks is 0.6 mg every 2 hours until the patient has relief; until intestinal symptoms, such as nausea or diarrhea, develop; or until a maximum dose of 6 mg has been given.[94] Dosages of anti-inflammatory medications vary. Indomethacin, one widely used drug, may be given in an initial dose of 50 to 75 mg and then in a dosage of 25 to 50 mg three or four times a day. For patients in whom colchicine and nonsteroidal anti-inflammatory medications are contraindicated, systemic or intra-articular administration of corticosteroids may be equally effective.[94,109,122] With proper treatment, most patients respond within 24 to 48 hours.[113] Hypouricemic agents, such as probenecid or allopurinol, should not be added or adjusted during an acute attack of gout as they may exacerbate the attack.[94,116] Surgery has no role in the management of acute gout.[124]

Pseudogout

Intrasynovial deposition of calcium pyrophosphate (CPP) crystals was discovered in 1961, during studies of patients who were believed to have gout.[125,126] Since then, similar crystalline deposition has been found in

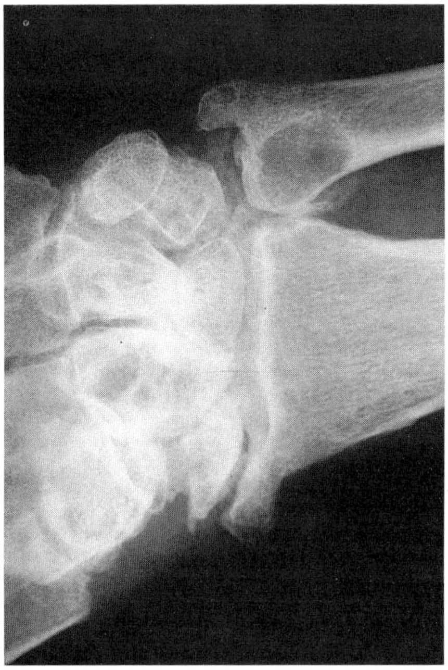

Fig. 9 Representative radiograph of a wrist with advanced calcium pyrophosphate deposition disease (pseudogout). There is prominent calcification within the triangular fibrocartilage complex and distal radioulnar joint, carpal and ulnar cysts, and advanced carpal collapse.

tendons, ligaments, and joint cartilage. Appropriately termed calcium pyrophosphate deposition disease, this clinical illness is also referred to as pseudogout. Radiographic evidence of crystal deposition in hyaline cartilage or fibrocartilage (Fig. 9) has led to the term chondrocalcinosis.

A pathologic study demonstrated CPP crystal deposits in 5% (32) of 598 cadaver specimens of patients who were an average of 72 years old at the time of death.[106] However, the prevalence of clinically symptomatic patients is much lower. Most studies have shown the prevalence of symptoms to be half that associated with gout, or about one in 1,000 patients.[127]

A patient history aids in the diagnosis. Most symptomatic patients are in at least the seventh decade of life. Many can describe previous episodes of pain and weakness in the affected joint.[106,127] Pseudogout may also be associated with metabolic diseases such as hemochromatosis, gout, hyperparathyroidism, and hypothyroidism.[127,128] As is the case for gout, surgery, trauma, or severe illness may precipitate acute attacks of pseudogout.[129-132] Occurrence in an ill patient may particularly raise the suspicion of an infectious process.

Pseudogout most commonly affects the knee. The wrist is the most common location in the upper extremity, with the lesion occurring less frequently in the metacarpophalangeal joints. Symmetrical involvement of joints is the rule; however, attacks are often unilateral.

Physical examination of the affected hand or wrist reveals the joint to be inflamed, with a mild or moderate effusion and a decreased range of motion. A pyarthrosis may be suspected on the basis of physical findings, but other methods of evaluation, including plain radiographs and arthrocentesis, aid in establishing the correct diagnosis. Pain on the ulnar side of the wrist may be particularly prominent since the triangular fibrocartilage complex (TFCC) is commonly involved. Radiographic evidence of chondrocalcinosis in the TFCC in a patient who has acute pain on the ulnar side of the wrist as well as an effusion is highly consistent with pseudogout. Attacks usually last about 1 week and may be accompanied by a low-grade fever. Acute compression of the median nerve, similar to that seen with infection of the carpal tunnel, may occur as a result of deposition of CPP.[133-136]

Screening for CPP deposition can be done with radiographs of the knees, hips, pubic symphysis, and wrists.[127,137,138] Additional study is unlikely to yield positive results if these areas are devoid of calcification. A presumptive radiographic diagnosis of pseudogout may be made on the basis of punctate or linear densities in articular or fibrocartilaginous tissues.

The definitive diagnosis is based on analysis of the synovial fluid. CPP crystals are usually irregular or rhomboid in shape, although needle-shaped crystals, as in gout, may be encountered. Unlike the negatively birefringent gouty crystals, the crystals in pseudogout are positively birefringent when viewed under a polarizing microscope.

CPP crystals cannot be removed from tissues. Treatment of associated diseases also has no proved effect on the progression of crystal deposition.[127] Symptomatic attacks in the hand may be treated with colchicine or with nonsteroidal medications, such as indomethacin. Injection of corticosteroids has proved useful in selected patients.[128,139] For lesions presenting as carpal tunnel syndrome, surgical release is the treatment of choice.[133]

Rheumatoid Arthritis

Rheumatoid arthritis, juvenile rheumatoid arthritis, and the seronegative spondyloarthropathies have many pathologic characteristics in common, including the ability to cause chronic progressive destruction of the hand and wrist. Confusion of an infectious condition with one of these inflammatory disorders is uncommon. However, when patients are seen because of the acute onset of monarticular inflammation or when the usual associated signs and symptoms are lacking, the specific diagnosis may be more difficult. Of the many autoimmune-related diseases, only rheumatoid arthritis and juvenile rheumatoid arthritis tend to present in this fashion.

While patients typically describe the insidious development of painful swollen joints in a symmetrical polyarticular fashion, confusion with an infectious process may occur when symptoms develop more acutely and in fewer joints. Acute onset has been found in 8% to 15% of patients.[140] The acute onset of rheumatoid arthritis is especially common in elderly patients.[141,142] In addition, many authors have noted monarthritis, usually of the knee or wrist, as the initial manifestation of rheumatoid arthritis.[143,144] Episodic attacks of monarticular arthritis, with periods of complete remission, also have been described. These attacks, termed palindromic arthritis, evolve into rheumatoid arthritis in approximately 33% of patients (218 of 653 in two studies).[145,146]

Complicating the diagnosis of rheumatoid arthritis is the potential coexistence of septic arthritis. Patients who have rheumatoid arthritis are more prone to joint infections.[147] Reasons for this may include the local and systemic effects of rheumatoid arthritis, the presence of other illnesses, or treatment with immunosuppressive medications.[147] Infection of the same joint may recur in as many as one third of patients, and polyarticular joint infections develop in many patients. In order to preserve function and to prevent recurrence, such infections necessitate more intensive treatment than do similar infections in otherwise healthy patients.[147-150]

In rheumatoid arthritis, physical examination of the digits reveals fusiform swelling, warmth, and a decreased range of motion of involved joints. Swelling on the volar aspect of the digits indicates inflammation of the flexor tendon sheaths. While involvement of the distal interphalangeal joint is less common, it does not exclude the diagnosis of rheumatoid arthritis.[151,152] Distinction from an infectious process may be impossible on the basis of physical examination alone.

Laboratory studies are frequently not helpful in the early diagnosis of rheumatoid arthritis. Initial laboratory analysis often reveals nonspecific elevations of the leukocyte count, the erythrocyte sedimentation rate, and the level of C-reactive protein. A positive rheumatoid factor is valuable as an indication, as 85% of patients with rheumatoid arthritis have a positive test for rheumatoid factor.[153] However, the rheumatoid factor may remain negative for 1 to 2 months after the onset of the disease.[146] Analysis of the synovial fluid for bacteria and crystals is negative. Also, the total white-blood-cell count in the synovial fluid is lower with rheumatoid arthritis (usually 2,000 to 75,000 cells/mm^3 [2×10^9 to 75×10^9 per liter]) than with septic arthritis (often more than 100,000 cells/mm^3 [100×10^9 per liter]).[154] Radiographs are usually not useful in the diagnosis of new-onset rheumatoid arthritis and reveal only evidence of soft-tissue swelling.[121]

Effective treatment of rheumatoid arthritis depends on interruption of the complex inflammatory process. Aspirin and nonsteroidal medications are first-line treatments. The trial of an agent at maximum dosage for 2 weeks appears to be the most accurate way to assess the efficacy of the drug.[155,156] Other medications, such as gold compounds, antimalarials, cytotoxic agents, or low-dose corticosteroids, are generally reserved for chronic progressive disease.[13,157-159] Surgery is not indicated in the treatment of acute rheumatoid arthritis.

Juvenile rheumatoid arthritis, like rheumatoid arthritis, is an autoimmune disease of unknown etiology. Unlike rheumatoid arthritis, juvenile rheumatoid arthritis has several distinct subtypes. In particular, monarticular juvenile rheumatoid arthritis may be confused initially with infection and occurs in 10% (33 of 316) to 31% (40 of 130) of patients.[14,160] Pauciarticular arthritis or polyarthritis may subsequently develop in children who initially have monarticular disease. However, there is no way to predict which children are at risk for more widespread disease.[161] Affected joints include the knees, ankles, elbows, and wrists.[161-163] The hips and small joints of the hand are often spared. Systemic signs and symptoms such as fever are rarely present.

The diagnosis of juvenile rheumatoid arthritis is frequently one of exclusion. Aspiration of the joint, with gram-staining and culture of synovial fluid, should be done for all patients to rule out infection. Serum blood tests for rheumatoid factor are rarely positive; however, antinuclear antibodies may be positive in as many as 85% of patients.[164,165] Radiographic evaluation frequently reveals only soft-tissue swelling.

As it does with rheumatoid arthritis, treatment centers on the reducing of inflammation of the involved joints. Aspirin and nonsteroidal medications are use to decrease inflammation, although not all anti-inflammatory drugs are approved for use in children.[166] Parents should be warned of the dangers of Reye syndrome in association with treatment with aspirin and should be told to briefly discontinue the use of aspirin during and after viral infections. Administration of corticosteroids systemically or by injection is contraindicated in most patients because of the potential for retarded skeletal growth.[166-168] Children who have monarticular or oligoarticular arthritis should be evaluated regularly by an ophthalmologist because of the occurrence of uveitis.[160,166,169]

In summary, despite the availability of an ever-enlarging technological armamentarium, the patient's history and physical examination remain pivotal with regard to arousing suspicion of an infection simulator. Once suspicion is raised, the diagnosis can usually be confirmed with simple laboratory tests or plain radiographs. Failure to include infection simulators in the differential diagnosis may lead to inappropriate medical or surgical treatment and may compromise the clinical outcome.

References

1. Cohen I: Calcareous deposit at the insertion of flexor carpi ulnaris tendon following trauma. *Am J Surg* 1924;38:172–173.
2. Carroll RE: Tumors of the hand skeleton, in Jupiter JB (ed): *Flynn's Hand Surgery*, ed 4. Baltimore, MD, Williams & Wilkins, 1991, pp 979–989.
3. Dilley DF, Tonkin MA: Acute calcific tendinitis in the hand and wrist. *J Hand Surg* 1991;16B:215–216.
4. Greene TL, Louis DS: Calcifying tendinitis in the hand. *Ann merg Med* 1980;9:438–440.
5. Moyer RA, Bush DC, Harrington TM: Acute calcific tendinitis of the hand and wrist: A report of 12 cases and a review of the literature. *J Rheumatol* 1989;16:198–202.
6. Selby CL: Acute calcific tendinitis of the hand: An infrequently recognized and frequently misdiagnosed form of periarthritis. *Arthritis Rheum* 1984;27:337–340.
7. Shaw JA: Acute calcific tendonitis in the hand. *Orthop Rev* 1986;15:482–485.
8. Yosipovitch G, Yosipovitch Z: Acute calcific periarthritis of the hand and elbows in women: A study and review of the literature. *J Rheumatol* 1993;20:1533–1538.
9. Carroll RE, Sinton W, Garcia A: Acute calcium deposits in the hand. *JAMA* 1955;157:422–426.
10. Millon SJ, Bush DC, Harrington TM: Acute calcific tendinitis in a child: A case report. *J Hand Surg* 1993;18A:592–593.
11. Phalen GS: Calcification adjacent to the pisiform bone. *J Bone Joint Surg* 1952;34A:579–583.
12. Phalen GS: Stenosing tenosynovitis: Trigger fingers, trigger thumb, and de Quervain's disease. Acute calcification in wrist and hand, in Jupiter JB (ed): *Flynn's Hand Surgery*, ed 4. Baltimore, MD, Williams & Wilkins, 1991, pp 439–447.
13. Gray RG, Tenenbaum J, Gottlieb NL: Local corticosteroid injection treatment in rheumatic disorders. *Semin Arthritis Rheum* 1981;10:231–254.
14. Cassidy JT, Brody GL, Martel W: Monarticular juvenile rheumatoid arthritis. *J Pediatr* 1967;70:867–875.
15. Russell FE, Waldron WG, Madon MG: Bites by the brown spiders Loxosceles unicolor and Loxosceles arizonica in California and Arizona. *Toxicon* 1969;7:109–117.
16. Young VL, Pin P: The brown recluse spider bite. *Ann Plast Surg* 1988;20:447–452.
17. Snyder CC, Leonard LG: Bites and stings of the hand, in Tubiana R (ed): *The Hand*. Philadelphia, PA, WB Saunders, 1988, vol 3, pp 894–895.
18. Foil LD, Norment BR: Envenomation by Loxosceles reclusa. *J Med Entomol* 1979;16:18–25.
19. Eichner ER: Spider bite hemolytic anemia: Positive Coombs' test, erythrophagocytosis, and leukoerythroblastic smear. *Am J Clin Pathol* 1984;81:683–687.
20. Wong RC, Hughes SE, Voorhees JJ: Spider bites. *Arch Dermatol* 1987;123:98–104.
21. Auer AL, Hershey FB: Proceedings: Surgery for necrotic bites of the brown spider. *Arch Surg* 1974;108:612–618.
22. Berger RS: The unremarkable brown recluse spider bite. *JAMA* 1973;225:1109–1111.
23. Fardon DW, Wingo CW, Robinson DW, et al: The treatment of brown spider bite. *Plast Reconstr Surg* 1967;40:482–488.
24. Jansen GT, Morgan PN, McQueen JN, et al: The brown recluse spider bite: Controlled evaluation of treatment using the white rabbit as an animal model. *South Med J* 1971;64:1194–1202.
25. King LE Jr, Rees RS: Dapsone treatment of a brown recluse bite. *JAMA* 1983;250:648.
26. Rees R, Campbell D, Rieger E, et al: The diagnosis and treatment of brown recluse spider bites. *Ann Emerg Med* 1987;16:945–949.
27. Rees RS, Altenbern DP, Lynch JB, et al: Brown recluse spider bites: A comparison of early surgical excision versus dapsone and delayed surgical excision. *Ann Surg* 1985;202:659–663.
28. Manus DA, Sherbert D, Jackson IT: Management considerations for the granuloma of pregnancy. *Plast Reconstr Surg* 1995;95:1045–1050.
29. Witthaut J, Steffens K, Koob E: Reliable treatment of pyogenic granuloma of the hand. *J Hand Surg* 1994;19B:791–793.
30. Cooper PH, McAllister HA, Helwig EB: Intravenous pyogenic granuloma: A study of 18 cases. *Am J Surg Pathol* 1979;3:221–228.
31. DiFazio F, Mogan J: Intravenous pyogenic granuloma of the hand. *J Hand Surg* 1989;14A:310–312.
32. Glicenstein J, Ohana J, Leclercq C (eds): *Tumours of the Hand: Part 4. Ungual Tumours*. Berlin, Germany, Springer-Verlag, 1988, pp 213–216.
33. Palmieri TJ: Vascular tumors of the hand and forearm. *Hand Clin* 1987;3:225–240.
34. Palmieri TJ: Common tumors of the hand. *Orthop Rev* 1987;16:367–378.
35. Popkin GL: Tumors of the skin: A dermatologist's viewpoint, in McCarthy JG, May JW Jr, Littler JW (eds): *Plastic Surgery: Tumors of the Head and Neck and Skin*. Philadelphia, PA, WB Saunders, 1990, vol 5, pp 3560–3613.
36. Allen RK, Rodman OG: Pyogenic granuloma recurrent with satellite lesions. *J Dermatol Surg Oncol* 1979;5:490–493.
37. Evans CD, Warin RP: Abstract: Pyogenic granuloma with local recurrences (2 cases). *Br J Dermatol* 1957;69:106.
38. Shall L, Stevens A, Saihan EM: Recurrent erythematous nodule on the sole of the foot. Recurrent pyogenic granuloma. *Arch Dermatol* 1991;127:1219–1223.
39. Warner J, Jones EW: Pyogenic granuloma recurring with multiple satellites: A report of 11 cases. *Br J Dermatol* 1968;80:218–227.
40. Callen JP, Taylor WB: Pyoderma gangrenosum: A literature review. *Cutis* 1978;21:61–64.
41. Holt PJ: The current status of pyoderma gangrenosum. *Clin Exper Dermatol* 1979;4:509–516.
42. Perry HO: Pyoderma gangrenosum. *Australas J Dermatol* 1982;23:53–61.
43. Schwaitzberg SD, Bradshaw MW, Williams TW Jr: Pyoderma gangrenosum: A possible cause of wound necrosis. *Arch Surg* 1982;117:363–367.
44. Brunsting LA, Goeckerman WH, O'Leary PA: Pyoderma (ecthyma) gangrenosum: Clinical and experimental observations in five cases occurring in adults. *Arch Dermatol Syphil* 1930;22:655–680.
45. Rand RP, Brown GL, Bostwick J III: Pyoderma gangrenosum and progressive cutaneous ulceration. *Ann Plast Surg* 1988;20:280–284.
46. Shore RN: New look at pyoderma gangrenosum. *Cutis* 1977;20:209–213;217–219.
47. Stolman LP, Rosenthal D, Yaworsky R, et al: Pyoderma gangrenosum and rheumatoid arthritis. *Arch Dermatol* 1975;111:1020–1023.
48. Wustrack KO, Zarem HA: Pyoderma gangrenosum: Recognition and management. *Plast Reconstr Surg* 1978;62:423–428.
49. Young VL, Fernando B, Tabas M, et al: A case study of pyoderma gangrenosum. *J Hand Surg* 1988;13A:259–262.

50. Papilion JD, Bergfield TG: Pyoderma gangrenosum complicating infection of the hand: A case report and review of the literature. *Clin Orthop* 1990;254:144–146.
51. Laurencin CT, Shoen SL: Pyoderma gangrenosum affecting the hand. *J Bone Joint Surg* 1994;76B:985–986.
52. Shands JW Jr, Flowers FP, Hill HM, et al: Pyoderma gangrenosum in a kindred: Precipitation by surgery or mild physical trauma. *J Am Acad Dermatol* 1987;16:931–934.
53. Ferlic DC: Pyoderma gangrenosum presenting as an acute suppurative hand infection: A case report. *J Hand Surg* 1983; 8A:573–575.
54. Brown RE, Lay L, Graham D: Bilateral pyoderma gangrenosum of the hand: Treatment with dapsone. *J Hand Surg* 1993; 18B:119–121.
55. Goldberg NS, Ottuso P, Petro J: Cyclosporine for pyoderma gangrenosum. *Plast Reconstr Surg* 1993;91:91–93.
56. Kerin R: Metastatic tumors of the hand: A review of the literature. *J Bone Joint Surg* 1983;65A:1331–1335.
57. Wu KK, Guise ER: Metastatic tumors of the hand: A report of six cases. *J Hand Surg* 1978;3B:271–276.
58. Rose BA, Wood FM: Metastatic bronchogenic carcinoma masquerading as a felon. *J Hand Surg* 1983;8A:325–328.
59. Amadio PC, Lombardi RM: Metastatic tumors of the hand. *J Hand Surg* 1987;12A:311–316.
60. Fragiadakis EG, Panayotopoulos G: Metastatic carcinoma of the hand. *Hand* 1972;4:268–272.
61. Mangini U: Tumors of the skeleton of the hand. *Bull Hosp Joint Dis* 1967;28:61–103.
62. Morris DM, House HC: The significance of metastasis to the bones and soft tissues of the hand. *J Surg Oncol* 1985;28: 146–150.
63. Cotran RS, Kumar V, Robbins SL (eds): *Robbins Pathologic Basis of Disease,* ed 4. Philadelphia, PA, WB Saunders, 1989, pp 39–86.
64. Cracchiolo A III, Goldberg L: Local and systemic reactions to puncture injuries by the sea urchin spine and the date palm thorn. *Arthritis Rheum* 1977;20:1206–1212.
65. Doig SG, Cole WG: Plant thorn synovitis: Resolution following total synovectomy. *J Bone Joint Surg* 1990;72B:514–515.
66. Ferreiro-Seoane JL: Foreign body synovitis, in Schumacher HR Jr, Klippel JH, Koopman WJ (eds): *Primer on the Rheumatic Diseases,* ed 10. Atlanta, GA, Arthritis Foundation, 1993, pp 294–295.
67. Ramanathan EBS, Luiz CPJ: Date palm thorn synovitis. *J Bone Joint Surg* 1990;72B:512–513.
68. Goldstein SA, Imbriglia JE: Erosion of the triquetrum and pisiform bones caused by a foreign body granuloma. *J Hand Surg* 1986;11A:899–901.
69. Morgan WJ, Leopold T, Evans R: Foreign bodies in the hand. *J Hand Surg* 1984;9B:194–196.
70. Reginato AJ, Ferreiro JL, O'Connor CR, et al: Clinical and pathologic studies of twenty-six patients with penetrating foreign body injury to the joints, bursae, and tendon sheaths. *Arthritis Rheum* 1990;33:1753–1762.
71. Fasanao FJ Jr, Hansen RH: Foreign body granuloma and synovitis of the finger: A hazard of ring removal by the sawing technique. *J Hand Surg* 1987;12A:621–623.
72. Goupille P, Fouquet B, Favard L, et al: Two cases of plant thorn synovitis: Difficulties in diagnosis and treatment. *J Rheumatol* 1990;17:252–254.
73. O'Connor CR, Reginato AJ, DeLong WG Jr: Foreign body reactions simulating acute septic arthritis. *J Rheumatol* 1988; 15:1568–1571.
74. Ettelson CD, Weeks PM: Thorn-induced tenosynovitis of the hand: Case report. *Missouri Med* 1984;81:257–259.
75. Piard F, Levillain P, Michiels R, et al: Tenosynovitis caused by a plant thorn. *Arch Anat Cytol Pathol* 1985;33:257–260.
76. Barry M, Maffulli N, Good C: The missed thorn. *Acta Orthop Belgica* 1992;58:468–470.
77. Russell RC, Williamson DA, Sullivan JW, et al: Detection of foreign bodies in the hand. *J Hand Surg* 1991;16A:2–11.
78. Marquis GP: Radiolucent foreign bodies in the hand: Case report. *J Trauma* 1989;29:403–404.
79. Hansson G, Beebe AC, Carroll NC, et al: A piece of wood in the hand diagnosed by ultrasonography. *Acta Orthop Scand* 1988;59:459–460.
80. Howden MD: Foreign bodies within finger tendon sheaths demonstrated by ultrasound: Two cases. *Clin Radiol* 1994;49: 419–420.
81. Lejeune A, Nizet M: Letter: Detection of foreign bodies in hand. *J Hand Surg* 1993;18A:166–168.
82. Levine WN, Leslie BM: The use of ultrasonography to detect a radiolucent foreign body in the hand: A case report. *J Hand Surg* 1993;18A:218–220.
83. Wendt JR, Ackley SM: Vascular complications of a foreign body in the hand of an asymptomatic patient. *Ann Plast Surg* 1995;34:92–94.
84. Kaplan HI, Sadock BJ, Grebb JA (eds): *Synopsis of Psychiatry: Behavioral Sciences, Clinical Psychiatry,* ed 6. Baltimore, MD, Williams & Wilkins, 1991, p 480.
85. Grunert BK, Sanger JR, Matloub HS, et al: Classification system for factitious syndromes in the hand with implications for treatment. *J Hand Surg* 1991;16A:1027–1030.
86. Friedman B, Yaffe B, Blankstein A, et al: Self-inflicted hand injuries: Diagnostic challenge and treatment. *Ann Plast Surg* 1988;20:345–350.
87. Louis DS, Lamp MK, Greene TL: The upper extremity and psychiatric illness. *J Hand Surg* 1985;10A:687–693.
88. Phelps DB, Buchler U, Boswick JA Jr: The diagnosis of factitious ulcer of the hand: A case report. *J Hand Surg* 1977; 2B:105–108.
89. Reading G: Secretan's syndrome: Hard edema of the dorsum of the hand. *Plast Reconstr Surg* 1980;65:182–187.
90 Smith RJ: Factitious lymphedema of the hand. *J Bone Joint Surg* 1975;57A:89–94.
91. Agris J, Simmons CW Jr: Factitious (self-inflicted) skin wounds. *Plast Reconstr Surg* 1978;62:686–692.
92. Drinker H, Knorr NJ, Edgerton MT Jr: Factitious wounds: A psychiatric and surgical dilemma. *Plast Reconstr Surg* 1972;50: 458–461.
93. Adams F (ed): *The Genuine Works of Hippocrates.* New York, NY, W Wood, 1886.
94. Kelley WN, Fox IH: Gout and related disorders of purine metabolism, in Kelley WN, Harris ED Jr, Ruddy S, et al (eds): *Textbook of Rheumatology,* ed 2. Philadelphia, PA, WB Saunders, 1985, vol 2, pp 1359–1398.
95. Terkeltaub R: Gout epidemiology, pathology, and pathogenesis, in Schumacher HR Jr, Klippel JH, Koopman WJ (eds): *Primer on the Rheumatic Diseases,* ed 10. Atlanta, GA, Arthritis Foundation, 1993, pp 209–213.
96. Kalia KK, Moossy JJ: Carpal tunnel release complicated by acute gout. *Neurosurgery* 1993;33:1102–1103.
97. Yu T, Yu TF: Milestones in the treatment of gout. *Am J Med* 1974;56:676–685.
98. Yu TF: Some unusual features of gouty arthritis in females. *Semin Arthritis Rheum* 1977;6:247–255.
99. Levinson DJ, Becker MA: Clinical gout and the pathogenesis of hyperuricemia, in McCarty DJ, Koopman WJ (eds): *Arthritis and Allied Conditions: A Textbook of Rheumatology,* ed 12. Philadelphia, PA, Lea & Febiger, 1993, vol 2, pp 1773–1805.
100. Macfarlane DG, Dieppe PA: Diuretic-induced gout in elderly women. *Br J Rheumatol* 1985;24:155–157.
101. Rogachefsky RA, Carneiro R, Altman RD, et al: Gout presenting as infectious arthritis: Two case reports. *J Bone Joint Surg* 1994;

76A:269–273.
102. Grahame R, Scott JT: Clinical survey of 354 patients with gout. *Ann Rheum Dis* 1970;229:461–468.
103. Abrahamsson SO: Gouty tenosynovitis simulating an infection: A case report. *Acta Orthop Scand* 1987;58:282–283.
104. Graff SN, Seiler JG III, Jupiter JB: Acute gout after carpal tunnel release. *J Hand Surg* 1992;17A:1031–1032.
105. Ho G Jr, DeNuccio M: Gout and pseudogout in hospitalized patients. *Arch Intern Med* 1993;153:2787–2790.
106. McCarty DJ: Calcium pyrophosphate dihydrate crystal deposition disease: 1975. *Arthrutis Rheum* 1976;19(suppl 3):275–285.
107. Moore JR, Weiland AJ: Gouty tenosynovitis in the hand. *J Hand Surg* 1985;10A:291–295.
108. Riordan DC: The hands in gout. *Am J Orthop* 1960;2: 256–259;266.
109. Straub LR, Smith JW, Carpenter GK, et al: The surgery of gout in the upper extremity. *J Bone Joint Surg* 1961;43A: 731–752.
110. Vukmir RB, Weiss L, Verdile VP: Polyarticular symmetric to phaceous joint inflammation as the initial presentation of gout. *Am J Emerg Med* 1990;8:43–45.
111. Kolba KS: The approach to the acute joint and synovial fluid examination. *Prim Care* 1984;11:211–218.
112. Newman JH: The differential diagnosis of septic arthritis in the elderly. *Compr Ther* 1984;10:29–34.
113. Lockie LM: Diagnosis of gouty arthritis. *Am J Orthop* 1960; 2:252–253.
114. Talbott JH: Diagnosis of gout. *Clin Orthop* 1970;71:23–27.
115. Preslar AJ III, Heckman JD: Emergency department evaluation of the swollen joint. *Emerg Med Clin North Am* 1984;2:425–440.
116. Tate GA, Schumacher HR: Gout clinical and laboratory features, in Schumacher HR Jr, Klippel JH, Koopman WJ (eds): *Primer on the Rheumatic Diseases,* ed 10. Atlanta, GA, Arthritis Foundation, 1993, p 213.
117. Hadler NM, Franck WA, Bress NM, et al: Acute polyarticular gout. *Am J Med* 1974;56:715–719.
118. Raddatz DA, Mahowald ML, Bilka PJ: Acute polyarticular gout. *Ann Rheum Dis* 1983;42:117–122.
119. Baer PA, Tenenbaum J, Fam AG, et al: Coexistent septic and crystal arthritis: Report of four cases and literature review. *J Rheumatol* 1986;13:604–607.
120. Smith JW: Infectious arthritis, in Mandell GL, Douglas RG Jr, Bennett JE (eds): *Principles and Practice of Infectious Diseases,* ed 3. New York, NY, Churchill Livingstone, 1990, pp 911–918.
121. Resnick D, Niwayama G: Gouty arthritis, in Resnick D (ed): *Diagnosis of Bone and Joint Disorders,* ed 3. Philadelphia, PA, WB Saunders, 1995, pp 1511–1555.
122. Emmerson BT: The management of gout. *N Engl J Med* 1996;334:445–451.
123. Wallace SL, Singer JZ: Therapy in gout. *Rheum Dis Clin North Am* 1988;14:441–457.
124. Brody GA, Chase RA, Hentz VR: The upper extremity in gout, in Jupiter JB (ed): *Flynn's Hand Surgery,* ed 4. Baltimore, MD, Williams & Wilkins, 1991, pp 429–438.
125. Kohn NN, Hughes RE, McCarty DJ, et al: The significance of calcium phosphate crystals in the synovial fluid of arthritic patients: The "pseudogout syndrome." II: Identification of crystals. *Ann Intern Med* 1962;56:738–745.
126. McCarty DJ, Hollander JL: Identification of urate crystals in gouty synovial fluid. *Ann Intern Med* 1961;54:452–460.
127. O'Duffy JD: Clinical studies of acute pseudogout attacks: Comments on prevalence, predispositions, and treatment. *Arthritis Rheum* 1976;19(suppl 3):349–352.
128. Howell DS: Diseases due to the deposition of calcium pyrophosphate and hydroxyapatite, in Kelley WN, Harris ED Jr, Ruddy S, et al (eds): *Textbook of Rheumatology,* ed 2. Philadelphia, PA, WB Saunders, 1985, vol 2, pp 1398–1416.
129. Esposito PW, O'Malley D, Litaker D: Acute pseudogout mimicking septic arthritis following urologic manipulation. *Orthop Rev* 1988;17:295–299.
130. Hamblen DL, Currey HL, Key JJ: Pseudogout simulating acute suppurative arthritis. *J Bone Joint Surg* 1966;48B: 51–55.
131. Masuda I, Ishikawa K: Clinical features of pseudogout attack: A survey of 50 cases. *Clin Orthop* 1988;229:173–181.
132. Wallace SL, Robinson H, Masi AT, et al: Preliminary criteria for the classification of the acute arthritis of primary gout. *Arthritis Rheum* 1977;20:895–900.
133. Chiu KY, Ng WF, Wong WB, et al: Acute carpal tunnel syndrome caused by pseudogout. *J Hand Surg* 1992;17A:299–302.
134. Goodwin DR, Arbel R: Pseudogout of the wrist presenting as acute median nerve compression. *J Hand Surg* 1985;10B: 261–262.
135. Monsivais JJ: Letter: Acute carpal tunnel syndrome due to pseudogout. *J Hand Surg* 1993;18B:409.
136. Rate AJ, Parkinson RW, Meadows TH, et al: Acute carpal tunnel syndrome due to pseudogout. *J Hand Surg* 1992;17B:217–218.
137. Genant HK: Roentgenographic aspects of calcium pyrophosphate dihydrate crystal deposition disease (pseudogout). *Arthritis Rheum* 1976;19(suppl 3):307–328.
138. Scutellari PN, Orzincolo C, Droghetti M: Crystalline calcium pyrophosphate dehydrate deposit disease. *Radiol Med* 1985; 71:129–134.
139. McCarty DJ: Calcium pyrophosphate dihydrate crystal deposition disease, in Schumacher HR Jr, Klippel JH, Koopman WJ (eds): *Primer on the Rheumatic Diseases,* ed 10. Atlanta, GA, Arthritis Foundation, 1993, pp 219–222.
140. Harris ED Jr: Rheumatoid arthritis: The clinical spectrum, in Kelley WN, Harris ED Jr, Ruddy S, et al (eds): *Textbook of Rheumatology,* ed 2. Philadelphia, PA, WB Saunders, 1985, vol 1, pp 915–950.
141. Corrigan AB, Robinson RG, Terenty TR, et al: Benign rheumatoid arthritis of the aged. *Br Med J* 1974;1:444–446.
142 Deal CL, Meenan RF, Goldenberg DL, et al: The clinical features of elderly-onset rheumatoid arthritis. A comparison with younger-onset disease of similar duration. *Arthritis Rheum* 1985;28:987–994.
143. David-Chaussé J, Ricard AM, Dehais J: 22 cases of rheumatic monoarthritis in adults (hips excluded). *Rev Rhum Mal Osteoartic* 1972;39:775–778.
144. Villiaumey J, Strauss J, Di Menza C, et al: Rheumatoid monoarthritis. *Rev Rhum Mal Osteoartic*1973;40:627–634.
145. Guerne PA, Weisman MH: Palindromic rheumatism: Part of or apart from the spectrum of rheumatoid arthritis. *Am J Med* 1992;93:451–460.
146. Schumacher HR: Palindromic onset of rheumatoid arthritis: Clinical, synovial fluid, and biopsy studies. *Arthritis Rheum* 1982;25:361–369.
147. Myers AR: Septic arthritis caused by bacteria, in Kelley WN, Harris ED Jr, Ruddy S, et al (eds): *Textbook of Rheumatology,* ed 2. Philadelphia, PA, WB Saunders, 1985, vol 2, pp 1507–1527.
148. Brancos MA, Peris P, Miro JM, et al: Septic arthritis in heroin addicts. *Semin Arthritis Rheum* 1991;21:81–87.
149. Goldenberg DL: Infectious arthritis complicating rheumatoid arthritis and other chronic rheumatic disorders. *Arthritis Rheum* 1989;32:496–502.
150. Myers AR, Miller LM, Pinals RS: Pyarthrosis complicating rheumatoid arthritis. *Lancet* 1969;2:714–716.
151. Halla JT, Fallahi S, Hardin JG: Small joint involvement: A systematic roentgenographic study in rheumatoid arthritis. *Ann Rheum Dis* 1986;45:327–330.
152. Jacob J, Sartoris D, Kursunoglu S, et al: Distal interphalangeal joint involvement in rheumatoid arthritis. *Arthritis Rheum*

1986;29:10–15.
153. Singer JM, Plotz CM: The latex fixation test: I. Application to the serologic diagnosis of rheumatoid arthritis. *Am J Med* 1956;21:888–892.
154. Schumacher HR: Synovial fluid analysis, in Kelley WN, Harris ED Jr, Ruddy S, et al (eds): *Textbook of Rheumatology,* ed 2. Philadelphia, PA, WB Saunders, 1985, vol 1, pp 561–568.
155. Brooks PM, Day RO: Nonsteroidal antiinflammatory drugs: Differences and similarities. *N Engl J Med* 1991;324:1716–1725.
156. Dromgoole SH, Furst DE, Paulus HE: Rational approaches to the use of salicylates in the treatment of rheumatoid arthritis. *Semin Arthritis Rheum* 1981;11:257–283.
157. Furst DE: Rational use of disease-modifying antirheumatic drugs. *Drugs* 1990;39:19–37.
158. Klippel JH: Winning the battle, losing the war? Another editorial about rheumatoid arthritis. *J Rheumatol* 1990;17:1118–1122.
159. McCarty DJ: Treatment of rheumatoid joint inflammation with triamcinolone hexacetonide. *Arthritis Rheum* 1972;15:157–173.
160. Bywaters EGL, Ansell BM: Monoarticular arthritis in children. *Ann Rheum Dis* 1965;24:116–122.
161. Blockey NJ, Gibson AA, Goel KM: Monarticular juvenile rheumatoid arthritis. *J Bone Joint Surg* 1980;62B:368–371.
162. Gristina AG, Kelsey WM, Green DL, et al: Pauciarticular juvenile arthritis. *South Med J* 1976;69:440–441.
163. Schaller J, Wedgwood RJ: Juvenile rheumatoid arthritis: A review. *Pediatrics* 1972;50:940–953.
164. Petty RE, Cassidy JT, Sullivan DB: Clinical correlates of antinuclear antibodies in juvenile rheumatoid arthritis. *J Pediatr* 1973;83:386–389.
165. Schaller JG, Johnson GD, Holborow EJ, et al: The association of antinuclear antibodies with the chronic iridocyclitis of juvenile rheumatoid arthritis (Still's disease). *Arthritis Rheum* 1974; 17:409–416.
166. Singsen BH: Nonarticular rheumatism, juvenile rheumatoid arthritis, juvenile spondylarthropathies, in Schumacher HR Jr, Klippel JH, Koopman WJ (eds): *Primer on the Rheumatic Diseases,* ed 10. Atlanta, GA, Arthritis Foundation, 1993, pp 171–175.
167. Lindsley CB: Pharmacotherapy of juvenile rheumatoid arthritis. *Pediatr Clin North Am* 1981;28:161–177.
168. Orozco-Alcala JJ, Baum J: Treatment of juvenile rheumatoid arthritis: A world survey. *J Rheumatol* 1974;1:187–189.
169. Hemady RK, Baer JC, Foster CS: Immunosuppressive drugs in the management of progressive, corticosteroid-resistant uveitis associated with juvenile rheumatoid arthritis. *Int Opthalmol Clin* 1992;32:241–252.

CHAPTER 9

Longitudinal Failure of Upper-Limb Formation

Paul R. Manske, MD

Failure of formation of the structures of the upper extremity presents as longitudinal or transverse deficiencies of the embryonic limb bud. The deficiencies that develop along longitudinal axes are classified as radial, central, or ulnar. Use of the once commonly employed terms preaxial and postaxial for describing longitudinal deficiencies is discouraged, as these terms do not include the concept of central defects.

It is tempting to speculate that these axially oriented failures of formation are the result of teratogenic insults or genetic influences that destroy cells at specific locations on the apical ectodermal ridge or the supporting mesoderm of the embryonic limb bud.[1] Although this is true for radial deficiencies, which characteristically affect only the structures on the radial border of the forearm and hand, the cause of ulnar and central deficiencies is not as clearly defined. Ulnar deficiency may include dysplasia of the thumb and the radial rays in addition to the ulnar structures. Central deficiency (cleft hand) is frequently associated with polydactyly (duplication) or syndactyly (failure of differentiation), or both, of the central digits. These more complex presentations suggest that the concept that deficiencies of the upper extremity are related to focal limb-bud-cell destruction is too simplistic. Nevertheless, it provides a basis for categorizing and discussing the clinical presentations.

Radial Deficiency

Radial deficiency describes a spectrum of osseous, musculotendinous, and neuromuscular dysplasias of the radial border of the upper limb.[2] Kato and associates[3] produced varying degrees of radial deficiency by administering Myleran (busulfan) to pregnant WKAH/Hkm rats at 9 to 11.5 days of gestation. The extent of the deficiencies was dose-related and resembled that seen in humans. Associated skeletal, hematologic, cardiac, renal, and gastrointestinal defects[4-10] may be overlooked initially because of the more obvious manifestations of radial dysplasia, most notably TAR (thrombocytopenia and absent radius) syndrome, VATER association, Holt-Oram syndrome, and Fanconi anemia.[4-10] It is important to identify these associated abnormalities, particularly the cardiac, hematologic, and renal defects, when a corrective surgical procedure is anticipated. I prefer to categorize these defects as those that may affect surgical intervention, skeletal abnormalities, and other abnormalities. Cardiac, hematologic, and renal abnormalities that may affect the surgical procedure must be identified and addressed before the operation. The surgeon or the pediatric orthopaedic colleague will be responsible for the treatment of skeletal abnormalities in the spine, lower limbs, or feet. The associated abnormalities of the other organ systems are of interest, but they are of less importance to the surgeon.

The dysplastic manifestations of radial deficiency range from the minimum finding of thenar muscle hypoplasia to the more severe anatomic and functional abnormalities of radial clubhand or an absent thumb. Radial dysplasia has occurred bilaterally in approximately two-thirds of patients in my experience (12 of 18 patients in a previous report).[11]

Radial Clubhand

Appearance The predominant characteristics of radial clubhand are defects of the radius, carpal bones, and radial rays, particularly the thumb. There is general hypoplasia of the upper extremity (including the humerus), shortening and bowing of the forearm, and radial angulation and displacement of the carpus with respect to the distal part of the ulna (Fig. 1).[12] A severely bowed ulna may contribute further to the clubbed appearance (Fig. 2).

Although the clubbed appearance of the hand is the result of a skeletal deficiency of the radius, it is important to note that the musculotendinous and neurovascular structures on the radial border of the upper extremity are also absent or abnormal. The elbow may have a fixed extension contracture because of capsular fibrosis, or it may have only passive flexion because of an absent biceps muscle and tendon. The muscles and tendons on the radial aspect of the forearm may form a firm fibrous structure that tethers the wrist and hand, preventing passive correction from the radially deviated position.

Classification Four types of radial clubhand have been recognized on the basis of the radiographic appearance of the radius.[13] In type I, the clubbing associated with the short distal radius is probably secondary to underdeveloped radial carpal bones (Fig. 3, *left*). Clubbing can also occur with a hypoplastic radius (type II), which provides insufficient support at the wrist (Fig. 3, *right*). In most patients, the radius is partially (type III) or completely absent (type IV), giving the forearm the appearance of a J-shaped club (Fig. 1). At times, it is not possible to distinguish between types III

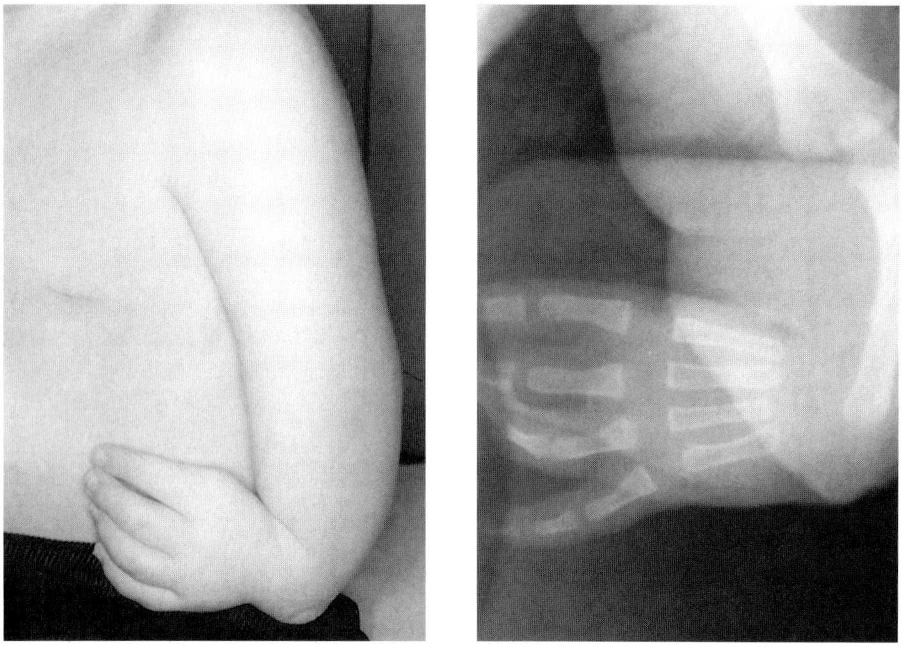

Fig. 1 **Left,** Radial clubhand, showing the clubbed appearance of the left upper extremity. **Right,** This patient has an absent radius and a lack of skeletal support. The carpal bones are angled and displaced radially with respect to the distal part of the ulna.

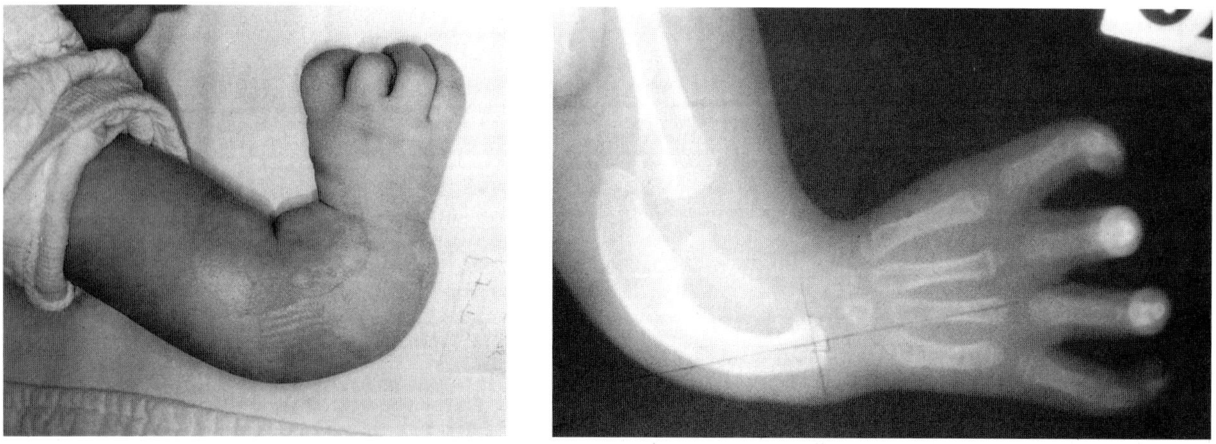

Fig. 2 **Left,** An apparent radial clubhand deformity secondary to severe ulnar bowing. **Right,** The same extremity, showing severe ulnar bowing with minimum angulation or displacement of the hand with respect to the distal part of the ulna. (Reproduced with permission from Manske PR, McCarroll HR Jr, Swanson K: Centralization of the radial clubhand: An ulnar surgical approach. *J Hand Surg* 1981;6A:423–433.)

and IV in an infant, as the small proximal remnant of the radius may not ossify until the child is older. Proximal radial defects with dislocation and migration of an underdeveloped radial head are rare; they are usually associated with only minimum clubbing and do not need treatment (Fig. 4).[14]

Function Although children who have radial clubhand deformity adapt adequately to this anomalous condition, there are obvious functional deficits that limit their activities. Motion of the elbow joint may be decreased or the joint may be fixed in extension. Motion of the wrist and fingers is frequently limited, with the deficit being most severe in the index finger and progressively less severe in the other fingers.[15] The factors contributing to the restricted motion are unclear but undoubtedly include defects in the articular surface as well as contracted capsular and ligamentous tissue in the more radial fingers.

Activities involving the use of two hands are difficult to perform when a normal hand must be brought to

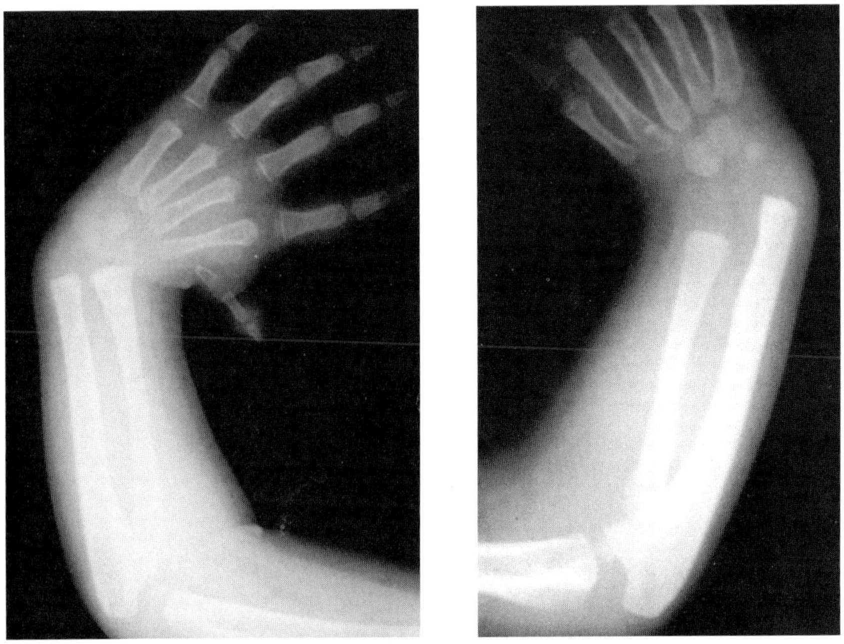

Fig. 3 **Left,** This extremity has a type-I clubhand deformity and a radius and ulna of equal length. The radial carpal bones have not yet ossified but are probably hypoplastic. Note the presence of a rudimentary thumb. **Right,** Radiograph of an extremity with a hypoplastic radius and a type-II clubhand deformity.

meet a shorter extremity. This discrepancy in the lengths of the forearms becomes more apparent as the extremity grows even though the percentage of the length deficit remains constant. When both extremities are involved, activities are greatly impaired by the absence of at least one upper extremity of normal length. In the presence of a severe radial deviation deformity, the fingers are located nearly in the antecubital fossa and objects are grasped in this fossa between the arm and the hand.

The carpus and the hand of patients who have radial clubhand deformity are unsupported on the radial side. As the wrist and the fingers are flexed, the flexion force results in radial deviation of the hand and volar displacement of the carpus; thus, the power available for flexion of the fingers is dissipated as the severity of the deformity increases. Patients who have a radial clubhand frequently have a hypoplastic or aplastic thumb. They often develop a side-to-side pinch between adjacent fingers that is useful for handling small objects but is ineffective for grasping large objects.

Surgical Treatment Since the anomaly of radial clubhand was described by Petit[16] in 1733, there has been considerable interest in its surgical correction. However, it has also been suggested that, because the results of surgical treatment are poor and not substantially better than the preoperative condition, surgical intervention is ill advised.[17] It is acknowledged that children adapt quite well to congenital deformities and develop patterns of activity that are quite functional. Lamb[15] documented

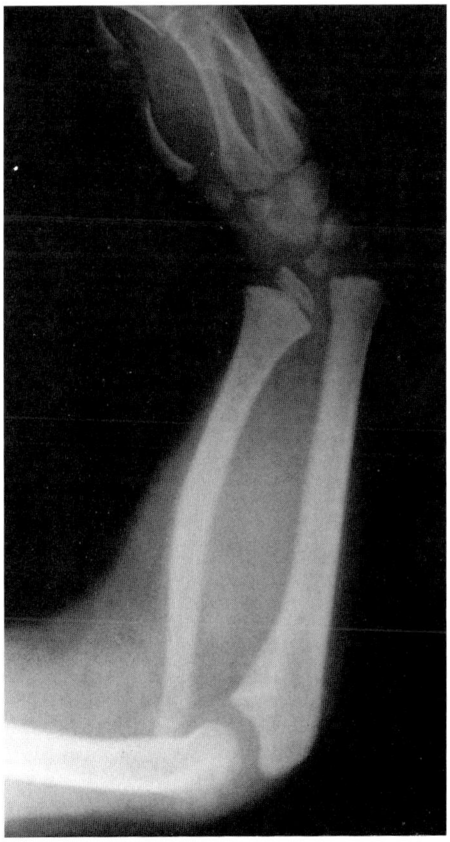

Fig. 4 Radiograph of an extremity with minimum clubbing because of a proximal radial deficiency and proximal migration of the radius.

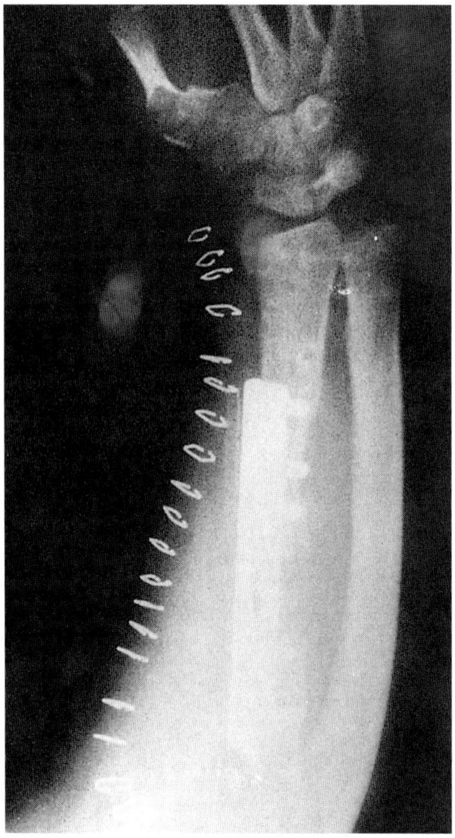

Fig. 5 Radiograph of the same extremity as seen in Fig. 3, *right*, after osteotomy and placement of a lengthening device. After an adequate distraction gap had been obtained, the defect was filled with bone graft and fixation was maintained with a plate and screws. The defect was subsequently bridged by callus, and osseous union was obtained.

little functional loss in patients who had a unilateral radial clubhand.

A primary objective of surgical treatment is to improve the appearance of the upper limb, as the deformity is unsightly and attracts considerable attention. There are also several functional objectives of surgical treatment. First, correction of the angled position and stabilization of the carpus on the forearm improves the mechanical advantage of the flexor muscles of the forearm. Alignment of the carpus and the forearm decreases the abnormal radial moment arm of the flexor muscle mass and minimizes the power lost to radial deviation of the unstable wrist. Theoretically, this increased mechanical advantage is manifested as increased digital motion or grip strength. Second, realignment of the hand in the direct line of the distal forearm can extend the length of the extremity. Third, when the forearm is in the clubbed position, reconstruction of a hypoplastic thumb or index finger pollicization is hindered by the close proximity of the hand to the radial side of the forearm or the antecubital fossa. If the hand is repositioned, such reconstructive procedures are more easily and effectively accomplished.

Not all of the manifestations of radial dysplasia can be corrected by surgery. Both the surgeon and the parents of the patient must understand that neither the appearance nor the function of the limb will be normal postoperatively. The extremity will always be relatively short, joint motion will be limited, grip strength will be diminished, and some degree of residual angulation of the hand and the forearm may continue. However, the current opinion of most hand surgeons is that surgical treatment by an experienced surgeon will considerably improve the function and appearance of the hand.

Type I Minimum clubbing of less than 10° to 15° may be seen with a short distal radius. This clubbing is not clinically important and does not require surgical correction. However, a substantial degree of clubbing may be associated with a short radius that is equal in length to the ulna (Fig. 3, *left*). The radial musculotendinous and capsular structures are usually tight, preventing passive correction of the hand. Treatment includes release of the tight radial capsule and other soft-tissue structures in addition to tendon transfers. The extensor carpi ulnaris is cut near its insertion; the extensor carpi radialis longus tendon is transferred to the distal stump of the extensor carpi ulnaris to facilitate ulnar deviation, and the proximal extensor carpi ulnaris tendon is transferred to the base of the third metacarpal to improve wrist dorsiflexion. This procedure corrects the clubbing and improves dorsiflexion of the wrist.

Type II The distal radius is 1 to 2 cm shorter than the distal ulna (Fig. 3, *right*). If the clubbing is clinically severe, radial lengthening should be considered. An osteotomy is performed at the mid-part of the radial shaft, an external fixator is applied, and the bone is lengthened as tolerated, at a maximum rate of 1 mm a day.[18] After the appropriate distraction length of a maximum of 20 mm has been achieved to equalize the lengths of the radius and the ulna, the fixator can be left in place until healing has occurred or until the osteotomy defect has been filled with bone graft and stabilized with a plate and screws (Fig. 5). Although the clubbing can be decreased with use of this technique, it may recur, making it necessary to repeat the bone-lengthening procedure after several years.

Types III and IV Surgical procedures have been used most frequently to correct radial clubhand deformity associated with complete absence or absence of a substantial portion of the distal radius. The operative approach has four components: (1) manipulation and soft-tissue stretching, (2) realignment and stabilization of the carpal bones, (3) tendon transfers, and (4) correction of the ulnar bowing.

Manipulation and stretching of the tight soft-tissue structures on the radial side of the forearm with use of serial casts has been suggested by many authors[13,19-21]

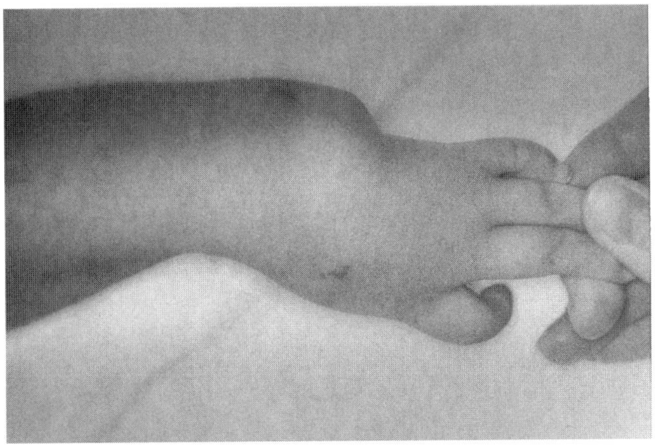

Fig. 6 Patient with absent radius whose angulation deformity was easily corrected to the neutral position without serial casting. Although the angulation has been corrected, the carpus remains radially positioned with respect to the prominent distal part of the ulna.

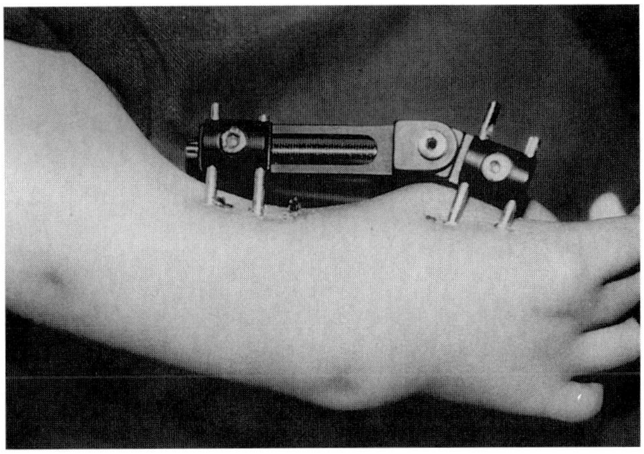

Fig. 7 Precentralization stretching of tight radial structures using an external fixator. The external fixator can also displace the hand distally with respect to the ulna.

for a preoperative period. The casts correct the abnormal angulation but not the abnormal position of the carpus with respect to the distal ulna. Preoperative casts are not necessary when the clubbed hand can be passively placed in a position of fully corrected longitudinal alignment (Fig. 6).

The sensation and movement of an unencumbered hand are important to growth and development in infants. Manipulation and stretching can begin in the neonatal period; however, if preoperative casts are used to obtain correction, it is recommended that (1) the treatment with the casts be instituted 6 to 8 weeks before the anticipated surgical procedure, (2) the digits be left as free and mobile as possible in the corrective casts, (3) the casts or splints be applied alternately rather than simultaneously when a patient has bilateral radial clubhand, and (4) removable splints rather than plaster casts be used to maintain a cast-corrected position.

Stretching of the tight radial tissues was recently accomplished with use of an external fixator for 6 to 8 weeks before surgical correction of the radial clubhand (Fig. 7).[22] This technique not only has improved the angulation of the deviated hand but also has distracted the hand distally, which should facilitate the subsequent centralization procedure. External fixation permits more unrestricted motion and activity of the digits than does a cast. Finally, surgical release of the radial fibrous tissue before soft-tissue stretching by cast manipulation or external fixation has also been suggested but not reported.

Historically, the second component of the surgical approach to radial clubhand deformity, realignment and stabilization of the carpal bones on the forearm, has been achieved with several methods. Surgical treatment of clubbing previously consisted primarily of soft-tissue releases and various types of ulnar osteotomies.[21,23-25] The improvement after these procedures was temporary, and the deformity frequently recurred. Several surgeons have attempted to construct an osse-ous support to replace the absent radius using a free fibular graft,[26] a portion of the distal ulna,[27-29] or the proximal fibula.[30] The principle of providing a radial support is mechanically sound; however, these procedures failed primarily because the grafted component did not grow. Provision of a radial support using microvascular techniques to transfer a vascularized bone graft with an open physis[31,32] may prove in time to be an effective method of treatment. Vilkki[33] performed free vascularized tissue transfer of the metatarsophalangeal joint as an articulated radial support structure and reported excellent early results. However, this technique has not yet been established and is not the standard procedure of choice. Arthrodesis of the carpal bones to the distal ulna improves the cosmetic appearance and stabilizes the wrist; however, this procedure is infrequently used by most surgeons except as a salvage for failed centralization.[34]

Centralization of the carpal bones on the distal ulna was one of the earliest described procedures and is currently the principal operation used to treat radial clubhand. In 1893, Sayre[21] placed a sharpened distal ulna into a notch created in the carpus by excising the lunate and the capitate. The original procedure has been modified by several authors.[14,15,18,35-37]

The traditional surgical approach to the wrist is through a longitudinal dorsal-radial incision that enables the surgeon to release the contracted soft tissue on the radial side. However, a transverse ulnar incision with a proximal longitudinal extension on the

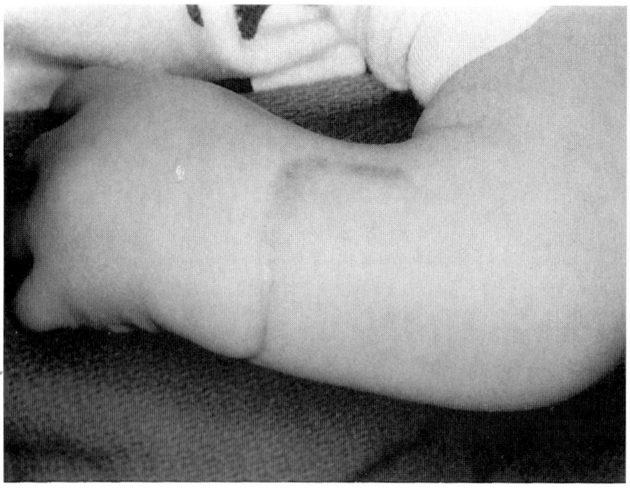

Fig. 8 Postoperative photograph showing my preferred incision for centralization. The transverse ulnar component allows excision of the excess skin and subcutaneous tissue, and the longitudinal extension on the radial side allows release of any tight or contracted tissue.

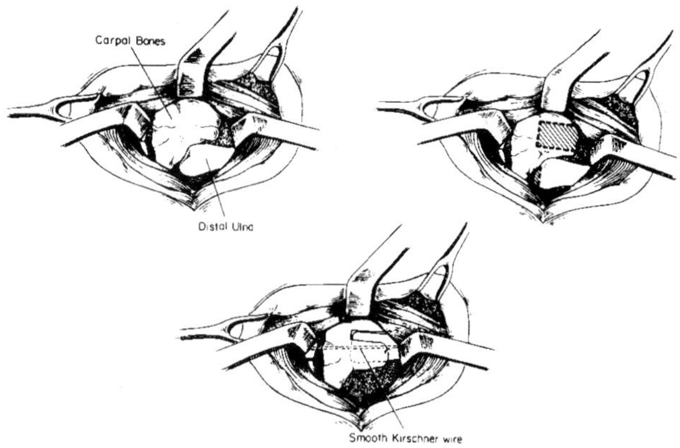

Fig. 9 Diagram showing a centralization procedure performed using an ulnar approach. (Reproduced with permission from Manske PR, McCarroll HR Jr, Swanson K: Centralization of the radial clubhand: An ulnar surgical approach. *J Hand Surg* 1981;6A:423–433.)

medial aspect of the forearm (Fig. 8) provides an easier approach to excision of the redundant mass of ulnar soft tissue and stabilization of the ulnar side of the wrist with capsulodesis.[12]

Centralization is usually accomplished by releasing the tight radial structures, excising a segment of the central carpal bones, and placing the distal ulna in the resultant notch (Fig. 9). The removal of a segment of the carpal bones is in effect a reduction osteotomy, which may also help to accommodate the tight radial soft-tissue structures. The distal end of the ulna may be quite large and may be surrounded by adherent fibrous tissue that prevents its placement into the carpal notch. The ulna must be carefully dissected free of this tissue and reduced in size by paring down the cartilage on the ulnar and radial sides; the surgeon must be careful to preserve the distal ulnar growth plate. Centralization has also been accomplished by placing the carpus on the distal ulna without forming a carpal notch.[37] In my experience, this construct is not as stable and may allow the deformity to recur. In an attempt to improve further the mechanical stability of the carpus on the distal end of the ulna, Buck-Gramcko[36] recommended a so-called radialization procedure, in which the carpus is positioned on the ulnar side of the ulna. The long-term results of this procedure are not available. Most surgeons have advocated temporary stabilization of the carpus on the distal end of the ulna with use of a longitudinal intramedullary Kirschner wire after centralization; the wire passes from the ulna across the carpus into the metacarpal of the long finger or the interspace between the index and long fingers. The wire is removed approximately 2 to 3 months after the operation.

In the third component of the surgical approach—tendon transfers—the extensor carpi ulnaris is the principal tendon that is advanced to provide an ulnar and dorsiflexion force to the wrist and the hand.[6,12,13,18] The flexor carpi ulnaris,[13] the flexor digitorum superficialis,[32] the flexor carpi radialis,[15] and the common mass of the radial flexor and extensor muscles[36] have also been used to contribute to the stability of the centralized hand. The importance of these transfers to the stability and function of the centralized hand should be emphasized. However, because of the variety of anomalous conditions, the tendons are not always available for transfer.

The fourth component of the surgical approach is correction of ulnar bowing. It is uncertain whether ulnar bowing is a progressive[13,15] or a static[12,35] deformity. It can be corrected by a single or multiple closing-wedge osteotomies at the time of centralization;[6,13,15,36] as many as three osteotomies may be needed to obtain a straight ulna. The procedure is most easily performed when the radius is absent or rudimentary. Although the procedure straightens the forearm, the closing wedges result in a reduction in the ulnar length. It has been my experience that, if corrective osteotomies are to be performed, they should be done at the time of centralization, before placement of the carpus on the distal ulna. If they are performed subsequently, the tightened radial structures cause the radial deviation to recur.

Results of Surgery Centralization primarily addresses the radial deviation; it does not effectively correct the volar flexion deformity. The anecdotal experience of surgeons involved in the long-term care of patients whose radial clubhand has been managed surgically has indicated that the wrist often has a flexed posture along with a limited range of motion; however, few reports have actually quantitated the long-term postoperative results.

Most authors have agreed that the appearance of the deformed upper extremity is improved by surgery (Fig. 10). Lamb[15] reported quantitative improvement from an average angle of radial deviation of 78° preoperatively to an average angle of 22° after centralization. In a previous study with colleagues,[12] I noted an average improvement of 26° in radial angulation, and carpal translation improved from an average of 10 mm radial to the longitudinal axis of the distal part of the ulna preoperatively to an average of 12 mm ulnar to the longitudinal axis, at an average of 34 months postoperatively, in 21 extremities. Buck-Gramcko[36] reported extension of the wrist ranging from neutral to 20° and flexion ranging from 40° to 90° in 30 extremities at an average of 46 months after the operation. Bora and associates[19] noted digital motion to be 54% of normal after centralization, compared with 27% of normal in patients who did not have surgery; however, those authors did not compare preoperative with postoperative motion.

Improvement of specific functional activities after centralization is difficult to document for a growing child because children generally adapt well to the limitations of congenital deformities. Lamb[15] noted no deterioration of the functional activities of 27 patients at an average of 5 years after centralization, and he emphasized the functional benefits of surgery for patients who had bilateral involvement.

There is the potential for decreased epiphyseal growth of the distal part of the ulna after centralization. Bora and associates[19] noted such a decrease in two of 13 patients. Lamb[15] noted a decrease in all seven of his patients who had surgery after they were 8 years old, whereas he found no decrease in eight patients who were 2 to 5 years old at the time of surgery.

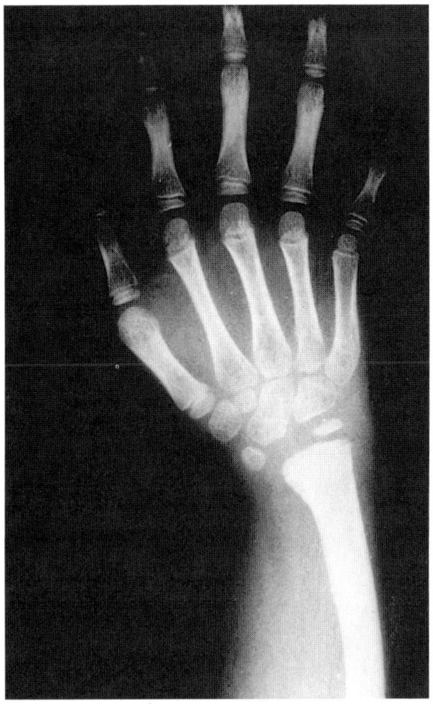

Fig. 10 Radiograph made 5 years after centralization of a radial clubhand. Note the corrected angulation and the position of the wrist and the hand with respect to the widened distal part of the ulna.

Table 1
Classification of hypoplasia of the thumb

Type	Characteristics
Type I	Minimum shortening and narrowing, mild hypoplasia of thenar muscles
Type II	Narrowing of web space between thumb and index finger, aplasia and hypoplasia of thenar intrinsic muscles, instability of metacarpophalangeal joint
Type III	Type-II features and:
Type IIIA	Abnormalities of extrinsic tendons, hypoplastic metacarpals, and stable carpometacarpal joint
	or
Type IIIB	Abnormalities of extrinsic tendons, partial aplasia of metacarpals, and unstable carpometacarpal joint
Type IV	*Pouce flottant*
Type V	Absent thumb

Hypoplastic Thumb

The hypoplastic thumb is characterized by a spectrum of abnormalities affecting the radial border of the upper extremity. The classification system[38-40] includes five categories that reflect the progressive severity of the condition (Table 1) and are helpful for identifying the progressive stages of arrested development. The features of each category are well defined, particularly the subclassification of type-III patterns according to the presence or absence of stability at the carpometacarpal joint.[40,41] The more subtle patterns (types I and II) in one extremity may go unrecognized by parents, pediatricians, and surgeons in the presence of more obvious manifestations of radial dysplasia, such as radial clubhand on the contralateral side. Therefore, it is very important to examine carefully both extremities of any patient who has unilateral radial deficiency.

Classification

Type I The thumb is decreased in size. The musculoskeletal and neurovascular components are present, but there may be mild hypoplasia of the intrinsic abductor pollicis brevis and the opponens pollicis muscles.

Type II There are three specific features: narrowing of

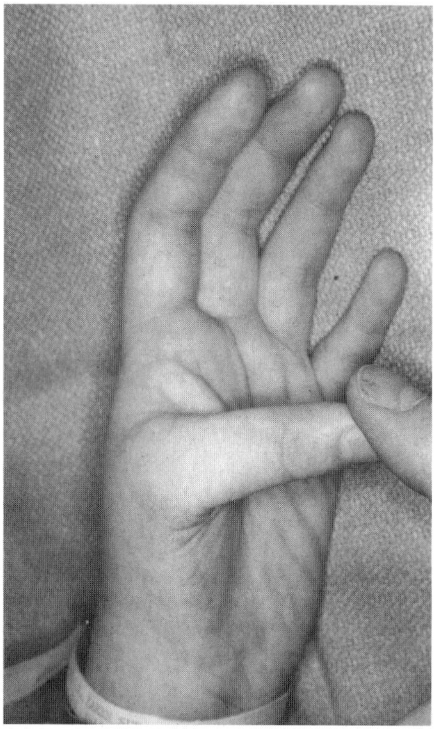

Fig. 11 Patient with absent thenar muscle mass and associated laxity of the ulnar collateral ligament of the metacarpophalangeal joint of the thumb (type-II hypoplasia).

the web space between the thumb and the index finger; aplasia or hypoplasia of the median innervated thenar intrinsic muscles (the abductor pollicis brevis and the opponens pollicis), usually sparing the deeper ulnar innervated muscles; and instability of the ulnar collateral ligament at the metacarpophalangeal joint (Fig. 11). (Global instability of the metacarpophalangeal joint is seen in more severe grades of hypoplasia.) Type-II hypoplasia causes a substantial functional deficiency for the child. The narrowed thumb web space and the unstable ulnar collateral ligament interfere greatly with the child's ability to pinch or grasp objects. The intrinsic muscle deficiency interferes with the child's ability to rotate the thumb in front of the fingers and also contributes to an inefficient pinch mechanism.

Type III Type-III hypoplastic thumbs are associated with more extensive deficiencies and functional deficits (Fig. 12, *left*). The three manifestations of the type-II thumb are present, usually in a more severe form. The narrow web space between the thumb and the index finger may present as a distal takeoff of the thumb from the hand, and the metacarpophalangeal instability may be more global, also involving the radial collateral ligament. There are two other potential deficiencies: abnormalities of the extrinsic tendons and osseous deficiencies of the first metacarpal base.[40] In type-IIIA hypoplasia, there are abnormalities of the extrinsic tendons, but the first metacarpal is present (although

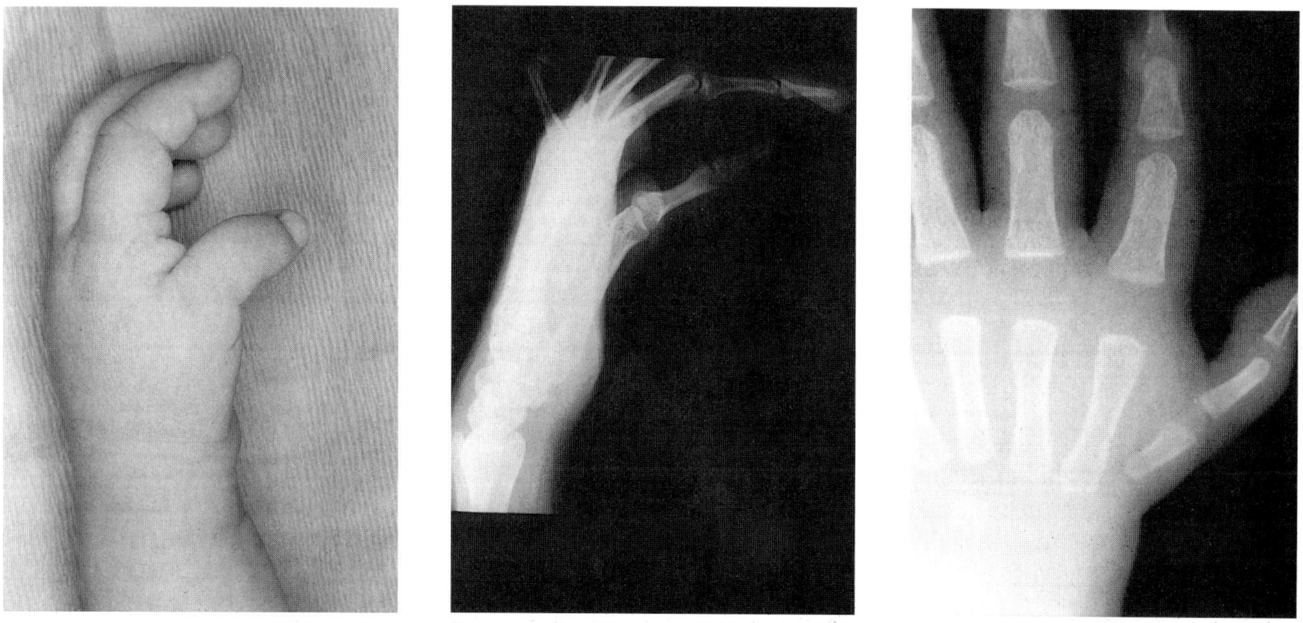

Fig. 12 Left, Type-III hypoplastic thumb. In addition to hypoplastic thenar muscles, an unstable ulnar collateral ligament at the metacarpophalangeal joint, and a narrow web space between the thumb and the index finger, there are abnormalities of the extrinsic tendons (an absent extensor pollicis longus and an aberrant flexor pollicis longus on the radial side of the thumb). The carpometacarpal joint is stable. **Center,** Type-IIIA hypoplastic thumb. The carpometacarpal joint is stable. **Right,** Type-IIIB hypoplastic thumb. The proximal aspect of the metacarpal is absent (that is, the base of the metacarpal is unstable).

hypoplastic) and the carpometacarpal articulation is stable (Fig. 12, *center*). In type-IIIB hypoplasia, there are abnormalities of the extrinsic tendons as well as absence of the first metacarpal base and an unstable basal (carpometacarpal) joint (Fig. 12, *right*). The most frequently observed musculotendinous abnormalities include an absent extensor pollicis longus, an absent or aberrant flexor pollicis longus, and a tendon interconnection between the flexor pollicis longus and the extensor aponeurosis; several deficiencies of the extrinsic tendons may be present in the same thumb. An increased awareness of type-III hypoplasia among hand surgeons may lead to identification of other abnormalities of the extrinsic tendons and additional anomalous muscles. The so-called pollex abductus thumb, described by Tupper[42] and others,[40] is a form of type-IIIA hypoplasia in which the thumb web space is narrowed; the intrinsic thenar muscles are hypoplastic; and there is aberrant placement of the flexor pollicis longus along the radial side of the thumb ray, which, in conjunction with laxity of the ulnar collateral ligament, causes marked abduction at the metacarpophalangeal joint.

Type IV Type-IV hypoplasia is the classic *pouce flottant* (Fig. 13). The thumb is attached to the hand only by soft tissue, primarily skin and neurovascular elements. There are essentially no musculotendinous structures, and there is no stable osseous unit between the thumb and the hand.

Type V Type-V hypoplasia is characterized by a complete absence of the thumb (Fig. 14). However, there may be rudimentary thumb muscles, tendons, or neurovascular structures along the radial border of the metacarpal of the index finger.

Reconstructive Procedures Reconstructive procedures are not usually indicated for type-I thumbs because of the generalized hypoplasia. Although a thumb-lengthening procedure could be considered for this condition, I have not yet had a patient who needed one.

When treating type-II thumbs, the three features of the hypoplasia must each be specifically addressed.[11,41] The narrow web space between the thumb and the index finger must be deepened, usually with a z-plasty and use of three or four flaps. On occasion, it may be necessary to increase the web space with use of a transposition or rotation flap from the dorsum of the hand or the thumb. I have never found it necessary to use a distant vascularized pedicle flap. The procedure should also include release of the deeper soft-tissue structures, particularly the fascia investing the adductor pollicis and the first dorsal interosseous muscles. Infrequently, the origin of these muscles must be released from the bone.

Stabilization of the metacarpophalangeal joint is also essential for the restoration of function of the type-II thumb. In a child, this can usually be accomplished by imbricating the ulnar capsule at the metacarpophalangeal joint and reinforcing it with the distal end

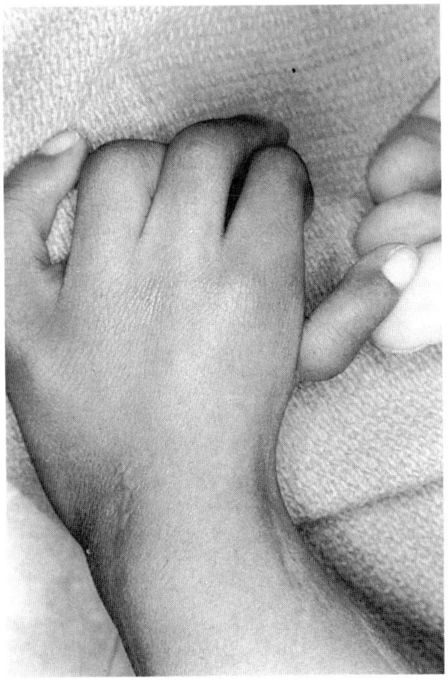

Fig. 13 Type-IV hypoplastic thumb (*pouce flottant*).

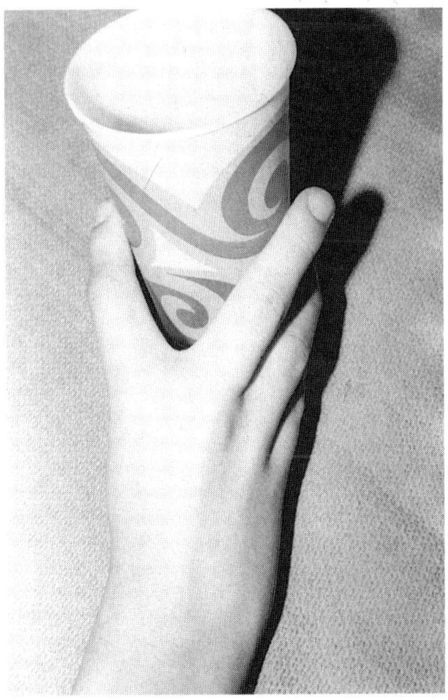

Fig. 14 Patient with absent thumb (type-V hypoplasia), demonstrating difficulty in grasping a large object.

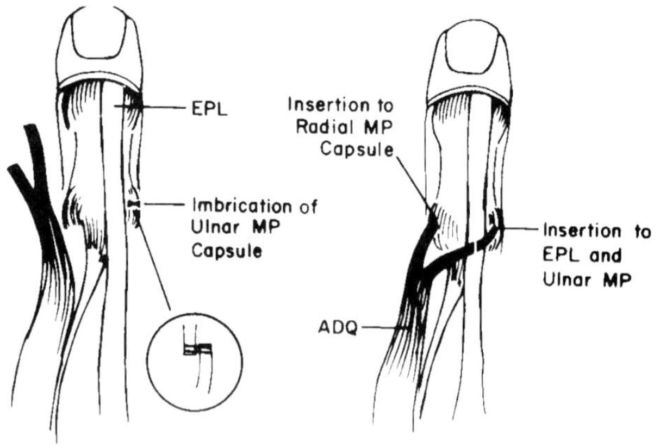

Fig. 15 Diagram demonstrating imbrication of the ulnar capsule of the metacarpophalangeal (MP) joint and insertion of the two parts of the tendon to obtain stability of the capsule at the joint. EPL = extensor pollicis longus and ADQ = abductor digiti quinti. (Reproduced with permission from Manske PR, McCarroll HR Jr: Abductor digiti minimi opponensplasty in congenital radial dysplasia. *J Hand Surg* 1978;3A:552–559.)

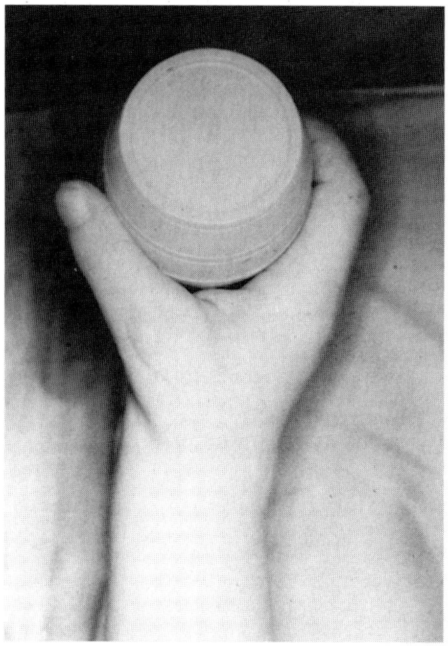

Fig. 16 Photograph made after opponensplasty of the abductor digiti minimi and stabilization of the ulnar collateral ligament of the metacarpophalangeal joint.

of the opponensplasty (Figs. 15 and 16).[11] When the radial collateral ligament is also deficient (as is usually seen in the more severe, type-III hypoplasia), stabilization of the radial aspect of the capsule may also be attempted but may not be adequate; a metacarpophalangeal epiphyseal arthrodesis[43] that preserves the growth plate may be necessary when procedures for stabilization of the collateral ligaments are not successful.

Finally, an opponensplasty, with use of either the abductor digiti minimi[11] or the flexor superficialis tendon of the ring finger, is necessary to restore opposition function. I prefer the abductor digiti minimi transfer (Fig. 17), described originally by Huber[44] and by Nicholaysen.[45] The procedure is a muscle transfer rather than a tendon transfer; consequently, a sufficient subcutaneous tunnel must be developed across the palm to accommodate the transposed muscle mass (Fig. 18). I prefer to leave the muscle origin attached to the pisiform as originally described by Huber[44] and by Nicholaysen,[45] as this osseous origin serves as a source of vascularization for the muscle.[46] The transferred abductor digiti minimi is as long and as strong as, and pulls in the direction of, the deficient opposition muscles that it replaces. It adds muscle mass to the thenar eminence and therefore also improves the aesthetic appearance of the thumb.

In the treatment of type-III hypoplasia, it is important to distinguish a type-IIIA from a type-IIIB thumb because the former is usually reconstructible[40,41] while the latter usually necessitates ablation and pollicization of the index finger. From a functional point of view, a reconstructed thumb has substantial advantages compared with a pollicized index finger. A reconstructed thumb is usually stronger than a pollicized digit. Additionally, the carpometacarpal joint of a reconstructed type-IIIA thumb has two axes of motion, flexion and extension and abduction and adduction, allowing full circumduction of that joint. In contrast, the basal joint of the pollicized index finger (the metacarpophalangeal joint) has only one primary axis of motion, in the plane of flexion and extension. This affects circumduction and limits the ability of the patient both to retract the pollicized digit and to flatten the palm.

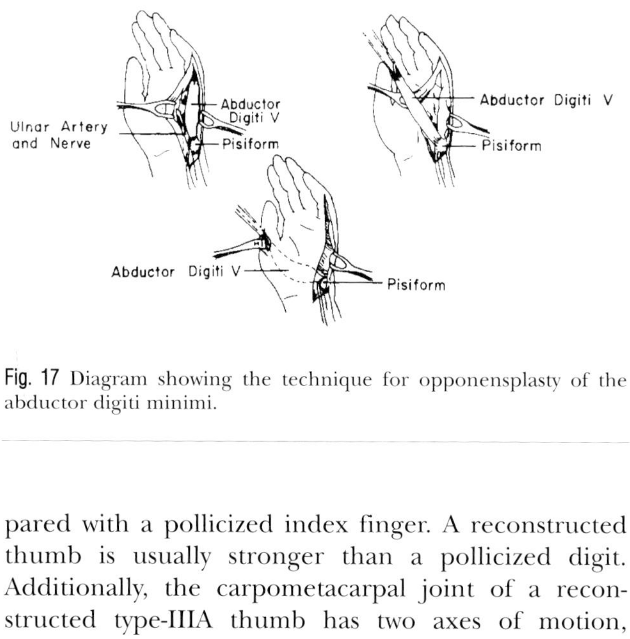

Fig. 17 Diagram showing the technique for opponensplasty of the abductor digiti minimi.

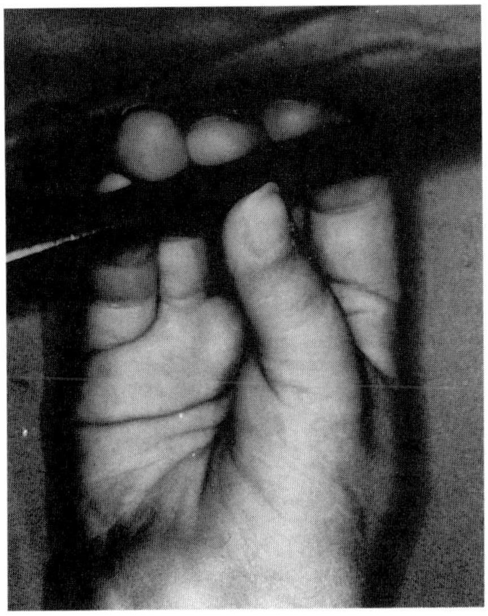

Fig. 18 Absent thenar musculature treated with opponensplasty of the abductor digiti minimi. The abductor digiti minimi at the base of the palm pulls the thumb into opposition for improved pinch.

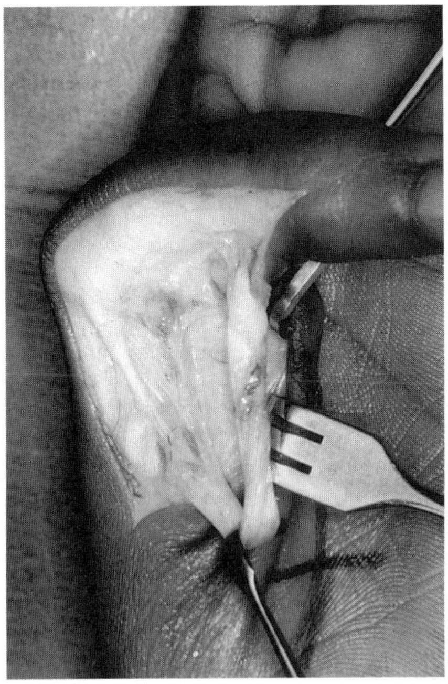

Fig. 20 Aberrant flexor pollicis longus tendon (under retraction) on the radial side of the thumb; the tendon contributes to the radial deviation deformity.

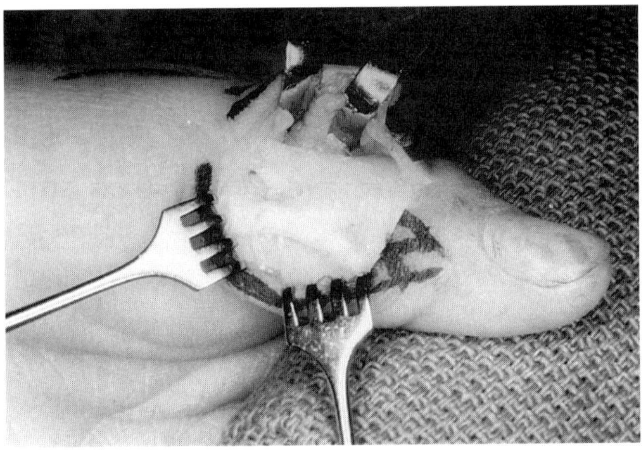

Fig. 19 Tendon interconnection between the flexor and extensor mechanism of the thumb; the interconnection must be released.

To reconstruct a type-III deformity, four conditions for adequate function of the thumb must be met, either by being inherently present in the thumb or by being accomplished surgically. First, there must be an adequate web space between the thumb and the index finger (as described previously for type-II deformity). Second, the length of the thumb must be sufficient to allow grasping and pinching activities. The tip of a normal thumb reaches the proximal interphalangeal joint of the adjacent digit; although the reconstructed thumb may be somewhat shorter, it should at least reach the mid-part of the proximal phalanx of the adjacent digit. Third, stability of the thumb ray must be achieved. Instability of the metacarpophalangeal joint can be treated with imbrication of the ligament, capsulodesis, or an epiphyseal arthrodesis[43] as noted earlier. If the carpometacarpal joint is not stable (as in type-IIIB hypoplasia), reconstruction is usually not possible. Fourth, musculotendinous units to extend, flex, abduct, and adduct the thumb must be present or must be provided by tendon transfer.

A type-IIIA deformity usually can be reconstructed to meet these requirements. The specific reconstructive procedures include those described already for type-II deformity—that is, deepening of the web space between the thumb and the index finger, stabilization of the metacarpophalangeal joint, and performance of an opponens transfer. In addition, the deficiencies of the extrinsic tendons must be addressed. The most straightforward procedures are releases of the tendons that cause deformities or limit motion. These include release of the tendon interconnection that tethers the flexor and extensor mechanisms (Fig. 19) and limits active flexion and extension of the interphalangeal joint as well as release of the aberrant flexor pollicis longus (Fig. 20) that contributes to the severe radial deviation at the metacarpophalangeal joint.

The more difficult procedures involve transfer of the extrinsic tendons to improve function. Limited or absent extension is usually treated with a transfer of the extensor indicis proprius. Limited or absent flexion can be addressed by rerouting the aberrant flexor pollicis longus to a more volar position on the thumb, by transferring the superficialis tendon of the ring finger and reconstructing the osseous pulleys, or by accepting the functional limitations of absent flexion of the interphalangeal joint and allowing the flexion force of the flexor pollicis brevis at the metacarpophalangeal joint to be sufficient. Abduction deficiency is treated by opponensplasty as described earlier. Adduction deficiency is rarely a problem as the adductor pollicis is usually present except in the most severely hypoplastic thumbs. (Those thumbs usually are not reconstructible.) These combined surgical procedures can be quite extensive, but function of the hand is usually improved substantially (Fig. 21).[40,41]

Particularly because of the instability at the carpometacarpal joint, type-IIIB hypoplastic thumbs usually do not meet the four conditions for adequate function. Therefore, unless there are social or cultural reasons for preserving five digits, the reconstruction of a type-IIIB thumb is not recommended. To obtain the best functional result, ablation of the hypoplastic thumb and pollicization of the index finger is the preferred treatment.

A child who has a type-IV or V (non-functioning or absent) thumb adapts quite well and becomes facile in using the remaining digits for picking up and manipulating small objects with a side-to-side pinch. This method of grasping usually involves the index and long fingers, but at times the long and ring fingers or the ring and small fingers are preferred if they are the better developed digits. Children frequently have a wide interdigital space and the ability to rotate the index finger almost 90° (autopollicization). The functional limitation associated with an absent or nonfunctioning thumb is much more notable when the person attempts to handle large objects (Fig. 14). There is insufficient space between the digits, and the absence of opposition results in a lack of power for grasping. This functional limitation is best treated by transposing the index finger, as the radial post, to the position of a thumb, a technique of pollicization that has been well described.[47-49]

Pollicization The standard surgical treatment for an absent or nonfunctioning thumb is pollicization of the index finger[47-49] in a single-stage transfer on its neurovascular pedicle to a position of opposition. The procedure has three primary objectives: to improve the ability to grasp large objects, to improve the appearance of the hand (a hand with a thumb and three fingers is a less noticeable abnormality than a four-fingered hand without a thumb), and to facilitate handshaking when the right hand is involved. Pollicization is indicated bilaterally when both hands are affected.

Pollicization is preferable to free-tissue transfer of a toe because the proximal osseous, musculotendinous, and neurovascular structures necessary for toe transfer are usually absent in patients who have congenital aplasia of the thumb. In addition, a child who does not have a thumb has no cerebral cortical representation for the absent thumb and, therefore, would not be likely to use the transferred toe for functional activities. In thumb

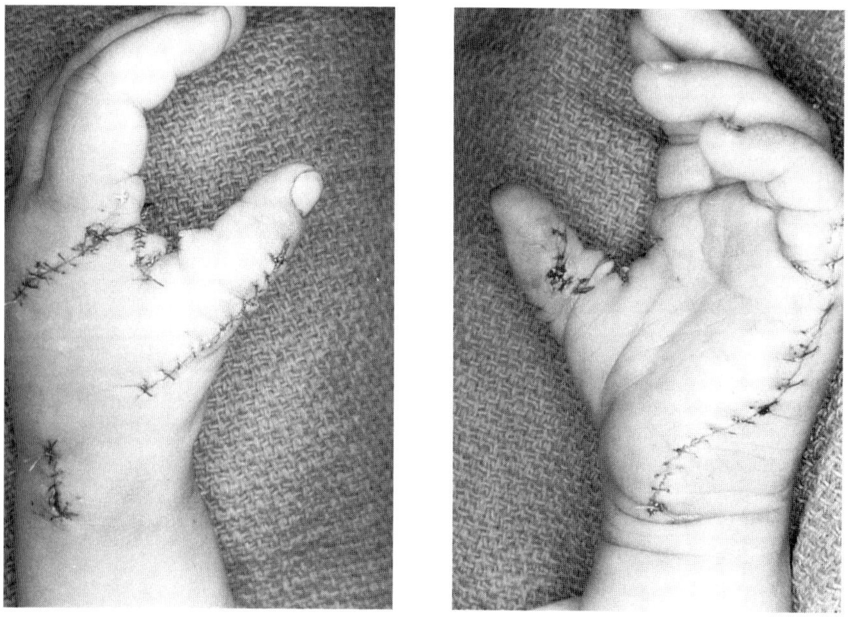

Fig. 21 Dorsal and palmar photographs made after reconstruction of the thumb shown in Fig. 12, *left*. The procedures included z-plasty of the web space between the thumb and the index finger, imbrication of the ulnar collateral ligament at the metacarpophalangeal joint, opponensplasty of the abductor digiti minimi, transfer of the extensor indicis proprius to the extensor hood, and rerouting of the aberrant flexor pollicis longus to a volar position.

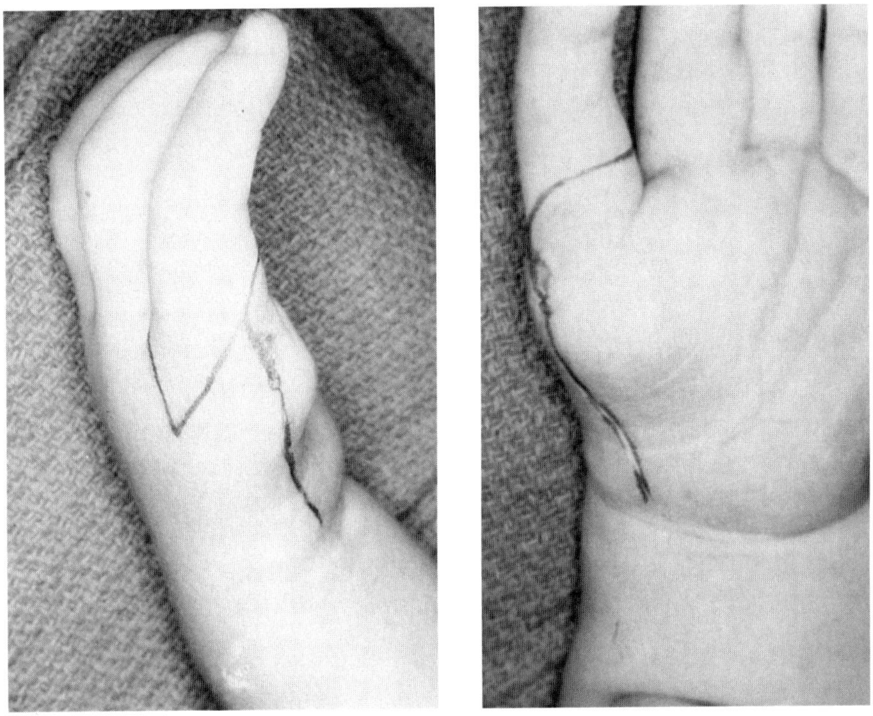

Fig. 22 Incisions for pollicization of the index finger. **Left,** Dorsal view. The apex of the circumferential racquet incision at the base of the index finger is located over the metacarpophalangeal joint. The longitudinal incision extends proximally along the radial mid-lateral line, ending near the base of the metacarpal of the index finger, on the palmar surface of the hand. **Right,** Volar view. The transverse portion of the circumferential racquet incision crosses the volar surface of the digit midway between the metacarpophalangeal and proximal interphalangeal flexion creases.

agenesis, the index finger is represented on the cerebral cortex as the most radial digit. Thus, repositioning this finger to a position of opposition by surgical pollicization presents no problem in cortical recognition.

The timing of surgery is somewhat controversial. It has been recommended that pollicization be performed when the patient is 9 to 12 months of age[47] because this is when cortical representation and awareness of the thumb develop in a normal child. However, in thumb agenesis, the index finger is cortically represented as the radial post and the timing of the surgical repositioning of this digit should not be age-dependent. A long-term study[50] of the functional activities of children who had pollicization between the ages of 9 months and 16 years showed no age-related differences in function. Early surgery is encouraged for social reasons related to restoring a more normal appearance to the hand rather than for the reason of enhancing the cortical representation of the digit as the thumb or for improving function.

The functional quality of the pollicized digit is related to the preoperative condition of the index finger, which has varying degrees of joint motion and tendon excursion. An index finger with little motion preoperatively does not function as effectively after transposition as does one with normal preoperative motion. Patients usually initiate motion and functional use of the hand by 3 to 4 months after surgery, but this can be delayed for as long as 2 years.

The technical procedure of pollicization has been well described.[41,47-49] The principles include skin incision, skeletal shortening, digital rotation, transfers of the intrinsic tendons to provide abductor and adductor pollicis function, and skin closure to give the appearance of a thumb.

A racquet incision is made circumferentially at the base of the index finger (Fig. 22). On the dorsal surface, the apex of the incision is located at the metacarpophalangeal joint. The incision passes distally from this point along the radial and ulnar sides of the metacarpophalangeal joint to cross the volar surface of the finger midway between the metacarpophalangeal and proximal interphalangeal flexion creases. This facilitates the subsequent skin closure that is carried out to give the pollicized digit the appearance of a thumb. A curved longitudinal incision proceeds proximally from the circumferential incision on the radial side of the metacarpophalangeal joint along the midlateral line, curving ulnarward to end near the base of the index metacarpal on the palmar surface of the hand.

The second principle, skeletal shortening, is accomplished with a reduction osteotomy in which the metacarpal diaphysis of the index finger is removed. The metacarpal head becomes the trapezium and the metacarpophalangeal joint becomes the carpometacarpal joint (Table 2). The distal osteotomy should pass through the growth plate so that longitudi-

Table 2
Pollicization

Index Finger		Pollicized Digit
Metacarpal head	→	Trapezium
Metacarpophalangeal joint	→	Carpometacarpal joint
Proximal phalanx	→	Metacarpal
Proximal interphalangeal joint	→	Metacarpophalangeal joint
Middle phalanx	→	Proximal phalanx
Distal interphalangeal joint	→	Interphalangeal joint
Distal phalanx	→	Distal phalanx

nal growth of the metacarpal head does not occur and create an excessively long pollicized digit. The amount of shortening should approximate the distance between the tip of the index finger and the proximal interphalangeal joint of the long finger; this will ensure that the length of the pollicized digit extends to the proximal interphalangeal joint of the adjacent digit.

Next, the digit is rotated 120° to 150° so that the pulp of the pollicized digit opposes the remaining digits. The metacarpal head is flexed and is secured to the metacarpal base with nonabsorbable sutures (not Kirschner wires). The specific position of the rotated digit is determined largely by the placement of the skin sutures and the hand-dressing.

To carry out the transfers of the intrinsic muscles, the first dorsal interosseous muscle is transferred to the radial lateral band at the proximal interphalangeal joint to function as an abductor, and the first volar interosseous muscle is transferred to the ulnar lateral band to function as an adductor. These muscles are not ideally positioned; their origin at the base of the transposed digit is not as mechanically effective for opposition and adduction as a more ulnar origin (as in a normal hand) would be. Furthermore, these muscles are often hypoplastic because of the radial deficiency. Nevertheless, they are the best available. Only if there is a complete absence of the first dorsal interosseous muscle is an opponensplasty performed at the time of pollicization.

When performing the skin closure, it is important to keep in mind that, as much as possible, the surgeon should make the transposed digit resemble a thumb (Fig. 23, *left*) rather than a finger projecting from the base of the palm (Fig. 23, *right*).[49] In the normal hand, the web space joins the thumb on the ulnar side at the metacarpophalangeal joint. Therefore, the web space should also join the pollicized digit at the metacarpophalangeal joint (which is actually the proximal interphalangeal joint of the transposed index finger). This can be accomplished by making a mid-lateral ulnar incision to reattach the first volar interosseous muscle. The incision is left open as an inverted V, and the resultant gap is filled with dorsal skin (Fig. 24). This web-space attachment improves the appearance of the transposed digit so that it better resembles a thumb (Fig. 23).

Before a patient has pollicization, the parents should be made aware that subsequent surgical procedures, including tenolysis, bone-shortening, or revision of the scar,[51] may be needed to maximize the results. In our previous report of the results of 46 index-finger pollicization procedures, 20 fingers required a subsequent operation and six needed more than one.[49] The additional procedures were needed most often in

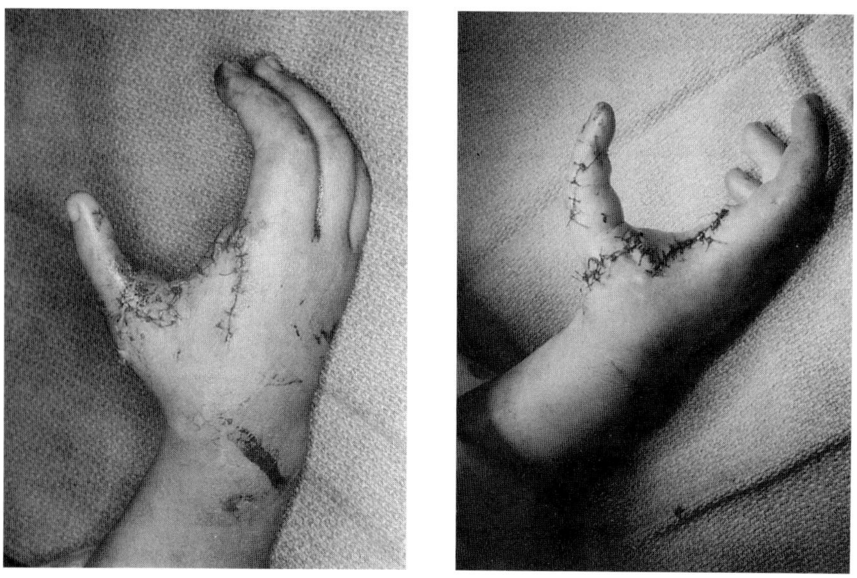

Fig. 23 **Left,** Post-pollicization of index finger that resembles a thumb. **Right,** Post-pollicization of index finger that resembles a finger projecting from the palm.

patients who had had more notable preoperative manifestations of radial dysplasia, such as radial clubhand, which presumably created a more severely affected index finger. An abductor digiti minimi opponensplasty was necessary in 18 patients even though the transferred first dorsal interosseous muscle was functioning after pollicization. Arthrodesis of an unstable or deformed interphalangeal joint was performed on four occasions. Shortening of the extensor tendons was not performed at the time of the initial pollicization, but it was subsequently necessary in four patients. We currently shorten the extensor tendons as a component of the initial pollicization because it positions the thumb in extension, which is more effective for early functional activities.

In general, the results of pollicization have been good, as reported by several authors.[47,48,52] In our experience,[49] there has been no loss of a pollicized digit because of vascular insufficiency and no evidence of altered sensibility. No patient has avoided using the pollicized digit. Patients who used the interspace between the long and ring or the ring and small fingers to grasp and manipulate small objects preoperatively continued to do so postoperatively; however, these patients all used the pollicized digit for grasping large objects. This suggests that the surgical procedure does not cause patients to alter previously established patterns of grasping that are functionally effective.

In a more detailed study,[50] the pollicized digit was noted to have approximately 50% of the range of motion of a normal thumb and approximately 25% of the pinch and grip strength of a normal thumb. It was used for about 85% of activities, more often for grasping large objects and less frequently for grasping small objects. Activities performed with this hand took 22% longer than did activities performed with a normal hand. These functions were improved when the pollicization had been done on an index finger with minimum deficiency: the pollicized digit was used for 93% to 99% of activities, and the activities were accomplished at a rate equal to that with use of a normal hand. The quality of function was not as good when the pollicization had been performed with use of a more deficient index finger (as in patients who had radial clubhand, mirror hand, or a five-fingered hand). Strength was approximately 15% that of a normal hand, the transposed digit was used for only 79% of activities, and it took an average of 33% longer to perform specific tasks.

Overview

In summary, radial deficiency presents as a spectrum of manifestations limited primarily to the radial border of the forearm and hand. Surgical procedures for the treatment of radial clubhand as well as the hypoplastic absent thumb have been effective in improving the appearance and function of the hand.

Central Deficiency

Central deficiency is characterized by failure of formation of at least one central ray of the hand. The deformity, first described in a 1770 report by the East India Trading Company on the status of its South American Dutch Guiana Colony,[53] was characterized as a crawfish claw and has subsequently been referred to as a lobster claw or split hand. Cleft hand is a less offensive term to describe this anomaly.

Although a soft-tissue cleft can occur alone without digital absence,[54-56] the defect usually includes varying

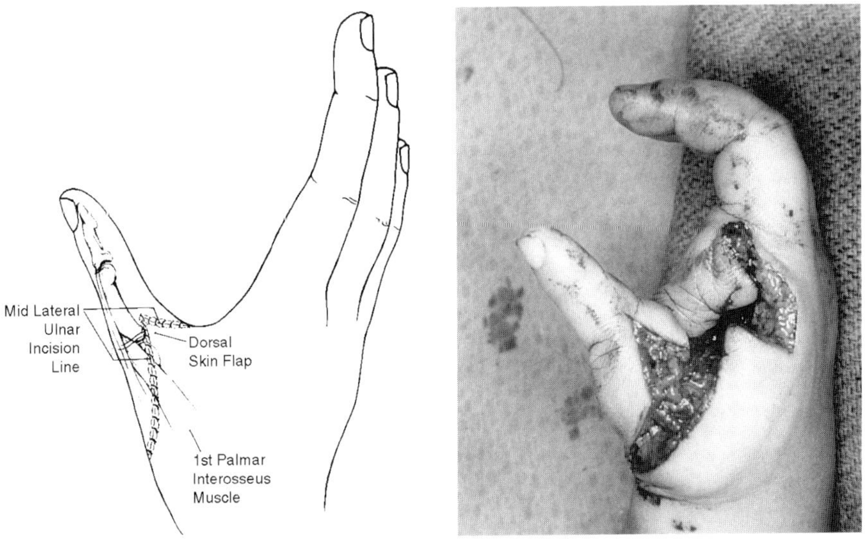

Fig. 24 Left, Drawing of the ulnar side of the transposed digit, showing the ulnar mid-lateral incision through which the palmar interosseous muscle was attached. The incision was not closed but was allowed to gap open, forming an inverted V. The dorsal skin was tailored to fit into the inverted V. (Reproduced with permission from Manske PR, McCarroll HR Jr: Index finger pollicization for a congenitally absent or nonfunctioning thumb. *J Hand Surg* 1985;10A:606–613.) **Right,** Ulnar midlateral incision on the pollicized digit through which the first volar interosseous muscle is attached to the lateral band. The dorsal skin was tailored to fit into the open inverted V.

degrees of suppression of the central rays (Fig. 25). An absent thumb and a monodactylous hand is considered the most severe form.[57-59] The defect has not been noted proximal to the wrist, although carpal coalescence and radioulnar synostosis are sometimes associated with central deficiency.[54]

Despite the obvious aesthetic problems associated with the cleft hand, there is little functional deficit related to the cleft itself.[60] The primary functional problem is related to the space between the thumb and the index finger, which frequently is narrowed to varying degrees.[61]

Cleft Hand, Polydactyly, and Syndactyly

Several investigators have noted that there is an association between cleft hand and syndactylized digits[61] or among cleft hand, central polydactyly, and syndactyly.[58,59,62,63] Ogino[64] observed this association experimentally by administering a teratogenic agent (Myleran) to pregnant female rats and producing a spectrum of anomalies of the central ray of the forepaw in the offspring. Analogous findings in identical human twins born with a spectrum of bilateral abnormalities of the central rays, including cleft hand, central polydactyly, and osseous syndactyly, have been reported (Fig. 26).[65]

The etiology of this spectrum of apparently dissimilar anomalies may be derived from the interrelationship between the cells of the apical ectodermal ridge and the underlying mesodermal cells. The viability of the cells of the apical ridge depends on the production of a maintenance factor by the underlying mesodermal cells. It is postulated that a severe teratogenic insult will kill the mesodermal cells, thereby eliminating the maintenance factor and destroying the overlying apical ectodermal ridge, resulting in central deficiency. A milder teratogenic insult may stimulate the cells and cause release of excess maintenance factor, resulting in the formation of extra digits.

Classification Various classification systems have been proposed, principally on the basis of the characteristics of the central deficiency. Initially, Barsky[66] distinguished between the typical and atypical cleft hand; the typical cleft featured deficiencies of the central rays with preservation of the normal marginal digits (Fig. 25), and the atypical cleft featured central rays that were reduced to nubbins with shortened and rudimentary marginal rays (Fig. 27). It is the prevailing opinion among hand surgeons who deal extensively with these anomalies that the so-called atypical cleft is not a central deficiency but rather a form of symbrachydactyly.[60,62,67,68] Therefore, the term atypical should not be used to describe central deficiencies of the hand.[69]

The common presentation of failure of formation, failure of differentiation, and formation of duplicated parts in genetically identical hands is not compatible with the standard classification system of the International Federation of Societies for Surgery of the Hand.[70] This classification system distinguishes among three different types of congenital malformation; it is important to note that the system primarily defines the presentation of abnormalities and not the in utero developmental pathomechanics. Other classification schemes have included the associated polydactyly and osseous syndactyly.[71]

Finally, several authors have classified the cleft according to the number of central osseous elements

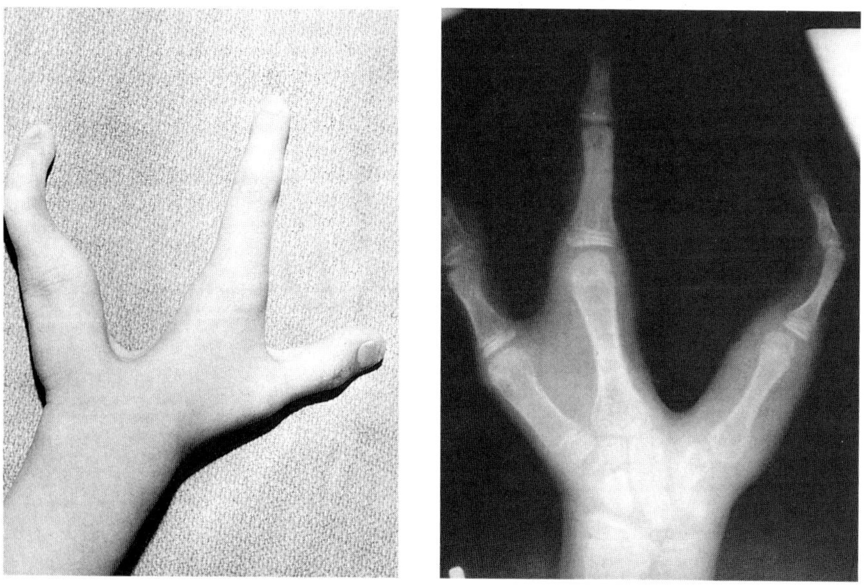

Fig. 25 **Left,** Photograph of a hand with a severe (type-IIB) central deficiency that includes absent long and ring fingers and a severely narrowed first web space. **Right,** Radiograph of a hand with a central deficiency that includes absent long and ring fingers. The configuration of the carpal bones is normal.

that are absent.[54-56,58,59] These classifications are based on the concept of progressive central deficiency, which Maisels[57] referred to as centripetal suppression. In a recent report, we proposed a classification system that reflects the progressive narrowing of the thumb web space,[61] which, as noted earlier, is functionally more important than the central defect. The value of this classification system is that it can be used to guide surgical treatment. It is of interest that progressive narrowing of the thumb web space is generally associated with progressive central deficiency (Fig. 28). In type I (a normal web), there is no narrowing (Fig. 29, *left*). In type II (a narrowed web), the web space is narrowed either mildly (type IIA; Fig. 29, *center*) or severely (type IIB; Fig. 25, *left*). In type III (a syndactylized web), the thumb and index rays are syndactylized (Fig. 29, *right*), with complete obliteration of the web space. In type IV (a merged web), the elements of the ray of the index finger are completely suppressed and the web space of the thumb is merged with the cleft (Fig. 30). In type V (an absent web), in association with the central deficiency, the thumb web space is no longer present; only the ulnar rays remain (Fig. 31).

We have noted that, as the thumb web space becomes progressively more narrowed, syndactylized, and finally, completely absent, the central deficiency progresses as well.[61] In type I, only the long ray is completely or partially deficient. In type IIA, the central ray is completely absent, the two ulnar digits are partially syndactylized, and the middle phalanx of the little fin-

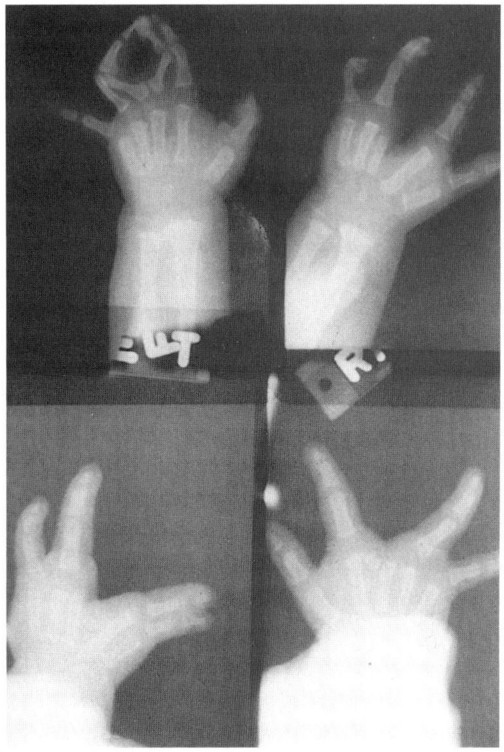

Fig. 26 Radiographs of both hands of identical twins, demonstrating a spectrum of anomalies, including cleft hand, central polydactyly, and osseous syndactyly. (Reproduced with permission from Manske PR: Letter: Cleft hand and central polydactyly in identical twins: A case report. *J Hand Surg* 1983;8A:907.)

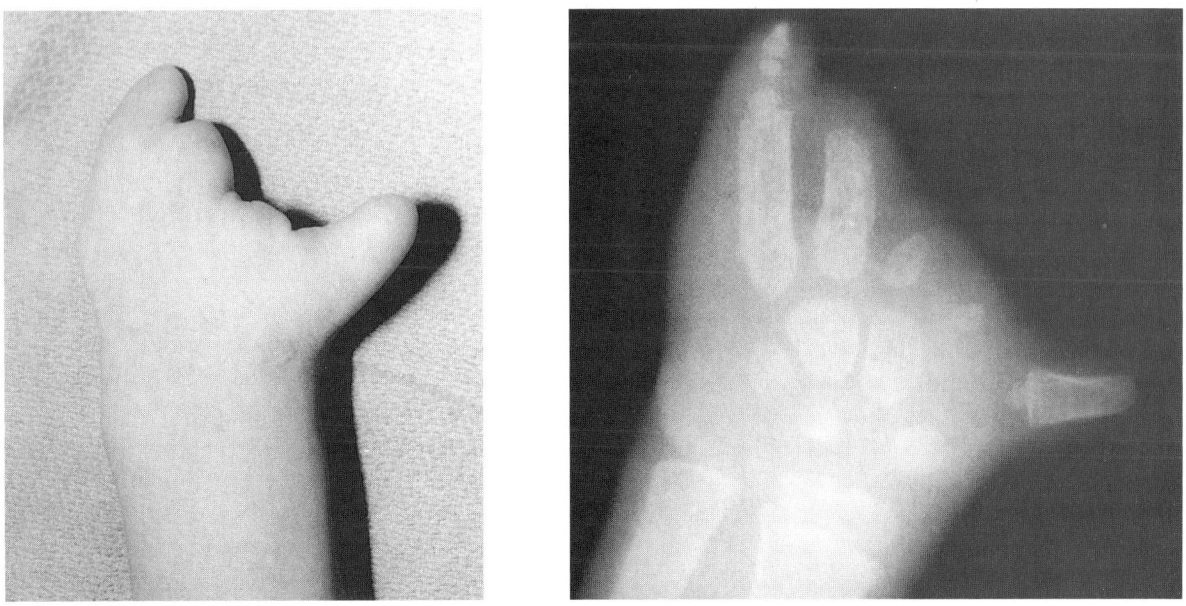

Fig. 27 Left, Photograph showing a form of symbrachydactyly formerly known as atypical cleft hand. The border digits are hypoplastic, and there is redundant skin in the central portion of the hand. **Right,** Radiograph of the same hand, showing small border digits and the potential block to pinching by the rudimentary central metacarpals.

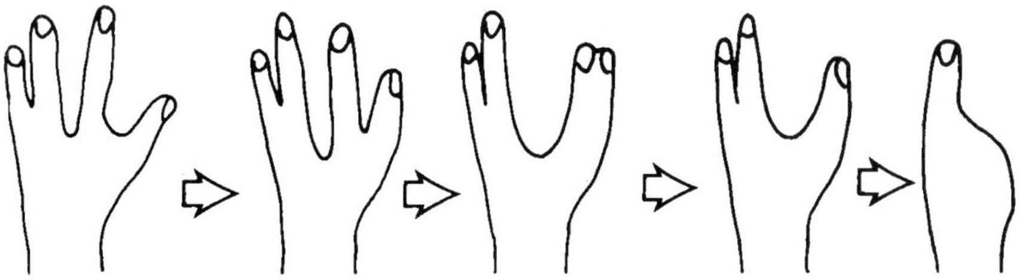

Fig. 28 Diagram showing the classification of central deficiency according to the progressive narrowing of the thumb web space.

Table 3
Surgical procedures for the treatment of central deficiency

Type	Thumb Web Space	Central Deficiency
Type I	None	Closure of cleft with local tissue Reduction of intermetacarpal space Circumferential tendon graft Attachment of local tissue to metacarpal heads Transposition of index metacarpal to base of third metacarpal Excision of polydactylous bone ossicles as needed
Type IIA	Local pedicle flap (z-plasty)	As described for type I
Type IIB	Dorsally or volarly based pedicle flap from cleft as needed	As described for type I
Type III	Release of syndactyly with skin grafts; dorsally or volarly based pedicle flap from cleft or excision of osseous elements from index finger	As described for type I, or excision of index ray
Type IV	None, or reduction of tissue and stabilization of metacarpophalangeal joint	None (cleft is web space)
Type V	Consider toe-to-hand transfer or lengthening of metacarpal	None

ger is somewhat hypoplastic. Type IIB represents a transition between the less involved type-IIA hands and the more extensively involved type-III hands. In type III, the long ray is absent and the index ray is syndactylized to the thumb, with suppressed development of the osseous structures; the ring finger is absent in about one half of hands. In type IV, the index and long rays are absent, with abnormal osseous structures or instability of the metacarpophalangeal joint in most hands. In type V, the long, index, and thumb rays are completely absent and there are associated deformities of the ulnar rays as well.

Surgical Treatment There are two components in the surgical treatment of the cleft hand. The first component is closure of the cleft. Although not functionally disabling, the cleft is so unusual in appearance that the patient often becomes the subject of social curiosity, and closure is appropriate for aesthetic reasons alone. The second component addresses the primary functional problem with the reconstruction of the thumb web space (Table 3).

The normal (type I) web space and the merged (type IV) web space are functionally stable and need essentially no reconstructive procedures; the only surgery for a type IV deficiency is stabilization of the metacarpophalangeal joint without reconstruction of the web space. Procedures for type IIA deficiencies involve reconstruction of a normal (type I) web space with use of local z-plasty flaps from the web itself. Procedures for type IIB deficiencies involve use of a dorsally or palmarly based transposition flap from the cleft to reconstruct a normal web space. Procedures for type III deficiencies involve reconstruction of a normal web space with use of a dorsally or palmarly based flap,

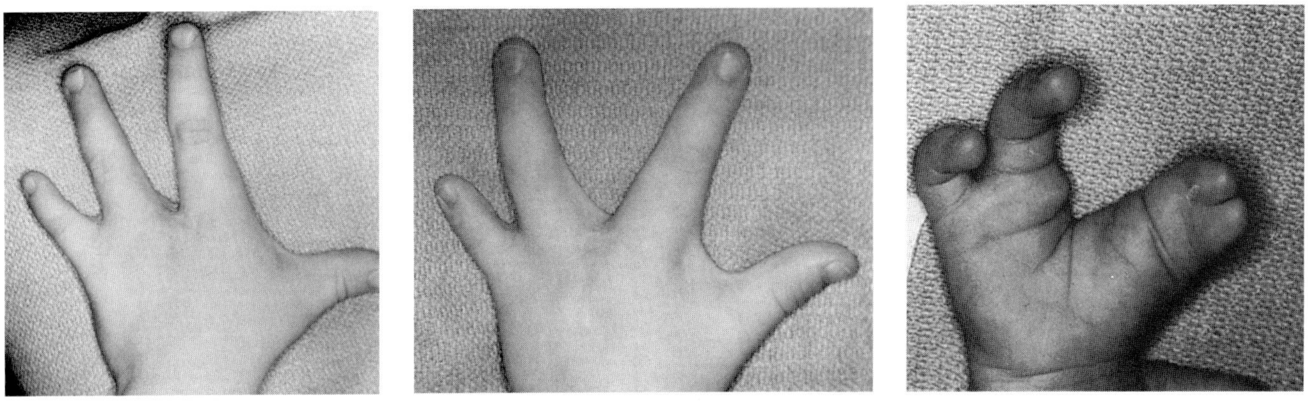

Fig. 29 Left, Type I central deficiency with a normal thumb web space. The long finger is absent, and the cleft has closed postoperatively. **Center,** Type IIA central deficiency with a mildly narrowed web space. The long finger is absent, and the cleft has closed postoperatively. **Right,** Type III central deficiency with a syndactylized web space between the thumb and the index finger.

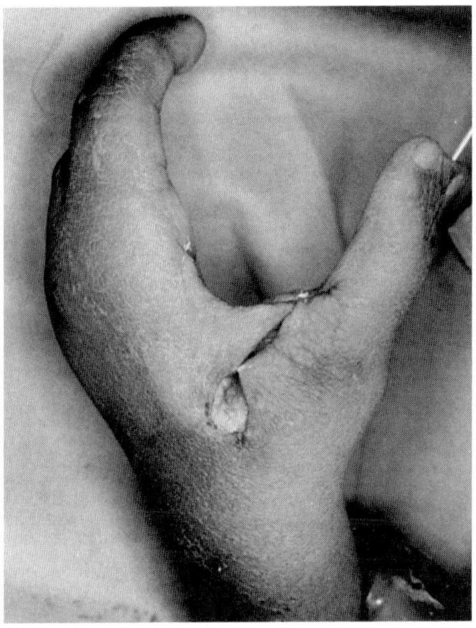

Fig. 30 Type IV central deficiency with merged thumb web and cleft. The index and long fingers are absent. The patient had excision of excess soft tissue and arthrodesis of an unstable metacarpophalangeal joint.

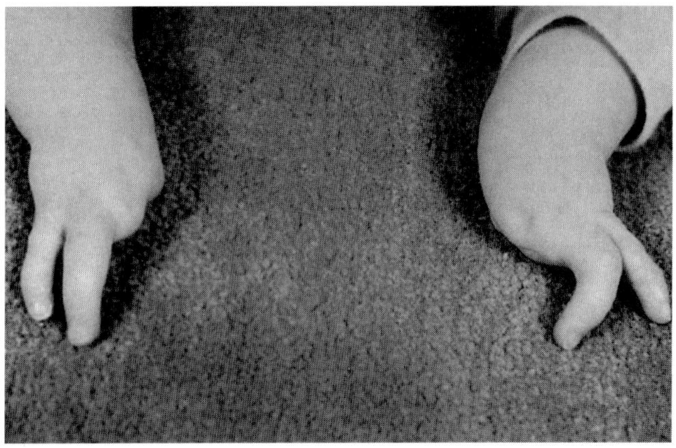

Fig. 31 Type V central deficiency with complete absence of thumb, index finger, and long finger. The web space is absent.

or both, from the cleft, along with release of the syndactyly and skin-grafting or, alternatively, reconstruction of a merged (type IV) web space by excising the index ray elements if they are rudimentary. Reconstruction of the type V cleft hand should be undertaken with caution as many patients function well despite the apparent deficiency; reconstruction of a thumb with use of a toe-to-hand free-tissue transfer[72,73] would result in a merged web space.

The first component of surgical treatment is closure of the cleft. Various skin incisions and local flaps have been proposed to accomplish this;[60,66,74] common to all is the elevation of the dorsal or the palmar skin, or both, to close the major portion of the cleft and the formation of a commissure with use of skin at the distal part of the cleft (Fig. 32). I elevate a dorsally based skin flap and a volarly based skin flap from the opposite side of the cleft, using a common vertical incision line at the depth of the cleft. Two short, distally based flaps are elevated at the distal part of both sides of the cleft, near the level of the metacarpophalangeal flexion crease, to form the interdigital commissure. The commissural flaps are sutured together to form the interdigital web, thereby narrowing the widened interdigital space. The dorsally and volarly based flaps are sutured to the volar and dorsal incision lines, thereby closing the cleft, and the excess skin from the flaps is excised.

In addition to closing the skin defect, the surgeon must narrow the palm by constructing a transverse metacarpal ligament (using local tissue attached to the metacarpals or a circumferential tendon graft) (Fig. 33, *left*) or must transpose the metacarpal of the index finger in an ulnar direction to the rudimentary base of the third metacarpal (Fig. 33, *right*). If the intermeta carpal space is not closed or stabilized, the digits will diverge over time and the deformity will recur within the closed skin envelope. As a general rule, reconstruction of the transverse metacarpal ligament is used for types I and IIA deficiencies whereas transposition of the metacarpal is used for more severely narrowed web spaces to facilitate reconstruction of the thumb web space. The technique for reconstruction of the thumb web space varies according to the type of central deficiency.

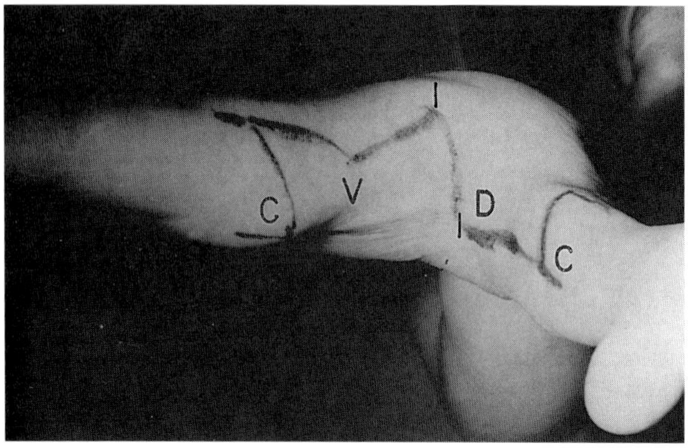

Fig. 32 Preoperative photograph showing the incisions used to create dorsal (D), volar (V), and commissural (C) flaps. The vertical incision (I) is at the base of the cleft.

Type IIA deficiencies Many standard techniques have been used to widen the mildly narrowed web space of the thumb, including the standard z-plasty or one of the four-flap or five-flap webplasties.[75,76]

Type IIB deficiencies When the web space is more severely narrowed, the amount of local skin is insufficient. Therefore, a dorsally based[77] (Fig. 34) or palmarly based[78] (Fig. 35) flap is transposed from the cleft into the web space. Split-thickness skin grafts are frequently needed. I prefer to transpose dorsal skin (Fig. 36), as it is more important to have pliable skin on the dorsal aspect of the web space than on the palmar side. At times, both dorsal and volar flaps are obtained from the cleft. Ulnar transposition of the metacarpal of the index finger facilitates deepening and widening of the web space between the thumb and the index finger.

Type III deficiencies Syndactyly of the thumb and the index finger is the most difficult pattern of central deficiency to treat. Priority is given to reconstructing the thumb web space; if this is not possible, the surgeon must consider excising the osseous elements of the index ray to form a merged space between the thumb

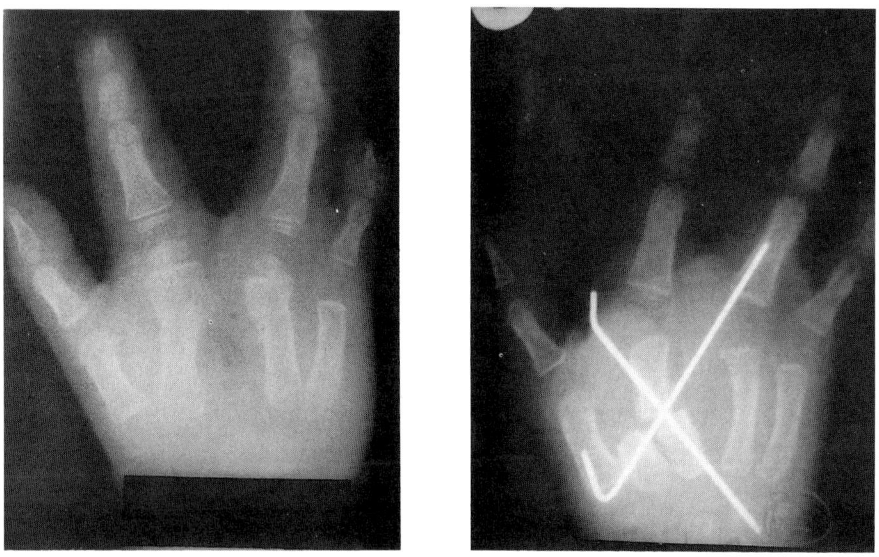

Fig. 33 **Left,** Postoperative radiograph after cleft closure and construction of a transverse metacarpal ligament using soft tissue dissected from the facing surfaces of the metacarpals of the index and ring fingers. The thumb web space is narrowed. **Right,** Postoperative radiograph after cleft closure and ulnar transposition of the second metacarpal to the base of the third metacarpal. The immobilizing pins were removed after the site of the osteotomy healed.

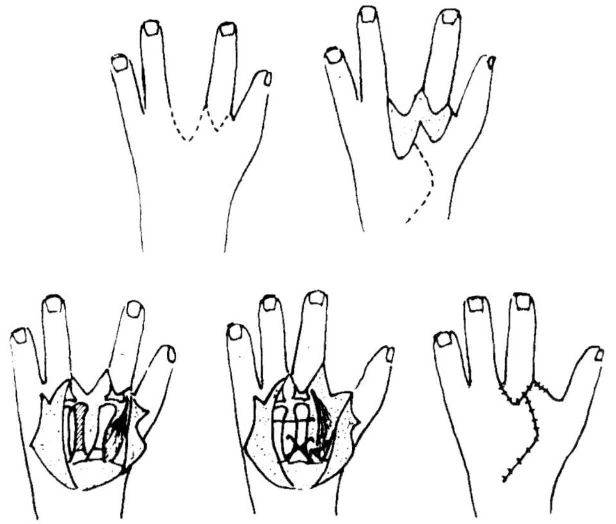

Fig. 34 Diagram showing closure of the cleft and release of the adducted thumb by transposition of a dorsal pedicle flap from the cleft to the web space between the thumb and the index finger. Ulnar transposition of the index ray to the base of the third metacarpal was also performed. (Reproduced with permission from Miura T, Komada T: Simple method for reconstruction of the cleft hand with an adducted thumb. *Plast Reconstr Surg* 1979;64:65-67.)

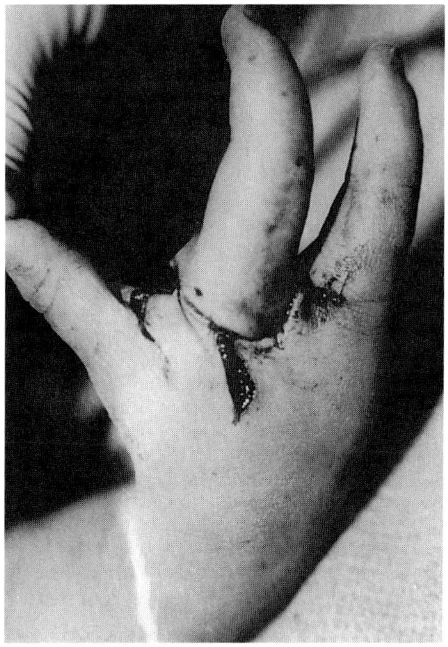

Fig. 36 Photograph made after closure of the cleft and transposition of the dorsal skin flap to the web space between the thumb and the index finger to release the adducted thumb.

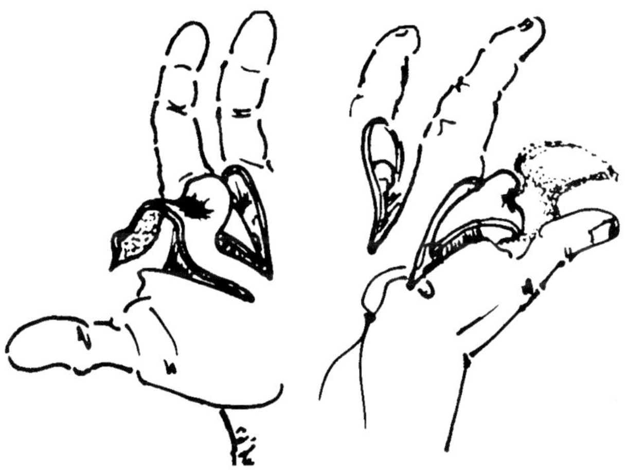

Fig. 35 Drawing showing release of the adducted thumb by transposition of a volarly based pedicle flap from the cleft to the web space between the thumb and the index finger. (Reproduced with permission from Snow JW, Littler JW: Surgical treatment of cleft hand, in Sanvenero-Rosselli G (ed): *Transactions of the Fourth International Congress of Plastic and Reconstructive Surgery*. Amsterdam, The Netherlands, Excerpta Medica Foundation, 1969, pp 888-893.)

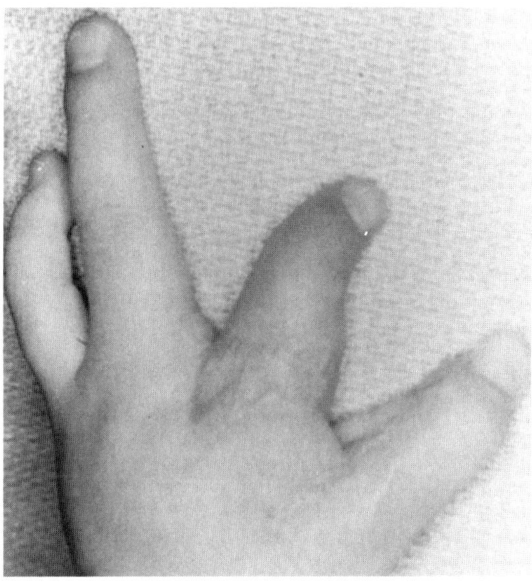

Fig. 37 Photograph of the same hand as seen in Fig. 29, *right*, after transposition of dorsal and volarly based flaps from the cleft.

web space and the cleft. Reconstruction involves separation of the syndactyly in addition to formation of the web space. A staged operation has been proposed in which the syndactylized digits are released initially and the web space is reconstructed later;[79] however, I prefer to accomplish both in a single operation. The syndactylized digits are released in a standard fashion, using skin grafts as necessary to fill in the uncovered areas. Both the palmar and the dorsally based flaps are often needed to create an adequate web space, and

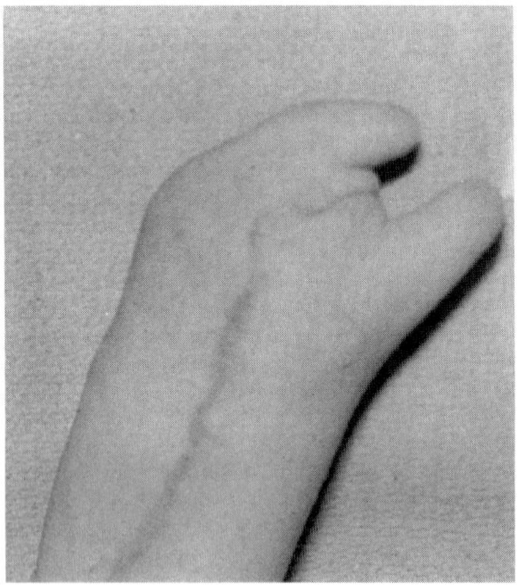

Fig. 38 Photograph of the same hand as seen in Fig. 27, after excision of the central metacarpals and the redundant skin to facilitate a pincer mechanism.

transposition of the index metacarpal to the middle metacarpal is usually necessary. The extensor or flexor tendons, or both, may be commonly joined and must be separated longitudinally; however, if they have a common muscle, independent function of the thumb and the index finger will be limited. Function is also impaired by the shortened index finger, which frequently has a delta-shaped middle phalanx that creates an inclination of the digit toward the thumb after the syndactyly has been separated (Fig. 37). Despite the persistent abnormalities, reconstruction of the thumb web space is considered worthwhile because it improves the appearance of the hand.

Type IV deficiencies Surgical procedures directed at the merged thumb web space and the cleft are usually not necessary, as the increased distance between the thumb and the ulnar digits is usually not a functional problem. If there is excess skin in the merged space, it can be reduced by excision. In a few hands, instability of the metacarpophalangeal joint of the thumb may necessitate an arthrodesis.

Type V deficiencies Toe-to-hand free-tissue transfer to provide an oppositional post for the monodactylous small finger may be considered. However, this procedure should be chosen with caution as many of these patients also have central deficiency of the feet, which precludes removal of the toes.

Treatment of the Symbrachydactyly-Cleft Hand Deformity In this condition (formerly known as atypical cleft hand), the central digits are absent and there are only remnants of the rays of the thumb and small finger on the radial and ulnar borders. The ability of these remnants to function as pincers may be blocked by interposed rudimentary metacarpals or skinfolds (Fig. 38). The surgeon should consider resection of the redundant skin, soft-tissue elements, and central rudimentary metacarpals to create a deeper cleft and facilitate the function of the border rays. Although the procedure may not make the hand more aesthetically attractive, it improves function. Microsurgical techniques now make it possible to transfer toes to lengthen the border digits or to provide additional central digits. Although it has not been established that such procedures provide any functional benefit, in time they may be recommended.

Ulnar Deficiency

Congenital ulnar deficiency includes a spectrum of developmental anomalies of the ulnar border of the upper limb. Although the abnormalities follow a longitudinal axis, ulnar deficiency is not the exact counterpart of radial deficiency. The anomalies in ulnar deficiency occur on both the ulnar and the radial side of the hand. Ulnar deficiency is the least common manifestation of failure of formation of the upper extremity. In an excellent review of ulnar deficiencies, Johnson and Omer[80] identified only 185 reported cases. Nearly one half of the patients had an anomaly (although not necessarily ulnar deficiency) of the contralateral hand, and almost one half had other musculoskeletal abnormalities. Associated hematologic, cardiac, gastrointestinal, and genitourinary anomalies occur only rarely.

Ogino and associates[3,81] produced ulnar deficiencies in pregnant Gunn-Wistar rats by administering Myleran, a teratogenic agent, at 8.5 to 10 days of gestation. The critical period for producing ulnar deficiencies was earlier than that for producing radial deficiencies and corresponded to higher rates of fetal mortality. This may explain the relative rarity of these deformities.

Five different classification systems for ulnar deficiency have been proposed,[82-87] based primarily the radiographic status of the ulna. I prefer the classification suggested by Bayne.[82] In this system (Fig. 39), type I indicates a hypoplastic ulna; type II, partial ulnar aplasia; type III, total ulnar aplasia; and type IV, radiohumeral synostosis. None of the classification systems corresponds to specific abnormalities of the hand. Furthermore, none includes the ulnar-deficient hand (a hand without the fourth and fifth rays) with a normal ulna (Fig. 40), which is the counterpart of the radial-deficient hand from which the thumb is absent and the radius is normal.

Ogino and Kato[81] classified the abnormalities of the hand according to the number of missing ulnar rays, but they did not describe the status of the deficient

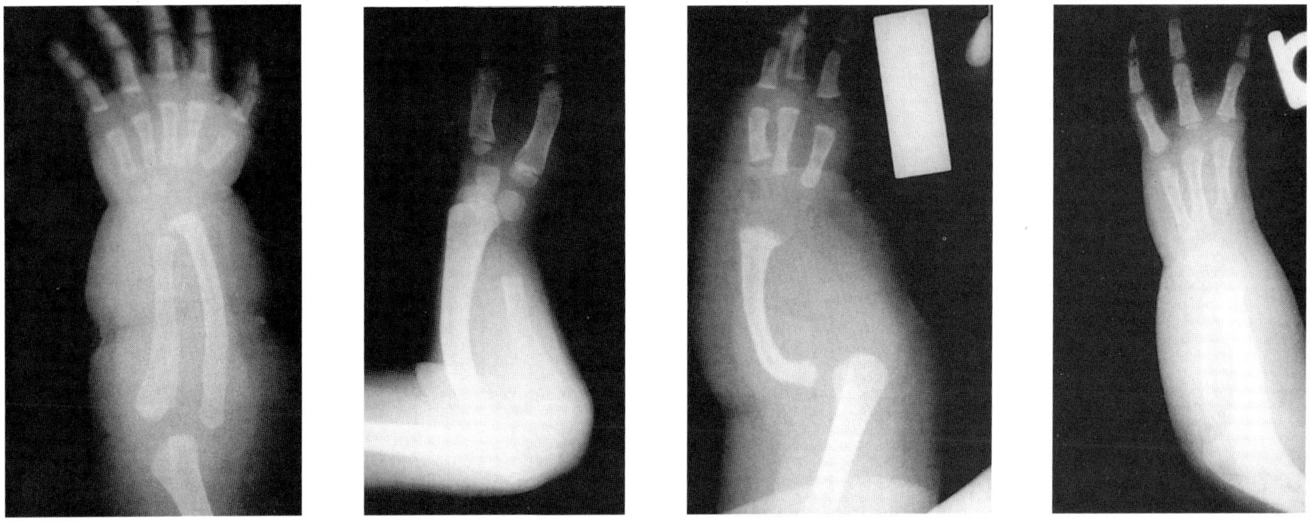

Fig. 39 **Left,** Type-I ulnar deficiency, characterized by hypoplasia of the distal part of the ulna in association with ulnar tilt of the distal radial epiphysis and probable dislocation of the radial head. The five-digit hand has a normal appearance. **Center left,** Type-II ulnar deficiency with partial aplasia of the ulna. There is bowing of the radius and dislocation of the radial head. The elbow has a limited range of motion but is stable. **Center right,** Type-III ulnar deficiency with total absence of the ulna. There is bowing of the radius and dislocation of the radial head. The elbow is stable. **Right,** Type-IV ulnar deficiency with a radiohumeral synostosis. A rudimentary ulna persists. Note the three-digit hand with absence of the thumb ray.

ulna to the same extent as have Bayne[82] and others,[83-87] nor did they include the absent thumb or other abnormalities of the hand.

Skeletal Abnormalities

Although the entire upper extremity may be hypoplastic, the most functionally limiting abnormalities are in the elbow, forearm, wrist, and hand.

The Elbow The appearance and function of the elbow vary considerably, depending on the position of the radial head. The range of motion may be normal or only slightly limited when there is a reduced radial head. The elbow may be stable but have limited motion because of a soft-tissue flexion contracture. In the most functionally limiting deformity, the elbow may be in a fixed position because of a radiohumeral synostosis (Fig. 39, *right*). Infrequently, the elbow is unstable because of a complete absence of the ulna.

The Forearm and the Wrist In congenital ulnar deficiency, the radius is always present, providing a stable articulation at the wrist. In a review of 185 cases in the literature, Johnson and Omer[80] reported that the ulna was completely absent in 22%, partially absent in 61%, and hypoplastic in 16%. Even when the ulna was hypoplastic or only partially absent, radial and ulnar growth occurred at relatively equal rates in eight patients. The extremity is usually shortened, and adequate motion of the wrist is retained, so that the shortened extremity can be used in conjunction with the contralateral extremity or to hold objects against the body.

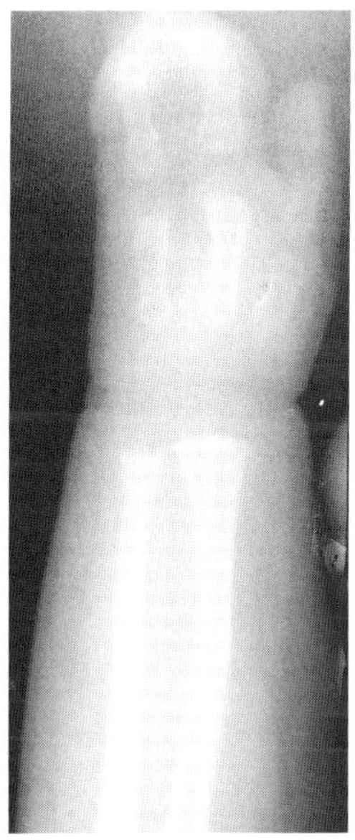

Fig. 40 Radiograph of an extremity that has deficient ulnar rays but a normal ulna. The classification systems currently in use do not describe this form of ulnar deficiency.

The most serious abnormality is marked rotation (pronation) or anterior bowing, or both, of the forearm, which orients the hand in an internally rotated or posterior direction, or both (Fig. 41). This condition usually occurs in patients who have a radiohumeral synostosis.

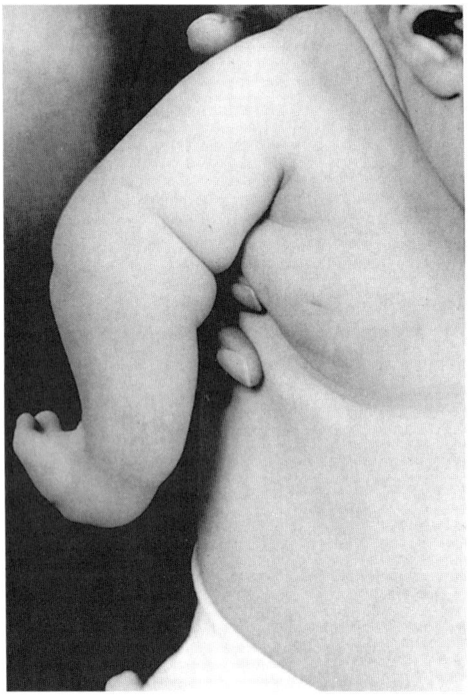

Fig. 41 Ulnar deficiency with anterior bowing and fixed pronation of the forearm. A corrective osteotomy was performed.

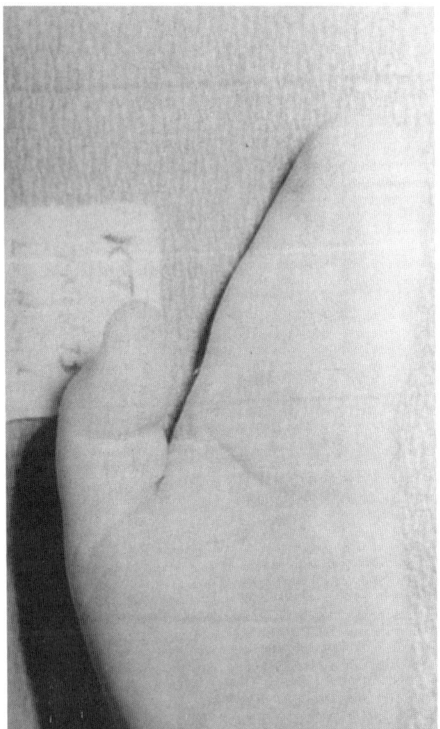

Fig. 42 Ulnar dysplasia characterized by absent ulnar rays and syndactyly of the remaining digits.

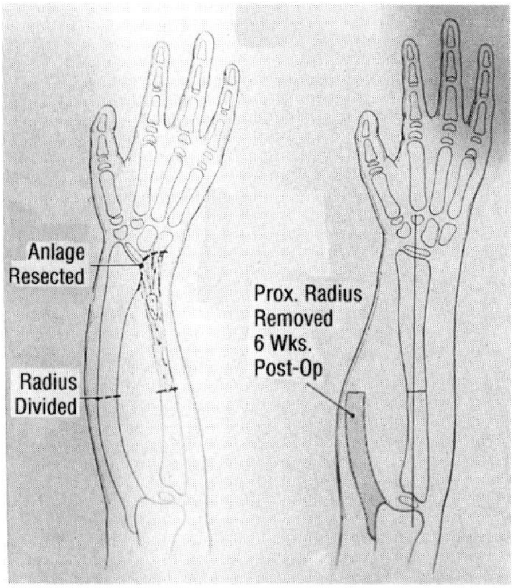

Fig. 43 The surgical procedure for the creation of a one-bone forearm with use of the radius and the partially deficient ulna. The procedure is recommended only if the forearm is unstable. (Reproduced with permission from Bayne LG: Ulnar club hand [ulnar deficiencies], in Green DP (ed): *Operative Hand Surgery*, ed 3. New York, NY, Churchill Livingstone, 1993, vol 1, p 303.)

The wrist is usually stable, but it may be deviated toward the ulna secondary to the absence of the ulnar carpal bones or secondary to ulnar tilt of the distal radial epiphysis, or both. The appearance of ulnar deviation may be accentuated by radial bowing. The ulnar deviation is thought to be nonprogressive and rarely results in a functional disability.

A fibrous cartilaginous anlage connects the distal part of the partially aplastic ulna to the distal radius and carpal bones.[60,85,88-90] Although the presence of the anlage is well recognized, its role in the creation of the various deformities of the forearm and the wrist has not been established conclusively. The anlage has been thought to act as a static tether that may be responsible for the decreased growth at the distal radial epiphysis, ulnar deviation of the wrist and the hand, bowing of the radius, or dislocation of the radial head. However, other investigators[80,84,91,92] have noted that these deformities are relatively static and have thought that the role of the anlage in their development is minimum.

The Hand The abnormalities frequently affect the ulnar side of the hand but may occur on the radial side as well. These abnormalities, which include complete digital absence, syndactyly, and digital malrotation, constitute the primary disability of patients who have ulnar deficiency. In their review of 185 cases, Johnson and Omer[80] found that syndactyly (Fig. 42) occurred in 34%; at least one absent digit, not necessarily restricted to the ulnar side of the hand, in 89%; and abnormalities of the thumb ray (an interesting observation with respect to developmental anatomy), in more than 50%.

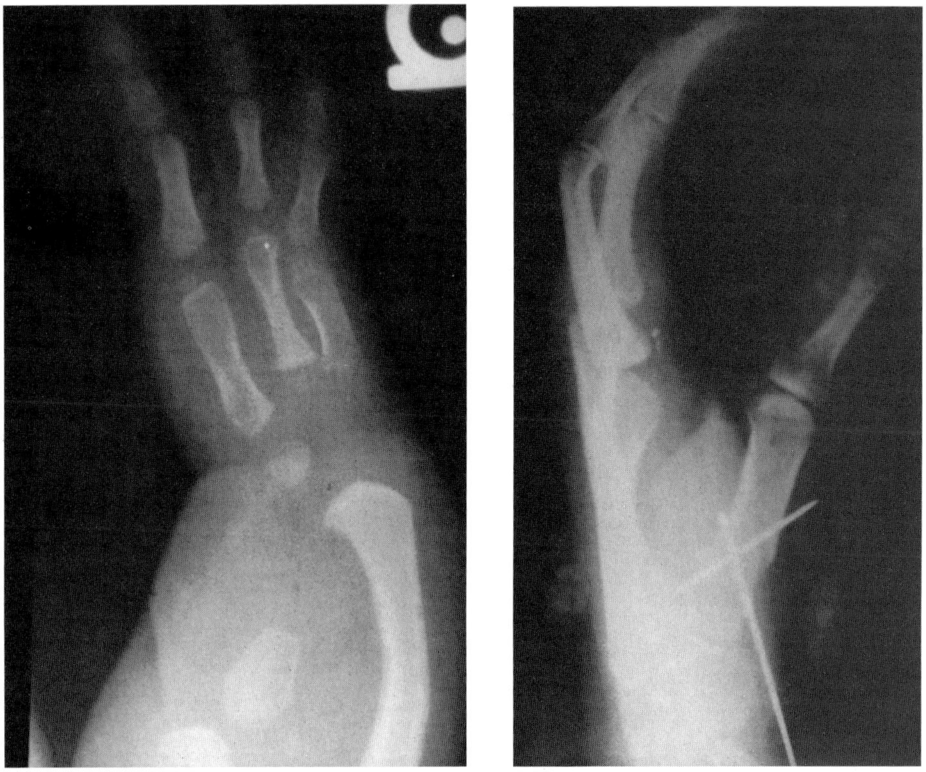

Fig. 44 Radiographs of a hand with absent ulnar rays. **Left,** Preoperative radiograph shows marked adduction of the thumb. **Right,** Postoperative radiograph, made after deepening of the web space between the thumb and the index finger and rotational osteotomy of the first metacarpal, shows that the thumb is now in opposition to the remaining digits.

Surgical Treatment

Despite the obvious deformities, patients with ulnar deficiency usually have few functional limitations[60,93] and surgery is infrequently indicated. However, several procedures for the forearm and the hand should be considered. Forearm procedures include corrective osteotomy of the radius, resection of the radial head, and construction of a one-bone forearm.

Corrective osteotomy of the radius is indicated when there is a severe anterior bow that positions the hand posteriorly (Fig. 41). The hand and the digits can be placed in a more functional position with use of multiple closing-wedge osteotomies.[84] Occasionally, a rotational osteotomy must also be performed to correct severe fixed pronation.

Resection[60,82] of a prominent, dislocated radial head is infrequently necessary because the elbow is usually stable and functions well despite the dislocation; resection alone does not usually improve motion because of the associated abnormalities of the forearm. The indications for resection of the radial head include complaints by the patient of pain or an unsightly appearance. The resection should preferably be performed at the time of skeletal maturity.

Construction of a one-bone forearm[82,88-90] or establishment of a proximal radioulnar synostosis[94] must also be considered in the unusual circumstance of forearm instability. I prefer the two-stage technique described by Bayne[82] (Fig. 43).

Resection of the fibrocartilaginous anlage has been strongly recommended by some authors[60,85,89,90] on the premise that the anlage has a tethering action on the radius and the carpal bones and is responsible for the evolution of the deformities. In previous studies,[80,84,91,92,95] notable functional improvement was not found after such resection, and no report, to my knowledge, has documented progressive deformity when the anlage has not been excised. Consequently, a more critical evaluation of this procedure is needed. Resection of the anlage is recommended only when progression of the deformity can be clearly documented.

Surgical procedures for a patient who has ulnar deficiency are more frequently performed to correct deformities of the hand, particularly abnormalities of the thumb or syndactylized digits. Release of syndactylized fingers using established techniques can increase the function of the limited number of digits that are present. Deepening of the web space between the thumb

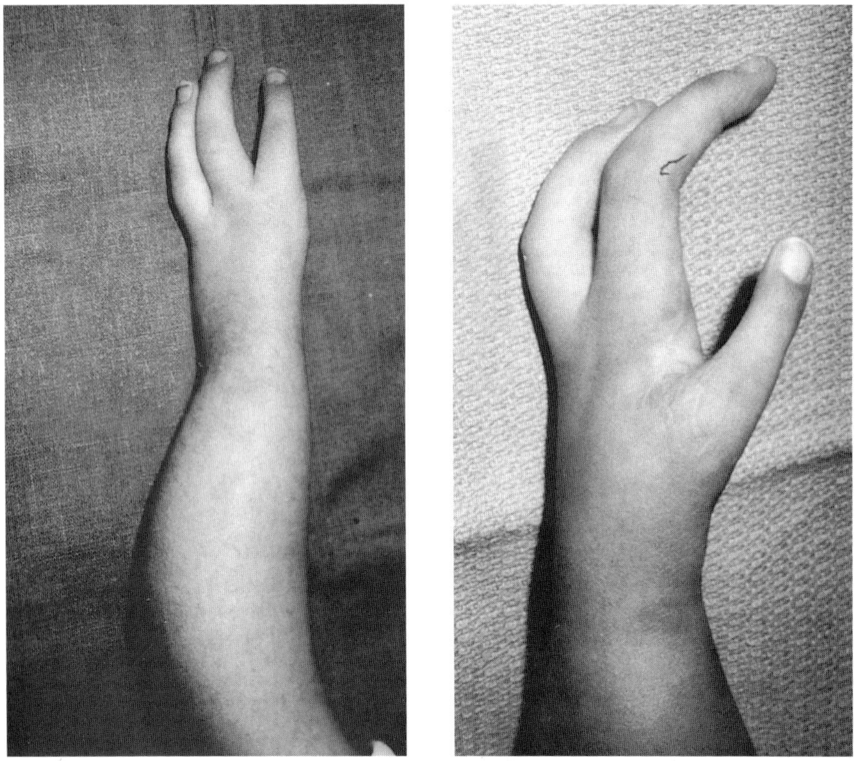

Fig. 45 Absent thumb ray. **Left,** Preoperative photograph shows three digits and an absent thumb ray. **Right,** Postoperative appearance of the hand after pollicization.

and the index finger and rotational osteotomy of the first metacarpal (Fig. 44) or pollicization (Fig. 45) can provide more effective opposition for grasping, and improved function after correction of the deformities can be anticipated.[60,80]

References

1. Beatty E: Upper limb tissue differentiation in the human embryo. *Hand Clin* 1985;1:391–403.
2. Pardini AG Jr: Letter: Radial dysplasia. *Clin Orthop* 1968; 57:153–177.
3. Kato H, Ogino T, Minami A, et al: Experimental study of radial ray deficiency. *J Hand Surg* 1990;15B:470–476.
4. Fanconi G: Familial constitutional panmyelocytopathy, Fanconi's anemia (F.A.): I. Clinical aspects. *Semin Hematol* 1967;4:233–240.
5. Goldberg MJ, Bartoshesky LE: Congenital hand anomaly: Etiology and associated malformations. *Hand Clin* 1985;1: 405–415.
6. Goldberg MJ, Meyn M: The radial clubhand. *Orthop Clin North Am* 1976;7:341–349.
7. Holt M, Oram S: Familial heart disease with skeletal malformations. *Br Heart J* 1960;22:236–242.
8. Quan L, Smith DW: The VATER association: Vertebral defects, Anal atresia, T-E fistula with esophageal atresia, Radial and Renal dysplasia: A spectrum of associated defects. *J Pediatr* 1973;82:104–107.
9. Schoenecker PL, Cohn AK, Sedgwick WG, et al: Dysplasia of the knee associated with the syndrome of thrombocytopenia and absent radius. *J Bone Joint Surg* 1984;66A:421–427.
10. Temtamy SA, McKusick VA, Bergsma D, et al (eds): *The Genetics of Hand Malformations.* New York, NY, Alan R Liss, 1978.
11. Manske PR, McCarroll HR Jr: Abductor digiti minimi opponensplasty in congenital radial dysplasia. *J Hand Surg* 1978;3A: 552–559.
12. Manske PR, McCarroll HR Jr, Swanson K: Centralization of the radial club hand: An ulnar surgical approach. *J Hand Surg* 1981;6A:423–433.
13. Bayne LG: Radial club hand (radial deficiencies), in Green DP (ed): *Operative Hand Surgery*, ed 2. New York, NY, Churchill Livingstone, 1988, vol 1, pp 261–275.
14. Skerik S, Flatt AE: The anatomy of congenital radial dysplasia: Its surgical and functional implications. *Clin Orthop* 1969;66: 125–143.
15. Lamb DW: Radial club hand: A continuing study of sixty-eight patients with one hundred and seventeen club hands. *J Bone Joint Surg* 1977;59A:1–13.
16. Petit JL: Remarques sur un enfant nouveau–né, dont les bras etaint difformes. *Mem Acad Roy Sci* vol 17, 1733.
17. Lloyd-Roberts GC (ed): *Orthopaedics in Infancy and Childhood.* New York, NY, Appleton-Century-Crofts, 1971.
18. Lidge RT: Abstract: Congenital radial deficient club hand. *J Bone Joint Surg* 1969;51A:1041–1042.
19. Bora FW Jr, Osterman AL, Kaneda RR, et al: Radial club-hand deformity: Long-term follow-up. *J Bone Joint Surg* 1981;63A: 741–745.
20. Kessler I: Centralisation of the radial club hand by gradual distraction. *J Hand Surg* 1989;14B:37–42.
21. Sayre RH: A contribution to the study of club-hand. *Trans Am Orthop Assn* 1893;6:208–216.
22. Cromack DT, Strecker WB, Manske PR: The presurgical treatment of the radial club hand. *Orthop Trans* 1995–1996; 19:833–834.
23. Bardenheuer B: Vorstellung von 4 Patienten, an welchen die totale Resektion des ganzen Hüftgelenkes ausgeführt worden war. *Ber Verh Deutsche Gesell Chir* 1894;23:105–107.

24. Hoffa A (ed): Lehrbuch der Orthopädischen Chirurgie, ed 4. Stuttgart, Germany, Ferdinand Enke, 1902.
25. Romano C: Grave mano torta congenita: Raddrizzamento mercè osteoectomia segmentaria trapezoidale del cubito e tenotomia del muscolo grande palmare. *Arch Ortop* 1894;11:80–93.
26. Albee FH: Formation of radius congenitally absent: Condition seven years after implantation of bone graft. *Ann Surg* 1928; 87:105–110.
27. Antonelli I: Sur un caso di mancanza congenita bilaterale del radio. *Gazz Med Italiana* 1904;55:501–513.
28. Define D: Treatment of congenital radial club hand. *Clin Orthop* 1970;73:153–159.
29. Kato K: Congenital absence of the radius: With review of literature and report of three cases. *J Bone Joint Surg* 1924;6:589–626.
30. Starr DE: Congenital absence of the radius: A method of surgical correction. *J Bone Joint Surg* 1945;27:572–577.
31. Tsai TM: Free epiphyseal transfer. *Orthop Trans* 1985;9:409–410.
32. Yamauchi Y: Vascularized epiphyseal transfers: Animal experiments and some clinical experiences. *Orthop Trans* 1985;9:409.
33. Vilkki SK: Distraction lengthening and microvascular bone transplantation in the treatment of radial club hand, in Canadell J, Forriol F, Lato-Zhikowsky J (eds): *The Congress Book of the 14th International Hoffmann External Fixation Conference.* Granada, Spain, 1992, pp 245–251.
34. Rayan GM: Ulnocarpal arthrodesis for recurrent radial club-hand deformity in adolescents. *J Hand Surg* 1992;17A:24–27.
35. Bora FW Jr, Nicholson JT, Cheema HM: Radial meromelia: The deformity and its treatment. *J Bone Joint Surg* 1970;52A:966–979.
36. Buck-Gramcko D: Radialization as a new treatment for radial club hand. *J Hand Surg* 1985;10A:964–968.
37. Watson HK, Beebe RD, Cruz NI: A centralization procedure for radial clubhand. *J Hand Surg* 1984;9A:541–547.
38. Blauth W, Schneider-Sickert F (eds): Numerical variations, in *Congenital Deformities of the Hand: An Atlas of Their Surgical Treatment.* Berlin, Germany, Springer-Verlag, 1981, pp 119–223.
39. Buck-Gramcko D: Hypoplasia and aplasia of the thumb, in Nigst H, Buck-Gramcko D, Millesi H, et al (eds): *Hand Surgery.* Stuttgart, Germany, Georg Thieme Verlag, 1988, vol 1, pp 12.93–12.94.
40. Manske PR, McCarroll HR Jr, James M: Type III-A hypoplastic thumb. *J Hand Surg* 1995;20A:246–253.
41. Manske PR, McCarroll HR Jr: Reconstruction of the congenitally deficient thumb. *Hand Clin* 1992;8:177–196.
42. Tupper JW: Pollex abductus due to congenital malposition of the flexor pollicis longus. *J Bone Joint Surg* 1969;51A:1285–1290.
43. Kowalski MF, Manske PR: Arthrodesis of digital joints in children. *J Hand Surg* 1988;13A:874–879.
44. Huber E: Hilfsoperation bei Medianuslähmung. *Deutsche Zeitschr Chir* 1921;162:271–275.
45. Nicolaysen J: Abstract: Transplantation du muscle abducteur du petit doigt, dans un cas d'incapacité de movement d'opposition du ponce. *Acta Chir Scand* 1923;55:183–184.
46. Dunlap J, Manske PR, McCarthy JA: Perfusion of the abductor digiti quinti after transfer on a neurovascular pedicle. *J Hand Surg* 1989;14A:992–995.
47. Buck-Gramcko D: Pollicization of the index finger: Method and results in aplasia and hypoplasia of the thumb. *J Bone Joint Surg* 1971;53A:1605–1617.
48. Littler JW: The neurovascular pedicle method of digital transposition for reconstruction of the thumb. *Plast Reconstr Surg* 1953;12:303–319.
49. Manske PR, McCarroll HR Jr: Index finger pollicization for a congenitally absent or nonfunctioning thumb. *J Hand Surg* 1985;10A:606–613.
50. Manske PR, Rotman MB, Dailey LA: Long-term functional results after pollicization for the congenitally deficient thumb. *J Hand Surg* 1992;17A:1064–1072.
51. Egloff DV, Verdan C: Pollicization of the index finger for reconstruction of the congenitally hypoplastic or absent thumb. *J Hand Surg* 1983;8A:839–848.
52. Lister G: Reconstruction of the hypoplastic thumb. *Clin Orthop* 1985;195:52–65.
53. Hartsinck JJ (ed): Beschryving van Guiana, of de Wilde Kust in Zuid-America. Amsterdam, The Netherlands, G Tielenburg, 1770, vol 2, pp 811–812.
54. Nutt JN III, Flatt AE: Congenital central hand deficit. *J Hand Surg* 1981;6A:48–60.
55. Ogino T: Cleft hand. *Hand Clin* 1990;6:661–671.
56. Saito H, Seki T, Suzuki Y, et al: Operative treatments for various types of the cleft hand. *Seikagaku* 1978;29:1551–1553.
57. Maisels DO: Lobster-claw deformities of the hand. *Hand* 1970;2:79–82.
58. Tada K, Yonenobu K, Swanson AB: Congenital central ray deficiency in the hand: A survey of 59 cases and subclassification. *J Hand Surg* 1981;6A:434–441.
59. Watari S, Tsuge K: A classification of cleft hands, based on clinical findings: Theory of developmental mechanism. *Plast Reconstr Surg* 1979;64:381–389.
60. Flatt AE (ed): *The Care of Congenital Hand Anomalies.* St. Louis, MO, CV Mosby, 1977, pp 265–285.
61. Manske PR, Halikis MN: Surgical classification of central deficiency according to the thumb web. *J Hand Surg* 1995; 20A:687–697.
62. Buck-Gramcko D: Cleft hands: Classification and treatment. *Hand Clin* 1985;1:467–473.
63. Egawa T, Horiki A, Senrui H, et al: Characteristic anatomical findings of the cleft hand: Its significance and classification. *Handchirurgie* 1978;10:3–8.
64. Ogino T: A clinical and experimental study on teratogenic mechanism of cleft hand, polydactyly and syndactyly. *Nippon Seikeigeka Gakkai Zasshi* 1979;53:535–543.
65. Manske PR: Letter: Cleft hand and central polydactyly in identical twins: A case report. *J Hand Surg* 1983;8A:906–908.
66. Barsky AJ: Cleft hand: Classification, incidence, and treatment. Review of the literature and report of nineteen cases. *J Bone Joint Surg* 1964;46A:1707–1720.
67. Blauth W, Gekeler J: Morphology and classification of symbrachydactylia. *Handchirurgie* 1971;3:123–128.
68. Ogino T, Minami A, Kato H: Clinical features and roentgenograms of symbrachydactyly. *J Hand Surg* 1989;14B: 303–306.
69. Manske PR: Letter: Symbrachydactyly instead of atypical cleft hand. *Plast Reconstr Surg* 1993;91:196.
70. Swanson AB: A classification for congenital limb malformations. *J Hand Surg* 1976;1A:8–22.
71. Sandzen SC Jr: Classification and functional management of congenital central defect of the hand. *Hand Clin* 1985;1: 483–498.
72. Gilbert A: Toe transfers for congenital hand defects. *J Hand Surg* 1982;7A:118–124.
73. May JW Jr, Smith RJ, Peimer CA: Toe-to-hand free tissue transfer for thumb construction with multiple digit aplasia. *Plast Reconstr Surg* 1981;67:205–213.
74. Kelikian H (ed): *Congenital Deformities of the Hand and Forearm.* Philadelphia, PA, WB Saunders, 1974, pp 467–489.
75. Hirshowitz B, Karev A, Rousso M: Combined double Z-plasty and Y-V advancement for thumb web contracture. *Hand* 1975;7:291–293.
76. Woolf RM, Broadbent TR: The four-flap Z-plasty. *Plast Reconstr Surg* 1972;49:48–51.
77. Miura T, Komada T: Simple method for reconstruction of the cleft hand with an adducted thumb. *Plast Reconstr Surg* 1979;64:65–67.
78. Snow JW, Littler JW: Surgical treatment of cleft hand, in Boggio-

Robutti G, Sanvenero–Rosselli G (eds): *Transactions of the Fourth International Congress of Plastic and Reconstructive Surgery, Rome, Italy, October 1967.* Amsterdam, The Netherlands, Excerpta Medica Foundation, 1969, pp 888–893.

79. Wood VE: The cleft hand (central deficiencies), in Green DP (ed): *Operative Hand Surgery,* ed 2. New York, NY, Churchill Livingstone, 1988, pp 275–291.
80. Johnson J, Omer GE Jr: Congenital ulnar deficiency: Natural history and therapeutic implications. *Hand Clin* 1985;1:499–510.
81. Ogino T, Kato H: Clinical and experimental studies on ulnar ray deficiency. *Handchir Mikrochir Plast Chir* 1988;20:330–337.
82. Bayne LG: Ulnar club hand (ulnar deficiencies), in Green DP (ed): *Operative Hand Surgery.* New York, NY, Churchill Livingstone, 1982, vol 1, pp 245–257.
83. Kummel W: Die Missbildungen der Extremitäeten durch defekt, Verwachsung und Ueberzahl. Cassel, Germany, TG Fisher, 1895, vol 3.
84. Miller JK, Wenner SM, Kruger LM: Ulnar deficiency. *J Hand Surg* 1986;11A:822–829.
85. Ogden JA, Watson HK, Bohne W: Ulnar dysmelia. *J Bone Joint Surg* 1976;58A:467–475.
86. Riordan DC: The upper limb, in Lovell WW, Winter RB (eds): *Pediatric Orthopaedics.* Philadelphia, PA, JB Lippincott, 1978, vol 2, pp 685–719.
87. Swanson AB, Tada K, Yonenobu K: Ulnar ray deficiency: Its various manifestations. *J Hand Surg* 1984;9A:658–664.
88. Carroll RE, Bowers WH: Congenital deficiency of the ulna. *J Hand Surg* 1977;2A:169–174.
89. Riordan DC, Mills EH, Alldredge RH: Abstract: Congenital absence of the ulna. *J Bone Joint Surg* 1961;43A:614.
90. Straub LR: Congenital absence of the ulna. *Am J Surg* 1965;109:300–305.
91. Broudy AS, Smith RJ: Deformities of the hand and wrist with ulnar deficiency. *J Hand Surg* 1979;4A:304–315.
92. Marcus NA, Omer GE Jr: Carpal deviation in congenital ulnar deficiency. *J Bone Joint Surg* 1984;66A:1003–1007.
93. Pardini AG Jr: Congenital absence of the ulna. *J Iowa Med Soc* 1967;57:1106–1112.
94. Lloyd-Roberts GC: Treatment of defects of the ulna in children by establishing cross-union with the radius. *J Bone Joint Surg* 1973;55B:327–330.
95. Blair WF, Shurr DG, Buckwalter JA: Functional status in ulnar deficiency. *J Pediatr Orthop* 1983;3:37–40

Spine

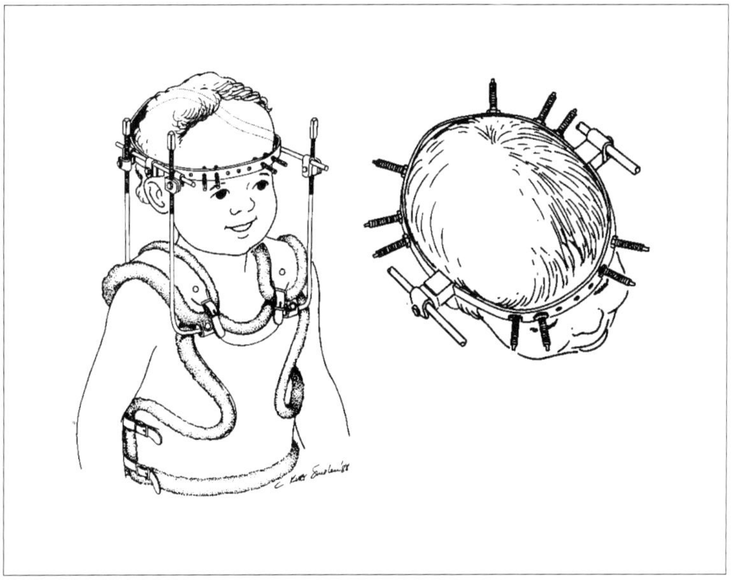

The Management of Acute Spinal Trauma: Prehospital and In-Hospital Emergency Care

Alexander R. Vaccaro, MD
Howard S. An, MD
Randal R. Betz, MD
Jerome M. Cotler, MD
Richard A. Balderston, MD

Prehospital Care

There are approximately 200,000 people in the United States presently living with some degree of spinal cord injury (SCI) resulting from trauma.[1,2] Of the 7,800 to 11,000 new cases each year, it is estimated that 4% to 14% of such injuries occur in children younger than 15 years of age, with a male-to-female ratio of 2.4:1.[3-6] The causes of spinal cord trauma in the adult are varied and include motor vehicle accidents (40%), falls (21%), acts of violence (15%), sports-related injuries (13%), and miscellaneous.[5] Etiologies for pediatric SCI parallel those in adults, with water-related injuries accounting for 13% of the cases and sports-related injuries composing 24% of cases.

In addition to the presence of SCI, 45% to 50% of patients may present with an associated injury, with 15% and 10% of patients having two or three related injuries, respectively.[7] These may include multiple appendicular skeletal fractures, closed head injury and facial fractures, cardiac and pulmonary contusions, thoracic rib fractures, and blunt abdominal injury, including viscus disruption and genitourinary dysfunction. Thoracolumbar and lumbar spine injuries secondary to lap belt injuries in the pediatric patients demand particular attention. Retroperitoneal injuries have been reported in 30% to 50% of patients presenting with these spine fractures,[8,9] and neurologic deficits occur in 4% to 39%.[10-12] The variance in neurologic deficits in the reported series can be attributed to whether the authors studied patients at a SCI center or patients were seen at random in an emergency room. Of pediatric spinal cord injuries, 25% to 50% may present with concomitant head trauma. Recognition of this head trauma is important because resulting perceptual, speech, and other associated deficits can significantly affect the rehabilitation process.[13,14] An additional complicating factor in the management of SCI patients is the presence of subtle noncontiguous spinal injuries, which may result in great morbidity if overlooked. Thus, individual patient morbidity is often greater than 100%, with each patient having one or more complications during the treatment phase.[15]

Aside from the substantial morbidity complicating SCI, significant patient mortality exists, is most pronounced during the initial hospitalization and treatment period, and is further increased in the elderly patient population.[16] Approximately 10% of patients die during the first year following their injury, with fulminant pneumonia (80%) being the most frequent cause of patient demise, followed by heart disease and septicemia.[5] Studies have shown that 1-year mortality rates for quadriplegic patients may range from 7.5% to 40%.[15] Also, patients who are older than 50 years of age have been found to have an overall mortality rate of 23% at 1 year following their accident.[17]

The successful long-term treatment of the patient with a SCI is contingent on early recognition of the injury, prompt medical resuscitation, mechanical stabilization of the injury, prevention of additional neurologic injury, and avoidance of complications. Therefore, effective care of the traumatized patient begins with a clear and comprehensive prehospital management protocol delivered by a well-organized emergency medical service working in tandem with an in-hospital multidisciplinary trauma team at a qualified receiving health care center.[7,15,18,19] The goal of in-field care is to maximize the potential for neurologic recovery from the scene of the accident to the time of patient arrival at the emergency room.[20] With the birth of qualified regional SCI centers over the last two decades, the ratio of incomplete to complete spinal cord injuries and normalization of life expectancy after the first year of injury has increased, largely as a result of improved sophistication of prehospital care givers and the birth of modern Emergency Medical Services (EMS) and Emergency Medical Technicians (EMT).[21,22]

Emergency Medical Services (EMS)

The principles of in-field resuscitation and stabilization of the patient with a SCI owe their development to the exposure of the deficiencies of prehospital care by a 1966 paper entitled, "Accidental Death and Disability—The Neglected Disease of Modern Society," released by the National Academy of Sciences National Research Council Committee on Shock and The Committee on Trauma.[21] Prior to this report, no organized means of prehospital care for multiple trauma victims existed in the United States. As a result of lack of suspicion of significant spinal injury and improper immobilization prior to transport, Toscano[20] reported a 26% incidence of major neurologic deterioration from the time of the accident prior to arrival to the emergency ward. Factors associated with a delay in diagnosis in the field include an altered state of consciousness, lack of suspicious soft-tissue injuries above the clavicle, and concurrent head trauma.[22] The awareness of the need for more efficient management of multiple trauma set in motion a series of recommendations on the national level, which eventually led to the passage of the National Highway Safety Act of 1966 and the Emergency Medical Services System Act of 1973 and its amendments in 1976. This legislation led to the development of the Division of Emergency Medical Services (DEMS), whose responsibility included the development of Regional Emergency Medical Service delivery systems. This agency was given the responsibility of creating public safety awareness and education programs, raising manpower and training, and developing effective communication systems, patient transfer mechanisms, and disaster planning to better care for medical emergency and multiple trauma patients, SCI, and burn victims, etc. As a result of these founding goals, the function of the emergency medical services regarding the management of patients with spinal cord injuries is to maintain and potentiate vital organ function, prevent further neurologic injury during transport, and provide rapid transportation to a well-qualified hospital center.[21] Today, despite difficulties with funding on the federal level, strong statewide and local programs continue to provide necessary training and in-field support for trauma care patients.

In-Field Personnel

In general, the initial responders to an injury scene are usually the police or fire services. These first responders are individuals who have been trained in general emergency procedures and have the ability to administer basic medical care, open an airway, and apply pressure to external bleeding sites. More highly trained and certified individuals, referred to as Emergency Medical Technicians-Basic (EMT-B), in addition provide basic life support and have been trained in basic extrication techniques, administration of oxygen, and patient immobilization and transport.[21] An EMT-P (paramedic) is a responder who is defined by attainment of certain educational objectives as opposed to the number of hours of training. The duties of these individuals include advanced life support, endotracheal intubation, intravenous line insertion, and administration of intravenous fluids and medications.[21,23]

The in-field responder, usually consisting of EMS personnel, in addition to providing immediate medical attention to the patient, must also make an immediate in-field assessment as to the security of the surrounding environment. After a determination is made as to the safety of the location for both the patient and the care giver, appropriate support personnel are summoned if necessary. Traffic may need to be averted, live electric wires may need to be controlled, and unruly crowds may have to be contained in order to effectively care for the injured. Concomitant with these responsibilities, an initial primary survey of the patient is conducted. This survey includes assessing the patient's airway patency and ventilation, checking for the presence of a pulse, and determining if the patient is conscious. Suspicion of a head or spinal injury may be derived directly, through communication with the patient, or indirectly, through observation of physical deformities or the mechanism of the injury. Definitive evidence of a potential SCI may exist if there is extremity weakness or paralysis, alteration of sensation, soft-tissue lacerations above the clavicle, tenderness on palpation of the spine, and loss of consciousness.

ABCs of EMS Management (Airway, Breathing, and Circulation)

Initially, the highest priority of medical intervention should be to establish a patent and secure airway.[7] Aside from the necessity of respiration, maintaining a patent airway helps prevent secondary injury to the spinal cord as a result of hypoxemia. Any manipulation of the cervical spine must be minimal to prevent injury to the cervical spinal cord in patients with neck trauma. A gentle chin lift or jaw thrust maneuver may prevent detrimental cervical flexion or extension while maintaining an open airway. Appropriate airway control also prevents aspiration of gastric contents, a leading cause of death in patients with SCI. Prior to their arrival at the hospital, frequent suctioning may be necessary in the event of emesis to avoid this complication. For airway control in an awake patient, a standard cutoff oral airway can be used to maintain an open airway and prevent gagging. Airway management in an unconscious patient requires the use of a standard oraltracheal or nasopharyngeal airway. Blinded nasotracheal intubation is a useful method of obtaining an airway while preventing hyperextension in a patient with an unstable cervical spine injury. These intubation techniques are equally safe, as long as all intubations are performed with in-line manual cervical immobilization.[7]

After a functioning airway is obtained, ventilation and, most importantly, oxygenation of the patient with a SCI is monitored. All such patients should be given supplemental oxygen (via mask or bag valve) while ventilating. If oxygenation is not monitored, the physiologic effects of SCI, including a loss of sympathetic tone with resultant neurogenic hypotension and decreased respiratory function, may mask the presence of tissue hypoxemia, a major cause of secondary neuronal injury.[22]

Active exsanguination of the patient with a SCI is managed with direct pressure to tamponade bleeding. Penetrating objects should not be removed from the neck or spine in the field to avoid the risk of excessive bleeding, but they should be managed definitively when appropriate operating room facilities and support personnel are available at the hospital.[15] Venous access must be obtained through the placement of two large 14- or 16-gauge peripheral venous catheters. Fluid resuscitation is commenced with strict attention to the patient's vital signs to prevent the signs of hypovolemia or fluid overload.

In the past, Military AntiShock Trousers (MAST), now called Pneumatic AntiShock Garments (PASG), were used frequently to prevent lower extremity pooling of venous blood by constricting the lower extremity vessels and by increasing peripheral vascular resistance. Use of the PASG also allowed for splinting of lower extremity and pelvic fractures and assisted in circulatory support by tamponading interstitial or retroperitoneal hemorrhaging in these fracture situations. Because of the not-so-infrequent reported side effects of these garments, which can include a detrimental increase in intra-abdominal and skeletal compartment pressures as well as increased peripheral ischemia and intracranial pressure as a result of lactic acid buildup, their use has fallen out of favor in many regional trauma centers. In addition, placement of a PASG may aggravate a neurologic injury if there is lower lumbar spinal instability.

Patient Extrication

Motor Vehicle Accident Before a patient can be extricated from an automobile, appropriate spinal immobilization is necessary to prevent neurologic injury during patient movement. Gentle stabilization in an axial direction is applied while a cervical collar is placed. Current recommendations state that the patient's head should be aligned with the axis of the body and in a neutral position for transport; however, this positioning, especially if forced, may result in further spinal cord compression in patients with specific injury patterns such as a cervical dislocation.[23] As a rule, patients should not be forced into a position that results in undue pain or results in a deformity different from their primary posture.[15] Great care must be afforded in the movement of unconscious patients, because 5% to 10% of these patients may have a significant cervical spine injury.[7] It is safest to assume the presence of SCI until proven otherwise.

Patient Immobilization The safest means of patient immobilization is to secure the patient in the supine position on a firm, rigid spine board that extends from the top of the head to the bottom of the buttocks, preferably one that also includes both lower extremities. Various means of patient transfer to a spine board have been investigated, including log-rolling techniques, the four-man lift, or a scoop stretcher, if one is available.[5] A cervical collar should be in place, and it should be one that is light and easily applied.[24] Cervical collars with an opening in the front are preferable for evaluation of tracheal deviation (in the case of tension pneumothorax) or to perform an emergent cricothyroidotomy if necessary.[21] The patient should be secured to the spine board by strapping of the forehead, thorax, and extremities. The chin should not be taped as the sole point for control of the head. In adults, occipital padding may be necessary to place the head in a neutral position as a result of the large trunk-to-head size ratio. In children, however, an occipital recess is usually necessary, to allow the head and neck to be in extension. In children up to 6 years of age, the head is disproportionately large in comparison to the torso, and placing the child flat on a spine board may flex the spine. Placement of a pad behind the child's shoulders and back should allow the cervical spine to be positioned in neutral.[25] Cervical and head side supports attached to the spine board, preferably with Velcro, further stabilize the cervical spine. Unsupported sand bags should not be used, because they can shift during transport and cause a loss in cervical spinal alignment.[21] Cervical traction should not be applied with free weights because they can cause overdistraction during acceleration of the transport vehicle. The principles of spinal immobilization are the same regardless of the setting. In cases of water trauma, patients should be floated flat on their back with the rescuers' hands supporting the victim's head, neck, and spine. The patient is then brought to the edge of the water and slowly floated onto a spine board, which is placed beneath the patient. In a helmeted patient, the patient is securely immobilized on a spine board without removing the helmet in the field, unless the patient's airway is threatened. In the case of a football injury, the shoulder pads should be left in place in order to maintain neutral spinal alignment. The mask or face shell may be removed in the field or in the emergency department, whenever the appropriate tools are present. The helmet shell may then be removed with the help of an assistant to immobilize the neck.

Transportation

If possible, patients should be transported safely to facilities that are equipped to provide a definitive contemporary standard of care.[26] Extra time during transport may be in the patient's best interest, if the patient's vital signs are stable, in order to bring a patient to a registered SCI center. The patient should be transported in the Trendelenburg position (20° to 40°) to maximize cardiovascular function and to avoid gastric aspiration. The feet forward position is the safest, especially in cases of frequent stops, to avoid undue harm to the patient with a cervical spine injury. As stated previously, the goal is to transfer a viable patient from the area of trauma to an emergency room with all systems stabilized in order to enhance the potential for maximal neurologic recovery. The choice of transport vehicle is largely determined by distance, but the patient's vital signs, traffic conditions, and the proximity of a suitable accepting institution must also be considered. In general, for distances less than 50 miles (81 km), an ambulance may be used for transportation; for distances between 51 and 150 miles (81 and 242 km) and during peak traffic for severe injuries, a helicopter; and for distances greater than 150 miles (242 km), a fixed-wing aircraft is useful.[22]

Emergency Room Evaluation

On arrival at the emergency room, a multisystem evaluation is again performed following resurveillance of the basic ABCs of trauma care (Airway, Breathing, and Circulation). A multidisciplinary team approach has been proven to be most effective in the definitive care of the patient with a SCI. Team members include the traumatologist or general surgeon, the orthopaedist, the neurosurgeon, the physiatrist, emergency room personnel, the anesthesiologist, and trained nursing and respiratory personnel. The initial goals are to normalize the patient's vital signs, administer oxygen and appropriate pharmacologic agents, and establish normal spine alignment. The presence of adequate airway patency and ventilation is monitored through arterial blood gases and pulse oximetry. Initially, patients with evidence of a SCI are administered a 40% oxygen humidity mask with a target $Pa{O_2}$ of 100 torr and a $Pa{CO_2}$ of less than 45 torr.[22] Patients with vital capacities less than 10 ml/kg or $Pa{O_2}/Pa{CO_2}$ ratios < 0.75 should be considered for semiurgent intubation.[7] Following this, appropriate laboratory studies are done, and a large-bore sump nasogastric tube is placed, if not already present, to decompress the stomach as well as to monitor gastric pH and provide a route of administration for antacids. A Foley catheter, again if not already present, is inserted to obtain a sample of urine as well as to monitor urine output and relieve pressure on a hypotense bladder.[26] If the patient presents with an open spinal wound, prophylactic wide-spectrum antibiotics and tetanus prophylaxis should be administered.

The Presence of Hypotension in the Patient With a SCI

During the initial evaluation and monitoring of the patient with a SCI, hypotension caused by either hypovolemia or autonomic dysfunction may be present.[4] It is important to differentiate between these two causes of hypotension, because they are managed differently. Neurogenic shock may be present in injuries above the T6 level, caused by disruption of descending sympathetic pathways with loss of the sympathetic inhibition of the parasympathetic effect of the vagus nerve. This leads to a loss of peripheral sympathetic tone, with increased vessel capacitance, lower extremity venous stasis, and decreased central venous return, resulting in hypotension, often accompanied by hypothermia.[7,22] This is usually accompanied by an increased cardiac output. Patients in neurogenic shock are hypotensive in the presence of bradycardia (pulse rate less than 60), unlike the patient in hypovolemic shock, who presents with a relative tachycardia in the setting of hypotension. In the setting of hemorrhagic shock, the patient's pulse is rapid and irregular; in neurogenic shock, the pulse is usually slow and regular.[22] The presence of hypotension should never be attributed to neurogenic shock in the patient with a spinal injury until occult internal hemorrhage has been ruled out. The treatment of neurogenic shock is similar to the initial resuscitation of hypovolemic shock, except that fluid replacement proceeds in a judicious manner to avoid fluid overload. Initially, these patients are relatively hypovolemic due to loss of peripheral vascular tone, and intravenous fluids resuscitation proceeds expediently. In addition to intravenous fluid replacement, the patient is initially placed in the Trendelenburg position (20° to 40°) to facilitate the central return of venous blood. This is followed, if necessary, by the administration of intravenous atropine (0.4 mg), used for its vagolytic effect, and cardiac pressors (dopamine), to increase peripheral vascular tone and cardiac output. Temporary cardiac pacing is rarely needed,[7] but fluid volume should be followed closely with the placement of a Swan-Ganz catheter.

History and Physical

Following the initial resuscitative phase, a complete history of the mechanism of injury and any prior history of spinal pathology, ie, a known diagnosis of ankylosing spondylitis, kyphoscoliosis, or preexisting central nervous system dysfunction, is obtained from the patient, family members, or emergency medical personnel.[4,15] The pre-injury neurologic status of the patient is invaluable to determine if any worsening of neurologic function has occurred as the result of the present injury. Also, record any change in the patient's clinical status that has occurred since the initial evaluation. Following the recording of an accurate history, the entire spine should be palpated in search of evidence of injury, including ecchymosis, an abrupt spinal step off, or spine tenderness. If a well-padded rotating bed is available, the patient should be placed on it to decrease the potential for sacral or heel ulcer formation, as well as to avoid further neurologic aggravation from repeated log rolling maneuver during patient care.[26]

The neurologic examination is performed with careful attention to the recording of accurate sensory and motor levels to determine the precise neurologic level of injury. In addition, cranial nerve function must be assessed as well as rectal tone and reflexes. There are 28 dermatomes in the sensory evaluation and 10 myotomes in the motor evaluation.[27] Muscle strength is graded on a 6-point scale: 0 for paralysis, 1 for palpable or visible contractions, 2 for active range of motion with gravity eliminated, 3 for active range of motion against gravity, 4 for active range of motion against moderate resistance, and 5 for active range of motion against full resistance. It should be remembered that children have different motor strengths, and what may be a motor strength of 5 in an adult may not be the same in a child. The sensory examination is determined by evaluation of pin prick and light touch for both sides of the body. There is a 3-point rating scale: 0 for absent, 1 for impaired, and 2 for normal, plus NT for not testable. Together, the numeric results of these tests determine the motor and sensory scores respectively. The presence of motor or pin prick sensation in the S4-S5 distribution carries a favorable prognosis for ambulation, unlike situations in which evidence of sacral sparing is absent after the resolution of spinal shock.

The ASIA (American Spinal Injury Association) impairment scale replaces the modified Frankel classification to which it is similar in many ways. A stands for a complete SCI with no sensory or motor function distal to the level of injury; B represents an incomplete SCI with preservation of sensation, but no motor function distal to the level of injury; C represents an incomplete SCI with motor function present below the level of injury with a motor grade of 3 or less; D represents an incomplete SCI with motor preservation greater than grade 3 below the level of injury, and E represents a normal neurologic examination.[27] In the zone of partial preservation, there are dermatomes or myotomes distal to the level of neurologic injury that remain partially innervated. This information should be recorded in patients with complete cord injuries.

Pathophysiology of SCI

Researchers have attempted to halt or reverse the secondary mechanisms of tissue injury after SCI by influencing the pathophysiologic consequence of tissue hypoxia. The most promising research, in animal models, has shown that only high-dose steroids and gangliosides were of benefit in prospective, randomized, placebo-controlled studies. To understand the potential effectiveness of the various agents being investigated, an overview of the pathophysiology of SCI is necessary.

Beginning with the initial insult, a cascading series of events occur related to both the disruption of blood flow and direct injury to the neuronal membrane. With a decrease in oxygen tension, local tissue metabolism switches from an aerobic to an anaerobic state, with a resultant decrease in local stores of adenosine triphosphate (ATP).[5,22,28] This, along with an increase in tissue lactic acid, and a decrease in intracellular pH, leads to the disruption of Ca^{+2}-dependent K^+ and Na^+ adenosine triphosphatase (ATPase), resulting in an influx of intracellular Ca^{+2} and an efflux of extracellular K^+. Rapid calcium accumulation within the cell causes dysfunction of Ca^{+2}-dependent mitochondrial electron transport, which uncouples oxidative phosphorylation and further depletes ATP stores. Destructive Ca^{+2}-dependent intracellular enzymes are activated, including phospholipases and various neutral proteinases, and this leads to neuronal and neurologic destruction.[5,22,28] In addition, there is a local increase in excitatory amino acid neurotransmitter (glutamate and aspartate), which also contributes to an increase in intracellular Ca^{+2} through specific activated ion channels. The activation of phospholipase A_2 leads, through enzymatic lipid hydrolysis, to the release of various membrane phospholipids, including arachidonic acid and other fatty acids, which are actively metabolized into various eicosanoids, including prostaglandins E_2 and $F_{2\alpha}$, prostacyclins, thromboxanes, leukotrienes, and various free radicals.[3] Specific leukotrienes and prostacyclins, in association with kinins and serotonin, all contribute to an increase in vascular permeability and endothelial wall disruption, leading to edema, polymorphonuclear cell infiltration, vessel thrombosis, and destruction of local neural tissue. The metabolites culminate in cellular destruction, inhibiting neurofilament release and promoting vascular constriction and the release of destructive lysosomes.[5,22,28]

With disruption of Ca^{+2}-dependent mitochondrial electron transport, destructive free radicals are produced, including superoxide anions, hydroxyl radicals, and hydrogen peroxide, which also break down cell membranes.[28] This process of oxidative degradation is referred to as free radical-induced lipid peroxidation and is evidenced by loss of membrane cholesterol with an increase in its auto-oxidation products (ie, 25-hydroxycholesterol) and with a concurrent decrease in tissue vitamin E. Free radicals are also generated from the breakdown of hemorrhagic products through the dislocation or decompartmentalization of intracellular iron complexes from blood components resulting in the release of hemoproteins and ferrous ions. The efflux of K+ itself results in membrane deplorization effectively blocking neurotransmissions. [5,22,28]

On a pathoanatomic level, the initial insult to the spinal cord is followed by the immediate (within minutes to hours) formation of small petechial hemorrhages. Caused by disruption of the microvasculature, these first appear in the central gray matter with eventual centrifugal spread into the surrounding white matter.[5,22] The endothelial lining of the spinal cord microvasculature is disrupted, which allows the deposition of platelets. Eventually, thrombi form and these contribute to further tissue ischemia and loss of vascular autoregulation. The small hemorrhagic foci eventually coalesce into a larger area of central necrosis. Contributing to the destruction of nervous tissue is the extravasation of polymorphonuclear leukocytes into the site of injury and subsequent phagocytosis.[5,22] Within the first few days, vasogenic edema progresses and is identified for up to 2 weeks after the initial insult.[5,22,28]

After 5 to 6 days, hemorrhagic debris is reabsorbed through phagocytosis. Activated glial cells deposit astrophytic fibers, which results in the formation, over the ensuing 3 to 6 months, of scar tissue or extensive gliosis as the result of wallerian degeneration of fiber tracts.[5,22,28]

Drug Therapy

The goal of drug treatment is to minimize the deleterious effects of secondary injury that occur as a result of neuronal hypoxemia and cellular dysfunction. The administration of steroids within 8 hours of SCI is now standard in all trauma centers. The dose of methylprednisolone is 30 mg/kg, given over 15 minutes, followed by a 5.4 mg/kg per hour dosage over 24 hours. The relative contraindications to the use of steroids include any patient with penetrating wounds, pregnancy, patients younger than 13 years of age, and patients with infection or diabetes. Steroid treatment aids neurologic recovery by increasing blood flow to the injured central nervous system, thereby increasing perfusion to the white matter. In addition, steroids reduce edema and inflammation, and they scavenge for oxygen free radicals. Importantly, this drug therapy suppresses the breakdown of cell membranes by inhibiting lipid peroxidation and hydrolysis at the site of injury, thus decreasing the extracellular calcium level. Phase 2 of the National Acute Spinal Cord Injury Study (NASCIS 2) noted the superiority of methylprednisolone over naloxone (an opiate antagonist).[4,22,28-31] In addition, it was noted that if steroids were given within less than 8 hours after SCI, motor scores as well as sensation to pin prick and light touch improved, both in patients with complete and those with incomplete injuries. Very little has been reported on injury modulation in children. Although most treating physicians use methylprednisolone in pediatric SCI, it should be noted that only 15% of the patients in the study by Bracken and associates[29] were aged 13 to 19 years, and the study included no data on patients younger than 13 years. Contrary to these findings, other studies have failed to show an improvement in neurologic function after high dose steroid use.[32]

In addition to steroids, GM-1 gangliosides have also been found useful in the treatment of patients with spinal cord injuries.[33,34] These drugs are complex acidic glycolipids found naturally in cells of the central nervous system. The mechanism of improvement is postulated to be related to an increased axonal survival rate at the site of injury. GM-1 gangliosides are also neurotopic, decrease retrograde neurologic degeneration, and modulate excitatory amino acid endotoxicity and destructive cell membrane enzymatic activity. In addition, these drugs may also reduce the anti-inflammatory effects of high-dose methylprednisolone, effects that can complicate their use when they are given with steroids.[22] Physicians should be aware that separate reports of acute motor neuropathy presenting as Guillain-Barré Syndrome have been noted as soon as 2 weeks after treatment with this drug.[35]

Oxygen free radical scavengers are also being investigated in the treatment of patients with spinal cord injuries. Vitamin E (alpha tocopherol), which functions as an antioxidant and phospholipid membrane stabilizer, and 21 amino steroids, a group of methylprednisolone analogs with antioxidant properties, are examples of extensively studied free radical scavengers. Tirilizad mesylate (U74006F), a 21 amino steroid drug, is currently in a phase-two clinical study, along with extended dose methylprednisolone therapy (48 versus 24 hours), as part of the NASCIS 3 study.

Potassium channel blocking agents, such as 4-aminopyridine (4-AP) are used to overcome the conduction blockades (Na/K ATPase disruption) that occur during the demyelination process in patients with spinal cord injuries.

Naloxone, an opiate receptor antagonist, has been used in the past for the initial treatment of patients with spinal cord injuries. As mentioned previously, no benefit was noted in the NASCIS 2 study. Still, studies indicate that high dosages of naloxone may benefit patients.[32] Naloxone increases spinal cord blood flow by blocking endogenous spinal cord opioid release and the associated systemic hypotension. Thyroid-releasing hormone (TRH), a partial opiate receptor antagonist, may also have the same effects as naloxone, while preserving the analgesic effects of endogenous opioids.[4,5]

Thromboxane inhibitors may increase spinal cord blood flow by reversing or preventing the vasoconstricting effects of thromboxane. The activation of phospholipase as a result of the cascade of SCI releases free fatty acids and arachidonic acid. These substances are metabolized to eicosanoid metabolites such as prostaglandins, thromboxanes, and leukotrienes. Thromboxanes are noted to deleteriously reduce the degree of spinal cord blood flow.

Ca^{+2} channel blockers, considered antihypertensive agents, may be useful in decreasing the post-injury influx of Ca^{+2} that occurs with membrane and enzymatic destabilization. Osmotic diuretics, including mannitol, glycerol, and low-molecular-weight dextran, have also been tried with varying success to decrease post-traumatic spinal cord edema and ischemia. Dimethylsulfoxide (DMSO), also a diuretic agent, contributes to membrane stabilization through free radical scavenging in addition to its anti-inflammatory and vasodilating properties.[4,5]

Medical Therapy

Aside from pharmacologic treatments, other medical modalities are being tested for patient care.[22] Decreasing the spinal cord temperature decreases the metabolic activity and oxygen requirements of the cord, thereby decreasing edema, hemorrhage, and local inflammatory processes. The effects of hypothermia have been reported in animal studies but have not been documented in humans. Direct current fields and functional electrical stimulation may assist in central nervous system fiber tract regeneration. Extracellular matrices are being investigated as a potential spatial framework for axonal migration. Finally, the transplantation of fetal tissues, as witnessed in the canine model, may provide function to compromised spinal cord tissue.

Spinal Imaging

The primary goal in the management of patients with spinal injuries with or without neural deficits is to realign the spinal elements in a position that will relieve abnormal pressure on the neural elements. This process begins in the emergency ward with radiographic documentation of the primary and secondary spinal lesions through anteroposterior and lateral plain radiographs of the entire space, including an odontoid view. Patients who are barrel-chested or have a short, wide neck may require arm traction or a swimmer's view to document the cervicothoracic junction. If this area cannot be documented by plain films, a computed tomographic (CT) scan with sagittal reconstruction may be obtained. A coronal CT reconstruction of the odontoid is useful in patients who are intubated and cannot provide an open mouth view of this region. Tomography may be extremely useful in documenting a transverse fracture of the odontoid or subtle lateral mass fractures. Such fractures may be missed on computed tomography, either because of the slice thickness of image or because the imaging is outside the plane of fracture.

In the pediatric patient with a known lap belt injury, the spine must be carefully evaluated radiographically, preferably before the patient is taken to the operating room. The flexion-distraction spine fracture secondary to a lap belt injury must be diagnosed on a plain radiograph. This fracture is extremely difficult to diagnose on CT scan, because the plane of the distraction of the spine injury is the same as the axial CT cut.[36] If the spine cannot be evaluated radiographically because the patient is unstable hemodynamically, it should be assumed that a fracture is present until it is detemined that it is not. Cases have been reported in which children who were previously neurologically intact have awakened paralyzed after an abdominal procedure. In such cases, the paralysis probably occurred during manipulation on the operating room table (Fig. 1). Oblique radiographs are helpful to confirm or rule out a facet or uncinate process fracture. In the neurologically intact but symptomatic patient (one with neck pain), flexion and extension lateral plain radiographs are deferred until cervical paraspinal muscle spasm subsides in order not to mask subtle instability patterns obscured by muscular guarding.

Careful scrutiny of the plain radiographs with a knowledge of normal radiologic skeletal relationships allows the treating physician to infer the primary and secondary force vectors of injury and to determine which anatomic structures are disrupted. A flexion force resulting in spinal injury will manifest as widening of the interspinous, interlaminar, and facet joint spaces with or without evidence of vertebral body subluxation or dislocation. The vertebral body may show evidence of asymmetric loss of height. On a lateral radiograph, compression is greater anteriorly than posteriorly, with associated loss of subadjacent disk space height.

An extension injury may reveal widening of the disk space anteriorly with or without a bony avulsion fracture. There may be evidence of retrolisthesis of the proximal vertebral body on the subadjacent vertebral body with bony failure of the posterior elements, including the pars interarticularis, lamina, or spinous process. A rotational injury will manifest as malalignment of the spinal column on an anteroposterior or lateral view. Above the level of injury, the spine appears to be out of plane from the spinal elements below the level of injury. Associated fractures or soft-tissue disruption may be present with this injury mechanism. A shear force is manifested as a displacement of the spinal elements at the level of injury in the direction of force application (horizontal with or without rotation), with complete disruption of the bony and soft-tissue elements at the level of injury.

Abnormal soft-tissue relationships, especially swelling in the paravertebral region, must be scrutinized, as they may be the only indication of a subtle vertebral body injury. During the radiographic assessment of the child, it is necessary to keep normal radiographic variants in mind. Pseudosubluxation of C2 on C3 is troublesome when seen on initial evaluation in the

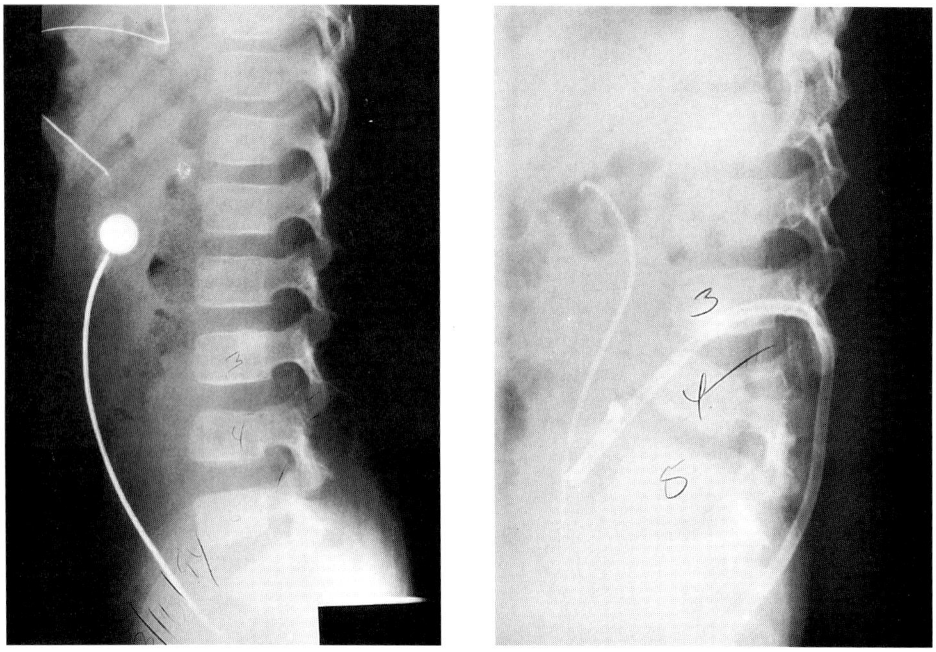

Fig. 1 **Left,** Lateral lumbar radiograph of a 4-year-old who was involved in a motor vehicle accident. She was in a lap belt in the back seat at the time of impact. She was hemodynamically unstable and was rushed to the operating room for repair of retroperitoneal lacerations. The lateral radiograph shows some suggestion of injury at L3-4. **Right,** Lateral radiograph of the same patient 24 hours after the first film was taken. Despite careful attempts at positioning this child because of suspected spinal injury, the fracture displaced further. This flexion-distraction injury was then stabilized using posterior interspinous wiring between L3 and L4.

emergency room, especially in a child who may have sustained neck trauma. If the posterior intralaminar line is not displaced, the pseudosubluxation seen is a normal variant[37] (Fig. 2). If the line is disrupted, it is pathologic (Fig. 3). Radiographs of the cranium may be necessary when head trauma is present in order to avoid missing a skull defect at the site of anticipated skeletal tong placement.

If a spinal lesion is identified, the treating physician must decide whether to pursue more advanced imaging studies, such as MRI, to exclude soft-tissue encroachment on the neural elements or to proceed immediately with attempted spinal realignment through closed traction techniques in the emergency ward. Eismont and associates[38] recommend using MRI before attempting closed reduction, because a high incidence of disk herniation is associated with cervical dislocations, and therefore there is a potential for neurologic worsening as a result of further spinal cord compression with cervical manipulation. A review of the case reports in which neurologic injury was associated with a closed reduction reveals that the reductions were performed under general anesthesia. On the other hand, if the reduction is performed in awake and alert patients, closed reduction is highly successful without reported neurologic complications.[39,40] Therefore, MRI is not mandatory prior to attempted closed reduction in appropriately selected patients. MRI is recommended in obtunded patients, those cases in which neurologic function deteriorates temporarily while adding weights during attempted closed reduction, and in any patient requiring open reduction. In all patients, MRI should be obtained after closed reduction is accomplished to rule out spinal cord compression by a herniated disk. If a herniated disk is found, anterior decompression should precede any posterior instrumentation or any attempt at reduction under general anesthesia.

Once patients are stabilized in the emergency ward, advanced spinal imaging such as MRI or CT scanning may be obtained if necessary. Flanders and associates[41] have documented, through MRI, that disk herniations of varying degrees occur in cervical dislocations and fracture subluxations 30% to 50% of the time. An interesting benefit of noninvasive MRI technology is the ability to evaluate the integrity of the extracranial circulation with MRI angiography. We prospectively evaluated 60 patients with cervical spine injuries at Thomas Jefferson University and identified 12 patients (20%) with vertebral artery disruptions. The clinical significance of these injuries is unclear, because only three of the patients manifested symptoms of vertebral artery insufficiency.

MRI following pediatric SCI can show problems not visible on plain radiographs. MRI also can be beneficial in delineating spinal column injury in difficult-to-see areas such as C7-T1 (Fig. 4).[42] SCIWORA (SCI without radiographic abnormality) has been reported in 10% to 20% of children with SCI.[43-46] In very young children (3 to 4 years of age), the association of SCIWORA with a Chiari malformation has been reported.[47] It is important to recognize the Chiari malformation because decompression of C1 and the foramen magnum has been reported to help with some recovery of function, especially when the lesion is incomplete.

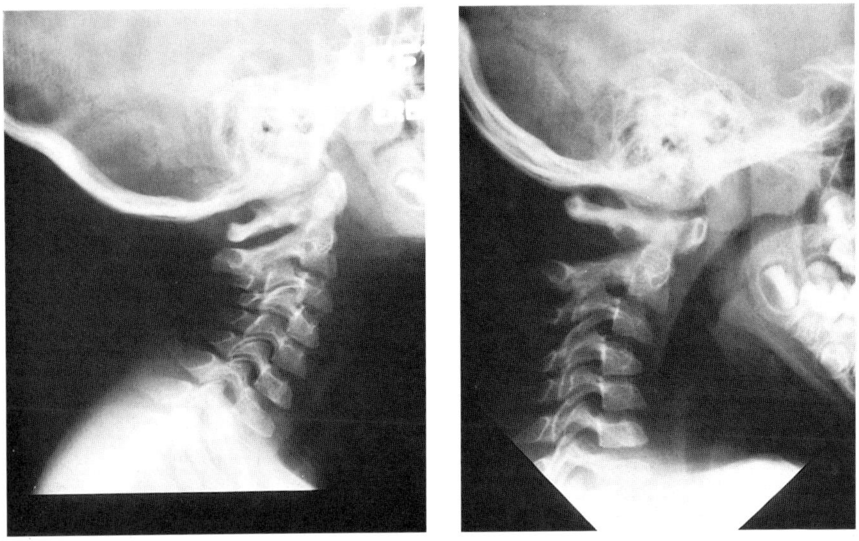

Fig. 2 **Left,** Lateral extension radiograph of the cervical spine. **Right,** Lateral flexion radiograph shows pseudosubluxation of the anterior vertebral body of C2-C3. The posterior intralaminar line (Line of Swichuk) is intact.

Growth plate injuries may be seen on MRI that may not be visible on plain radiographs, and any external dural compression caused by the fragments may be relieved by removing them.[48-50]

Technique of Closed Cervical Reduction for Cervical Facet Dislocations

The goals of closed cervical reduction are to restore anatomic alignment of the spine, thereby restoring the space for the spinal cord. In order to maximize neurologic recovery, closed reduction is performed as quickly and safely as possible, usually within 2 to 3 hours after the patient is brought to the emergency room.

Following the general trauma evaluation, the patient is placed in the supine position on a Stryker frame (Stryker Corp, Kalamazoo, MI). Gardner-Wells tongs (Zimmer, Inc, Warsaw, IN) are usually applied without removing the patient's hair. The areas are thoroughly prepped, and tongs are inserted using local anesthesia. For straight traction, pins are inserted 1 cm superior to the middle of the pinna of the ear. The pins should be tightened until the pressure indicator protrudes 1 mm. For a flexion moment, pins may be inserted slightly posterior to the pinna. A further flexion moment may be added by removing the bed springs caudal to the injury. If an extension moment is desired, the pins may be inserted slightly anterior to the pinna. A small pad may be placed under the upper back between the scapulae if more extension of the neck is needed. The mean pull-out strength of stainless steel Gardner-Wells tongs is up to 300 pounds, whereas MRI-compatible titanium tongs fail at an average of 75 pounds.[51] For this reason, stainless steel tongs are recommended for closed reduction, particularly if high weight reduction is anticipated.

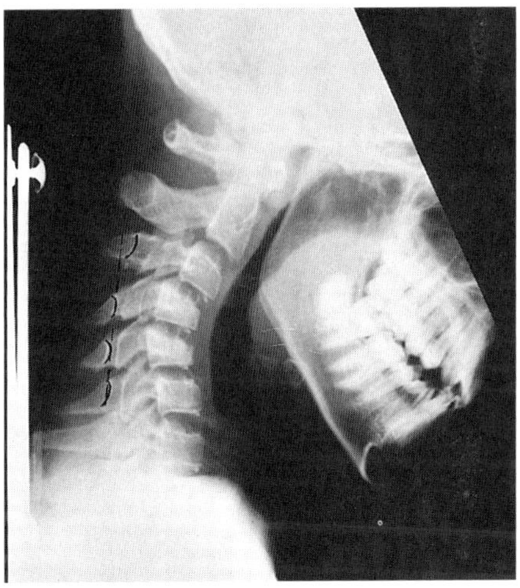

Fig. 3 Lateral flexion cervical radiograph shows subluxation after C3-C4. Posterior interlaminar line is disrupted to confirm that this is true instability.

The initial amount of traction applied should be 10 pounds, to rule out upper cervical spine injuries. Weight is added sequentially, in 10-pound increments every 10 or 15 minutes, until reduction is obtained. Immediately after each application of weight, a neurologic examination is performed and a lateral radiograph is obtained. As weight exceeds 50 pounds, the Stryker bed should be placed in a reverse Trendelenburg position to provide some countertraction. Up to 140 pounds of traction can be used to reduce dislocations in awake and cooperative patients.[39] Once the facets have been unlocked, reduction usually occurs spontaneously. When the tips of the facets are perched,

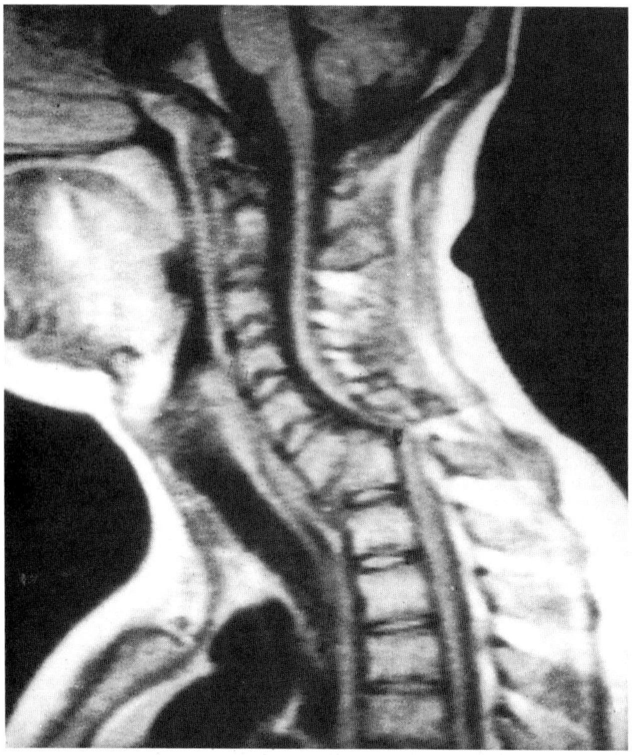

Fig. 4 Sagittal cervical magnetic resonance image of a football player with a T7 complete spinal cord injury. Radiographs were indeterminate in defining the spinal column injury.

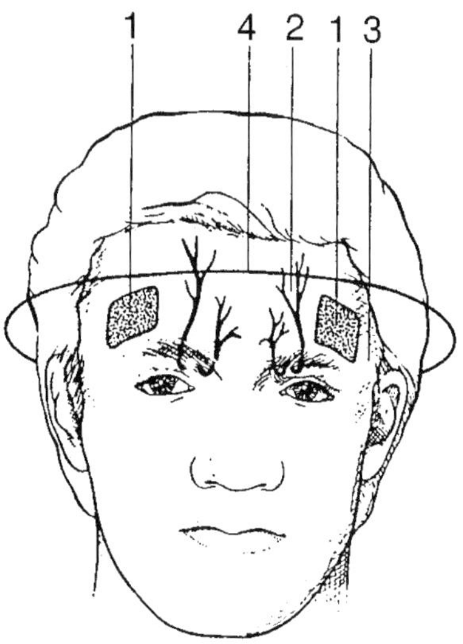

Fig. 5 (1) Safety zones for the anterior pin sites. (2) Medially, over the medial one third of the orbit are the supraorbital and supratrochlear nerves and artery. (3) The temporal fossa has very thin bone, which should be avoided. (4) The pins are inserted below the equator line or the largest circumference of the skull. (Reproduced with permission from Mubarak SJ, Camp JF, Vuletich W, et al: Halo application in the infant. *J Pediatr Orthop* 1989;9:612–614.)

a gentle manual reduction maneuver may help reduction. Once reduction is confirmed with a lateral radiograph, 10 to 15 pounds of traction is retained to maintain reduction. In 200 consecutive patients, this technique of closed reduction was success-ful in approximately 90% of cases with no permanent worsening or progressive neurologic deficit.[52] Even if complete reduction is not achieved, at least the canal's volume has been increased and a significant degree of cord decompression obtained. After the closed reduction, the patient may undergo surgery while still in traction or a halo-vest may be applied.

Cervical traction in children younger than 12 years of age is associated with greater risk than in adults, and primary halo traction may be preferred. Martinez-Lage and associates[53] reported dural leaks with Crutchfield tongs in patients younger than 12 years.

Halo Vest Application

The advantages of preoperative halo vest immobilization include increased ease and safety of patient transfer and transport, improved pulmonary care, and facilitation of MRI. At surgery, either the anterior or posterior bars of the halo vest may be taped to the Stryker frame and the opposite vest and bars removed for either an anterior or posterior cervical approach.

Additionally, the halo vest may be used for nonoperative management in patients with C1 fractures (Jefferson's fracture), C2 hangman's fractures, odontoid fractures, stable compression fractures, axial loading burst fractures, and flexion-compression fractures with minimal ligamentous disruption in the absence of a neurologic deficit. The halo vest is frequently used for adjunctive support following surgical stabilization with nonrigid internal fixation as in long segment anterior cervical corpectomies and plating or posterior wiring procedures for the upper and lower cervical spine.

There are many varieties of Halo rings and vests available on the market (Outline 1). A posteriorly opened ring gives surgical access to the occiput and upper cervical spine and is easy to apply with the patient in the supine position. Lightweight and MRI-compatible rings are preferred. Appropriate pin site placement is crucial. Anterior pins are placed anterolaterally approximately 1 cm above the orbital rim, below the equator of the skull and cephalad to the lateral two thirds of the orbit (Fig. 5). Posterior pins should be directly opposite the anterior pins. Anterior pins should be tightened with the patient's eyes closed. Structures that are at risk anteriorly during pin placement include the frontal sinus, which usually is located centrally cephalad to the bridge of the nose but which can extend to a variable extent above the medial aspect of the orbit.[54] Medially, over the medial one third of the orbit are the supraorbital and supratrochlear nerves

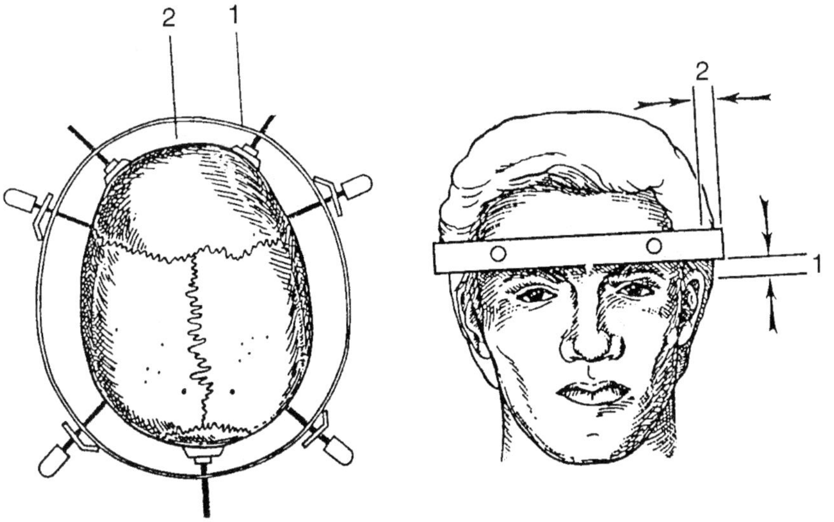

Fig. 6 Proper positioning of the halo ring. **Left,** (1) Top view showing the ring with 1 cm clearance around the circumference of the skull. (2) Temporary positioning posts. **Center,** (1) Front view showing the ring about 1 cm above the ear and eyebrows and (2) 1 cm clearance from the skull. **Right,** The ring is placed about 1 cm above the ears, and the anterior ring is slightly more cephalad than the posterior ring so that the head is slightly extended. The ring of the halo should be inferior to the equator or widest diameter of the skull.

and artery. Laterally, cephalad to the orbital ridge and eyebrow over the lateral one half of the orbit, there are no significant structures and, therefore, this is the optimum location for pin placement. The temporal fossa has very thin bone that may fracture or be penetrated by a pin that is too tightly torqued. Additionally, muscles of mastication are located in the temporal fossa. Posterior to the temporal fossa there are no significant anatomic structures of risk and this area is an acceptable alternative pin placement site (Fig. 6). The torque of insertion should be 8 in/lb, applied at increments of 2 in/lb with opposite pins being tightened alternatively.[54] Pins should be retightened once to 8 in/lb at 24 hours later. Following halo ring application, a well-fitting vest is applied. The posterior vest is applied first by log rolling or raising the patient's trunk to 30°. The connection mechanism between the halo ring and upright posts may allow for additional flexion-extension, anterior-posterior translation, or compression-traction manipulation. Halo fixators can safely be used in children,[55] but the number of pins must be increased to 8 or 10 and the torques reduced to 2 pounds instead of 8. If standard halo rings are used, additional holes must be drilled in them (Fig. 7).[56,57] For children younger than 6 years of age, CT scans of the head are recommended to help determine the best pin sites.[58,59] Should the halo become loose, or if for some reason it cannot be applied, a Minerva type of cervico-thoracic-lumbar-sacral orthosis (CTLSO) may be an option.

Outline 1
Ten steps of halo vest application in the adult patient

1. Have patient lie supine over the edge of the table or bed.
2. Determine the correct ring and vest size. The ring is placed about 1 cm above the ears, and the anterior ring is slightly more cephalad than the posterior ring so that the head is slightly extended. The ring of the halo should be inferior to the equator or widest diameter of the skull.
3. Identify the pin site locations by holding the ring in place. A 3 cm by 3 cm hair trim, shave, and prep is carried out just superior and posterior to the ear. The halo ring is positioned, using temporary positioning posts.
4. Prepare pin sites with povidone-iodine solution and 1% lidocaine. Approximately 5 cc is injected down to and including the periosteum of the skull.
5. Insert the pins and tighten to 8 in/lb at 2 in/lb increments.
6. Apply the posterior vest first by log rolling or raising the patient's trunk to 30°.
7. Apply the anterior vest and connect it to the posterior vest.
8. Apply four upright posts and tighten linkages.
9. Obtain cervical spine radiographs to check reduction and alignment.
10. Retighten the pins to 8 in/lb and recheck all nuts and screws 24 hours later.

In conclusion, successful management of the patient with a SCI requires a multidisciplinary team approach beginning with an organized emergency medical service and effective utilization of regional centers that specialize in the care of these devastating injuries. As further research defines the precise pathophysiology of acute SCI as well as reinjury from the secondary

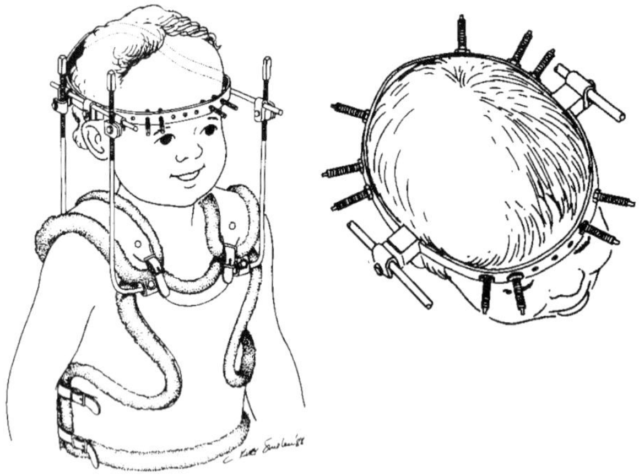

Fig. 7 Schematic of halo placement in an infant. Note the increased number of pins from 4 to 8 or 10. Use 2 lb/in of torque instead of 8. (Reproduced with permission from Mubarak SJ, Camp JF, Vuletich W, et al: Halo application in the infant. *J Pediatr Orthop* 1989;9: 612–614.)

byproducts of tissue dysfunction, more selective pharmacologic and physical modulations may be chosen to improve the overall neurologic prognosis. It is imperative that patients with spinal injury be immobilized and stabilized as quickly and safely as possible in order to maximize their neurologic function and rehabilitation.

References

1. DeVivo MJ, Fine PR, Maetz HM, et al: Prevalence of SCI: A reestimation employing life table techniques. *Arch Neurol* 1980;37:707–708.
2. Harvey C, Rothschild BB, Asmann AJ, et al: New estimates of traumatic SCI prevalence: A survey-based approach. *Paraplegia* 1990;28:537–544.
3. Burke DC: Injuries of the spinal cord in children, in Vinken PJ, Bruyn GW, Braakman R, et al (eds): *Handbook of Clinical Neurology: Injuries of the Spine and Spinal Cord. Part 1.* Amsterdam, The Netherlands, North Holland Publishing, 1976, vol 25, pp 175–195.
4. Maroon JC, Abla AA: Classification of acute spinal cord injury, neurological evaluation, and neurosurgical considerations. *Crit Care Clin* 1987;3:655–677.
5. Sonntag VK, Douglas RA: Management of spinal cord trauma. *Neurosurg Clin North Am* 1990;1:729–750.
6. Kewalramani LS, Taylor RG: Multiple non-contiguous injuries to the spine. *Acta Orthop Scand* 1976;47:52–58.
7. Cohen M: Initial resuscitation of the patient with spinal cord injury. *Trauma Quarterly* 1993;9:38–43.
8. Glassman SD, Johnson JR, Holt RT: Seatbelt injuries in children. *J Trauma* 1992;33:882–886
9. Rumball K, Jarvis J: Seat-belt injuries of the spine in young children. *J Bone Joint Surg* 1992;74B:571–574.
10. Gumley G, Taylor TK, Ryan MD: Distraction fractures of the lumbar spine. *J Bone Joint Surg* 1982;64B:520–525.
11. Rizzolo SJ, Piazza MR, Cotler JM, et al: Intervertebral disc injury complicating cervical spine trauma. *Spine* 1991;16(suppl 6):S187–S189.
12. Womack MS, Kehl DK, Baggett A, et al: Pediatric spine injuries associated with lap seat belts. Proceedings of the American Academy of Orthopaedic Surgeons 60th Annual Meeting, San Francisco, CA. Rosemont, IL, American Academy of Orthopaedic Surgeons, 1993, p 140.
13. Desmond J: Paraplegia: Problems confronting the anaesthesiologist. *Can Anaesth Soc J* 1970;17:435–451.
14. Nand S, Goldschmidt JW: Abstract: Hypercalcemia and hyperuricemia in young patients with spinal cord injury. *Arch Phys Med Rehabil* 1976;57:553.
15. Green BA, Eismont FJ, O'Heir JT: Spinal cord injury: A systems approach. Prevention, emergency medical services, and emergency room management. *Crit Care Clin* 1987;3:471–493.
16. Spivak JM, Weiss MA, Cotler JM, et al: Cervical spine injuries in patients 65 and older. *Spine* 1994;19:2302–2306.
17. Alander DH, Andreychik DA, Stauffer ES: Early outcome in cervical spinal cord injured patients older than 50 years of age. *Spine* 1994;19:2299–2301.
18. Green BA, Eismont FJ, Klose KJ: Management of cervical cord lesions including advances in rehabilitative engineering, in Camins MB, O'Leary PF (eds): *Disorders of the Cervical Spine.* Baltimore, MD, Williams & Wilkins, 1992, pp 351–367.
19. Green BA, Klose KJ, Eismont FJ, et al: Immediate management of the spinal cord injured patient, in Lee BY, Ostrander LE, Cochran GVB, et al (eds): *The Spinal Cord Injured Patient: Comprehensive Management.* Philadelphia, PA, WB Saunders, 1991, pp 24–33.
20. Toscano J: Prevention of neurological deterioration before admission to a spinal cord injury unit. *Paralegia* 1988;26: 143–150.
21. Ramzy AI, Parry JM, Greenberg J: Head and spinal injury: Prehospital care, in Greenberg J (ed): *Handbook of Head and Spine Trauma.* New York, NY, Marcel Dekker, 1993, pp 29–44.
22. Slucky AV, Eismont FJ: Treatment of acute injury of the cervical spine. *J Bone Joint Surg* 1994;76A:1882–1896.
23. Crosby LA, Lewallen DG (eds): *Emergency Care and Transportation of the Sick and Injured*, ed 6. Rosemont, IL, American Academy of Orthopaedic Surgeons, 1995.
24. Chandler DR, Nemejc C, Adkins RH, et al: Emergency cervical-spine immobilization. *Ann Emerg Med* 1992;21:1185–1188.
25. Fielding JW: Fractures of the spine: Part I. Injuries of the cervical spine, in Rockwood CA Jr, Wilkins KE, King RE (eds): *Fractures in Children.* Philadelphia, PA, JB Lippincott, 1984, pp 683–705.
26. Pasarin GA, Green BA: Emergency room assessment and stabilization of spinal injury, in Greenberg J (ed): *Handbook of Head and Spine Trauma.* New York, NY, Marcel Dekker, 1993, pp 413–425.
27. American Spinal Injury Association International Medical Society of Paraplegia: *International Standards for Neurological and Functional Classification of Spinal Cord Injury.* Chicago, IL, American Spinal Injury Association, 1992.
28. Anderson DK, Hall ED: Pathophysiology of spinal cord trauma. *Ann Emerg Med* 1993;22:987–992.
29. Bracken MB, Shepard MJ, Collins WF, et al: A randomized controlled trial of methylprednisolone or naloxone in the treatment of acute spinal-cord injury: Results of the Second National Acute Spinal Cord Injury Study. *N Engl J Med* 1990;322: 1405–1411.
30. Bracken MB, Shepard MJ, Collins WF Jr, et al: Methylprednisolone or naloxone treatment after acute spinal cord injury: 1-year follow-up data. Results of the Second National Acute Spinal Cord Injury Study. *J Neurosurg* 1992;76:23–31.
31. Bracken MB: Pharmacological treatment of acute spinal cord injury: Current status and future projects. *J Emerg Med* 1993;

11(suppl 1):43–48.
32. Segal JL: Clinical pharmacology of spinal cord injury, in Young RR, Woolsey RM (eds): *Diagnosis and Management of Disorders of the Spinal Cord.* Philadelphia, PA, WB Saunders, 1995, pp 414–438.
33. Geisler FH, Dorsey FC, Coleman WP: GM-1 ganglioside in human spinal cord injury. *J Neurotrauma* 1992;9(suppl 2): S517–S530.
34. Geisler FH, Dorsey FC, Coleman WP: Past and current clinical studies with GM-1 ganglioside in acute spinal cord injury. *Ann Emerg Med* 1993;22:1041–1047.
35. Nobile-Orazio E, Carpo M, Scarlato G: Gangliosides: Their role in clinical neurology. *Drugs* 1994;47:576–585.
36. Taylor GA, Eggli KD: Lap-belt injuries of the lumbar spine in children: A pitfall in CT diagnosis. *Am J Roentgenol* 1988;150: 1355–1358.
37. Swischuk LE: Anterior displacement of C2 in children: Physiologic or pathologic? A helpful differentiating line. *Radiology* 1977;122:759–763.
38. Eismont FJ, Arena MJ, Green BA: Extrusion of an intervertebral disc associated with traumatic subluxation or dislocation of cervical facets: Case report. *J Bone Joint Surg* 1991;73A:1555–1560.
39. Cotler JM, Herbison GJ, Nasuti JF, et al: Closed reduction of traumatic cervical spine dislocation using traction weights up to 140 pounds. *Spine* 1993;18:386–390.
40. Star AM, Jones AA, Cotler JM, et al: Immediate closed reduction of cervical spine dislocations using traction. *Spine* 1990;15: 1068–1072.
41. Flanders AE, Tartaglino LM, Friedman DP, et al: Magnetic resonant imaging in acute spinal injury. *Semin Roentgenol* 1992; 27:271–298.
42. Betz RR, Gelman AJ, DeFilipp GJ, et al: Magnetic resonance imaging (MRI) in the evaluation of spinal cord injured children and adolescents. *Paraplegia* 1987;25:92–99.
43. Anderson JM, Schutt AH: Spinal injury in children: A review of 156 cases seen from 1950 through 1978. *Mayo Clin Proc* 1980;55:499–504.
44. Hadley MN, Zabramski JM, Browner CM, et al: Pediatric spinal trauma: Review of 122 cases of spinal cord and vertebral column injuries. *J Neurosurg* 1988;68:18–24.
45. Pang D, Wilberger JE Jr: Spinal cord injury without radiographic abnormalities in children. *J Neurosurg* 1982;57:114–129.
46. Yngve DA, Harris WP, Herndon WA, et al: Spinal cord injury without osseous spine fracture. *J Pediatr Orthop* 1988;8:153–159.
47. Bondurant CP, Oro JJ: Spinal cord injury without radiographic abnormality and Chiari malformation. *J Neurosurg* 1993;79: 833–838.
48. Keller RH: Traumatic displacement of the cartilagenous vertebral rim: A sign of intervertebral disc prolapse. *Radiology* 1974; 110:21–24.
49. Lawson JP, Ogden JA, Bucholz RW, et al: Physeal injuries of the cervical spine. *J Pediatr Orthop* 1987;7:428–435.
50. Ogden JA (ed): Spine, in *Skeletal Injury in the Child.* Philadelphia, PA, Lea & Febiger, 1982, pp 385–422.
51. Blumberg KD, Catalano JB, Cotler JM, et al: The pull-out strength of titanium alloy MRI-compatible and stainless steel MRI-incompatible Gardner-Wells tongs. *Spine* 1993;18: 1895–1896.
52. Rizzolo SJ, Vaccaro AR, Cotler JM: Cervical spine trauma. *Spine* 1994;19:2288–2298.
53. Martinez-Lage JF, Perez-Espejo MA, Masegosa J, et al: Bilateral brain abscesses complicating the use of Crutchfield tongs. *Childs Nerv Syst* 1986;2:208–210.
54. Botte MJ, Garfin SR, Byrne TP, et al: The halo skeletal fixator: Principles of application and maintenance. *Clin Orthop* 1989; 239:12–18.
55. Garfin SR, Botte MJ, Waters RL, et al: Complications in the use of the halo fixation device. *J Bone Joint Surg* 1986;68A:320–325.
56. Botte MJ, Byrne TP, Garfin SR: Application of the halo device for immobilization of the cervical spine utilizing an increased torque pressure. *J Bone Joint Surg* 1987;69A:750–752.
57. Mubarak SJ, Camp JF, Vuletich W, et al: Halo application in the infant. *J Pediatr Orthop* 1989;9:612–614.
58. Garfin SR, Roux R, Botte MJ, et al: Skull osteology as it affects halo pin placement in children. *J Pediatr Orthop* 1986;6:434–436.
59. Letts M, Kaylor D, Gouw G: A biomechanical analysis of halo fixation in children. *J Bone Joint Surg* 1988;70B:277–279.

CHAPTER 11

Minimally Invasive Approaches to the Spine

John J. Regan, MD
Hansen Yuan, MD
Geoffrey McCullen, MD

Development of Endoscopic Surgery

Endoscopic surgery began with the invention of the cystoscope in 1806 by Bozzini.[1] He is recognized as the father of endoscopy for the development of the first endoscopic instrument, the *lichtleiter*, in which candlelight was used to illuminate multiple orifices including the vulva, urethra, and rectum. Bozzini was censured by the surgical academy for "undue curiosity." He died at age 35 in 1809, and his epitaph reads:

"In memory of the devout, deceased soul of Phillip Bozzini, medical doctor. He, German born, was the first who tried to look into the hollow cavities of the human body by ingeniously conducted light."[2]

Introduction, History, and Benefits

Surgeons have been looking through tubes into the thoracic cavity since 1910 when Jacobaeus[3] reported his use of thoracoscopy for the division of tuberculous adhesions. Applications of this technique remained limited because of visualization problems, and no significant advances were recorded until the advent of video-assisted technology. Dr. Ralph Lewis of New Brunswick, New Jersey, first recognized the importance of employing video-assisted technology to look into the thoracic cavity, and from the time of his first reports in 1991,[4,5] a vital new technical branch of surgery—video-assisted thoracic surgery (VATS)—has developed. Since then, a number of thoracic procedures, including sympathectomy, lung biopsy and resection, pericardiectomy, mediastinal tumor excision, and esophageal procedures have been performed employing this technology.[6-11]

In 1993, Landreneau and associates[12] reported reduced postoperative pain, improved shoulder girdle function, and shortened hospital stays in 106 patients undergoing VATS for peripheral lung lesions when these patients were compared to patients who underwent thoracotomy.

The technique of VATS for spinal disease or injury was first reported in 1993 by Mack and associates.[13] In this initial series, in vivo porcine experiments led to the development of specialized equipment initially used in March 1991 to perform diagnostic tissue biopsy and subsequent drainage of a thoracic paravertebral abscess. Since then, VATS has been applied to numbers of cases of thoracic disk herniation, spinal deformity requiring anterior release, osteotomy and bone grafting, and corpectomy for vertebral body tumor.[14] Subsequent reports of cadaver studies, in vivo animal studies, and early clinical experience have documented the efficacy of this procedure for the excision of thoracic disk herniation.[15,16] Although VATS is in its infancy, minimal complications have been reported in a combined series of 50 patients treated by VATS spinal techniques in three separate centers.[17] The considerable benefit of hindsight makes one wonder why it took our specialty so long to recognize the value of video-assisted spinal surgery, considering that its principles have been applied by gynecologists since 1974, by abdominal surgeons since 1987, and by orthopaedic surgeons for arthroscopy since 1977.[18-21]

Advantages and Disadvantages

There are several advantages of video-assisted spinal surgery over conventional transthoracic open procedures. The enhanced visualization provided to the operating team, including the anesthesiologist, results in more interest and participation in the case. Two surgeons may work side by side allowing standard instruments to be inserted while visualization is preserved, in spite of minimal incisions. The option of using 30° and 0° endoscopes allows extensive visualization of the thoracic spine anatomy, exceeding that possible with an open incision. The result is less vertebral body excision required to visualize and excise the disk herniation. Because the rib resection or the spreading of ribs associated with open thoracotomy is avoided with VATS, there is a reduction in incisional pain, chest tube drainage, respiratory problems, and shoulder girdle dysfunction, problems commonly associated with open procedures.[22] Decreased blood loss and decreased potential for infection result from the minimal incisions made in a relatively closed body cavity, as opposed to the large incisions required with rib distraction and its associated trauma. The scars from the three or four incisions measuring 1 to 2 cm are also cosmetically more appealing than the conventional long curvilinear thoracotomy scar. Reduced postoperative pain leads to improved perioperative ventilation, decreased intensive care unit time, decreased blood loss, shorter hospitalization, and shorter rehabilitation time with a resultant decrease in overall medical costs.[23] As with laparoscopic cholecystectomy,[24] it is expected that more patients will opt for video-assisted thoracic spine surgery rather than suffer intractable pain, given the unattractive alternative of thoracotomy.

The primary obstacle to video-assisted spinal surgery is the technical skill that must be acquired to employ endoscopic methods. Surgeons must look straight ahead at a monitor while coordinating their hand movements. Endoscopic techniques in general require the surgeon to develop facility in a two-dimensional environment and to relinquish the tactile sense used in open procedures. Orthopaedic surgeons with experience in arthroscopy quickly overcome this limitation, and recent evaluations of three-dimensional endoscopic camera systems indicate that they are primarily advantageous to the surgeon with little experience in endoscopic surgery and do not save time for the surgeon experienced in two-dimensional endoscopy. Placing the surgeon and the primary assistant on the ventral side of the patient facilitates the orientation and coordination process. Nonetheless, a period of practice with in vivo laboratory and cadaver specimens is indispensable for adapting to this new method. The addition of a skilled endoscopic thoracic surgeon, although it adds manpower to the procedure, is a necessity early on, for it provides optimal results while the spine surgeon gains the considerable experience needed.

In order for the procedure to be successful, the ipsilateral lung must be deflated. Technical difficulty, which occurs more commonly in pediatric and young adolescent patients because of their small airways and the necessity to use bronchial blockers, may result in reinflation or incomplete deflation of the lung, which can seriously impair visualization. Although vascular injury presents a potential problem, most situations can be managed without resorting to open incision. Incidental durotomy, which has not occurred in our first 50 cases,[15] would require open repair or lumbar spinal fluid drainage depending on the injury.

Bony work requires skilled manipulation of sharp spinal instruments at a distance averaging 24 cm from the spine. Visualization, as the instrument passes into the closed thoracic cavity, and two-handed control of the instrument are required. It is even more crucial that instruments used to cut or curette bone remain sharp to avoid slipping. The addition of a surgical drill system has improved the removal of bone, but needs further modification to become safer and more effective. A further disadvantage is that, at this time, there is no internal fixation device for the anterior thoracic spine that can be placed endoscopically. Currently, investigation is underway that may resolve this problem. As with any procedure that requires a skill vastly different from everyday open surgery, the success of VATS as a treatment for spinal disorders will in large part be determined by the frequency with which particular surgeons perform anterior thoracic spinal surgery in their practices.

Indications and Contraindications

In general, thoracoscopy is indicated for patients who require anterior approaches to the thoracic spine (Table 1).[25-30] Patients at high risk for thoracotomy may be better candidates for thoracoscopy. Many physiologic sequelae, which are detrimental to high-risk patients, occur following thoracotomy. These include decrease in functional residual capacity as well as documented incidence of postoperative atelectasis, secondary to chest wall splinting from pain.[31-34] Thoracoscopy is less traumatic than open thoracotomy or muscle-sparing thoracotomy incisions, and it results in less postoperative pain, improved shoulder girdle function, and less morbidity.[12,22]

Table 1
Indications: Spinal Thoracoscopy

Infection	Tumor	Degenerative Disk Disease	Spinal Deformity	Trauma
Biopsy, debridement Drainage of spinal abscess	Biopsy, tumor excision Corpectomy and grafting internal fixation (future)	Excision of thorcic herniated disk Fusion for diskogenic pain Interbody instrumentation (future)	Anterior release for rigid scoliosis > 75° Anterior release, fusion for Scheuermann's kyphosis > 90° Anterior epiphysiodesis in skeletally immature patients at risk of developing crankshaft phenomena Congenital spinal anomalies requiring anterior arthrodesis Neuromuscular deformity requiring anterior arthrodesis	Decompression/ fusion Internal fixation (future)

Patients with chronic obstructive pulmonary disease or interstitial fibrosis have abnormal pulmonary function preoperatively and obviously fit into the high risk category. Because these patients do not tolerate the physiologic effects of thoracotomy as well as those with normal lung function, thoracoscopy is an appropriate alternative. Patients with cardiac disease who require cardiac medications for either hypertension or mild congestive heart failure are considered high risk for the postoperative sequelae of thoracotomy.

Diagnostic and therapeutic biopsy of vertebral body tumors, osteomyelitis, and paravertebral abscesses are straightforward indications for thoracoscopy. Degenerative disk disease from T4-5 to T12-L1 can be approached from the left or right side depending on the location of the lesion. Patients who have undergone previous thoracic disk surgery from costotransversectomy or thoracotomy with retained disk material can be approached from the contralateral side. The endoscope provides a clear view across to the contralateral retained disk, which can be excised without going through scar tissue from previous surgery.

Thoracoscopy has been performed for pulmonary disease in children with ages ranging from 5 months to 17 years.[35] The pediatric patient with neuromuscular scoliosis and at-risk pulmonary status would most likely benefit from a less traumatic operative approach than the open approach. Rigid idiopathic deformities greater than 75° with associated restrictive lung disease are suitable candidates for thoracoscopic anterior release.[36] Skeletally immature patients who are at risk for developing crankshaft phenomena[37] are also candidates for anterior VATS epiphysiodesis, and VATS excision of neurofibromatosis has been amply described in the literature.[9] Hemivertebra resection using VATS has also been reported (GD Picetti, MD, Sacramento, CA, personal communication, 1995).

Thoracoscopy offers considerable advantages in cases of spinal deformity in adults whose treatment involves complex surgical procedures that require two or more stages. Anterior release can be performed in a shorter time, and, if a third stage is required, bone graft can be inserted thoracoscopically into the osteotomy defect without requiring a separate anesthetic. For example: A patient with severe kyphosis required anterior osteotomy followed by posterior osteotomy and correction of spinal deformity (Fig. 1, *left* and *center*). In stage three of the procedure, a rib strut graft harvested through the endoscope was placed in the anterior osteotomy. At 22-month follow-up, tomograms demonstrated fusion of the rib graft across the osteotomy defect (Fig. 1, *right*).

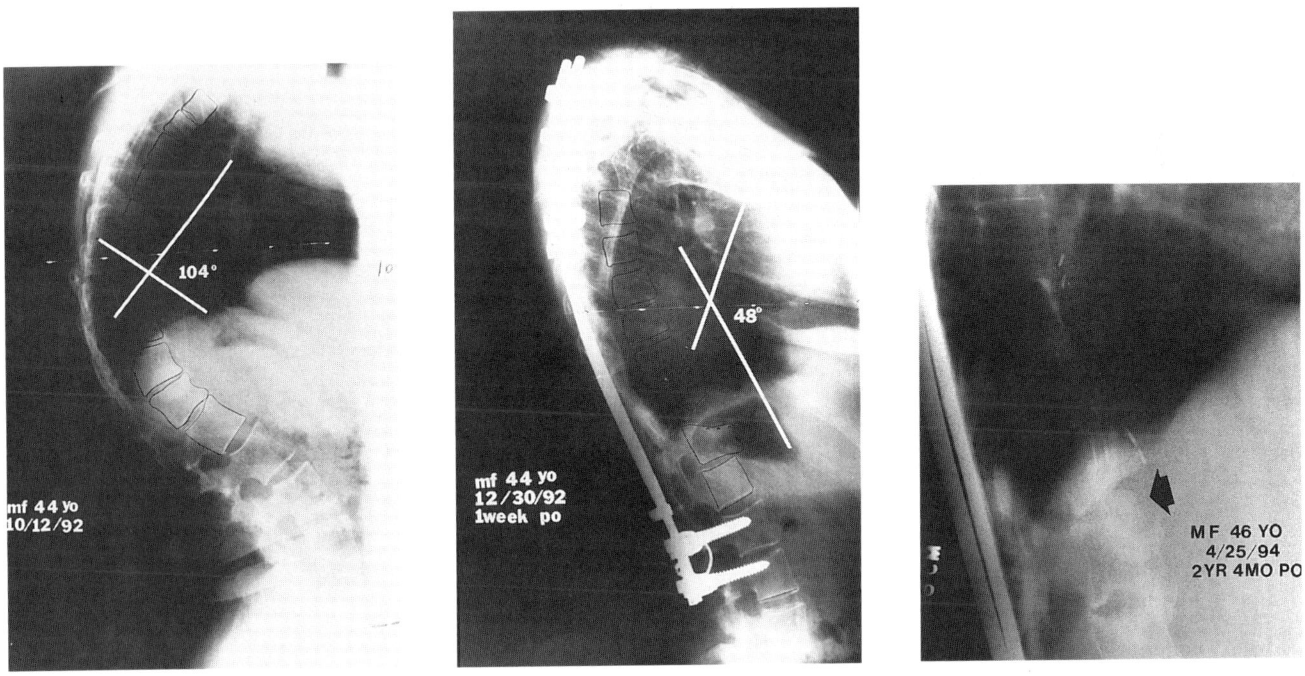

Fig. 1 **Left,** This 44-year-old female presented with 104° Scheuermann kyphosis following two previous unsuccessful attempts at correction with Harrington rods. **Center,** Under the same general anesthesia, video-assisted thoracic surgery (VATS) anterior spinal osteotomy was performed, followed by posterior osteotomy and correction of the deformity to 48° using the Isola System. **Right,** In a third stage performed 1 week following the initial two-stage procedure, a rib strut graft harvested endoscopically was placed into the anterior osteotomy site using VATS. The 22-month follow-up tomogram demonstrates solid fusion across the osteotomy defect.

Corpectomy for fracture and tumor has been successfully performed in ten cases using endoscopic technology. Rib strut grafts followed by posterior stabilization have been necessary to complete the reconstruction. The development of endoscopic anterior internal fixation should replace the necessity for posterior surgery. One additional category of patient for whom thoracoscopy may provide a benefit is the highly infectious patient with AIDS or hepatitis. In addition to minimizing risk to the surgical team, thoracoscopy may be the best alternative for immunocompromised patients who often have poor postoperative pulmonary function as a result of their underlying disease.

Thoracoscopic surgery is not indicated for all patients. VATS is contraindicated in patients with an inability to tolerate single lung ventilation, severe or acute respiratory insufficiency, high airway pressures with positive pressure ventilation, and pleural symphysis. Relative contraindications include previous tube thoracostomy or previous thoracotomy. Patients who require anterior internal fixation are not yet candidates for this procedure, although it is expected that future developments will rectify this problem.

Specialized Technology

In the past, thoracoscopy was performed bedside, primarily for diagnosis of pleural disease or in the treatment of a collapsed lung as a result of tuberculosis. Early experience with spinal VATS included the biopsy of vertebral body lesions and paravertebral masses. These biopsies and the more complex procedures of anterior spinal surgery should be performed in an operating room with equipment and personnel available to convert to open thoracotomy if that becomes necessary.

Operating Room Setup, Personnel, and Basic Equipment

Spinal VATS should be performed in a standard operating room that has monitors for assessing patients receiving general anesthesia and equipment available for open thoracotomy. Some modifications of the standard thoracoscopy setup are necessary for spinal procedures. After the anesthesiologist has set in place a double-lumen endotracheal tube, the patient is positioned in the lateral decubitus position and held securely in an Olympic positioner. It is vital to orient the patient in a straight lateral position to avoid confusion about the exact orientation of the spine, especially when work is to be done in the spinal canal. The hips and lower extremities may be gently brought down out of the way, but the extreme jack-knife position should be avoided as this may stretch an already compromised spinal cord. The patient should be fully prepared for a standard posterolateral thoracotomy with the iliac crest available if additional bone graft is needed. For approaches to the upper thoracic spine, the arm should be flexed slightly above 90° and the axilla draped out. The anesthesiologist must be prepared to set the table in an anterior tilt (Fig. 2) and apply Trendelenburg or reverse Trendelenburg as needed to permit the atelectatic lung to fall away from the dorsal spine.

In addition to the standard operating room setup, two video monitors are optimal. Unlike standard thoracoscopic procedures, the surgeon and first assistant stand on the same side—the abdominal side of the patient—viewing the monitor on the opposite side of the table when performing spinal VATS. Because two-handed control of the orthopaedic instruments is essential, a third assistant is necessary, especially when continuous fan retraction on the lung is required. The third assistant stands at the back side of the patient facing the opposite monitor (Fig. 3). Heads up display, a newer technology, will alleviate the problem of viewing interference, which can occur when operating personnel on the opposite side of the table from the surgeons block their view. Currently, dual monitors are placed at the head of the table in cases involving the mid and upper thoracic spine (Fig. 3). For surgery of the lower thoracic spine, in proximity to the diaphragm, a monitor is placed at the foot of the table so the surgeon can

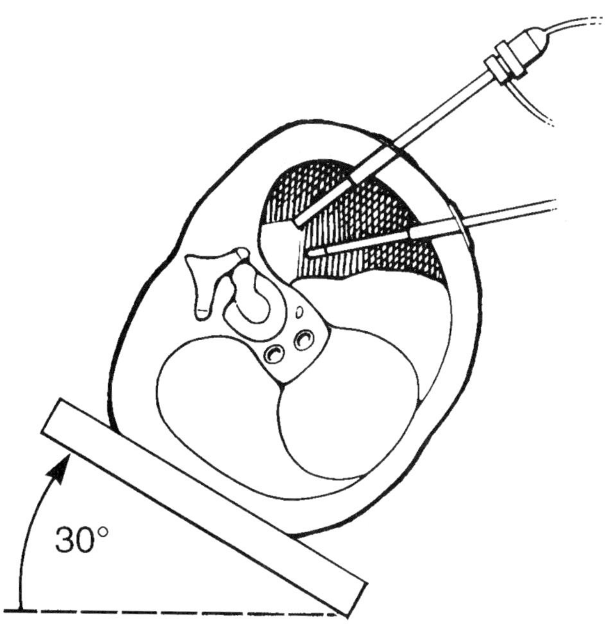

Fig. 2 Thoracoscopic approach to the dorsal spine with an operating table anterior-tilt 20° to 30°, allowing the lung to fall away from the spine. (Reproduced with permission from Regan JJ, McAfee PC, Mack MJ (eds): *Atlas of Endoscopic Spine Surgery*. St. Louis, MO, Quality Medical Publishers, 1995.)

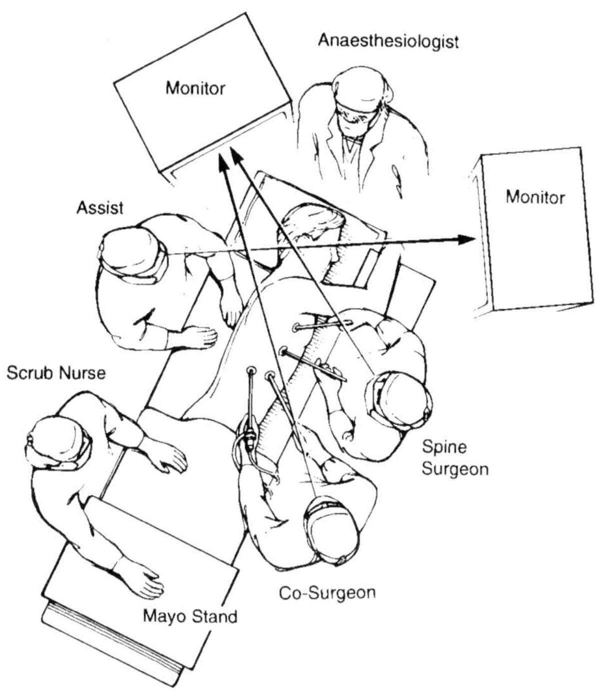

Fig. 3 Usual operating room (OR) setup, including location of OR personnel for approach to thoracic spine. (Reproduced with permission from Regan JJ, McAfee PC, Mack MJ (eds): *Atlas of Endoscopic Spine Surgery*. St. Louis, MO, Quality Medical Publishers, 1995.)

look toward the lower dorsal spine and take in the monitor at the same time. This orientation—the surgeon and camera facing the monitor—avoids mirror imaging, which occurs when the camera faces the surgeon. This orientation of camera and monitor is also the most comfortable working setup for the surgeon.

Extra personnel are usually required for spinal thoracoscopy, an equipment intensive surgery. The spinal surgeon is usually assisted by a thoracic surgeon with experience in thoracoscopy until the spine surgeon has gained considerable experience. The thoracic surgeon provides and maintains the exposure, holding the camera and operating the suction-irrigator or grasper. In many cases, the spine surgeon must use two hands to safely control the orthopaedic instruments. The third assistant may be another surgeon, a surgical resident, a medical student, a physician assistant, or a scrub nurse. This third assistant may be called upon to hold the camera, retract the lung, or assist in the suction or removal of disk or bony debris.

Maintaining the camera focus on the operating field is a challenging yet crucial task; thus, it helps if the third assistant has had arthroscopic experience. When working in the spinal canal, close-up camera work is required without obstructing the path of the instruments. Often, the individual holding the camera must gently zoom out of view an incoming instrument, then follow it with appropriate magnification, close to the spinal canal without changing the camera angle.

Camera, Monitors, Insufflator, and Video Recorder

With few exceptions, the equipment required for spinal thoracoscopy is similar to that used for general thoracoscopy. The basic equipment required for spinal VATS procedures includes telescopes, light sources, cameras, monitors, video recorders, and insufflators. The 30° angled telescope is used almost exclusively for spinal procedures because it allows visualization of safe passage of an instrument behind a structure at various angles. It also allows the visualization of the tip of an instrument around a corner, which occurs when disk material is being removed from the spinal canal. In adults, the 10-mm, 15-inch end-viewing scope is preferred; in pediatric cases, a 5-mm scope may be preferred. Although the smaller scope does not provide the same magnitude of illumination and resolution as the 10-mm scope, it is usually adequate and avoids the intercostal nerve injury that can occur with the larger scope. Telescopes with lens-washing and site irrigation systems are available, and are useful in defogging and cleansing the end of the scope. These features save the time that would otherwise be required to remove and clean the scope. Removing the scope to clean it can become a nuisance when working close to bleeding bone or adjacent oozing epidural veins.

Thoracoscopic Instruments

The vast array of instruments designed for use in general thoracoscopy may also be used in spinal VATS procedures. Instruments ranging from endoscopic Duvall lung clamps to endoscopic stapling devices must be available if pleural adhesions are encountered or if inadvertent injury to the lung occurs in the process of accessing the dorsal spine. See the *Atlas of Thoracoscopic Surgery* for a more detailed description of general thoracoscopic techniques and equipment.[38]

Trocars Trocars provide access into the chest for the surgical instruments and the camera. Because no CO_2 insufflation is required, an airtight seal is not necessary. We commonly use three to four 10.5-mm trocars in adults, and the same number of 5.5-mm trocars in children. Flexible trocars are now available (Flexipath Trocars, Ethicon, Cincinnati, OH). These can be cut to a desired length and are particularly helpful in patients with a thick chest wall. Soft trocars are purported to cause less intercostal nerve irritation than stiff trocars, but this observation has yet to be proven. In fact, the collapsing wall of the flexible catheter may sometimes impede ease of insertion and manipulation of the modified orthopaedic instruments needed for delicate spinal work.

Graspers One of the most commonly used instruments in spinal thoracoscopy is the grasper. This instrument is designed to hold, retract, palpate, and dissect tissue. Multiple configurations are available, but the most commonly used grasper for spinal procedures is the curved tip dissector, used to palpate disk, anulus, and rib, and to dissect around the segmental vessels. Right-angled dissectors are also useful in elevating segmental vessels off the periosteum. Bullet-tipped graspers aid in retracting the pleura and azygos vein away from the anterior spine to facilitate the surgical release in cases of scoliosis. Graspers may be either disposable or reusable. Most come with "pistol grip" handles, but there are some versions that have an axial control mechanism. These instruments come with unipolar cautery attachments. The insulated shaft of a grasper, especially a reusable one, should always be checked before using it with cautery. Conduction of a current through a defect in the instrument's insulation has been reported to cause bowel injury, and has the potential to cause cardiac fibrillation if the current arcs to the conduction system of the myocardium. Furthermore, electrical stimulation of the vagus nerve can produce bradycardia.

Endoscopic Scissors Endoscopic scissors are available in disposable and reusable versions. Although reusable instruments are generally more economical, the reusable shears tend to dull after multiple uses. The reticulating endoscopic disposable shears, which come with a curved tip and unipolar cautery, are especially useful for endoscopic dissection of pleura and sectioning of ligated segmental vessels.

Endoscopic Retractors There are a number of retractors on the market, both disposable and reusable. We have found the Endotract II (US Surgical Corporation, Norwalk, CT) fan retractor (Fig. 4) to be the most useful in retracting the atelectatic lung. The articulating arm is especially helpful for gently depressing the diaphragm, which is necessary for exposures to the lower dorsal spine.

Suction Irrigation Systems A variety of suction irrigation systems are available for use. A system that combines suction, irrigation, and unipolar cautery is the most useful for minimizing the need for several working portals. Employing an end-suction instrument like a Frazier tip suction device, smaller than 5 mm in diameter, that will not become clogged with bone or disk fragments is one of the challenges of performing spinal endoscopic procedures. A suction-irrigation system with monopolar cautery (Fig. 5) accomplishes a three-function goal, allowing the surgeon to suction the smoke at the point of coagulation to keep the field clear. This device must frequently be irrigated and often removed from the chest to clear bone and disk material from the device tip. Suction devices with sponge tips avoid the problem of plugging but prevent removal of debris. Further technologic development is expected to result in a more suitable device for suctioning and bone or disk removal.

Endoscopic Clip Appliers Clip appliers are used for hemostasis and for ligation of blood vessels before they are divided. This commonly occurs in the sectioning of segmental vein and artery. The position of segmental vessels in the trough of the vertebral body sometimes renders end-clipping devices obsolete. We have employed graspers and right-angled clamps to elevate vessels for end-clipping. We have also used right-angled vascular clip appliers with some success. The ideal clip applier for endoscopic spinal surgery has not yet been manufactured .

Modified Spinal Instruments The single advance that has made spinal endoscopy possible is the modification of instruments that are commonly used for open procedures of the spine (Fig. 6). These instruments have

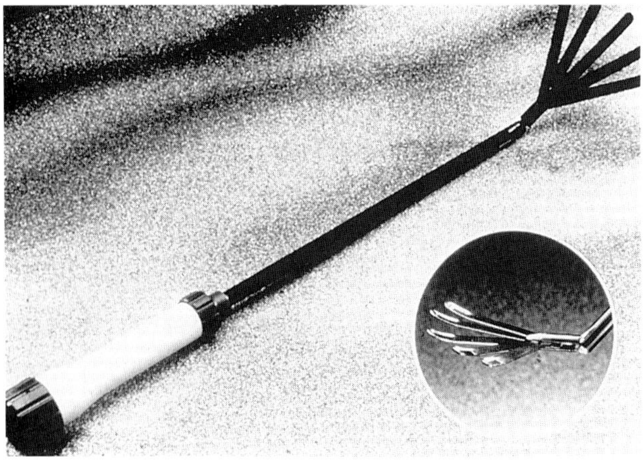

Fig. 4 Variable angled fan retractor used for lung retraction (Endotract II, USSC, Norwalk, CT).

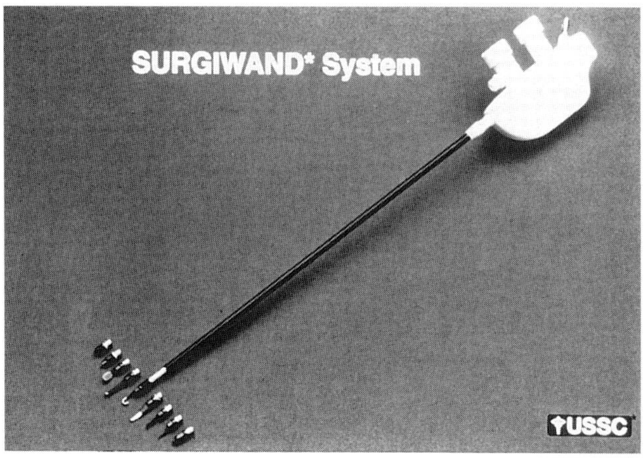

Fig. 5 Suction, irrigation, and unipolar cautery system with "Frazier-tipped" suction device useful in delicate spinal procedures (Surgiwand, USSC, Norwalk, CT).

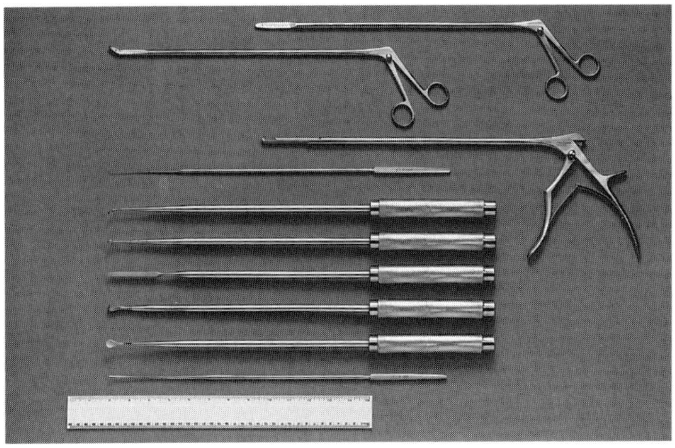

Fig. 6 Modified thoracoscopic instruments used in spinal video-assisted thoracic surgery: Cobb elevator, straight and angled pituitary rongeurs, Kerrison rongeurs, nerve probe and Penfield elevator, and angled curette.

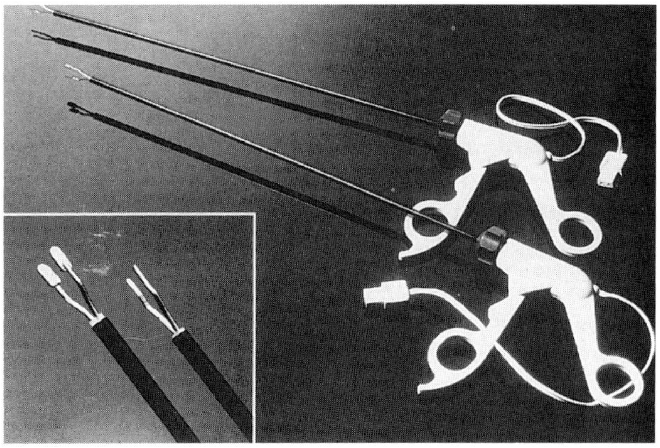

Fig. 7 Two endoscopic bipolar systems. The fine-tip bipolar is most commonly used in spinal procedures (Origin Medsystems, Menlo Park, CA).

been lengthened, and a uniform cylindrical diameter compatible with the 5-mm and 10-mm portals has been added for working in either gasless environments, eg, during thoracoscopy, or in instances requiring sealed gas environments, eg, most laparoscopic spinal procedures. In addition, a stiffer metal has been used for instrument shafts so they will not deflect when working at a distance to curette or remove bone. Modified Cobb elevator handles, osteotomes, and curettes have also been improved to provide room for two-hand control at a distance of approximately 24 cm from the spine.

Cobb elevators, straight and angled curettes, and pituitary and Kerrison rongeurs are the most commonly used modified spinal instruments. Long Penfield elevators and ball-tipped nerve hooks, used for probing the spinal canal for disk herniation or tumor, are made with thin shafts for more delicate proprioceptive control. Modified osteotomes are occasionally used to create a rib osteotomy, but their role is becoming limited with the application of the power drill to the procedure. Often, they may be used as an adjunct to complete an osteotomy started with a burr.

Bipolar Cautery Devices Bipolar cautery is an essential part of any procedure that involves work near the spinal canal. Epidural vessels must sometimes be cauterized, and this calls for an instrument with delicate hand control and fine tip to control small bleeders. These devices come in disposable (Origin Medsystems, Menlo Park, CA) (Fig. 7) and reusable varieties, with the Kleppinger forceps being the most widely available device used commonly in gynecologic procedures. Unfortunately, most Kleppinger forceps have a spatula tip that is too large for the delicate work required in spinal procedures.

Drill Systems Power systems have not yet been fully developed for use in thoracic or lumbar endoscopic procedures and are therefore considered investigational at this time. The ideal drill system will allow the surgeon to work at a distance and still maintain control over the drill. Some of the high RPM systems such as the Ultra Power Drill System (Zimmer Ultrapower, Hall Surgical, Carpinteria, CA) come in varying sizes that permit work at a hand-holding distance averaging 16 cm from the spine. The grip allows adequate control of the drill and the high RPM minimizes skipping on the bone. Side-cutting burrs are used to increase the safety while working near the spinal canal. Unfortunately, these drills do not yet come with a long enough tapered drill to optimize visualization. This, in addition to a drill guard, useful in rib resection, should add a measure of safety and facilitate procedures such as corpectomy or thoracoplasty.

Intervertebral Fusion Cages Endoscopic fusion systems are currently under investigation and are therefore considered experimental at this time. Instrumentation is currently being developed to facilitate the efficient removal of intervertebral disk, the preparation of the bony end plate, and the subsequent endoscopic insertion of a device that will both distract and provide internal fixation of the disk level to be fused.

Surgical Technique

Thoracoscopic procedures are performed under general anesthesia with a double-lumen endotracheal tube inserted for ipsilateral lung collapse and single lung ventilation. A bronchial blocker may be necessary in the pediatric spinal patient, but we have found this difficult to place with problems of spontaneous reinflation occurring during the procedure as a result of dislodging of the bronchial blocker. The univent tube is especially helpful in the pediatric patient.

Patient Positioning

Patients are placed in the lateral decubitus position, similar to that used for thoracotomy, using an axillary roll and the Olympic positioner (Fig. 3). The patient is subsequently tilted anteriorly to allow the atelectatic ipsilateral lung to fall away from the dorsal spine (Fig. 2). A Trendelenburg position is then used when approaching the lower thoracic spine, while reverse Trendelenburg is used to improve visualization of the apical thorax and dorsal spine. In many cases, appropriate positioning combined with a brief period of CO_2 thoracic cavity inflation at 8 cm H_2O will result in sufficient atelectasis to permit surgery without the need to manually retract the lung.

Trocar Insertion Techniques

Before discussing strategy specific to spinal thoracoscopy, basic principles of endoscopy must be accomplished regardless of the specific location of each trocar site: (1) Trocar sites must be placed at a distance from the lesion to achieve a panoramic view and to provide room to manipulate instruments. (2) Instrument crowding, which results in "fencing," comes from portals placed too near to each other. (3) Avoid mirror imaging by positioning instruments in a 180° arc, with instruments and camera facing in the same direction toward the lesion. (4) Instruments should be manipulated only when seen through the thoracoscope. Sharp orthopaedic instruments must be visualized at all times. (5) Avoid random simultaneous movement of camera and instruments. In close-up situations, move the camera slowly back to pick up an incoming instrument and then slowly zoom in without changing the camera angle.

The primary operative strategy in spinal cases is to orient the instruments and camera facing the spine. This is accomplished by placing the operating surgeon and co-surgeon, usually a thoracic surgeon, on the abdominal side of the patient facing the monitor on the opposite side of the table (Fig. 3). In situations where decompression of the spinal canal is necessary, ie, thoracic disk herniation, trocar sites are placed near the anterior axillary line. In scoliosis deformity the spine is rotated toward the apex of the curve making optimal trocar placement in the midaxillary line. Regardless of the location of pathology, the initial portal for the thoracoscope is placed at the sixth or seventh intercostal space to avoid perforation of the diaphragm and provide the best location for inspection of the thoracic cavity.

After initial exploratory thoracoscopy is completed, a second portal is placed three intercostal spaces above or below this depending on the location of the pathology. If resorptive atelectasis has not occurred at this point, a brief period of carbon dioxide insufflation of up to 8 cm H_2O can be temporarily added to facilitate lung collapse. Gravity is then used to enhance visualization by tilting the patient forward (Fig. 2) and using Trendelenburg or reverse Trendelenburg depending on the location of the spine to be visualized. A fan retractor can be inserted and the ipsilateral lung open to atmosphere to facilitate the completion of this process by gentle pressure on the lung with the fan retractor.

Once the thoracic spine is well-visualized through the parietal pleura, the correct level is identified by counting the ribs as seen through the endoscope. The first rib, which takes off at a more acute angle than the second rib, often is not visualized but can be palpated. Once the correct level is identified, a localizing Veress needle or 10-inch spinal needle is directed from the anterior axillary line on the skin directly across to the desired disk space, avoiding any significant angulation. After radiographic confirmation, a third trocar site, the

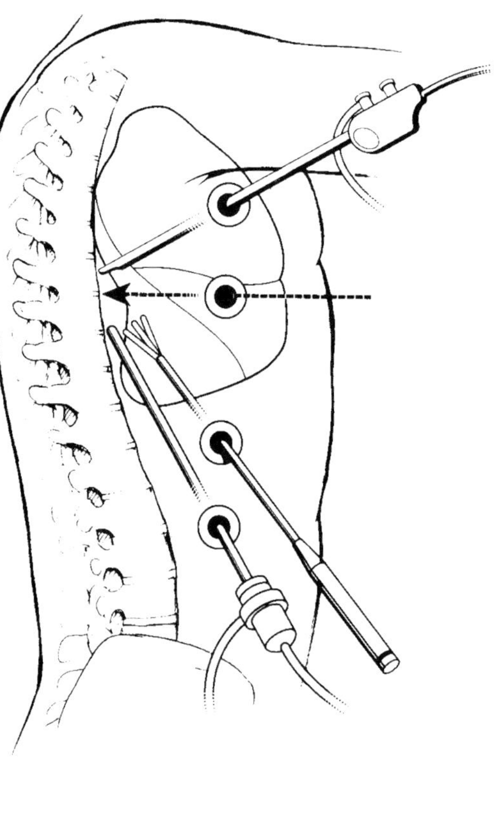

Fig. 8 Right thoracoscopic approach to mid-thoracic spine with typical positioning of instruments and camera for an approach to herniated disk at the T8-9 disk space. (Reproduced with permission from Regan JJ, McAfee PC, Mack MJ (eds): *Atlas of Endoscopic Spine Surgery.* St. Louis, MO, Quality Medical Publishers, 1995.)

primary working portal, can be placed here. If necessary, a fourth portal can be placed for suction and irrigation, and this is usually placed toward the posterior axillary line opposite the disk space targeted (Fig. 8).

In spinal deformity, four trocar sites are established, all in the midaxillary line. In thoracic disk herniations, trocar sites form a diamond in the mid thoracic region and an "L" in lesions of the upper or lower dorsal spine. We have been able to successfully approach thoracic disk herniations from T4-5 to T12-L1 using these principles. The thoracolumbar disk, situated at or just above the diaphragm, is approached by placing a fan retractor in the anterior axillary line just above the diaphragm so that the diaphragm can be depressed. In the upper dorsal spine, the arm is flexed slightly beyond 90° without putting the brachial plexus on stretch. With the axilla prepared, portal placements can be made as high as the third intercostal space.

Thoracic Disk Herniation

If a procedure is being performed to excise a disk herniation, the rib head and proximal 2 to 3 cm are removed after cauterizing the parietal pleura over the appropriate rib. In the case of T8-9 herniation, the head of the ninth rib is removed. In disk herniations at T11-12 it is not necessary to remove the rib, because it inserts below the disk space. In the case of T12-L1 herniations, the pleural reflection of the diaphragm is sectioned and the L1 pedicle clearly identified before disk removal.

Once the rib head is removed, using an osteotome or drill, the pedicle is identified and subsequently the superior portion is removed with a curette or an angled Kerrison rongeur. Once the superior pedicle is removed, the dura can be identified and the process of disk excision is begun with an angled curette. Nuisance epidural bleeding may occur at this time necessitating the use of bipolar cautery. Small amounts of oozing are common during these procedures and continuous suction is usually required during work around the dura. Excessive epidural bleeding can be controlled with Endoavitene (MedChem Products, Waburn, MA) followed by insertion of a surgical sponge. A brief period of tamponade should result in hemostasis, allowing the surgeon to continue. The cell-saver system should not be used during Avitene installation. Prior to terminating the operation, Avitene should be irrigated away from the dura to prevent the possibility of an epidural hematoma, which can form under this hemostatic plug. Segmental vessels, which usually are not sacrificed during this procedure, require endoscopic clips.

Anterior Release for Spinal Deformity

Multiple level anterior disk releases can be performed in cases of kyphosis and scoliosis (GD Picetti, Sacramento, CA, personal communication, 1995). The intervertebral disk space is entered by cauterizing the anulus pulposus. After thorough disk removal, using pituitary rongeurs, the release can proceed anteriorly. A grasper is used to elevate the pleura and azygos vein away from the anterior longitudinal ligament and the concave aspect of the anulus. Following this, a rongeur is used to complete the resection until anterior instability is produced. In this manner, five or six levels can be released in many cases with minimum sacrifice of the segmental vessels. Subsequently, morcellated rib graft or iliac graft can be placed in the intervertebral disk spaces prior to terminating the procedure. Following the anterior release procedure, the patient is turned in the prone position for definite curve correction, stabilization, and fusion.

Corpectomy for Excision of Tumor or Fracture

The procedure for corpectomy is very similar to diskectomy with the exception that the entire pedicle is removed to visualize the dura. Once this is performed, diskectomy above and below the vertebra to be excised is accomplished. Using angled curettes and rongeurs, tumor or bone fragment are then pulled away from the cord into a trough made by excising the bulk of the vertebral body, similar to open techniques of corpectomy (Fig. 9). After the dura has been sufficiently decompressed, strut grafting with allograft or autograft can be performed through the endoscope. Anterior internal fixation has recently been performed at several medical centers (P McAfee, MD, D Rosenthal, MD, J Regan, MD, personal communication, 1995). This has been possible using a slightly larger incision to place a vertebral replacement cage followed by internal fixation using a thoracic Z-plate. (Danek, Memphis) (Fig. 10). Posterior internal fixation may be necessary if further stabilization is felt to be necessary.

Laparoscopic Approach to the Lumbar Spine

This approach requires the combined and coordinated efforts of a general surgeon well-versed in laparoscopic surgery and the orthopaedic surgeon. Specific training is required prior to beginning such cases. Preparation before the surgery is perhaps the most important step. Necessary instruments include C-arm fluoroscopy, CO_2 insufflation equipment, a 30° endoscope, laparoscopic trocars with adaptors, and two television monitors.

The patient is placed in a supine position on a radiolucent table. An elevated kidney rest or a roll may be placed beneath the lumbar region to maintain lordosis. Knees are flexed to 20°. Padded shoulder-restraining devices are used to stabilize the patient when the steep

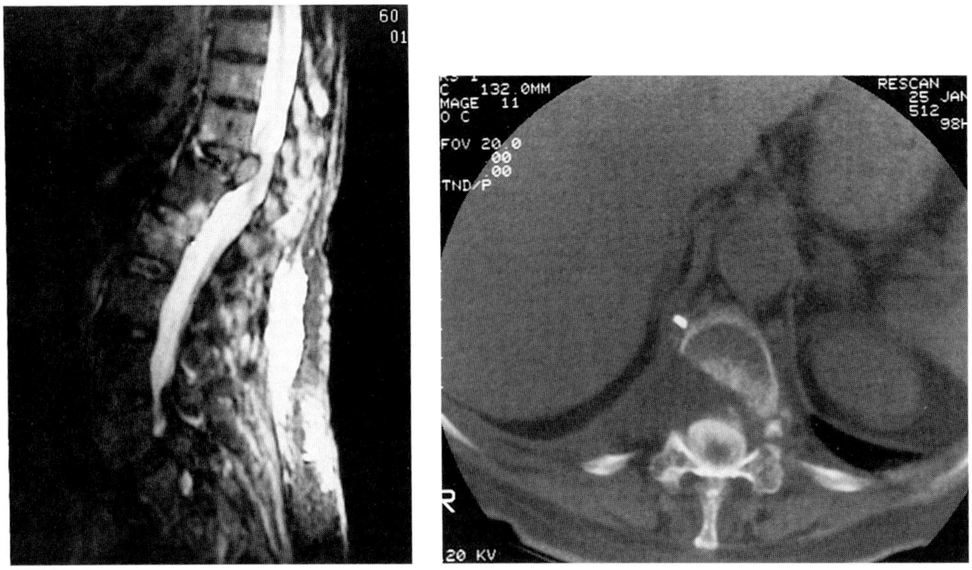

Fig. 9 Top Left, Successful corpectomy was performed using video-assisted thoracic surgery in this 61-year-old female with cord compression secondary to osteoporotic burst fracture at T11. **Top right,** Postoperative computed tomography scan demonstrates satisfactory decompression of thecal sac. **Bottom left,** Endoscopic photograph and **Bottom right,** drawing depict decompression of thecal sac and excellent visualization of dural tube and nerve root. (Reproduced with permission from Regan JJ, McAfee PC, Mack MJ (eds): *Atlas of Endoscopic Spine Surgery.* St. Louis, MO, Quality Medical Publishers, 1995.)

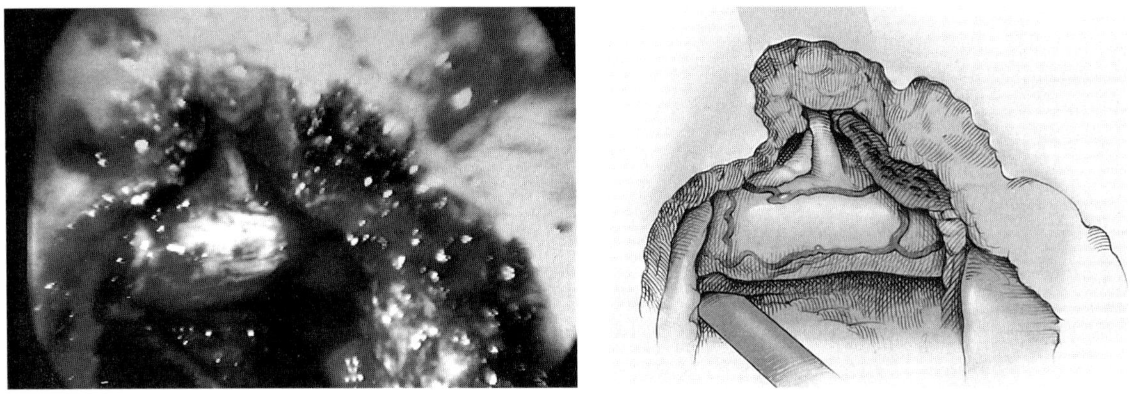

Trendelenburg position is used to mobilize the bowel from the pelvis. The entire chest, abdomen, and proximal thighs are prepped and widely draped to allow for emergency access to the great vessels, if necessary, to gain both proximal and distal control.

The first portal is most typically placed at the umbilicus. The "Hassan" technique uses an open incision with direct visualization of the peritoneum. Alternatively, a camera placed in an "optiport" trocar allows visualization as retractable cutting blades proceed through successive layers of the anterior abdominal wall. Insufflation is performed to 15 mm Hg through a port on this trocar. The scope then can be safely entered. Inspection of the abdominal wall lateral to the epigastric vessels reveals satisfactory entry sites for the working portals. A single left trocar is placed under direct endoscopic visualization. Through this a fan retractor or Babcock is placed and used to mobilize the sigmoid colon from right to left. Retraction is performed to tension the peritoneal reflection. Two right-sided trocars are placed, separated so as to avoid instrument crowding. Monopolar endoshears are then used to incise the peritoneum along this reflection. The drop-off at the sacral promontory is visualized.

Access to L5-S1 requires a blunt, spreading technique with Kitners to expose the aortic bifurcation and the middle sacral artery and vein. These latter vessels are mobilized, ligated with hemoclips, and divided. During this dissection, care must be taken not to injure the underlying bifurcation of the inferior vena cava that is typically drawn tight, like a ribbon, across the L5 vertebral body. The inferior hypogastric sympathetic plexus is best protected through the use of gentle, blunt tissue handling with complete avoidance of monopolar coagulation. In males, inadvertent injury to this plexus may cause retrograde ejaculation.

For exposure of L4-5, a left to right mobilization of the left common iliac vein and artery is performed. The large, ascending segmental vein on the left must first be identified, ligated, and divided. Hyperlordosis

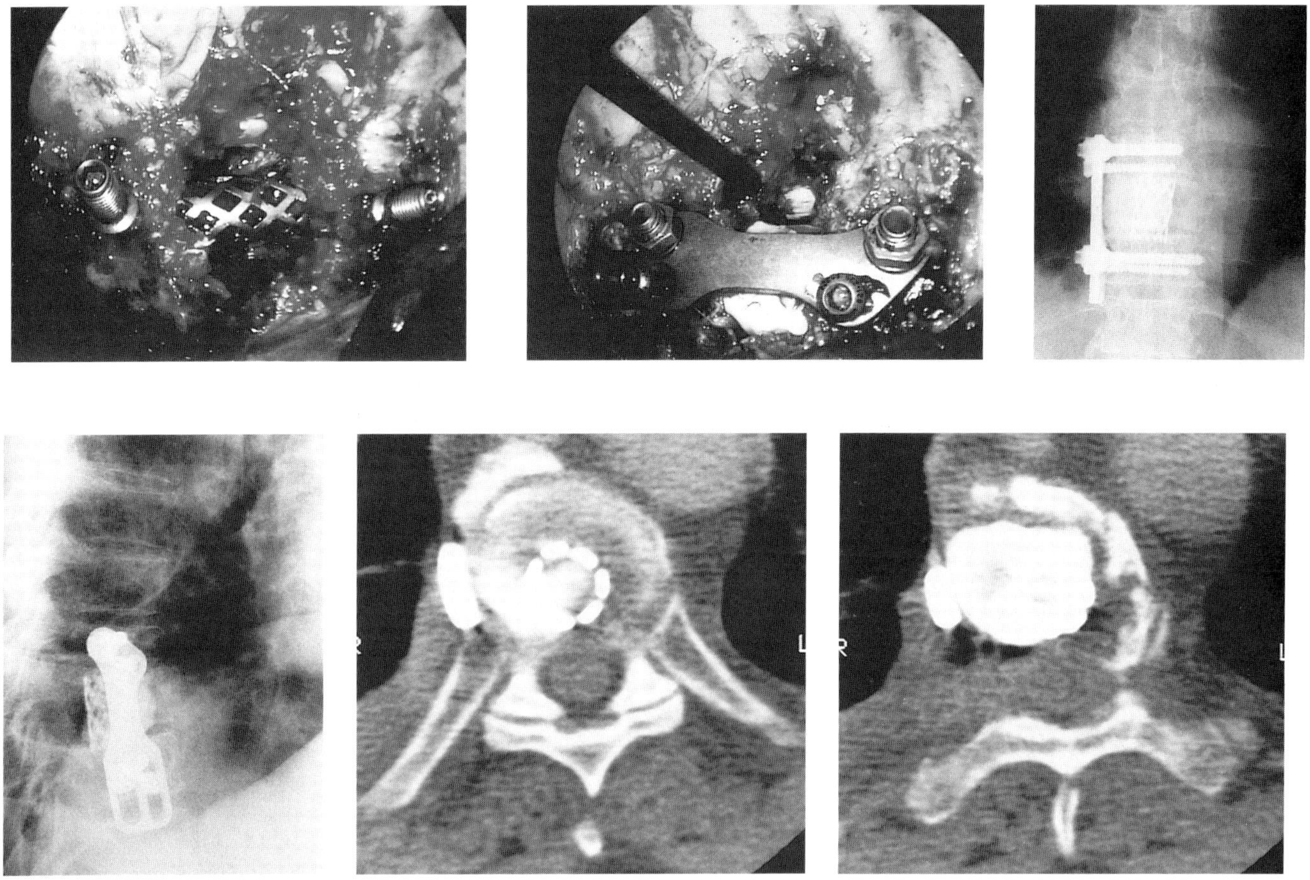

Fig. 10 This 51-year-old female with metastatic breast cancer at T8 presented with paraparesis. Using video-assisted thoracic surgery, corpectomy was accomplished. Subsequently a Hairms cage was inserted into the vertebral body defect **(top left)** followed by application of a Z-plate with polymethylmethacrylate utilized to fill the cage **(top center).** Postoperative anteroposterior and lateral radiographs **(top right** and **bottom left)** and CT scan **(bottom center** and **right)** demonstrate satisfactory fixation with a Z-plate. The patient was discharged on the fourth postoperative day with improving neurologic function.

causes this vein to be stretched over the spine. It may be necessary to lower the kidney rest. Fan retractors then maintain exposure.

Two-plane fluoroscopic imaging confirms a parallel and central approach to the disk space via a cannula placed in the midline suprapubically. Through this fifth portal site, a starter drill enters the disk space. Serial dilation of the interbody space ensues with placement of progressively larger "bullets." A hand drill provides end-plate exposure and decortication for a successful interbody fusion. Under sagittal plane fluoroscopic imaging, a laparoscopic pituitary disk rongeur completes the process of disk debridement. An interbody cage packed with cancellous bone or a dowel graft is placed.

At completion, to obtain optimal inspection for bleeding, the Trendelenburg position is reversed and the insufflation pressure is decreased. The peritoneum may be electively closed with suture or approximated with clips. Each trocar site is inspected for bleeding as the trocar is removed. The fascia and skin are closed with an absorbable suture.

Mobilization of the patient is begun as soon as possible, usually within 1 day of the surgery. No oral intake is allowed until bowel sounds and flatus return. Postoperative ileus may occasionally last 3 to 4 days.

As described, the laparoscopic approach allows safe access to the L4-5 and L5-S1 interspaces. The majority of cases have been for degenerative disk disease at these levels. Ongoing research is seeking to expand these current limits to include upper lumbar levels via endoscopy of the retroperitoneum. An expandable balloon is used to first dilate this potential space; insufflation follows. An anterolateral view of the disk is allowed. Interbody fusion with a cage or dowel graft is possible. As instrumentation improves, the scope of available interventions will widen and will include decompression and stabilization for tumor, infection, and fracture.

Preliminary Results

The first reported clinical series of VATS spinal surgery demonstrated the efficacy of this technique in managing a variety of thoracic spinal problems that otherwise require open thoracotomy.[13,14] Anterior release and fusion for deformity, biopsy of vertebral body lesions, drainage of paravertebral abscess, internal thoracoplasty, and thoracic diskectomy were all successfully accomplished in this initial series of 12 patients. When compared to thoracotomy, times required for the procedures were comparable, and blood loss, intensive care unit stay, narcotic usage, and hospitalization were reduced by almost 50%.[23]

The most extensive experience of the VATS technique in spine has been for transthoracic excision of herniated thoracic disks.[39] A variety of techniques, such as costotransversectomy[40] have been used as effective surgical methods of diskectomy, while laminectomy has fallen out of favor as a result of increased neurologic morbidity.[41]

Transthoracic diskectomy, using either standard or muscle-sparing thoracotomy incision[42] or the extrapleural transthoracic approach,[43] has the advantage of a direct approach to the anteriorly located disk herniation. Bohlman and Zdeblick[44] reported improved results of transthoracic technique when this was compared to posterior techniques. It seems clear that anterior approaches to the thoracic disk provide a more direct approach to all but the laterally oriented disk herniations.

The advent of thoracoscopy has provided the next evolutionary step in managing this problem by the most direct method with a minimally invasive technique. In our initial experience, 28 consecutive patients with thoracic disk herniation treated by VATS techniques between March 1991 and February 1993 were reviewed.[14] All patients presented with at least 6 months of thoracic central and/or radicular pain, with the exception of three patients who presented with progressive myelopathy. Three patients had previously undergone unsuccessful costotransversectomy and presented with persistent symptoms as a result of a retained disk herniation. Diagnosis was established by magnetic resonance imaging (MRI) or computed tomography (CT) myelogram demonstrating flattening of the spinal cord by the disk herniation.

Mean operative time for the 28 patients was 2.6 hours, down from 4.2 hours for the first five patients to 2.1 hours for the last five patients in the series. The thoracic aorta did not prove to be a problem, because 50% of the patients were approached from the left side as a result of the location of the lesion. One patient, with persistent disk herniation following a posterior procedure, had to be converted to an open thoracotomy as a result of difficulty defining appropriate landmarks through the thoracoscope. Two other patients, with persistent disk herniation following costotransversectomy, were successfully approached using VATS techniques from the contralateral side to avoid problems of scarring. The location of disk herniations ranged from T4-5 to T12-L1, with the majority at or below T8-9. Lower thoracic disk herniation and thoracolumbar disk herniation were successfully excised by inserting a fan retractor to depress the diaphragm. In the case of the T12-L1 herniation, posterior fibers of the diaphragm were divided to provide access to this disk space.

Rib head resection was necessary to visualize the spinal canal in all cases except T11 and T12 where the rib inserts below the disk space. Successful disk removal was determined by visual inspection of the dura with the scope and obtaining a cross-table anteroposterior thoracic radiograph with a Penfield probe to ensure adequate removal. Postoperative CT or MRI scans were also obtained in the first 15 patients to determine adequacy of decompression (Fig. 11). Blood loss, which averaged 800 cc in the earlier experience, has been reduced to 250 cc in the most recent cases. Use of intensive care has been eliminated except for elderly patients or those medically compromised before the surgery. Chest tube duration averaged 24 hours. A #24 French tube was used to minimize postoperative discomfort. In the last ten cases, chest tube drainage diminished to less than 150 cc as a result of experience gained with techniques of securing hemostasis.

Hospitalization, which averaged 7 days early in the series, was reduced to 3.2 days in the last five patients, with the best case leaving the hospital after 24 hours. Minimum 6-month follow-up indicates 86% improvement or resolution of preoperative symptoms. As with open series, poor results occurred in patients with longer than 2 years' duration of symptoms and workers' compensation cases with litigation pending.

In this series of the first 28 cases of thoracic disk herniation treated with VATS techniques, there were no cases of neurologic deterioration following the surgery. No dural lacerations occurred in spite of calcified disk herniations in almost 50% of patients and posterior osteophytes requiring resection in three patients. Pulmonary complications were minimal, with an isolated case of persistent pleural effusion and one of asymptomatic pneumothorax, which resolved spontaneously.

In another multicenter study of the first 50 consecutive cases of endoscopic anterior thoracic spinal reconstructive surgery; which included 27 thoracic diskectomies, 17 scoliosis anterior releases, and six anterior vertebral corpectomies for trauma, tumor, or infection;[17] one case of perforation of the diaphragm with a trocar occurred. This points out the necessity for endoscopic visualization of all instrument and trocar placements during the surgery. There were no cases of permanent neurologic deficit. One patient, an adult with a 120° thoracic scoliosis undergoing anterior release

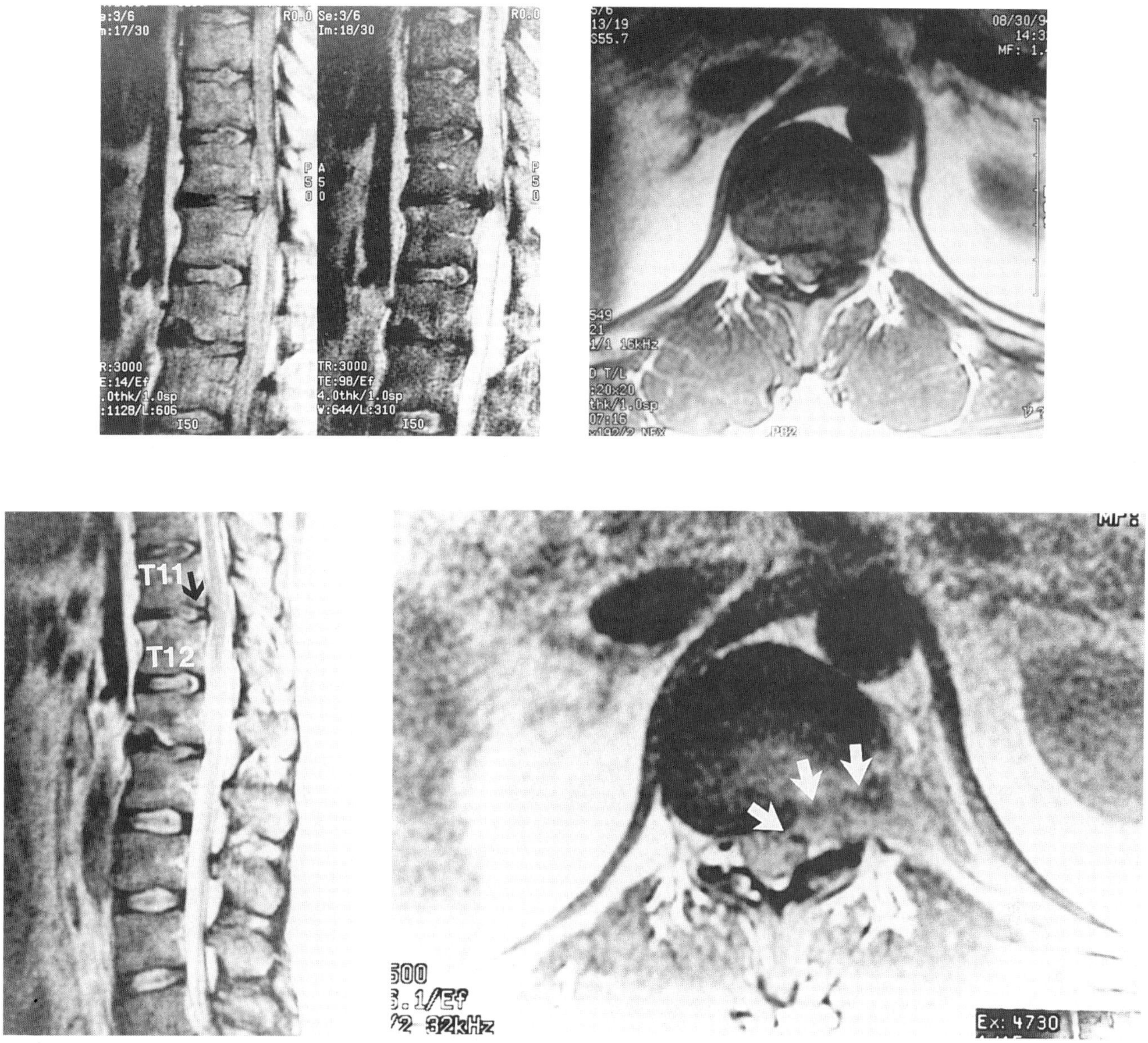

Fig. 11 **Top,** This 35-year-old male presented with paraparesis following a water-skiing accident. Magnetic resonance imaging (MRI) demonstrates left paracentral disk herniation at T11-12. Following thoracoscopic diskectomy, MRI demonstrates removal of herniation **(bottom left)** with minimal resection of normal disk and end plate **(bottom right)** as indicated by arrows.

from T4 to T12, developed transient paraparesis secondary to focal stenosis not recognized preoperatively. This complication was felt to be secondary to intraoperative jack-knife positioning of the patient. There were no wound infections, no dural lacerations, and no injury to major blood vessels. The most common area of complications was pulmonary. There was one case of prolonged intubation in a patient with prior lobectomy for adenocarcinoma, two cases of atelectasis that resolved spontaneously in 5 days, and one case of loculated effusion that resolved in 1 month. Intercostal neuralgia occurred in four instances, with all but one resolving in 6 weeks and the last taking 4 months to resolve.

Conclusion

Recently, video-assisted thoracic surgical techniques for the treatment of thoracic spinal disease have been performed successfully for a variety of conditions ranging from biopsy to corpectomy and anterior reconstruction using internal fixation. As with knee arthroscopy, it will take time and technical improvements before this technique will be widely accepted and demonstrate clear advantages over open techniques, especially for complex procedures such as anterior spinal reconstruction and instrumentation. This technique presently provides minimal incisional and approach related trauma while affording excellent visualization of the thoracic spine, sometimes superior to that of open approaches. This affords the basis to achieve the ultimate goal of spinal surgical care, which is to direct the treatment specifically to the pathology with minimal impact on normal anatomic structures. It is with improvements in surgical skill and technology that we will eventually achieve the goal of restoring the spine to near normal function without the injuries to ligamentous, muscular, and bony structures that result in prolonged and sometimes incomplete recovery following open spinal surgical procedures.

Acknowledgments

The authors thank Scott Bodell for his very fine medical illustrations and Sandra Pinkerton, PhD, for reading and editing the manuscript at different stages prior to submission. The authors also thank the publications staff of the Institute for Spine and Biomedical Research for their help with literature searches and for manuscript production. Finally, the authors thank Schelle Browning for her untiring support in preparing the manuscript.

References

1. Bozzini P: Lichtleiter, eine Erfindung zur Anschung innerer Theile und Krankheiten nebst Abbidung. *Pract Arzekunde* 1806;24:107.
2. Bush RB: Leonhardt H, Bush IV, et al: Dr. Bozzini's Lichtleiter: A translation of his original article (1806). *Urology* 1974; 3:119–123.
3. Jacobaeus HC: Possibility of the use of cystoscope for the investigation of the serous cavities. *Munch Med Wochenschr* 1910; 57:2090–2092.
4. Lewis RJ, Caccavale RJ, Sisler GE: Special report: Video-endoscopic thoracic surgery. *N J Med* 1991;88:473–475.
5. Lewis RJ, Caccavale RJ, Sisler GE: Imaged thoracoscopic surgery: A new thoracic technique for resection of mediastinal cysts. *Ann Thorac Surg* 1992;53:318–320.
6. Landreneau RJ, Mack MJ, Hazelrigg SR, et al: Video-assisted thoracic surgery: Basic technical concepts and intercostal approach strategies. *Ann Thorac Surg* 1992;54:800–807.
7. Landreneau RJ, Hazelrigg SR, Ferson PF, et al: Thoracoscopic resection of 85 pulmonary lesions. *Ann Thorac Surg* 1992; 54:415–420.
8. Landreneau RJ, Dowling RD, Castillo WM, et al: Thoracoscopic resection of an anterior mediastinal tumor. *Ann Thorac Surg* 1992;54:142–144.
9. Landreneau RJ, Dowling RD, Ferson PF: Thoracoscopic resection of a posterior mediastinal neurogenic tumor. *Chest* 1992;102:1288–1290.
10. Coltharp WH, Arnold JH, Alford WC Jr, et al: Videothoracoscopy: Improved technique and expanded indications. *Ann Thorac Surg* 1992;53:776–779.
11. Mack MJ, Aronoff RJ, Acuff TE, et al: Present role of thoracoscopy in the diagnosis and treatment of diseases of the chest. *Ann Thorac Surg* 1992;54:403–409.
12. Landreneau RJ, Hazelrigg SR, Mack MJ, et al: Postoperative pain-related morbidity: Video-assisted thoracic surgery versus thoracotomy. *Ann Thorac Surg* 1993;56:1285–1289.
13. Mack MJ, Regan JJ, Bobechko WP, et al: Application of thoracoscopy for diseases of the spine. *Ann Thorac Surg* 1993; 56:736–738.
14. Regan JJ, Mack MJ, Picetti GD III: A technical report on video-assisted thoracoscopy in thoracic spinal surgery: Preliminary description. *Spine* 1995;20:831–837.
15. Horowitz MB, Moossy JJ, Julian T, et al: Thoracic discectomy using video assisted thoracoscopy. *Spine* 1994;19:1082–1086.
16. Rosenthal D, Rosenthal R, de Simone A: Removal of a protruded thoracic disc using microsurgical endoscopy: A new technique. *Spine* 1994;19:1087–1091.
17. McAfee PC, Regan JR, Zdeblick T, et al: The incidence of complications in endoscopic anterior thoracolumbar spinal reconstructive surgery: A prospective multicenter study comprising the first 100 consecutive cases. *Spine* 1995; 20:1624–1632.
18. Marlow J: History of laparoscopy, optics, fiberoptics, and instrumentation. *Clin Obstet Gynecol* 1976;19:261–275.
19. Wheeless CR Jr: Abstract: The status of outpatient tubal sterilization by laparoscopy. Improved technics and review of 1000 cases. *Obstet Gynecol* 1972;39:635–636.
20. Reddick EJ, Olsen DO: Laparoscopic laser cholecystectomy: A comparison with mini-lap cholecystectomy. *Surg Endosc* 1989;3:131–133.
21. Watanabe M: Editorial: Development of arthroscope. *Ryumachi* 1977;17:371–372.
22. Ferson PF, Landreneau RJ, Dowling RD, et al: Comparison of open versus thoracoscopic lung biopsy for the diagnosis of diffuse infiltrative lung disease. *J Thorac Cardiovasc Surg* 1993; 106:194–199.
23. Regan JJ, Mack MJ, Picetti GD III, et al: A comparison of video-assisted thoracoscopic surgery (VATS) with open thoracotomy in thoracic spinal surgery. *Today's Therapeutic Trends* 1994; 11:203–218.
24. McKernan JB, Saye WB: Laparoscopic general surgery. *J Med Assoc Ga* 1990;79:157–159.
25. Bradford DS: Adult scoliosis: Current concepts of treatment. *Clin Orthop* 1988;229:70–87.
26. Byrd JA III, Scoles PV, Winter RB, et al: Adult idiopathic scoliosis treated by anterior and posterior spinal fusion. *J Bone Joint Surg* 1987;69A:843–850.
27. Dwyer AF: Experience of anterior correction of scoliosis. *Clin Orthop* 1973;93:191–214.
28. Dwyer AF, Schafer MF: Anterior approach to scoliosis: Results of treatment in fifty-one cases. *J Bone Joint Surg* 1974;56B:218–224.
29. Lobosky JM, Hitchon PW, McDonnell DE: Transthoracic anterolateral decompression for thoracic spinal lesions. *Neurosurgery* 1984;14:26–30.
30. Johnson JR, Holt RT: Combined use of anterior and posterior surgery for adult scoliosis. *Orthop Clin North Am* 1988;19: 361–370.
31. Tarhan S, Moffitt EA, Sessler AD, et al: Risk of anesthesia and surgery in patients with chronic bronchitis and chronic obstructive pulmonary disease. *Surgery* 1973;74:720–726.
32. Logas WG, el-Baz N, el-Ganzouri A, et al: Continuous thoracic epidural analgesia for postoperative pain relief following thoracotomy: A randomized prospective study. *Anesthesiology* 1987;67:787–791.

33. Harman E, Lillington G: Pulmonary risk factors in surgery. *Med Clin North Am* 1979;63:1289–1298.
34. Ponn RB, Ferneini A, D'Agostino RS, et al: Comparison of late pulmonary function after posterolateral and muscle-sparing thoracotomy. *Ann Thorac Surg* 1992;53:675–679.
35. Rogers DA, Philippe PG, Lobe TE, et al: Thoracoscopy in children: An initial experience with an evolving technique. *J Laparoendosc Surg* 1992;2:7–14.
36. Bradford DS: Techniques of surgery, in Bradford DS, Lonstein JE, Moe JH, et al (eds): *Moe's Textbook of Scoliosis and Other Spinal Deformities*, ed 2. Philadelphia, PA, WB Saunders, 1987, pp 135–189.
37. Dubousset J, Herring JA, Shufflebarger H: The crankshaft phenomenon. *J Pediatr Orthop* 1989;9:541–550.
38. Krasna M, Mack MJ (eds): *Atlas of Thoracoscopic Surgery*. St. Louis, MO, Quality Medical Publishing, 1994, p 216.
39. Regan JJ, Ben-Yishay A, McAfee P: Excision of herniated thoracic disc utilizing video-assisted thoracoscopy: Technique and results in the first 36. *J Spine Disord*, in press.
40. Hulme A: The surgical approach to thoracic intervertebral disc protrusions. *J Neurol Neurosurg Psychiatry* 1960;23:133–137.
41. Arseni C, Nash F: Thoracic intervertebral disc protrusion: A clinical study. *J Neurosurg* 1960;17:418–430.
42. Hazelrigg SR, Landreneau RJ, Boley TM, et al: The effect of muscle-sparing versus standard posterolateral thoracotomy on pulmonary function, muscle strength, and postoperative pain. *J Thorac Cardiovasc Surg* 1991;101:394–401.
43. Otani K, Nakai S, Fujimura Y, et al: Surgical treatment of thoracic disc herniation using the anterior approach. *J Bone Joint Surg* 1982;64B:340–343.
44. Bohlman HH, Zdeblick TA: Anterior excision of herniated thoracic discs. *J Bone Joint Surg* 1988;70A:1038–1047.

CHAPTER 12

Minimally Invasive Arthroscopic Spinal Surgery

Parviz Kambin, MD
Geoffrey McCullen, MD
Wesley Parke, PhD
John J. Regan, MD
Jonathan L. Schaffer, MD
Hansen Yuan, MD

Introduction

Medical practice is an ever-evolving art. Perhaps nowhere is this fact more dramatically illustrated than in the burgeoning field of minimally invasive surgery. With recent technological advances, the spine surgeon faces a welcome challenge posed by the variety of available approaches and exposures. Throughout this evolution, the ultimate challenge for surgeons, more important than mastery of a new technique, will remain the same. When do we choose a given method for a specific patient?

The options now available for addressing lumbar spine pathology include the anterior (transperitoneal and retroperitoneal), posterior, and posterolateral approaches. A minimally invasive procedure via endoscopy makes it possible to achieve decompression with less scar formation, shorter hospitalization, and more rapid recovery. With minimal soft-tissue and bony dissection, this approach avoids iatrogenic disruption of the intrinsic stabilizers and decreases the likelihood that the intervention will contribute to biomechanical change. To best assess the "state of the art" and to guide the course of future advances, a detailed analysis of past successes and failures is required.

A little more than 60 years ago, patients presenting with back and leg pain as a result of "sciatica" were a diagnostic and therapeutic enigma for their treating physicians. In 1929, Walter Dandy[1] reported that "tumors" of diskal origin could produce sciatica by direct compression. With a major breakthrough in 1932, William Mixter and Joseph Barr[2] correctly identified the herniated disk as the culprit and proved that mechanical decompression by disk excision could lead to symptom resolution. The original technique called for a posterior midline incision, laminectomy, and longitudinal durotomy. By 1939, Love[3] developed a technique for extradural removal of the disk. Armstrong,[4] in 1951, assessed possible reasons for the failures occasionally seen after disk excision. For analysis, these failures can be divided into three groups: failure of identification, failure of technique, and failure due to natural causes.

Failures Following Disk Excision

Failures of Identification Failures of identification have decreased significantly in recent years, due in large part to advances in computed tomography (CT) and magnetic resonance imaging (MRI). Foraminal and extraforaminal disk herniations, lateral recess stenosis, and double lesions were often missed during early surgical exploration and were frequently the prime offenders in causing continued pain.[5] Improvements in radiologic techniques have allowed the surgeon to pursue a more defined and limited approach.

Failures of Technique Failures of technique arise as a direct consequence of the surgical intervention and its adverse effects on the neural or structural elements of the spine. For adequate exposure, the posterior laminotomy technique may require excision of the medial one third of the facet, leading directly to articular damage and indirectly to subsequent stress fractures of the inferior articular process.

Battered root syndrome may result from direct handling or over-retraction of the nerve, especially near the dorsal root ganglion. Manipulation of the epidural space may disrupt nerve root venous outflow, causing intraneural edema, secondary ischemia, and an indirect neural injury.[6] Such a vascular abnormality can lead to permanent periradicular fibrosis.[7]

In 1974, LaRocca and McNab[8] described, in an experimental model, the laminectomy membrane. A subfascial hematoma accumulates immediately after a posterior laminectomy. Within 6 weeks, this hematoma is serially replaced, first by granulation and ultimately by well-formed fibrous tissue. This scar has been found to extend laterally through the neuroforamen with the exiting nerve root. Without an annular incision, no scar forms within the ventral canal. However, with an annular injury or incision, a scar can form circumferentially around the dura.[9] Not all such scar formation is directly symptom causing.[10] However, by decreasing both the nerve root excursion and venous outflow and by increasing the technical demands during revision surgery, scar formation ultimately results in a greater susceptibility to future nerve injury. Therefore, the search for the optimal interposition membrane and methods to limit the initial hematoma, such as minimally invasive surgery, are ongoing.

Failures Due to Natural Causes Natural causes of failure include those factors that might possibly be successfully reduced, but not altogether eliminated, by improvements in technique. This category includes recurrent disk herniations, infections, and arthritis of the intervertebral joint with end plate sclerosis.

Biomechanical change within the motion segments undergoing diskectomy is inevitable. Subtotal diskectomy induces significantly less instability than total diskectomy in all loading modes.[11] The segment adjacent to the diskectomy site is also affected, irrespective of the amount of disk that is removed. The resulting disk degeneration leads to a reduction in intervertebral disk height and a concomitant increase in pressure borne across the facet joints. Progressive intervertebral disk space narrowing has been appreciated radiographically, occurring within years of a diskectomy.[12] Spondylosis of the triple joint complex follows, occasionally progressing to a degenerative spondylolisthesis and local stenosis from reactive hypertrophy. As many as 14% to 30% of patients will have significant long-standing back pain after diskectomy.[13,14]

Unseen physiologic mechanisms of radicular pain must also be considered. These include vascular, immunologic, chemical, and inflammatory causes of continuing pain. A more than 1,000-fold increase occurs in phospholipase A2, a key enzyme in the formation of prostaglandins within degenerative and herniated disks.[15] The immunogenic and inflammatory capacity of the unsheltered nucleus has also been identified.[16] Despite these disadvantages, the posterior laminotomy technique remains the gold standard to which newer techniques are compared.

Technical Developments

Kambin, in 1973, combined laminotomy and posterolateral nuclear decompression. Subsequently, a Craig biopsy cannula was used to perform percutaneous posterolateral nucleotomy.[17,18] In Japan, Hijikata[19] independently developed a percutaneous method that used straight instruments. Later advances included instruments to perfect nuclear debridement: an automated mechanical cutting device and a laser. Arthroscopic visualization and development of a deflecting rongeur improved safety while substantially broadening the scope of application for the minimally invasive technique.[20,21] Direct access to foraminal and extraforaminal herniations, possible through a triangular working zone (TWZ), obviates the need for a passage through the epidural space.[21-23]

Automated percutaneous nucleotomy successfully accomplishes intranuclear decompression and, ideally, achieves indirect reduction of a contained disk herniation. No effort is made to reach the posterior aspect of the disk space or to excise an offending fragment directly.[24]

Clinical results have been good to excellent in 37% to 87% of cases.[25-28] Reoperation rates vary from 8% to 33%.[25-28] Debulking the center of a disk does not always lead to a decompressive shift of the bulge away from the neural elements. In a degenerative disk, a portion of the nucleus may remain trapped between successive layers of the posterior anulus[29] and is not effectively mobilized by decreasing intranuclear pressure. Therefore, the external geometry of the anulus is not altered.[30]

The biportal technique, which uses two cannulas placed within the TWZ, permits direct observation through one site while tools for direct decompression are inserted through the second site. Articulating instruments[3] can now be deflected more than 90° posteriorly to retrieve central, extraligamentous fragments that have not migrated cranially or caudally from the disk space. Such fragments can be grasped by one end, pulled to within the disk space, and then removed through the cannula.

A laparoscopic lumbar diskectomy was first reported by Obenchain[31] in 1991. Like the posterolateral approach, the anterior approach avoids direct manipulation of the epidural space. Posterior stabilizing structures are maintained.

Degenerative disk disease leads to collapse of the anterior column and a reduction in the neuroforaminal opening. Anterior interbody fusions allow reconstruction of the anterior column, while interbody distraction may allow restoration of the neuroforaminal dimensions. A fusion cage was originally developed by Bagby for use in the treatment of cervical spondylosis in horses, and Bagby and Kuslich modified this cage for human application. Initially, the cage was placed anteriorly by an open, retroperitoneal approach. Then, in 1993, when laparoscopic fusion instruments were developed, it was inserted with laparoscopic visualization. By 1995, several authors had published encouraging preliminary reports.[32-34]

The major disadvantage of an anterior approach is the interference of anatomic structures that overlie the ventral spine. The great vessels and the sympathetic chain (inferior hypogastric plexus) must be effectively but gently mobilized. Other disadvantages include the inability to confirm the extent of the neural decompression. Lateral recess stenosis cannot be addressed.

Diagnostic thoracoscopy has been available for more than 80 years.[35] Beginning in 1992, complex therapeutic spinal interventions became possible. Through the use of video, video-assisted thoracoscopic surgery (VATS) provides enhanced illumination, magnification, and three-dimensional capability. VATS obviates

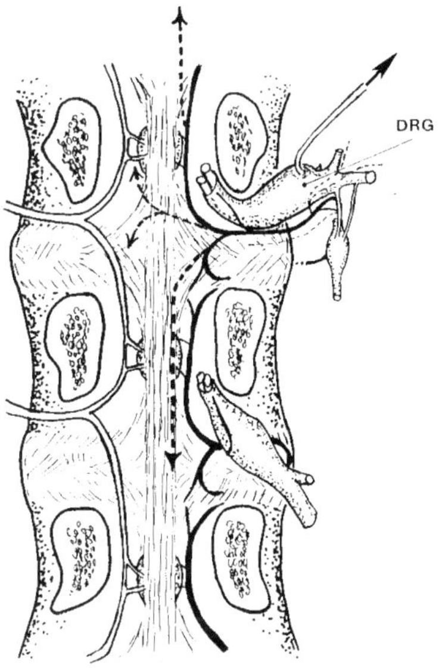

Fig. 1 A schematic drawing showing the sources of the sinuvertebral nerves and the arteries serving the dorsal aspects of the vertebral bodies and their associated connective tissues. A dorsal root ganglion (DRG) has been retracted to illustrate the sinuvertebral nerve connections to the segmental spinal nerve and the related sympathetic ganglion. Black lines indicate the major nerve ramifications, and dotted lines show the extended branches.

the need for a broad incision with rib excision. Thus, there is reduced postoperative pain, improved respiratory capacity, and early shoulder function, culminating in a shorter hospitalization.[36-37] The technique has found application in the treatment of thoracic spinal abscess, tumor, and disk herniation, and in anterior release for spinal deformity.

Arthroscopic Posterolateral Approach to the Lower Thoracic and Lumbar Spine

Gross Anatomy of Periannular Structures

Spinal Nerve and Triangular Working Zone As a common consequence of degenerative conditions in the intervertebral disk, the herniated nucleus pulposus (HNP) is a frequent cause of symptoms referable to mechanical alterations in the relationships of several features of the spinal motion segment unit (MSU). The peripheral migration of nuclear material may produce localized pain by direct disruption of nerves in the periannular connective tissues and/or radicular pain by the compression of the regionally related spinal nerve roots.

Anatomy of Diskogenic Pain The connective tissues most intimately involved in the distortions produced by a HNP are the laminae of the anulus and the overlying fibers of the posterior longitudinal ligament (PLL) that receive branches from the sinuvertebral nerve (of Luschka). Although the general distribution of this medial branch of the dorsal ramus of the spinal nerve to the ligaments, periosteum, meninges, and vasculature within the spinal canal has been known for over a century, the recognition of its involvement in the production of back pain has recently stimulated serious inquiries concerning the nature of its terminal ramifications. There is much controversy concerning the extent of innervation of the intervertebral disk, but there is agreement that the nucleus pulposus is without nerves and at least the outer layers of the laminae of the anulus may contain nerve endings. However, the overlying lateral expansions of the PLL, for their relative thickness, are the most highly innervated tissues within the MSU, showing both complex encapsulated receptors and numerous free nerve endings with little myelination that are usually regarded as nocioceptors. The lateral expansion of the PLL extends laterally through the intervertebral foramen, covering all of the dorsal and most of the dorsolateral aspects of the disk. Undoubtedly, the elevation of this thin, highly innervated strap of connective tissue may provide a significant component of the pain associated with acute disk herniations. Because the PLL lateral expansion is firmly attached to the disk at its edges, a HNP will stretch or actually disrupt its nerve fibers.

Cross-sections of a sinuvertebral nerve show its complex composition of variously myelinated fibers. The fewest but largest of these (10 μm in diameter) are most likely involved with proprioception. Of the smaller fibers, many are undoubtedly postganglionic sympathetics that supply the smooth muscle of the radiculomedullary blood vessels. However, Groen and associates,[38] using a stain (acetylcholinesterase) specific for cholinergic fibers, recently demonstrated an extensive plexus of sensory nerves leading to the connective tissues on the ventral surface of the spinal canal. Although the PLL receives contributions from the sinuvertebral nerve at every segment, the distribution of fibers from a single level may extend several segments up or down the spinal canal as well as to contralateral tissues (Fig. 1). Thus the poor localization of the source of diskogenic pain may be caused by the rather generous distribution of the individual sinuvertebral nerves.

Anatomy of Radicular Compression Reports by Parke and associates[39-41] and Garfin and associates[42] have indicated that the radicular pain associated with HNP most likely involves compressive neuroischemic phenomena. Vascular injections have demonstrated that the intrinsic tissues of the spinal nerve roots receive their arterial supply from both their proximal and distal ends through several parallel radicular arteries that maintain a rather consistent caliber throughout their course. As in the cerebral circulation, the arteries and veins within the nerve roots do not course in close approximation to each other although they are

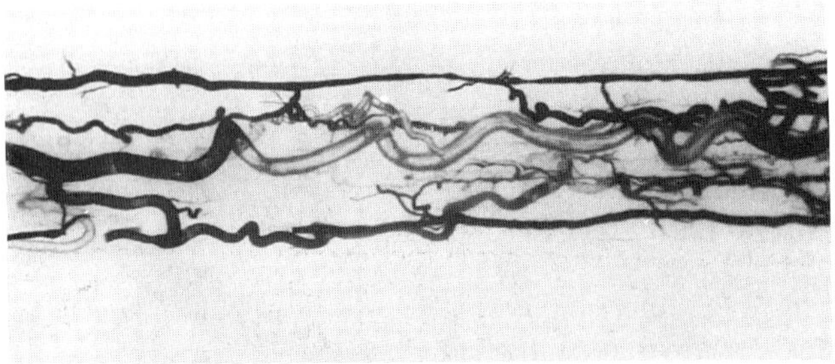

Fig. 2 A photograph of a section of an injected and cleared lumbar spinal nerve root. The intrinsic radicular arteries are shown coursing along the root periphery while a major radicular vein (inflated with hydrogen peroxide) runs through the center. Note the conspicuous arteriovenous anastomosis on the left side of the picture.

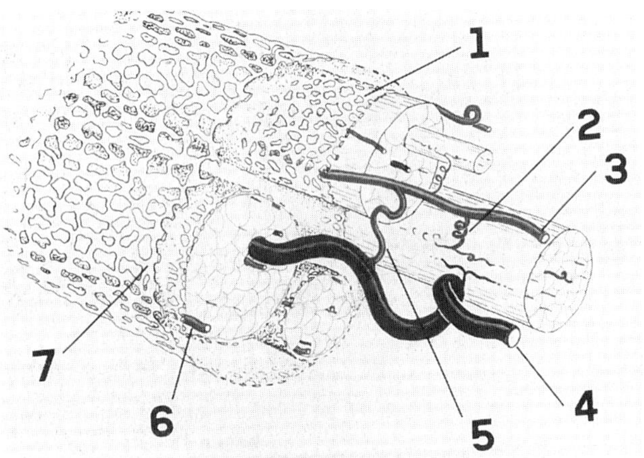

Fig. 3 A graphic compilation showing the structure of a typical lumbar nerve root derived from data obtained by injection studies and scanning electron microscopy. The gauze-like pia-arachnoid membranes permit cerebrospinal fluid to percolate into nerve tissues and assist metabolic support. Shown are: 1, fascicular pia; 2, inter- and intrafascicular arteries; 3, longitudinal radicular artery; 4, large radicular vein; 5, arteriovenous anastomosis; 6, collateral radicular, artery; and 7, gauze-like pia-arachnoid.

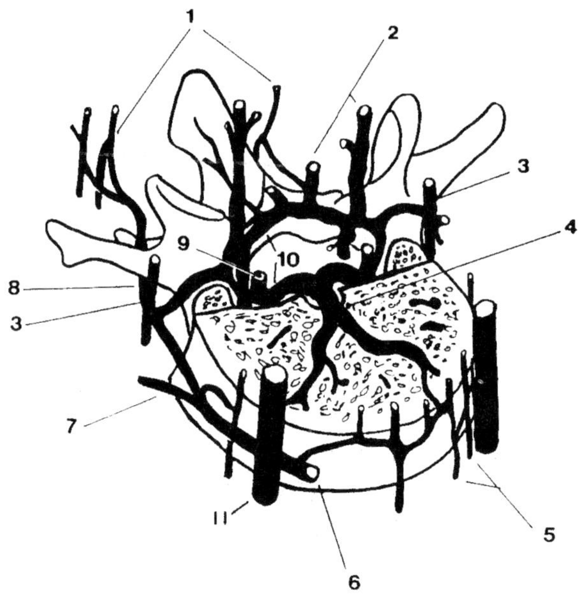

Fig. 4 A schematic drawing showing the venous relations of the lumbar vertebrae. Shown are: 1, dorsal external vertebral plexus; 2, dorsal epidural plexus; 3, intersegmental lumbar veins; 4, basivertebral vein; 5, ventral external vertebral plexus; 6, lumbar segmental veins; 7, muscular vein; 8, musculovertebral branch of external vertebral plexus; 9, longitudinal sinuses of epidural plexus; 10, circumferential sinuses of epidural plexus; and 11, iliolumbar vein.

connected by numerous arteriovenous anastomoses (Figs. 2 and 3). Scanning electron microscopy has revealed that the pia-arachnoid membranes enveloping the nerve roots and their fascicles are open-meshed or gauze-like (Fig. 3). This feature is of considerable importance since Rydevik and associates[43] demonstrated that approximately 50% of the nerve root nutrition is dependent on the percolation of metabolites from the cerebrospinal fluid (CSF), a fact that makes this route of nutrition very vulnerable to pathologic thickenings of these meninges. Chronic nerve root compression has indicated that the radicular venous drainage is more sensitive to local compressive forces and alterations in the extraradicular vascular pressure gradients than is the arterial side of the system. As the radicular veins drain into components of the epidural sinus system, these thin-walled, low-pressure vessels (Fig. 4) are easily constricted by external forces. These compressions may be caused by local space-taking lesions (HNP) or by more generalized peripheral constrictions such as occur in spinal stenoses.

Periradicular Fibrosis Hoyland and associates[44] have reported that periradicular fibrosis is often a consequence of the localized venous obstruction associated with an HNP. Their findings indicated that HNP, mediated by compression of surrounding epidural fat in the intervertebral foramen, chronically interfered with the segmental venous drainage and resulted in fibrotic changes in the periradicular and intraradicular pia-arachnoid. Thus, in addition to directly interfering with radicular vascular flow, the thickening of the periradicular meninges would compound the problem by reducing the free percolation of the metabolite-laden CSF to the root tissues. Recent techniques in spinal phlebography have supported the contentions of Hoyland and associates by showing that the interruption of venous flow in the epidural veins is closely associated with an HNP.

Spinal Stenosis The increased resistance to radicular venous drainage that accompanies a segmental spinal stenosis would also compromise the nutrition of the involved components of the cauda equina in a dual manner. In 1981, Magnaes[45] noted an elevated CSF pressure associated with the segmental dural constriction that resulted when a stenosis isolated the distal cauda equina within a section of the dural sac. He directly measured the increased fluid pressure on the distal roots by a manometer needle inserted into the isolated dural sac and recorded the gradients of introduced fluid pressure required to force past the dural constriction, which he then termed the "spinal block pressure" (Fig. 5). It was reasoned that this increased intradural pressure interfered with the intrinsic radicular circulation, causing intermittent neurogenic claudication. As Magnaes[45] reported prior to the publication of Rydevik and associates,[43] he did not note that stagnation of the confined CSF also reduced this source of radicular nutrition. He did, however, note that the spinal block pressure was reduced when the spine was flexed—an explanation for the sitting and flexing maneuver common to patients seeking to relieve the pain of their neuroischemic claudication.

Further emphasis on the significance of venous drainage impairment on neuroischemic radiculopathy is provided by an illustrated case of an anomalous arteriovenous arterialization of a medullary vein discovered in an injected cadaver. Antemortem records indicated that the patient developed the symptoms of claudication whenever his arterial pressure was raised by exertion, although there was no evidence of any other significant spinal pathology. The general lability of the radiculomedullary venous drainage was additionally indicated by the "vesper's curse" of LaBan.[46] He recorded that patients with already compromised radiculomedullary circulation due to stenosis, who subsequently developed decreased cardiopulmonary compliance with congestive heart failure, reported an increased neuroischemic pain during nocturnal recumbency. LaBan claimed that this was caused by a venous hypertensive engorgement of the epidural sinuses.

Anatomy of the Triangular Working Zone The triangular working zone (TWZ) of Kambin[20] is the site of surgical access to the anulus that is used in arthroscopic microdiskectomy (AMD) procedures. It is anatomically described as a right triangle over the dorsolateral aspect of the intervertebral disk. The hypotenuse of the triangle is formed by the spinal nerve, and its base (width) is defined by the horizontal superior border of the next inferior vertebral body. The height of the triangle, which runs parallel to the axis of the vertebral

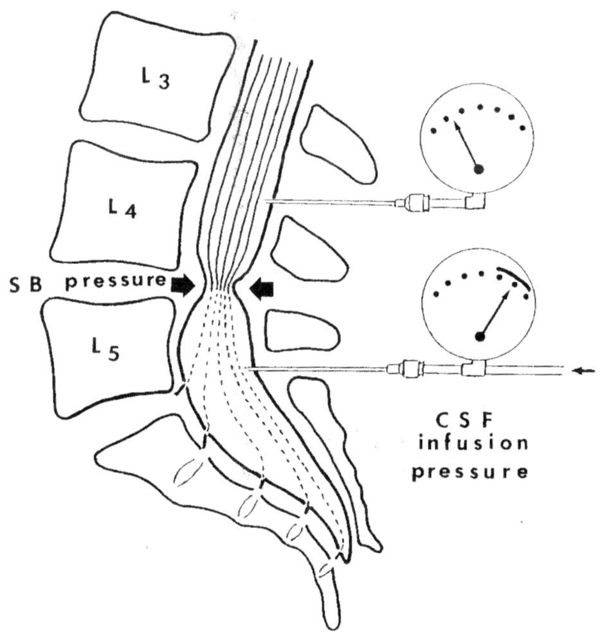

Fig. 5 Schematic drawing derived from Magnaes[45] showing how he determined the pressure required to force past constriction of a stenosis (spinal block pressure). This also demonstrates how lower sac cerebrospinal fluid can become stagnant and less nutritive to root elements caudal to the level of stenosis.

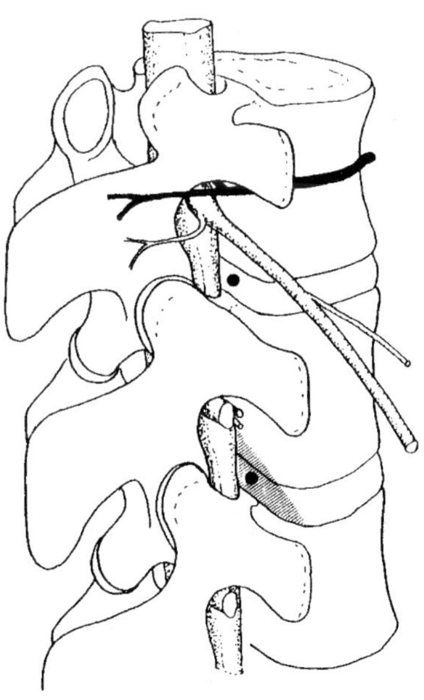

Fig. 6 Schematic drawing of a posterior oblique view of a generic (no specific level intended) lumbar vertebrae showing the major anatomic relations of Kambin's triangular working zone (TWZ). The shaded triangle shows the area of the TWZ as defined in the text. The black circle indicates the target point for annular fenestration in arthroscopic microdiskectomy procedures.

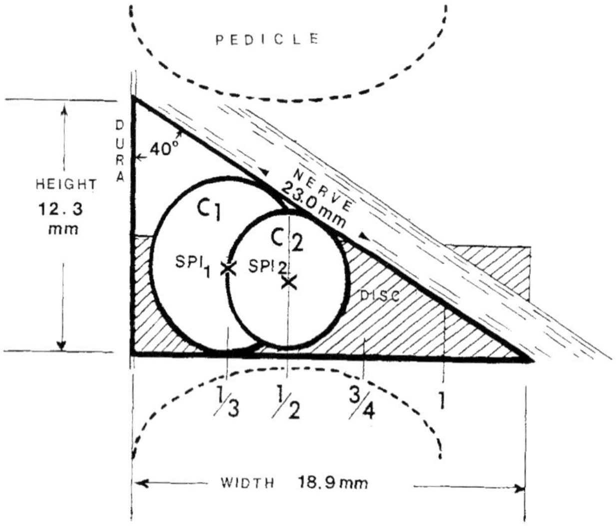

Fig. 7 A composite schematic drawing derived from the data of Mirkovic and associates[24] and Cohen and associates[47] showing the average dimensions of the lumbar TWZ. Using the 1/3 and 1/2 reference points of the related pedicles, Mirkovic and associates determined the safe point of insertion (SPI) for larger cannulas (C1) and smaller cannulas (C2).

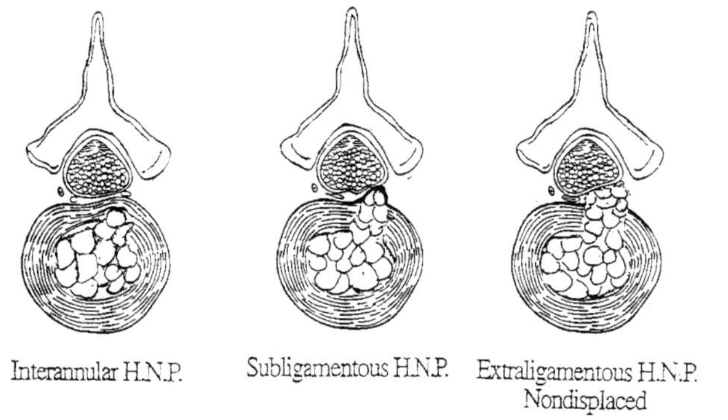

Fig. 8 Illustration of the Graduate Hospital Disk Herniation Classification System for HNP in the transverse orientation. With the exception of cases in which an extraligamentous herniated nucleus pulposus (HNP) has migrated vertically, all of these HNP configurations can be corrected by posterolateral diskectomy.

column, is formed by the structures dorsal to the intervertebral foramen (but actually may be considered to be formed by the dura), and its superior angle is formed by the axilla of the exiting spinal nerve (Fig. 6).

Because the major segmental artery, sinuvertebral nerve, and spinal nerve hug the inferior border of the superior foraminal pedicle, the major area of the TWZ that lies dorsolateral to the anulus is devoid of significant structures. The dimensions of the TWZ show a surprising uniformity throughout the lumbar region. Here the spinal nerves and their thecal extensions leave the lumbar dura at a remarkably consistent angle that ranges from 37° to 41°, with a mean angulation of 40° (Fig. 7).[47] Because the major components of other transforaminal structures, namely the vertebromedullary branches of the segmental arteries and the sinuvertebral nerve, lie superior to the apex of the axillary angle, only some of the smaller ubiquitous channels connecting the radiculomedullary veins with the epidural sinuses traverse the TWZ. In addition to this angular consistency, Mirkovic and associates[24] showed that the average TWZ (they called it the "safe zone") is 18.9 mm wide and 12.5 mm high, with a hypotenuse measuring 23 mm. They then determined that the "safe point" for the insertion of the larger cannulas (5.0 mm to 10.0 mm) lies along a vertical line, projected over the dorsolateral anulus, that connects points located on the medial third of the adjacent foraminal pedicles. For cannulas of 4.0 mm to 8.9 mm, a safe point of insertion corresponds to the midline points on the pedicles (Fig. 7).

Disk Herniation Classification

Because of the current plethora of terms used to describe the degree and position of HNPs, the use of a classification system has been proposed to enhance uniformity in communications concerning AMD procedures.[48] This system labels the transverse orientations of HNP as intra-annular, subligamentous, extraligamentous, and extraligamentous-migrated (Fig. 8) and the sagittal orientations as central, paramedian, foraminal, and extraforaminal.

Because simple debulking of the central substance of the anulus fibrosus (central nucleotomy) may yield uncertain results, a posterolateral diskectomy, in which the instrumentation is directed so as to remove the actual offending mass of the HNP, is here favored by most of the anatomic considerations. This approach effectively removes herniated nuclear material in all of the transverse orientations of an HNP with the exception of those in which the herniated substance has migrated vertically. This procedure avoids any threat to the contents of the spinal canal and will not compromise any significant components of the foraminal vasculature.

Arthroscopic Anatomy, Surgical Technique, and Treatment of Lumbar Spine Disorders

Arthroscopic visualization and identification of the anatomic structures of the lumbar spine remain the cornerstone of minimally invasive spinal surgery. Although nuclear debulking procedures[49-55] traditionally have been performed under fluoroscopic control, selective removal of posterior and posterolateral herniated fragments under arthroscopic control[20,21,56-58] requires protection of neurovascular tissues and demands clear arthroscopic visualization.

Arthroscopic visualization of intradiskal or foraminal structures requires proper fluid management and a high resolution arthroscope. When performing surgery adjacent to the neural structures, constant inflow and outflow of saline solution insures the protection of these structures against the excessive heat generated by the light source of the Videodiscoscope. Adequate fluid management is also essential for removal from the surgical site of debris that presents an obstruction to clear visualization of anatomic and pathologic structures. When performing intradiskal surgery through biportal access, the inflow tube of saline solution is connected to the Videodiscoscope irrigation sheath while the outflow is attached to a cannula inserted into the opposite portal. To prevent periannular leakage and to stabilize the medial end of the cannula during the bilateral biportal approach, the cannulas are engaged into the annular fibers, thus the establishment of inflow and outflow of saline solution does not pose any difficulty and is safe.

The TWZ (Figs. 6 and 7) is the area situated on the posterolateral anulus where it is safe to perform an annulectomy for intradiskal and foraminal surgery. Arthroscopic visualization of the TWZ, foramen, and spinal canal[21,58] through foraminal access requires instrumentation that contains channels for the insertion of the Videodiscoscope and inflow and outflow of saline solution through a single cannula. When performing extra-annular surgery (foraminal and extraforaminal herniations), one should make certain that most of the injected saline solution is retrieved via the outflow channel. The use of high negative pressure adjacent to the neural structures is also potentially hazardous. Usually a negative pressure of about 6 to 8 in of mercury is adequate to control the rate at which the saline solution flows into the surgical field. (The negative pressure of wall suction is about 12 in of mercury in most operating rooms.)

Generally, it is difficult to establish inflow and outflow of saline solution inside the intervertebral disk through a single cannula. The swollen nuclear tissue and nuclear debris obstruct the outflow channel of the arthroscope. However, low negative pressure (gravity) may be used in conjunction with an oval cannula for simultaneous visualization and extraction of disk fragments.

Arthroscopic Visualization of Myoligamentous Structures

When the posterolateral approach is used, the instruments are passed through the skin, subcutaneous adipose tissue, thoracolumbar fascia, and paraspinal muscles under fluoroscopic control. However, the operating surgeon should become familiar with the arthroscopic appearance of these structures. As the instrument passes through the skin and subcutaneous adipose tissue, it meets with resistance when it reaches the thoracolumbar fascia. The fascia attaches to the iliac crest distally, to the spinal process of the lumbar segment and the medial crest of the sacrum medially, and joins posteriorly to the intracostal fascia. The superficial layer of the thoracolumbar fascia is seen through the Videodiscoscope as a heavy band of avascular fibrous tissue. As soon as the instrument penetrates the thoracolumbar fascia, it passes through the sacrospinalis, quadratus lumborum, and psoas major muscles. The muscular tissue is readily identified as red semielastic fibers.

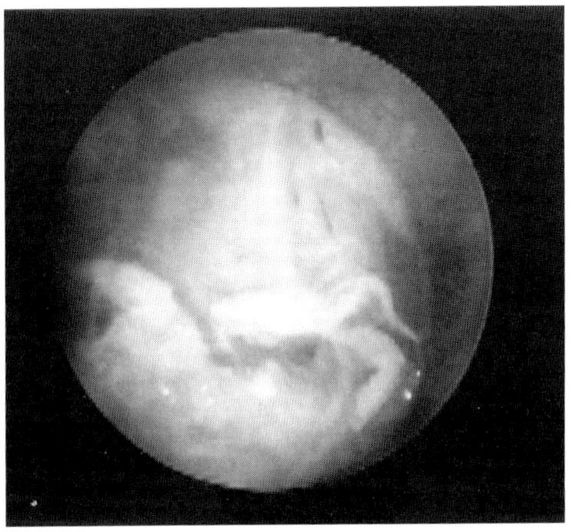

Fig. 9 Intraoperative arthroscopic view of the annular surface at the TWZ. Note the adipose tissue in the lower part of the photo.

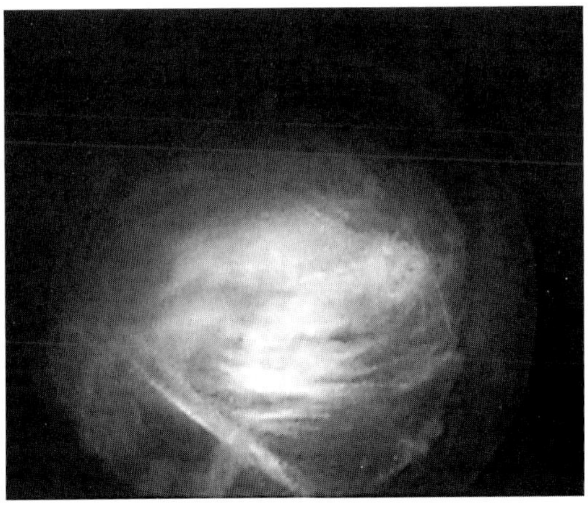

Fig. 10 The coarse annular fibers are visualized following extraction of the adipose tissue from the annulotomy site.

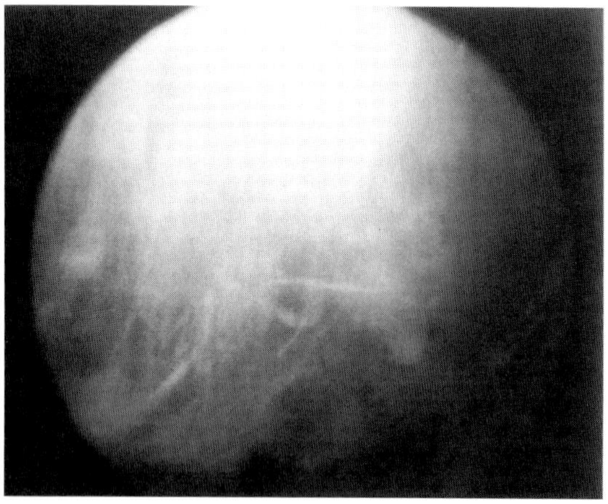

Fig. 11 A bursal type of tissue is covering the surface of the anulus in the TWZ.

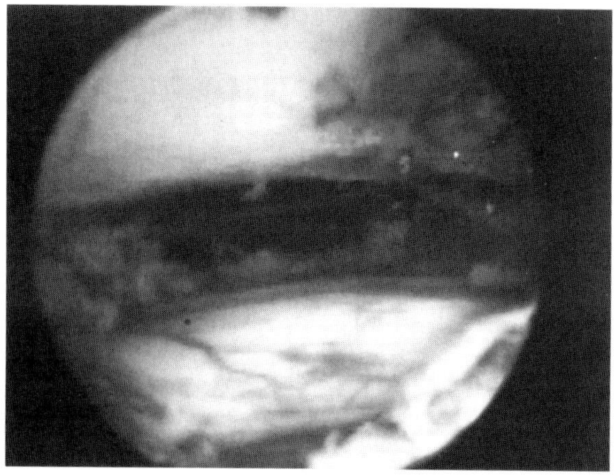

Fig. 12 Arthroscopic view of the spinal canal. A 30° arthroscope is passed under the pars interarticularis for inspection of the spinal canal. Note the traversing nerve root at the bottom of the photo and the dural sac at the top.

Arthroscopic Visualization of the Triangular Working Zone

The TWZ is covered with loosely woven adipose tissue that usually extends into the neural foramen (Fig. 9). When this adipose tissue is extracted with the aid of forceps under arthroscopic control, the fibers of the superficial layer of the posterolateral anulus and the annu-lotomy site are easily seen through the Videodiscoscope (Fig. 10). If the skin entry point is inadvertently made too far laterally, the medial end of the access cannula may be positioned against epidural adipose tissue. The fat globules in epidural adipose tissue are usually larger and more abundant than periannular fat. In addition, some of the annular fibers are invariably seen behind the fat globules that cover the TWZ. At times, particularly when the medial end of the cannula has been laterally positioned, one may observe a loosely woven, bursal type tissue on the annular surface (Fig. 11). Although the spinal nerve is not usually observed during the posterolateral approach, in extremely rare occasions an abnormal extrapedicular communication may be identified between the proximal and distal spinal nerve. This must be protected during surgery.

Arthroscopic Visualization of Neurovascular Structures

While the medial end of the Videodiscoscope cannula assembly is resting on the anulus in the TWZ, the operating surgeon tilts the instrument slightly laterally and cephalad in order to visualize the exiting root as it departs from the foramen. At times, bleeding or perineural adipose tissue may prevent clear visualization of the latter structures. The 30° Videodiscoscope cannula assembly may be further medialized and passed under the pars interarticularis for inspection of the traversing nerve root, dura, and the contents of the spinal canal (Fig. 12). The roots are seen as pale yellow, multifiber structures with fine vessels on their surface. The pulsating spinal artery adjacent to the exiting root as it passes under the pedicular notch may also be observed through a 30° Videodiscoscope.

Spencer and associates[59] have described the dural ligament as a structure that fixes the dura and nerve roots at their exit from the dural sac to the PLL and the periosteum of the vertebral bodies. These structures may be observed by an extra-annular arthroscopic examination of the spinal canal. Hofmann ligaments are seen as fibrous bands that extend from the ventral and lateral dura to the posterior longitudinal ligament. Here, too, it should be noted that at times large quantities of epidural adipose tissue and massive bleeding can interfere with clear visualization of these structures. In addition, undue manipulation of the access cannula or working channel scope in the lateral recess may cause neural injury.

Arthroscopic Visualization of the Intervertebral Disk

In children, one can observe a clear transitional zone between the anulus and the nucleus pulposus. At this stage the nucleus consists of a soft gelatinous structure that is contained by annular fibers. Arthroscopic examination of nuclear tissue in young individuals demonstrates a soft whitish structure with a cotton-ball appearance, and annular fibers are readily seen and identified as a thick fibrous bundle.

In older individuals, dehydration of the nucleus pulposus associated with the development of nuclear clefts and disruption of the collagenized annular fibers alter the arthroscopic appearance of the nucleus and the anulus. However, even in the fourth and fifth decades of life, it is not uncommon to observe a combina-

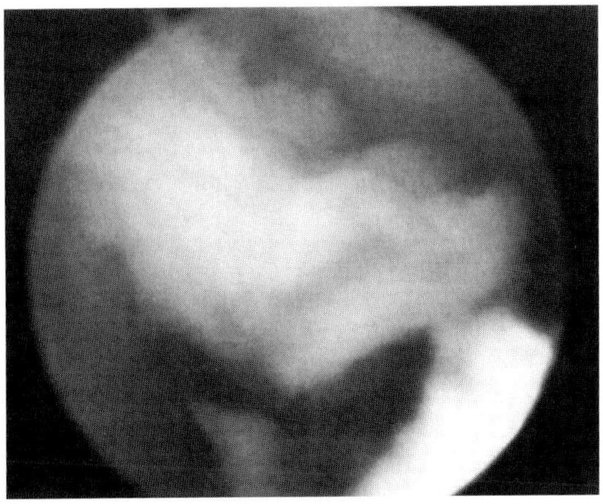

Fig. 13 Intradiskal view of the tail of a large subligamentous herniated nucleus pulposus.

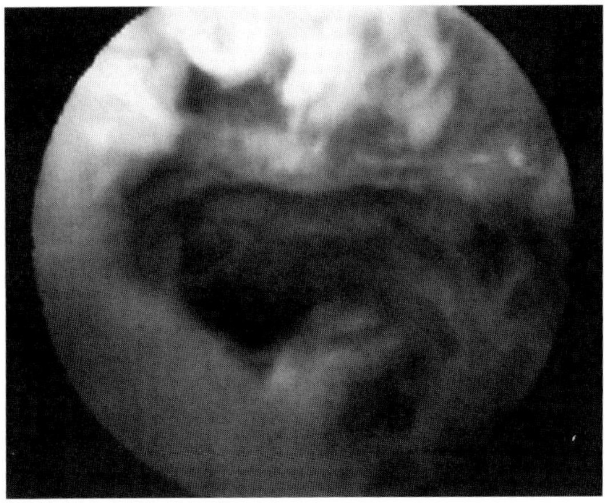

Fig. 14 Intradiskal arthroscopic view of a large tear in the posterior longitudinal ligament (PLL) following retrieval of a sequestered fragment. Note the bleeding from the ventral dura at the center of the photo.

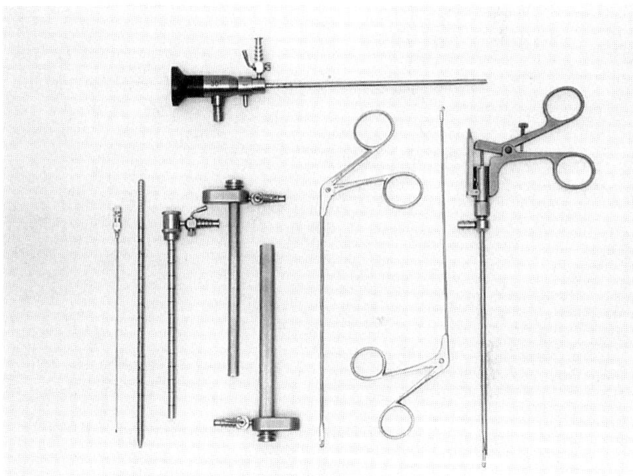

Fig. 15 Instruments. **Top,** 30° arthroscope; **Bottom,** (from left to right) 18-gauge needle, cannulated obturator, universal access cannula and suction irrigation valve, 5 × 8 mm I.D. oval cannula, 5 × 10 mm I.D. oval cannula, straight forceps, upbiting forceps, deflecting suction forceps.

tion of soft whitish nuclear tissue and collagenized fibrous nuclear fragments within a given intervertebral disk.

Occasionally, collagenized nuclear tissue is seen as a free disk fragment within the intervertebral disk (internal disk sequestration).[60] At times the arthroscopic differentiation between collagenized nuclear tissue and thickened, torn annular fibers is difficult in patients between 30 and 50 years of age. The tail of a subligamentous or extraligamentous posterior herniated fragment may be identified during intradiskal arthroscopy (Fig. 13). Fibers of the PLL run in a direction different from that of the annular fibers (cephalocaudad) and may be identified with a 70° arthroscope.

Following retrieval of an extraligamentous sequestered fragment, the ventral dura may be clearly visualized with the aid of a 70° arthroscope (Fig. 14). The ventral dura voids adipose tissue. However, exposure of the ventral dura is invariably associated with bleeding that may be controlled by hydrostatic pressure or use of Avitene® (MedChem Products, Woburn, MA) plunge that is introduced through the inserted access cannula.

Surgical Technique for Posterolateral Intradiskal and Extra-Annular Access to the Spinal Canal

For the retrieval of herniated fragments and decompression of a compromised nerve root, intervertebral disks of the lumbar spine may be accessed through an intradiskal, a subligamentous, or an extra-annular foraminal approach. Arthroscopic intradiskal access has been the subject of a number of clinical studies and publications.[21,61-64] However, surgery performed inside the spinal canal via an extra-annular foraminal access is tedious and often difficult, and it remains experimental. Epidural adipose tissue and bleeding may impede adequate visualization and satisfactory completion of the surgical procedure.

Instruments

Many instruments are available for the performance of arthroscopic disk surgery via a posterolateral approach. An 18-gauge needle or blunt-end Kirschner wire is usually used for localization of the annulotomy site under anteroposterior and lateral C-arm fluoro-

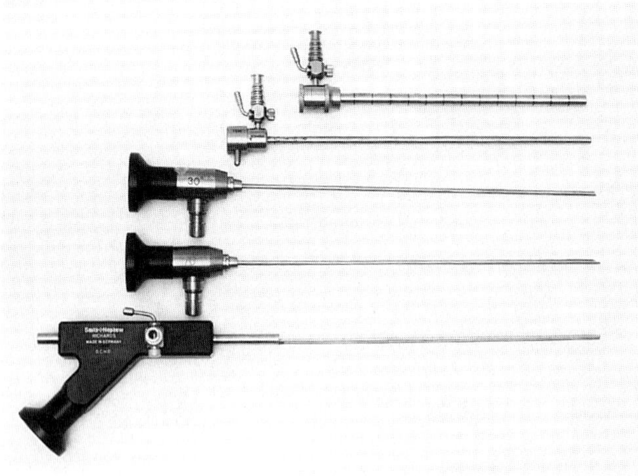

Fig. 16 From top to bottom: universal access cannula and suction irrigation valve, arthroscope irrigation valve, 30° rigid arthroscope, 70° rigid arthroscope, working channel scope.

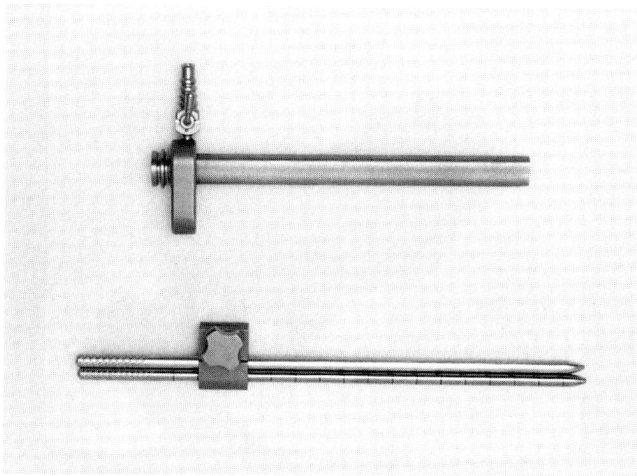

Fig. 17 **Top,** 5 × 10 mm oval cannula. **Bottom,** Two cannulated obturators are passed through the lumen of the cannular jig in preparation for insertion of the oval cannula.

scopy. This step is then followed by introduction of a single soft-tissue dilator[18,26,65] (Fig. 15) or series of sequential cannulas[19,66] and final positioning of an access cannula on the anulus.

Kambin[20,21,49,58] has emphasized the importance of arthroscopic visualization of the TWZ prior to annulotomy. Arthroscopic visualization of periannular structures is achieved either with a working channel scope or an arthroscope and arthroscope sheath that is introduced into the lumen of the access cannula. Three rigid arthroscopes (0°, 30°, and 70°) with long shafts are used for arthroscopic disk surgery (Fig. 16). At the present time, the flexible disposable scopes do not provide high enough resolution and the clear visibility necessary for inspection and protection of neural tissue during surgery. A variety of instruments, including trephines, knife blades, forceps, and curettes that may be used in conjunction with a working channel scope or independently through the access cannula, are also required for satisfactory performance of arthroscopic spinal surgery. The working scope contains channels for inflow and outflow of saline solution. A separate channel of 2.5 mm I.D. limits the size of instruments that may be inserted for removal of herniated disk tissue. Articulating instruments with ample deflection are necessary for intradiskal retrieval of posterior and posterolateral herniated disk fragments under arthroscopic control.

Two sizes of oval cannulas, 5 × 8 mm I.D. and 5 × 10 mm I.D., are used for unilateral biportal arthroscopic disk surgery. Two specific jigs are used to convert a uniportal access to a unilateral biportal approach. The combination of a universal obturator (4.9 mm O.D.) with a half-moon obturator permits the insertion of a 5 × 8 mm I.D. oval cannula, while the combination of a universal obturator and a circular obturator allows the positioning of a 5 × 10 mm I.D. oval cannula (Fig. 17). Broad decorticating blades provides access to the concave surface of the vertebral plate in preparation for arthroscopic intrabody arthrodesis.

Intradiskal Approach

The lumbar intervertebral disk may be approached posterolaterally by insertion of a single access cannula into the intervertebral disk from a distance of about 9 to 11 cm from the midline. Bilateral biportal access requires insertion of two cannulas, one from the right and one from the left side. This arrangement permits triangulation inside of the intervertebral disk while providing uninterrupted visualization and extraction of the posterior herniated fragments, and exposure of the PLL and the contents of the spinal canal.

Unilateral biportal access permits the ipsilateral positioning of two parallel cannulas into the TWZ. The TWZ accommodates the placement of an oval cannula into the intervertebral disk. In the absence of degenerative narrowing of the intervertebral disk and facet arthropathy, the TWZ can accommodate a 7 to 8 mm O.D. cannula at the midpedicular region. The inferior boundary of the TWZ is wide enough to accommodate the positioning of an oval cannula at this site.

Uniportal Intradiskal Access Surgery must be performed with the patient in a prone position. When the surgery is being performed under local anesthesia, this positioning makes it possible to reposition patients if they move. It also permits reproducible intraoperative imaging studies and allows the conversion of a uniportal approach to a biportal access when it is deemed necessary. Patients are placed on a radiolucent frame and

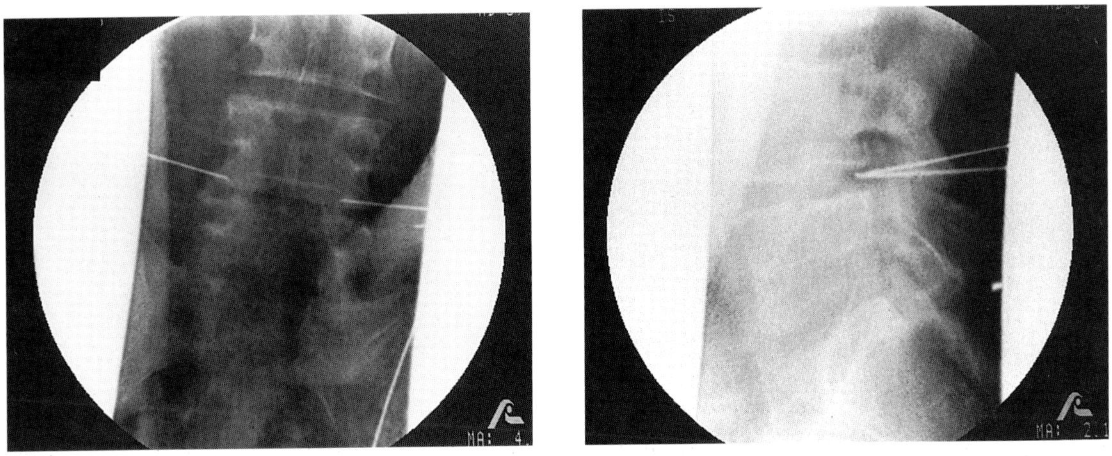

Fig. 18 Left, Intraoperative fluoroscopy. Note the proper positioning of the tip of the needle at the midpedicular region. **Right,** Lateral fluoroscopic view.

table. In order to reduce lumbar lordosis and expand the posterior height of the intervertebral disk at the index level, the operating table is maintained in slight flexion. Depending upon the size of the patient and the site of herniation, the skin entry point is selected 9 to 11 cm from the midline. Local anesthesia is usually sufficient for uniportal surgery. However, an anesthesiologist must be available to provide systemic analgesics if it is deemed necessary.

The tip of the needle is properly positioned on the anulus when it is seen at the midpedicular line on an anteroposterior fluoroscopic examination and is adjacent to the posterior annular fibers in the lateral roentgenogram (Fig. 18). When an attempt is being made to decompress an extraforaminal herniation, the tip of the needle may have to be positioned on the lateral pedicular line in an anteroposterior fluoroscopic examination. The positioning of the tip of the needle at the medial pedicular line requires further lateralization of the skin entry point. At times, articular facets of segments adjacent to the index level prevent adequate medialization of the tip of the inserted needle. This is usually observed in elderly patients who display radiographic evidence of facet arthropathy. Facet joints in the upper lumbar and thoracolumbar regions are smaller in size and the operating surgeon must exercise great caution to prevent inadvertent placement of the needle in the spinal canal. In addition, a vertical skin entry, close to the midline, may position the tip of the inserted guide wire or needle anterior to the intertransverse ligament, which can cause neurovascular complications.

Prior to full insertion of the cannulated obturator, it is advisable to withdraw the guide wire. This allows the blunt end of the cannulated obturator to bypass the spinal nerve and reach the annular surface. This step is then followed by positioning of a 5 mm I.D. cannula in the TWZ (Fig. 19). The access cannula may be positioned adjacent to the traversing nerve root for extraction of a subligamentous or small intracanalicular sequestered fragment. In this case, the operating surgeon should not use a trimmer blade or other power-driven instrumentation. Surgery must be performed under clear arthroscopic magnification and illumination by using a working channel scope or an oval cannula that permits simultaneous insertion of a 30° arthroscope and manual instruments.

A thorough arthroscopic inspection and examination of the annulotomy site with the aid of a working channel scope or 0° or 30° arthroscope is mandatory. Adipose tissue on the surface of the anulus may be wiped off with a cottonoid or removed under direct visualization with a forceps inserted into the working channel scope. The firm surface of the anulus may be examined with a small hook or a blunt-tip probe. The dura and the contents of the spinal canal display minimal resistance to probing and present a different palpatory consistency. Removal of adipose tissue may be associated with venous bleeding from the annular surface. A radio-frequency probe may be used via a working channel scope for coagulation of these veins. We have also used Avitene® plunge for the same purpose. Periannular bleeding should be controlled to prevent the development of postoperative pain or causalgic type of symptoms.

The annular surface in the TWZ is enriched by a nerve supply through the expansion of the PLL. When the surgical procedure is being performed under local anesthesia, the anulus must be anesthesized either by application of topical anesthetics delivered through the

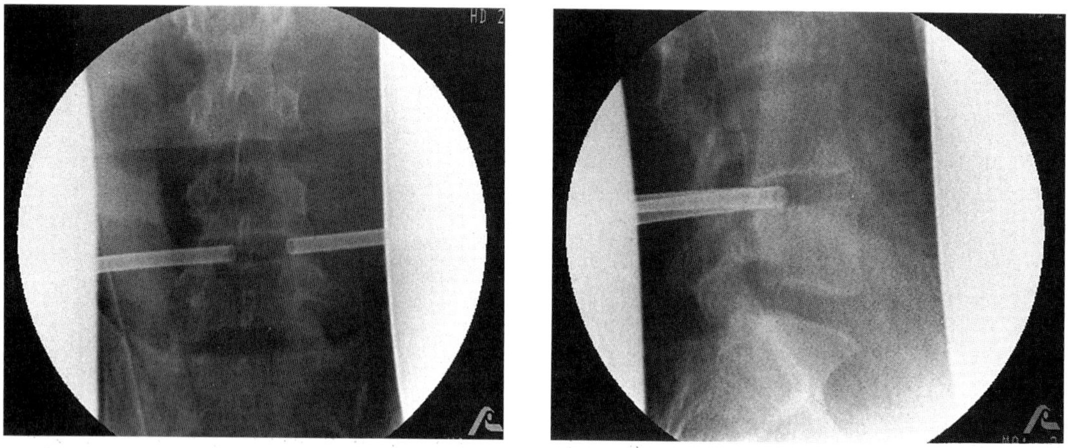

Fig. 19 **Left,** Biportal access to the L4-5 intervertebral disk. The cannulas are positioned to access a right paramedial herniation. **Right,** This lateral intraoperative radiograph of the photo shown at left shows the posterior positioning of the instruments to provide easy access to the spinal canal.

inserted cannula or by local infiltration of the anulus with a xylocaine solution.

The annulotomy may be accomplished under arthroscopic control via a working channel scope. Alternatively, while holding the access cannula firmly against the annular surface, a trephine may be used to fenestrate the anulus. At this stage of the surgery, it is advisable to use manual instruments to access and remove disk fragments that may have been dislodged to the periphery and are within the reach of the straight or upbiting manual forceps. Power-driven instruments should not be used until the universal access cannula is engaged and seated into the annular fibers and the nuclear tissue is identified by arthroscopic examination.

A trimmer blade may be used to create a cavity behind the inner fibers of the posterior anulus. The 5 mm I.D. access cannula may be replaced by a 5 × 8 mm I.D. oval cannula in order to gain a broader access to the intervertebral disk. Broader access permits simultaneous insertion of a 30° arthroscope and an upbiting forceps for visualization and extraction of herniated disk fragments (Fig. 20).

Bilateral Intradiskal Access Bilateral access to the intervertebral disk is necessary for uninterrupted visualization of the instruments inserted from the opposite portal and the tissue that is being extracted. The bilateral biportal approach is generally employed for removal of large subligamentous or extraligamentous nonmigrated herniations and when arthroscopic interbody arthrodesis is being attempted. Biportal access is more time-consuming than the uniportal approach. When arthroscopic interbody fusion with or without instrumentation is being performed, the use of general or spinal anesthesia becomes necessary. The familiarity of the operating surgeon with the arthroscopic anatomy of the spine is a prerequisite for performing these procedures.

Positioning of the patient on the operating table and needle insertion for biportal access is similar to that described under uniportal approach. Needles should be positioned on the right and left side of the patient at the onset of the procedure. Otherwise, the cannulated obturator or cannula that has been positioned from the opposite side may interfere with clear visualization of the tip of the inserted needle in the lateral fluoroscopic examination. In addition, communication between the two portals is at times difficult and time consuming. The relation between the instruments inserted from the left and right should be inspected with an anteroposterior fluoroscopic examination to make certain that the instruments reach, and do not bypass, one another. If the needles and instruments on both sides are not inserted at equal angles, the tips of the instruments will tend to bypass one another. Trimmer blades or radio-frequency coagulator probes may be used in normal saline solution to remove fine nuclear tissue that may lie between the arthroscope and instruments that have been introduced from the opposite portal.

In contrast to uniportal access, the bilateral biportal approach provides for an adequate inflow and outflow of saline solution through the intervertebral disk at the index level. This permits clear visualization of nuclear tissue, the PLL, ventral dura, and, at times, the ventral surface of the traversing nerve root.

Unilateral Biportal Access A unilateral biportal approach permits insertion of an oval cannula into the interver-

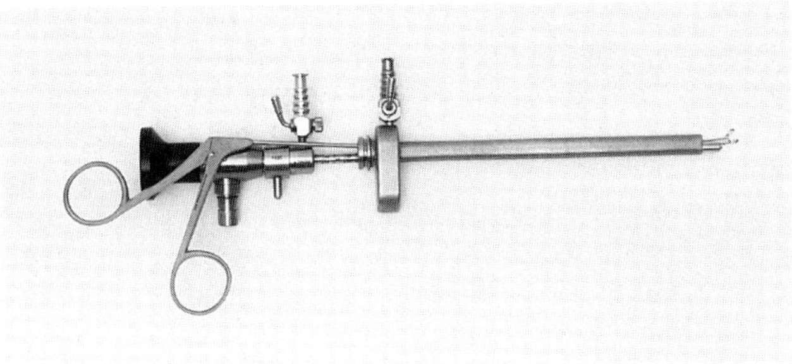

Fig. 20 A 30° arthroscope and upbiting forceps are inserted into the lumen of the oval cannula for direct visualization and extraction of a paramedial disk herniation.

tebral disk, providing a broader access to the herniation site and the intervertebral plates. A 5 × 8 mm I.D. oval cannula is useful for retrieval of intracanalicular paramedial or extracanalicular foraminal and extraforaminal herniations. A larger oval cannula (5 × 10 mm I.D.) is generally used for arthroscopic interbody fusion.

To convert a uniportal approach to unilateral biportal access, a cannular jig and auxiliary obturator are used (Fig. 17). Combination of a half-moon auxiliary obturator with a universal obturator permits the insertion of a 5 × 8 mm oval cannula. Positioning of a 5 × 10 mm oval cannula requires use of the jig that permits insertion of a universal obturator (4.9 mm O.D.) and a circular obturator.

The insertion of an oval cannula first requires the establishment of a uniportal access to the intervertebral disk. The needle positioning, introduction of the cannulated obturator, insertion of the access cannula, inspection of the annulotomy site, and fenestration of the anulus have been described previously. The cannulated obturator is reinserted into the universal access cannula and passed through the annular fenestration and positioned in the center of the intervertebral disk. This maneuver will firmly stabilize the inserted cannula in the intervertebral disk. At this time the obturator jig is attached to the proximal end of the inserted obturator and secured in place by tightening the knob on the jig. The auxiliary obturator is passed through the jig, skin incision, subcutaneous tissue, lumbar fascia, paravertebral muscles, and the annular fenestration. The proper position of the auxiliary obturator inside the intervertebral disk is documented with C-arm fluoroscopy. The gradually beveled tip of the auxiliary obturator permits dilatation of the annular fibers and protects the exiting root at the annulotomy site. This step is followed by withdrawal of the jig and introduction of the oval cannula over the two cannulated obturators.

Subligamentous Approach

Subligamentous approach to the herniation site eliminates the need for entry to the spinal canal while allowing closer access to the herniation site. The 5 × 8 mm oval cannula is most suitable for performing this procedure. Following the positioning of the oval cannula in the TWZ under direct arthroscopic control, the operating surgeon medializes the inner end of the cannula by forcing the cannula slightly toward a horizontal plane. This permits visualization of epidural fat and the traversing nerve root. Annulotomy is then performed adjacent to the traversing root, permitting the introduction of straight and upbiting forceps under the PLL for removal of herniated disk fragments (Fig. 20).

Extra-Annular Arthroscopic Approach

The extra-annular approach is commonly used for decompression and evacuation of foraminal and extraforaminal herniations. Extra-annular access may also be used for arthroscopic visualization of the contents of the spinal canal and, at times, evacuation of a paramedial sequestered fragment. Extra-annular access to the spinal canal requires further lateralization of the skin entry point so that the medial opening of the cannula is positioned under the pars interarticularis of the proximal lumbar segment, adjacent to the dural sac and the traversing nerve root. Intracanalicular surgery using an extra-annular approach must be performed under strict, uninterrupted arthroscopic visualization with the aid of a working channel scope. Operating surgeons are warned to avoid undue manipulation of the contents of the spinal canal or excess use of fluid to gain clear visualization during surgery.

Posterolateral Arthroscopic Treatment of Disorders of the Lumbar Spine

Since introduction of the modified arthroscope for visualization of periannular, foraminal, and intradiskal structures and the extraction of herniated disk fragments, there have been ongoing investigations to identify and treat other spinal disorders through a posterolateral arthroscopic approach.

Lumbar Diskectomy and Posterior Fragmentectomy

The arthroscopic posterolateral approach may be used to retrieve disk fragments from extraforaminal, foraminal, or intracanalicular regions. The perceived simplicity of this procedure should not influence decision making and appropriate patient selection. The operating surgeon must adhere to indications and guidelines that have been described in the literature for surgical treatment of herniated lumbar disks.

Arthroscopic microdiskectomy should not be used to treat low back pain if there is no associated radiculopathy. The patients' radicular pain should be more severe than their back pain and should have dematomal root distribution. Patients must have the benefit of a well-planned and executed nonsurgical management prior to surgical consideration. These individuals should demonstrate an unequivocal positive tension sign preoperatively. Tests for these signs should be performed and recorded while the patient is in the supine position, sitting, and under physiologic loading.[21] A thorough neurologic examination must be conducted. Motor, sensory, and reflex abnormalities are found and documented. Correlative imaging studies are prerequisites for arthroscopic disk surgery. Both MRI and CT scanning may be necessary during the preoperative phase of patient evaluation. CT scanning will provide additional information concerning the presence or absence of bony lateral stenosis, osteophytosis, and calcification within the annular fibers or PLL. Preoperative myelography may be reserved for individuals who are claustrophobic or whose obesity precludes optimal MRI studies. CT myelography may also provide additional information in individuals who have had previous lumbar surgery and those with scoliosis and deformities.

Accessibility of the herniation site via a uniportal or biportal approach must be determined preoperatively by plain anteroposterior and lateral roentgenograms of the lumbar and lumbosacral spine. Biportal access to the L5-S1 intervertebral disk in individuals with high iliac crests is extremely difficult. Patients who present with imaging evidence of a large central subligamentous or extraligamentous sequestered herniation at the L5-S1 level should be treated with an open laminotomy.

Although in the past it was not possible to retrieve extraligamentous and nonmigrated sequestered herniated fragments through the intradiskal approach, in skilled hands these fragments may be retrieved via an intradiskal bilateral biportal approach. Individuals presenting with bony lateral stenosis and facet arthropathy and those with migrated sequestered herniations are not considered for arthroscopic disk surgery at this state of the art.

Patients presenting with a symptomatic extraforaminal, foraminal, or paramedial intracanalicular herniation may be treated through a single 5 × 5 mm I.D. universal cannula or 5 × 8 mm I.D. oval cannula positioned into the intervertebral disk at the index level. However, individuals with large central or paramedial subligamentous or extraligamentous herniations require a bilateral biportal approach.

Under direct arthroscopic control, the torn and scarred posterior annular fibers are grasped and removed. The herniated fragment is identified and extracted.

Lateral Recess Stenosis

Our limited experience with arthroscopic decompression of lateral recess stenosis in properly selected patients has been encouraging. Patients presenting with severe facet arthropathy associated with narrowing of the intervertebral disk and posterior osteophytosis are not suitable candidates for arthroscopic decompression via a 5 mm I.D. access cannula. Individuals with imaging evidence of a symmetrical or asymmetrical circumferential bulging disk[1] that is deemed to be responsible for compression of the exiting root in the lateral recess may undergo arthroscopic annular resection. Small posterolateral osteophytes arising from the vertebral plate may also be extracted with a trephine under arthroscopic visualization and illumination. To accomplish this, a 5 × 5 mm I.D. or 5 × 8 mm I.D. cannula is placed in the midpedicular region in accordance with the surgical technique described previously. Annular resection and extraction are accomplished with the aid of a working channel scope or insertion of an arthroscope-arthroscope sheath assembly and a 0° or 30° arthroscope into the lumen of the oval cannula. A radio-frequency coagulator or laser may also be used via a working channel scope with ample inflow and outflow of saline solution for final debridement and removal of fibrotic annular tissue.

Arthroscopic Debridement of Disk-Space Infection

The development of disk-space infection following arthroscopic disk surgery, open or closed diskectomy procedures, and diskography is not uncommon. Invariably, the diagnosis of bacterial diskitis is delayed. Radiographic changes such as end plate erosion may not appear until 4 to 6 weeks postoperatively, although MRI may provide information at earlier stages of diskitis.[67] Cultures may be negative in the presence of active infection. An early diagnosis may be made by arthroscopic visualization of necrotic and discolored nuclear tissue in the intervertebral disk. A 5 × 5 mm I.D. cannula may be positioned into the intervertebral disk through a posterolateral approach. Following extraction of tissue for culture and sensitivity testing, debridement of the nucleus and annular fibers is accomplished with the aid of manual instruments and the trimmer blade. Following removal of necrotic tissue, the disk space is irrigated with ample saline solution containing antibiotics effective against both gram-negative and gram-positive organisms. This step is then followed by external immobilization and 6 weeks of appropriate intravenous antibiotic therapy.

Posterolateral Arthroscopic Interbody Fusion

Arthroscopic interbody fusion may be performed with or without augmentation by pedicular fixators. In the early and mid 1980s,[68] our inability to access the vertebral plates, leading to inadequate decortication,

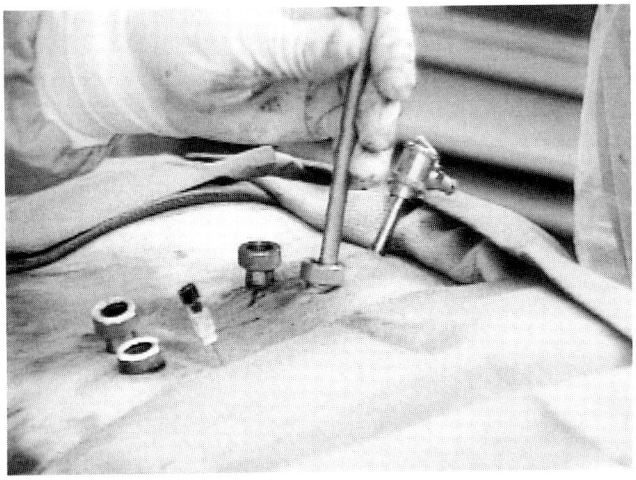

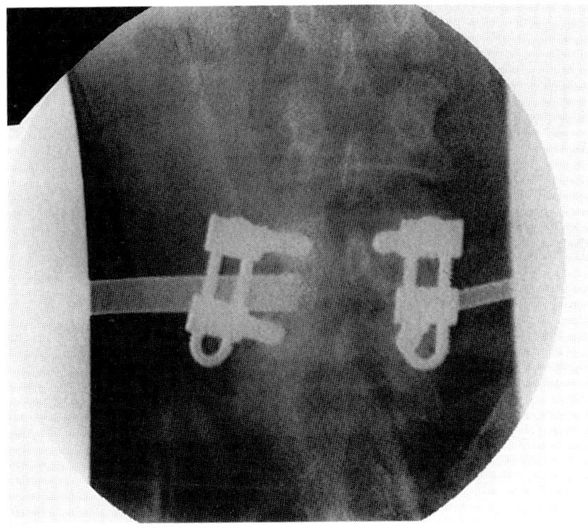

Fig. 21 **Left,** Four cannulas are inserted percutaneously and positioned over the pedicles in preparation for insertion of pedicular bolts. Note two access cannulas that are inserted into the intervertebral disk from the right and left side of the patient and are used for nucleotomy, decortication of the vertebral plates, and insertion of the bone grafts. **Right,** Postoperative anteroposterior and lateral roentgenograms demonstrating an oval cannula inserted from the left and a universal cannula inserted from the right side into the intervertebral disk. The pedicular bolts and subcutaneous plates have also been properly positioned.

may have been in part responsible for a high rate of postoperative pseudarthrosis. Introduction of the oval cannula that permitted insertion of an aggressive bone decorticator combined with the use of removable pedicular bolts and subcutaneous plates have enhanced the development of bony union in our more recently treated patients.[69,70] A bilateral biportal access to the intervertebral disk is necessary for meticulous extraction of the nuclear material, decortication of the vertebral plates, and insertion of autogenous bone grafts.

Percutaneous insertion of pedicular screws and external fixators was first described by Magerl.[71,72] In contrast to this technique, we insert the pedicular bolts through a pedicular cannula that is positioned over the pedicles under fluoroscopic control (Fig. 21). This is accomplished by first inserting rigid guide pins into the medullary canal of pedicles of segments adjacent to the surgical site under fluoroscopic guidance. While the patient is lying prone on a radiolucent table and frame, the C-arm is tilted 20° away from the pedicle that is being instrumented. A 6-inch guide pin is held with a long forceps or a jig. The pin is then maneuvered until its entire length is visualized as a bull's eye in the center of the pedicle. The pin is then drilled or hammered into the medullary canal of the pedicle.

A cannulated pedicular obturator is then used for soft-tissue dilatation. This step is then followed by introduction of pedicular cannulas (10 mm I.D.). The pedicles are tapped and examined with a sound that is inserted through the previously positioned pedicular cannula. Pedicular bolts of appropriate lengths and diameters are then used and inserted through the previously tapped medullary canal of the pedicles into the vertebral bodies. The pedicles of all of our patients who have undergone arthroscopic arthrodesis at L3-L4, L4-L5, and L5-S1 have been able to accommodate 7 mm O.D. pedicular bolts. Extension bars are then attached to the proximal end of the pedicular bolts. This permits extension of the bolts to the subcutaneous region where plates, washers, and nuts are inserted (Fig. 21). Arthroscopic interbody fusion and insertion of removable pedicular bolts and subcutaneous plates are currently under an investigational device exemption feas-ibility study in our institution.

Inclusion criteria for arthroscopic interbody fusion and fixation are similar to those described in the literature for spinal stabilization. Individuals with elevated iliac crests who require stabilization of the L5-S1 spinal unit are not suitable candidates for arthroscopic interbody fusion through the posterolateral approach.

Diagnostic Fixation of Lumbar Motion Segments

A number of diagnostic measures, including pain-provocation testing and local blocks with anesthetics,[73] have been used to identify a painful symp-tomatic lumbar motion segment. External fixators,[71,72] originally designed for fixation of thoracolumbar fractures, have been used to predetermine the necessity and expected outcome of spinal fusion in some patients.[74]

We have used removable pedicular bolts and subcutaneous plates for diagnostic purposes. However, the efficacy of this approach for selection of the surgical site is unclear at this time.

Arthroscopic Biopsy of Vertebral Bodies in the Lumbar and Lower Thoracic Spine

Vertebral bodies of the lower thoracic and lumbar spine may be accessed via a 5 × 5 mm I.D. access cannula, either through an intradiskal or transpedicular approach. For the intradiskal approach, the cannula is inserted into the intervertebral disk in accordance with the surgical technique described previously. The inserted cannula is then tilted cephalad or caudad and placed adjacent to the vertebral plates of the proximal or distal segment, and a trephine is inserted to penetrate the vertebral plates. A forceps is then passed into the lumen of the cannula and an ample amount of bone and tissue is removed from the vertebral bodies for pathologic examination.

The transpedicular approach to the vertebral bodies requires insertion of a guide wire into the medullary canal of the pedicle of the vertebra under fluoroscopic guidance as described previously. This step is followed by insertion of a cannulated obturator and positioning of a pedicular cannula over the pedicle. The medullary canal of the pedicle is then enlarged with the aid of a cannulated tap and an access cannula is positioned inside the pedicle. Straight and upbiting forceps may be inserted through the cannula for removal of tissue from the vertebral body for pathologic examination.

Discussion

Valls and associates,[75] Ottolenghi and associates,[76] and Craig[77] first described the posterolateral approach to the lumbar and lower thoracic vertebrae to obtain tissue for pathologic examination. A modified version of this technique and instrumentation were used for mechanical nucleotomy and central debulking of the intervertebral disk by Kambin and Hijikata in the early and mid 1970s.[17-19,26,78] Schreiber and Suezawa used the arthroscope for visualization and resection of central nuclear tissue via a percutaneous approach.[66,79] The subsequent availability of small-caliber arthroscopes and articulating instruments permitted intradiskal and periannular visualization and extraction of offending herniated disk fragments under arthroscopic illumination and magnification.[20,21,56] Arthroscopic identification of periannular anatomic structures combined with radiographic landmarks of the dorsolateral aspect of the anulus paved the way for safe positioning of the instruments and the use of the biportal approach and insertion of a larger oval cannula that provided broader access to the intervertebral disk.

Prior to the introduction of a modified arthroscope for visualization of intradiskal, extra-annular, and intracanalicular structures,[20,21,56] percutaneous retrieval of a large subligamentous and extraligamentous herniation was not possible. A distinction must be made between the surgical technique which places emphasis on nuclear debulking[19,50,52,53] and those that provide the capability of retrieving the posterior herniated fragments or even extracting a nonmigrated sequestered herniation. During the clinical evaluation process, the role of nonsurgical care for the treatment of symptom-producing herniated lumbar disks should not be discounted. The majority of patients respond satisfactorily to partial bed rest, the use of nonsteroidal anti-inflammatory medications, physical therapy and supervised exercise programs, or, at times, although they are controversial, epidural steroid injections.

It has been demonstrated that prolonged compression of the neural elements can interfere with venous drainage of the nerve root and cause chronic neural edema and fibrosis.[6,7] In addition to this, the progression of the neurologic deficit also calls for surgical intervention. As the preoperative imaging studies are evaluated, the spatial position and orientation of the osseous and soft-tissue anatomic structures must be noted. The surgical approach to the posterolateral corner of the intervertebral disk space critically depends on the initial placement of a needle in the TWZ of the anulus.[21,54,56,58] Parke and Watanabe[39-41] have demonstrated that the major transforaminal structures, the vertebromedullary branches of the segmental arteries and the sinuvertebral nerve, are located superior to the TWZ, and thus are clear of the path to the TWZ. There are low pressure venous branches that do, however, cross the TWZ. Fortunately, these branches are of little consequence as they are quite small; they have been arthroscopically visualized during the approach so that avoidance of them is possible.

Although plain radiographs of the lumbar spine do not yield much significant information in younger patients, the success of a minimally invasive approach dictates that the bony anatomy be evaluated completely to ensure that access to the disk space is possible. All patients have anteroposterior and lateral radiographs of the lumbar spine and pelvis that are helpful in preoperative planning for posterolateral arthroscopic access to the lumbar intervertebral disks. The anatomic position of the iliac crest and its relation to the intervertebral disk at the index level should be studied in order to determine whether the height of the iliac crest permits pass-age of the instruments to the herniation site. In addition to this, the height of the intervertebral disk, presence or absence of posterolateral osteophytosis, and the size and anatomic position of the transverse process will provide additional information in the preoperative planning stage. The presence or absence of kyphosis, scoliosis, congenital anomalies, and degenerative joint disease is recorded. The degenerated, narrowed intervertebral disks are usually associated with spinal stenosis. These patients will not respond to arthroscopic decompression. Also the narrowed disk spaces may not accommodate the 6.4 mm O.D. universal cannula. A broad transverse process, particlarly the transverse process of L5, may interfere with the passage of instruments to the L5-S1 intervertebral disk.

If the patient remains symptomatic after a period of nonsurgical care and surgical intervention is contemplated, further imaging evaluation is undertaken. MRI or myelography and postmyelography CT are both acceptable modalities to evaluate the disk herniation and surrounding anatomy.

An MRI study of the lumbar spine will provide ample information with regard to the degenerative status of the lumbar and lower thoracic intervertebral disks and is capable of demonstrating the presence or absence of extradural defects at the suspected site. The MRI study should be complemented by a CT from the index level, particularly in individuals who are older than 50 years of age. The CT provides information regarding the presence or absence of calcified tissue and will confirm that the herniation found in the MRI study does not represent osteophytosis. Myelography, which may not be necessary for routine preoperative evaluation, should be reserved for obese and claustrophobic patients whose MRIs are of suboptimal quality. In addition to this, patients who have undergone multiple previous spine procedures and those with deformities may require preoperative myelography.

The evaluation for arthroscopic microdiskectomy (AMD) strives to identify those anatomic abnormalities that would preclude a successful result. Extreme care should be exercised to exclude patients with a cauda equina syndrome, sequestered migrated disk herniation, spinal stenosis (including bony lateral recess stenosis), facet impingement, or pedicle-induced nerve root kinking. Those patients with developmental anomalies or tumors and those patients with reherniation following laminectomy or chemonucleolysis are not candidates for this procedure because of the potential for anatomic distortion. Each patient is carefully evaluated for the presence of psychosocial problems. Those patients who could be considered unstable, those with secondary gains, and those patients who are incapable of cooperating with the postoperative functional re-storation program are not candidates for arthroscopic microdiskectomy.

Minimally invasive spine surgery is not to be considered in patients who otherwise would not be eligible for surgery by traditional methods and represent a subset of those being considered for laminectomy or laminotomy and diskectomy.[21,56,58] Open laminotomy technique for the decompression of neural elements remains an acceptable and time-tested method for the treatment of herniated lumbar disks and spinal stenosis. The selection of arthroscopic or open technique depends largely on the patient's condition, and the surgeons must choose whichever technique will obtain the best result for that patient.

References

1. Dandy WE: Loose cartilage from intervertebral disk simulating tumor of the spinal cord. *Arch Surg* 1929;19:660–672.
2. Mixter WJ, Barr JS: Rupture of the intervertebral disc with involvement of the spinal canal. *N Engl J Med* 1934;211:210–215.
3. Love JG: Removal of protuded intervertebral disks without laminectomy. *Proc Staff Meet Mayo Clin* 1939;14:800.
4. Armstrong JR: The causes of unsatisfactory results from the operative treatment of lumbar disc lesions. *J Bone Joint Surg* 1951;33B:31–35.
5. Macnab I: Negative disc exploration: An analysis of the causes of nerve-root involvement in sixty-eight patients. *J Bone Joint Surg* 1971;53A:891–903.
6. Parke WW: The significance of venous return impairment in ischemic radiculopathy and myelopathy. *Orthop Clin North Am* 1991;22:213–221.
7. Cooper RG, Freemont AJ, Hoyland JA, et al: Herniated intervertebral disc-associated periradicular fibrosis and vascular abnormalities occur without inflammatory cell infiltration. *Spine* 1995;20:591–598.
8. LaRocca H, Macnab I: The laminectomy membrane: Studies in its evolution characteristics, effects and prophylaxis in dogs. *J Bone Joint Surg* 1974;56B:545–550.
9. Songer MN, Rauschning W, Carson EW, et al: Analysis of peridural scar formation and its prevention after lumbar laminotomy and discectomy in dogs. *Spine* 1995;20: 571–580.
10. Annertz M, Jonsson B, Stromqvist B, et al: No relationship between epidural fibrosis and sciatica in the lumbar postdiscectomy syndrome: A study with contrast-enhanced magnetic resonance imaging in symptomatic and asymptomatic patients. *Spine* 1995;20:449–453.
11. Goel VK, Goyal S, Clark C, et al: Kinematics of the whole lumbar spine: Effect of discectomy. *Spine* 1985;10:543–554.
12. Kambin P, Cohen LF, Brooks M, et al: Development of degenerative spondylosis of the lumbar spine after partial discectomy: Comparison of laminotomy, discectomy, and posterolateral discectomy. *Spine* 1995;20:599–607.
13. Hanley EN Jr, Shapiro DE: The development of low-back pain after excision of a lumbar disc. *J Bone Joint Surg* 1989;71A: 719–721.
14. Weir BK, Jacobs GA: Reoperation rate following lumbar discectomy: An analysis of 662 lumbar discectomies. *Spine* 1980; 5:366–370.
15. Saal JS, Franson RC, Dobrow R, et al: High levels of inflammatory phospholipase A2 activity in lumbar disc herniations. *Spine* 1990;15:674–678.
16. Spiliopoulou I, Korovessis P, Konstantinou D, et al: IgG and IgM concentration in the prolapsed human intervertebral disc and sciatica etiology. *Spine* 1994;19:1320–1323.
17. Kambin P: History of disc surgery, in Kambin P (ed): *Arthroscopic Microdiscectomy: Minimal Intervention in Spinal Surgery*. Baltimore, MD, Urban & Schwarzenberg, 1991, pp 3–8.
18. Kambin P, Gellman H: Percutaneous lateral discectomy of the lumbar spine: A preliminary report. *Clin Orthop* 1983;174: 127–132.

19. Hijikata S: Percutaneous nucleotomy: A new concept technique and 12 years' experience. *Clin Orthop* 1989;238:9–23.
20. Kambin P: Posterolateral percutaneous lumbar discectomy and decompression: Arthroscopic microdiscectomy, in Kambin P (ed): *Arthroscopic Microdiscectomy: Minimal Intervention in Spinal Surgery*. Baltimore, MD, Urban & Schwarzenberg, 1991, pp 67–100.
21. Kambin P: Arthroscopic microdiscectomy. *Arthroscopy* 1992; 8:287–295.
22. Kambin P: Percutaneous lumbar discectomy: Current practice. *Surg Rounds Orthop* 1988;2:31–35.
23. Kambin P: Posterolateral percutaneous lumbar discectomy and decompression: Arthroscopic microdiscectomy, in Kambin P (ed): *Arthroscopic Microdiscectomy: Minimal Intervention in Spinal Surgery*. Baltimore, MD, Urban & Schwarzenberg, 1991, pp 67–100.
24. Mirkovic SR, Schwartz DG, Glazier KD: Anatomic considerations in lumbar posterolateral percutaneous procedures. *Spine* 1995;20:1965–1971.
25. Kahanovitz N: Percutaneous diskectomy. *Clin Orthop* 1992;284: 75–79.
26. Kambin P, Schaffer JL: Percutaneous lumbar discectomy: Review of 100 patients and current practice. *Clin Orthop* 1989;238:24–34.
27. Onik G, Mooney V, Maroon JC, et al: Automated percutaneous discectomy: A prospective multi-institutional study. *Neurosurgery* 1990;26:228–233.
28. Revel M, Payan C, Vallee C, et al: Automated percutaneous lumbar discectomy versus chemonucleolysis in the treatment of sciatica: A randomized multicenter trial. *Spine* 1993;18:1–7.
29. Kambin P, Nixon JE, Chait A, et al: Annular protrusion: Pathophysiology and roentgenographic appearance. *Spine* 1988; 13:671–675.
30. Delamarter RB, Howard MW, Goldstein T, et al: Percutaneous lumbar discectomy: Preoperative and postoperative magnetic resonance imaging. *J Bone Joint Surg* 1995; 77A:578–584.
31. Obenchain TG: Laparoscopic lumbar discectomy: Case report. *J Laparoendosc Surg* 1991;1:145–149.
32. Bagby GW: Arthrodesis by the distraction-compression method using a stainless steel implant. *Orthopedics* 1988;11:931–934.
33. Zucherman JF, Zdeblick TA, Bailey SA, et al: Instrumented laparoscopic spinal fusion: Preliminary results. *Spine* 1995; 20:2029–2035.
34. Mathews HH, Evans MT, Molligan HJ, et al: Laparoscopic discectomy with anterior lumbar interbody fusion: A preliminary review. *Spine* 1995;20:1797–1802.
35. Jacobaeus HC: The practical importance of thoracoscopy in surgery of the chest. *Surg Gynecol Obstet* 1922;34: 289–296.
36. Landreneau RJ, Hazelrigg SR, Mack MJ, et al: Postoperative pain-related morbidity: Video-assisted thoracic surgery versus thoracotomy. *Ann Thorac Surg* 1993;56:1285–1289.
37. Regan JJ, Mack MJ, Picetti GD III: A technical report on video-assisted thoracoscopy in thoracic spinal surgery: Preliminary description. *Spine* 1995;20:831–837.
38. Groen GJ, Baljet B, Drukker J: Nerves and nerve plexuses of the human vertebral column. *Am J Anat* 1990;188:282–296.
39. Parke WW, Watanabe R: The intrinsic vasculature of the lumbosacral spinal nerve roots. *Spine* 1985;10:508–515.
40. Parke WW: Applied anatomy of the spine, in Rothman RH, Simeone FA (eds): *The Spine*, ed 3. Philadelphia, PA, WB Saunders, 1992, vol 1, pp 35–87.
41. Watanabe R, Parke WW: Vascular and neural pathology of lumbosacral spinal stenosis. *J Neurosurg* 1986;64:64–70.
42. Garfin SR, Rydevik B, Lind B, et al: Spinal nerve root compression. *Spine* 1995;20:1810–1820.
43. Rydevik B, Holm S, Brown MD, et al: Diffusion from the cerebrospinal fluid as a nutritional pathway for spinal nerve roots. *Acta Physiol Scand* 1990;138:247–248.
44. Hoyland JA, Freemont AJ, Jayson MI: Intervertebral foramen venous obstruction: A cause of periradicular fibrosis? *Spine* 1989;14:558–568.
45. Magnaes B: Clinical recording of pressure on the spinal cord and cauda equina. *J Neurosurg* 1982;57:48–63.
46. LaBan MM: "Vesper's Curse" night pain: The bane of Hypnos. *Arch Phys Med Rehabil* 1984;65:501–504.
47. Cohen MS, Wall EJ, Brown RA, et al: Cauda equina anatomy: II. Extrathecal nerve roots and dorsal root ganglia. *Spine* 1990;15:1248–1251.
48. Schaffer JL, Kambin P: Minimally invasive spine surgery, in *Textbook of Rheumatology*. Philadelphia, PA, WB Saunders, 1993, pp 1–12.
49. Kambin P: Arthroscopic microdiscectomy laser nucleolysis. *Philadelphia Med* 1991;87:548–549.
50. Smith L, Garvin PJ, Gesler RM, et al: Enzyme dissolution of the nucleus pulposus. *Nature* 1963;198:1311–1312.
51. Onik G, Helms CA, Ginsburg L, et al: Percutaneous lumbar diskectomy using a new aspiration probe. *Am J Roentgenol* 1985;144:1137–1140.
52. Onik G, Maroon J, Davis GW: Automated percutaneous discectomy at the L5-S1 level: Use of a curved cannula. *Clin Orthop* 1989;238:71–76.
53. Ascher PW, Holzer P, Sutter B: Laser denaturation of the nucleus pulposus of herniated intervertebral discs, in Kambin P (ed): *Arthroscopic Microdiscectomy: Minimal Intervention in Spinal Surgery*. Baltimore, MD, Urban & Schwarzenberg, 1991, pp 137–140.
54. Cummings RS, Progoehl JA, Hermantin FU, et al: Percutaneous laser discectomy using a flexible endoscope: Technical considerations, in Sherk HH (ed): *Laser Discectomy*. Philadelphia, PA, Hanley & Belfus, 1993, pp 37–40.
55. Javid MJ, Nordby EJ, Ford LT, et al: Safety and efficacy of chymopapain (Chymodiactin) in herniated nucleus pulposus with sciatica: Results of a randomized, double-blind study. *JAMA* 1983;249:2489–2494.
56. Schaffer JL, Kambin P: Percutaneous posterolateral lumbar discectomy and decompression with a 6.9-millimeter cannula: Analysis of operative failures and complications. *J Bone Joint Surg* 1991;73A:822–831.
57. Kambin P: Arthroscopic microdiscectomy of the lumbar spine. *Clin Sports Med* 1993;12:143–150.
58. Kambin P: Arthroscopic microdiscectomy: Lumbar and thoracic, in White AH, Schofferman JA (eds): *Spine Care*. St. Louis, MO, Mosby-Year Book, 1995, vol 2, pp 1002–1016.
59. Spencer DL, Irwin GS, Miller JA: Anatomy and significance of fixation of the lumbosacral nerve roots in sciatica. *Spine* 1983;8:672–679.
60. Kambin P: Gross and arthroscopic anatomy of the lumbar spine, in McGinty JB, Caspari RB, Jackson RW, et al (eds): *Operative Arthroscopy*, ed 2. Philadelphia, PA, Lippincott-Raven, 1996, pp 1207–1214.
61. Kambin P, Schaffer JL, Zhou L: Incidence of complications following percutaneous posterolateral arthroscopic disc surgery. *Clin Orthop*, in press
62. Kambin P: Arthroscopic microdiscectomy: Laser nuclear ablation, in Sherk HH (ed): *Laser Discectomy*. Philadelphia, PA, Hanley & Belfus, 1993, pp 95–101.
63. Savitz MH: Same-day microsurgical arthroscopic lateral-approach laser-assisted (SMALL) fluoroscopic discectomy. *J Neurosurg* 1994;80:1039–1045.

64. Hochschuler SH: Posterior lateral arthroscopic microdiskectomy. *Semin Orthop* 1991;6:113–114.
65. Kambin P, Sampson S: Posterolateral percutaneous suction-excision of herniated lumbar intervertebral discs: Report of interim results. *Clin Orthop* 1986;207:37–43.
66. Schreiber A, Suezawa Y, Leu H: Does percutaneous nucleotomy with discoscopy replace conventional discectomy? Eight years of experience and results in treatment of herniated lumbar disc. *Clin Orthop* 1989;238:35–42.
67. Boden SD, Davis DO, Dina TS, et al: Postoperative diskitis: Distinguishing early MR imaging findings from normal post-operative disk space changes. *Radiology* 1992;184: 765–771.
68. Kambin P: Posterolateral percutaneous lumbar interbody fusion, in Kambin P (ed): *Arthroscopic Microdiscectomy: Minimal Intervention in Spinal Surgery*. Baltimore, MD, Urban & Schwarzenberg, 1991, pp 117–121.
69. Kambin P, Schreiber A, Sheppherd J, et al: Minimal intervention surgical techniques in spinal surgery. *Orthop Trans* 1993;17:1132.
70. Kambin P: Arthroscopic lumbar interbody fusion, in White AH, Schofferman JA (eds): *Spine Care*. St. Louis, MO, Mosby-Year Book, 1995, vol 2, pp 1055–1066.
71. Magerl FP: Stabilization of the lower thoracic and lumbar spine with external skeletal fixation. *Clin Orthop* 1984;189: 125–141.
72. Magerl F: External skeletal fixation of the lower thoracic and the lumbar spine, in Uhthoff HK, Stahl E (eds): *Current Concepts of External Fixation of Fractures*. Berlin, Germany, Springer-Verlag, 1982, pp 353–366.
73. Derby R, Bogduk N, Kine G: Precision percutaneous blocking procedures for localizing spinal pain: Part 2. The lumbar neuroaxial compartment. *Pain Digest* 1993;3:175–188.
74. Esses SI, Botsford DJ, Kostuik JP: The role of external spinal skeletal fixation in the assessment of low-back disorders. *Spine* 1989;14:594–601.
75. Valls J, Ottolenghi CE, Schajowicz F: Aspiration biopsy in diagnosis of lesions of vertebral bodies. *JAMA* 1948;136:376–382.
76. Ottolenghi CE: Diagnosis of orthopaedic lesions by aspiration biopsy: Results of 1,061 punctures. *J Bone Joint Surg* 1955; 37A:443–464.
77. Craig FS: Vertebral-body biopsy. *J Bone Joint Surg* 1956;38A: 93–102.
78. Hijikata S, Yamagishi M, Nakayama T, et al: Percutaneous diskectomy: A new treatment method for lumbar disk herniation. *J Toden Hosp* 1975;5:5–13.
79. Schreiber A, Suezawa Y: Transdiscoscopic percutaneous nucleotomy in disk herniation. *Orthop Rev* 1986;15:35–38.

Knee

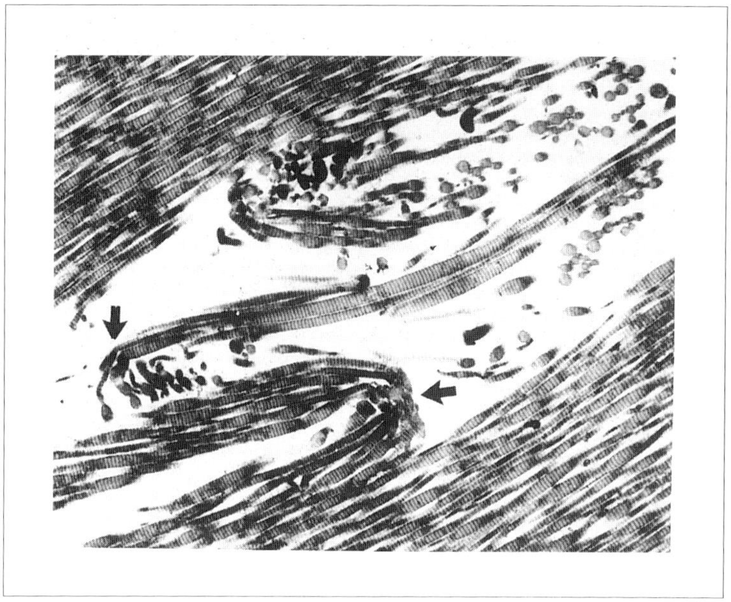

CHAPTER 13

Wound Complications in Total Knee Arthroplasty

Douglas A. Dennis, MD

Primary wound healing is critical for the success of any total knee arthroplasty (TKA). Any delay in wound healing risks infection and arthroplasty failure.[1] Prevention of soft-tissue problems through the proper selection of skin incision, an understanding of vascular anatomy and patient risk factors, and prompt management should wound problems arise, is imperative to achieve desired results.

Vascular Anatomy

The blood supply to the soft tissues of the anterior aspect of the knee is completely random, with contributions from multiple vessels.[2-8] This blood supply arises predominantly from the terminal branches of the peripatellar anastomotic arterial ring. This anastomotic ring has numerous contributing arterial branches, including the medial and lateral superior genicular arteries, the medial and lateral inferior genicular arteries, the supreme genicular artery, the anterior tibial recurrent artery, and a branch of the profunda femoris artery (Fig. 1). In contrast to the skin circulation of the thigh proximal to the knee, there is no underlying muscle or intermuscular septa directly anterior to the knee to provide a direct pathway for arterial perforators.[2,5] Skin circulation in this area is dependent on the dermal plexus, which originates directly from arterioles traveling within the subcutaneous fascia. Any surgical dissection performed superficial to this subcutaneous fascia disrupts the arterial supply to the skin and increases the possibility of skin necrosis. Elevation of skin flaps about the anterior aspect of the knee requires dissection deep to the subcutaneous fascia to preserve the perforating arteriolar network between the subcutaneous fascia and dermal plexus.[2]

Choice of Skin Incision

Analysis of vascular anatomy about the knee suggests that choice of a midline skin incision is less disruptive to the arterial network.[2] Medial peripatellar skin incisions are undesirable, because they create a large, laterally based skin flap, which has been associated with higher wound complication rates.[2] Transcutaneous oxygen measurements, both before and after skin incisions about the knee, have demonstrated reduced oxygenation of the lateral skin region.[9,10] The further medially the skin incision is made, the larger the lateral skin flap. A larger lateral skin flap has a lower oxygen tension, which increases the risk of wound complications. Placement of the skin incision slightly lateral to the midline will assist in eversion of the patella, particularly in obese patients in whom a large and bulky lateral skin flap resists patellar eversion.

For patients in whom a previous skin incision is present, utilization of the previous skin incision is generally recommended. Although it is usually safe to ignore previous short medial or lateral peripatellar skin incisions, one should beware of wide scars with thin or absent subcutaneous tissue, as damage to the underlying dermal plexus is likely, increasing the risk of wound necrosis.[2] Problems with placement of a longitudinal incision crossing a transverse incision previously used for high tibial osteotomy are uncommon.[11,12]

If long parallel skin incisions exist, choice of the lateral-most skin incision is favorable to avoid a large lateral skin flap which has been previously compromised at the time of the initial lateral skin incision. In com-

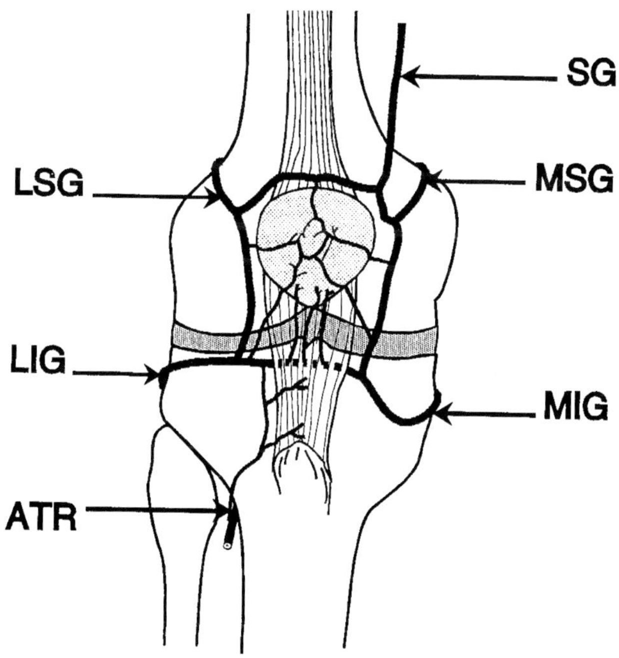

Fig. 1 Diagram demonstrating the extraosseous peripatellar anastomotic ring supplied by six main arteries (LSG = lateral superior genicular; MSG = medial superior genicular; MIG = medial inferior genicular; LIG = lateral inferior genicular; SG = supreme genicular; ATR = anterior tibial recurrent). (Reproduced with permission from Dennis DA: Patellofemoral complications in total knee arthroplasty: A literature review. *Am J Knee Surg* 1992;5:156-166.)

plex situations, such as knees with multiple skin incisions or previously burned or irradiated skin, consideration of plastic surgical consultation is wise, both for the design of the upcoming skin incision as well as for consideration of preoperative muscle flap procedures if the risk of skin necrosis is substantial. In selected complex situations, wound problems can be reduced by using a staged technique. A "pre-revision" skin incision to the depth of the subcutaneous fascial layer is made and is then closed. If this incision heals without difficulty, one can later proceed with TKA through this incision with much greater confidence.

Soft-tissue expansion techniques have been used successfully in cases of contracted soft tissues from previous skin incisions or exposure of the skin to irradiation or burns.[13-18] These techniques involve implantation, usually subcutaneously, of an expandable reservoir, into which saline can be intermittently injected to expand the surface area of the skin. Studies have shown that this technique maintains epidermal thickness. Although some dermal thinning is encountered, actual dermal collagen synthesis is increased. Complications with soft-tissue expansion have been minimal and include hematoma formation, reservoir deflation, infection, and skin necrosis from overly vigorous soft-tissue expansion.

Technical Factors

A thorough preoperative vascular examination of the limb is necessary to minimize the risk of wound-healing difficulties. The skin incision for TKA should be of adequate length to avoid excessive tension on the wound edges, particularly when the knee is in extremes of flexion. Gentle retraction of the skin edges is necessary to avoid disruption of perforating arterioles originating in the subcutaneous fascial layer. It is best to attempt to avoid undermining large areas of skin. If undermining of skin flaps is required, it must be done in the subfascial plane to preserve the blood supply to the skin, which originates in the dermal plexus.[2,5] Numerous studies have demonstrated that a lateral retinacular release decreases lateral skin oxygenation and increases the subsequent risk of wound complications.[19-22] If a lateral retinacular release is required, attempts should be made to preserve the lateral superior geniculate artery. Meticulous wound hemostasis is required to avoid postoperative hematomas. Routine use of suction drainage will reduce pain and postoperative ecchymosis. Lastly, wound closure without tension is imperative to minimize the risk of skin necrosis.

Patient Risk Factors

Numerous reports suggest an increased incidence of wound-healing difficulties in patients who chronically use corticosteroids.[2,23-30] Corticosteroid use has been shown to decrease fibroblast proliferation, which is necessary for proper wound healing.[24] Chronic corticosteroid use also reduces collagenase clearance from the healing wound, which results in diminished collagen accumulation at the wound healing site and a subsequent decrease in wound tensile strength.[23,29,30] An increased incidence of wound complications in patients with rheumatoid arthritis has been well documented. Although the specific cause of this association is not known, it may be related to the increased long-term use of corticosteroids in many of these patients.[31 36]

Patients with substantial obesity demonstrate increased wound complication rates.[26,35,37,38] Extreme obesity can create exposure difficulties in TKA, necessitating more vigorous retraction of skin flaps and the subsequent risk of soft-tissue devascularization. Additionally, in heavier patients with a thick adipose layer, the skin is less adherent to its underlying vascular supply, which increases the risk of separation of the dermis from the subcutaneous layer during skin retraction.[2]

Malnutrition, represented by albumin levels less than 3.5 g/dl and total lymphocyte counts less than 1500 cells/mm^3, has been associated with poor healing of Syme amputation stumps and may play a role in wound healing following TKA.[38,39] The damaging effects of cigarette smoking have been well documented and are related to the systemic vasoconstriction resulting from nicotine use.[40-44]

While the exact relationship is unclear, the increased frequency of wound problems in patients with diabetes mellitus may be secondary to delayed collagen synthesis and delayed wound tensile strength. Early capillary ingrowth into the healing wound is also reduced.[2,38,45-47] Use of high-dose nonsteroidal anti-inflammatory drugs inhibits the acute inflammatory response, which is an important step in the early phases of wound healing. Inhibition of this early, acute inflammatory response may exacerbate wound healing difficulties.[48] Patients on chemotherapy may be similarly at risk for delayed wound healing. The routine need to discontinue methotrexate in preoperative patients with rheumatoid arthritis is unclear. Bridges and associates[49] found a slight increase in the incidence of infection in ten patients treated with methotrexate when compared with patients with rheumatoid arthritis in whom methotrexate had been discontinued more than 1 month preoperatively. Other larger comparison studies have demonstrated no increase in wound-healing complications with continuance of methotrexate perioperatively in patients with rheumatoid arthritis.[50,51]

Adequate hydration is necessary for satisfactory wound healing. Hypovolemia can delay wound healing due to reduced oxygen delivery to the healing soft tissues.[2] Reduction in transcutaneous oxygen levels has been documented to increase wound healing complications following lateral retinacular release in TKA[20] and to decrease wound healing after soft-tissue flap transfers.[52] Use of continuous passive motion beyond 40° has been shown to reduce transcutaneous oxygen tension measured in the healing wound edges, especially during the initial 3 days following TKA. Continuous passive motion should be limited to less than 40° during the early postoperative period.[53,54] Additional risk factors for wound complications following TKA include those knees in which the anterior skin has previously been irradiated or suffered severe scarring from previous burns.

Wound Complication Management

Various types of wound complications can occur, including prolonged postoperative drainage, superficial soft-tissue necrosis, and full-thickness soft-tissue necrosis, in which the prosthetic components are usually exposed. All three types of wound problems require immediate attention, as delay in treatment risks deep infection and subsequent failure of the TKA.

Prolonged Serous Drainage

If the TKA wound is chronically draining yet the wound does not exhibit substantial erythema or purulence, immobilization and local wound care can be attempted. In the author's experience, if drainage persists beyond 5 to 7 days despite immobilization and local wound care, spontaneous cessation of drainage is unlikely and surgical debridement is indicated. Subcutaneous hematomas or large intra-articular hemarthroses are commonly encountered in cases of persistent wound drainage. Hematomas threaten the wound by increasing soft-tissue tension, releasing toxic breakdown products of hemoglobin, and serving as a healthy medium for bacterial growth.[2]

Scientific data are lacking to clearly support surgical drainage rather than observation of the nondraining hematoma. We recommend treating the nondraining hematoma nonsurgically through close observation as long as no signs of impending skin necrosis from excessive soft-tissue tension are present. An additional consideration for surgical drainage is a large hematoma that substantially limits knee range of motion. Drainage procedures should be performed in the operating theater with perioperative antibiotic prophylaxis.

The incidence of prolonged drainage in patients who eventually develop culture-proven infected TKA ranges from 17% to 50%.[55-57] Weiss and Krackow,[55] in a retrospective review of 597 TKA procedures, found eight patients (1.3%) with persistent wound drainage. All were treated with surgical irrigation and debridement and parenteral antibiotics. All cases healed without infection despite the fact that two patients (25%) had positive cultures at the time of irrigation and debridement. The authors suggest that prompt surgical management in these cases may prevent chronic drainage problems from becoming established infections.

Superficial Soft-Tissue Necrosis

Necrotic tissue generally requires surgical debridement. Small necrotic areas less than 3 cm in diameter may heal with local wound care or delayed secondary closure.[28] Larger areas of superficial necrosis should be debrided and covered by split-thickness skin grafting or fasciocutaneous flaps.[58,59]

Full-Thickness Soft-Tissue Necrosis

Full-thickness soft-tissue necrosis is usually associated with exposed prosthetic components and requires immediate, aggressive debridement. Simple secondary closure procedures are often unsuccessful, and some type of flap reconstruction is usually required. Various types of flaps have been used, including cutaneous,[60] fasciocutaneous,[58,59] and myocutaneous flaps.[60-67] Bengtson and associates[61] reported on treatment of ten TKAs with full-thickness skin loss and exposed prosthetic components. Delayed closure failed in six of six cases in which it was attempted. Split thickness skin grafting failed in both cases in which it was tried. In contrast, coverage with gastrocnemius myocutaneous flaps proved successful and was recommended as the treatment of choice in these cases. Gerwin and associates[67] reviewed 12 patients with full-thickness skin necrosis and exposed prostheses, six of whom had positive deep cultures. All patients were treated with aggressive debridement and closure with medial gastrocnemius myocutaneous flaps. Eleven of 12 patients (92%) obtained excellent results, with ten (82%) retaining their prosthetic components or having a successful reimplantation.

The medial head of the gastrocnemius muscle is often the preferred type of flap reconstruction. It is both larger and 2 to 3 cm longer than the lateral gastrocnemius muscle. Furthermore, because it does not have to traverse the fibula, it therefore has a larger arc of rotation. It provides excellent soft-tissue coverage in the region of the patella and tibial tubercle, the area where the incidence of skin necrosis is the highest. Free myocutaneous flaps may also be used,[2,68] but they are reserved for cases with full-thickness necrosis which cannot be covered with gastrocnemius or other local flap reconstructions.

Antibiotic Use

Parenteral antibiotics are often required in cases with persistent drainage and wound necrosis, but they should not be used indiscriminately. Unnecessary use of antibiotics risks alteration of bacterial flora and sensitivities, should deep infection occur.[2] Joint aspiration for culture is suggested before initiation of antibiotic therapy in order to maximize culture results. Cultures of superficial drainage are often spurious with little correlation with deep infecting organisms.[2,28,69]

Summary

Wound problems are a dreaded complication following TKA and the ideal is to avoid them. Preventive measures include proper choice of the skin incision, gentle handling of the soft tissues, meticulous hemostasis, and wound closure without excessive tension. Should persistent wound drainage or soft-tissue necrosis occur, early intervention is imperative, because delay risks deep infection and failure of the TKA. Cases associated with full-thickness soft-tissue necrosis often require transfer of well-vascularized tissue, such as a medial gastrocnemius myocutaneous flap reconstruction.

References

1. Poss R, Thornhill TS, Ewald FC, et al: Factors influencing the incidence and outcome of infection following total joint arthroplasty. *Clin Orthop* 1984;182:117–126.
2. Klein NE, Cox CV: Wound problems in total knee arthroplasty, in Fu FH, Harner CD, Vince KG, et al (eds): *Knee Surgery*. Baltimore, MD, Williams & Wilkins, 1994, vol 2, pp 1539–1552.
3. Müller W (ed): *The Knee: Form, Function and Ligament Reconstruction*. Berlin, Germany, Springer–Verlag, 1983, pp 158–167.
4. Scapinelli R: Studies on the vasculature of the human knee joint. *Acta Anat* 1968;70:305–331.
5. Craig SM: Soft tissue considerations in the failed total knee arthroplasty, in Scott WN (ed): *The Knee*. St. Louis, MO, Mosby-Year Book, 1994, vol 2, pp 1279–1295.
6. Abbott LC, Carpenter WF: Surgical approaches to the knee joint. *J Bone Joint Surg* 1945;27:277–310.
7. Björkström S, Goldie IF: A study of the arterial supply of the patella in the normal state, in chondromalacia patellae and in osteoarthrosis. *Acta Orthop Scand* 1980;51:63–70.
8. Waisbrod H, Treiman N: Intra-osseous venography in patellofemoral disorders: A preliminary report. *J Bone Joint Surg* 1980;62B:454–456.
9. Johnson DP: Midline or parapatellar incision for knee arthroplasty: A comparative study of wound viability. *J Bone Joint Surg* 1988;70B:656–658.
10. Johnson DP, Houghton TA, Radford P: Anterior midline or medial parapatellar incision for arthroplasty of the knee: A comparative study. *J Bone Joint Surg* 1986;68B:812–814.
11. Ecker ML, Lotke PA: Wound healing complications, in Rand JA (ed): *Total Knee Arthroplasty*. New York, NY, Raven Press, 1993, pp 403–407.
12. Windsor RE, Insall JN, Vince KG: Technical consideration of total knee arthroplasty after proximal tibial osteotomy. *J Bone Joint Surg* 1988;70A:547–555.
13. Mahomed N, McKee N, Solomon P, et al: Soft-tissue expansion before total knee arthroplasty in arthrodesed joints: A report of two cases. *J Bone Joint Surg* 1994;76B:88–90.
14. Argenta LC, Marks MW, Pasyk KA: Advances in tissue expansion. *Clin Plast Surg* 1985;12:159–171.
15. Manders EK, Oaks TE, Au VK, et al: Soft-tissue expansion in the lower extremities. *Plast Reconstr Surg* 1988;81:208–219.
16. Manders EK, Schenden MJ, Furrey JA, et al: Soft-tissue expansion: Concepts and complications. *Plast Reconstr Surg* 1984;74:493–507.
17. Radovan C: Tissue expansion in soft-tissue reconstruction. *Plast Reconstr Surg* 1984;74:482–492.
18. Riederman R, Noyes FR: Soft tissue skin expansion of contracted tissues prior to knee surgery. *Am J Knee Surg* 1991;4:195–198.
19. Clayton ML, Thirupathi R: Patellar complications after total condylar arthroplasty. *Clin Orthop* 1982;170:152–155.
20. Johnson DP, Eastwood DM: Lateral patellar release in knee arthroplasty: Effect on wound healing. *J Arthroplasty* 1992;7(suppl):427–431.
21. Kayler DE, Lyttle D: Surgical interruption of patellar blood supply by total knee arthroplasty. *Clin Orthop* 1988;229:221–227.
22. Scuderi G, Scharf SC, Meltzer LP, et al: The relationship of lateral releases to patella viability in total knee arthroplasty. *J Arthroplasty* 1987;2:209–214.
23. Craig SM: Soft tissue considerations, in Scott WN (ed): *Total Knee Revision Arthroplasty*. Orlando, FL, Grune & Stratton, 1987, pp 99–112.
24. Green JP: Steroid therapy and wound healing in surgical patients. *Br J Surg* 1965;52:523–525.
25. McNamara JJ, Lamborn PJ, Mills D, et al: Effect of short-term pharmacologic doses of adrenocorticosteroid therapy on wound healing. *Ann Surg* 1969;170:199–202.
26. Nelson CL: Prevention of sepsis. *Clin Orthop* 1987;222:66–72.
27. Petty W, Bryan RS, Coventry MB, Peterson LF: Infection after total knee arthroplasty. *Orthop Clin North Am* 1975;6:1005–1014.
28. Sculco TP: Local wound complications after total knee arthroplasty, in Ranawat CS (ed): *Total Condylar Knee Arthroplasty: Technique, Results, and Complications*. New York, NY, Springer–Verlag, 1985, pp 194–196.
29. Wahl LM: Hormonal regulation of macrophage collagenase activity. *Biochem Biophys Res Commun* 1977;74:838–845.
30. Werb Z: Biochemical actions of glucocorticoids on macrophages in culture: Specific inhibition of elastase, collagenase, and plasminogen activator secretion and effects on other metabolic functions. *J Exp Med* 1978;147:1695–1712.
31. D'Ambrosia RD, Shoji H, Heater R: Secondarily infected total joint replacements by hematogenous spread. *J Bone Joint Surg* 1976;58A:450–453.
32. Garner RW, Mowat AG, Hazleman BL: Wound healing after operations on patients with rheumatoid arthritis. *J Bone Joint Surg* 1973;55B:134–144.
33. Grogan TJ, Dorey F, Rollins J, et al: Deep sepsis following total knee arthroplasty: Ten-year experience at the University of California at Los Angeles Medical Center. *J Bone Joint Surg* 1986;68A:226–234.
34. Thomas BJ, Moreland JR, Amstutz HC: Infection after total joint arthroplasty from distal extremity sepsis. *Clin Orthop* 1983;181:121–125.
35. Wilson MG, Kelley K, Thornhill TS: Infection as a complication of total knee-replacement arthroplasty: Risk factors and treatment in sixty-seven cases. *J Bone Joint Surg* 1990;72A:878–883.
36. Wong RY, Lotke PA, Ecker ML: Factors influencing wound healing after total knee arthroplasty. *Orthop Trans* 1986;10:497.
37. Cruse PJ, Foord R: A five-year prospective study of 23,649 surgical wounds. *Arch Surg* 1973;107:206–210.
38. Ecker ML, Lotke PA: Postoperative care of the total knee patient. *Orthop Clin North Am* 1989;20:55–62.
39. Dickhaut SC, DeLee JC, Page CP: Nutritional status: Importance in predicting wound-healing after amputation. *J Bone Joint Surg* 1984;66A:71–75.
40. Craig S, Rees TD: The effects of smoking on experimental skin flaps in hamsters. *Plast Reconstr Surg* 1985;75:842–846.
41. Benowitz NL, Kuyt F, Jacob P III: Influence of nicotine on cardiovascular and hormonal effects of cigarette smoking. *Clin Pharmacol Ther* 1984;36:74–81.

42. Mosely LH, Finseth F, Goody M: Nicotine and its effect on wound healing. *Plast Reconstr Surg* 1978;61:570–575.
43. Rees TD, Liverett DM, Guy CL: The effect of cigarette smoking on skin-flap survival in the face lift patient. *Plast Reconstr Surg* 1984;73:911–915.
44. Kaufman T, Eichenlaub EH, Levin M, et al: Tobacco smoking: Impairment of experimental flap survival. *Ann Plast Surg* 1984;13:468–472.
45. Goodson WH III, Hunt TK: Studies of wound healing in experimental diabetes mellitus. *J Surg Res* 1977;22:221–227.
46. Goodson WH III, Hunt TK: Wound healing and the diabetic patient. *Surg Gynecol Obstet* 1979;149:600–608.
47. McMurry JF Jr: Wound healing with diabetes mellitus: Better glucose control for better wound healing in diabetes. *Surg Clin North Am* 1984;64:769–778.
48. McGrath MH: The effect of prostaglandin inhibitors on wound contraction and the myofibroblast. *Plast Reconstr Surg* 1982;69:74–85.
49. Bridges SL Jr, Lopez Mendez A, Tracy I, et al: Should methotrexate be discontinued prior to total joint arthroplasty in rheumatoid arthritis patients? *Arthritis Rheum* 1989;32(suppl 4):543.
50. Kasden ML, June L: Postoperative results of rheumatoid arthritis patients on methotrexate at the time of reconstructive surgery of the hand. *Orthopedics* 1993;16:1233–1235.
51. Perhala RS, Wilke WS, Clough JD, et al: Local infectious complications following large joint replacement in rheumatoid arthritis patients treated with emthotrexate versus those not treated with methotrexate. *Arthritis Rheum* 1991;34:146–152.
52. Achauer BM, Black KS, Litke DK: Transcutaneous PO_2 in flaps: A new method of survival prediction. *Plast Reconstr Surg* 1980;65:738–745.
53. Goletz TH, Henry JH: Continuous passive motion after total knee arthroplasty. *South Med J* 1986;79:1116–1120.
54. Johnson DP: The effect of continuous passive motion on wound-healing and joint mobility after knee arthroplasty. *J Bone Joint Surg* 1990;72A:421–426.
55. Weiss AP, Krackow KA: Persistent wound drainage after primary total knee arthroplasty. *J Arthroplasty* 1993;8:285–289.
56. Bengtson S, Knutson K, Lidgren L: Treatment of infected knee arthroplasty. *Clin Orthop* 1989;245:173–178.
57. Insall J, Aglietti P: A five to seven-year follow-up of unicondylar arthroplasty. *J Bone Joint Surg* 1980;62A:1329–1337.
58. Hallock GG: Salvage of total knee arthroplasty with local fasciocutaneous flaps. *J Bone Joint Surg* 1990;72A:1236–1239.
59. Lewis VL Jr, Mossie RD, Stulberg DS, et al: The fasciocutaneous flap: A conservative approach to the exposed knee joint. *Plast Reconstr Surg* 1990;85:252–257.
60. Lian G, Cracchiolo A III, Lesavoy M: Treatment of major wound necrosis following total knee arthroplasty. *J Arthroplasty* 1989;4(suppl):S23–S32.
61. Bengtson S, Carlsson A, Relander M, et al: Treatment of the exposed knee prosthesis. *Acta Orthop Scand* 1987;58:662–665.
62. Eckardt JJ, Lesavoy MA, Dubrow TJ, et al: Exposed endoprosthesis: Management protocol using muscle and myocutaneous flap coverage. *Clin Orthop* 1990;251:220–229.
63. Greenberg B, LaRossa D, Lotke PA, et al: Salvage of jeopardized total-knee prosthesis: The role of the gastrocnemius muscle flap. *Plast Reconstr Surg* 1989;83:85–89;97–99.
64. Hemphill ES, Ebert FR, Muench AG: The medial gastrocnemius muscle flap in the treatment of wound complications following total knee arthroplasty. *Orthopedics* 1992;15:477–480.
65. Salibian AH, Anzel SH: Salvage of an infected total knee prosthesis with medial and lateral gastrocnemius muscle flaps: A case report. *J Bone Joint Surg* 1983;65A:681–684.
66. Sanders R, O'Neill T: The gastrocnemius myocutaneous flap used as a cover for the exposed knee prosthesis. *J Bone Joint Surg* 1981;63B:383–386.
67. Gerwin M, Rothaus KO, Windsor RE, et al: Gastrocnemius muscle flap coverage of exposed or infected knee prostheses. *Clin Orthop* 1993;286:64–70.
68. Gordon L, Levinsohn DG: Versatility of the latissimus and serratus anterior muscle transplants in providing cover for exposed hardware and endoprostheses. *Orthop Trans* 1992;16:68.
69. Insall J, Scott WN, Ranawat CS: The total condylar knee prosthesis: A report of two hundred and twenty cases. *J Bone Joint Surg* 1979;61A:173–180.

CHAPTER 14

Extensor Mechanism Problems in Total Knee Arthroplasty

Douglas A. Dennis, MD

Long-term evaluations of total knee arthroplasty (TKA) have demonstrated that these procedures provide excellent relief of pain, improved function, and superior durability.[1-4] Improvements in prosthetic design have resulted in increased range of motion and functional capabilities, yet problems with the patellofemoral joint persist.[1,5-23] Many of the early total knee prostheses failed to provide for resurfacing of the patellofemoral joint. Anterior knee pain, in as many as half the cases, has been reported when patellar resurfacing was not done.[20,22,24-42] Design modifications that allow resurfacing of the patella have produced superior functional results with a reduction in patellofemoral pain,[29-31,38,39,43-49] but additional complications have emerged, including patellofemoral instability, fracture, loosening, component failure, patellar clunk syndrome, and tendon rupture.[9,11,18,24,50-57] Rates of complications resulting from patellofemoral resurfacing have ranged from 5% to 55%,[9,15,20-22,24,29,35,39,44,51,53,55,58,59] and have accounted for up to 50% of revision TKA procedures performed.[60-62] The patellofemoral complications encountered have been attributed to errors in surgical technique, inferior prosthetic design, and excessive patellofemoral loads. Numerous studies of patellofemoral joint reaction forces have demonstrated compressive loads of one half to one times body weight during level gait, increasing to three to four times body weight with stair climbing and as much as seven to eight times body weight during squatting.[40,63,64]

The purpose of this chapter is to review the patellofemoral complications associated with TKA and methods for their prevention and management.

Patellofemoral Instability

The incidence of patellar subluxation following TKA has been reported to be as high as 29%.[65] Failure to obtain satisfactory patellofemoral tracking can result in patellofemoral pain and crepitus as well as component wear, failure, loosening, and/or fracture, and can jeopardize the result of an otherwise successfully functioning TKA.[1,9,20,24,35,39,40,52,53,61,66-69]

Numerous causes of patellofemoral instability have been documented (Outline 1). Instability most commonly results from extensor mechanism imbalance with excessive tightness of the lateral retinaculum and associated weakness of the vastus medialis muscle.[9,20,39] Placement of prosthetic components in an excessively valgus position increases the Q-angle and results in an increased lateral force vector on the patella, predisposing to subluxation.[9,44,53,67] Disruption of the capsular repair, either through hemarthrosis, overly aggressive physiotherapy, or trauma, can result in patellofemoral instability.

The normal patella is asymmetric in contour with the thickness of the medial facet greater than that of the lateral facet. Resection of equal amounts of bone from both the medial and lateral facets retains the asymmetry of the patella. Asymmetric patellar resection (typically, resecting too much from the lateral facet) can lead to patellar tracking problems.[66,67,70] Minimal lateral facet resection, usually flush with its subchondral bone, is recommended for optimal function (Fig. 1).

Malposition of the femoral, tibial, or patellar components also can predispose to patellofemoral instability.[9,39,44,53,67,71,72] Internal rotation or medial shift of the femoral component places the trochlear groove at a greater distance from the patella, leaving the patella laterally positioned relative to the femoral component (Fig. 2). If the tibial component is placed so that it is internally rotated relative to the cut surface of the tibial plateau, the tibia will be externally rotated relative to the femur. Such rotation results in lateralization of the tibial tubercle and an increase in the Q-angle, which predisposes to lateral patellar subluxation (Fig. 3). Medial shift of the tibial component on the cut tibial plateau surface similarly results in lateralization of the tibial tubercle. Lateral placement of the patellar component on the patella also creates problems with the patella being captured into the trochlear groove of the femoral component.

Outline 1
Factors associated with patellofemoral instability

- Extensor mechanism imbalance
- Capsular repair disruption
- Asymmetric patellar resection
- Component malposition (femoral, tibial, patellar)
- Component design
  - Rotationally unconstrained
  - No axial rotation (rigid hinge)

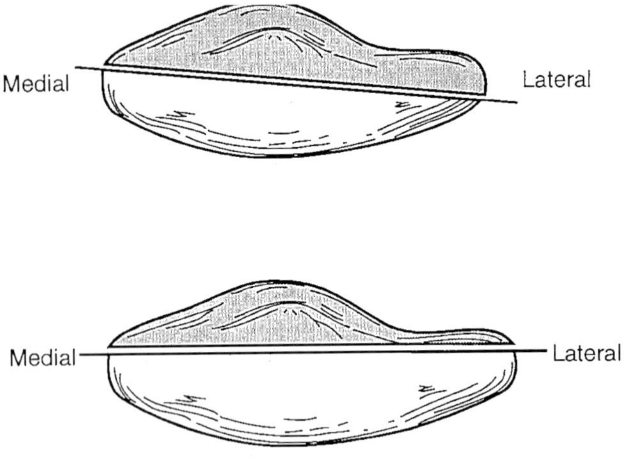

Fig. 1 The top diagram shows the asymmetric facet thickness of the normal patella. Resection of an equal thickness of bone from both the medial and lateral facets retains this asymmetry in the remaining patella. The lower diagram shows the recommended level of resection, removing minimal bone from the lateral facet. (Reproduced with permission from Dennis DA: Patellofemoral complications in total knee arthroplasty: A literature review. *Am J Knee Surg* 1992;5:156-166.)

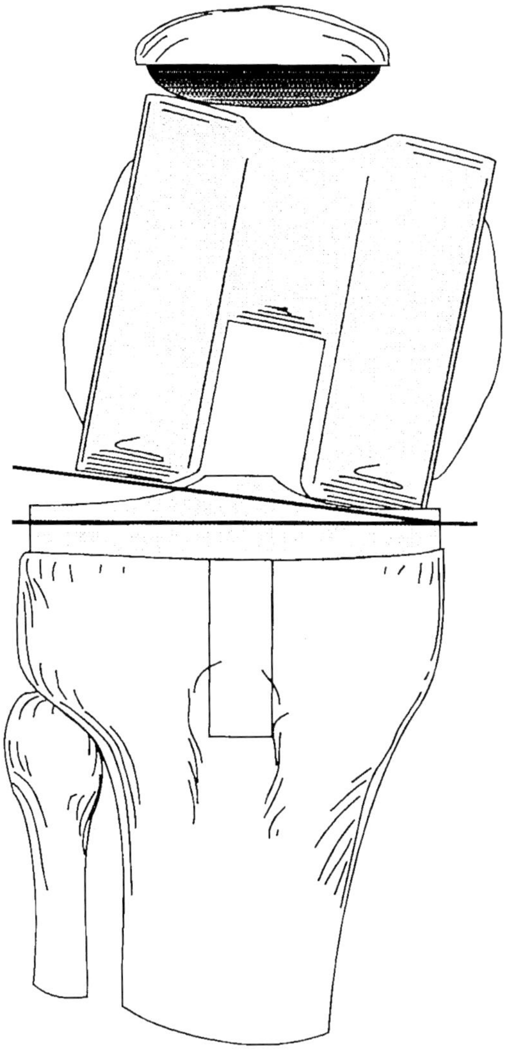

Fig. 2 Internal rotation of the femoral component distances the trochlear groove medially away from the patella. (Reproduced with permission from Dennis DA: Patellofemoral complications in total knee arthroplasty: A literature review. *Am J Knee Surg* 1992;5:156-166.)

Certain prosthetic designs predispose to patellar tracking problems. In the presence of extensor mechanism imbalance, rotationally unconstrained implants may allow excessive external rotation of the tibia and lateralization of the tibial tubercle.[67,73] Rand and associates[74] have reported a 22% incidence of patellofemoral instability with use of the kinematic rotating hinge prosthesis. A similar situation may exist in the TKA with posterior cruciate and collateral ligamentous instability.[75,76] Alternatively, prostheses that allow no axial rotation, such as rigid hinges, have also demonstrated increased rates of patellofemoral instability.[35,77-79] In the normal knee, up to 20° of internal rotation occurs during early knee flexion. With rigid hinge prostheses, this internal tibial rotation does not occur, forcing the tibial tubercle to assume a lateralized position during flexion, increasing the laterally directed forces on the patella.

To minimize this complication, intraoperative assessment of patellar tracking is critical. To assess true patellofemoral alignment, tourniquet release is recommended to eliminate the tourniquet's binding effect on the extensor mechanism.[1] Should the patella sublux laterally as the knee is flexed (before capsular closure) without additional medially directed stabilization by the surgeon's thumb (the no-thumb technique), a lateral retinacular release is advised.[40,72]

Management of patellofemoral instability is based on etiology. Nonsurgical measures include aggressive quadriceps rehabilitation, external patellofemoral bracing, and avoidance of activities, such as squatting or stair climbing, that heavily load the patellofemoral joint. In cases of extensor mechanism imbalance that do not respond to these nonsurgical measures, a lateral retinacular release, often combined with advancement of the vastus medialis muscle (proximal realignment) is indicated.[72] Capsular repair is required in cases with initial central patellar tracking reverting to immediate lateral subluxation following a traumatic event. In some cases, a capsular defect is palpable, which is useful to further confirm this diagnosis. Medial transfer of the tibial tubercle by an osteotomy should be considered in cases of more severe malalignment because of the inherent risk of nonunion and subsequent complicated salvage options.[80] Revision of

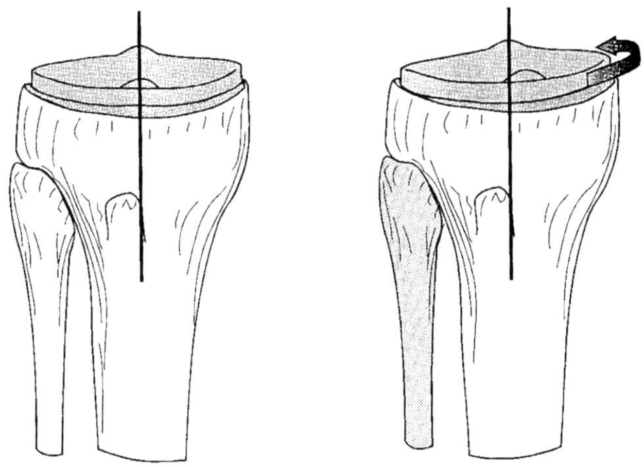

Fig. 3 Internal rotation of the tibial component on the proximal tibia causes lateralization of the tibial tubercle. (Reproduced with permission from Dennis DA: Patellofemoral complications in total knee arthroplasty: A literature review. *Am J Knee Surg* 1992;5:15–166.)

prosthetic components is performed for those patients with substantial component malposition that is not amenable to simpler realignment procedures.

Patellar Fractures

Patellar fractures are an infrequent complication of TKA,[81-83] although an incidence as high as 21% has been reported.[65] Various etiologies for patellar fracture have been proposed (Outline 2).[9,21,24,39,44,59,65,66,82-87] An increased incidence of patellar fracture associated with patellofemoral malalignment is supported by biomechanical studies which demonstrate that contact forces substantially increase with patellofemoral malalignment.[88] Both the eccentricity and magnitude of patellofemoral loads increase with patellar subluxation,[89] enhancing the risk of patellar fracture.

Excessive, asymmetric, or inadequate patellar resection all increase the probability of patellar fracture. Excessive patellar resection, especially if the subchondral bone is resected,[90] predisposes to patellar fracture. Reuben and associates[91] have demonstrated that a patellar osteotomy resulting in an osseous patellar thickness of less than 15 mm substantially increases anterior patellar strain. Conversely, minimal patellar resection, resulting in thickening of the patella-patellar component composite, increases patellofemoral joint reaction forces and tension within the quadriceps tendon. Use of femoral components with an excessive anteroposterior diameter or implantation of femoral components in a flexed position increases patello-femoral joint reaction forces and the probability of fracture.[39,69] Asymmetric patellar resection can also result in

Outline 2
Factors associated with patellar fractures

Trauma
Patellar subluxation
Improper patellar resection
Vascular compromise
Component design
Component malposition
Increased flexion
Thermal necrosis
Revision TKA

impaired mechanical strength of the patella, particularly if the lateral facet is over-resected. Finally, when the patella is prepared for component fixation, it has been shown that the creation of a large central peg hole increases anterior patellar strain more than smaller peripheral peg designs, thereby enhancing the risk of fracture.[67,92]

Surgical disruption of patellar blood supply, resulting in avascular necrosis, has been associated with patellar fracture.[21,44,61,67,83] Analyses of patellar blood supply have demonstrated both extraosseous and intraosseous vascular systems.[93-96] The extraosseous system comprises a peripatellar anastomotic ring, supplied by six main arteries (Fig. 4, *left*). The superior portion of the vascular ring passes anterior to the quadriceps tendon, while the inferior portion passes posterior to the patellar tendon through the fat pad. The intraosseous system comprises the midpatellar, polar, and quadriceps tendon blood supplies (Fig. 4, *right*). The midpatellar vessels penetrate anteriorly through the middle one third of the patella, branching into both the proximal and distal poles. The polar vasculature passes through the proximal fat pad, posterior to the patellar tendon, entering and supplying the inferior pole of the patella. Scapinelli[95,96] observed minimal vascular penetration into the superior pole and periphery of the patella while Bjorkstrom and Goldie[93] have demonstrated a superior vascular supply via the quadriceps tendon.

Substantial disruption of patellar vascular systems occurs during routine TKA.[21,24,31,44,61,65,76,82,83,94,97-99] The medial superior and inferior genicular arteries and supreme genicular arteries are divided during a medial peripatellar arthrotomy. Damage to the lateral inferior genicular artery is common during lateral meniscectomy or fat pad excision. The lateral superior genicular artery is at risk when a lateral retinacular release is performed. The intraosseous vascular system can be compromised during creation of fixation holes, particularly the large central type. Technetium bone scan studies following TKA have demonstrated reduced patellar vascularity if a lateral retinacular release has been performed.[98,99] McMahon and associates[97] also found

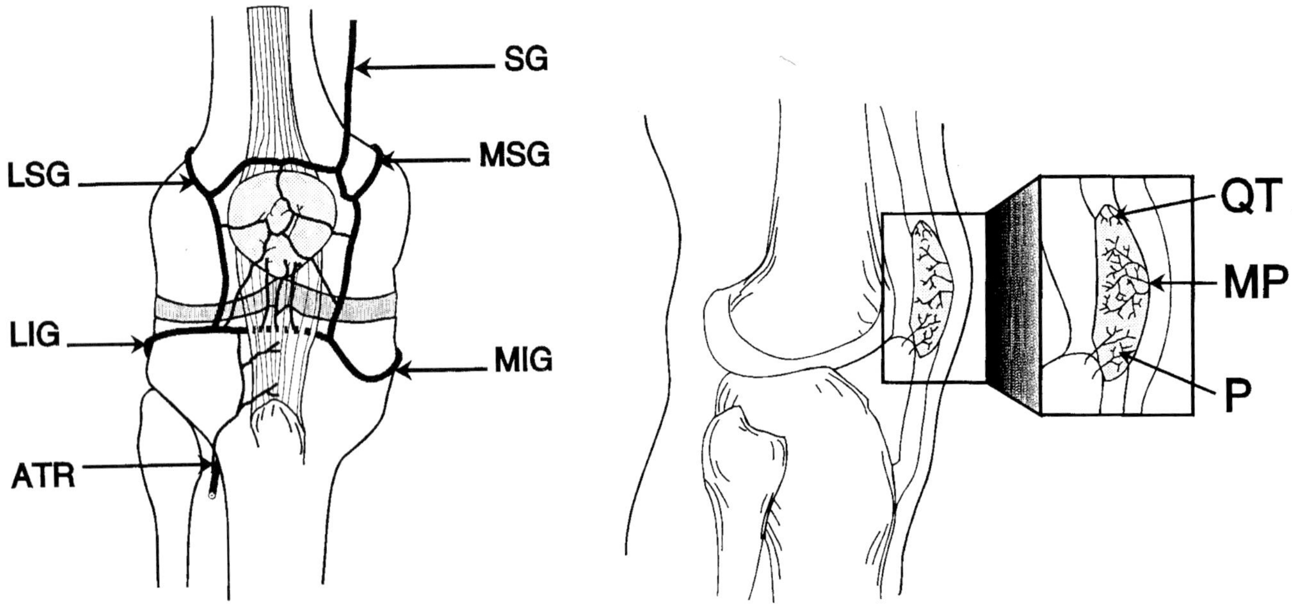

Fig. 4 **Left,** The extraosseous peripatellar anastomotic ring is supplied by six main arteries (LSG = Lateral Superior Genicular; MSG = Medial Superior Genicular; MIG = Medial Inferior Genicular; LIG = Lateral Inferior Genicular; SG = Supreme Genicular; ATR = Anterior Tibial Recurrent). **Right,** This diagram shows the midpatellar (MP), polar (P), and quadriceps tendon (QT) intraosseous blood supplies of the patella. (Reproduced with permission from Dennis DA: Patellofemoral complications in total knee arthroplasty: A literature review. *Am J Knee Surg* 1992;5:156–166.)

reduced patellar vascularity following lateral retinacular release, but determined that fat pad excision has no detrimental effect. Histologic evaluations of patellar specimens following patellar fracture have documented the presence of osteonecrosis.[21,31]

Component malposition can affect the incidence, type, severity, and prognosis of patellar fractures.[82,100] Errors in joint line position, lower extremity alignment, or patellar coverage by the prosthesis may risk fracture. Cases associated with major malalignment have been associated with more complex fracture patterns and a worse prognosis.

Additional risk factors for patellar fracture include increased flexion following TKA, thermal necrosis, and revision TKA. Windsor and associates[101] have reported that patients with flexion greater than 95° generate increased patellofemoral compression forces and frequently have higher activity levels. The heat of polymerization of the polymethylmethacrylate (reported to be as high as 80° to 90°C in total hip arthroplasty) may, therefore, exceed the coagulation temperature of tissue proteins, causing thermal necrosis of bone.[97,102-105] Grace and Sim[103] reported that the incidence of patellar fracture following primary TKA (0.12%) was much less than after revision TKA (0.61%).

Patellar Component Loosening

Loosening of cemented patellar components in TKA has been uncommon, with a reported incidence of less than 2% in most studies.[9,24,38,39,66] The incidence of loosening following cementless patellar resurfacing has been higher, yet variable, with reported loosening rates of 0.6% to 13.5%.[9,24,38,39,66,106] Factors associated with loosening of patellar components include cementing the prosthesis into deficient bone, component malposition, patellar subluxation or fracture, patellar osteonecrosis, osteoporosis, asymmetric bone resection, loosening of other prosthetic components, and failure of bone ingrowth in porous-coated designs.[61,67] Reduction of the rate of patellar loosening requires improved bone preparation and cementing techniques,[38] proper patellar resection, avoidance of asymmetric or excessive bone removal, and assurance of central patellar tracking.

Treatment options for patellar component loosening include component revision, component removal and patellar arthroplasty (smoothing of the remaining patella without resurfacing) if remaining bone stock is unsatisfactory, and patellectomy. Some patients are asymptomatic and require no treatment, although Brick and Scott[61] noted that 75% were eventually symp-

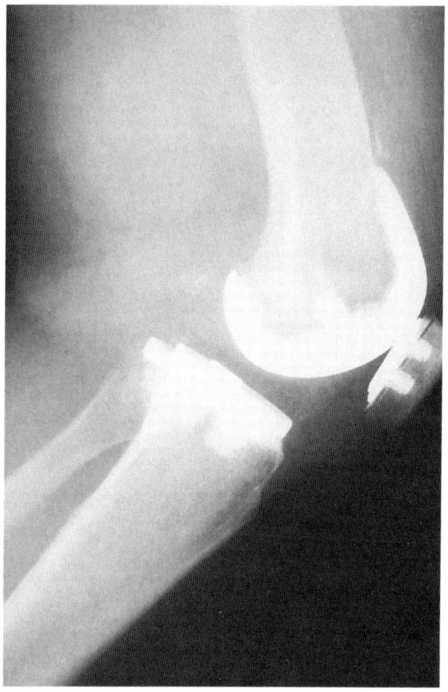

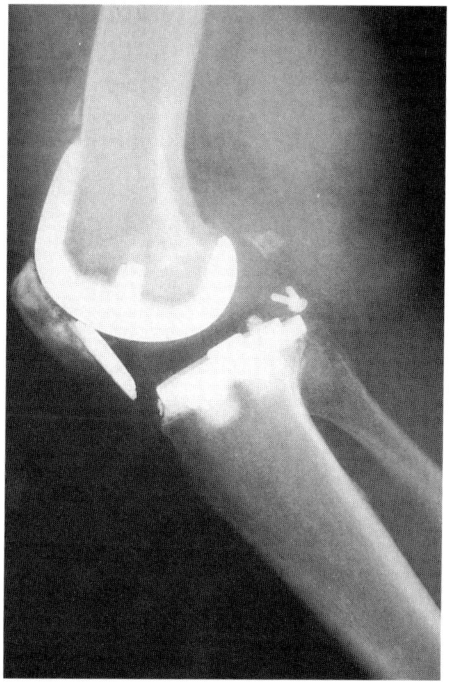

Fig. 5 Left, This lateral radiograph shows early peg angulation of a metal-backed patellar component. **Right,** The later lateral radiograph shows fracture of the peg-plate. (Reproduced with permission from Dennis DA: Patellofemoral complications in total knee arthroplasty: A literature review. *Am J Knee Surg* 1992;5:156–166.)

tomatic enough to require revision TKA. It should be noted that total dislodgment of the component, most commonly inferiorly, can lead to erosion of the posterior surface of the overlying patellar tendon, risking patellar tendon disruption.

Patellar Component Failure

Although failure of polyethylene patellar components has been reported,[107,108] this complication has primarily been a problem of metal-backed designs.[60,68,69,109] Metal-backed designs were adopted with the proposed advantages of decreasing patellar surface strains,[92] supporting the overlying polyethylene, thereby lessening deformation, and allowing for cementless patellar component fixation. Failure modes of these designs have included polyethylene wear and fracture, polyethylene-metal plate dissociation, peg-plate dissociation, and metal plate fracture.[60,68,109]

Patellar component polyethylene wear is not unexpected. Cepulo and associates[110] observed that peak patellofemoral contact pressures far exceed the yield strength of polyethylene. Wright and Bartel[111] reported enhanced polyethylene degradation in retrieved tibial components with less polyethylene thickness. The addition of metal backing to patellar components results in reduction of polyethylene thickness, which may predispose to enhanced wear rates. Also, with metal-backed designs, less wear is required before catastrophic failure occurs from wear-through of the polyethylene to the underlying metal plate. Polyethylene thickness as minimal as 2.4 mm at the periphery of the metal plate has been reported in some metal-backed designs.[69] In most designs, the metal-backing does not totally extend to the edge of the polyethylene. Therefore, as the peripheral polyethylene is loaded, it deforms over the rim of the metal plate and may be severed by the sharp nondeforming edge of the metal plate.[69]

Dissociation of the polyethylene from the metal plate may result in cases of excessive polyethylene wear or fracture. In most designs, the polyethylene is attached to the metal backing by means of a mechanical gripping of the plate periphery by the polyethylene without the presence of a chemical bond between the two materials. With advanced peripheral polyethylene wear, the integrity of the polyethylene-plate attachment may be disrupted, allowing the polyethylene to dissociate.[69]

Fracture of patellar component fixation pegs at their attachment to the metal plate can occur because of high sheer stresses at this site. Due to the eccentric loads normally placed on the patella, substantial sheer stresses can occur at the peg-plate junction.[68] These sheer stresses are increased in cases of patellofemoral malalignment.[34] Retrieval analyses of cementless patellar components have shown that osseous ingrowth into the anchoring pegs does occur.[112] If osseous ingrowth into the fixation pegs occurs without accompanying bony ingrowth into the metal plate itself, a high sheer load is placed at the peg-plate junction, risking peg fracture (Fig. 5). Rosenberg and associates,[68] who reviewed 122 TKAs with cementless metal-backed patellar components, observed 12 fatigue fractures at the peg-plate junction. In all 12 cases, there was good osseous ingrowth into the fixation pegs but no ingrowth into the porous plate.

Risk factors for patellar component failure include excessive body weight, enhanced postoperative knee flexion (greater than 115°), high activity levels, and male sex.[60,68,69,109] Additional factors associated with increased patellofemoral loading and subsequent component failure include patellar malalignment, increased patella-patellar component composite thickness, use of oversized femoral components, flexion malposition of the femoral component, and failure to restore the prosthetic joint line to anatomic levels. Failure of metal-backed patellar components often occurs early, with most reviews reporting failure within two years following TKA.[60,68,69,109]

Clinical signs of patellar component failure include effusion and crepitus, which is occasionally audible. Clinical symptoms often appear suddenly, following activities that load the patellofemoral joint heavily, such as climbing stairs, squatting, or arising from a seated position. Intraoperative findings frequently include black staining of the synovium with metal debris and wear or fragmentation of the polyethylene. Femoral component wear may be present, observed in 11 of 25 cases of failed metal-backed patellar components reported by Bayley and associates.[60] Loose porous-coated beads or titanium fiber mesh fragments may be found imbedded within the polyethylene of the patellar and tibial components. Therefore, if revision is required for failure of a metal-backed patellar component, the surgeon must always be prepared to revise all three components.[113]

Patellar Clunk Syndrome

Patellar clunk syndrome is a condition resulting from development of a fibrous nodule at the junction of the posterior aspect of the quadriceps tendon and proximal pole of the patella. With knee flexion, this nodule enters the intercondylar notch of the femoral prosthesis. As the knee is extended, the nodule becomes entrapped within the notch as the quadriceps tendon and patella migrate proximally. At 30° to 45° from full extension, enough tension is placed on the fibrous nodule to cause it to clunk out of the intercondylar notch (Fig. 6).[50,114]

Proposed etiologies for this condition include the use of femoral components with a sharp anterior edge at the superior aspect of the intercondylar notch, malpositioning of the patellar component beyond the proximal border of the patella, postoperative scarring, and alterations of the joint line, patellar height, or patellar thickness.

Recommended treatment includes debridement of the fibrous nodule, either openly or arthroscopically,[56] with or without revision of the patellar component if it is malpositioned superiorly.

Tendon Rupture

Rupture of the quadriceps or patellar tendon is an infrequent complication of TKA, with a reported incidence of 0.17%[54] to 2.5%.[66] Quadriceps tendon ruptures occur more frequently in cases in which a lateral retinacular release has been performed. This occurrence may be due to tendon devascularization or to extension of the release too far anteriorly, disrupting tendinous fibers of the quadriceps.[66] Results of surgical repair are often suboptimal, with extensor lag and weakness or limited range of motion resulting.

The risk of patellar tendon rupture following TKA is enhanced in patients who have had previous knee operations and in those who have undergone partial patellar tendon release to enhance exposure at the time of TKA. Additional risk factors include closed knee manipulation and tibial tubercle osteotomy for extensor mechanism realignment.[54] Numerous methods of treatment have been employed, including casting; tendon suture; fixation with wires, staples, or screws; tendon augmentation; and extensor mechanism allografts.[115] No single reconstructive procedure has provided consistently satisfactory results. Persistent tendon rupture following attempted treatment is common, occurring in 11 of 18 cases reported by Rand and associates.[54] Tendon rupture remains one of the most dreaded complications of TKA with difficult and often unsatisfactory salvage options. Prevention via meticulous surgical technique is imperative.[113]

Surgical Technique

If the accuracy of techniques for femoral and tibial component preparation is compared with the precision of present methods of patellar preparation and component placement, it is logical to relate today's patellar problems, in some part, to surgical technique. Essential surgical goals include accurate patellar resection, maintenance of patellar vascularity, proper positioning of prosthetic components, avoidance of soft-tissue impingement, and assurance of central patellar tracking.

The amount of patellar bone excised should ideally be equal to the thickness of the patellar component to be inserted (usually about 10 mm), thereby restoring the preoperative patellar thickness.[39,67,70,116] Patellar resection must result in a symmetric patellar remnant with equal medial and lateral facet thicknesses.

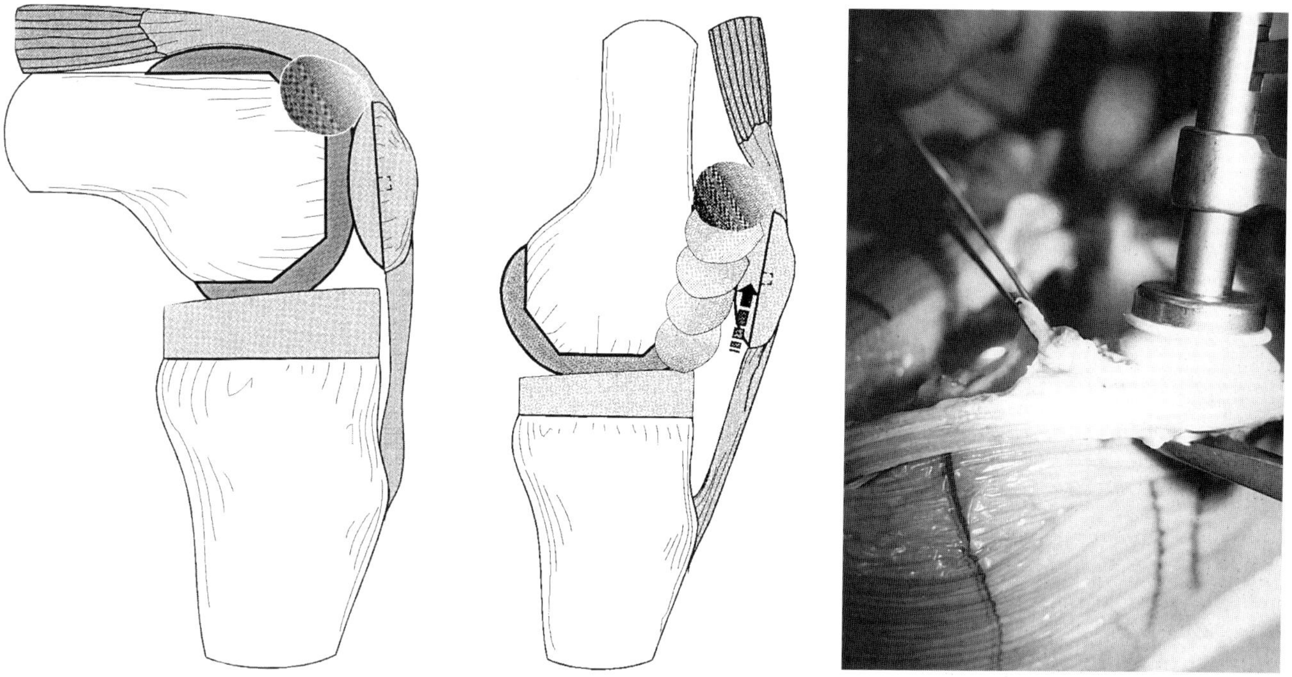

Fig. 6 Left, A suprapatellar fibrous nodule has become entrapped within the intercondylar notch during knee flexion. **Center,** The fibrous nodule clunks out of the intercondylar notch when the knee is extended to 30° to 45°. **Right,** This intraoperative photograph shows the suprapatellar fibrous nodule. (Reproduced with permission from Dennis DA: Patellofemoral complications in total knee arthroplasty: A literature review. *Am J Knee Surg* 1992;5:156–166.)

Efforts to preserve patellar vascularity include maintaining the fat pad,[1,24,93,117] preservation of the lateral superior genicular artery during lateral retinacular release,[1,21,24,67,118] and the lateral release performed 2 cm posterior to the patella in order to maintain peripheral vessel penetration of the patella.[67,86] Avoidance of patellar components with large central fixation pegs will help preserve the intraosseous blood supply.[24]

Accurate positioning of all three TKA components is critical. Medial shift and internal rotation of both femoral and tibial components, as well as lateral positioning of the patellar component, must be avoided to prevent patellar maltracking.[35,71] After release of the tourniquet, central patellar tracking must be obtained using the no-thumb technique described previously.[40,53,72] If patellar subluxation is present, realignment procedures are performed until a balanced extensor mechanism is obtained.

Isolated patellar component revision has been associated with higher than expected complication rates, including patellar fractures, instability, polyethylene wear-through, infection, peroneal nerve palsy and extensor lag.[117] Removal of well-fixed, metal-backed patellar components with osseous ingrowth into the anchoring pegs can be difficult but is facilitated by disruption of the peg-plate junction with a diamond-edge saw to gain direct access to the bone-peg interface.[112]

Numerous patellofemoral complications associated with patellar resurfacing have rekindled enthusiasm to avoid patellar resurfacing. While most surgeons agree that it is necessary to resurface the patella in patients with rheumatoid arthritis to minimize the antigenic response of retained articular cartilage,[21,118] controversy exists over whether to resurface the patella in patients with osteoarthritis and good remaining articular cartilage. Similar results with and without patellar resurfacing have been reported in some studies. Other reports have determined increased patellofemoral problems without patellofemoral resurfacing, resulting in anterior knee pain in as many as 30% of patients.[4,30,39,46,47,119] Boyd and associates[119] reviewed 891 TKAs with and without patellar resurfacing reported complication rates of 4% and 12%, respectively. Results of secondary patellar resurfacing proved inferior to results of cases in which the patella was resurfaced at the time of primary TKA. If the surgeon elects not to resurface the patella, ideal patients are those with osteoarthritis, but with excellent remaining articular cartilage, and those in whom central patellar tracking can be assured at the time of arthroplasty.

The best results in TKA will be obtained with maximum attention to accurate patellar resection, maintenance of patellar vascularity, assurance of central patellar tracking, and avoidance of metal-backed patellar components.

References

1. Dennis DA, Clayton ML, O'Donnell S, et al: Posterior cruciate condylar total knee arthroplasty: Average 11-year follow-up evaluation. *Clin Orthop* 1992;281:168–176.
2. Goldberg VM, Figgie HE III, Figgie MP: Technical considerations in total knee surgery: Management of patella problems. *Orthop Clin North Am* 1989;20:189–199.
3. Insall JN, Binazzi R, Soudry M, et al: Total knee arthroplasty. *Clin Orthop* 1985;192:13–22.
4. Ranawat CS, Rose HA: Total-condylar knee arthroplasty: A three- to eight-year follow-up. Proceedings of the American Academy of Orthopaedic Surgeons 50th Annual Meeting, Los Angeles, CA. Park Ridge, IL, American Academy of Orthopaedic Surgeons, 1983.
5. Bandi W: Chondromalacia patellae and femoro-patellar arthrosis: Etiology, clinical aspects and therapy. *Helv Chir Acta* 1972;39(suppl 11):1–70.
6. Bryan RS, Peterson LF: Polycentric total knee arthroplasty: A prognostic assessment. *Clin Orthop* 1979;145:23–28.
7. Cracchiolo A III, Benson M, Finerman GA, et al: A prospective comparative clinical analysis of the first-generation knee replacements: Polycentric vs. geometric knee arthroplasty. *Clin Orthop* 1979;145:37–46.
8. Deburge A, Guepar: GUEPAR hinge prosthesis: Complications and results with two years' follow-up. *Clin Orthop* 1976;120: 47–53.
9. Doolittle KH II, Turner RH: Patellofemoral problems following total knee arthroplasty. *Orthop Rev* 1988;17:696–702.
10. Ficat RP, Hungerford DS (eds): *Disorders of the Patello-femoral Joint.* Baltimore, MD, Williams & Wilkins, 1977, pp 29–32.
11. Freeman MA, Samuelson KM, Bertin KC: Freeman-Samuelson total arthroplasty of the knee. *Clin Orthop* 1985;192:46–58.
12. Gschwend N: The GSB knee prosthesis: Basic considerations and results. *Aktuelle Probl Chir Orthop* 1981;15:24–31.
13. Gschwend N, Loehr J: The Gschwend-Scheier-Bahler (GSB) replacement of the rheumatoid knee joint. *Reconstr Surg Traumatol* 1981;18:174–194.
14. Gschwend N, Scheier HJ, Bahler A, et al: The GSB knee arthroplasty. *Int Orthop* 1980;3:281–284.
15. Hassenpflug J, Holland C, Heupel R, et al: Patellar changes during long-term observations on the Blauth knee joint endoprosthesis. *Z Orthop* 1984;122:185–197.
16. Hofmann GO, Hagena FW: Pathomechanics of the femoropatellar joint following total knee arthroplasty. *Clin Orthop* 1987;224:251–259.
17. Insall JN, Ranawat CS, Aglietti P, et al: A comparison of four models of total knee-replacement prostheses. *J Bone Joint Surg* 1976;58A:754–765.
18. Insall J, Tria AJ, Scott WN: The total condylar knee prosthesis: The first 5 years. *Clin Orthop* 1979;145:68–77.
19. Kohler G, Mohing W, Richter R: Experiences with reoperations after partial and total prosthetic treatment of the knee joint. *Aktuelle Probl Chir Orthop* 1981;15:84–90.
20. Moreland JR, Thomas RJ, Freeman MA: ICLH replacement of the knee: 1977 and 1978. *Clin Orthop* 1979;145:47–59.
21. Scott RD, Turoff N, Ewald FC: Stress fracture of the patella following duopatellar total knee arthroplasty with patellar resurfacing. *Clin Orthop* 1982;170:147–151.
22. Sledge CB, Ewald FC: Total knee arthroplasty experience at the Robert Breck Brigham Hospital. *Clin Orthop* 1979;145:78–84.
23. Thornhill TS, Dalziel RW, Sledge CB: Alternatives to arthrodesis for the failed total knee arthroplasty. *Clin Orthop* 1982; 170:131–140.
24. Clayton ML, Thirupathi R: Patellar complications after total condylar arthroplasty. *Clin Orthop* 1982;170:152–155.
25. Eftekhar NS: Total knee-replacement arthroplasty: Results with the intramedullary adjustable total knee prosthesis. *J Bone Joint Surg* 1983;65A:293–309.
26. Enis JE, Gardner R, Robledo MA, et al: Comparison of patellar resurfacing versus nonresurfacing in bilateral total knee arthroplasty. *Clin Orthop* 1990;260:38–42.
27. Evanski PM, Waugh TR, Orofino CF, et al: UCI knee replacement. *Clin Orthop* 1976;120:33–38.
28. Ewald FC, Thomas WH, Poss R, et al: Duo-patella total knee arthroplasty in rheumatoid arthritis. *Orthop Trans* 1978;2:202.
29. Freeman MA, Todd RC, Bamert P, et al: ICLH arthroplasty of the knee: 1968-1977. *J Bone Joint Surg* 1978;60B:339–344.
30. Insall JN, Lachiewicz PF, Burstein AH: The posterior stabilized condylar prosthesis: A modification of the total condylar design. Two to four-year clinical experience. *J Bone Joint Surg* 1982; 64A:1317–1323.
31. Insall J, Scott WN, Ranawat CS: The total condylar knee prosthesis: A report of two hundred and twenty cases. *J Bone Joint Surg* 1979;61A:173–180.
32. Kaufer H, Matthews LS: Spherocentric arthroplasty of the knee: Clinical experience with an average four-year follow-up. *J Bone Joint Surg* 1981;63A:545–559.
33. Kettlekamp DB, Pryor P, Brady TA: Selective use of the variable axis knee. *Orthop Trans* 1979;3:301–302.
34. Matthews LS, Sonstegard DA, Henke JA: Load bearing characteristics of the patello-femoral joint. *Acta Orthop Scand* 1977; 48:511–516.
35. Mochizuki RM, Schurman DJ: Patellar complications following total knee arthroplasty. *J Bone Joint Surg* 1979;61A:879–883.
36. Murray DG, Webster DA: The variable-axis knee prosthesis: Two-year follow-up study. *J Bone Joint Surg* 1981;63:687–694.
37. Picetti GD III, McGann WA, Welch RB: The patellofemoral joint after total knee arthroplasty without patellar resurfacing. *J Bone Joint Surg* 1990;72A:1379–1382.
38. Rae PJ, Noble J, Hodgkinson JP: Patellar resurfacing in total condylar knee arthroplasty: Technique and results. *J Arthroplasty* 1990;5:259–265.
39. Ranawat CS: The patellofemoral joint in total condylar knee arthroplasty: Pros and cons based on five- to ten-year follow-up observations. *Clin Orthop* 1986;205:93–99.
40. Scott RD: Prosthetic replacement of the patellofemoral joint. *Orthop Clin North Am* 1979;10:129–137.
41. Sledge CB, Stern P, Thomas WH, et al: Two year follow-up of the duo-condylar total knee replacement. *Orthop Trans* 1978;2:193.
42. Vanhegan JA, Dabrowski W, Arden GP: A review of 100 Attenborough stabilised gliding knee prostheses. *J Bone Joint Surg* 1979;61B:445–450.
43. Insall J, Tria AJ, Aglietti P: Resurfacing of the patella. *J Bone Joint Surg* 1980;62A:933–936.
44. Leblanc JM: Patellar complications in total knee arthroplasty: A literature review. *Orthop Rev* 1989;18:296–304.
45. Levai JP, McLeod HC, Freeman MA: Why not resurface the patella? *J Bone Joint Surg* 1983;65B:448–451.
46. Ranawat CS, Insall J, Shine J: Duo-condylar knee arthroplasty: Hospital for Special Surgery design. *Clin Orthop* 1976;120:76–82.
47. Ranawat CS, Rose HA, Bryan WJ: Technique and results of replacement of the patellofemoral joint with total condylar knee arthroplasty. *Orthop Trans* 1982;6:88.
48. Scott WN, Rozbruch JD, Otis JC, et al: Clinical and biomechanical evaluation of patella replacement in total knee arthroplasty. *Orthop Trans* 1978;2:203.
49. Soudry M, Mestriner LA, Binazzi R, et al: Total knee arthroplasty without patellar resurfacing. *Clin Orthop* 1986;205:166–170.
50. Hozack WJ, Rothman RH, Booth RE Jr, et al: The patellar clunk syndrome: A complication of posterior stabilized total knee arthroplasty. *Clin Orthop* 1989;241:203–208.
51. Hungerford DS, Krackow KA: Total joint arthroplasty of the knee. *Clin Orthop* 1985;192:23–33.
52. Mazas FB: Guepar total knee prosthesis. *Clin Orthop* 1973;

94:211–221.
53. Merkow RL, Soudry M, Insall JN: Patellar dislocation following total knee replacement. *J Bone Joint Surg* 1985;67A:1321–1327.
54. Rand JA, Morrey BF, Bryan RS: Patellar tendon rupture after total knee arthroplasty. *Clin Orthop* 1989;244:233–238.
55. Simison AJ, Noble J, Hardinge K: Complications of the Attenborough knee replacement. *J Bone Joint Surg* 1986;68B: 100–105.
56. Vernace JV, Rothman RH, Booth RE Jr, et al: Arthroscopic management of the patellar clunk syndrome following posterior stabilized total knee arthroplasty. *J Arthroplasty* 1989;4:179–182.
57. Webster DA, Murray DG: Complications of variable axis total knee arthroplasty. *Clin Orthop* 1985;193:160–167.
58. Habermann ET: Revision arthroplasty for failed total knee replacements, in Hungerford DS, Krackow KA, Kenna RV (eds): *Total Knee Arthroplasty: A Comprehensive Approach*. Baltimore, MD, Williams & Wilkins, 1984, pp 219–257.
59. Thompson FM, Hood RW, Insall J: Patellar fractures in total knee arthroplasty. *Orthop Trans* 1981;5:490–491.
60. Bayley JC, Scott RD, Ewald FC, et al: Failure of the metal-backed patellar component after total knee replacement. *J Bone Joint Surg* 1988;70A:668–674.
61. Brick GW, Scott RD: The patellofemoral component of total knee arthroplasty. *Clin Orthop* 1988;231:163–178.
62. Thomas WH, Ewald FC, Poss R, et al: Duopatella total knee arthroplasty. *Orthop Trans* 1980;4:329–330.
63. Hungerford DS, Barry M: Biomechanics of the patellofemoral joint. *Clin Orthop* 1979;144:9–15.
64. Reilly DT, Martens M: Experimental analysis of the quadriceps muscle force and patello-femoral joint reaction force for various activities. *Acta Orthop Scand* 1972;43:126–137.
65. Cameron HU, Fedorkow DM: The patella in total knee arthroplasty. *Clin Orthop* 1982;165:197–199.
66. Lynch AF, Rorabeck CH, Bourne RB: Extensor mechanism complications following total knee arthroplasty. *J Arthroplasty* 1987;2:135–140.
67. Rand JA, Gustilo RB: Technique of patellar resurfacing in total knee arthroplasty. *Tech Orthop* 1988;3:57–66.
68. Rosenberg AG, Andriacchi TP, Barden R, et al: Patellar component failure in cementless total knee arthroplasty. *Clin Orthop* 1988;236:106–114.
69. Stulberg SD, Stulberg BN, Hamati Y, et al: Failure mechanisms of metal-backed patellar components. *Clin Orthop* 1988;236: 88–105.
70. Gomes LS, Bechtold JE, Gustilo RB: Patellar prosthesis positioning in total knee arthroplasty: A roentgenographic study. *Clin Orthop* 1988;236:72–81.
71. Figgie MP, Goldberg VM, Figgie HE, et al: Salvage of the symptomatic patellofemoral joint following cruciate substituting total knee arthroplasty. *Am J Knee Surg* 1988;1:48.
72. Insall JN: Disorders of the patella, in Insall JN (ed): *Surgery of the Knee*. New York, NY, Churchill Livingstone, 1984, pp 119–260.
73. Buchanan JR, Greer RB III, Bowman LS, et al: Clinical experience with the variable axis total knee replacement. *Orthop Trans* 1982;6:367.
74. Rand JA, Chao EY, Stauffer RN: Kinematic rotating-hinge total knee arthroplasty. *J Bone Joint Surg* 1987;69A:489–497.
75. Scott WN, Rubinstein M: Posterior stabilized knee arthroplasty: Six years' experience. *Clin Orthop* 1986;205:138–145.
76. Scott WN, Rubinstein M, Scuderi G: Results after knee replacement with a posterior cruciate-substituting prosthesis. *J Bone Joint Surg* 1988;70A:1163–1173.
77. Jones EC, Insall JN, Inglis AE, et al: GUEPAR knee arthroplasty results and late complications. *Clin Orthop* 1979;140:145–152.
78. Ranawat CS, Wilde AH, Rovere GD: Experience with the GUEPAR total-knee prosthesis. *Orthop Rev* 1976;5:47–53.
79. Sheehan JM: Arthroplasty of the knee. *Clin Orthop* 1979;145: 101–109.
80. Kirk P, Rorabeck CH, Bourne RB, et al: Management of recurrent dislocation of the patella following total knee arthroplasty. *J Arthroplasty* 1992;7:229–233.
81. Tria AJ Jr, Harwood DA, Alicea JA, et al: Patellar fractures in posterior stabilized knee arthroplasties. *Clin Orthop* 1994;299: 131–138.
82. Goldberg VM, Figgie HE III, Inglis AE, et al: Patellar fracture type and prognosis in condylar total knee arthroplasty. *Clin Orthop* 1988;236:115–122.
83. Hozack WJ, Goll SR, Lotke PA, et al: The treatment of patellar fractures after total knee arthroplasty. *Clin Orthop* 1988;236: 123–127.
84. Ahmed AM, Burke DL, Hyder A: Force analysis of the patellar mechanism. *J Orthop Res* 1987;5:69–85.
85. Dupont JA, Baker SA: Complications of patellofemoral resurfacing in total knee arthroplasty. *Orthop Trans* 1982;6:369.
86. Rand JA: Patellar resurfacing in total knee arthroplasty. *Clin Orthop* 1990;260:110–117.
87. Roffman M, Hirsh DM, Mendes DG: Fracture of the resurfaced patella in total knee replacement. *Clin Orthop* 1980;148: 112–116.
88. Kaufer H: Mechanical function of the patella. *J Bone Joint Surg* 1971;53A:1551–1560.
89. Huberti HH, Hayes WC: Patellofemoral contact pressures: The influence of q-angle and tendofemoral contact. *J Bone Joint Surg* 1984;66A:715–724.
90. Josefchak RG, Finlay JB, Bourne RB, et al: Cancellous bone support for patellar resurfacing. *Clin Orthop* 1987;220:192–199.
91. Reuben JD, McDonald CL, Woodard PL, et al: Effect of patella thickness on patella strain following total knee arthroplasty. *J Arthroplasty* 1991;6:251–258.
92. Goldstein SA, Coale E, Weiss AP, et al: Patellar surface strain. *J Orthop Res* 1986;4:372–377.
93. Bjorkstrom S, Goldie IF: A study of the arterial supply of the patella in the normal state, in chondromalacia patellae and in osteoarthrosis. *Acta Orthop Scand* 1980;51:63–70.
94. Kayler DE, Lyttle D: Surgical interruption of patellar blood supply by total knee arthroplasty. *Clin Orthop* 1988;229:221–227.
95. Scapinelli R: Blood supply of the human patella: Its relation to ischaemic necrosis after fracture. *J Bone Joint Surg* 1967;49B: 563–570.
96. Scapinelli R: Studies on the vasculature of the human knee joint. *Acta Anat* 1968;70:305–331.
97. McMahon MS, Scuderi GR, Glashow JL, et al: Scintigraphic determination of patellar viability after excision of infrapatellar fat pad and/or lateral retinacular release in total knee arthroplasty. *Clin Orthop* 1990;260:10–16.
98. Scuderi G, Scharf SC, Meltzer LP, et al: The relationship of lateral releases to patella viability in total knee arthroplasty. *J Arthroplasty* 1987;2:209–214.
99. Wetzner SM, Bezreh JS, Scott RD, et al: Bone scanning in the assessment of patellar viability following knee replacement. *Clin Orthop* 1985;199:215–219.
100. Figgie HE III, Goldberg VM, Figgie MP, et al: The effect of alignment of the implant on fractures of the patella after condylar total knee arthroplasty. *J Bone Joint Surg* 1989;71A:1031–1039.
101. Windsor RE, Scuderi GR, Insall JN: Patellar fractures in total knee arthroplasty. *J Arthroplasty* 1989;4(suppl):S63–S67.
102. Berman AT, Reid JS, Yanicko DR Jr, et al: Thermally induced bone necrosis in rabbits: Relation to implant failure in humans. *Clin Orthop* 1984;186:284–292.
103. Grace JN, Sim FH: Fracture of the patella after total knee arthroplasty. *Clin Orthop* 1988;230:168–175.
104. d'Hollander A, Burny F, Monteny E, et al: Extraosseous variations of temperature during polymerization of acrylic cement in hip arthroplasties. *Acta Orthop Scand* 1976;47:186–188.
105. Willert HG, Ludwig J, Semlitsch M: Reaction of bone to methacrylate after hip arthroplasty: A long-term gross light

microscopic and scanning electron microscopic study. *J Bone Joint Surg* 1974;56A:1368–1382.
106. Firestone TP, Teeny SM, Krackow KA, et al: The clinical and roentgenographic results of cementless porous-coated patellar fixation. *Clin Orthop* 1991;273:184–189.
107. Conway WF, Gilula LA, Serot DI: Breakage of the patellar component of a kinematic total knee arthroplasty: A case report. *Orthopedics* 1986;9:532–534.
108. Wasilewski SA, Frankl U: Fracture of polyethylene of patellar component in total knee arthroplasty, diagnosed by arthroscopy. *J Arthroplasty* 1989;4(suppl):S19–S22.
109. Bayley JC, Scott RD: Further observations on metal-backed patellar component failure. *Clin Orthop* 1988;236:82–87.
110. Cepulo AJ, Stahurski TM, Moran JM, et al: Mechanical characteristics of patello-femoral replacements. *Trans Orthop Res Soc* 1983;8:41.
111. Wright TM, Bartel DL: The problem of surface damage in polyethylene total knee components. *Clin Orthop* 1986;205:67–74.
112. Dennis DA: Removal of well-fixed cementless metal-backed patellar components. *J Arthroplasty* 1992;7:217–220.
113. Dennis DA: Patellofemoral complications in total knee arthroplasty: A literature review. *Am J Knee Surg* 1992;5:156–166.
114. Beight JL, Yao B, Hozack WJ, et al: The patellar "clunk" syndrome after posterior stabilized total knee arthroplasty. *Clin Orthop* 1994;299:139–142.
115. Emerson RH Jr, Head WC, Malinin TI: Reconstruction of patellar tendon rupture after total knee arthroplasty with an extensor mechanism allograft. *Clin Orthop* 1990;260:154–161.
116. Dorr LD, Boiardo RA: Technical considerations in total knee arthroplasty. *Clin Orthop* 1986;205:5–11.
117. Berry DJ, Rand JA: Isolated patellar component revision of total knee arthroplasty. *Clin Orthop* 1993;286:110–115.
118. Steinberg J, Sledge CB, Noble J, et al: A tissue-culture model of cartilage breakdown in rheumatoid arthritis: Quantitative aspects of proteoglycan release. *Biochem J* 1979;180:403–412.
119. Boyd AD Jr, Ewald FC, Poss R, et al: Long-term complications of the resurfaced and unsurfaced patella in total knee arthroplasty. Proceedings of the American Academy of Orthopaedic Surgeons 58th Annual Meeting, Anaheim, CA. Rosemont, IL, American Academy of Orthopaedic Surgeons, 1991, p 107.

CHAPTER 15

Neurovascular Complications Following Total Knee Replacement: Causes, Treatment, and Prevention

Norman A. Johanson, MD

Introduction

Total knee replacement has been found to be safe and effective in well over 90% of patients who undergo the procedure. Although they are rare, neurovascular complications are serious problems, particularly in high-risk patients with complex deformities or in patients who have undergone previous surgical procedures and have multiple scars around the knee. Awareness of the risk of various neurovascular injuries facilitates the development of preventive strategies, as well as the opportunity to provide the patient with valuable information prior to undergoing this elective procedure.

Peroneal Nerve Palsy

The incidence of peroneal nerve palsy has been reported as being between 0.5% and 1%,[1-3] but the actual incidence probably varies with the severity of the case mix for a given surgeon or institution. The mechanism of nerve injury may be by traction during correction of a deformity, ischemia when the surrounding soft tissue is stretched causing small vessel occlusion, or by compression by a tight dressing or splint.[3]

Associated conditions that are thought to have an increased incidence of peroneal nerve injury are a valgus deformity or flexion contracture greater than 20° or a complex biplanar (flexion and valgus) deformity.[2,3] Factors that have been found not to have an association with nerve palsy are age, type of arthritis, gender, or tourniquet time.[3]

Peroneal nerve palsy is most commonly diagnosed within 2 days of knee replacement. In a study of 22 patients with a peroneal nerve palsy, all were found to have motor deficits in both the extensor hallucis longus and tibialis anterior, with peroneus longus weakness being reported in nine of the 22 patients (39%) and a sensory deficit in 20 of 22 (87%).[3] While the prognostic effectiveness of electromyograms and nerve conduction studies remains unclear, confirmatory electrophysiologic tests should be scheduled for at least 3 weeks from surgery.[2] The purpose of the test is primarily for documentation of the extent and location of the nerve lesion.

Early treatment of peroneal nerve injury is directed primarily at preventing further injury. As soon as it is diagnosed, all dressings should be loosened and the knee should be allowed to flex to 20° or 30°.[3] These measures resulted in partial sensory and motor recovery in two of eight patients whose injuries were recognized early. The role of early surgical exploration and decompression of the peroneal nerve has not been established, and, for this reason, patients should be observed unless there is clear evidence of a compressive hematoma that could be drained surgically.

The chronic treatment of peroneal palsy consists of the fabrication of a foot drop brace and the institution of passive exercises to prevent an equinus deformity. Complete recovery from this injury is rare.[2,3] If a dense neurologic deficit persists at 3 months postoperatively, there may be some benefit in surgical decompression of the peroneal nerve. Krackow and associates[2] reported complete or nearly complete resolution of neurologic deficits in five patients who underwent decompression from 5 to 45 months after total knee replacement. On further follow-up (12 to 72 months), 30 of 31 patients treated with surgical decompression of the peroneal nerve had some degree of functional and neurologic recovery, whereas this occurred in only three of nine patients treated nonsurgically. This study underscores the need for close follow-up postoperatively in patients with nerve palsy to determine if there is any improvement within 3 months. It strongly supports surgical intervention if no recovery is noted during this period.[4]

Preventive strategies in patients at high risk for developing nerve injury include the following: (1) resect an adequate amount of bone, especially in flexion or valgus deformities, to prevent excessive bowstringing of the peroneal nerve; (2) avoid tight dressings; (3) avoid plaster splints; and (4) allow knee flexion in the recovery room. There has been no demonstrated advantage in exploring and prophylactically releasing the peroneal nerve at the time of knee replacement surgery in high risk cases.[3]

Wound-Healing Problems

Causative Factors

The viability of the wound margins after a total knee replacement is an important determinant of a satisfactory outcome. Localized ischemia and necrosis is a common cause of delayed wound healing and prolonged hospitalization. Wound-healing problems have been reported in from 10% to 20% of patients undergoing knee replacement, but the seriousness of these problems is highly variable.[1] In its least serious form, wound necrosis occupies a zone 2 mm or less extending for a variable distance along the wound, usually in the prepatellar or suprapatellar region. The lateral skin is more commonly affected, but simultaneous medial involvement can occur. The necrotic tissue forms a firm eschar, which ultimately separates to reveal a fresh bed of granulation tissue or newly formed epithelium. The actual depth of necrosis is difficult to determine, but as the surface zone becomes wider, the necrosis tends to extend deeper into the subcutaneous fat. Larger areas of necrosis that extend more than 1 cm from the wound margin are usually associated with significant deep necrosis and may require surgical debridement. Massive skin necrosis is a rare but devastating complication that is usually associated with previous vascular compromise in a patient who has had multiple surgical procedures. This situation requires prompt aggressive surgical intervention.

Proper wound healing requires that adequate oxygenation be maintained in the marginal soft tissues.[5] Mechanical tension on the skin caused by postoperative swelling and flexion of the knee during therapy can compromise small vessel blood flow. In a cadaver study, Johnson and associates[6] found that mechanical tension on the skin margins of a midline incision was higher than in a medial parapatellar incision. Johnson[7] also studied the oxygen tension in the marginal soft tissues in the postoperative period. Oxygen tension is lowest during the first 3 days, especially in the lateral flap. This decrease in oxygen tension is exacerbated by continuous passive motion above 40°. These findings are the basis of protocols that use a medial parapatellar incision and limit flexion during the early period, but no clinical data are available to support such regimens.

Superficial wound infection is a significant inhibitor of wound healing.[8] The spread of infection may be potentiated by wound ischemia and necrosis, which impairs antibiotic delivery to the affected area.

Scars around the knee from previous surgical procedures are the most serious risk factor for major wound-healing problems.[9] The presence of a medial or lateral plate on the tibia or femur represents an obstacle that necessitates thorough preoperative planning. If at all possible, previous scars should be incorporated into the surgical incision. Perpendicular scars may generally be safely crossed, but parallel incisions should be avoided. The development of the lateral and medial subvastus approaches to the knee has facilitated the incorporation of a wider variety of preexisting scars.[10,11]

Other conditions that can affect wound healing but do not in themselves constitute contraindications for performing total knee replacement are diabetes, peripheral vascular disease, corticosteroid use, and heavy smoking. These factors should be taken into account when informing the patient of the risks of surgery.

Diagnosis

In high-risk patients the wound should be evaluated on the first postoperative day for signs of ischemia or necrosis. It is often difficult to distinguish ecchymosis from necrosis during the early period, and the wound should be observed for a blackening at the center of the ecchymotic zone, which is suggestive of necrosis. Marginal wound necrosis usually appears within the first 3 days. This should be observed closely for evidence of an enlarging zone of necrosis. Early drainage from around the eschar, or liquefaction of the eschar itself, is an indication of impending infection. Copious amounts of drainage may signal the presence of a direct communication with the joint.

Treatment

In cases of severe wound necrosis (marginal necrosis greater than 1 cm wide or localized necrosis greater than 2 cm in diameter), range of motion should be severely restricted until a definitive plan has been reached. Use of any device for immobilization that could cause excessive pressure on the wound must be avoided.

Marginal wound necrosis without deep extension to the joint may be treated with primary excision and wound closure with uniformly good results. At the time of excision, deep wound cultures should be obtained. Closure is performed using the least number of subcutaneous sutures needed to eliminate dead space, and the skin is closed with monofilament simple sutures that incorporate the skin and subcutaneous tissues. Intravenous broad-spectrum antibiotics should be used for at least 48 hours, or until the wound is benign in appearance. If deep wound cultures are positive, antibiotic treatment should be continued for 2 weeks.

Wound necrosis that extends more than 2 cm from the skin margin, or a remote zone of necrosis greater than 2 cm in diameter, may require excision and filling of the defect with a gastrocnemius flap.[9,12] This technique has been refined so that prompt recognition of major necrosis and aggressive intervention may lead to a satisfactory outcome with no more functional impairment than in an uncomplicated total knee replacement.[13]

In the nonsurgical treatment of wound necrosis following total knee replacement there is frequent uncertainty as to the extent of necrosis in the deep tissues. Vascular compromise to the skin may be associated with ischemic injury to such important deep structures as the quadriceps tendon, the patellar tendon, and the patella. In general, the size of the skin necrosis correlates with the extent of deep necrosis, but in multiply operated knees, particularly those requiring extensive dissection to mobilize the knee, there is added risk for massive deep necrosis even with relatively mild or no evidence of skin necrosis. Several weeks may pass before increasing pain, swelling, erythema, or spontaneous drainage signal the late effects of important deep necrosis.[9] Careful follow-up of high-risk patients, early recognition of the problem, and aggressive surgical debridement of necrotic tissue are essential elements in the prevention of secondary infection and permanent loss of the implant. Ischemic wound healing problems are prevented primarily by recognition of risk factors, combined with gentle handling of soft tissues, avoidance of closing the skin under excessive tension, and the minimizing of wound pressure from postoperative dressings.

Preoperative vascular evaluation should include a thorough inspection of the skin in the lower extremity. The location of surgical or traumatic scars, skin color, temperature variations, capillary refill, and the presence of ulcerations should be noted. The strength of the dorsalis pedis and posterior tibial pulsations should be documented by palpation or, if necessary, by Doppler. The ankle/brachial pressure index has been a valuable index of the extent of peripheral vascular disease. An index of less than 0.5 should alert the surgeon to possible risk of vascular compromise and the need for preoperative consultation with a vascular surgeon. The measurement of transcutaneous oxygen tension has been reported to be an objective indicator of skin viability, and has been used clinically to select the level of amputation for ischemic disease.[5] Normal volunteers were found to have oxygen pressures between 45 and 95 mm of mercury, while patients with peripheral vascular disease were found to have decreasing levels depending on the severity of their disease.

Arteriography as a preoperative evaluation should be reserved for patients who may be candidates for vascular bypass prior to total knee replacement, or those who are undergoing reconstruction for a severe posttraumatic condition or a tumor.

Absolute vascular contraindications for performing total knee replacement include the presence of verified vascular claudication with minimal or no activity, active skin ulcerations secondary to arterial insufficiency or venous stasis, and ischemia or frank necrosis in the toes. If the peripheral pulses are not palpable, and there is no potential for vascular bypass, the surgery should be done without inflating the tourniquet, as the tourniquet could cause thrombosis of the atherosclerotic femoral artery.[14]

Direct Injury to Vascular Structures Around the Knee

Structures at Risk

Direct injury to vascular structures adjacent to the knee can be prevented using a knowledge of knee anatomy combined with careful surgical technique.[15] The location of the critical vascular structures can be correlated with points on a clock face. At the joint line of the left knee, the popliteal vein is directly posterior (12 o'clock position) with the tibial nerve lying medial (11 o'clock) and the popliteal artery lying lateral to the vein (1 o'clock). All three of these structures are vulnerable to penetrating injury through the posterior capsule during meniscal resection, removal of the posterior cruciate ligament, or capsular release. Below the joint line, the popliteal artery bifurcates to form the posterior and anterior tibial arteries (2 o'clock). The common peroneal nerve lies against the fibula below the joint line at the 3 o'clock position. Damage to all structures between the 11 o'clock and 3 o'clock positions can occur when excessively long screws are used in this zone for fixation of cementless tibial components.[15]

Diagnosis

Any suspicion of vascular injury should be followed up with deflation of the tourniquet prior to implantation of the components. The joint and popliteal region should be carefully inspected and the return of distal arterial pulsations should be confirmed. An expanding popliteal mass, copious posterior bleeding into the joint, or the loss of distal pulses is an indication for intraoperative arteriograpy and a vascular surgery consultation.

Treatment

In the case of all confirmed vascular damage, a vascular surgery consultation should be obtained. A small vascular perforation may be treated with simple suture. Transection of a vessel may be repaired directly, if there is no tension on the anastomosis with the knee in full extension. Vascular grafting may be necessary for extensive vessel damage or when there is tension on the direct repair, as in the setting of significant (> 20°) preoperative flexion contracture.

Prevention

During resection of the medial and lateral menisci, there is a risk of penetrating injury to the popliteal vessels. Therefore, it is helpful to perform as much resection as possible with the scalpel blade parallel to the posterior tibia, pulling the meniscus anteriorly during this procedure. Laterally, the popliteal artery is protected at the joint line by the belly of the popliteus muscle. After the resection of the lateral meniscus back to the hiatus of the popliteus tendon, the meniscus should be drawn forward and removed completely without violating the muscle belly of the popliteus.

During the notch cut for a cruciate-substituting design, aggressive resection of the posterior cruciate ligament may lead to an entry into the popliteal fossa, where the popliteal vein lies directly behind the knee joint in the midline. Leaving a stump of posterior cruciate ligament behind will reduce the risk of vascular injury.

The division of the posterior capsule at the joint line when correcting a flexion contracture requires special care to avoid injury to the popliteal vessels and tibial nerve. A safer approach is to elevate the capsule from the back face of the tibia and distal femur, making sure to stay on the bone with the scalpel or elevator.

References

1. Huo MH, Sculco TP: Complications in primary total knee arthroplasty. *Orthop Rev* 1990;19:781–788.
2. Krackow KA, Maar DC, Mont MA, et al: Surgical decompression for peroneal nerve palsy after total knee arthroplasty. *Clin Orthop* 1993;292:223–228.
3. Rose HA, Hood RW, Otis JC, et al: Peroneal-nerve palsy following total knee arthroplasty: A review of the Hospital for Special Surgery experience. *J Bone Joint Surg* 1982;64A:347–351.
4. Mont MA, Dellon AL, Chen F, et al: The operative treatment of peroneal nerve palsy. *J Bone Joint Surg* 1996;78A:863–869.
5. Dowd GS, Linge K, Ross R, et al: Abstract: The transcutaneous measurement of oxygen in normal and abnormal skin. *J Bone Joint Surg* 1982;64B:248–249.
6. Johnson DP, Houghton TA, Radford P: Anterior midline or medial parapatellar incision for arthroplasty of the knee: A comparative study. *J Bone Joint Surg* 1986;68B:812–814.
7. Johnson DP: The effect of continuous passive motion on wound-healing and joint mobility after knee arthroplasty. *J Bone Joint Surg* 1990;72A:421–426.
8. Johnson DP, Bannister GC: The outcome of infected arthroplasty of the knee. *J Bone Joint Surg* 1986;68B:289–291.
9. Lian G, Cracchiolo A III, Lesavoy M: Treatment of major wound necrosis following total knee arthroplasty. *J Arthroplasty* 1989; 4(suppl):S23–S32.
10. Hofmann AA, Harlow ML: Submedialis approach, in Lotke PA (ed): *Knee Arthroplasty*, ed 1. New York, NY, Raven Press, 1995, pp 15–24.
11. Buechel FF: Lateral approach, in Lotke PA (ed): *Knee Arthroplasty*, ed 1. New York, NY, Raven Press, 1995, pp 25–39.
12. LaRossa D: The management of skin necrosis, in Lotke PA (ed): *Knee Arthroplasty*, ed 1. New York, NY, Raven Press, 1995, pp 241–252.
13. Sanders R, O'Neill T: The gastrocnemius myocutaneous flap used as a cover for the exposed knee prosthesis. *J Bone Joint Surg* 1981;63B:383–386.
14. Rush JH, Vidovich JD, Johnson MA: Arterial complications of total knee replacement. *J Bone Joint Surg* 1987;69B:400–402.
15. Rubash HE, Berger RA, Britton CA, et al: Avoiding neurologic and vascular injuries with screw fixation of the tibial component in total knee arthroplasty. *Clin Orthop* 1993;286:56–63.

CHAPTER 16

Thromboembolic Disease

Vincent D. Pellegrini, Jr, MD

Historical data from large series of patients undergoing total knee replacement have demonstrated a prevalence of deep vein thrombosis in the absence of prophylaxis of 70% to 80%.[1] Additionally, although considerably less than that following total hip replacement, the risk of subsequent pulmonary embolism is real, but this complication often escapes the attention of the operating surgeon, as it most frequently occurs weeks following hospital discharge.[1-5] Thromboembolic disease following total knee arthroplasty has been studied less systematically than that after total hip arthroplasty and, as such, remains an area fertile for organized prospective clinical investigation.

Epidemiologic Considerations

Thromboembolic disease following total knee replacement has a considerably different profile than that noted after total hip arthroplasty. There is a strong propensity for deep vein thrombosis in vessels of the calf, with 85% to 90% of thrombi after knee replacement noted to occur distal to the trifurcation of the popliteal vein, in the paired anterior tibial, posterior tibial, and peroneal veins.[1,2,6] In contrast to patients following total hip replacement, proximal vein thrombosis is infrequent after total knee replacement. Only 10% to 15% of patients experience femoropopliteal vein thrombosis after knee arthroplasty and, when present, proximal thrombosis is most frequently noted to be a continuous extension from a concurrent calf thrombosis.[2,3,6,7] Rarely is segmental discontinuous femoral thrombosis noted in the total knee replacement patient, again a situation quite distinct from that observed after hip arthroplasty.

There is evidence for a systemic diathesis and hypercoagulability playing a role in the prevalence of deep vein thrombosis in this patient population. Bilateral deep vein thrombosis is noted in 10% to 15% of patients and, specifically, deep vein thrombosis is identifiable in the nonoperated leg in 10% to 15% of patients following unilateral total knee arthroplasty.[1,6] Hypercoagulability is likely secondary to instrumentation of the intramedullary canal with embolization of marrow fat and other materials that activate the endogenous clotting cascade. Stasis in both the operated and the nonoperated lower extremities further adds to this systemic diathesis in producing venous thrombosis. The effect of the pneumatic tourniquet has been difficult to characterize definitively. Conflicting evidence exists that identifies both beneficial and detrimental effects of the tourniquet.[8-10] Beyond the obvious detrimental influence in the promotion of venous stasis distal to the tourniquet, a stimulation of the fibrinolytic system by the vascular endothelium has been observed following tourniquet release.[8,10] This latter effect may actually contribute to reducing the risk of venous thrombosis, but it clearly is not the predominant effect, in view of the high prevalence of thrombi in patients without prophylaxis.

The impact of adjunctive nonpharmacologic measures is supported by circumstantial evidence. Perhaps most interesting among these measures is the use of regional and, specifically, continuous epidural, anesthesia, which is associated with a decreased frequency of deep vein thrombosis.[11] The effects of regional anesthesia on lower extremity hemodynamics are more definitively understood than is its direct impact on thromboembolic disease. Most evident is an increase in venous flow and blood return to the central circulation, based on a sympathectomy effect and decreased resistance in the capacitance vessels of the lower extremity following administration of an epidural anesthetic. Additionally, there is evidence for increased fibrinolysis secondary to activity of the vascular endothelium and a decreased platelet adhesiveness as a possible direct effect of the local anesthetic agent. The net clinical impact of a regional anesthetic is a reported decrease in frequency of deep vein thrombosis.[11-14] Further analysis suggests a selective effect in reducing calf vein thrombosis with relatively little impact on thrombosis in the larger more proximal femoropopliteal vessels. Unfortunately, the message is not entirely clear, due to the heterogeneous nature of the studies providing evidence concerning deep vein thrombosis. The exact type of anesthetic, spinal versus epidural for operation versus epidural maintained postoperatively for pain control, the patient population undergoing surgery, the diagnosis of hip fracture, hip replacement, or knee replacement, and the use of only local anesthetic agents contrasted with a mixture of narcotics or even general anesthesia serve to confuse the interpretation of these studies. Therefore, the true beneficial component of regional anesthesia in reducing frequency of deep venous thrombosis remains to be identified.

Continuous passive motion machines have offered a theoretical advantage in potentially reducing stasis in the calf veins.[15,16] However, there is no documented beneficial effect of their reducing the incidence of venous thrombi following total knee arthroplasty. Similarly, the concept of early mobilization and shorter hospital stay provides an intuitive benefit, but the scientific basis of this approach is somewhat questionable. Demonstration of beneficial effects of this management strategy has been "soft" and documented by nonvenogram screening studies, which suffer from lack of sensitivity in identifying calf thrombi.

Impact of Chemoprophylaxis

In general, the impact of anticoagulant prophylaxis on the prevalence of deep vein thrombosis after total knee replacement has been considerably less profound than that observed after chemoprophylaxis following total hip replacement. The reasons for the difference in effectiveness of anticoagulants following these two procedures remain to be elucidated. Warfarin is currently the agent for deep vein thrombosis prophylaxis most commonly employed by those orthopaedic surgeons who routinely use prophylaxis. A lack of popularity of this method in past years was attributed to the historical recommendation to maintain the prothrombin time index at two times control (INR 3 to 4), which resulted in prothrombin times in excess of 20 seconds, and bleeding complication rates of 8% to 10%.[17-19] More recently, it has been recognized that anticoagulation with warfarin, whether intended as prophylaxis or as specific treatment for identifiable venous thrombosis, is quite effective when the prothrombin time index is maintained between 1.3 and 1.5 (INR 2.0 to 2.5), resulting in prothrombin times of 15 to 18 seconds and considerably lower rates of bleeding, in a range of less than 2%.[6,17-20] Routine use of warfarin as a prophylactic agent after total knee replacement has decreased the overall prevalence of deep vein thrombosis to 30% to 40% and has not affected the distribution of thrombi proximally to distally.[1,2,6] Although representing a considerable reduction in the prevalence of deep vein thrombosis over those patients not receiving prophylaxis, the rates of deep vein thrombosis with warfarin prophylaxis are felt to be still unacceptably high and have prompted a continued search for better methods of prevention.

Low molecular weight dextran enjoyed a transient phase of popularity, particularly following hip replacement, but more recently its effectiveness has been shown only to be comparable to placebo.[21,22] Moreover, it is associated with considerable risk of volume overload and congestive heart failure in elderly patients and an occasional allergic reaction, both of which have led to its fall from favor as a prophylactic agent. Aspirin, in contrast, has relatively few adverse effects and acts to decrease platelet adhesiveness. Numerous studies have been designed comparing aspirin to other agents and placebo, but none have definitively demonstrated an advantage of aspirin over placebo as a prophylactic agent against deep vein thrombosis after total knee replacement.[1,15,23] Meta-analyses have suggested a possible beneficial affect, but the National Institutes of Health consensus conference on thromboembolic disease in 1986 considered aspirin to be ineffective for this purpose. Even so, aspirin remains a frequently employed prophylactic agent after hip and knee arthroplasty, largely enjoying popularity because of its low complication profile.[1,2,15]

Pneumatic compression devices have enjoyed recent enthusiasm and indeed are intuitively attractive for total knee replacement patients, considering that calf thrombosis is the prevalent location for thrombi and their formation is likely secondary to stasis.[15,24,25] Thigh-length sleeves are awkward to use after knee arthroplasty, because they cover the surgical incision. In contrast, calf-length sleeves have been more practical and shown to reduce the prevalence of calf vein thrombosis after knee arthroplasty; calf compression stimulates fibrinolytic activity through activation of mediators produced by the vascular endothelium.[15] More recently, plantar impulse pads have become popular. They are more convenient to use and work by a slightly different mechanism. They deliver a high impact compression to the sole of the foot, resulting in high velocity pulsatile flow in the femoral vein. Recently published results from a single study of plantar impulse pads suggest a decrease in prevalence of deep vein thrombosis when compared with aspirin prophylaxis in the total knee replacement population.[26] With an essentially nonexistent bleeding complication profile, compressive devices are inherently attractive to the orthopaedic surgeon and it is hoped that they will be definitively proven as effective in preventing deep vein thrombosis.

Fractionated heparin has also enjoyed recent popularity. This smaller, more homogeneous heparin molecule, with a molecular weight of approximately 5,000 d, is characterized by a more favorable binding affinity profile to activated factor X than to factor II. This affinity results in an antithrombotic effect exerted earlier in the clotting cascade with a theoretical decrease in risk of concurrent bleeding complications as compared with unfractionated heparin. Coagulation times do not need to be monitored, but parenteral subcutaneous administration is required. Although fractionated heparin has been shown to be extremely effective in reducing deep vein thrombosis following total hip replacement to less than 10% overall,[27,28] like warfarin, it has enjoyed consid-erably less efficacy following total knee arthroplasty.[29,30] Overall deep vein thrombosis rates of 20% to 30% following total knee replacement have been reported, but the overall bleeding rates range from 8% to 10%, which is statistically significantly greater than that associated with low-dose warfarin in prospective controlled studies.[27-30] Bleeding complications are more frequent with use of fractionated heparin, both at the surgical wound and at the injection site, but wound bleeding may be reduced by beginning the medication no sooner than 12 hours postoperatively. Recent information has incriminated fractionated heparin in epidural hematomas and associated neurologic deficit when used in conjunction with regional anesthesia or indwelling postoperative epidural catheters. In the setting of outpatient treatment, self injection is required for administration of the drug. While offering great promise in reduction of rates of thromboembolic disease following total joint arthroplasty, the fractionated heparins remain to be definitively proven as superior prophylaxis without an unacceptable increase in perioperative bleeding risk.

Current Prophylaxis: A Rational Approach

Assimilation of available information concerning prevalence of deep vein thrombosis with contemporary prophylaxis allows several comparisons between thromboembolic disease after hip and knee arthroplasty. The prevalence of deep vein thrombosis is two to four times greater after knee than hip arthroplasty, occurs with a strong predisposition for calf vein thrombosis after knee arthroplasty, and has a much lower risk of pulmonary embolism following knee than hip arthroplasty despite the greater prevalence of deep vein thrombosis after knee replacement. Additionally, there is less wound tolerance for postoperative bleeding complications after knee replacement, considering the thinner soft-tissue envelope with less muscle cover over the knee.

It would appear that the mechanism of deep vein thrombosis following any musculoskeletal operative procedure includes a hypercoagulable state resulting from intramedullary instrumentation and activation of the clotting cascade. Moreover, stasis would appear to be a primary factor in the development of calf thrombosis after knee replacement, with proximal thrombosis in this patient population largely the result of contiguous thrombosis resulting from proximal propagation of calf disease. This contrasts considerably with the segmental proximal vein thrombosis evident following hip replacement, felt to be secondary to manipulation and torsion of the femoral vein during retraction and positioning.

It then follows that flow augmentation by any one of a number of means is intuitively attractive in reducing the stasis thought to be important in calf vein thrombosis after knee replacement. Compression devices, either calf sleeves or a plantar foot pump, offer promise but remain to be proven as effective agents. Regional anesthesia is also associated with a decrease in calf vein thrombosis, but the specifics of type and duration of the regional anesthetic have yet to be delineated. Finally, a plan of early mobilization, frequently the byproduct of shorter lengths of stay and contemporary health care reform, also contribute to a reduction in calf vein thrombosis in a way that is difficult to define or to quantitate precisely.

The ideal pharmacologic agent for prophylactic anticoagulation likewise has not been identified. Clearly the superior agent should have a low frequency of bleeding complications, particularly after knee replacement, because the tolerance for wound hematoma is quite small given the threat to viability of the overlying skin envelope. Warfarin, aspirin, and fractionated heparin all enjoy some popularity at the present time, and each has its advantages and disadvantages. While usage of fractionated heparin remains to be further characterized, at this time warfarin possesses the better efficacy/safety profile with reasonable effectiveness and a very low risk of concomitant bleeding complications. In the current environment, with prevalence rates of deep vein thrombosis of 30% to 40%, even with the best available prophylactic agents, easy outpatient application of continued anticoagulant therapy is important for patient acceptance and effective outpatient treatment of recognized thrombi.

Perhaps the most provocative question is the duration of chemoprophylaxis in the setting of an average hospital stay of 4 to 5 days following knee replacement. Two strategies have been proposed. Extended prophylaxis for all patients, consisting of warfarin or fractionated heparin for 6 to 12 weeks after operation, has the advantage of not requiring routine surveillance to identify deep vein thrombosis. As such, it is also very effective in prevention of deep vein thrombosis and complicating pulmonary embolism. Unfortunately, given prevalence rates of 30% to 40% deep vein thrombosis after knee replacement, such extended anticoagulant exposure is unnecessary in 60% to 70% of patients. This "unnecessary" fraction of treated patients only increases with improved efficacy of anticoagulant agents. Furthermore, exposure of the entire postoperative population to outpatient anticoagulant use increases the likelihood of bleeding complications. Alternatively, a strategy of routine surveillance for deep vein thrombosis followed by selective treatment of identified venous disease may be adopted. In this setting, routine surveillance testing for deep vein thrombosis is conducted to identify venous thrombi in need of further treatment. Unfortunately, noninvasive screening modalities, such as color flow Doppler or duplex ultrasound, are relatively blind to identifying disease in the calf, which is the most prevalent location for deep vein thrombosis after total knee arthroplasty.[7,31] The contrast venogram remains quite sensitive in the identification of calf thrombi, but it is an invasive test that is accompanied by modest morbidity.[6,31,32] If the inconvenience of venogram screening is accepted, the postoperative population of patients exposed to outpatient anticoagulation is reduced to 20% to 40% with identified venous thrombi. Although the screening studies add to in-hospital costs, the reduced outpatient exposure to anticoagulant agents considerably lowers the effective risk of bleeding and associated rehospitalization and proves the strategy of routine surveillance to be more cost effective than that of extended prophylaxis for all patients.[4,33] With the advent of better noninvasive studies for identification of deep vein thrombosis, the most promising among which is magnetic resonance venography,[34] the author believes that this strategy of routine surveillance and selective treatment will become the favored approach in managing the patient at risk for thromboembolic disease following total knee replacement.

Treatment of Thromboembolic Disease

Critical to formulation of any treatment plan for identified thromboembolic disease is the notion that the treatment should not be accompanied by greater risks than the disease being treated. In the postoperative joint replacement population, the risk involved is clearly that of bleeding in the face of anticoagulant therapy. Therefore, the risk of morbidity and mortality due to thromboembolic disease must continuously be weighed against the risk of hemorrhage while on anticoagulant therapy.[2]

Proximal thrombosis, involving the femoropopliteal veins, is managed by bed rest and intravenous heparin therapy for 5 days or until the prothrombin time on warfarin becomes therapeutic, whichever is greater. Caution should be exercised in the initiation of parenteral heparin therapy; a conservative loading bolus, or preferably none at all, should be used to avoid overshooting the therapeutic range of the partial thromboplastin time. Major complications of bleeding have been demonstrated in 35% of the postoperative joint replacement population when full heparin therapy is initiated within 5 days postoperatively. Heparin is followed by warfarin, continued on an outpatient basis, to maintain the prothrombin time index at 1.5 times control for 3 months, extending to 6 months if the initial course was complicated by pulmonary embolism. Deep vein thromboses in the calf vessels, those distal to the popliteal trifurcation, do not require heparin. In this scenario, the bleeding risk with heparin outweighs the therapeutic benefit. However, the use of no heparin is not synonymous with no treatment; rates of proximal thrombi propagation and pulmonary embolism ranging from 17% to 25% have been reported following untreated deep vein thrombosis in the calf.[3,33] Outpatient warfarin therapy is administered for 6 to 12 weeks to maintain the prothrombin time index at 1.5 times control; no patients under this management scheme have returned with symptomatic pulmonary embolism. Superficial thrombi, or those involving the muscular perforating veins, have no demonstrated propensity to proximal propagation and require no specific therapy.

References

1. Stulberg BN, Insall JN, Williams GW, et al: Deep-vein thrombosis following total knee replacement: An analysis of six hundred and thirty-eight arthroplasties. *J Bone Joint Surg* 1984;66A:194–201.
2. Lotke PA, Ecker ML, Alavi A, et al: Indications for the treatment of deep venous thrombosis following total knee replacement. *J Bone Joint Surg* 1984;66A:202–208.
3. Oishi CS, Grady-Benson JC, Otis SM, et al: The clinical course of distal deep venous thrombosis after total hip and total knee arthroplasty, as determined with duplex ultrasonography. *J Bone Joint Surg* 1994;76A:1658–1663.
4. Pellegrini VD Jr, Clement D, Lush-Ehmann C, et al: The natural history of thromboembolic disease following hospital discharge after total hip arthroplasty: The case for routine surveillance. *Clin Orthop*, in press.
5. Sikorski J, Hampson W, Staddon G: The natural history and etiology of deep vein thrombosis after total hip replacement. *J Bone Joint Surg* 1981;63B:171–177.
6. Francis CW, Pellegrini VD Jr, Leibert KM, et al: Comparison of two-step vs. night before warfarin prophylaxis of deep venous thrombosis following total knee arthroplasty. *Thromb Haemost* 1996;75:706–711.
7. Grady-Benson JC, Oishi CS, Hanson PB, et al: Postoperative surveillance for deep venous thrombosis with duplex ultrasonography after total knee arthroplasty. *J Bone Joint Surg* 1994;76A:1649–1657.
8. Fahmy N, Patel D: Hemostatic changes with postoperative deep vein thrombosis asssociated with use of a pneumatic tourniquet. *J Bone Joint Surg* 1981;63A:461–465.
9. Kroese A, Stiris G: The risk of deep vein thrombosis after operations on a bloodless lower limb: A venography study. *Injury* 1976;7:271–273.
10. Larsson J, Risbert B: Fibrinolytic activity in human legs in tourniquet ischemia. *Thromb Res* 1977;11:817–825.
11. Dalldorf PG, Perkins FM, Totterman S, et al: Deep venous thrombosis following total hip arthroplasty: Effects of prolonged postoperative epidural anesthesia. *J Arthroplasty* 1994;9:611–616.
12. Jorgensen L, Rasmussen L, Nielsen P, et al: Anti-thrombic efficacy of continuous extradural analgesia after knee replacement. *Br J Anaesth* 1991;66:8–12.
13. Nielsen P, Jorgensen L, Albrecht-Beste E, et al: Lower thrombosis risk with epidural blockade in knee arthroplasty. *Acta Orthop Scand* 1990;61:29–31.
14. Thorburn J, Louden J, Vallance R: Spinal and general anesthesia in total hip replacement: Frequency of deep vein thrombosis. *Br J Anaesth* 1980;52:1117–1120.
15. Haas SB, Insall JN, Scuderi GR, et al: Pneumatic sequential-compression boots compared with aspirin prophylaxis of deep-vein thrombosis after total knee arthroplasty. *J Bone Joint Surg* 1990;72A:27–31.
16. Lynch AF, Bourne RB, Rorabeck CH, et al: Deep-vein thrombosis and continuous passive motion after total knee arthroplasty. *J Bone Joint Surg* 1988;70A:11–14.
17. Hirsch J: Therapeutic range for the control of oral anticoagulant therapy. *Arch Intern Med* 1985;145:1187–1188.
18. Hirsch J: The optimal intensity of oral anticoagulant therapy. *JAMA* 1987;258:2723–2726.
19. Hirsch J: Oral anticoagulant drugs. *N Engl J Med* 1991;324:1865–1875.
20. Francis C, Marder V, Evarts C, et al: Two-step warfarin therapy. *JAMA* 1983;249:374–378.
21. Francis C, Pellegrini VD Jr, Harris C, et al: Antithrombin III prophylaxis of venous thromboembolic disease after total hip or knee replacement. *Am J Med* 1989;87:3(suppl):615–665.

22. Francis C, Pellegrini VD Jr, Marder V, et al: Prevention of venous thrombosis after total hip arthroplasty: Antithrombin III and low-dose heparin compared with dextran-40. *J Bone Joint Surg* 1989;71A:327–335.
23. McKenna R, Galante J, Bachmann F: Prevention of venous thromboembolism after total knee replacement by high dose aspirin or intermittent calf and thigh compression. *Br Med J* 1980;280:514–517.
24. Francis C , Pellegrini VD Jr, Marder V, et al: Comparison of warfarin and external pneumatic compression in prevention of venous thrombosis after total hip replacement. *JAMA* 1992; 267:2911–2915.
25. Hull R, Raskob G, Geut M, et al: Effectiveness of intermittent pneumatic leg compression for preventing deep vein thrombosis after total hip replacement. *JAMA* 1990;263:2313–2317.
26. Westrich G, Sculco T: Prophylaxis against deep venous thrombosis after total knee arthroplasty: Pneumatic plantar compression and aspirin compared with aspirin alone. *J Bone Joint Surg* 1996;78A:826–834.
27. Colwell C, Spiro T, Trombridge A, et al: Use of enoxaparin, a low molecular weight heparin and unfractionated heparin for the prevention of deep venous thrombosis after elective hip replacement. *J Bone Joint Surg* 1994;76A:3–14.
28. Turpie AGG: Enoxaparin prophylaxis in elective hip surgery. *Acta Chir Scand* 1990;556(suppl):103–107.
29. Leclerc JR, Geerts W, Desjardins L, et al: Prevention of deep vein thrombosis after major knee surgery: A randomized double-blind trial comparing a low moleculaar weight heparin fragment (enoxaparin) to placebo. *Thromb Haemost* 1992;67: 417–423.
30. RD Heparin Arthroplasty Group: RD heparin computed with warfarin in prevention of venous thromboembolic disease following total hip or knee arthroplasty. *J Bone Joint Surg* 1994; 76A:1174–1185.
31. Wells PS, Lensing AW, Davidson BL, et al: Accuracy of ultrasound for the diagnosis of deep venous thrombosis in asymptomatic patients after orthopaedic surgery: A meta-analysis. *Ann Intern Med* 1995;122:47–53.
32. Rabinov K, Paulin S: Roentgen diagnosis of venous thrombosis in the leg. *Arch Surg* 1992;104:134–144.
33. Pellegrini VD Jr, Langhans MJ, Totterman S, et al: Embolic complications of calf thrombosis following total hip arthroplasty. *J Arthroplasty* 1993;8:449–457.
34. Larcom P, Lotke P, Holland G, et al: Comparison of MR venography to standard contrast venography in the diagnosis of deep venous thrombosis after total hip and knee surgery. *Orthop Trans* 1996;20:149.

CHAPTER 17

The Stiff Total Knee Replacement: Causes, Treatment, and Prevention

Norman A. Johanson, MD

Introduction and Definitions

The term stiffness as it relates to total knee replacement (TKR) has several different meanings that are essentially observer dependent. From the surgeon's perspective, stiffness has meant inadequate or less than expected range of motion (ROM) when measured in a standardized fashion on the examining table. Active or active-assisted ROM measured under optimal conditions is routinely documented during the patient's recovery period, and the norms for motion following TKR have been generated from this sort of data.[1-4] Functional capacity is also evaluated to confirm that the clinically derived ROM corresponds to an appropriate level of function (walking, sitting, stairs, etc).[3,5] A patient whose knee by clinical examination has 90° of flexion and comes to within 10° of full extension and who has no complaints of pain or functional difficulties is not considered to have a stiff knee. However, a patient 1 year after TKR who has clinically acceptable motion but who complains of knee stiffness, has difficulty getting out of a chair, has pain on climbing stairs, and walks with an observably stiff-knee gait should be further evaluated for underlying knee problems.

From the patient's point of view, the problem of stiffness has different dimensions that should be integrated into the overall clinical picture. Although it is closely related to pain, stiffness has a wider application to the patient's experience while attempting to move the knee, particularly during the early postoperative period. Stiffness is therefore closely related to the patient's own motivation to gain a functional ROM, and his or her willingness to endure pain to achieve that goal. For example, a patient who has minimal supportive care at home and has to get out of bed for every need will probably complain of more stiffness in the knee than someone who is receiving total support from family members or nursing facility staff, even though the reported pain levels may be similar. This little-studied phenomenon may have significant implications for the patient's final ROM and functional capacity.

Stiffness, which is nearly always present during the early postoperative period, gradually decreases over time, and is, therefore, a valuable marker of improvement throughout the recovery period. Surgical pain is the most important cause of early knee stiffness. It results in both quadriceps and hamstring guarding and makes passive flexion and extension difficult to perform. This factor has formed the theoretical basis for implementation of in-hospital continuous passive motion (CPM).[6,7] The CPM device cradles the leg while slowly moving it through its prescribed range, minimizing the guarding response. Whether or not it actually does minimize the guarding response, CPM has not been conclusively demonstrated either to shorten the hospital stay or to provide significantly increased ROM in a population of TKR patients. For these reasons, its value in the early postoperative period is questionable in view of its cost. In addition, CPM has no capacity to promote knee extension because of the difficulties in securing the leg to apply an extension force to the prepatellar area. Nevertheless, CPM may be beneficial in selected cases, and it has been generally well accepted within the hospital environment, even to the point of being expected as standard treatment by many patients. CPM should not be viewed as a substitute for the persistence and encouragement of an experienced physical therapist.[2,5] In addition to using their expertise to obtain the desired ROM and functional capacity, physical therapists serve in an educational capacity and are positioned well for picking up early problems with motivation and compliance. This is particularly important as hospital length of stay continuously shrinks. The unpredictable quality and the lack of direct supervision of home or outpatient physical therapy within the managed care environment demands that patients at high risk for developing knee stiffness be identified within the first 4 postoperative days, before they leave the hospital.

Postoperative knee stiffness usually subsides within 6 to 8 weeks. Knee ROM generally improves steadily through the first 3 months, and then less rapid progress may be seen for an additional 9 months or more.[2,3] If a limited or deteriorating ROM occurs, the following complications should be considered: (1) infection, (2) mechanical complications related to the implant or soft tissue, (3) impending arthrofibrosis, and (4) reflex sympathetic dystrophy (if associated with severe pain and vasomotor skin changes).[5]

The late onset of knee stiffness following a relatively symptom-free period may be suggestive of one of the following conditions: (1) infection, (2) overuse synovitis or tendinitis (particularly in the younger, more active patient), (3) synovitis secondary to rheumatoid arthritis, particulate wear debris, or recurrent hemarthrosis, and (4) implant loosening or breakage.[8]

Causes of TKR Stiffness

Infection

Early infection (within the first 6 weeks) is characterized by increasing swelling, erythema, and generalized pain, with or without wound drainage. All of these findings may also be present in a noninfected knee during the immediate postoperative period. The progressive nature of the signs and symptoms, especially after a period of 2 to 3 days of rest and immobilization, should stimulate early recognition of infection.

Late infection is more easily recognized, because it follows a relatively asymptomatic period, although an aspiration and culture may be required to distinguish an indolent infection from other causes of synovitis listed above.

Mechanical Problems (Implant/Soft Tissue)

Because of the wide variety of available implant designs and the rarity of severely stiff TKR's in published series, the overall problem remains enigmatic. However, it is probable that each implant has certain design features which carry a definable margin of safety for variations from the prescribed method of bone cuts and the treatment of ligaments. It is in these poorly defined safety zones that the majority of stiff TKR's would find their etiology.[1,5,8-10] Dorr and associates[11] found that patients who had obtained excellent clinical results following either posterior cruciate (PCL) retaining or sacrificing designs continued to walk with a stiff-knee gait 2 years postoperatively. These findings suggest that TKR rarely produces a completely normal gait, and that some degree of stiffness is present even with an excellent result. The right balance between motion, strength, and stability is the surgical goal for a good functional result. Inadequate bone resection combined with persistent ligamentous imbalance or tightness may result in knee stiffness. If, during trial reduction, asymmetric or symmetric tightness is recognized, it can be corrected by either revising the bone cuts, releasing the ligaments, or a combination of the two. If a flexion contracture is present, more distal femur should be resected and/or a posterior capsular release performed. If the residual contracture is severe (> 15°), some additional bone may be removed from the proximal tibia, provided that doing so does not make the flexion gap too wide. However, if tibial resection is essential and the flexion gap threatens stability in flexion, the femoral component could be set more posteriorly with augmentation, either by cutting more bone anteriorly or by using a larger size femoral component.

The approach to bone resection in TKR is highly dependent on the plan to preserve or to sacrifice the posterior cruciate ligament (PCL).[5,12,13] When the PCL is to be preserved, the femur is usually cut first in order to preserve the level of the joint line and, hence, more closely approximate the normal kinematics of the knee. Variable amounts of tibia must be resected to provide the proper alignment and stability while preserving and balancing the tension of the PCL in both flexion and extension. A potentially dangerous pitfall during this procedure is reversing the tilt of the tibia in the sagittal plane. This will cause tightening of the PCL in flexion if the rollback mechanism functions according to design. Alternatively, as has been reported, the tibia may actually drop back, compromising the patellofemoral mechanics.[13] The problem of tightness in flexion is most important from the standpoint of postoperative knee stiffness. If tightness is recognized intraoperatively, PCL recession can be considered or the tibia can be cut again at neutral or with a 5° posterior slope. If there is excessive posterior instability that results from laxity of the PCL, a cruciate-substituting design may be used. Hirsch and associates[12] reported that the clinical results achieved with use of a PCL-sacrificing device did not differ from those achieved using a PCL-retaining device.

The selection of an oversized femoral component or the posterior placement of the component can lead to a disproportionately narrow flexion gap. It is difficult to manage this problem by resecting more tibia, especially if the extension gap is adequate, because resection of additional tibia may lead to an unacceptable amount of laxity in extension. Downsizing the femoral component and resecting more posterior femur will expand the flexion gap without affecting stability in extension.

Inadequate release of tight capsular and ligamentous structures is an important cause of the stiff TKR, but is difficult to measure. Poor flexion and extension may result from inadequate release or recession of a tight PCL. Flexion contractures most commonly result from inadequate posterior capsular release in conjunction with insufficient bone resection. The medial collateral ligament in varus deformities, and the lateral collateral ligament and iliotibial band in valgus deformities often require release to prevent asymmetric implant wear and to promote optimal range of knee motion. External rotation of the femoral component has been recommended to enhance ligament bal-ancing in flexion and to facilitate optimal patellar tracking.[14-17]

Although not necessarily a causative problem in TKR stiffness, patellofemoral dysfunction may cause pain that may promote stiffness because of disuse.[17-19] Conversely, patellofemoral pain may result from knee stiffness, particularly with flexion contractures. The following patellar conditions should be considered when evaluating the stiff TKR: (1) patella not resurfaced, (2) inadequate lateral release, (3) asymmetrical cutting of the patella, (4) excessive elevation of the joint line, (5) internal rotation of the femoral component, (6) the formation of intra-articular adhesions that tether the patella to surrounding structures, thereby altering the normal tracking mechanism,[20,21] (7) patellar fracture, and (8) patellar component loosening. All of these problems may be clinically evident by either loss of ROM or by patient complaints of stiffness.

The generation of an excessive volume of wear debris over a given period of time causes synovitis, with pain, stiffness, and swelling being the usual result. Poor quality polyethylene, high patient weight and activity level, failure to remove cement and bone debris from knee joint, or implant design factors (contact stresses, poly distribution) are possible causative factors.[8]

Patient-Related Factors

The availability and efficiency of in-hospital physical therapy has been thought to have a significant impact on the outcome of TKR.[2,5] With shorter hospital stays, there is an increasing reliance on outpatient and home physical therapy services, services that are frequently not under the direct supervision of the operating surgeon. The impact of this relatively rapid change on the incidence of knee stiffness and the long-term outcome of TKR has not been thoroughly studied. An important factor in the process is the patient's motivation to achieve a good clinical result. In addition the patient must be willing to undergo a rigorous rehabilitation program.

Patient preferences, expectations, and satisfaction with elective procedures such as TKR have received recent attention as being important indicators as to the likelihood of obtaining good outcomes from surgery. Preoperative patient education is an important tool for guiding the patient into an understanding of his or her own goals in light of the actual risks and benefits of surgery. The educational process gives the surgeon an opportunity to recognize patients with unrealistic expectations or who lack the motivation to comply with the postoperative regimen. Patients with potential problems that may require additional services should be identified as soon as possible, so that hospital use review panels and insurers can be notified of the additional needs that may arise.

Host factors that promote arthrofibrosis in and around the replaced knee joint are not well understood, but they should be further studied as a rare but important causes of knee stiffness. It is apparent that certain patients are predisposed to develop early knee stiffness and unusual amounts of pain and swelling in the absence of infection, bleeding, or mechanical complications.[22]

Diagnostic Considerations

Physical Examination

The most important diagnostic tool in the evaluation of the stiff TKR is the physical examination. At least two examinations should be done within the first 6 weeks to assure acceptable progress with ROM and functional status. Patients who are having problems should be seen more frequently. Unexpected restriction of ROM should be assessed in light of other findings, such as swelling, effusion, erythema, skin viability, and drainage.

Radiographic Evaluation

Plain radiographs should be ordered within the first 6 weeks, and repeated if stiffness and pain increases. Anteroposterior, lateral, and tangential patellar views should be obtained. Findings associated with knee stiffness may include one or more of the following: (1) inadequate bone resection, (2) oversized femoral implant, (3) evidence of ligamentous imbalance resulting from asymmetric cement pressurization if components were cemented simultaneously,[23] and (4) gross maltracking or subluxation of the patella.

A bone scan is indicated in late cases of stiffness that follow an asymptomatic period. Bone scans are less useful during the early recovery period and throughout the first year postoperatively, when they normally demonstrate increased uptake around the implants. Cementless implants tend to increase bone scan activity for an even longer period of time.[8]

Aspiration and Culture

In early cases of progressive stiffness, pain, and swelling, infection should be ruled out with an aspiration and culture of the joint fluid. A negative culture, however, does not absolutely rule out infection. If suspicion of infection is high, an arthrotomy may be necessary to obtain tissue for a positive culture. If symptoms develop after a relatively asymptomatic period of 1 year or more, the joint aspirate should also be examined under polarized microscopy for evidence of polyethylene wear debris.

Treatment Alternatives

Physical Therapy

In a stiff, noninfected, radiographically satisfactory TKR, the most important initial treatment is an adequately supervised course of sustained intensive physical therapy, which may last from 3 to 6 months, depending on the initial results. If some progress is being made with therapy and the patient is able to tolerate the discomfort, conservative management should be continued.

Manipulation

If, during the first 3 months, a plateau in ROM is reached, manipulation of the knee under regional or general anesthesia should be considered. Manipulation is not necessary within the first postoperative month. Fox and Poss[4] found that a group of patients whose knees had been manipulated 2 weeks postoperatively could not be distinguished from those whose knees had not, when ROM was assessed 1 year postoperatively. Moreover, there was a significant loss of motion during the week following manipulation. Preoperative ROM is an important predictor of the resulting ROM following TKR.[1,2] Parsley and associates[1] reported that 17 knees with less than 75° of preoperative flexion gained a mean of 16° (from 61° to 77°). Two hundred fifty-seven knees with preoperative flexion greater than 95° lost a mean of 6° (from 115° to 109°). Therefore, although poor preoperative flexion may yield a better improvement in flexion, the final flexion angle achieved is generally inferior. Knowledge of preoperative flexion should assist the surgeon and the patient in formulating the goals for motion and in postoperatively identifying a reasonable threshold for manipulation.

Debridement

If manipulation of the knee does not obtain a sustained acceptable improvement in ROM, an exploration and debridement of the knee may be performed, using either open or arthroscopic techniques. Good results have been reported in arthroscopic debridement for localized tethering of the patella or fibrous nodules that cause clunking of the patella over the anterior flange of the femoral component.[20,21] These conditions, however, are not usually associated with significant loss of motion. Results of arthroscopic treatment of generalized arthrofibrosis following TKR have not been as good.[22,24] In one report of seven patients, two had undergone knee arthrodesis and another two were scheduled to have this salvage operation.[24] The results of either open or arthroscopic debridement for a stiff TKR are probably related primarily to the extent of the intra-articular fibrosis.

Revision Surgery

The exchange of a modular tibial polyethylene spacer in conjunction with a capsular or ligamentous release may provide improvement in ROM, particularly when done to correct a flexion contracture. Intraoperatively, the deformity should be completely corrected with a new trial spacer in place. If complete correction cannot be achieved, revision of the tibial and/or femoral components should be performed after making new bone cuts that provide optimal flexion and extension gaps. In all cases, when both components are revised for a stiff TKR, a PCL-substituting design should be used. This type of design more readily accommodates alterations in the joint line caused by the revision bone cuts, and it has the inherent stability to allow generous flexion and extension gaps and ligament release.[5,25,26]

During revision for TKR stiffness, it is very important to fully release all structures that may have contributed to the condition, including the following: (1) the quadriceps tendon and vastus intermedius adhesion to the femur and suprapatellar pouch, (2) the medial and lateral gutters, (3) the collateral ligaments, and (4) the lateral patellar retinaculum. Several or all of these releases are usually necessary for exposure of the stiff knee.[27] In severe cases, the integrity of the extensor mechanism must be carefully guarded. Avulsion of the patellar tendon from the tibial tubercle is a potentially devastating complication that can be prevented by a systematic approach to the knee that uses the releases noted above and by suturing or reinforcing the tendon insertion when appropriate.[19,28]

Prevention of the Stiff TKR

The most fundamental consideration for the prevention of TKR complications in general and stiffness in particular is the selection of an implant and instrumentation system that is complex enough to allow flexibility, yet simple enough to minimize the chances for technical error. The selection should be based on a published track record of satisfactory implant performance over a period of 5 to 10 years, and the technical difficulty should be compatible with the proficiency and experience of the surgeon. Like a normal knee, a TKR design will have tolerances for tightness (stability) and laxity (flexibility) throughout a given ROM. In general, a design with less inherent stability or constraint will require more exacting bone cuts and ligament balancing to deliver an acceptable result. This requirement applies to many PCL-sparing designs, particularly those that use cementless fixation. Cemented cruciate-substituting designs have more inherent stability and will better tolerate the aggressive ligament releases required to correct severe varus or valgus deformities. Elevation of the joint line is also better tolerated in PCL-substituting implants.[17,26] Therefore, for the surgeon who performs an occasional TKR, the PCL-substituting designs offer at least a theoretically wider margin of safety. The definitive answer to this problem can only be addressed through the implementation of a broad-based outcome database for TKR.

Knowledge of patient expectations, goals, and motivations is essential for early detection of potential problems with stiffness following TKR. A poorly motivated patient with little or no preoperative education combined with a short hospital stay and marginally delivered home or outpatient physical therapy constitutes a dangerous mix that may result in a less than optimal surgical result. More research is needed on this scenario and the compromising influences that are brought to bear on it by the managed care environment. A strategy of early identification of problems should be formulated, and appropriate treatment pathways for these outliers should be constructed and tested with the goal of ultimately preventing the harmful and costly long-term effects of stiffness following TKR.

References

1. Parsley BS, Engh GA, Dwyer KA: Preoperative flexion: Does it influence postoperative flexion after posterior-cruciate-retaining total knee arthroplasty? *Clin Orthop* 1992;275:204–210.
2. Schurman DJ, Parker JN, Ornstein D: Total condylar knee replacement: A study of actors influencing range of motion as late as two years after arthroplasty. *J Bone Joint Surg* 1985;67A: 1006–1014.
3. Ritter MA, Campbell ED: Effect of range of motion on the success of a total knee arthroplasty. *J Arthroplasty* 1987;2:95–97.
4. Fox JL, Poss R: The role of manipulation following total knee replacement. *J Bone Joint Surg* 1981;63A:357–362.
5. Moreland JR: Mechanisms of failure in total knee arthroplasty. *Clin Orthop* 1988;226:49–64.
6. Colwell CW Jr, Morris BA: The influence of continuous passive motion on the results of total knee arthroplasty. *Clin Orthop* 1992;276:225–228.
7. Romness DW, Rand JA: The role of continuous passive motion following total knee arthroplasty. *Clin Orthop* 1988;226:34–37.
8. Berman AT, Coutts RD, Engh GA, et al: Symposium: The painful total knee replacement and the influence of component design. *Contemp Orthop* 1994;28:523–545.
9. Edwards E, Miller J, Chan K–H: The effect of postoperative collateral ligament laxity in total knee arthroplasty. *Clin Orthop* 1988;236:44–51.
10. Rorabeck CH, Bourne RB, Nott L: The cemented kinematic II and the non-cemented porous-coated anatomic prostheses for total knee replacement: A prospective evaluation. *J Bone Joint Surg* 1988;70A:483–490.
11. Dorr LD, Ochsner JL, Gronley J, et al: Functional comparison of posterior cruciate-retained versus cruciate-sacrificed total knee arthroplasty. *Clin Orthop* 1988;236:36–43.
12. Hirsch HS, Lotke PA, Morrison LD: The posterior cruciate ligament in total knee surgery: Save, sacrifice, or substitute? *Clin Orthop* 1994;309:64–68.
13. Insall JN: Presidential address to The Knee Society: Choices and compromises in total knee arthroplasty. *Clin Orthop* 1988; 226:43–48.
14. Laskin RS: Flexion space configuration in total knee arthroplasty. *J Arthroplasty* 1995;10:657–660.
15. Rhoads DD, Noble PC, Reuben JD, et al: The effect of femoral component position on the kinematics of total knee arthroplasty. *Clin Orthop* 1993;286:122–129.
16. Anouchi YS, Whiteside LA, Kaiser AD, et al: The effects of axial rotational alignment of the femoral component on knee stability and patellar tracking in total knee arthroplasty demonstrated on autopsy specimens. *Clin Orthop* 1993;287:170–177.
17. Scuderi GR, Insall JN, Scott WN: Patellofemoral pain after total knee arthroplasty. *J Am Acad Orthop Surg* 1994;2:239–246.
18. Fern ED, Winson IG, Getty CJ: Anterior knee pain in rheumatoid patients after total knee replacement: Possible selection criteria for patellar resurfacing. *J Bone Joint Surg* 1992;74B:745–748.
19. Lynch AF, Rorabeck CH, Bourne RB: Extensor mechanism complications following total knee arthroplasty. *J Arthroplasty* 1987;2:135–140.
20. Lintner DM, Bocell JR, Tullos HS: Arthroscopic treatment of intraarticular fibrous bands after total knee arthroplasty: A followup note. *Clin Orthop* 1994;309:230–233.
21. Thorpe CD, Bocell JR, Tullos HS: Intra-articular fibrous bands: Patellar complications after total knee replacement. *J Bone Joint Surg* 1990;72A:811–814.
22. Sprague NF III, O'Connor RL, Fox JM: Arthroscopic treatment of postoperative knee fibroarthrosis. *Clin Orthop* 1982;166: 165–172.
23. Sambatakakis A, Wilton TJ, Newton G: Radiographic sign of persistent soft–tissue imbalance after knee replacement. *J Bone Joint Surg* 1991;73B:751–756.
24. Bocell JR, Thorpe CD, Tullos HS: Arthroscopic treatment of symptomatic total knee arthroplasty. *Clin Orthop* 1991;271: 125–134.
25. Stiehl JB, Anouchi Y, Dennis DA, et al: Symposium: Revision total knee replacement. *Contemp Orthop* 1995;30:249–276.
26. Becker MW, Insall JN, Faris PM: Bilateral total knee arthroplasty: One cruciate retaining and one cruciate substituting. *Clin Orthop* 1991;271:122–124.
27. Ranawat CS, Flynn WF Jr: The stiff knee: Ankylosis and flexion, in Lotke PA (ed): *Knee Arthroplasty*, ed 1. New York, NY, Raven Press, 1995, pp 141–159.
28. Johanson NA: Extensor mechanism failure: Treatment of patella fracture, dislocation, and ligament rupture, in Lotke PA (ed): *Knee Arthroplasty*, ed 1. New York, NY, Raven Press, 1995, pp 219–240.

CHAPTER 18

Supracondylar Fracture of the Distal Femur Proximal to a Total Knee Replacement

David C. Ayers, MD

A fracture of the distal femur proximal to a total knee replacement (TKR) presents a challenging problem to the treating orthopaedic surgeon. Historical data documenting the results of these fractures illustrate this challenge.[1-12] Thirteen articles are present in the orthopaedic literature from 1981 to 1989 that report the results of treatment of supracondylar fractures of the distal femur proximal to a TKR. Of the 173 patients included in these 13 studies, 78 were treated surgically and 95 were treated nonsurgically. Good to excellent results were reported in 69% of the patients treated surgically and in 68% of the patients treated nonsurgically. Complications of treatment included malalignment, loss of motion of the knee replacement, nonunion, infection, and the complications associated with prolonged immobilization. Proponents of internal fixation believe that surgical treatment provides the best restoration of mechanical alignment to the limb, permits early mobilization to avoid the complications of prolonged bed rest, and may maximize healing potential in a region where blood supply is already compromised by providing stable fixation.[13,14] Current treatment recommendations include the appropriate use of both surgical and nonsurgical treatment of supracondylar fractures proximal to a TKR.

Incidence

The incidence of supracondylar fracture after TKR is approximately 1%, with reported rates ranging from 0.5% to 2.0%.[1-3,8,12] Conditions that are associated with these fractures include rheumatoid arthritis, chronic steroid therapy, and other conditions that result in osteopenia of the distal femur (Fig. 1). Also, arthrofibrosis of a TKR can predispose to fracture by producing increased stress in the distal femoral metaphysis, particularly at the time of manipulation.[3] The association between notching of the anterior aspect of the distal femur during total knee replacement and subsequent supracondylar fracture has been debated. Aaron and Scott[1] retrospectively reviewed a series of 12 patients with supracondylar fractures and found that, in five of the 12, notching of the anterior cortex of the distal femur had occured during TKR. They concluded that notching of the distal femur predisposed the patient to subsequent supracondylar fracture. Ritter and associates[10] disagree. They reviewed a series of 180 patients who had anterior femoral notching following TKR and found that only one patient had a subsequent supracondylar fracture. Most authors agree, however, that notching of the anterior femur during TKR is to be avoided and is probably of more clinical importance in osteopenic bone.

Treatment

The goals of treating a supracondylar fracture proximal to a total knee arthroplasty are to obtain union of the fracture and return the patient to prefracture function while maintaining knee range of motion. Current treatment recommendations include the appropriate use of surgical and nonsurgical treatment.

Indications for Nonsurgical Treatment

Nonsurgical treatment is recommended for fractures that are nondisplaced and for minimally displaced fractures in which alignment of the fracture and the mechanical axis of the limb is easily achieved and maintained by closed reduction (Fig. 2).[15,16] Patients treated without surgery are placed in a long leg cast for 3 weeks and are allowed to bear weight as tolerated on the affected limb during this period. Three weeks following the fracture, the patient is placed in a cast

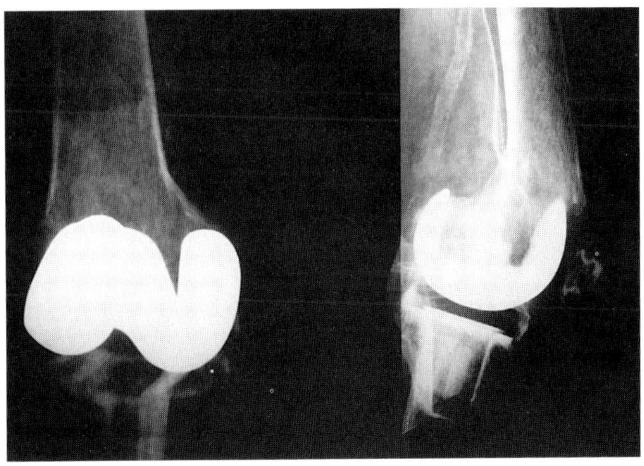

Fig. 1 Anteroposterior and lateral radiographs of a supracondylar fracture in a patient with osteopenic bone.

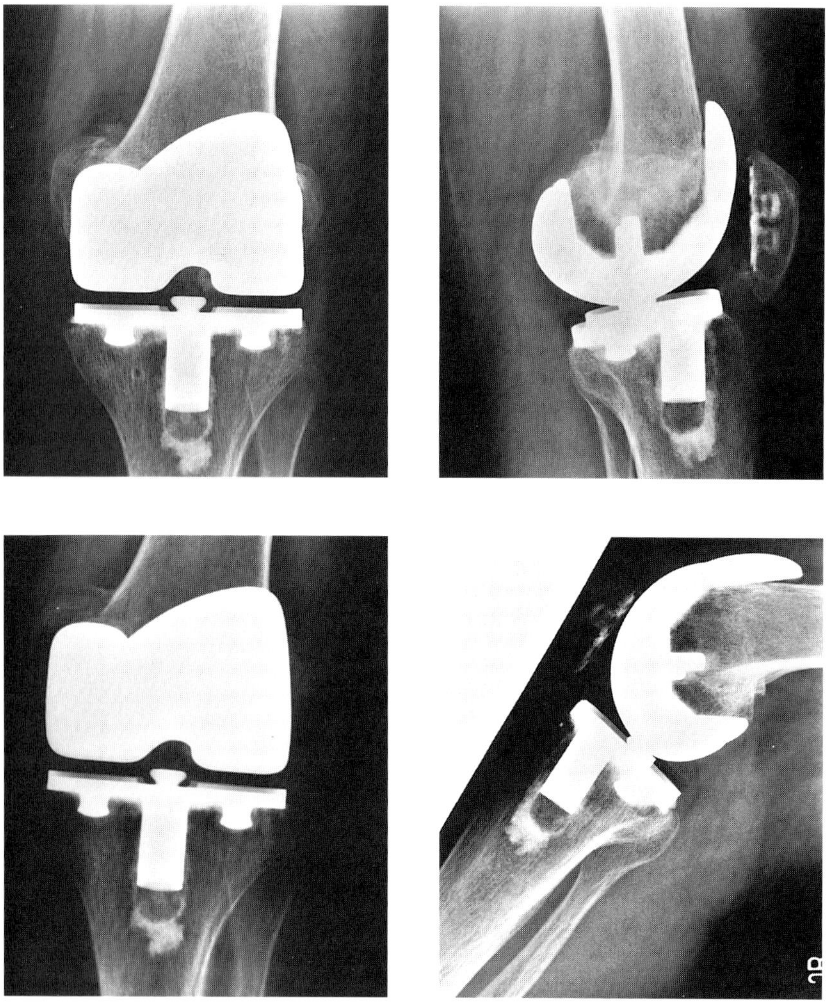

Fig. 2 **Top,** Anteroposterior and lateral radiographs of an impacted supracondylar fracture above a TKR in a patient with rheumatoid arthritis. **Bottom,** Radiographs following conservative treatment show an excellent result.

brace and range of motion exercises are begun. The patient is maintained in a cast brace until there is radiographic evidence of callus and the fracture is healed clinically.

Indications for Surgical Treatment

Surgical treatment of supracondylar fractures above a TKR is indicated in displaced fractures if satisfactory alignment cannot be achieved or maintained by closed reduction (Fig. 3), or if there is radiographic evidence of prosthetic loosening. Surgical treatment should be considered to be elective, and timing of the surgery should allow for a thorough medical evaluation of the patient preoperatively. This includes optimal medical management of any of the many conditions that may have led to the patient's fall, such as a cardiac arrhythmia or electrolyte imbalance. High quality anteroposterior and lateral radiographs must be obtained preoperatively. Prior to beginning internal fixation, it is advisable to have instruments and implants available for both internal fixation of the fracture and long-stem revision TKR. Revision knee replacement may become necessary if stable internal fixation of the fracture cannot be obtained or if previously unrecognized loosening of the implant is discovered intraoperatively.

Choice of Internal Fixation Device

Multiple choices are available to provide secure internal fixation of supracondylar fractures of the distal femur. The supracondylar blade plate and the condylar compression screw and side plate have been used successfully for many years to treat these fractures.[13,14] These devices work best when there is minimal comminution of the distal fragment and for more proximal fractures. The condylar buttress plate is preferable when there is comminution of the distal fragment, because it allows the use of multiple screws to fix the distal fragment. It is thereby more versatile than the condylar blade plate and condylar compression screw systems, which provide a single point of fixation in the

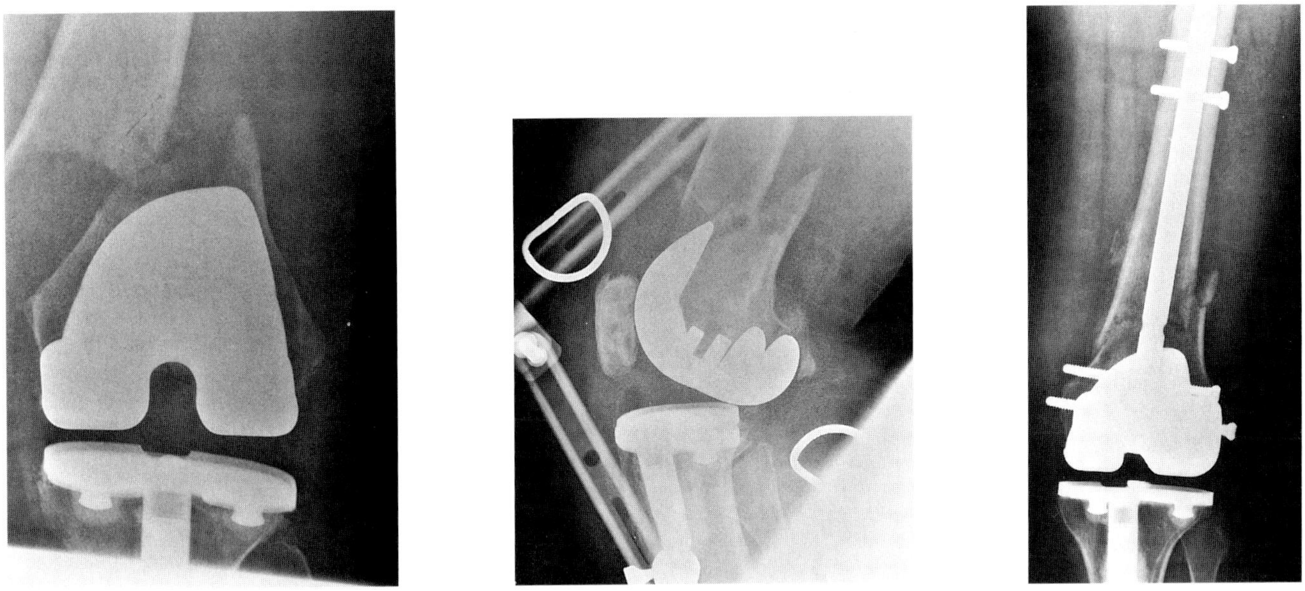

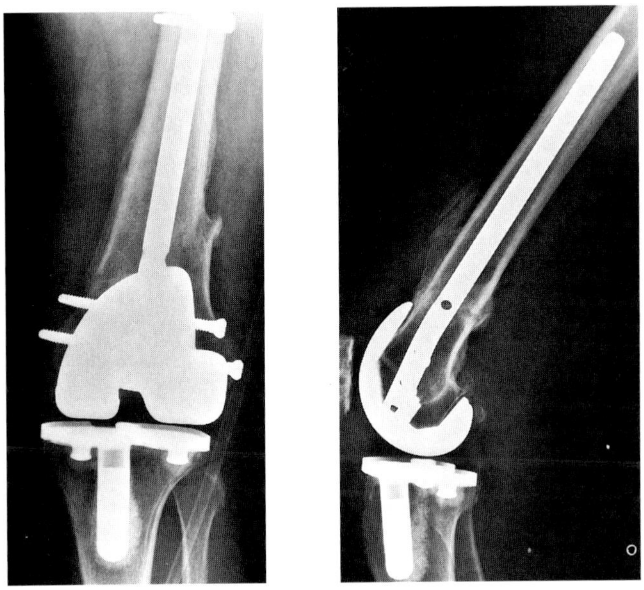

Fig. 3 **Top left** and **center,** Anteroposterior and lateral radiographs of a displaced supracondylar distal femur fracture in a 68-year-old patient 2 years following total knee replacement. **Top right,** Anteroposterior radiograph 6 weeks after surgical stabilization with a locked supracondylar rod. **Bottom,** Anteroposterior and lateral radiographs 6 months after surgery.

distal fragment. Such versatility also makes the condylar buttress plate the preferred device for fixation of the more distal supracondylar femur fractures, and for fractures that may extend into the intercondylar region that are not amenable to internal fixation using the blade plate or condylar compression screw alone.

Internal fixation with an intramedullary rod inserted in a retrograde manner through the knee joint is a new method that has been used successfully to treat supracondylar fractures above knee replacements.[15,17-20] Intramedullary fixation provides an attractive alternative to lateral plate fixation because both the surgical technique and the instrumentation system used for rod insertion are comparatively simple. In addition, intramedullary fixation is biomechanically stronger and less prone to failure than is lateral plate fixation, which has higher bending moments. Intramedullary rods are load-sharing devices that may have some inherent advantages, particularly in treating these patients, who typically have osteopenia of the distal femoral metaphysis with poor cortical bone quality.

Surgical Technique

Lateral Plating

The surgical technique for successful internal fixation of supracondylar femur fractures using a lateral plate and screws is exacting. Anteroposterior and lateral radiographs of high quality must be available preoperatively, and the surgeon should carefully assess the

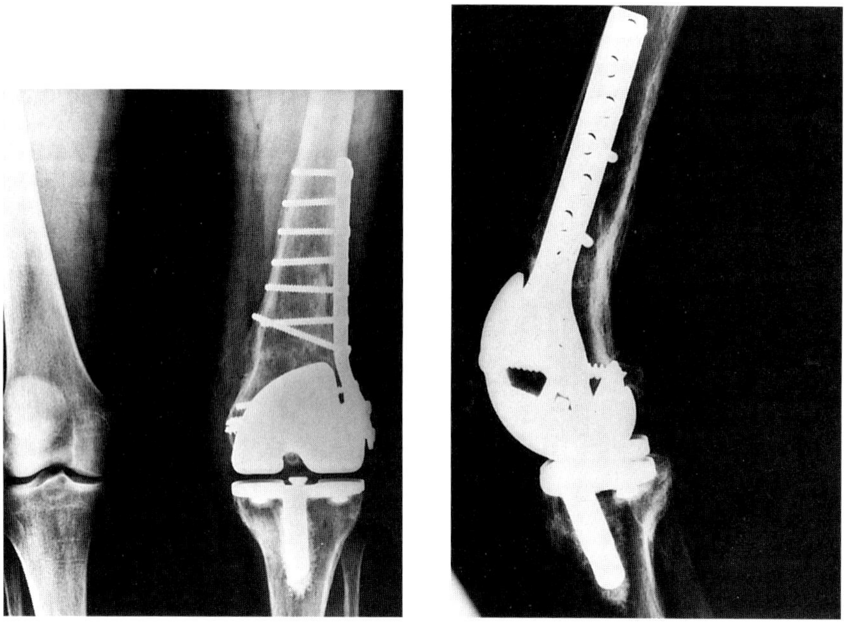

Fig. 4 Anteroposterior and lateral radiographs following open reduction and internal fixation of a supracondylar fracture of the distal femur using a condylar buttress plate.

level of the fracture, the degree of comminution, and the quality of the cortical bone before choosing the type of lateral plate and screw system to be used. The condylar buttress plate is more versatile than the condylar blade plate or the condylar compression screw because multiple screws are used for fixation of the distal fragment. This is of particular benefit for these patients, who have osteopenia of the distal femur and marked comminution of the fracture, which can extend into the intercondylar region.

The patient is positioned in the supine position on a radiolucent operating table to allow use of the C-arm image-intensifier intraoperatively. A hip roll is placed beneath the hip to internally rotate the lower extremity. A sterile tourniquet and an anterior midline incision, which uses the previous total knee scar, are recommended. Extending the midline incision laterally and proximally and continuing in the midline off the tibial crest distally provides excellent exposure. A separate lateral incision, typically used in patients without previous knee replacement, places the soft-tissue blood supply at risk in the tibial tubercle region where the lateral incision comes in close proximity to the anterior knee replacement scar.

An indirect reduction technique must be used for reduction of these fractures intraoperatively.[21] Medial dissection of soft tissues can disrupt this important blood supply and is to be avoided.[21,22] Use of a femoral distractor is beneficial in achieving an anatomic reduction using an indirect reduction technique.[23] If a femoral distractor is not available, an external fixator can be applied temporarily to provide the distraction necessary to successfully carry out an indirect reduction. A Steinmann pin placed into the distal fragment can be used as a joy stick to manipulate the fragment. Once reduction is achieved, the Steinmann pin can be driven across the fracture to provide preliminary fixation until the plate and screws are applied and while the adequacy of the indirect reduction is assessed radiographically via C-arm image-intensifier or plain radiographs. Use of autogenous iliac crest cancellous bone graft is recommended if there is marked comminution of the fracture (Fig. 4).

Locked Intramedullary Rod

Locked supracondylar rods are becoming increasingly popular to treat supracondylar fractures proximal to a total knee replacement (TKR) because of the simplicity of the instrumentation and the simplicity of the surgical technique when compared to lateral plate and screws.[15,17-20] The patient is positioned in the same manner as previously described for lateral plating, supine on a radiolucent table with a hip roll. A nonsterile tourniquet is routinely applied. High quality radiographs must be available preoperatively and the surgeon must know the distance between the prosthetic femoral condyles of the femoral prosthesis. A minimum intercondylar distance of 12 mm is required for use of an intramedullary nail (Table 1). Care must be taken when treating a supracondylar fracture above a posterior stabilized knee replacement to ascertain if the intercondylar box is closed or open. If the in-

Table 1
Intercondylar distances of femoral prostheses

Manufacturer	Prosthesis	Intercondylar Distance
Biomet (Warsaw, IN)	AGC	18 mm
Depuy (Warsaw, IN)	AMK	20 mm
Howmedica (Rutherford, NJ)	PCA	18 mm
Johnson and Johnson (New Brunswick, NJ)	PFC	20 mm
Osteonics (Allendale, NJ)	Omnifit	19 mm
Smith and Nephew-Richards (Memphis, TN)	Genesis	20 mm
Zimmer (Warsaw, IN)	IB-II	15 mm

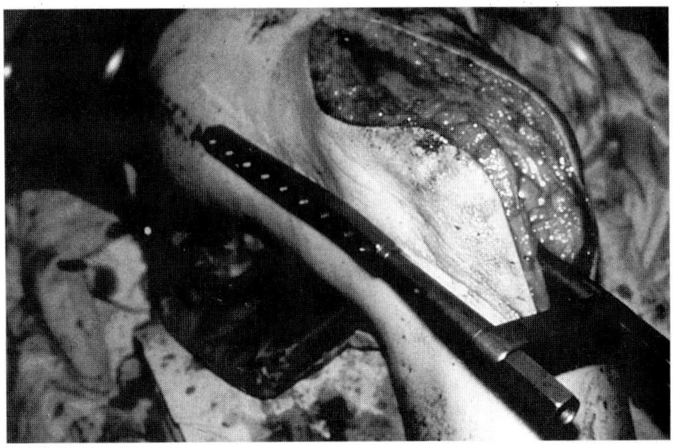

Fig. 5 Insertion of an intramedullary rod to treat a patient with a supracondylar fracture of the distal femur.

tercondylar box is closed, use of a retrograde nail is contraindicated, because there is no access to the medullary canal.

A routine revision total knee exposure is performed using the anterior midline scar. Care should be taken not to dissect the medial or lateral soft tissues attached to the fracture, but to remain directly anterior. The knee is flexed 45° to 55° over a sterile bolster. An open reduction is achieved through the fracture, using a bone hook to correct the typical recurvatum deformity and reduction forceps to achieve reduction in the coronal plane. Provisional reduction is then obtained by the surgeon, who places one hand behind the proximal border of the tibia and pulls forward, a maneuver similar to that used when performing an anterior drawer test. The reduction is verified by C-arm image-intensifier. The medullary canal is then entered at a point midway between the condyles. This is the same starting point used for intramedullary instrumentation during TKR surgery. The medullary canal is progressively reamed over a guide wire in 0.5-mm increments to a diameter 1.0 to 1.5 mm larger than the selected supracondylar nail. Nail diameters typically range from 11 to 13 mm, and are available in a variety of lengths. Use of preoperative templates aids in selection of the nail diameter and length. A larger diameter nail is preferred, and use of the 25-cm or longer nail will help to centralize the nail within the femoral diaphysis and minimize varus or valgus malalignment of the fracture. The intramedullary nail is then assembled to the guide bar used for insertion of the interlocking screws on the back table and the alignment rod is placed through the most proximal and then the most distal interlocking hole in the intramedullary rod to check that the assembly procedure has been properly performed. The rod is inserted over the guidewire, while performing the anterior drawer reduction maneuver, and is advanced by hand pressure until the proximal aspect of the nail is 2 mm beneath the articular surface (Fig. 5). Multiple 5.0 locking screws are then placed percutaneously, using the guide system; typically, two screws are placed in the distal fragment and two in the proximal fragment (Fig. 6). The option of using bolts with nuts is available for patients with marked osteopenia of the distal fragment.

Revision Total Knee Replacement

Revision TKR using a long-stem femoral component is recommended for all patients who have loosening of the femoral component associated with the supracondylar femur fracture. Because it may be difficult to accurately predict femoral component stability from preoperative radiographs, it is recommended that instruments and prosthetic components necessary for revision TKR be available at the time that internal fixation is undertaken. During revision TKR for supracondylar fracture, one must retain the collateral ligaments and avoid cement extrusion into the fracture. In instances in which there is severe comminution in the region of the origin of the collateral ligament, a modular metaphyseal femoral replacement (tumor type of prosthesis) or a combination of a distal femoral allograft and a revision femoral component with an intramedullary stem may be used.[23]

Treatment Results

The results of surgical treatment of supracondylar fractures proximal to TKRs using the techniques and devices described here, which were developed during the 1990s, have demonstrated markedly improved results over those of earlier studies. Healy and associ-

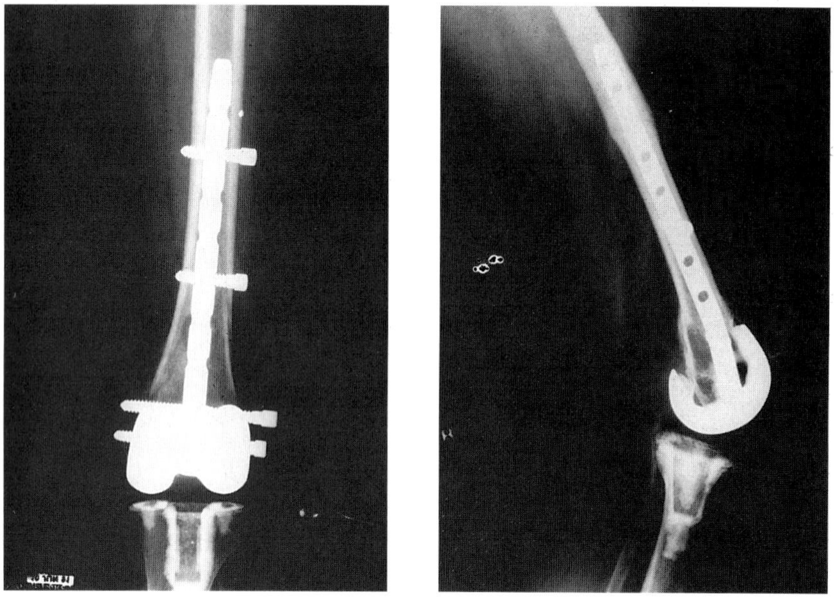

Fig. 6 Anteroposterior and lateral radiographs 6 months after placement of a locked intramedullary rod to treat a fracture of the distal femur above a total knee replacement.

ates[16] reported the results of a series of 20 patients treated by open reduction, bone grafting (15 of the 20), and internal fixation using a lateral plate. In these 20 patients, seven were treated with a condylar blade plate, seven with a condylar compression plate, and six with a condylar buttress plate. Union was achieved in 18 of the 20 patients (90%) without additional surgery at an average of 16 weeks (range 6 to 26 weeks). Nonunion requiring additional surgery was found in two of the 20 patients (10%). Union was achieved in both of these patients after a second surgery, which included autologous bone grafting. Ten of the 20 patients had delayed union, requiring greater than 4 months to have radiographic signs of union. McLaren and associates[20] reported on seven patients with supracondylar fractures proximal to a TKR that were treated with a supracondylar nail. This report documented radiographic evidence of union by 6 weeks in six of the seven patients. Complete union had occurred in all seven patients by 12 weeks. Subsequent studies of fractures treated by locked supracondylar nail have reported radiographic union by 12 weeks, with low rates of delayed or nonunion. In a large multicenter series[17] that reported on 41 such fractures internally fixed with a locked intramedullary rod, delayed union occurred in three patients (7.2%), and a nonunion in one patient (2.4%). The mean time to union was 13 weeks for the remaining 38 patients.

Successful surgical treatment of supracondylar fractures of the distal femur proximal to a TKR requires meticulous surgical technique and careful attention to detail. Nondisplaced fractures or minimally displaced fractures that can be reduced closed are best treated nonsurgically. Displaced supracondylar fractures in which closed reduction cannot be achieved or maintained are best treated surgically, using lateral plating or a locked intramedullary rod. The simplicity of the surgical technique and the simplicity of the instrumentation for intramedullary fixation using a locked intramedullary rod is a significant advantage in comparison with internal fixation with a lateral plate and screws. Surgical treatment of displaced supracondylar fractures with locked supracondylar rods has reduced the incidence of delayed union and nonunion,[4,5,16,17] as well as the incidence of surgical revision, when compared with internal fixation using a lateral plate. For these reasons, the use of locked supracondylar rods is worthy of consideration for treatment of these challenging fractures.

References

1. Aaron RK, Scott R: Supracondylar fracture of the femur after total knee arthroplasty. *Clin Orthop* 1987;219:136–139.
2. Bogoch E, Hastings D, Gross A, et al: Supracondylar fractures of the femur adjacent to resurfacing and MacIntosh arthroplasties of the knee in patients with rheumatoid arthritis. *Clin Orthop* 1988;229:213–220.
3. Culp RW, Schmidt RG, Hanks G, et al: Supracondylar fracture of the femur following prosthetic knee arthroplasty. *Clin Orthop* 1987;222:212–222.
4. Figgie MP, Goldberg VM, Figgie HE III, et al: The results of treatment of supracondylar fracture above total knee arthroplasty. *J Arthroplasty* 1990;5:267–276.
5. Hirsh DM, Bhalla S, Roffman M: Supracondylar fracture of the femur following total knee replacement: Report of 4 cases. *J Bone Joint Surg* 1981;63A:162–163.
6. Insall JN, Haas SB: Complications of total knee arthroplasty, in Insall JN, Windsor RE, Scott WN, et al (eds): *Surgery of the*

Knee, ed 2. New York, NY, Churchill Livingstone, 1993, vol 2, pp 891–934.

7. Lotke PA, Ecker ML: Influence of positioning of prosthesis in total knee replacement. *J Bone Joint Surg* 1977;59A:77–79.
8. Merkel KD, Johnson EW Jr: Supracondylar fracture of the femur after total knee arthroplasty. *J Bone Joint Surg* 1986;68A:29–43.
9. Nielsen BF, Petersen VS, Vanmarken JE: Fracture of the femur after knee arthroplasty. *Acta Orthop Scand* 1988;59:155–157.
10. Ritter MA, Faris PM, Keating EM: Anterior femoral notching and ipsilateral supracondylar femur fracture in total knee arthroplasty. *J Arthroplasty* 1988;3:185–187.
11. Sanders R, Regazzoni P, Ruedi TP: Treatment of supracondylar-intracondylar fractures of the femur using the dynamic condylar screw. *J Orthop Trauma* 1989;3:214–222.
12. Sisto DJ, Lachiewicz PF, Insall JN: Treatment of supracondylar fractures following prosthetic arthroplasty of the knee. *Clin Orthop* 1985;196:265–272.
13. Schatzker J: Supracondylar fractures of the femur, in Schatzker J, Tile M (eds): *The Rationale of Operative Fracture Care.* Berlin, Germany, Springer-Verlag, 1987, pp 255–273.
14. Zehntner MK, Ganz R: Internal fixation of supracondylar fractures after condylar total knee arthroplasty. *Clin Orthop* 1993; 293:219–224.
15. Rolston LR, Christ DJ, Halpern A, et al: Treatment of supracondylar fractures of the femur proximal to a total knee arthroplasty: A report of four cases. *J Bone Joint Surg* 1995;77A:924–931.
16. Healy WL, Siliski JM, Incavo SJ: Operative treatment of distal femoral fractures proximal to total knee replacements. *J Bone Joint Surg* 1993;75A:27–34.
17. Henry SL, Busconi B, Gold S, et al: Management of supracondylar femur fractures proximal to total knee prostheses with the GSH supracondylar intramedullary nail. *Orthop Trans* 1995; 19:153.
18. Henry SL, Booth RE Jr: Management of supracondylar fractures above total knee prostheses. *Tech Orthop* 1995;9:243–252.
19. Jabczenski FF, Crawford M: Retrograde intramedullary nailing of supracondylar femur fractures above total knee arthroplasty: A preliminary report of four cases. *J Arthroplasty* 1995;10:95–101.
20. McLaren AC, Dupont JA, Schroeber DC: Open reduction internal fixation of supracondylar fractures above total knee arthroplasties using the intramedullary supracondylar rod. *Clin Orthop* 1994;302:194–198.
21. Mast J, Jakob R, Ganz R: Reduction with plates, in Mast J, Jakob R, Ganz R (eds): *Planning and Reduction Technique in Fracture Surgery.* Berlin, Germany, Springer-Verlag, 1989, pp 48–129.
22. Schatzker J: Screws and plates and their application, in Müller ME, Allgöwer M, Schneider R, et al (eds): *Manual of Internal Fixation: Techniques Recommended by the AO-ASIF Group.* Berlin, Germany, Springer-Verlag, 1991, pp 179–290.
23. Kraay MJ, Goldberg VM, Figgie MP, et al: Distal femoral replacement with allograft/prosthetic reconstruction for treatment of supracondylar fractures in patients with total knee arthroplasty. *J Arthroplasty* 1992;7:7–16.

CHAPTER 19

Polyethylene Wear and Osteolysis Following Total Knee Replacement

David C. Ayers, MD

Polyethylene wear and osteolysis following total knee replacement (TKR) surgery may result from many factors, such as surgical technique, patient selection, and choice of implant design, which directly impact the polyethylene wear rate. Surgical technique is intimately associated with polyethylene wear; particularly the thickness of the polyethylene insert, the postoperative mechanical axis of the limb, and the alignment of the tibial component in the coronal plane (Fig. 1). Patient selection is important because patient body weight and activity level have been shown to correlate with polyethylene wear rate. Prosthetic design also plays a role in polyethylene wear, because femoral-tibial contact areas, peak contact forces, and surface topography of the polyethylene are important considerations. Polyethylene quality and method of sterilization are also important. Wear of polyethylene is one source of particulate debris following TKR. Phagocytosis of the particulate debris by macrophages occurs at the prosthesis-bone interface. The macrophages produce inflammatory mediators in response to the particulate debris. Inflammatory mediators, such as interleukin-1 (IL-1), tumor necrosis factor (TNF), interleukin-6 (IL-6), and prostaglandin E_2 (PGE_2), act at the failed interface to effect bone resorption and produce osteolysis.

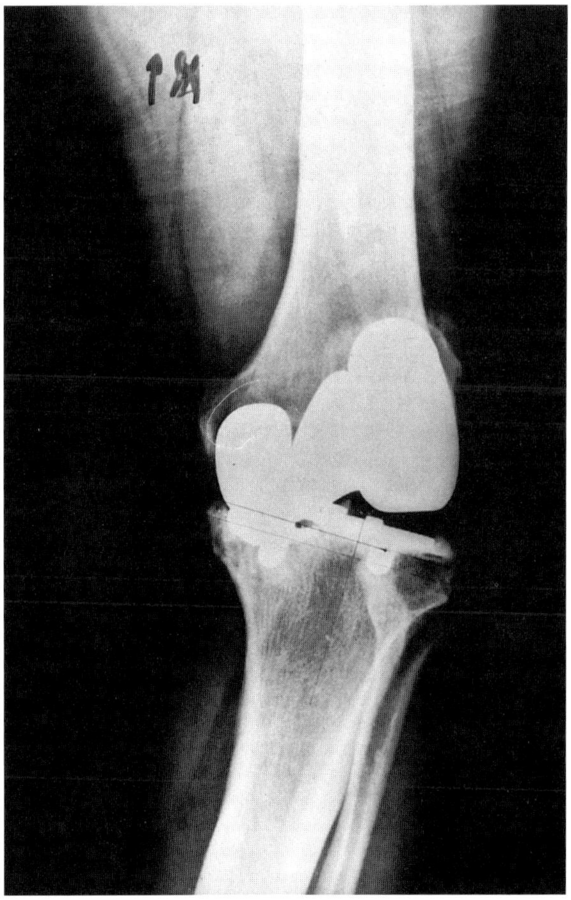

Fig. 1 Catastrophic wear of the polyethylene insert in a 55-year-old, active, overweight male patient with varus postoperative limb alignment following total knee replacement and varus coronal position of the tibial component.

Incidence of Polyethylene Wear Following TKR

A high incidence of accelerated polyethylene wear was reported by Kilgus and associates[1] in 1991. A series of 176 porous-coated anatomic (PCA) TKRs performed between 1981 and 1987 with a mean follow-up of 60 months was evaluated retrospectively. The average postoperative mechanical axis of the limb in this series was neutral. Greater than 30% of the patients showed radiographic evidence of polyethylene wear. Ten percent of the patients underwent revision surgery due to severe polyethylene wear or fracture of the polyethylene insert.

Tsao and associates[2] reviewed 487 PCA TKRs performed by a single surgeon between 1982 and 1989. There were 32 clinical failures (7%) caused by severe wear of the surfaces of the tibial and patellar polyethylene components. Thirty of these patients underwent revision, and the average time to failure was 4.5 years. Significant predictors of an increased risk of failure were thin polyethylene tibial inserts, increased patient weight, and decreased patient age. Examination of the retrieved tibial components revealed extensive delamination caused by fracture of the polyethylene at a depth of about 1 mm below the articular surface. The accelerated rate of polyethylene wear in this series and the series of Kilgus and associates[1] may be attributed to heat treatment of the polyethylene, use of thin polyethylene tibial components, relatively low femoral-tibial contact areas, and high maximal contact stresses.

Wasielewski and associates[3] examined 55 tibial polyethylene components retrieved at revision total knee arthroplasty for evidence of wear after a mean implan-

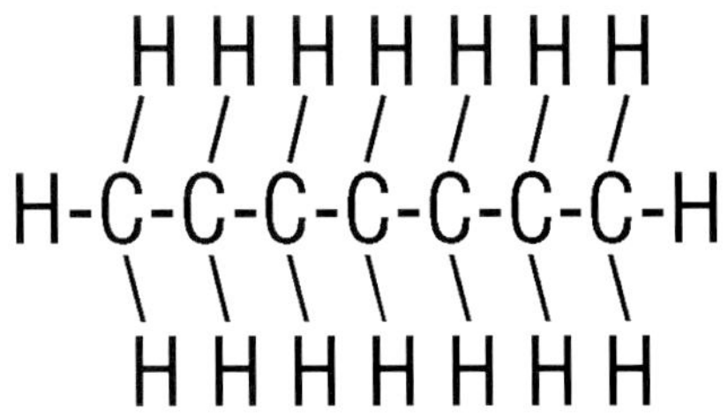

Fig. 2 Linear chemical structure of polyethylene.

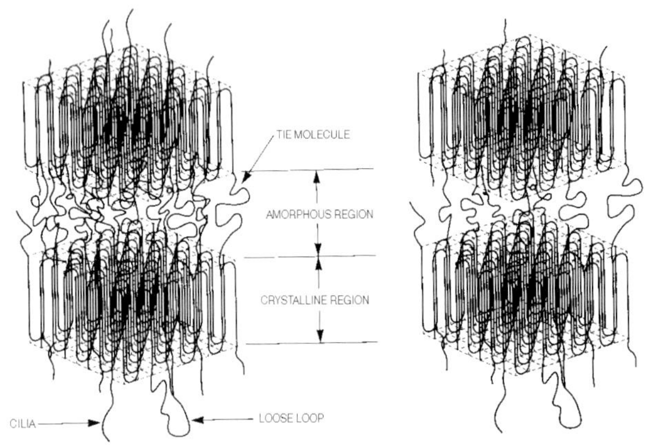

Fig. 3 **Left,** Molecular structure of ultra-high molecular weight polyethylene (UHMPWE). **Right,** Molecular structure of high-density polyethylene. (Reproduced with permission from *Overview and Fundamentals of UHMWPE.* Rutherford, NJ, Howmedica, 1994, p 3.)

tation of 34.2 months. Twenty tibial components retrieved were ultra-high molecular weight polyethylene (UHMWPE) and 35 were carbon-reinforced polyethylene. Severe generalized articular wear was seen in inserts with three-body wear from metal and cement debris. Severe localized delamination wear was seen in inserts with rotational-subluxation patterns of wear. Preoperative varus was found to be related to the occurrence of posteromedial cold flow of polyethylene into tibial tray screw holes. Increasing tibial insert posterior slope was associated with increasingly posterior articular wear track location. Articular wear and cold flow into screw holes tended to be greater in the tightest pre-arthroplasty compartment—medial in varus knees and lateral in valgus knees. The authors concluded that wear patterns and the severity of UHMWPE wear in unconstrained tibial components may be associated with clinical and mechanical factors under the surgeon's control, including component size and position, knee alignment, and ligament balance.[3]

A total of 665 patients underwent revision TKR at the Mayo Clinic from July 1983 to November 1990.[4] In 24 of these 665 patients (3.6%), revision arthroplasty was performed following gross failure of the UHMWPE insert. Although there were multiple styles of knee replacements in this series of 24 polyethylene failures, there are three features common to this group of patients. In all 24 patients, the tibial component was positioned in varus, resulting in varus postoperative alignment of the limb, and the UHMWPE thickness of the tibial component was equal to or less than 9 mm. Because this measurement typically included the metal backing of the tibial component, the actual thickness of the UHMWPE itself ranged between 4 and 7 mm in the thinnest area of the insert. Of these 24 patients, 12 (50%) exceeded their ideal body weight by more than 20%.[4]

One may conclude from these clinical studies that the problem of polyethylene wear is a multifactorial problem in knee replacement surgery and involves such diverse factors as patient selection, surgical technique, and UHMWPE quantity and quality. To better understand how UHMWPE quantity and quality relate to UHMWPE wear, it is necessary to review the molecular structure of polyethylene, how it is manufactured and sterilized, and biomechanical studies investigating how UHMWPE functions as a weightbearing material.

Structure of Polyethylene

Polyethylene is a long-chain polymer composed of a carbon chain backbone with hydrogen subgroups (Fig. 2). Polyethylene grades differ primarily on the basis of molecular weight and the number of branches that make up the polymer chain. Medical grade UHMWPE, which accounts for approximately 0.1% of the annual production of polyethylene, has a molecular weight greater than 1 million. As is typical of semicrystalline polymers, UHMWPE has a microstructure consisting of crystalline regions that are highly ordered, as well as amorphous or disordered regions (Fig. 3). Surrounding and connecting the crystalline regions are the bridging tie molecules. One major difference between the morphology of UHMWPE and that of regular high-density polyethylene (HDPE) is the higher number of tie molecules in the UHMWPE. These tie molecules act as cross-links between the crystalline regions and provide improved load bearing, stress transfer, and chemical and physical strength. Despite current concerns regarding wear, UHMWPE, when used properly, remains the best polymer available for use in TKR today because of its unique material properties, which include high impact resistance, high ductility, high abrasion resistance and good chemical resistance, and biocompatibility when compared to other polymers.[5]

Three methods are currently used to make medical grade UHMWPE devices. In direct compression molding, polyethylene powder is placed into a mold, which

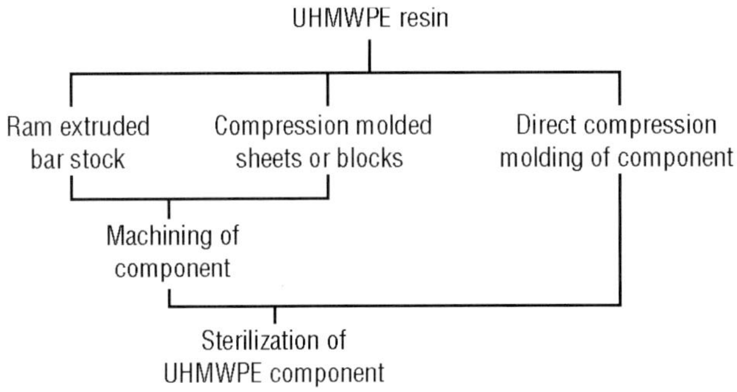

Fig. 4 The manufacturing process for ultra-high molecular weight polyethylene (UHMWPE) surgical implants.

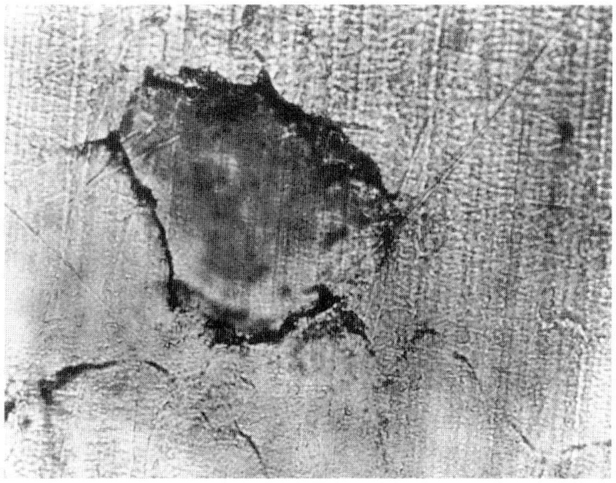

Fig. 5 Photomicrograph of typical fusion defect found in ultra-high molecular weight polyethylene. (Reproduced with permission from Li S, Burstein AH: Ultra-high molecular weight polyethylene: The material and its use in total joint implants. *J Bone Joint Surg* 1994;76A:1080–1090.)

is then heated under pressure to compress it into the final shape of the device. Devices made in this manner have no external machining lines. A second method is ram-extrusion of the powder into cylindrical bar stock. The implant is then machined from the bar stock. A third method involves compression molding of large sheets of UHMWPE. The implant is then machined from the sheet (Fig. 4).[5]

UHMWPE Quality

The quality of the UHMWPE affects the wear characteristics of a UHMWPE component. Authors have reported the presence of defects in UHMWPE tibial components. These defects have been observed with the unaided eye, as well as by means of x-ray defraction and optical analyses (Fig. 5).[6-10] Impurities, also called inclusions, have also been found within the UHMWPE. The most common inclusion is calcium stearate. Inclusions have been found to be closely associated with fusion defects within the UHMWPE (Fig. 6).[10] Fusion defects are areas within the UHMWPE component where there are areas of polyethylene powder that did not consolidate completely during the manufacturing process. Fusion defect areas are highly susceptible to damage after implantation when the UHMWPE is subjected to stress. In an implant retrieval study, Wrona and associates[10] showed a statistically significant correlation between fusion defects and UHMWPE component total wear, delamination, and cracking.

UHMWPE Sterilization

Sterilization of UHMWPE devices can cause structural changes that alter the mechanical properties of the device and lead to rapid wear and early failure of the implant. The majority of UHMWPE implants are currently sterilized by gamma radiation. Typically, 2.5 Mrad is used. Gamma radiation in air causes oxidation of the UHMWPE, which alters the physical structure of the material by scission of individual polymer chains.[11] Chain scission produces free radicals, which, in an air environment, combine with oxygen to cause oxidative degradation. Oxidative degradation decreases the molecular weight of the UHMWPE, and the resultant increased mobility of the shortened polyethylene chains allows for a change in orientation and an increase in the percentage of the material that is crystalline.[12,13] Oxidative degradation of the UHMWPE continues during the shelf life of the implant.[11] The shelf life is defined as the time elapsed between the sterilization and implantation of the implant. Alternate methods of sterilization are currently being explored to sterilize UHMPE without causing oxidation. Gamma radiation in an inert, nonoxygen environment and use of ethylene oxide are two methods currently being tested.

UHMWPE In Vivo Degradation

Oxidative degradation also occurs in vivo after implantation of a UHMWPE component.[11,13] The greatest changes occur on the surface of the implant, because oxidative degradation is a diffusion-controlled process. Measured changes are highest at the articulating surface because the degradative process appears to be accelerated, through an as yet unknown process, by the mechanical forces transmitted across the articular surface. Wrona and associates[10] have studied the oxidative changes that occur in vivo following sterilization by gamma radiation. Oxidative changes are typically seen grossly as a "white band" at the edge of the UHMWPE.

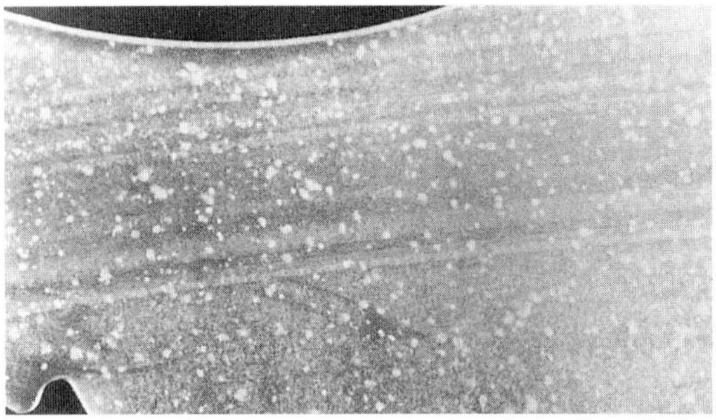

Fig. 6 Fusion defects within ultra-high molecular weight polyethylene (UHMWPE). These are areas of unconsolidated UHMWPE particles. (Reproduced with permission from Li S, Burstein AH: Ultra-high molecular weight polyethylene: The material and its use in total joint implants. *J Bone Joint Surg* 1994;76A:1080–1090.)

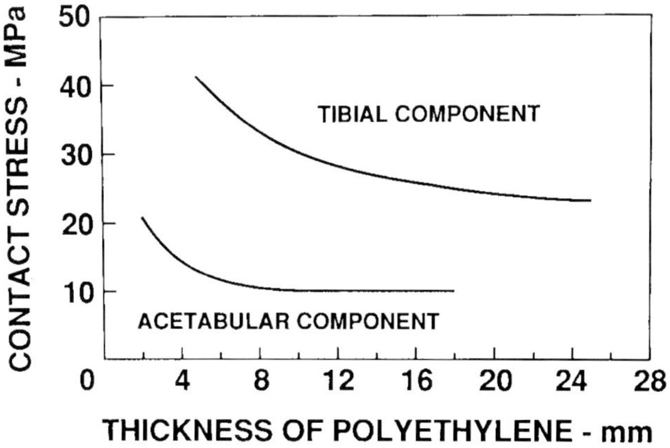

Fig. 7 As the thickness of a polyethylene component decreases, the contact stress perpendicular to the surface increases. Because it is a less conforming surface, the stresses are greater for the tibial component of a total knee replacement at all thicknesses of polyethylene than they are for the acetabular component. A minimum thickness of 8 mm of true polyethylene should be chosen for tibial components. (Reproduced with permission from Bartel DL, Rimnac CM, Wright TM: Evaluation and design of the articular surface, in Goldberg VM (ed): *Controversies of Total Knee Arthroplasty*. New York, NY, Raven Press, 1991, pp 61–73.)

UHMWPE Thickness

Polyethylene thickness is an important determinant of contact stress distribution within a UHMWPE component and the associated UHMWPE damage. Bartel and associates[14] in 1985 delineated the relationship between polyethylene thickness and contact stress in metal-backed UHMWPE implants. The authors showed that the contact stresses increase exponentially when the thickness of the UHMWPE decreases (Fig. 7). Based on their studies, which used a relatively dished articular geometry, they recommended that a minimum of 8 to 10 mm of UHMWPE thickness be used in knee replacements.

Widespread use of metal-backed tibial components in knee replacement surgery has resulted in a potential dilemma for surgeons; they must either resect more bone from the proximal tibia to accommodate the metal backing or use a thinner polyethylene component. Advantages of metal-backed tibial components are that the metal backing stiffens the overall structure and allows more even distribution of load transfer to the supporting bone. Metal backing also prevents gross deformation of the UHMWPE. The disadvantage of the metal-backed tibial component is that as the metal backing is added, the thickness of the UHMWPE is often decreased. Manufacturers often include the thickness of the metal backing with the thickness of the UHMWPE when labeling a polyethylene insert. If the true thickness of the UHMWPE falls below the 8- to 10-mm limit recommended by Bartel and associates,[14] the device becomes more susceptible to surface damage, deformation, and catastrophic failure.

Surgeons may incorrectly emphasize preserving proximal tibial bone by minimizing resection of the proximal tibia during TKR. Goldstein and associates[15] demonstrated that the mechanical strength of the proximal tibia bone diminishes with increasing distance from the articular surface. Fixation of the tibial component in weaker bone could theoretically result in increased potential for implant loosening. Thus the surgeon must choose whether to preserve bone of the proximal tibia in order to fix the component in the strongest supportive bone possible, which requires use of a thinner UHMWPE insert, or to remove the correct amount of proximal tibia necessary to allow use of a tibial insert of at least 8 to 10 mm of true UHMWPE thickness in addition to the metal backing. Because the mechanical performance of UHMWPE as a weight-bearing material depends directly on the thickness of the UHMWPE, it is strongly recommended that adequate bone resection of the proximal tibia be performed to allow use of 8 to 10 mm of true UHMWPE at the tibial component articulating surface.

UHMWPE Damage Following TKR

Polyethylene damage of tibial components in TKR has been extensively studied.[1,6-9,16] Retrieval studies have correlated the duration of implantation and patient body weight with the extent of UHMWPE damage. In one study, the three most common modes of damage were found to be abrasive wear, adhesive wear, and delamination.[9] Landy and Walker,[8] in an implant retrieval study, found a high incidence of three-body wear resulting from the entrapment of a third body, such as a bone or polymethylmethacrylate fragment, between the femoral condyle and the UHMWPE. Delamination, consisting of complete breakup of material

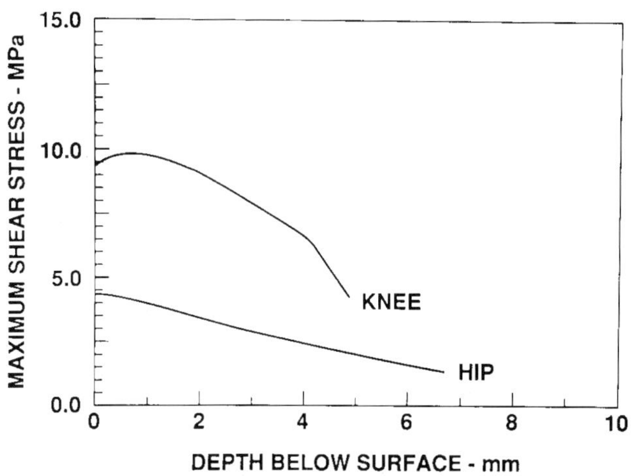

Fig. 8 The magnitude and location of the maximum shear stress for knee and hip replacements (28-mm head). (Reproduced with permission from Bartel DL, Rimnac CM, Wright TM: Evaluation and design of the articular surface, in Goldberg VM (ed): *Controversies of Total Knee Arthroplasty*. New York, NY, Raven Press, 1991, pp 61–73.)

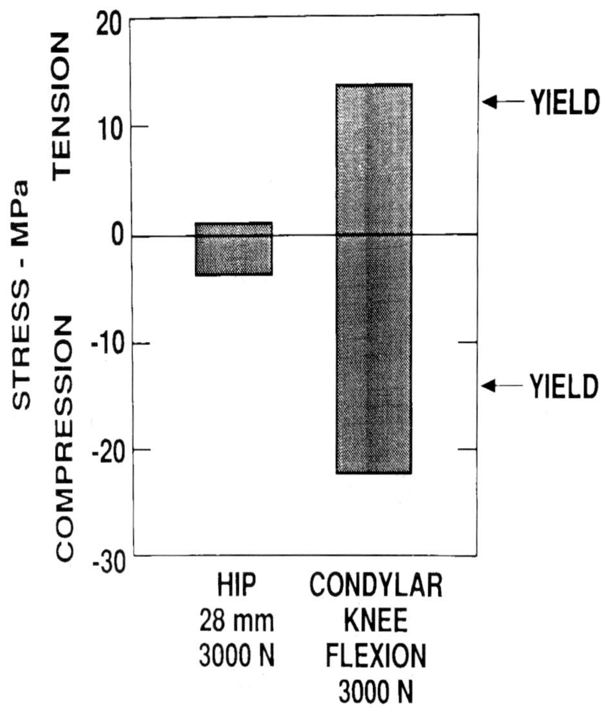

Fig. 9 The range of maximum principal stress for knee replacements and hip replacements (28-mm femoral head) in extension and flexion. The values below the axis represent compressive stress. (Reproduced with permission from Bartel DL, Rimnac CM, Wright TM: Evaluation and design of the articular surface, in Goldberg VM (ed): *Controversies of Total Knee Arthroplasty*. New York, NY, Raven Press, 1991, pp 61–73.)

in flakes and particles, was also observed and appeared to be initiated by intergranular fusion defects within UHMWPE. These defects were propagated by the subsurface shear stresses beneath the contact zone (Fig. 8). Maximum shear stresses in the UHMWPE occur at a depth of 1 to 2 mm beneath the articular surface. In vivo testing to 10 million cycles demonstrated that if the location of contact between the prosthetic femoral condyles and the UHMWPE remained constant, some surface deformation was observed but surface damage was minimal.[4] However, if sliding was allowed in the sagittal plane, severe delamination and numerous subsurface cracks developed. Blunn and associates[17] have concluded that minimization of sliding and maintenance of relatively localized contact area minimizes UHMWPE wear.

In vitro testing and finite element analysis have demonstrated that compressive and tensile stresses that exceed the endurance of the UHMWPE exist in tibial components of TKRs.[18,19] The yield stress of UHMWPE is approximately 15 MPa. Contact stresses in conforming total knee designs have been shown to vary from 25 MPa compression to 15 MPa tension (Fig. 9). These stresses are significantly higher than the contact stresses that are present in hip replacements, where the articular surface is more conforming. These findings are consistent with implant retrieval studies that show that the less conforming tibial components from TKRs experienced greater surface UHMWPE damage than did acetabular components from total hip replacements. Conformity is an important consideration in TKR prosthetic design. Conformity in the coronal plane has been shown to have a greater effect on contact stresses than conformity in the sagittal plane (Fig. 10).[18] The effects of large compressive and tensile maximum stresses are compounded in TKR's because the contact area size and location change during flexion and extension. The UHMWPE of the tibial component is thus subjected to cyclic stresses that are an order of magnitude greater than the cyclic stresses that the acetabular component is subject to. Posterior cruciate-retaining designs typically have a less conforming, or flatter, UHMWPE tibial sagittal geometry to permit roll back and function of the posterior cruciate ligament. Studies have been conducted that compare the surface contact areas and areas of maximum contact stresses between various posterior cruciate-retaining knee implants and between various posterior cruciate-sacrificing implants.[20] More conforming surfaces have been associated with a lower incidence of UHMWPE wear in clinical use.[21] Plante-Bordeneuve and Freeman[22] studied UHMWPE wear following TKR in 27 patients with up to 9-year follow-up. The design of the components gave a nominal contact area of 320 mm^2 on each condyle. For the tibial component, the

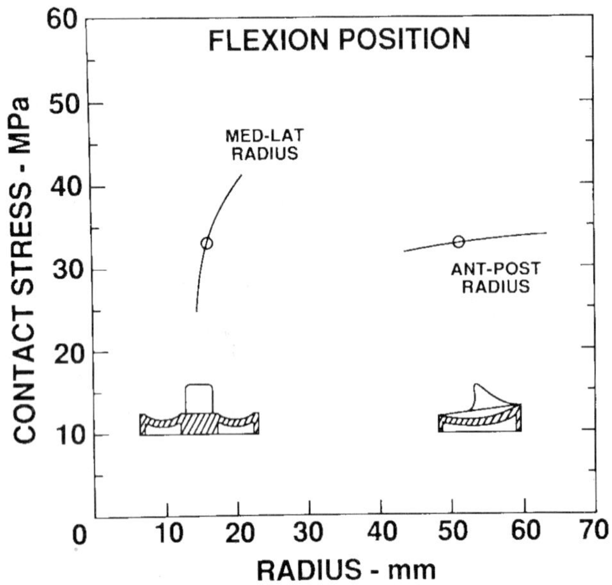

Fig. 10 Compressive contact stress on the tibial component polyethylene as a function of the geometry of the contact surfaces. Note that conformity in the coronal plane has a greater effect on contact stress than conformity in the sagittal plane. (Reproduced with permission from Bartel DL, Rimnac CM, Wright TM: Evaluation and design of the articular surface, in Goldberg VM (ed): *Controversies of Total Knee Arthroplasty*. New York, NY, Raven Press, 1991, pp 6–73.)

UHMWPE was at least 6 mm thick and was not heat-treated. The average wear rate was 0.025 mm/year. The relative wear in the medial and lateral compartments was related to the axis of the leg. None of the retrieved components showed any severe disruption of their surface. The authors concluded that the rate of wear of UHMWPE in a conforming tibiofemoral bearing with a fixed tibial component is slow enough to be safe for use in clinical practice.[22]

Prevalence of Osteolysis Following TKR

The prevalence of tibial osteolysis in cementless TKRs was reported by Peters and associates[23] after a review of 174 consecutive cementless TKR patients. Twenty-seven of these patients (16%) were found to have radiographic evidence of osteolysis at an average of 35 months after the procedure. Of the 27 patients with osteolysis, 15 underwent revision surgery after an average of 45 months. The medial aspect of the tibial metaphysis was the most common radiographic site for osteolysis, being affected in 24 of the 27 patients with osteolysis. Sequential radiographs demonstrated progressive extension of the osteolytic process around the tibial base plate, from which it extended distally into the tibial metaphysis along the screw-bone interface. The average age of the patients who had osteolysis was 63 years, and their average weight was 76 kg. Mechanical failure of the thin, modular polyethylene insert and excessive abrasion of the prominent polyethylene tibial eminence resulted in secondary wear and impingement of the pin on the femoral component. This failure mechanism was believed to contribute to the extensive amount of polyethylene debris generated by this prothesis, which resulted in the osteolysis in the tibial metaphysis.

Cadambi and associates[24] reported an 11.1% incidence of femoral osteolysis in a series of 271 primary TKRs (30 cases of osteolysis in 28 patients). Femoral osteolysis was observed in 26 Synatomic and 4 PCA knees. The average time to the diagnosis of the femoral osteolysis was 31 months (range, 7 to 96 months). All of the femoral components with osteolysis had cementless implantation. Wear of the thin tibial inserts and patellar components were two sources of particulate polyethylene. The authors postulate that histiocytic granuloma gained access to the proximal femur primarily via the unbonded interface between the smooth metal and bone. Statistically significant factors associated with femoral osteolysis included male gender, younger age, increased patient weight, the presence of tibial osteolysis, a preoperative diagnosis of osteoarthritis, and increasing length of time in situ.

Kim and associates[25] reported the incidence of osteolysis in the femur, tibia, and patella of 60 consecutive cementless PCA TKRs in 44 patients. At a mean follow-up of 7 years, radiographs revealed osteolysis in the tibial plateau of 90% of the patients and the patella of 80%. No osteolysis was reported in the distal femur. The average wear of the polyethylene liner was 2.5 mm in the medial compartment and 1.7 mm in the lateral compartment. The authors concluded that fixation of the tibial and patellar components without cement fails to seal the interface between bone and prosthesis and allows the migration of polyethylene particulate debris, which causes osteolysis.

Robinson and associates[26] reviewed 185 revision TKRs over a 16-year period in London, Ontario. Seventeen of these 185 patients (9.2%) were identified as having severe osteolysis. The average age was 62.7 years and the average weight was 90.8 kg. The average time interval from the index surgery to radiographic evidence of osteolysis was 56 months. Radiographic review showed gross polyethylene wear in ten patients, loose tibial implants in eight patients, fractured tibial baseplates in two patients, and evidence of a metallic synovitis in two patients. Retrieved polyethylene liners had an average thickness of 7 mm and none were conforming. Eight of these patients had cementless implants, four had cemented implants, and five had hybrid implants. The authors concluded that younger, overweight patients seem to be at higher risk of implant failure and that osteolysis is not restricted to cementless implants. They also stated that review of the radiographs led to a consistent underestimation of the osteolytic defect found to be present at revision surgery.

Ezzet and associates[27] reviewed 88 total knee arthroplasties performed at a single university hospital. Their study was conducted specifically to discover the presence of osteolysis. The incidence of osteolysis varied significantly with the method of component fixation. The highest incidence of osteolysis (30%) was seen when the tibial component was fixed with cement and screws and the femoral component was implanted without cement. When the tibial component was fixed with cement and screws and the femoral component was cemented, the incidence of osteolysis was 13% (2 of 13). When the femoral component was press fit and the tibia was cemented without screws, the incidence of osteolysis was 10% (1 of 10). When the femoral and tibial components were cemented and no screws were used, the incidence of osteolysis was 0 (0 of 12). The authors concluded that the use of screws with cement to fix the tibial component is associated with a high incidence of osteolysis and cannot be recommended. This study questions whether use of a press-fit femoral component may contribute to a higher incidence of osteolysis.[9]

Lewis and associates[28] studied 217 cementless total knee replacements 4 years after surgery to look at the radiographic appearance of the screw-bone interface. There were 102 Miller-Galante I prostheses, 59 Miller-Galante II prostheses, and 56 Anatomic Modular Knee prostheses. Two hundred sixty-five of the 851 screws that were studied showed some evidence of osteolysis at the screw-bone interface, with 185 (21.7%) of the screws showing a cavitary appearance (Fig. 11). The Anatomic Modular Knee prosthesis showed a higher incidence of cystic and cavitary change. Design of the components, and particularly the polyethylene attachment mechanism, was postulated to be responsible for the differences in the frequencies of osteolysis as observed by the authors.

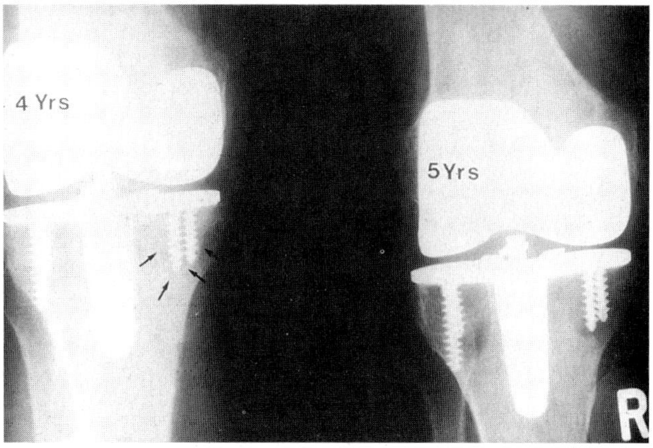

Fig. 11 Anteroposterior radiographs illustrating the osteolysis at the screw-bone interface 4 and 5 years after total knee replacement. Note the cavitary appearance around the screws in the medial and lateral tibial plateau.[28]

Pathophysiology of Osteolysis

Osteolysis has been observed in cemented and cementless TKR patients around well-fixed and loose components. The pathophysiology of osteolysis centers on the role of the macrophage and its response to particulate debris. Particulate debris from the prosthetic replacement gains access to the bone-cement or the bone-prosthesis interface and elicits formation of a fibrous tissue membrane that contains macrophage and foreign body giant cells.[29] The foreign body debris is phagocytosed by the macrophages. In response, the macrophages produce inflammatory mediators, such as cytokines (IL-1, TNF, IL-6) and prostinoids (PGE_2, PGF_{2a}), that result in the stimulation of osteoclasts to effect bone resorption. In order for this complex biologic cascade to proceed, the particulate debris must have access to the interface. The bone-cement interface, or alternatively the prosthesis-bone interface in cementless implants, is included as part of the effective joint space.[30] The pressure generated within the joint is sufficient to act as a hydraulic pump to circulate the particulate debris throughout the effective joint space.

A number of factors influence the biologic response to particulate debris; the number of particles present, the size of the particles, the surface chemistry of the particles, and the type of particulate material. Studies have demonstrated that the size distribution of the particles obtained from the inflammatory membrane retrieved from TKR patients with osteolytic defects differs from the size of particulate debris from total hip replacement patients with osteolytic defects.[31] Particulate polyethylene debris retrieved from total hip replacement patients has a higher percentage of particulate material that is larger in size than the debris obtained from total hip replacement patients.[31] Conversely, particulate debris retrieved from total hip replacement patients with osteolysis has a higher percentage of particles in the submicron range. It has been hypothesized that the small, submicron particles may be a greater stimulus to the macrophage to produce inflammatory mediators that result in osteolysis.[31]

Treatment of Osteolysis

Current recommendations to treat osteolytic lesions in TKR patients include the following measures. (1) Removal of the source of the particulate debris. Typically, this includes the removal of the worn or fractured UHMWPE tibial insert and screws that may have

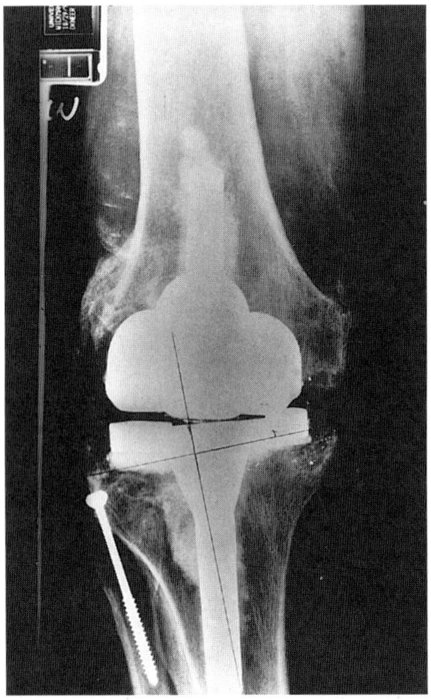

Fig. 12 Anteroposterior radiograph of polyethylene wear following variable axis total knee replacement (TKR). In addition to the polyethylene wear, this patient also has varus positioning of the tibial component and osteolysis present at the tibial interface. Exchange of the ultra-high molecular weight polyethylene liner alone is insufficient to treat this patient, and revision TKR is recommended.

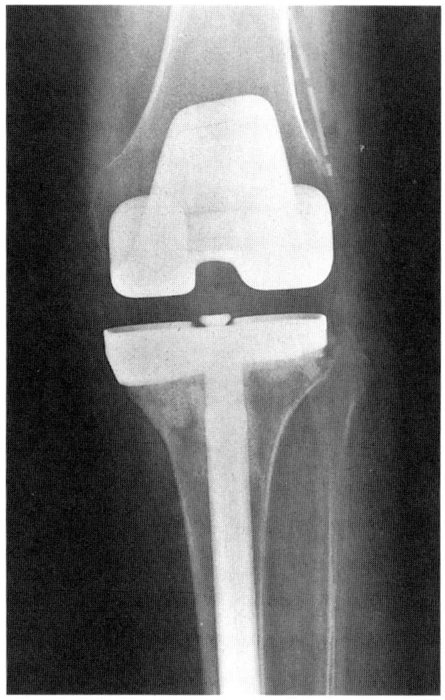

Fig. 13 Anteroposterior radiograph of revision total knee replacement with metal wedge to correct peripheral structural defect of medial tibial plateau. Methylmethacrylate was used to bond and seal the tibial plateau. The tibial stem was press fit.

been used to help fix the tibial component. Removal of the source of the debris is rarely sufficient by itself; the surgeon must also correct the cause of polyethylene wear and debris generation (Fig. 12). (2) Meticulous removal of the inflammatory soft-tissue membrane present at the failed interface. Because this membrane is effecting the osteolytic process, a meticulous debridement is necessary to ensure removal of all the inflammatory membrane at the failed interface. (3) Correction of the mechanical axis of the limb. Removal of malpositioned components, typically a varus tibial component, is necessary to correct the mechanical axis of the limb. This is of the utmost importance. Ligamentous balancing is carried out simultaneously. (4) Morcellized bone graft is used to fill contained metaphyseal bone defects, using an impaction grafting technique. (5) Structural bone grafts or metal wedges are used to correct peripheral structural defects. (6) Long-stemmed revision components are used for biomechanical protection of the bone-grafted region. The surface of the bone is typically sealed with methylmethacrylate to fix the prosthesis to the tibial plateau, whereas the stems may be either press-fit or cemented (Fig. 13).

Prevention of Osteolysis

Current recommendations to prevent osteolysis include the following measures. (1) Cement the tibial component to prevent access of particulate debris to the intramedullary space. Avoid screw fixation of the tibial component, because the screw-bone interface provides an access channel for the egress of debris into the tibial metaphysis. (2) Use a tibial UHMWPE insert with a thickness of at least 8 mm of true polyethylene to allow proper biomechanical function of the UHMWPE as a weightbearing material. This dictates that an equal amount of bone is resected from the proximal tibia using a measured resection technique from the less affected tibial plateau. (3) Select a prosthesis that will maximize surface contact areas and minimize contact stresses. Optimize UHMWPE quality, minimize oxidative damage during the sterilization process, and minimize shelf-life prior to implantation. (4) Ensure proper mechanical axis of the limb and neutral coronal positioning of the tibial component. (5) Remove all bone and polymethylmethacrylate debris that could be a potential source of three-body wear. Finally, remember that in the prevention of osteolysis, as in the prevention of complications in general, there is no substitute for good surgical technique and careful patient selection.

References

1. Kilgus DJ, Moreland JR, Finerman GA, et al: Catastrophic wear of tibial polyethylene inserts. *Clin Orthop* 1991;273:223–231.
2. Tsao A, Mintz L, McRae CR, et al: Failure of the porous-coated anatomic prosthesis in total knee arthroplasty due to severe polyethylene wear. *J Bone Joint Surg* 1993;75A:19–26.
3. Wasielewski RC, Galante JO, Leighty RM, et al: Wear patterns on retrieved polyethylene tibial inserts and their relationship to technical considerations during total knee arthroplasty. *Clin Orthop* 1994;299:31–43.
4. Rand JA: Revision total knee arthroplasty: Techniques and results, in Morrey BF (ed): *Joint Replacement Arthroplasty*. New York, NY, Churchill Livingstone, 1991, pp 1093–1111.
5. Li S, Burstein AH: Ultra-high molecular weight polyethylene: The material and its use in total joint implants. *J Bone Joint Surg* 1994;76A:1080–1090.
6. Collier JP, Mayor MB, McNamara JL, et al: Analysis of the failure of 122 polyethylene inserts from uncemented tibial knee components. *Clin Orthop* 1991;273:232–242.
7. Hood RW, Wright TM, Burstein AH: Retrieval analysis of total knee prostheses: A method and its application to 48 total condylar prostheses. *J Biomed Mater Res* 1983;17:829–842.
8. Landy MM, Walker PS: Wear of ultra-high-molecular-weight polyethylene components of 90 retrieved knee prostheses. *J Arthroplasty* 1988;3(suppl):S73–S85.
9. Wright TM, Bartel DL: The problem of surface damage in polyethylene total knee components. *Clin Orthop* 1986;205:67–74.
10. Wrona M, Mayor MB, Collier JP, et al: The correlation between fusion defects and damage in tibial polyethylene bearings. *Clin Orthop* 1994;299:92–103.
11. Streecher RM: Localizing irradiation for sterilization and modification of high molecular weight polyethylenes. *Plast Rubber Process Applicat* 1988;10:221–229.
12. Rimnac CM, Klein RW, Betts F, et al: Post-irradiation aging of ultra-high molecular weight polyethylene. *J Bone Joint Surg* 1994; 76A:1052–1056.
13. Rose RM, Crugnola A, Ries M, et al: On the origins of high in vivo wear rates in polyethylene components of total joint prostheses. *Clin Orthop* 1979;145:277–286.
14. Bartel DL, Burstein AH, Toda MD, et al: The effect of conformity and plastic thickness on contact stresses in metal-backed plastic implants. *J Biomech Eng* 1985;107:193–199.
15. Goldstein SA, Wilson DL, Sonstegard DA, et al: The mechanical properties of human tibial trabecular bone as a function of metaphyseal location. *J Biomech* 1983;16:965–969.
16. Landy M, Walker PS: Wear in condylar replacement knees: A 10-year follow up. *Trans Orthop Res Soc* 1985;10:96.
17. Blunn GW, Walker PS, Joshi A, et al: The dominance of cyclic sliding in producing wear in total knee replacements. *Clin Orthop* 1991;273:253–260.
18. Bartel DL, Bicknell VL, Wright TM: The effect of conformity, thickness and material on stresses in UHMW components for total joint replacement. *J Bone Joint Surg* 1986;68A:1041–1051.
19. Bartel DL, Rimnac CM, Wright TM: Evaluation and design of the articular surface, in Goldberg VM (ed): *Controversies of Total Knee Arthroplasty*. New York, NY, Raven Press, 1991, pp 61–73.
20. Statler KD, Werner FW, Ayers DC, et al: Contact surface areas in cruciate sparing knee replacements. *Trans Orthop Res Soc* 1992; 17:331.
21. Colizza WA, Insall JN, Scuderi GR: The posterior sterilized total knee prosthesis: Assessment of polyethylene damage and osteolysis after a ten-year minimum follow-up. *J Bone Joint Surg* 1995;77A:1713–1720.
22. Plante-Bordeneuve P, Freeman MA: Tibial high-density polyethylene wear in conforming tibiofemoral prostheses. *J Bone Joint Surg* 1993;75B:630–636.
23. Peters PC Jr, Engh GA, Dwyer KA, et al: Osteolysis after total knee arthroplasty without cement. *J Bone Joint Surg* 1992;74A: 864–876.
24. Cadambi A, Engh GA, Dwyer KA, et al: Osteolysis of the distal femur after total knee arthroplasty. *J Arthroplasty* 1994;9: 579–594.
25. Kim YH, Oh JH, Oh SH: Osteolysis around cementless porous-coated anatomic knee prostheses. *J Bone Joint Surg* 1995;77B: 236–241.
26. Robinson EJ, Mulliken BD, Bourne RB, et al: Catastrophic osteolysis in total knee replacement. *Clin Orthop* 1995;321:98–105.
27. Ezzet KA, Garcia R, Barrack RL: Effect of component fixation method on osteolysis in total knee arthroplasty. *Clin Orthop* 1995;321:86–91.
28. Lewis PL, Rorabeck CH, Bourne RB: Screw osteolysis after cementless total knee replacement. *Clin Orthop* 1995;321: 173–177.
29. Mirra JM, Marder RA, Amstutz HC: The pathology of failed total joint arthroplasty. *Clin Orthop* 1982;170:175–183.
30. Schmalzried TP, Jasty M, Harris WH: Periprosthetic bone loss in total hip arthroplasty: Polyethylene wear debris and the concept of the effective joint space. *J Bone Joint Surg* 1992;74A:849–863.
31. Chiba J, Schwendeman LJ, Booth RE Jr, et al: A biochemical, histologic, and immunohistologic analysis of membranes obtained from failed cemented and cementless total knee arthroplasty. *Clin Orthop* 1994;299:114–124.

CHAPTER 20

Management of the Patient With an Infected Knee Arthroplasty

Vincent D. Pellegrini, Jr, MD

While successful total joint replacement offers dramatic and lasting improvement in quality of life, deep sepsis as a complication of prosthetic joint replacement represents the most feared outcome of this procedure, threatening joint function, limb preservation, and, on occasion, even the life of the patient. Since the inception of prosthetic joint replacement, total knee arthroplasty has been associated with a greater infection rate than its sister operation, total hip replacement. Various factors have been held responsible for this difference. With the Guepar prosthesis, various reports documented the prevalence of deep sepsis as ranging from 6% to 40%. In this specific device with metal-on-metal bearing and fixed hinge, there was generation of considerable metallic debris, which has been shown to impair active phagocytosis of particulate debris by the macrophage. Beyond this characteristic of the metal hinge device, the knee lies superficially beneath the skin and fascial envelope, covered by a limited amount of well vascularized muscle, and with a watershed area of vascular supply to the skin lying directly anteriorly in the position of the typical skin incision. Although many advances have considerably lowered the rate of infection associated with knee replacement, there remain anatomic risk factors inherent to the knee that contribute to an infection rate that will likely always remain higher than that associated with total hip arthroplasty.

Prevalence of Deep Sepsis

Published rates of deep infection complicating contemporary total knee replacement range from 1.1% to 2.8% with a greater risk of infection associated with implants that provide more mechanical constraint between components.[1,2] This observation would appear to be a holdover of the extremely high infection rates observed in association with the hinged devices. In contrast, no meaningful difference in rate of infection has been associated with differences in component fixation-cemented to cementless devices. This significant reduction in contemporary infection rate compared with that of hinged implants is attributable to several factors, most notably the routine use of parenteral antibiotic prophylaxis around the time of operation. While time intervals of antibiotic administration vary among surgeons, the most important dose would appear to be that administered immediately preoperatively, so that antibiotic levels are present in the hematoma that accumulates following surgery; good data exist only to support use of prophylactic antibiotics for 24 hours following operation, beginning with an immediate preoperative dose of a first-generation cephalosporin that provides excellent staphylococcus coverage.[3–5] There is additional evidence to support the use of one additional adjunctive measure, contributing a further reduction in the infection rate of nearly an order of magnitude. Ultraviolet lights[6,7] and closed air exhaust suits[8,9] are the most popular measures used in conjunction with prophylactic antibiotics. The use of clean air systems remains controversial; increasing evidence[10,11] suggests that horizontal laminar flow may actually contribute to an increased infection rate in total knee replacement due to the frequent interposition of operating room personnel between the source of air and the open surgical wound. Therefore, vertical laminar systems are preferable. Common operating room conditions usually place members of the surgical team looking down on the open knee wound, in contrast to the total hip wound which is at eye or shoulder level of the operating surgeon, thereby reducing the risk of contamination by fallout of shed particulate debris. The most prevalent organisms remain gram positive in nature: *Staphylococcus aureus* accounting for 50% to 65%, *Staphylococcus epidermidis* for 25% to 30%, and the remaining 10% to 15% including other gram positive and negative organisms in addition to fungi and mycobacteria.[1,12] A trend of increasing prevalence of *Staphylococcus epidermidis* as a pathogenic organism in prosthetic joint infection has been observed.

Various factors have been associated with an increased risk of infection in total knee replacement; some are inherent to the host and are not subject to alteration, while others may be reduced or eliminated by meticulous preoperative screening of the patient. The diagnosis of rheumatoid disease (independent of the associated use of steroids), the presence of open skin lesions on the affected extremity, previous operation about the knee leaving behind scars of old incisions, and a history of prior infection all carry with them a statistically significant increase in rate of deep infection.[12–14] While three of these factors cannot be altered by the surgeon, the presence of open skin lesions should be noted preoperatively and treatment addressed toward obtaining closure of these wounds prior to elective surgery. It is the author's preference for a 3-month interval of intact dermis over prior ulcerations, such as venous stasis ulcers, before embarking on elective total knee replacement. The greatest risk of infection is associated with a prior history of sepsis in the knee, resulting in an observed rate of 7% deep infection following knee replacement.[1] Less convincingly proven by statistical methods, the presence of recurrent urinary tract infection, diabetes mellitus, systemic steroid use, and obesity have been suggested as being associated with trends toward increased infection rates after knee replacement.[1] Among these, the presence of urinary tract infection can certainly be identified preoperatively. When a structural cause of recurrent urinary tract infections is identified, it should be corrected prior to knee replacement; patients with chronic incorrectable urinary tract infection should be placed on lifelong antibiotic suppression to minimize the risk of immediate postoperative infection as well as late hematogenous seeding of the prosthesis. Rheumatoid disease, in addition to being associated with the risk of acute infection, is also associated with a risk of late infection secondary to hematogenous bacterial seeding of the prosthesis. The risk of late infection is as high as 50% during the lifetime of the patient.[1]

Routine dental cleaning and extraction produces bacteremia in nearly all patients. Conventional wisdom has suggested that antibiotic prophylaxis is appropriate around the time of dental manipulation, but the subject remains controversial.[15] Most orthopaedists agree that the guidelines[16] developed by the American Heart Association for the prophylaxis of infection of prosthetic heart valves are sound, sensible, and cost effective and may reasonably be extended to the prophylaxis of patients with prosthetic joint replacements.

Diagnosis

The patient with an infected prosthetic knee device usually presents with a painful, warm, stiff, swollen, and tender knee joint. Among the differential diagnoses of a painful knee replacement in the absence of mechanical loosening is reflex sympathetic dystrophy, heterotopic ossification, and arthrofibrosis. Beyond physical examination and plain radiographs, which may demonstrate no pathologic findings early but later often show evidence of marginal body resorption, erosion, and loosening of the prosthetic components, the keystone of diagnosis is aspiration of the joint and analysis of the Gram stain, cell count, and differential of the fluid obtained. The joint should be aspirated under meticulous sterile conditions with surgical preparation of the skin to minimize risk of contamination of the specimen with skin flora. An erythrocyte sedimentation rate provides a baseline for serial follow-up analysis of response to treatment. The use of various nuclear medicine techniques has received a great deal of attention, ranging from the traditional technetium bone scan to indium-labeled white cell scan. Sequential and differential application of these two techniques has reportedly yielded an 84% accuracy rate, but these results remain highly dependent on both the technique and the institution in which it is used.[17] Occasionally all efforts at definitive identification of an infecting organism are fruitless despite a very suspicious and often convincing clinical course with painful, loose components of the prosthesis. In this setting, it is not uncommon that staged reconstruction is undertaken, based on clinical presentation and symptoms in the absence of identification of the offending organism, and it is only following removal of the suspected components with direct culture of the metallic device or cement fragments that identification of an organism is obtained.

Management

Once a deep-seated infection is established, the greatest challenge to the managing physician is the conflict between treatment of the patient and treatment of the prosthetic infection. It is important to treat the patient rather than an isolated knee joint, and the orthopaedic physician must weigh the balance of quality and anticipated longevity of life and function against the desire to eradicate the infection. Systemic factors for consideration include chronologic and physiologic age of the patient, concurrent medical illness—most notably insulin-dependent diabetes mellitus, rheumatoid disease, or other related immunosuppressive conditions—and the functional demands of the patient. Local conditions that influence the treatment decision are the nature of the infecting organism and its sensitivity to available antibiotics, the integrity of the extensor mechanism, the adequacy and integrity of the skin and soft-tissue envelope, and the adequacy of adjacent bone stock. It is clear that with eradication of infection as the primary goal of treatment, the entire infected prosthetic joint should be removed to optimize the chance of cure of the infection.[18,19] In the elderly and infirm patient with a mechanically secure knee replacement, the morbidity associated with prosthesis removal is often considerably greater than that associated with chronic antibiotic suppression with preservation of the knee joint, even though the prospect for eradication of the infection is remote in the latter circumstance. Therefore in placing the priority of treatment of the patient above that of aggressive treatment of the knee infection, retention of a secure prosthesis in conjunction with chronic antibiotic suppression often offers greater function to the elderly patient. When progression of infection contributes to mechanical loosening and knee joint symptoms, surgical removal becomes a more practical, functional, and less destructive treatment course.

Prosthesis Retention

In the setting of acute infection, defined as onset within 10 to 21 days of the surgery, and no evidence for mechanical loosening of components, efforts have been advanced to preserve the prosthesis with treatment by parenteral antibiotics alone. When antibiotic therapy is instituted within 48 hours of onset, and the infecting organism is a susceptible gram-positive bacteria (most commonly streptococcus or pneumococcus), success rates ranging from 6% to 10% have been reported.[2,3,12,13,20] The likelihood of successful retention of the acutely infected prosthesis may be increased by debridement, preferably by open technique with radical synovectomy, when the infection occurs within 21 days of the initial knee replacement operation. Success rates of 23% to 28% have been reported with this approach, which necessitates lifelong antibiotic suppression in an effort to indefinitely contain the infection and reduce the chance of systemic bacteremia.[12,14] It is generally accepted that this approach in the setting of late infection (onset more than 21 days from initial implantation) is associated with a lesser chance of success. Surgical debridement followed by short-term parenteral antibiotics and then indefinite oral antibiotic suppression has been associated with less than a 25% success rate for retention of the implant at 5 years, but in selected circumstances in the elderly and infirm patient this remains a viable treatment option. Recent reports concerning the use of rifampin in combination with a fluoroquinone antibiotic for suppression of prosthetic joint infection have been encouraging, and this technique may gain a place in the management of these patients when prosthesis removal is believed not to be in their overall best interest.[21]

Prosthesis Removal

It is widely accepted that with eradication of infection as a primary treatment goal in the majority of patients, removal of the infected prosthesis is a mandatory part of the overall treatment plan. Definitive resection arthroplasty following prosthesis removal is infrequently selected as an end point in patient management. However, in selected patients with multiple joint involvement, such as those with rheumatoid disease, those with limited functional goals and a prospect for ambulation only with assistance of a walker, and those with local risk factors precluding reoperation about the knee, definitive resection arthroplasty remains a viable treatment option.[22] In this patient population, there is preservation of modest motion for activities of daily living, often in the range of 45°, usually with a need for external brace support for ambulation. Overall patient satisfaction approaches 80%, with most having good to excellent pain relief despite the persistence of a sinus tract in 11% of patients.

Alternatively, arthrodesis of the knee provides a more durable lower extremity while increasing the energy expenditure of ambulation. After arthrodesis, the ability to walk independently is dependent on good function of the neighboring lower extremity joints. This procedure, however, is complicated by a 30% nonunion rate,[2,14,23] which has prompted the use of various techniques to obtain a sound arthrodesis. Intramedullary nailing has evolved to be the preferred procedure for knee arthrodesis.[23-26] When employed in a staged fashion with debridement of the infected knee prosthesis first, followed at a later date by placement of an intramedullary nail, solid arthrodesis has been reported in more than 90% of patients.[23] The risk of intramedullary spread of quiescent sepsis in the knee joint space remains present but is considerably reduced by staging of the debridement and reconstructive portions of the treatment plan. The mean time to bony arthrodesis is 6 months, with a nonunion rate of 10% to 20%, for the intramedullary arthrodesis approach. In return for the greater rate of successful arthrodesis, complication rates as high as 56% have been reported in association with intramedullary techniques and include spread of infection by an intramedullary route to previously unaffected areas of the bone. Various devices have been advanced for this particular indication, but the ideal implant remains to be designed. Alternatively, arthrodesis by application of external fixator is reported to have a 70% to 80% rate of successful fusion.[1,27] This method is indicated in the setting of a particularly virulent organism with a considerable risk of intramedullary metastasis of infection or in cases involving an arthritic hip or ipsilateral total hip replacement above the infected knee, which precludes passing of the intramedullary device. Fusion with the external fixator can be accomplished in a single surgical setting, allows delayed skin coverage for management of the deficient skin envelope, and is associated with a complication rate of 36%, largely consisting of pin tract infections and related problems that resolve with removal and replacement of the offending pin.

In the instance of a particularly virulent or resistant organism, amputation may be considered. While fortunately only infrequently required in the setting of life-threatening sepsis refractory to antibiotic therapy, gross bone deficiency, or an irretrievably incompetent soft-tissue envelope, amputation may provide the most expeditious resolution of a very difficult problem. Unfortunately, a poor functional result is the rule, with only one third of patients retaining the ability to ambulate, even with assistive devices, and two thirds remaining confined to a wheelchair.[28]

Prosthesis Exchange

Single stage exchange is largely of historic interest only at this time, with prior reported success rates ranging from 50% to 75%. It is now commonly accepted that if the treatment goal is a durable and functional prosthetic knee joint free of infection, staged debridement followed at a later date by reimplantation is the preferred treatment plan.[2,18,19] In order for such a course of staged reimplantation to be successfully pursued, several requisite conditions must be met. Skin coverage must be adequate; the presence of multiple old incisions or myofascial flaps for prior closure of the wound increase the risk of subsequent failure of the soft-issue envelope. An intact extensor mechanism-patellar ligament complex is essential for independent functional use of the knee. Adequate bone stock to support the revision implant is likewise required, and need for allograft reconstruction of bone deficiency carries with it an increased risk of infection and failure. The infecting organism must have an antibiotic sensitivity profile that offers the therapeutic option of several antibiotic agents. Finally, the systemic health of the host must provide a competent immune system, preferably in the absence of diabetes mellitus, rheumatoid disease, or other systemic conditions associated with relative immunodeficiency. The existence of problems in any two of these five areas of critical concern considerably increases the likelihood of failure of reimplantation of the prosthetic knee joint; it is the author's preference that prosthetic reimplantation be avoided in the patient with deficiencies in three of these critical prerequisites.

When pursuing a course of staged reimplantation following infection, all foreign material, including the implant and all methylmethacrylate, must be removed at the initial debridement. The bone is cleansed meticulously, and an antibiotic-impregnated methylmethacrylate spacer block is interposed between femur and tibia, both to preserve the joint space for later reimplantation and to allow stability with weightbearing across the resected knee joint. Vancomycin (500 mg) and tobramycin powder (1.2 g) are usually added to each 40-g bag of methylmethacrylate. Often, two to three packs of cement are necessary for a block of sufficient size to fill a large defect. Appropriate parenteral antibiotics are continued for 6 weeks as directed by the sensitivity profile of the offending organism. The subsequent use of oral antibiotics is variable, but it is the preference of the author to continue oral antibiotics for an additional 6 weeks, to total 3 months of systemic antimicrobial therapy. This is followed by a drug-free interval of a minimum of 4 to 6 weeks and subsequent reaspiration of the knee pseudarthrosis. Reimplantation can be considered if the culture of the aspirate is negative. It is critically important to assess the readiness of the soft-tissue envelope to undergo an additional surgical procedure; continued induration, dermal edema, or a woody character to the wound are relative contraindications to proceed with reimplantation of a knee prosthesis. It is best to embark on the delayed reimplantation when the wound is soft, supple, and free of edema and induration. Reimplantation, therefore, is carried out between 12 weeks and 1 year following the initial debridement. While a negative aspiration of the pseudarthrosis does not guarantee against the recurrence of infection after reimplantation, a confirmed positive culture is a contraindication to reimplantation of a prosthetic device. A posterior cruciate-replacing implant is always used in this setting and partial patellectomy is occasionally helpful to obtain skin closure in difficult cases with a marginal skin envelope. Antibiotic-impregnated methylmethacrylate (prepared as above) is routinely employed for prosthetic fixation, with antibiotic agents selected according to the sensitivity profile of the previously cultured organism(s). Chronic antibiotics are generally not used, but rather are discontinued after return of all intraoperative cultures reported as clear of infection. While staged reimplantation is fraught with numerous potential problems and is dependent on meticulous patient management and surgical technique, the careful surgeon is rewarded with an 80% to 97% success rate as measured by freedom from infection in the functioning prosthetic knee joint.[18,19,29]

References

1. Wilson MG, Kelley K, Thornhill TS: Infection as a complication of total knee-replacement arthroplasty: Risk factors and treatment in sixty-seven cases. *J Bone Joint Surg* 1990;72A:878–883.
2. Windsor RE, Bono JV: Infected total knee replacements. *J Am Acad Orthop Surg* 1994;2:44–53.
3. Friedman RJ, Friedrich L, White R, et al: Antibiotic prophylaxis and tourniquet inflation in total knee arthroplasty. *Clin Orthop* 1990;260:17–23.
4. Hill C, Flamant R, Mazas F, et al: Prophylaxis cefazolin vs. placebo in total hip replacement: Report of a multicentre double-blind randomized trial. *Lancet* 1981;1:795–796.
5. Mauerhan DR, Nelson CL, Smith DL, et al: Prophylaxis against infection in total joint arthroplasty: One day of cefuroxime compared with three days of cefazolin. *J Bone Joint Surg* 1994;76A: 39–45.
6. Berg M, Bergman B, Hoborn J: Ultraviolet radiation compared to an ultraclean air enclosure: A comparison of air bacteria counts in operating rooms. *J Bone Joint Surg* 1991;73B:811.
7. Berg-Perier M; Cederbald A, Persson U: Ultraviolet radiation and ultra-clean enclosures in operating rooms. *J Arthroplasty* 1992;7:457–463.
8. Charnley J, Eftekar N: Postoperative infection in total prosthetic replacement arthroplasty of the hip joint with special reference to the bacterial content of the air of the operating room. *Br J Surg* 1969;56:641–649.
9. Lidwell O, Lowbury E, Whyte W, et al: Effect of ultraclean air in operating rooms on deep sepsis in the joint after total hip or knee replacement: A randomized study. *Br Med J* 1982;284: 10–14.
10. Fitzgerald RH: Total hip arthroplasty sepsis: Prevention and diagnosis. *Orthop Clin North Am* 1992;232:259–264.
11. Salvati E, Robinson R, Zeno SM, et al: Infection rates after 3175 total hip and total knee replacements performed with and without a horizontal unidirectional filtered air-flow system. *J Bone Joint Surg* 1982;64A:525–535.

12. Schoifet SD, Morrey BF: Treatment of infection after total knee arthroplasty by debridement with retention of the components. *J Bone Joint Surg* 1990;72A:1383–1390.
13. Bengtson S, Knutson K: The infected knee arthroplasty: A 6-year follow-up of 357 cases. *Acta Orthop Scand* 1991;62:301–311.
14. Rand JA: Evaluation and management of infected total knee arthroplasty. *Semin Arthroplasty* 1994;5:178–182.
15. Cawson R: Antibiotic prophylaxis for dental treatment: For hearts but not for prosthetic joints. *Br Med J* 1992;304:933–934.
16. Imperiale T, Horwitz R: Does prophylaxis prevent postdental infection endocarditis? A controlled evaluation of protective efficacy. *Am J Med* 1990;88:131–136.
17. Rand J, Brown M: The value of Indium-III leukocyte scanning in the evaluation of painful or infected total knee arthroplasties. *Clin Orthop* 1990;259:179–182.
18. Rand JA, Bryan RS: Reimplantation for the salvage of an infected total knee arthroplasty. *J Bone Joint Surg* 1983;65A:1081–1086.
19. Windsor RE, Insall JN, Urs WK, et al: Two-stage reimplantation for the salvage of total knee arthroplasty complicated by infection: Further follow-up and refinement of indications. *J Bone Joint Surg* 1990;72A:272–278.
20. Johnson D, Bannister G: The outcome of infected arthroplasty of the knee. *J Bone Joint Surg* 1986;68B:289–291.
21. Drancourt M, Stein A, Argenson JN, et al: Oral rifampin plus ofloxacin for treatment of Staphylococcus-infected orthopedic implants. *Antimicrob Agents Chemother* 1993;37:1214–1218.
22. Falahee MH, Matthews LS, Kaufer H: Resection arthroplasty as a salvage procedure for a knee with infection after a total arthroplasty. *J Bone Joint Surg* 1987;69A:1013–1021.
23. Ellingsen DE, Rand JA: Intramedullary arthrodesis of the knee after failed total knee arthroplasty. *J Bone Joint Surg* 1994;76A:870–877.
24. Donley B, Matthews L, Kaufer H: Arthrodesis of the knee with an intramedullary nail. *J Bone Joint Surg* 1991;73A:907–913.
25. Puranen J, Kortelainen P, Jalovaara P: Arthrodesis of the knee with intramedullary nail fixation. *J Bone Joint Surg* 1990;72A:433–442.
26. Wilde A, Stearns K: Intramedullary fixation for arthrodesis of the knee after infected total knee arthroplasty. *Clin Orthop* 1989;248:87–92.
27. Rand J, Bryan R, Chao E: Failed total knee arthroplasty treated by arthrodesis of the knee using the Ace-Fisher apparatus. *J Bone Joint Surg* 1987;69A:39–45.
28. Pring DJ, Marks L, Angel JC: Mobility after amputation for failed knee replacement. *J Bone Joint Surg* 1988;70B:770–771.
29. Booth R, Lotke P: The results of spacer block technique in revision of infected total knee arthroplasty. *Clin Orthop* 1989;248:57–60.

CHAPTER 21

Surgical Exposure in Revision Total Knee Arthroplasty

Leo A. Whiteside, MD

The standard surgical approach to total knee replacement is seldom adequate for use in revision arthroplasty. Nevertheless, the standard approach is generally the first attempt at exposure, with final exposure achieved through an extension of the standard approach. All approaches to knee arthroplasty use the anterior route, and violate the quadriceps mechanism to some extent. The extensions of this approach all endanger quadriceps function, and must be used with caution. The skin and subcutaneous tissues also are often compromised from previous surgical procedures, and special techniques are required to avoid skin and fat necrosis. Obesity is one factor that impedes exposure of the knee in primary arthroplasty and causes even more problems with revision arthroplasty. Scarred subcutaneous tissue and overlying skin, a fibrotic quadriceps mechanism, and a shortened patellar tendon necessitate extensile exposure. In the non-obese patient whose subcutaneous tissue is not scarred densely to the underlying capsule, the quadriceps mechanism can be turned laterally for extensile exposure without extensive undermining. However, in the obese patient, the thick fibrotic adipose tissue layer that is directly adherent to the capsule and skin prevents the quadriceps mechanism from being folded laterally. This difficulty can be circumvented if subcutaneous undermining can be safely performed to allow placement of the quadriceps mechanism into a secure, subcutaneous pocket so that the entire wall of fat is not forcefully stuffed under the patella and quadriceps mechanism during exposure (Fig. 1).

The subfascial dissection technique makes exposure of the knee both safe and effective in obese patients. Subcutaneous fat receives its blood supply from vessels penetrating from the subdermal plexus and through anastomotic channels from vessels that penetrate through the deep investing fascia of the lower extremity.[1] These anastomotic channels can be severely disrupted during dissection into the subcutaneous fat for creation of a flap for exposure of the knee. Extensive subcutaneous fat necrosis can result, and dissection into this plane can cause overlying skin necrosis as well. However, dissection in the subfascial plane between the deep investing fascia of the lower extremity and the capsule of the knee is relatively safe. Fairly extensive dissection can be done in this plane without significantly devascularizing the subcutaneous fat or overlying skin.[1] Exposure is achieved by incising directly through the subcutaneous tissue and deep investing fascia of the leg. Then, the dissection is directed laterally between the fascia and capsule of the knee approximately three finger breadths past the lateral edge of the patella (Fig. 1). The patella is turned under the subcutaneous flap and into this pocket (Fig. 2).

Quadriceps Transection Exposure

Exposure in the presence of quadriceps contracture and fibrosis of the capsule and patellar tendon often requires additional surgical procedures as well as more extensive subfascial exposure. The classic exposure for extensive intra-articular work on the knee is the quadriceps turndown or V-Y plasty.[2] In this procedure the quadriceps incision is extended proximally with a downward incision across the top of the patella and through the lateral retinaculum to the joint line (Fig. 3). The patella and patellar tendon then become a distally based flap (Fig. 4). Excellent exposure can be achieved with this procedure, but extension lag is almost always reported in series' results of the turndown or classic Coonse-Adams approach to the knee.[3]

The more commonly used transquadriceps approach to the knee is the so-called "quadriceps snip" procedure.[4] The standard incision is extended proximally along the main rectus tendon and then

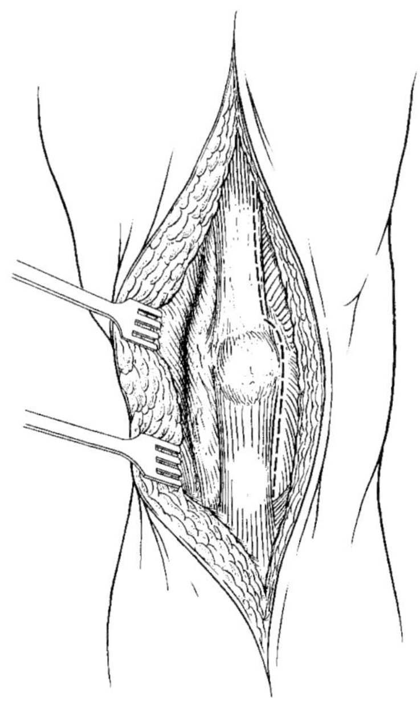

Fig. 1 Lateral subfascial dissection creates a pocket for the patella.

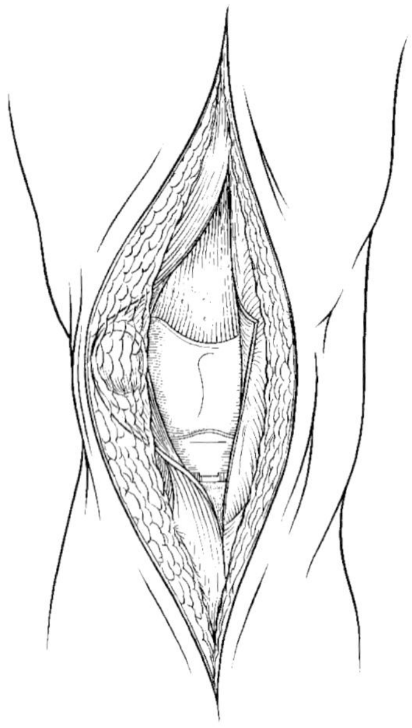

Fig. 2 Exposure of the obese knee. The patella is turned laterally into the subfascial pocket.

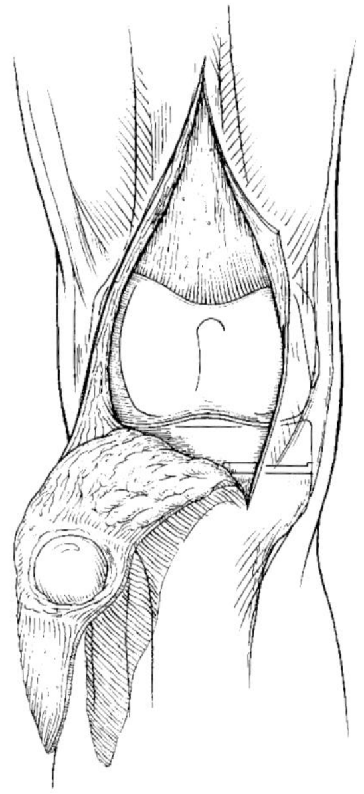

Fig. 4 Exposure of the knee with quadriceps turndown. Anterior knee exposure is excellent. The patella, patellar tendon, and fat pad form a large, poorly vascularized, distally based flap.

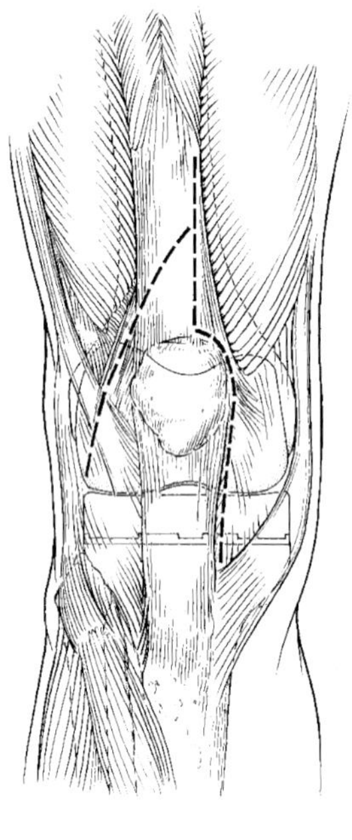

Fig. 3 Outline for the quadriceps turndown (Coonse-Adams) approach to the knee. The standard medial parapatellar quadriceps-splitting approach is made, and then a lateral extension of the incision is made from above the patella to the joint line.

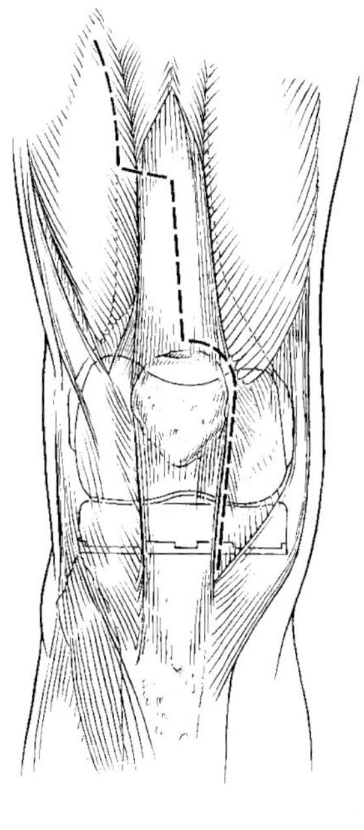

Fig. 5 Outline of the "quadriceps snip" for exposure of the knee. The quadriceps tendon is split in the initial approach. To gain further exposure, the remaining portion of the tendon is cut and the incision is allowed to extend further into the vastus lateralis.

transversely into the vastus lateralis (Fig. 5). As the knee is flexed, the ends of the tendon and muscle fibers separate so that more slack is created in the quadriceps mechanism, and the patella can be retracted laterally more easily (Fig. 6). Complications with this procedure are few, and extension lag is uncommon. Normal rehabilitation can be prescribed, and splinting usually is not necessary. Because this procedure requires proximal extension along the quadriceps tendon, it cannot be used when a more medial approach has been made, such as the vastus medialis splitting or subvastus approach.

Tibial Tubercle Osteotomy

Osteotomy of the tibial tubercle for extensile exposure into the knee is especially effective when extensive exposure to the lateral half of the knee is required, and when a vastus medialis splitting or subvastus approach has been made. This procedure offers the

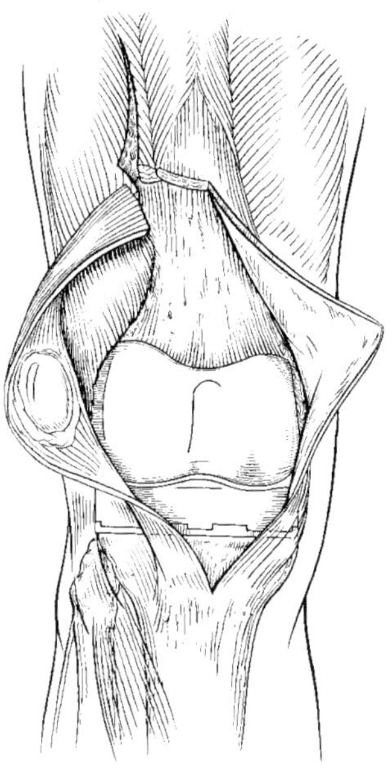

Fig. 6 Exposure of the knee with the quadriceps snip approach. The entire quadriceps, except for a portion of the vastus lateralis, has been transected.

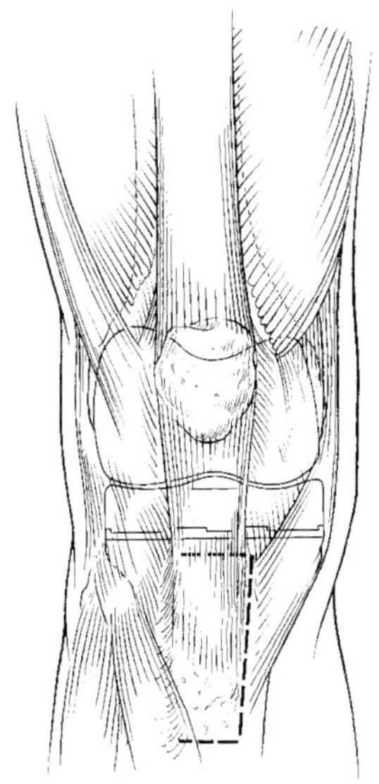

Fig. 7 Outline of the tibial tubercle osteotomy. The distal portion of the osteotomy is made with a saw, and the medial, superior, and lateral portions are made with a curved osteotome. Lateral soft-tissue attachments are left intact.

most extensive exposure to the knee in patients with severe quadriceps contracture, and it is especially useful in patients with fibrous ankylosis and with takedown of knee fusion.

A flap approximately 4 cm long, measured from the top of the tibial tubercle, is elevated through a medial osteotomy that is carried transversely under the tubercle through the lateral cortex (Fig. 7). A flap of bone 4 cm long, 2 cm wide, and 1 cm thick is elevated. The lateral attachments of the muscles and the periosteum are left intact (Fig. 8). The stress riser effect of the osteotomy is minimized by making an oblique saw cut at the distal end of the osteotomized segment. The soft-tissue attachments between the fat pad and anterior tibia must be severed, and a small amount of the anterolateral capsular attachment of the tibia must be released to allow the quadriceps mechanism to turn laterally. Where there is dense contracture of the quadriceps group, an extended incision proximally is necessary (Fig. 8).

When the tubercle osteotomy is used for exposure of the knee, it is not necessary to transect the main rectus tendon. Instead, the proximal incision is allowed to follow the line of the vastus medialis fibers above the vastus medialis obliquus (Fig. 9). The nerves and blood supply to the vastus medialis enter from the posterior edge, so the muscle-splitting incision does not compromise healing and function of the muscle. Often the quadriceps mechanism is tightly adherent to the anterior aspect of the femur, and must be dissected carefully from the bone to allow the quadriceps to be turned laterally; however, it is not necessary to transect any of the lateral aspect of the quadriceps mechanism. The

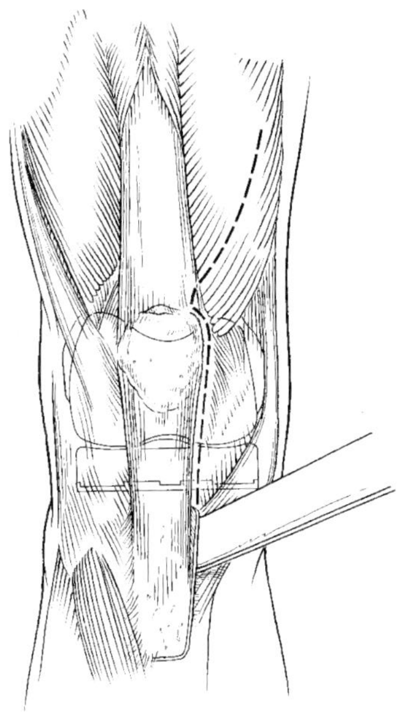

Fig. 8 Outline of the incision used with tibial tubercle osteotomy exposure of the knee. The incision can be placed medially to the main quadriceps tendon, and can be allowed to extend proximally in line with the fibers of the vastus medialis. The osteotomy is made from the medial side to maintain the lateral soft-tissue hinge.

lateral soft-tissue attachments to the tibial tubercle allow the bone flap to turn laterally while maintaining its blood supply. These fibers also maintain attachment of the bone fragment and prevent its proximal migration.

Careful reattachment of the tibial tubercle osteotomy will avoid fracture of the proximal pole of the osteotomized fragment. Because the lateral, soft-tissue hinge has been left intact, the lateral edge does not need to be fixed. However, the medial edge

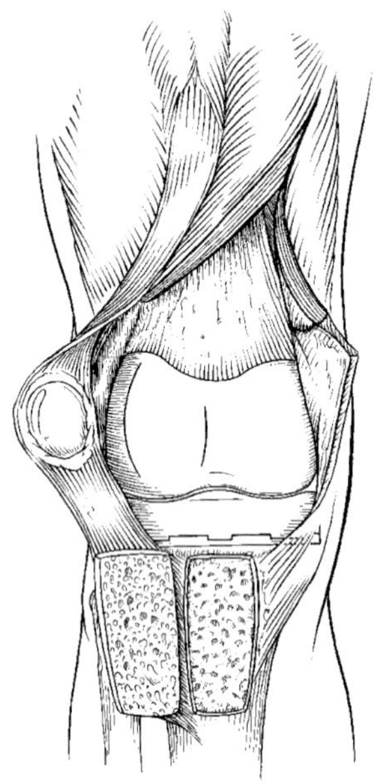

Fig. 9 Exposure of the knee with tibial tubercle osteotomy. The interval between the vastus medialis and vastus medialis obliquus has been split in line with the muscle fibers. The lateral soft-tissue attachments to the tibial tubercle are oriented longitudinally, so the bone fragment does not slip proximally.

requires firm attachment to bone. When screws are used to reattach this segment, they must be placed through the central or medial aspect of the fragment to be effective. Drill holes in this area significantly weaken the bone fragment, and often cause fractures. The proximal screw hole, placed in the soft cancellous bone of the tubercle, is especially vulnerable to fracture. Severe extension lag can result if a fracture occurs through the proximal pole, and surgical repair is difficult. Fixation of the tibial tubercle with wires, however, is highly effective and is safe from fracture. The drill holes are placed along the lateral edge of the tibial tubercle and matching drill holes—offset approximately 1 cm distally—place the wires so that they pull obliquely downward across almost the entire width of the tibial tubercle. When these wires are twisted and tightened, semirigid fixation of the tubercle is achieved. Despite the less-than-rigid fixation, healing occurs in virtually all cases. Fracture of the proximal pole of the tubercle has not occurred in more than 200 surgical exposures with this technique, and only minimal, clinically insignificant slippage of the tubercle fixation has occurred in a few cases.[5,6] Fracture of the tibia, however, has occurred, and is associated with a tibial tubercle bone segmentof longer than 4 cm.[6,7] When a short stem is used on the tibial component, the tibial tubercle osteotomy causes concentration of stress in the anterior tibial cortex, and increases the risk of fracture. However, too short an osteotomy fragment often can be associated with fracture of the tubercle fragment itself.[8] A tubercle segment measuring about 4 cm is recommended.

Exposure of the Posterior Recess

Thorough debridement of the knee and complete ligament reconstruction usually requires full exposure of the posterior capsule and debridement of the posterior recess, which can be achieved by applying a rake retractor to the distal end of the femur and elevating the femoral shaft. With the knee flexed 90°, posterior capsular structures are readily visible. They should be dissected directly from the femoral attachment distally, leaving at least half the thickness of the capsule to maintain posterior ligamentous integrity. In cases of infection, the entire posterior capsule should be resected to extirpate infectious material. Access to the posterior recess behind the tibia can be obtained when the femur is released and the tibia is pulled directly forward. This exposes the posterior recess for thorough cleaning and debridement. The central portion of the capsular structures must be dissected with great care because the popliteal artery lies directly adjacent to the capsule and can be injured if complete capsulectomy is done.

Intraosseous Exposure

When infection is present, or on rare occasions in which long stems have been cemented into the femur and tibia, intraosseous exposure must be achieved to remove the implants and to debride thoroughly. Anterior exposure of the distal half of the femur can be achieved easily through the quadriceps split approach described earlier. Once subperiosteal exposure is achieved, the anterior cortex is drilled to outline an anterior slot osteotomy. The bone segment is removed with a straight osteotome and lifted directly anteriorly. This direct approach to the cemented stem and polymethylmethacrylate allows safe removal of the implant and thorough debridement of the bone. The bone is then repaired by replacing the removed segment and securing it with circumferential cables to create a strong construct that can accept a tight-fitting stem and withstand early weightbearing loads.

Extended intraosseous tibial exposure can be achieved through the tibial tubercle osteotomy, and through extensions of this osteotomy distally. Cable reconstruction of the anterior tibial slot is more difficult, because passing wires and cables around the tibia is more dangerous than the same procedure done with the femur. A long stem that completely bypasses the tibial osteotomy creates a safer construct for early load bearing.

Closure

Management of skin closure after revision total knee replacement is sometimes the most challenging aspect of this surgical procedure. A thin subcutaneous or subcuticular closure over implants is inadequate surgical technique, and will result in a high rate of deep infection. In instances of severe loss of skin and subcutaneous tissue, medial and lateral gastrocnemius flaps are necessary to secure adequate vascularized coverage of the capsule and underlying implants.

Summary

Extensile exposure is one of the crucial skills for managing the challenges presented by revision total knee arthroplasty. Full exposure is necessary to perform the intricate bone and ligament work, and short incisions combined with a timid approach to the quadriceps mechanism will result in inadequate reconstruction of the knee. Repair and reconstruction of the fascial, subcutaneous, and cutaneous tissues to achieve closure are separate and equally important skills.

Acknowledgment

The author appreciates the editorial assistance of Diane Morton in the preparation of this manuscript.

References

1. Hallock GG: Salvage of total knee arthroplasty with local fasciocutaneous flaps. *J Bone Joint Surg* 1990;72A:1236–1239.
2. Coonse K, Adams JD: A new operative approach to the knee joint. *Surg Gynecol Obstet* 1943;77:344–347.
3. Trousdale RT, Hanssen AD, Rand JA, et al: V-Y quadricepsplasty in total knee arthroplasty. *Clin Orthop* 1993;286:48–55.
4. Garvin KL, Scuderi G, Insall JN: Evolution of the quadriceps snip. *Clin Orthop* 1995;321:131–137.
5. Whiteside LA: Exposure in difficult total knee arthroplasty using tibial tubercle osteotomy. *Clin Orthop* 1995;321:32–35.
6. Whiteside LA, Ohl MD: Tibial tubercle osteotomy for exposure of the difficult total knee arthroplasty. *Clin Orthop* 1990;260:6–9.
7. Ritter MA, Carr K, Keating EM, et al: Tibial shaft fracture following tibial tubercle osteotomy. *J Arthroplasty* 1996;11:117–119.
8. Wolff AM, Hungerford DS, Krackow KA, et al: Osteotomy of the tibial tubercle during total knee replacement: A report of twenty six cases. *J Bone Joint Surg* 1989;71A:848–852.

CHAPTER 22

The Management of Bone Defects in Revision Total Knee Arthroplasty

Gerard A. Engh, MD
Nancy L. Parks, MS

Introduction

Revision total knee surgery encompasses a wide variety of procedures because of the variable amount of damage to soft tissues and bone from arthritis, total knee implant failure, and repetitive surgery. Bone defects, which occasionally are present in revision cases, can be repaired with polymethylmethacrylate or bone graft, or the defect can be resected and replaced by a custom or hinged implant. Primary implants are not appropriate for revision cases with damaged metaphyseal bone because they do not provide for joint line restoration and stable component fixation in such circumstances.

Today, revision total knee implants are available for difficult total knee reconstructions with bone loss and ligament damage. Most contemporary revision knee components have canal-filling stems, designed to enhance implant stability and reduce stress on the damaged metaphyseal bone. Fixed or modular augments are available to replace lost bone, to restore the joint line level, and to correct condylar malrotation. Large bone defects, however, may exceed the size options available with component augments. Structural allografts provide a seemingly attractive material for addressing revision cases with extensive bone loss. In this chapter we will present the surgical techniques and discuss the clinical results that have been achieved with allograft reconstruction of major bone defects in revision total knee arthroplasty.

Causes of Bone Defects

Some bone loss occurs when a stable implant is revised after total knee surgery. An error in judgment or surgical technique during the index arthroplasty is often evident as a cause of early failures. In most cases, a nominal amount of bone was removed at the time of the primary knee replacement. A small amount of bone is also lost during component revision, but a good cancellous bed is usually retained for cement interdigitation. The revision of early failed total knees with stable components, therefore, usually results in only minor bone defects that can be managed with primary total knee implants.

Prosthetic-Induced Bone Remodeling

It is important to recognize the reduced strength of metaphyseal bone when performing a revision total knee arthroplasty. Bone beneath a prosthetic device even without osteolysis may be friable and soft. This bone can often be indented with the light pressure of a finger. Decreased bone strength occurs with both cemented and cementless implants. Long-stemmed implants should be used to reduce stress on the damaged bone that is frequently present at revision arthroplasty and that must support the components.

The strength of the metaphyseal bone of the distal femur is reduced through bone remodeling in response to an altered mechanical environment created by the presence of a total knee implant. Bone loss occurs primarily within the first postoperative year and is independent of the mode of fixation or type of implant used.[1] Using three-dimensional finite element analysis, it has been calculated that the rigid femoral component reduces stress to the anterior distal femur by one order of magnitude.[2] This dramatic stress shielding effect following total knee arthroplasty correlates with a clinically and radiographically observed area of osteopenia at the anterior distal femur.[3]

In a similar fashion, metal backing of the tibial component reduces stress on proximal tibial bone. A decrease in load to the proximal tibia has been measured in laboratory tests, using a metal-backed tibial component with a 60-mm central stem.[4] In another laboratory study, a metal stem and tibial tray reduced maximum compressive stresses in the underlying bone by 16 to 39%.[5]

Debris-Generated Osteolytic Defects

Late failure of total knee implants with aseptic loosening is usually associated with particulate debris, component migration, and osteolysis. Although mechanical factors can contribute to late loosening, they cannot cause a device that has been stable for many years to become loose. The more extensive bone loss encountered in such cases is primarily a biologic response to particulate wear products. Willert[6] described the pathomechanics of this process in the classic monograph entitled "Reaction of the Articular Capsule to Wear Products of Artificial Joint Prostheses."

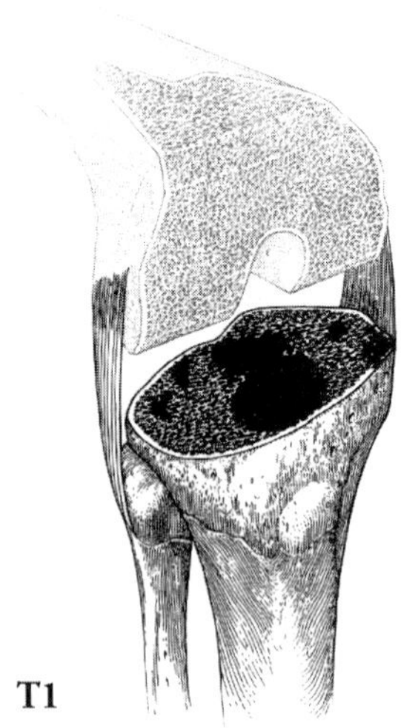

Fig. 1 Type T1 tibial defect: healthy cancellous bone at a normal joint line level. (Reproduced with permission from Engh GA, McAuley J: Allografts in revision surgery, in Engh GA, Rorabeck CH (eds): *Revision Total Knee Arthroplasty*. Baltimore, MD, Williams & Wilkins, in press.)

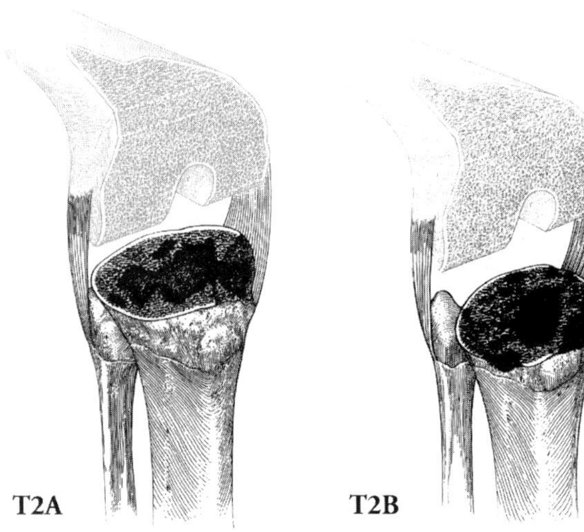

Fig. 2 **Left,** Type T2A tibial defect: damaged metaphyseal bone in one plateau. **Right,** Type T2B tibial defect: damaged metaphyseal bone in both plateaus. (Reproduced with permission from Engh GA, McAuley J: Allografts in revision surgery, in Engh GA, Rorabeck CH (eds): *Revision Total Knee Arthroplasty*. Baltimore, MD, Williams & Wilkins, in press.)

A total knee implant is a low-friction wear couple with debris generated by asperities of the contacting surfaces that abrade with knee motion. Most of the micron- and submicron-sized debris is phagocytized by the synovial lining and transported through the lymphatic system to regional lymph nodes. Particles that are not phagocytized migrate along the path of least resistance. Debris gains access to bone adjacent to the components.[7] A pumping action occurs with cyclic loading and unloading of the knee.[7-9] Once debris gains access to the bone-cement interface, the host biologic response to wear debris weakens the mechanical bond established at the time of surgery between the implant and host bone.[10-13]

Bone Loss With Implant Loosening

The tissue response at the fixation interface changes if the implant moves. Motion between an implant and bone stimulates the formation of synovial-like tissue. Motion generates additional sources of debris by fragmenting methacrylate and the underlying bone. The local tissue response to an increasing volume of particulate is overwhelmed, cell damage occurs, and high levels of digestive enzymes are released from this activated membrane. An enzymatic destruction of surrounding bone creates bone defects that will require repair at the time of revision surgery.

A Bone Defect Classification for Revision Total Knee Surgery

When planning revision surgery, surgeons find a classification of bone defects is helpful to determine the relative difficulty of reconstructing the failed total knee. The severity of bone loss dictates the type of prosthesis, the need for bone graft material, and any special equipment requirements. The preoperative radiographs must be carefully scrutinized for bone defects.

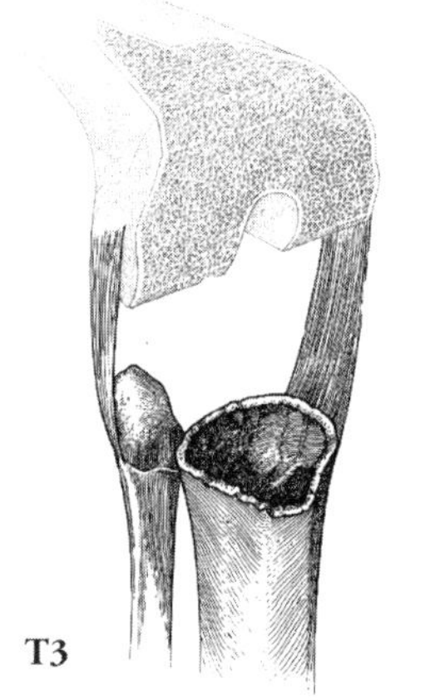

Fig. 3 Type T3 tibial defect: deficient metaphyseal bone. (Reproduced with permission from Engh GA, McAuley J: Allografts in revision surgery, in Engh GA, Rorabeck CH (eds): *Revision Total Knee Arthroplasty*. Baltimore, MD, Williams & Wilkins, in press.)

The surgeon should anticipate the worst-case scenario, because the defects often turn out to be more severe than predicted from the radiographs. Equipment should be ordered to perform the reconstruction efficaciously.

The surgeon determines whether the defect will be easy, moderate, or difficult to reconstruct by classifying bone defects from the preoperative radiographs. Arrangements can be made to have allografts of the appropriate size available when needed to reconstruct a damaged bone segment. Reconstructions with bulk allografts require skill, experience, and extra preparation. Surgeons approaching such procedures for the first time should practice on laboratory sawbone models.

A bone defect classification categorizes cases into

groups of comparable difficulty. A classification that is easy to understand is a useful method for evaluating the clinical outcome achieved with the many different surgical treatment options available. Articles on revision total knee arthroplasty should include a bone defect classification of the reported cases. The evaluation of a surgical technique or implant type is valid when the reader has full knowledge of the severity of bone damage at the time of revision. Outcome studies should then demonstrate improved clinical results and superior implant durability for the more difficult revision cases, thus justifying the added expense of the newer, modular revision implant systems.

In developing the Anderson Orthopaedic Research Institute (AORI) bone defect classification, we applied the following criteria: (1) The classification should be simple and easy to understand. (2) The similarities in metaphyseal bone of the femur and tibia should be recognized. The same terminology should be employed to define the femoral and tibial defects. (3) The definition of bone defects as central or peripheral, cortical or cancellous, contained or uncontained, which are used in most defect classifications, should be eliminated because of the absence of cortical bone in the metaphyseal segments of the distal femur and proximal tibia. (4) Definitions that eliminate ambiguity are needed. (5) A minimal number of bone defect types permits clinical investigators to accumulate enough cases to allow meaningful statistical comparisons. (6) The classification should permit retrospective categorization of cases through intraoperative information and postoperative radiographs.

We used these criteria to establish the following bone defect classification. In the type 1 defect, the metaphyseal bone is intact, and only minor bone defects are present that do not compromise the component stability (Fig. 1). In the type 2 defect, the metaphyseal bone is damaged, and there is loss of cancellous bone in the metaphyseal segment that necessitates an area of cement fill, augments, or bone graft to restore a reasonable joint line level. Type 2 bone defects (Fig. 2) can occur in one femoral condyle or tibial plateau (type 2A), or in both condyles or plateaus (type 2B). In the type 3 defect, the metaphyseal segment is deficient, and there is bone loss that compromises a major portion of either condyle or plateau. These severe defects are occasionally associated with collateral or patellar ligament detachment and usually require bone grafts or custom implants (Fig. 3).

We call this scheme The Anderson Orthopaedic Research Institute (AORI) Bone Defect Classification. Every revision total knee arthroplasty is initially classified from preoperative radiographs for an anticipated bone deficiency. At the time of surgery, the final defect classification is assigned. No defect is assigned when a component is retained. The bone defect classification is applied separately to the femur (F) and tibia (T). In a revision of both the femoral and tibial components, defects of both the femur and tibia are classified, taking into consideration any bone loss from the previous arthroplasty.

Preoperative radiographs, intraoperative findings, implant type, method of reconstruction, and inspection of the postoperative films are considered when determining defect type. The femoral epicondyles, the posterior femoral condyles, and location of the patella relative to the joint line may be used as landmarks to differentiate femoral defects. The fibular head and the tibial tubercle should be used as landmarks for tibial defects.

Joint line elevation is usually recognized by a reduction in the dimensions of the metaphyseal segment of the femur or tibia. Therefore, the main criteria for classifying a bone deficiency from postoperative radiographs is reduction in the profile and dimensions of the metaphyseal segments of the femoral condyles and/or the tibial plateau. The metaphyseal segments of the femur and tibia have a distinct appearance on both anteroposterior (AP) and lateral radiographs. The condylar length-to-width relationship of the metaphyseal regions of the femur and tibia is similar. The distance from the epicondylar region to the end of the femur varies according to an individual's bone structure, but this distance is proportional to all other dimensions of the bone. When a bone defect is present, this relationship is altered. A distal bone defect that has not been repaired with bone graft or augment will appear on an AP radiograph as a shortened distance from the epicondyle and metaphyseal flare to the end of the femoral component. If the bone defects were reconstructed with cement, augments, or grafts and the joint line restored, the reconstructed segment should be visible on postoperative radiographs or evident from a review of the patient's operative note. The metaphyseal bone segment should not appear as a shortened segment, with an augmented component or bone graft filling the deficient area.

In any classification scheme, some cases will fall on the borderline. Information from the surgical reconstruction and postoperative radiographs is used to categorize borderline cases. If a primary component was used, no bone defect has been addressed in the operative note, and the postoperative radiographs demonstrate no joint line elevation, a type 3 defect would not apply. If a structural bone graft, major cement fill, or a hinged component with condylar resection was used in the revision, we conclude that the patient had a type 2 or type 3 bone defect.

Using a bone defect classification system requires discipline. The process becomes progressively easier with each case. Using all available information, including preoperative and postoperative radiographs and

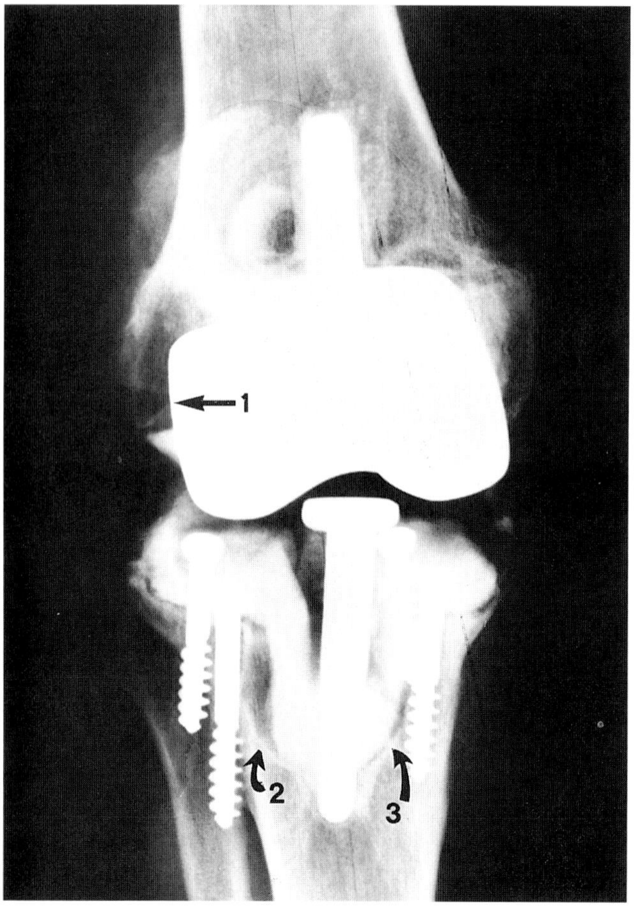

Fig. 4 AP radiograph showing failure of reinforced bone cement with screws (arrows). Bone screws do not improve the bone-cement bond, and should not be used for large bone defects. (Reproduced with permission from Engh GA, McAuley J: Allografts in revision surgery, in Engh GA, Rorabeck CH (eds): *Revision Total Knee Arthroplasty*. Baltimore, MD, Williams & Wilkins, in press.)

intraoperative information, makes the task much easier and the results much more consistent. In general, an F1-T1 classification is applied when cancellous bone is present at a normal joint line level, which permits the use of standard nonstemmed implants. F2-T2 categories include cases with damaged cancellous bone that require augmentation or repair to restore joint line and knee stability. The F3-T3 category should be reserved primarily for severe cases in which the damaged metaphyseal segment of bone must be repaired with major bone grafts, custom components, or hinges in order to reconstruct the damaged bone.

Options for Reconstruction of Major Bone Deficiencies

Currently accepted options for reconstructing a large bone defect in revision knee arthroplasty include bone cement, modular or custom components, autograft, and allograft.

Polymethylmethacrylate and Screw-Reinforced Polymethylmethacrylate

Bone cement has been a valuable material in reconstructive orthopaedic surgery. The major advantage of bone cement used to fill the irregular architecture of damaged bone is that it conforms to the shape of the defect. However, it is a nonphysiologic material that lacks the potential for union and incorporation of bone. It also lacks the necessary biomechanical properties even when reinforced with cortical or cancellous bone screws that limit its durability in large defect reconstruction (Fig. 4).

Modular and Custom Components

Modular implants have enhanced our ability to reconstruct many of the bone deficiencies encountered in revision knee arthroplasty. However, a bone deficiency in revision knee surgery often exceeds the sizes of available augments, which limits the surgeon's ability to restore an appropriate joint line level. Other methods of reconstruction must be available in such cases.

Autografts

Autograft is the optimum biologic material for reconstructing a bone defect. If the graft has not been frozen, the viable osteoblasts have osteogenic potential. Therefore autograft has osteoinductive capabilities not present with allograft bone. This property makes autograft healing to host bone more rapid and predictable than that of allograft. An important additional advantage of autograft use is the absence of disease transmission. Some structural defects, however, are often not amenable to autograft reconstruction because they are too large, because of architectural dissimilarities between the donor site and the recipient site, and because of the limited quantity of bone available without considerable donor site morbidity.

Allograft

Allograft bone is a "physiologic" material that is structurally similar to host bone. A most important advantage of allograft is the ability of host bone to heal to the graft. A strong bond can develop between the host bone and the graft in an area where good cancellous bone is usually absent at the base of a large bone defect. A strong bond with polymethylmethacrylate is often not possible in this location.

Another major advantage of allograft reconstruction is the ability to rebuild the defect with material of similar biomechanical properties as the recipient bone. Restoration of major bone defects is possible because the amount of allograft available is relatively unlimited. Allografts are a cost-effective alternative that provide intraoperative flexibility compared with custom prostheses.

It has been estimated that more than 200,000 bone allografts are performed annually in the United

States.[14] "Allograft bone" encompasses a wide range of structural and morsellized grafts, which have undergone variable harvesting, processing, and utilization techniques. In order to optimize results when reconstructing type 3 femoral and tibial bone deficiencies during revision total knee arthroplasty, it is essential to have a clear understanding of biological principles and allograft reconstructive techniques.

Allograft bone is a necrotic material with the potential for osteoconduction, particularly if the material has been processed to decrease its immunogenicity. Allograft cortical bone incorporates by an osteoclastic response, not an osteoblastic one as occurs in cancellous bone, which significantly weakens the cortical construct.[15] The slower osteoclastic and revascularization response in allograft cortical and subchondral bone may be advantageous in the short term.

The role of immunologic factors in allograft incorporation remains unclear. There is a higher potential for graft resorption, nonunion, and infection than with autograft. The aims of allograft preparation are to diminish the exposure of the recipient to donor cells. Efforts must be made to eliminate the marrow elements, which are the most potent source of immunologic sensitization. Thorough cleansing and flushing should be standard in graft preparation.

The foremost disadvantage to allograft is the potential for necrotic cortical bone to undergo fatigue failure. The potential for this complication exists until the graft revascularizes and remodels with the host bone. A graft fractures as a result of fatigue failure.[16] This probably accounts for the failure of acetabular allografts that had not revascularized in revision total hip arthroplasty.[17] The surgeon should consider the mechanical loads and the necessary support and protection that a graft needs, keeping in mind that incorporation and remodeling may take years.

The potential for disease transmission still exists with allografts, particularly when the source is cadaveric bone. Retesting of the donor and eliminating this risk is one advantage to the use of femoral heads removed at the time of total hip arthroplasty as a source of allograft bone.

Mechanical factors are more important than immunologic factors in graft outcome.[18] Allograft bone is used in two ways, either as a structural graft, in which some cortical and subchondral bone is present, or as morcellized pieces of cancellous bone. Intact structural bone behaves as an anisotropic material, whereas morcellized bone is isotropic. The ability of the graft to withstand stresses will depend on the strength, direction, and type of loading it encounters. Allograft is strongest in compression, as is living bone.

The method used to preserve allograft bone affects its strength. The most common method is freezing. Maintaining stored bone segments at -70° to -80°C minimizes enzymatic degradation.[19] Freezing has little effect on torsional or bending strength. Freeze drying produces minimal change in compression strength,[19] but torsional and bending strength is markedly diminished, up to 90%.[20] Freeze drying is appropriate if a piece of bone will be used purely under compressive loads.

Osteoarthritic femoral heads removed and frozen at the time of total hip arthroplasty provide excellent allograft bone for revision knee arthroplasty. Pelker and Freidlaender[19] report that 70% to 85% of graft strength is maintained in bone from patients in their 70s, and they believe that the size and geometry of the graft are more important than age considerations. They challenged the usual guidelines of excluding elderly patients for structural grafts,[19] and the exclusion of elderly female bone. They reported that male and female segments are comparable in strength if the sizes of the segments are equivalent. However, the use of very osteopenic elderly patients' femoral heads for repairing large bone defects is not recommended.

Techniques for Allograft Reconstruction in Revision Knee Arthroplasty

Host Bone Preparation

In revision surgery, the use of allograft bone for treatment of septic failure remains a subject of debate. Therefore, before allograft bone is used, sepsis must be ruled out as a contributing factor in the total knee arthroplasty failure. Preoperative blood work should include complete blood count, erythrocyte sedimentation rate, and C-reactive protein. Aspirations and the use of three-phase technetium-99 bone and gallium or indium-111 scans are means of detecting suspected infection. As in total hip arthroplasty, sepsis can be difficult to confirm. Multiple tissue cultures should always be obtained during the revision surgery.

Prepare the host base of the bone defect as if it were a delayed union or nonunion fracture site. Remove all residual cement debris, membranous tissue, and nonviable sclerotic bone to provide a bleeding bed at the allograft-host junction. Make an effort to preserve the host bone. Preserve any shell of bone contributing to ligament origin or insertion. A viable, vascularized host interface must be created to allow allograft to host bone healing and subsequent remodeling.

Graft Preparation

Open the allograft in a sterile fashion and obtain cultures. Frozen bone is brittle and should be completely thawed before it is reamed or cut. The bone can be thawed in saline or saline with Betadine solution, a process that takes about 60 minutes depending on the size of graft. Soft tissue should be removed from the

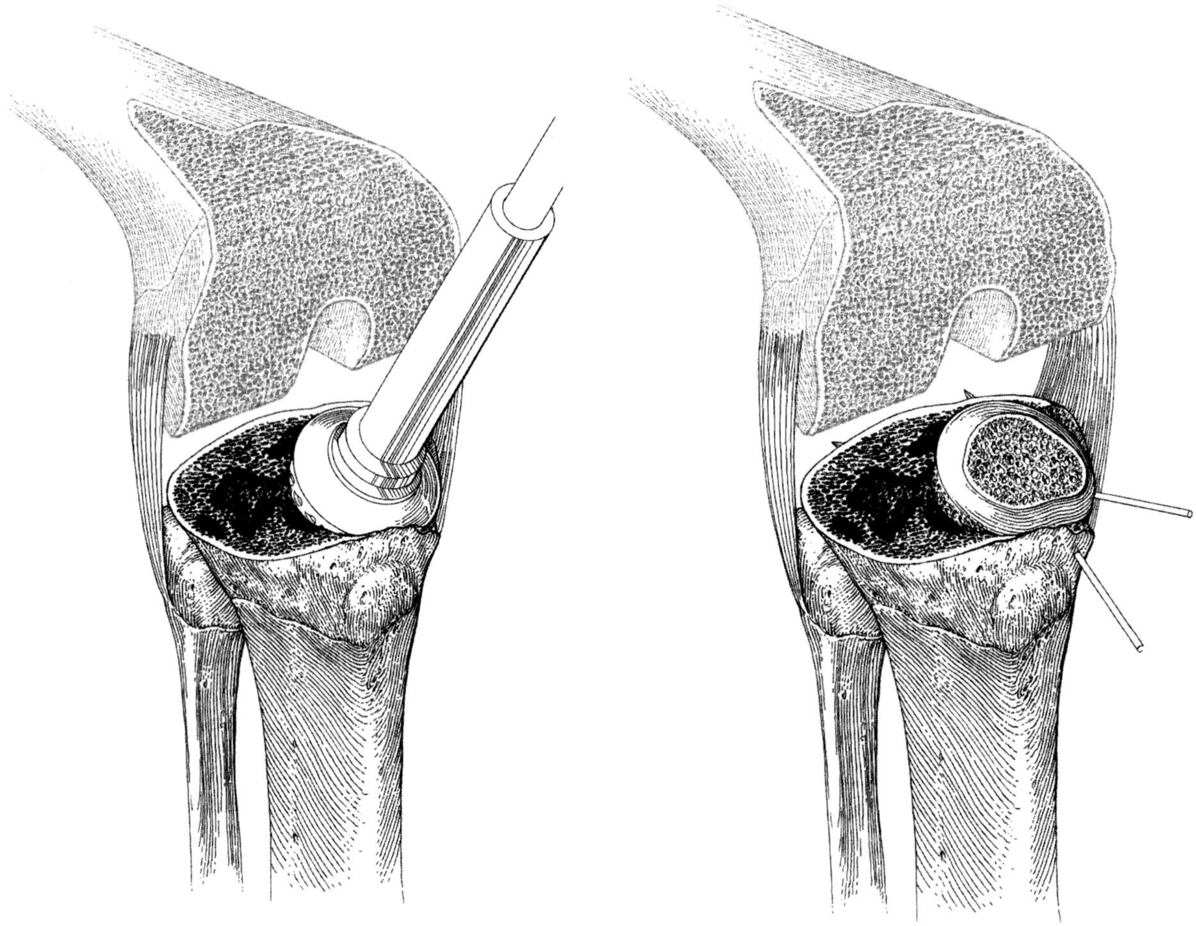

Fig. 5 **Left,** Acetabular reamers are used to create hemispherical shapes from irregularly shaped tibial defects. Reaming is continued to viable cancellous bone. **Right,** The femoral head allograft has been prepared with a female reamer, slightly larger than the bone defect. An interference fit of the graft is achieved, and the graft is temporarily secured with K-wires. (Reproduced with permission from Engh GA, McAuley J: Allografts in revision surgery, in Engh GA, Rorabeck CH (eds): *Revision Total Knee Arthroplasty*. Baltimore, MD, Williams & Wilkins, in press.)

graft. Flush out marrow elements or tissue with saline solution to decrease the immunologic response to the graft. Prepare the graft with the best trabecular orientation for the graft in vivo. Avoid making unnecessary screw holes or perforations in cortical graft because they are stress risers and increase the potential for early revascularization, resorption, and graft collapse.

Graft Fixation

Whenever possible, create an interference fit of the graft. As in a fracture repair situation, endeavor to obtain union between the allograft-host junction by selecting an optimum fixation mode. Internal fixation, with cortical or cancellous screws, can be added to stabilize the graft to host bone, particularly at the allograft-host interface. The resected graft itself provides an excellent cancellous surface for cement interdigitation that further stabilizes the graft to the implant. It is important to remember that union to allograft bone occurs more slowly than to autograft bone.

Prosthetic Stability

When a structural allograft is required, select a stemmed component with a stem diameter that fills the intramedullary canal to enhance stability through contact with diaphyseal bone. Cement should not be allowed access to the allograft-host interface because it mechanically blocks bone healing. Use cement beneath the component for fixation unless good host cancellous bone is available to permit adequate ingrowth. There is no potential for bone ingrowth from the exposed allograft surface to a porous-coated surface. Stem fixation is an unresolved issue and can be left to the individual surgeon's preference. However, a fully cemented stem is indicated when a varus-valgus or more constrained articulation is selected and the stem of the component does not fill the patient's intramedullary canal.

Femoral Head Allograft Reconstruction

Most type 3 bone defects in the proximal tibia and distal femur are irregular in shape as a result of oste-

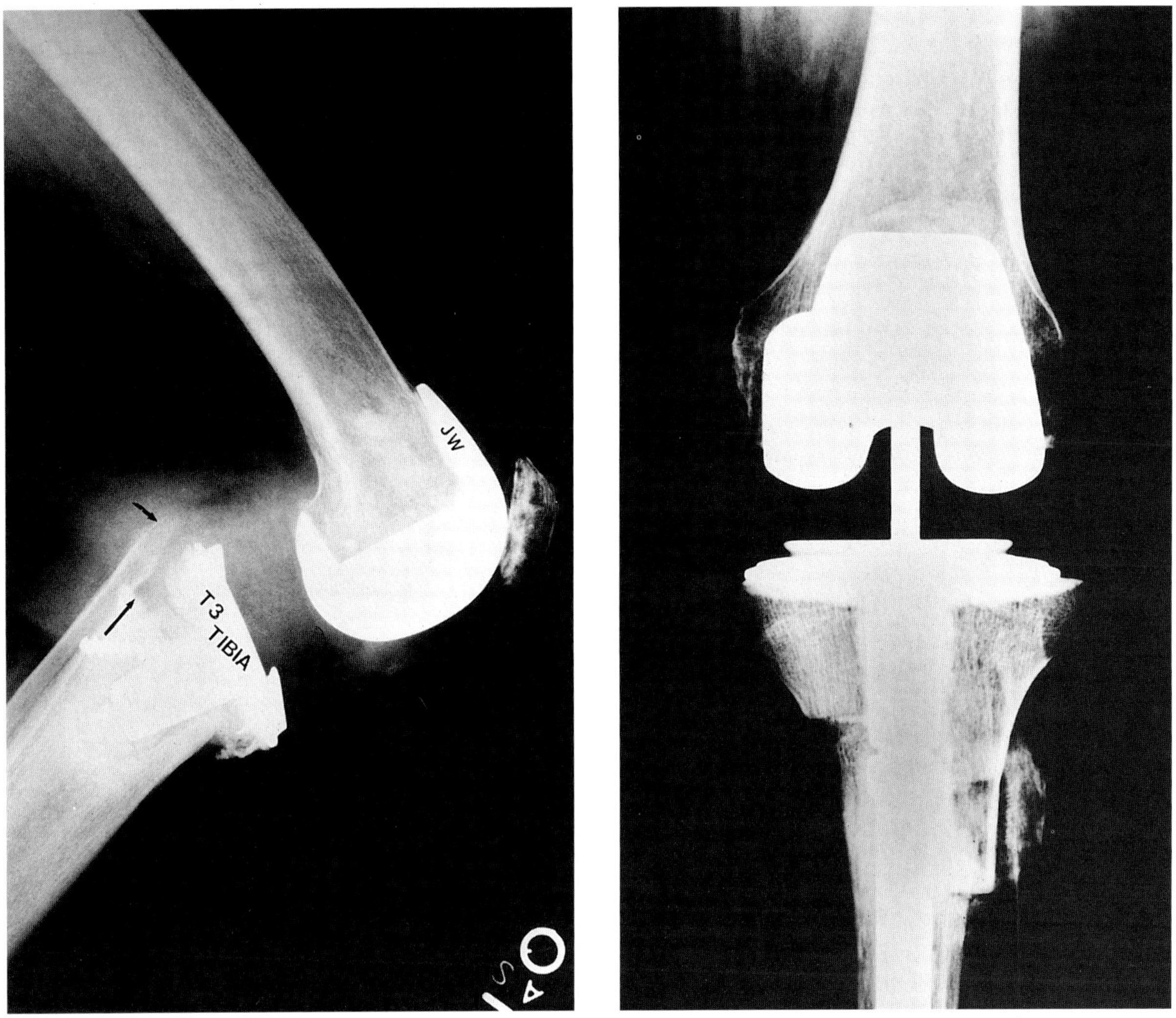

Fig. 6 **Left,** Lateral radiograph of a T3 defect before revision. Bone loss extends well below the fibular head. A high-riding patella suggests disruption of the extensor mechanism. **Right,** AP radiograph of a composite allograft to the proximal tibia. The step cut provides rotational stability. The extensor mechanism was maintained as part of the allograft construct.

olytic bone destruction and cement removal, and they have an intact peripheral rim of bone. The defects are the result of a combination of component subsidence and osteolytic destruction from particulate debris. The flared metaphysis of the femur and tibia provides considerable cancellous bone adjacent to most defects. A straightforward way to repair such a defect is to convert the irregular cavity to a hemispheric shape with a male acetabular reamer, and prepare a femoral head allograft to match the reamed defect with a corresponding female reamer.

A bone-holding device is useful for stabilizing the graft during reaming with hemispherical reamers. Insert the threaded post of a device such as the "Allogrip" (DePuy, Warsaw, Indiana) into a drill hole in the femoral neck and mount the graft on the platform. Select a female reamer that approximates the diameter of the femoral head allograft. Ream the graft until cancellous bone is exposed in the areas of the graft that will juxtapose host bone in the defect.

Prepare the defect in the host bone with a male (acetabular) reamer, preferably one that is 2 mm smaller than the prepared head to allow an interference fit. Reaming should follow the axis of loading only until a bed of viable host bone is created to accept the graft. Preserve the peripheral rim of bone and ligament attachments. (Fig. 5, *left*)

Position the graft and secure it to the host bone with K-wires, placed so as not to impinge on the stem of the component. Trim the protruding wire, leaving enough for subsequent removal. (Fig. 5, *right*)

The final step is to prepare the allograft-host bone construct to receive the revision femoral or tibial component. Trim the protruding neck or portions of the femoral head in such a way that guides for the appropriate size revision implant system can be positioned and secured to prepare the exposed surface of the graft and adjacent metaphyseal bone. Adhere to the principles of balanced flexion-extension gaps with correct bone preparation. Use the least constrained prosthetic interface necessary for knee stability. Once the components are in place, remove the K-wires. In essence, the graft is now captured between the component and host bone and is secured to the component with cement.

A cadaveric distal femur or proximal tibia is an alternative graft source for metaphyseal bone defects. Because the anatomy is similar, a distal femoral or proximal tibial allograft can be osteotomized to provide a piece of bone corresponding to the size and shape of a defect. Interfragmentary fixation screws are ideal to hold the allograft in place. Carefully position the screws to avoid broaching the likely path of the stem. Once the graft is held in place with appropriate interfragmentary fixation, proceed with bone preparation. Cement the femoral component to the cut allograft surface to provide immediate fixation between the prosthesis and the graft. In repairing all defects, it is important to maintain host bone contributing to ligament origin or insertion. It is equally important to use revision components with canal-filling intramedullary stems to reduce load on the allograft and damaged host bone. This minimizes the risk of fatigue fracture of the graft or loosening of the component.

Allograft Prosthetic Composite Reconstruction

Large composite grafts are needed to revise failed hinged knee implants that sacrifice metaphyseal bone, supracondylar fractures that are not amenable to fracture fixation, and cases in which there is extensive osteolysis and implant migration. Using a whole distal femoral or proximal tibial allograft for the more extensive T3 or F3 defect is relatively straightforward because it involves reconstructing a deficiency with bone of a similar shape and structure.

When the failed implant is removed, maintain as much continuity as possible in the capsular elements and ligaments surrounding the knee. For additional exposure, osteotomize the epicondyles, preserving proximal-to-distal continuity with capsular, periosteal, and tendinous structures. Step cut the patient's distal femur or proximal tibia to retain as much bone as possible. The step cut provides rotational stability for the composite and should be long enough to apply two cerclage wires to the step-cut segment of bone.

To prepare the allograft, stabilize the graft in a bone-holding device and perform an arthroplasty on the allograft with a long-stemmed trial revision knee component. Ideally the allograft should be the size of the patient's contralateral femur. Step cut the cortical end of the allograft to mate with the step cut of the patient's femur or tibia. Advance the stem of the component, protruding from the end of the allograft, into the intramedullary canal of the patient. Attain flexion-extension stability with a femoral allograft composite by achieving knee stability in flexion with a trial implant and shortening the cortical end of the allograft until the knee can be extended to neutral.

A press-fit, canal-filling stem is desirable to reduce stress on the allograft and the component/bone interfaces, particularly when more constrained varus-valgus stabilized implants are necessary. Plate fixation can be used, but doing so may be difficult in the presence of a large intramedullary stem. A fully cemented stem is undesirable because cement might interfere with healing of the host-allograft junction or transfer desirable compressive load from the graft-host junction to the cemented stem interface.

Composite reconstruction of T3 bone deficiencies with proximal tibial allografts is analogous to that of distal femoral reconstructions. Proximal tibial grafts are relatively easy to use because of the familiar bony anatomy, trabecular orientation, and cortical structure. If possible, preserve the patellar tendon insertion to the patient's tibial tubercle or release it with an extended tibial tubercle osteotomy that can be reattached to the allograft with multiple cerclage wires, or cortical or cancellous screws. In cases of severe bone deficiency with loss of the extensor apparatus, the allograft can include an intact patellar tendon-patella-quadriceps tendon complex to reconstruct the extensor mechanism (Fig. 6).

Clinical Results of Allografts in Revision Total Knee Arthroplasty

The largest clinical results and outcome studies of knee reconstructions with allografts have been in tumor reconstructions. The 10% to 20% incidence of early failures in this young patient population from opportunistic infection and graft fracture was caused primarily by compromise of the host from tumor, radiation, and chemotherapy.

The clinical results of allograft revision of total knee arthroplasties have generally been favorable. Stockley and associates[16] reported allograft reconstruction of 32 grafts in 20 revision knees having an average 4.2-year follow-up. There were 16 distal femoral reconstructions, 12 with large structural grafts, three morcellized grafts, and one strut graft. There were 16 proximal tibial reconstructions, 11 with bulk structural grafts, four morcellized grafts, and one strut graft.

Seven hinged and 13 semiconstrained prostheses were used for these reconstructions. Failure was defined as an increase in the preoperative knee score of less than 20 points or reoperation. There were three clinical failures secondary to infections. Two grafts fractured, but these cases still had successful outcomes and have not been revised. Subsidence occurred in one case in which morcellized graft was inappropriately used for axial support of the knee replacement. Seventeen of the 20 patients had good results at 4.2-year follow-up. The number of cases was inadequate to comment on prosthetic selection for these deficiencies.

Recommendations from this series are to avoid plate and screw fixation if not clinically necessary, and use interfragmentary fixation, even for fairly large structural grafts. An obvious conclusion was that morcellized grafts cannot tolerate load.

Whiteside[21] reported a series of 56 total knee revisions in which he used long-stemmed components with morcellized allograft reconstruction. The prostheses were seated on the rim of the femur and tibia, and stability between the prostheses and the host bone was obtained using stemmed components and screws to the host bone. The bone was planed down so that a minimum of 25% of the peripheral rim supported the prosthesis. Posterior stabilized components were used. At 2-year follow-up one component had migrated, and there were three recurrent tibial-femoral dislocations, three patellar dislocations, and four revisions for pain without evidence of loosening. Subsidence may have contributed to the instability problems. Although this technique has yielded 80% successful results, there is limited capacity for restoration of the joint line using morcellized grafts.

Mnaymneh and associates[22] reviewed 10 patients with massive allograft reconstructions during revision arthroplasty. There were 14 large grafts, 12 of which were invaginated in the remaining shell of the femur. The other two were segmental grafts held in place with plate and screw fixation. Union occurred in 12 of the 14 cases, and in two cases grafts developed a nonunion and fracture after a mean 40-month follow-up. Nonunion of an allograft-ligament interface led to instability problems in two knees. There was one dislocation in this series and no sign of infections.

Wilde and associates[23] reported a series of 12 allografted tibial defects with 32-month follow-up. Constrained total condylar prostheses were used. There were seven uncontained defects rebuilt with bulk allografts, and five contained defects with morcellized grafts. They reported no graft collapse or fracture, but there was one revision for nonunion of a graft. By 23 months, a variety of imaging techniques showed all grafts had signs of incorporation. A notable finding of this paper was that two revisions of previously infected arthroplasties had successful outcome with allograft reconstruction.

Kraay and associates[24] reported a series of seven distal femoral allograft reconstructions in treating supracondylar fractures in patients with total knee arthroplasty. Open reduction and internal fixation were not felt to be appropriate for these fractures. Care was taken to preserve the soft-tissue envelope and collateral ligaments. All cases had stemmed semiconstrained components, which were fully cemented, including cement plugs. Three were treated with rotating hinges, and four with long-stemmed revision condylar design components. At a mean 44-month follow-up they report no graft resorption or failures. Complications included one dislocation and two cases of persistent instability that required brace stabilization. They used cement to stabilize the allograft/prosthesis composite to host bone and found one case with full and one with partial union, despite autografting the host/graft junctions.

Harris and associates[25] reported 14 patients with large composite allograft reconstructions with total knee arthroplasty. They made no attempt to maintain or repair the collateral ligaments. Constrained condylar prostheses were cemented to the graft in all cases. Stem length and fixation to host bone varied. The authors avoided exposing cancellous surfaces on the graft and autografted the allograft-host junctions.

With 43-month average follow-up they reported extensor lags of 10° to 75° in five patients. Two of these were among the six patients who had an osteotomy of the tubercle as part of the exposure. In five cases, the tibial tubercle was fixed to the allograft and the tubercle subsequently united to the graft. Seven patients had excellent clinical scores, six had good, and one failed. One septic failure was also described. None of the patients required bracing.

The Anderson Clinic experience with femoral head reconstructions consists of 21 patients with 23 grafts with an average follow-up of 51 months. There were 14 tibial and nine femoral reconstructions. The components consisted primarily of modular and custom stemmed implants. No hinged components were used. Four of the custom implants with canal-filling stems were placed in a press-fit mode. Three of the tibial revisions with femoral head allografts used a Synatomic tibial component with a 70-mm tapered stem, and one metal-backed total condylar tibial component with a 35-mm stem.

There have been no revisions or reoperations to date and none are pending. When responding to a patient satisfaction questionnaire all 21 patients reported mild or no pain. Three of the four press-fit components subsided in the first 2 years and then developed a reactive line and endosteal hypertrophy adjacent to the stem. These patients describe mild pain with walking and have worse pain and function scores compared with cemented revisions that averaged 87 on the Knee Society Score (67-99).

Summary

The number of failed total knees with large bone defects is increasing. This is related to the large number of total knee arthroplasty procedures that are being performed in an increasingly active patient population. Long-term results are needed to compare clinical outcome and survivorship of allograft reconstruction versus custom prosthetic components. A benefit to using allograft reconstruction is that the bone deficiency is not increased as occurs with custom devices, and may be decreased with incorporation of the graft.

In our current economic climate there are advantages to using allografts, despite costs as high as $1,600 for processing of a proximal or distal femur.[26] In comparison, custom prostheses are not as cost effective. A material that can unite and gradually incorporate with host bone increases the potential for long-term success.

Allograft may be used as part of a reconstructive armamentarium for total knee arthroplasty. Allografts are not implants and must be used as physiologic material. The early results are comparable or superior to traditional methods of reconstruction. The augmented bone stock in allograft knees remains a theoretical advantage and may facilitate subsequent revisions.

References

1. Mintzer CM, Robertson DD, Rackemann S, et al: Bone loss in the distal anterior femur after total knee arthroplasty. *Clin Orthop* 1990;260:135–143.
2. Angelides M, Chan KH, Ahmed AM, et al: Effect of porous coating distribution on stress shielding of the distal femur following total knee arthroplasty. *Orthop Trans* 1988;12:394–395.
3. Cameron HU, Cameron G: Stress-relief osteoporosis of the anterior femoral condyles in total knee replacement: A study of 185 patients. *Orthop Rev* 1987;16:449–456.
4. Reilly D, Walker PS, Ben-Dov M, et al: Effects of tibial components on load transfer in the upper tibia. *Clin Orthop* 1982; 165:273–282.
5. Bartel DL, Burstein AH, Santavicca EA, et al: Performance of the tibial component in total knee replacement. *J Bone Joint Surg* 1982;64A:1026–1033.
6. Willert HG: Reaction of the articular capsule to wear products of artificial joint prostheses. *J Biomed Mater Res* 1977;11:157–164.
7. Schmalzried TP, Jasty M, Harris WH: Periprosthetic bone loss in total hip arthroplasty: Polyethylene wear debris and the concept of the effective joint space. *J Bone Joint Surg* 1992;74A:849–863.
8. Anthony PP, Gie GA, Howie CR, et al: Localised endosteal bone lysis in relation to the femoral components of cemented total hip arthroplasties. *J Bone Joint Surg* 1990;72B:971–979.
9. Hendrix RW, Wixson RL, Rana NA, et al: Arthrography after total hip arthroplasty: A modified technique used in the diagnosis of pain. *Radiology* 1983;148:647–652.
10. Peters PC Jr, Engh GA, Dwyer KA, et al: Osteolysis after total knee arthroplasty without cement. *J Bone Joint Surg* 1992;74A: 864–876.
11. Wroblewski BM: Wear of high-density polyethylene on bone and cartilage. *J Bone Joint Surg* 1979;61B:498–500.
12. Dannenmaier WC, Haynes DW, Nelson CL: Granulomatous reaction and cystic bony destruction associated with high wear rate in a total knee prosthesis. *Clin Orthop* 1985;198:224–230.
13. Nolan JF, Bucknill TM: Aggressive granulomatosis from polyethylene failure in an uncemented knee replacement. *J Bone Joint Surg* 1992;74B:23–24.
14. Horowitz MC, Friedlaender GE: The immune response to bone grafts, in Friedlaender GE, Goldberg VM (eds): *Bone and Cartilage Allografts: Biology and Clinical Applications.* Park Ridge, IL, American Academy of Orthopaedic Surgeons, 1991, pp 85–101.
15. Goldberg VM, Stevenson S, Shaffer JW: Biology of autografts and allografts, in Friedlaender GE, Goldberg VM (eds): *Bone and Cartilage Allografts: Biology and Clinical Applications.* Park Ridge, IL, American Academy of Orthopaedic Surgeons, 1991, pp 3–12.
16. Stockley I, McAuley JP, Gross AE: Allograft reconstruction in total knee arthroplasty. *J Bone Joint Surg* 1992;74B:393–397.
17. Hooten JP, Engh CA, Heekin RD, et al: Structural bulk allografts in acetabular reconstruction: Analysis of two grafts retrieved post-mortem. *J Bone Joint Surg* 1995;78B:270–275.
18. Zukor DJ, Paitich B, Oakeshott RD, et al: Reconstruction of post-traumatic articular surface defects using fresh small-fragment osteochondral allografts, in Aebi M, Regazzoni P (eds): *Bone Transplantation.* Berlin, Germany, Springer-Verlag, 1989, pp 293–305.
19. Pelker RR, Friedlaender GE: Biomechanical considerations in osteochondral grafts, in Friedlaender GE, Goldberg VM (eds): *Bone and Cartilage Allografts: Biology and Clinical Applications.* Park Ridge, IL, American Academy of Orthopaedic Surgeons, 1991, pp 155–162.
20. Triantafyllou N, Sotiropoulos E, Triantafyllou JN: The mechanical properties of the lyophylized and irradiated bone grafts. *Acta Orthop Belg* 1975;41(suppl):35–44.
21. Whiteside LA: Cementless revision total knee arthroplasty. *Clin Orthop* 1993;286:160–167.
22. Mnaymneh W, Emerson RH, Borja F, et al: Massive allografts in salvage revisions of failed total knee arthroplasties. *Clin Orthop* 1990;260:144–153.
23. Wilde AH, Schickendantz MS, Stulberg BN, et al: The incorporation of tibial allografts in total knee arthroplasty. *J Bone Joint Surg* 1990;72A:815–824.
24. Kraay MJ, Goldberg VM, Figgie MP, et al: Distal femoral replacement with allograft/prosthetic reconstruction for treatment of supracondylar fractures in patients with total knee arthroplasty. *J Arthroplasty* 1992;7:7–16.
25. Harris AI, Poddar S, Gitelis S, et al: Arthroplasty with a composite of an allograft and a prosthesis for knees with severe deficiency of bone. *J Bone Joint Surg* 1995;77A:373–386.
26. Spire B, Dormont D, Barre-Sinoussi F, et al: Inactivation of lymphadenopathy-associated virus by heat, gamma rays, and ultraviolet light. *Lancet* 1985;1:188–189.

CHAPTER 23

Cost Effectiveness of Revision Total Knee Replacement

Cecil H. Rorabeck, MD, FRCSC
Paraic Murray, MSc, MCh(Orth), FRCS Ed(Orth)

Introduction

In an attempt to reduce cost in a managed care environment, a number of initiatives have evolved, the net effect of which has been to shorten hospital stay. These initiatives have included cost reduction in the purchase of implants,[1] as well as demand matching of implants to patient, reduction in surgical fee, and other improved efficiencies within the system.[2,3] Lavernia and associates[2] have noted that orthopaedic surgeons have experienced a major fee reduction for total knee replacement from an estimated $2,436 (1992) to $1,825 (1995). Barrack and associates[4] predict a reduction in reimbursement for revision total knee replacement of 46%. This is based on the actual reimbursement for 1991-1992 at $3,361 and the Medicare estimated 1996 reimbursement at $1,825. The challenge facing managed care therefore is to insure that quality of care and outcome of a given procedure as well as the cost effectiveness will not be impacted adversely by these cost reductions (savings).

Thus, when one considers a patient with a failed primary knee replacement for which a revision procedure is felt to be indicated, a number of questions arise. For example, if the primary knee has failed because the metal-backed patella has worn through, should the patient have a revision of the patellar component only or should the entire knee be revised? Similarly, in a patient with an infected total knee, would it be less expensive and equally effective to revise the infected knee in one stage or should the gold standard continue to be a two-stage revision? With a move toward modularity in the industry, should a patient with a worn modular liner have only the liner exchanged in an attempt to control cost? Similarly, one could ask whether primary components should be used in revision total knee replacement in order to save money. To date, longitudinal studies have not been done to demonstrate the cost of revision total knee replacement, or its cost effectiveness compared to primary total knee replacement. This is a necessary prerequisite before contemplating cost reduction for revision total knee replacement with the potential risk of sacrificing the quality of the result. It will be the purpose of this chapter to define the cost incurred in revision total knee replacement, and to assess its cost effectiveness.

Materials and Methods

A longitudinal study of 68 consecutive patients who had revision total knee replacement in 1994 and who were operated on by a single surgeon forms the basis of this review. A detailed cost analysis, encompassing preoperative costs, in-hospital costs, and postoperative costs in the first year following surgery, was done. The costs for those patients undergoing revision total knee replacement were compared to costs for a group of 35 consecutive primary total knee joint replacements also done in 1994 by the same surgeon, subjected to the same costing analysis.

Fully allocated hospital costs were done for each patient in the two groups. These were costs and not charges. The cost per minute of operating time was analyzed, as were the anesthetics and surgeon cost and the cost associated with the postoperative management in the recovery room. In addition, each physiotherapy visit was costed, and the various laboratory tests, including biochemistry, hematology, microbiology, and pathology, were assigned fully allocated costs. An analysis of radiology costs examined the cost of in-hospital radiographs, the use of doppler ultrasound, scans, etc, and the cost of the radiologist's fee to analyze these tests. Any costs incurred in pharmacy were included, as were costs attributed to psychology, nutrition, social work, and other ancillary costs as, for example, if a patient needed an endoscopy during the hospital stay. This detailed cost analysis makes it possible to determine the in-hospital cost of a patient having a revision total knee replacement as compared to a primary total knee replacement, and also to examine the efficacy and cost-effectiveness of revision total knee replacement compared to primary total knee replacement.

Results

Table 1 demonstrates a comparative cost analysis of primary total knee replacement versus revision total knee replacement. It can be seen from this table that all items analyzed, with the exception of physiotherapy, are slightly more expensive for patients undergoing revision total knee replacement than for those undergoing primary total knee replacement. Much of this is related to the fact that the patients who underwent revision total knee replacement stayed in the hospital an

Table 1
Comparative cost analysis of primary total knee replacement versus revision total knee replacement

Service	Department	Individual Primary Cost $	Total Primary Cost $	Individual Revision Cost $	Total Revision Cost $
PACU*			305.00		350.00
In-patient ward	4th floor		4,027.24		4,588.00
Surgery	Operating room and implant	3,733.64		5,967.00	
	Anesthesia	168.86		264.00	
	Surgeon's fee	657.50		771.00	
	Recovery room	100.57		143.00	
Total Surgery Cost			4,660.57		7,145.00
Radiology			702.87		909.30
Physiotherapy			514.31		458.00
Laboratory			403.56		576.00
Pharmacy			167.68		325.00
Cardiac investigation			38.00		38.00
Other			32.71		38.57
Family doctor	Suture removal		16.25		16.25
Total			10,868.19		14,444.12

*PACU, Preadmission Acute Care Unit

average of 11 days, whereas those who underwent primary knee replacement were discharged after an average of 7.9 days. Thus, the costs of ward care, radiology, laboratory, pharmacy, etc, were all increased. Other cost increases assigned to revision total knee replacement are related to the duration of the operation, the cost of the implant, and the complexity of the operation, which is reflected in a higher surgeon's fee. The total of all in-hospital costs for patients undergoing primary total knee replacement in 1994 was $10,868 as compared to $14,444.12 for a patient undergoing a revision total knee replacement during the same period of time. On average, the implant costs for a revision total knee replacement were $1,200 more expensive. An analysis of the surgeon's fee as a percentage of the implant cost reveals a greater discrepancy in patients undergoing revision knee replacement (Table 1). A comparative cost analysis in patients undergoing total knee replacements was carried out to determine the difference in cost between those undergoing revision for aseptic loosening as opposed to patients undergoing revision for septic loosening or patients having an isolated patellar revision for wear-through of a metal-backed patella. Table 2 demonstrates the large variations in cost. Patients undergoing revision for sepsis cost the system over $6,934 at the time of removal of the implant and a further $12,471.57 on the occasion of their second admission for reimplantation, for a total cost of almost $19,405.57. Conversely, a patient having an isolated revision of a patellar button for wear-through cost the system $6,293, considerably less than the cost for a patient having a complete revision for aseptic loosening ($14,444.12).

Preoperative Cost

In addition to in-hospital cost, a detailed analysis of preadmission clinic costs was done comparing those patients awaiting revision total knee replacement with those scheduled for primary total knee replacement. Table 3 demonstrates a slightly increased cost in those patients being seen preoperatively for revision total knee replacement, with most of the cost increase being related to knee aspiration and bacteriologic assessment to rule out sepsis.

Postoperative Cost in Year 1

In an attempt to determine the costs incurred by our health care system after these patients had left the acute care institution, a study was done analyzing the costs incurred during the first year postoperatively. Patients were asked to keep a diary of all visits to family physicians, outpatient clinics, physiotherapy, and laboratories, and a detailed cost analysis was performed. A patient undergoing revision total knee replacement cost the health care system approximately $1,304 the first year postoperatively as opposed to a patient having undergone a primary total knee replacement, who in-curred costs of $1,126. The major difference between the two groups was in the amount of physiotherapy performed in patients with revision total

Table 2
Variations in cost

	Revision of Patellar Prosthesis	One Stage Revision	Two Stage Revision
First operation	$ 6,293.00	$14,444.12	$ 6,934.00
Second operation			$12,471.57
Total	$ 6,293.00	$14,444.12	$19,405.57

knee replacement, which accounted for the majority of the increased cost associated with a revision knee replacement.

Cost Effectiveness of Primary Versus Revision Total Knee Replacement

The total cost incurred by a patient undergoing primary total knee replacement as compared with a patient undergoing revision total knee replacement during the same time period in the same institution in 1994 is shown in Table 4. When the preadmission cost, the cost incurred during the hospital stay, and the cost incurred after the patient leaves the hospital in the first year are added together, it is evident that revision total knee replacement costs $15,748.12 as opposed to $11,994.19 for a patient undergoing primary knee replacement.

A comparative analysis of Knee Society clinical rating scores between primary and revision knee replacement is shown in Table 5. Preoperatively, the Knee Society scores were approximately the same, suggesting that both patient groups were equally disabled. The preoperative score for a patient waiting for a primary knee replacement was 71 as opposed to 75 for a patient waiting for a revision knee replacement. Six months postoperatively the primary knee replacement had achieved the clinical rating score of 152 as opposed to 135 for revision. At one year, the primary had obtained a score of 156 as opposed to 136 for the patient with revision knee replacement. An analysis of the cost effectiveness of primary versus revision total knee replacement may be expressed as the cost incurred for each 10-point change in the Knee Society rating score. Using that as a parameter, $1,411.08 were spent for each 10-point increase in the clinical rating score for those patients undergoing primary knee replacement as opposed to $2,581.66 for each 10-point increase in patients undergoing a revision total knee replacement (Table 6).

Discussion

Cost reduction programs designed to control the cost of primary knee replacements have been carried out successfully. Barber and Healy[3] demonstrated a reduction in length of hospitalization time from 17 days in 1980 to 9.3 days in 1991. These cost reduction programs have also succeeded in reducing the costs for a hospital room, radiology, blood bank, and operating room, as well as hospital stay; however, the cost reduction programs have been less successful in reducing implant cost, physiotherapy and occupational therapy cost, and costs incurred with the use of drugs. In addition, while the hospital administrators and bureaucrats are implementing cost reduction programs within each institution, the orthopaedic community needs to insure that the quality of patient care is not being sacrificed on the altar of cost containment. To this end, we need to develop positions on such concerns as single versus staged procedures for the infected total knee, the role of isolated patellar revision for a failed metal-backed patella, and the place of primary implants in revision total knee replacement. If data are not forthcoming in these areas, it may well be that managed care organizations will mandate certain clinical pathways, which could impact adversely on quality of patient care.

This study has demonstrated that two-stage revision for infected total knee is extremely expensive. On the other hand, if it reduces the readmission rate, and if the failure rate is lessened with a two-stage revision, then the cost effectiveness of two-stage revision can be sustained unequivocally. On the other hand, if the readmission rate following a two-stage revision rate is no different from the readmission rate following a

Table 3
Preoperative costs in patients awaiting primary/revision total knee replacement

	Primary Total Knee Replacement	Revision Total Knee Replacement
Preadmit clinic cost	$305.00	$305.00
Knee aspiration		$ 45.00

Table 4
Cost effectiveness of primary versus revision total knee replacement

	Primary Total Knee Replacement	Revision Total Knee Replacement
In-patient costs	$10,868.19	$14,444.12
Cost for year 1	$ 1,126.00	$ 1,304.00
Total	$11,994.19	$15,748.12

Table 5
Comparative analysis of Knee Society clinical rating scores between primary and revision knee replacement

Time	Primary Total Knee Replacement	Revision Total Knee Replacement
Preoperative	71	75
6 months	152	135
1 year	156	136

Table 6
An analysis of the cost effectiveness of primary versus revision total knee replacement

	Primary Total Knee Replacement	Revision Total Knee Replacement
Improvement in KSCRS	85	61
Total cost	$11,994.19	$15,748.12
Cost per 10-point increase in KSCRS	$ 1,411.08	$ 2,581.66

one-stage revision, then managed care providers are in a strong position to criticize this practice. Conversely, this study has demonstrated that isolated patellar revision for patients with worn metal-backed patella is relatively inexpensive, costing our health care system approximately $6,000, less than half the amount required for a patient having a revision for aseptic loosening. However, an analysis of these patients has demonstrated an extraordinarily high complication rate associated with isolated patellar revision.[5] Other authors have reported similarly high failure rates in patients undergoing isolated patellar component revision.[6] Thus, while it may seem attractive to managed care bureaucrats to encourage isolated patellar revision within a well-established clinical pathway, this practice is clearly not cost effective in many cases because of the high readmission rate, between 19% and 34% within the first 2 years. These data emphasize the importance of not only analyzing in-hospital cost but also performing longitudinal studies on these patients and analyzing readmission rates. Based on these data, it is our practice now to revise all components with failed metal-backed patella, particularly if a titanium femoral component has been used or if there is any significant burnishing or grooving of the femoral component. The exception is in the low-demand elderly patient in whom isolated patellar revision is still felt to be cost effective.

These data have demonstrated that revision total knee replacement is extremely effective in improving function and improving quality of life. Within the first postoperative year it is not as effective as primary total knee replacement, but, nevertheless, there is still a dramatic improvement in function as well as patient satisfaction following the revision procedure. If one compared only those patients undergoing revision for aseptic loosening and eliminated patients with infected total knees, the cost effectiveness of revision knee replacement would more closely approximate that of primary knee replacement. Revision of a failed knee replacement would appear to be highly cost effective when it is compared with the cost to society of revising a failed liver transplant or perhaps a failed coronary artery bypass. Nevertheless, it is incumbent upon the orthopaedic community to devise techniques of ensuring improved longevity of our primary total knee replacements. In addition, all of us as health care providers need to develop a strategy for cost containment. Notwithstanding that, this study has demonstrated that revision total knee replacement is extremely cost effective in improving the patient's quality of life.

References

1. Healy WL: Economic considerations in total hip arthroplasty and implant standardization. *Clin Orthop* 1995;311:102 –108.
2. Lavernia CJ, Drakeford MK, Tsao AK, et al: Revision and primary hip and knee arthroplasty: A cost analysis. *Clin Orthop* 1995;311:136 –141.
3. Barber TC, Healy WL: The hospital cost of total hip arthroplasty: A comparision between 1981 and 1990. *J Bone Joint Surg* 1993;75A:321 –325.
4. Barrack RL, Hoffman GJ, Tejeiro WV, et al: Surgeon work input and risk in primary versus revision total joint arthroplasty. *J Arthroplasty* 1995;10:281 –286.
5. Kim P, Bourne RB, Rorabeck CH, et al: Is isolated patellar revision of failed metal-backed patellar components in total knee arthroplasty effective? Proceedings of the American Academy of Orthopaedic Surgeons 63rd Annual Meeting, Atlanta, GA. Rosemont, IL, American Academy of Orthopaedic Surgeons, 1996, p 320.
6. Berry DJ, Rand JA: Isolated patellar component revision of total knee arthroplasty. *Clin Orthop* 1993;286:110–115.

CHAPTER 24

Patella Infera Syndrome: An Analysis of the Patellar Tendon Pathology

Edward M. Wojtys, MD
Barry Oakes, MD
Thomas N. Lindenfeld, MD
Bernard R. Bach, Jr, MD

Introduction

Developmental patella infera is a devastating syndrome most frequently seen in the postoperative knee.[1-6] Although the cascade of events responsible for its development is somewhat variable, both extrinsic and intrinsic mechanisms can play a role. Extrinsic mechanisms such as quadriceps muscle dysfunction secondary to pain or joint effusion at the knee can begin this process.[6] Intrinsic mechanisms involving abnormal collagen response to injury are also key factors to consider.[7-18] Regardless of which mechanism is at work, the time sequence involved is of utmost importance. Initially, there is a short period of time (approximately 3 months), during which the condition can be treated successfully with at least a partial return to normal patellar position.[4] However, if the descended position of the patella as well as the contracted state of the peripatellar soft tissues is not corrected, adaptive changes can occur on the patella femoral articular interface secondary to abnormal loading of the patellofemoral joint.[6,19] Failure to recognize and appropriately treat this condition in its early stage of development can lead to a situation in which a good result is no longer possible and only a salvage procedure can be done.[6]

Van Eijden and associates[20] studied the effects of a shortened patellar tendon in a mathematical model and found increased anterior translational forces on the tibia near full extension when the patellar tendon is shortened. At terminal extension, an increased quadriceps force was needed to generate the same extension moment. This increase in force transmitted through the extensor mechanism will increase the contact force between the patella and femur. This increase in loading could contribute to the deterioration of a patellofemoral interface already compromised by disuse, immobilization, peripatellar contracture, and/or trauma.

An important factor to consider in this sequence of events is: When does the lowered position of the patella become permanent? Clinically, this occurs when reversal can no longer be accomplished either by soft-tissue manipulation in therapy or by soft-tissue release at surgery. If all fibrotic and contracted soft tissues are released, and if active quadriceps function is achieved, normal patella position should be attainable. If the patella remains in the lower position despite adequate soft-tissue release and an active quadriceps, attention should be directed to the patellar tendon.[21,22]

Until this investigation, claims that the lowered position of the patella can become permanent were based on radiographic and surgical observations, and on the frustration experienced by clinicians who had to deal with the chronic cases postoperatively after a thorough soft tissue release had been performed.[2-4,6] Those who are unfamiliar with this syndrome usually claim that the patellar tendon is merely kinked or folded on itself, and all that is needed to attain normal patellar position is adequate soft tissue release. The idea of actual tendon shortening is not readily accepted. Yet there is good evidence to believe that the phenomenon can and does occur.[2,11,13] Burks and associates[23] have shown that the patellar tendon is capable of shortening when the central third is removed for anterior cruciate ligament (ACL) replacement in dogs. This occurred even when the central defect in the patellar tendon was not closed and when there was no postoperative immobilization. We believe that immobilization and the lack of active quadriceps contraction providing tension to the patellar tendon further encourage shortening of this collagenous structure.[21,22,24,25] Previous investigators have reported on the negative effects of decreasing the forces transmitted through tendons.[26,27]

Intrinsic mechanisms by which collagenous tissues shorten in scar tissue during wound healing and also in the palmar fascia affected by Dupuytren's contracture are well-recognized clinical phenomena that need to be considered in this syndrome. The collagen shortening in these conditions, as well as in patella infera, may in some cases be caused by the active contraction of "myofibroblasts" within the collagen matrix, producing direct mechanical traction on the collagen fibrils.[13]

Biopsy and histologic examination of the patellar tendons involved with patella infera syndrome appeared to be the best way to resolve the question of whether or not these patellar tendons had undergone ultrastructural cellular and/or matrix changes resulting in shortening. In this study, particular attention has been directed to quantitative analyses of collagen fibril population profiles in four patients with patella infera;

these profiles are compared with the collagen fibril profiles found in the normal patellar tendon.

Materials and Methods

The patellar tendons of four patients in various stages of developmental patella infera were biopsied. Specimens were prepared according to the following protocol.[28] Small blocks of tissue (2 mm x 1 mm) from the central third fibers of six normal patellar tendons (from patients aged less than 30 years) and four patients with patella infera were obtained at surgery. These were initially fixed in 4% buffered glutaraldehyde and then in formaldehyde-glutaraldehyde and picric acid buffered at pH 7.4 with 0.2 m sodium cacodylate.[29] The blocks were post fixed in 1% osmium tetroxide for 4 hours and were then dehydrated and embedded and oriented in Epon-Araldite in the usual way.

Thin sections were cut at exactly 90° to the longitudinal axis of the tendon blocks and three random micrographs taken and enlarged to 80k. Then, collagen fibers were manually analyzed over a constant area using a digitizing pen coupled to a Leitz-ASM image analysis system. A calibration grating was used and a separate micrograph was taken of this as a reference for collagen fibril quantitative analysis.

Quantitative Ultrastructural Collagen Fibril Analysis

Using the image analysis system described, a histogram was plotted of the number of fibers in 15 diameter groupings ranging from 0 to 200 nm. The percentage area occupied for the number of fibers in each diameter grouping was also calculated[30-33] in order to determine the "mass" of collagen represented for each diameter group. The mass of collagen gives a better correlation with the mechanical properties of the tissue than the diameter alone, because the tensile strength of collagen is related to its total cross-sectional area. The histograms shown in Figure 1, which compare these patellar tendons with normal ones, were calculated from means of the number of fibrils in each diameter group from each patient, which in turn reflected the mean on at least three separate micrographs. Specimens were also examined qualitatively with the following areas of particular interest in mind: (1) size of collagen fibrils, (2) cross-sectional area of the distribution of collagen fibrils, (3) viability and distribution of fibroblasts, (4) evidence of neovascularity and inflammation, (5) elastin content, and (6) evidence of active myofibroblasts.

Results

The five parts of Figure 1, lettered *A* through *E*, show the size distribution and percentage of area occupied by each fiber size as compared to normal patellar tendon (*A*) for each of the four patients (*B* through *E*). The five photomicrographs in Figure 1 show typical regions of normal patellar tendon (*A*) and of the tendon of each of the four patients (*B* through *E*).

Normal and Ultrastructure Collagen Fibril Population of the Patellar Tendon

The normal patellar tendon is composed of large fasciculi of tightly packed collagen fibrils. The fibroblasts, found in and between the fasciculi, are elongated cells with long thin cell processes which branch and extend in between the collagen fibrils and fasciculi. Bundles of actin filaments are not prominent in these cells.

The normal collagen fibril population profile (which is a mean of six patients aged less than 30 years) demonstrates a maximum number of large diameter fibrils greater than 100 nm diameter (Fig. 1, *A, left*) which is best seen in Figure 1, *A, right,* where the small number of large diameter fibrils occupies about 50% of the cross-sectional area of the patellar tendon.[34] The profile just described was remarkably similar and consistent between patients for the central region of the patellar tendon, indicating that regional variation in collagen fibril profiles may not be a problem.

Clinical Histories

Patient 1 This patient, a 38-year-old male coal miner, sustained a work-related knee injury. His initial surgery (March, 1986) consisted of open lateral meniscectomy and medial meniscus repair. Postoperatively, he was placed in a cast in flexion for 2 weeks and developed a flexion contracture at the knee. An arthroscopy and successful manipulation was performed. Postoperatively, despite aggressive physical therapy, the flexion contracture redeveloped. At that time, patella infera was noted on a lateral radiograph of the knee and at physical examination. The range of knee motion was 20° to 110°. Significant quadriceps atrophy was present, along with moderate patellofemoral crepitus. An arthroscopic lysis of adhesions was performed and a patellar tendon biopsy was obtained. Grade IIB Outerbridge[35] changes were noted on the patellar articular surface and IIA changes on the medial femoral condyle. This patient continued to complain of patellofemoral pain, and a Maquet osteotomy was performed. The patient did not improve, required a cane for walking, and subsequently considered total knee replacement.

The collagen fibril population profile of this patient is shown in Figure 1, *B.* This micrograph demonstrates many small diameter fibrils and also some large fibrils. The inset at left shows this distribution of a large number of small diameter fibrils less than 75 nm,

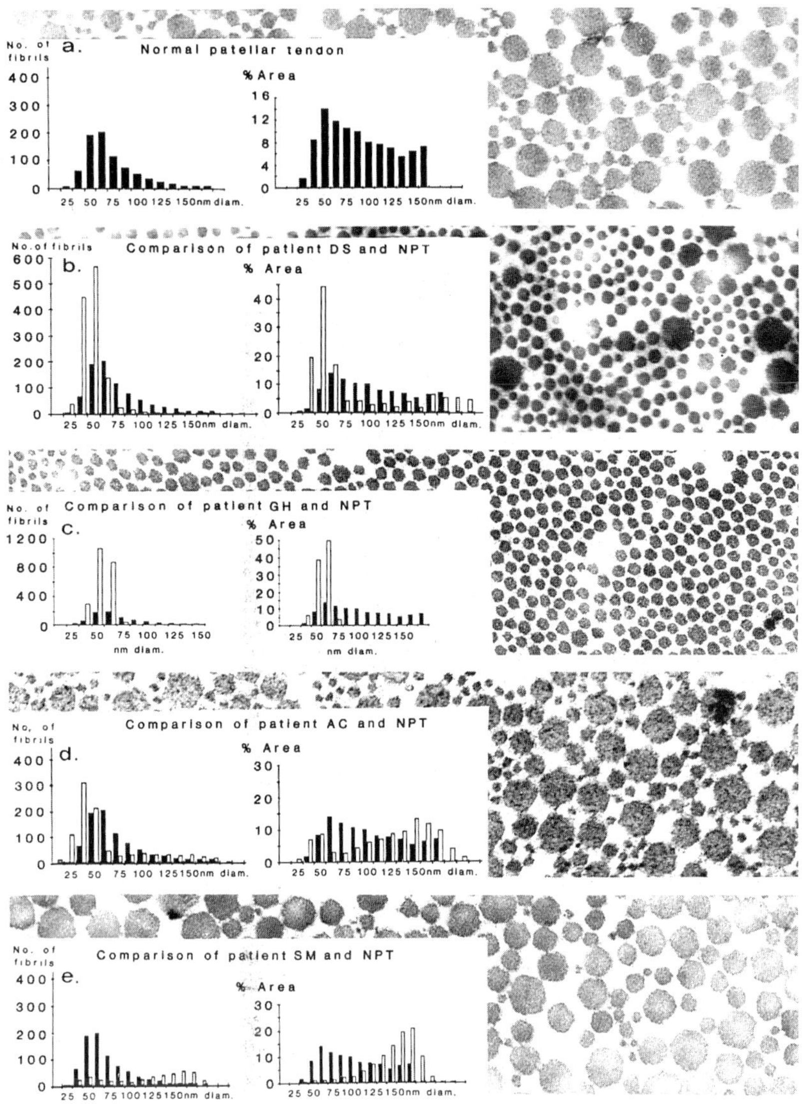

Fig. 1 **A,** A representative electromicrograph of a normal patellar tendon (male, age 26 years) and a histogram of mean collagen fibril profiles of six normal patellar tendons from individuals aged 30 years. At left is shown the number of fibrils versus diameter (nm) and at right is the percent area occupied per diameter group. Note that the small number of large diameter fibrils (> 100 nm) account for nearly 50% of the total collagen cross-sectional area. **B,** A representative micrograph of one of the patients. The histograms compare the collagen fibril profiles of this patient (open bars) with normal patellar tendon profile (closed black bars) as in (**A**) above. Note the large number of small diameter fibrils in the micrograph as well as in the histogram. **C,** A representative micrograph of the second patient. As in b, the histograms compare the collagen fibril profiles of this patient (open bars) with normal patellar tendon profile (closed black bars). Note the very large number of small diameter fibrils in the micrograph as well as the histogram. Very few large fibrils are present. (Note the scale of vertical axis of left histogram). **D,** A representative micrograph of the third patient. Once again, the histograms compare the collagen fibril profiles of this patient (open bars) with normal patellar tendon profile (closed black bars). Note the increased number of small diameter fibrils in the micrograph as well as the histogram and the presence of large diameter fibrils. **E,** Representative micrograph of the fourth patient. Here, too, the histograms compare the collagen fibril profiles of the patient (open bars) with normal patellar tendon profile (closed black bars). Note the few small diameter fibrils and the persistence of large diameter fibrils in micrograph, also seen in the histogram.

and the right side shows that this group of fibers occupies about 85% of the total cross-sectional area of collagen.

Patient 2 This patient, a 28-year-old male, underwent an ACL reconstructive procedure in July of 1986. Following the reconstruction, he was immobilized in a cast for 3 weeks and then began a range of motion exercise program. The knee range of motion was described as poor. Three manipulations were performed under anesthesia between November, 1986, and April, 1987. These attempts failed. Patella infera was then noted on the lateral radiograph of the knee and on physical examination. Range of motion of the knee was from 10° to 90° with mild patellofemoral crepitus noted. Arthroscopy was recommended, and, at the time of the surgery, an extensive release of contracted soft tissues, including medial and lateral retinaculum, was performed, along with fat pad resection and biopsy of the patellar tendon. Postoperatively, an extension cast was employed for 1 week, and a range of motion from 0° to 95° was subsequently achieved. Unfortunately, the patient continued to have problems with knee flexion and pain. He returned to the operating room for a repeat arthroscopy, medial/lateral release, and hardware removal. At the time of his last evaluation (January, 1989) a range of motion of 0° to 105° was noted, along with no improvement in his patellofemoral symptoms.

The collagen fibril population profile of this patient is shown in Figure 1, *C*. The collagen fibril profile again was characterized by a large number of small diameter fibrils with few large fibrils greater than 100 nm remaining. Most of the fibrils were less than 75 nm diameter.

Patient 3 This patient, a 20-year-old female, noted the onset of pain in her left knee in November of 1982, with no apparent history of trauma. Because of her continued complaints of pain, she underwent an arthroscopy and arthrotomy with total medial meniscectomy in March, 1983. Physician notes indicate that the patient was "most reluctant regarding her exercises, really not doing her quads at all." By May, 1983, the patient had "barely any quadriceps activity at all." A question concerning psychological problems surfaced at that time.

This patient complained of pain, swelling, and giving way with activities of daily living. Physical examination at that time showed severe quadriceps weakness, a minimal amount of patellofemoral crepitus, and fat pad swelling. A lateral radiograph of the knee showed bone density changes compatible with disuse (Fig. 2). After 1 year of conservative treatment consisting of intense physical therapy, there was a lack of progress and problems continued. An arthroscopy, lateral release, exploration of the patellar tendon, patellar chondroplasty, and neuroma excision of the infrapatellar branch of the saphenous nerve were then performed. Postoperatively, poor quadriceps function was again noted. Postoperatively, patella infera was diagnosed on a lateral radiograph of the knee. By this time, severe patellofemoral crepitus was present on physical examination. A month later, the quadriceps function had deteriorated further with active extension beyond 30° unattainable. Despite these problems, the patient continued to work up to 12 hours a day as a waitress. Three months later, a repeat arthroscopy, lateral release, and patellaplasty were performed, during which grade IIb changes were noted throughout the patellar articular surface. Lateral radiographs of both knees showed the severe infera position on the left knee with loss of 80% of the patellar tendon length (Fig. 3). Subsequently, a Maquet osteotomy and lengthening of the patellar tendon with fascia lata graft along with a patellar realignment were performed (Fig. 4). For the next 12 months, extensive physical therapy was stressed, which included inpatient treatment, extension casting, psychological evaluation, and hypnosis: all treatments were designed to improve quadriceps function, all without success. The newly lengthened patellar tendon shortened a second time and the patella resumed its lowered position (Fig. 5). The next year, the wire used in the patellar tendon lengthening procedure was removed and a biopsy of the patellar tendon was performed. Postoperatively, the patient was evaluated by a neurologist; no lower motor neuron dysfunction was found. Treatment for reflex sympathetic dystrophy was begun using Dilantin and Elavil, followed by sympathetic blocks at a pain clinic. All failed to decrease pain or improve function.

The collagen ultrastructure of this patient is shown in Figure 1, *D*. Viable cells (Fig. 6) containing many intermediate filaments on longitudinal section and small diameter collagen fibrils amongst the larger collagen fibrils were confirmed on quantitative analysis. Abrupt kinking of both large and small collagen fibrils was also evident (Fig. 7).

Patient 4 This patient was a 15-year-old female when she underwent a medial meniscectomy after a twisting injury while cheerleading. This operation was followed by 8 weeks of immobilization and no physical therapy. One year later, some type of tendon transfer was performed along with patellar chondroplasty via arthrotomy; no rehabilitation program was performed postoperatively. Three years later, an ACL reconstruction was

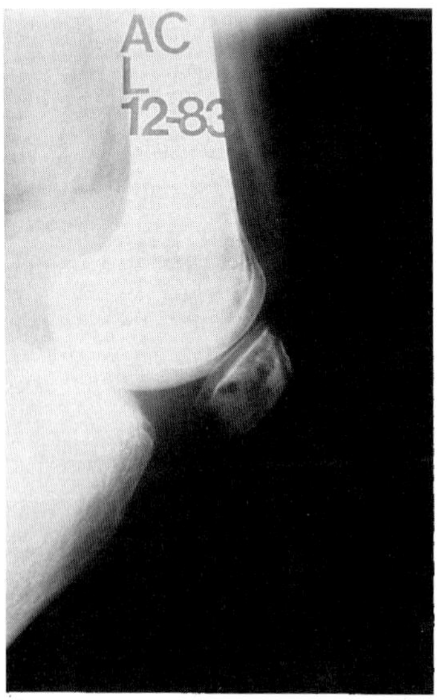

Fig. 2 Lateral radiograph of the involved knee of patient 3 taken 1 year after the onset of symptoms. Note the density changes in the patella.

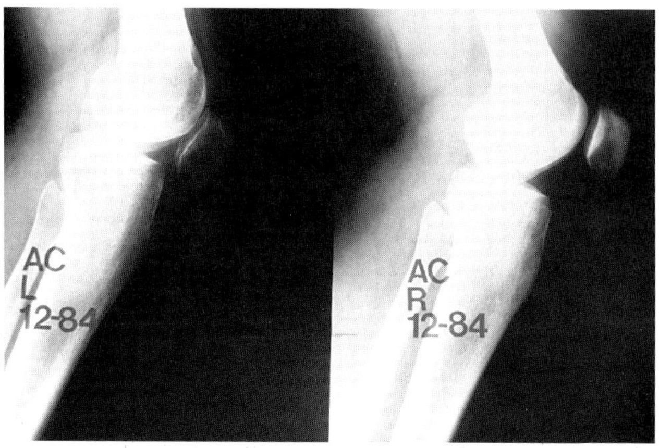

Fig. 3 Lateral radiograph (**left**) of patient 3 taken 2 years after the onset of symptoms compared to the normal side (**right**). Note the descended position of the patella on the left.

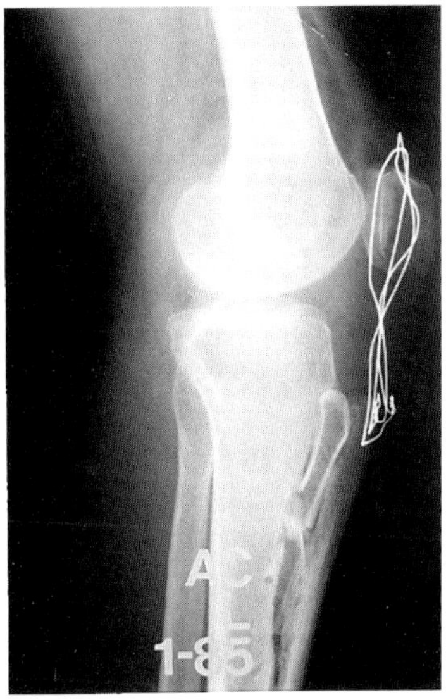

Fig. 4 Lateral radiograph of the knee of patient 3 taken immediately after Maquet tibial osteotomy and lengthening of the patellar tendon.

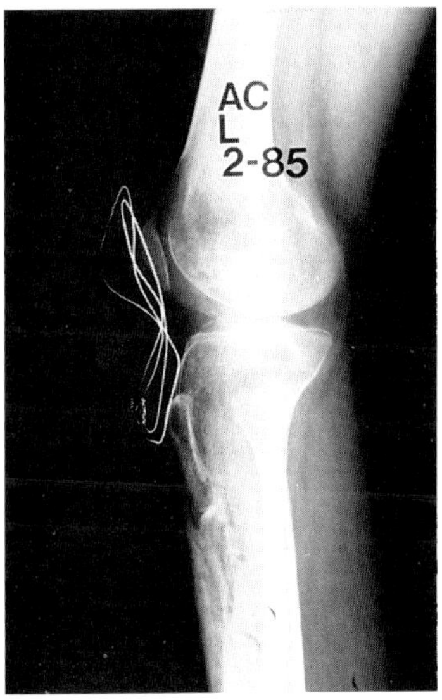

Fig. 5 This lateral radiograph of the knee of patient 3 taken 6 weeks postoperatively demonstrates shortening of the recently lengthened patellar tendon.

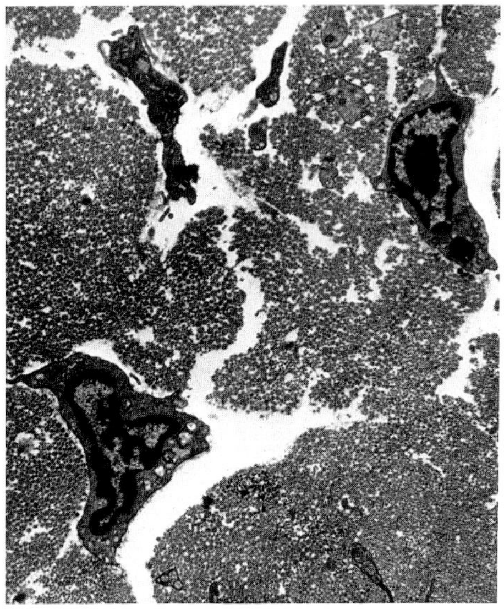

Fig. 6 Low-power transverse section electromicrograph of patellar tendon biopsy of patient 3. Note the viable cells and both large and small diameter fibrils.

performed, followed by 8 weeks of immobilization. The following year, a medial collateral ligament reconstruction was performed followed by a "ligament tightening." Two years later, an arthroscopic partial medial meniscectomy, and arthroplasty of the femoral condyles, patella, and tibial plateaus for grade II hyaline cartilage changes was performed. Later that year, a posterior cruciate ligament reconstruction, using the semitendinosus and gracilis tendons, was performed for grade IV posterior cruciate insufficiency. The patella was "olecronized" with a Steinmann pin, and the lower extremity was immobilized with a cast for 4 weeks. Subsequent deterioration in the patellofemoral joint occurred, and a Maquet osteotomy was performed in October, 1984, to relieve debilitating patellofemoral pain. The allograft bone used for the Maquet procedure did not unite and, at the time of exploration, a patellar tendon biopsy was performed on both the medial and lateral sides. Subsequently, the patient's complaints of pain decreased when swimming was introduced in physical therapy. She is now the mother of two children, unable to perform regular physical therapy because of time limitations, and is experiencing significant patellofemoral pain.

The collagen ultrastructure of this patient is shown in Figure 1, *E*. Using light microscopy and low power electromicroscopy, 2 nm sections showed the cells of the patellar tendon on both the medial and lateral sides were not viable as evidenced by clear cytoplasm with loss of organelles and rounded pyknotic nuclei (Figs. 8 and 9). Definite buckling and folding of collagen fiber bundles and individual fibrils are also seen (Figs. 10, 11, and 12). Figure 10 and its inset show collagen fiber bundle buckling. Capillaries are full of red blood cells with endothelial cells, which are necrotic.

The collagen fibril population of this patient is shown in Figure 1, *E*. This was the only patient in this group who did not demonstrate an increase in the number of small diameter fibrils. However, there was an apparent increase in the number of large diameter fibrils.

Discussion

The light microscopy, ultrastructure, and quantitative ultrastructural collagen fibril analyses of the four

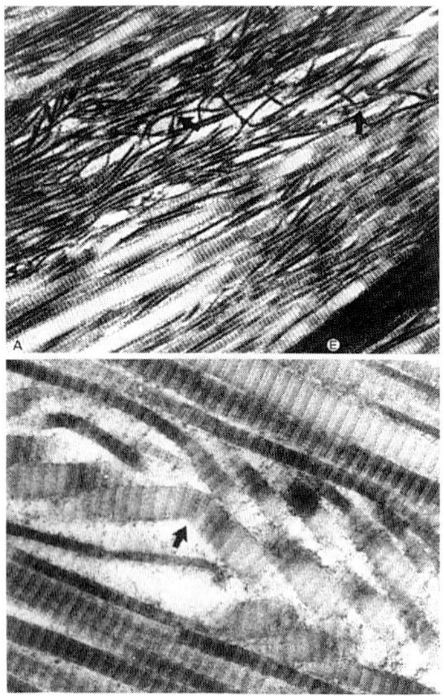

Fig. 7 **Top,** Low-power longitudinal section of patellar tendon biopsy of patient 3. Note both large and small diameter fibrils and acute buckling of some of the fibrils (arrows); electron dense elastic fiber (E). **Bottom,** Acute buckling of large diameter fibrils (arrows) in the same biopsy.

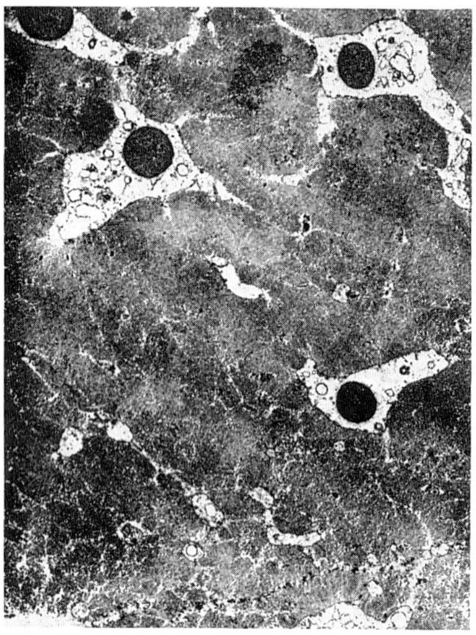

Fig. 8 Low power transverse section electronmicrograph of patellar tendon biopsy of patient 4. Note all cells are effete with pyknotic nuclei but adjacent collagen matrix is essentially intact.

patellar tendon biopsies were abnormal when compared to the normal patellar tendon.[34] In the first three, there was a marked increase in the number of small diameter fibrils present, which was also evident in the cross-sectional area occupied by these small diameter fibrils (Figs. 1, *B*, *C*, and *D*). This predominance of small diameter fibrils appears to be at the expense of the large diameter fibrils, especially in patients 1 and 2. This population pattern of small diameter fibrils in patellar tendon is also seen at 3 months postoperatively, when patellar tendon is used as an ACL auto- or allograft.[34,36] With the ACL grafts, we believe the rapid appearance and predominance of these small diameter fibrils reflect the rapid collagen remodeling and collagen neosynthesis process, which occurs almost immediately after ACL reconstruction.[37] It is probable that a similar neosynthesis of small diameter collagen fibrils occurred in patients 1, 2, and 3.

Of interest is that in patients 3 and 4, the large fibrils remain even as the newer smaller fibrils are produced. This is not the expected profile for active collagen synthesis occurring during the process of repair. In fact, the biopsy of patient 4 shows no viable cells (Figs. 8 and 9); this appeared to be a devascularized tendon. In order to put these two patient biopsies into perspective, it is important to note that both of these biopsies were obtained after the Maquet osteotomies of the tibial tubercle had been performed. These osteotomies may have partially devascularized the tibial end of the patellar tendon. In patient 4, this was further complicated by a nonunion that occurred at the Maquet osteotomy site, which necessitated further bone grafting. Because the Maquet osteotomy elevates the tibial end of the patella tendon, it may compromise both the soft-tissue and tibial blood supply to the tendon. It is clear that in patient 4, many or most of the patellar tendon fibroblasts at biopsy (3 months post-Maquet) probably died from ischemia (Figs. 8 and 9). This could account for the persistence of the large diameter fibrils without any evidence of neocollagen synthesis in the form of small diameter fibrils.

It is also of interest that in patient 4 collagen fiber bundles and individual fibrils were folded back twice on one another (180°) (Figs. 11 and 12). This suggests the possibility that collagen fiber bundles and fibrils slipped over one another. This could occur if the patellar tendon was compressed or unloaded axially by contracted soft tissues outside the patellar tendon, or if myofibroblasts within the tendon were capable of any myofibroblast "active" actin-mediated cell contraction. This former mechanism has been postulated by Brickley-Parsons and associates,[8] as a means of shortening the collagen in Dupuytren's contracture of the palmar fascia (Figs. 13 and 14). This may have occurred in patient 4. The ultrastructural mechanism of shortening of the patellar tendon in the other patients remains unclear, because no quantitative analysis of contractile intracellular myofilaments within the fibroblasts of these patellar tendon biopsies was performed.

Acute collagen bundle folding is not a new concept in a biological context and has been previously reported in specialized elastic ligaments.[38] Cyclical collagen bundle folding probably occurs in the ligamentum nuchae and flavum with vertebral extension and subsequent relaxation of the posterior spinal ligaments. In these unique elastic tissues, the elastic fibers are in a state of "pre-stress" when the spine is not in the extended position. Because of this unique attachment of collagen to elastin, a considerable amount of buckling and

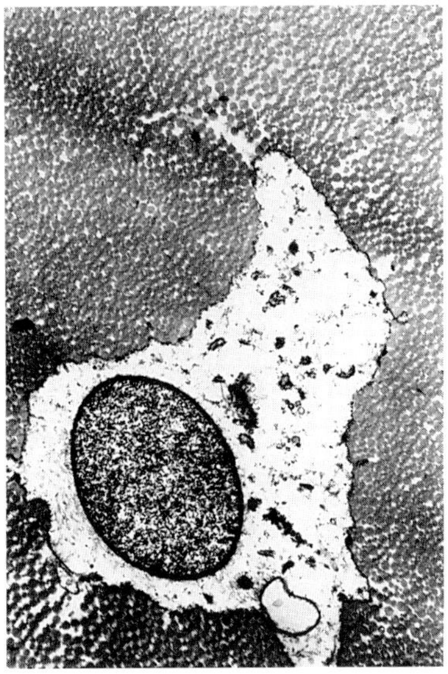

Fig. 9 Transverse section electromicrograph of patellar tendon biopsy of patient 4 showing detail of an effete cell with surrounding intact collagen matrix composed mainly of large diameter fibrils.

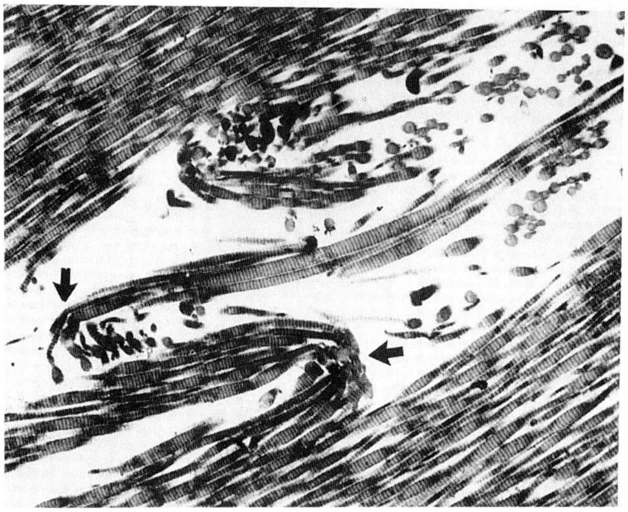

Fig. 11 Detail of collagen fibril acute buckling (arrows) in patient 4.

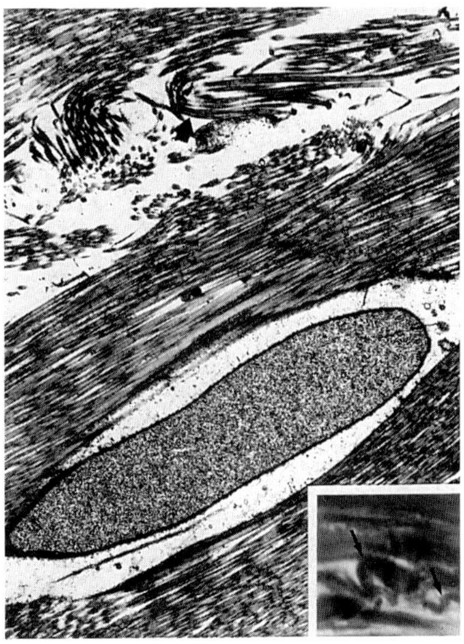

Fig. 10 Longitudinal section electromicrograph of patellar tendon biopsy of patient 4 demonstrating an effete cell as well as collagen fibril acute buckling (large arrow). The inset is a light micrograph showing collagen fiber bundle buckling (arrows) between collagen fasciculi.

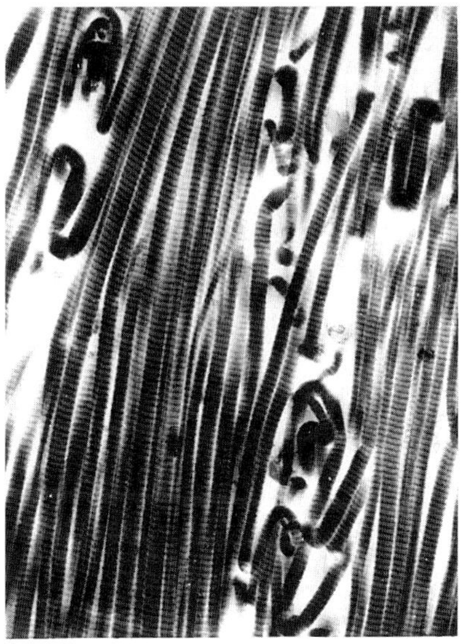

Fig. 12 Detail of acute buckling observed of individual collagen fibrils within patellar tendon biopsy of patient 4.

folding of collagen fibers in the ligament is possible during extension.

The de novo shortening of collagenous tissue such as the patellar tendon is not a well-accepted concept. However, in the last two decades focused research on the phenomenon of wound contraction has provided evidence that this process may be cell mediated via "myofibroblasts."[13] James and Taylor [39] were first to demonstrate that fibroblasts could exert tension in vitro. Hay [40] later showed condensations of actin fibers within the involved cells. Ippolito and associates,[41] in 1977, reported actin within tendon fibroblasts and, more recently, Dahners and associates,[11] 1986, have demonstrated the presence of actin within ligament fibroblasts.

In 1980, Gelberman and associates[14] were also able to confirm the presence of myofibroblasts in seven out of 24 patients with Dupuytren's nodules in their palmar fascia. In Gelberman's study, there was also an increased number of type III small diameter collagen

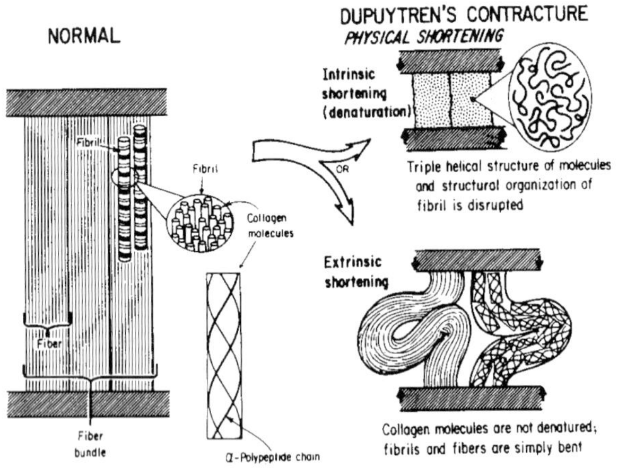

Fig. 13 Two possible mechanisms in which a physical shortening of collagen might occur and thus account for the shortening of the palmar tissue in Dupuytren's disease: **(top right)** by intrinsic changes within the collagen—that is, by denaturation, and **(bottom right)** by plication or folding of the fibrils, fibers, fiber bundles, and higher-ordered structural elements. Neither of these explanations accounts satisfactorily for the gross shortening or contracture of the palmar fascia in Dupuytren's disease. (Reproduced with permission from Brickley-Parsons D, Glimcher M, Smith R, et al: Biochemical changes in the collagen of the palmar fascia in patients with Dupuytren's disease. *J Bone Joint Surg* 1981;63A:787–797.)

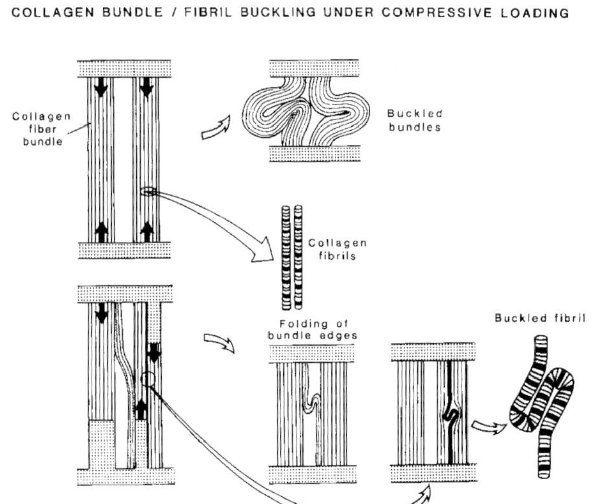

Fig. 14 Possible mechanisms of collagen fiber bundle shortening in the patella infera syndrome. **Top left,** Two collagen fiber bundles fixed at either end may undergo "extrinsic" shortening and cause fiber bundles to buckle as shown top right and in Figure 13, which was not observed in this study. **Bottom left,** Collagen fiber bundle may undergo selective remodeling at either end of one bundle and/or at both ends of the same bundle but in differing locations as indicated by the cross-hatched areas. Collagen fibrils were observed linking between two bundles as shown at **top left**. If collagen remodeling occurs as indicated in the two bundles shown "interbundle" folding will occur as shown at **bottom center,** with folding of fibrils along the edges of the two bundles as shown in actual micrographs in Figures 10 and 11. **Bottom right,** Shows intrabundle folding of collagen fibrils as the two areas of collagen remodeling occur in the same bundle (**right**) but from each end opposite one another as shown in an actual micrograph in Figure 12.

fibrils in the palmar nodules. It would appear that in two of our patients examined ultrastructurally (patients 1 and 2), where obvious large amounts of "new" small diameter collagen fibrils were present, that intrinsic tendon contraction, via fibronectin, is a possible mechanism mediated by myofibroblasts attaching to the collagen fibril matrix. Myofilaments and intermediate fibrils were identified in these patients, but their detailed morphometric quantification was beyond the scope of this study.

Data correlating collagen age, fibril size, mechanical loading and tensile strength have been reported by Parry and Craig,[31-33] who used collagen fibril diameter studies from a large number of tissues in various species. This concept has been supported by Shadwick[42] who correlated the tensile strength of hind limb flexor and extensor tendons of immature swine with collagen fibril populations. The mechanically weaker extensor tendons had collagen fibril population profiles that showed much smaller average diameter fibrils than the much stronger flexor tendons.

In several collagen fibril profile studies from a number of tissues, including rat ACL remodeling in response to a vigorous exercise program, remodeling of human ACL patellar tendon autografts[34] and ACL allografts,[36] and in chronic human Achilles tendonitis,[43] there is no evidence that collagen remodeling and repair processes can produce the high-tensile-strength large collagen fibrils. Hence, the small collagen fibril profile seen in the biopsies of patients 1 and 2 is probably the result of neocollagen synthesis. This process seems to be quite vigorous, suggesting a similarity to wound repair.

Intrinsic mechanisms may be the etiology for the patellar tendon shortening seen in patients 1 and 2, which raises the important question of whether there is a balance of forces involved in determining the definitive adult length of the patellar tendon. Extrinsic quadriceps muscle tension on the patellar tendon may be balanced by intrinsic, "myofibroblast" actin-mediated, mechanical traction on the collagen matrix via fibronectin. This theory has been explored recently in animal models.[26,27] Clinically, there is a well-defined but thankfully small group of patients who with ACL knee reconstructive surgery experience excessive intra-articular collagen neosynthesis with subsequent joint contracture (arthrofibrosis). These unfortunate patients can experience unusual amounts of pain and stiffness, as did the patients in this study. The biological mechanisms involved with this excessive intra-articular collagen biosynthesis are also poorly understood.[44]

Initially, when the patella infera syndrome is suspected, quadriceps muscle dysfunction and soft-tissue contracture around the knee should be treated nonsurgically, with vigorous supervised daily physical therapy.[24] However, the soft-tissue reaction can soon progress to arthrofibrosis if range of motion exercises and patellar mobilization techniques are not successful. If this maturation of collagen occurs, surgical release of the contracted medial and lateral retinaculum, resection of the fat pad, debridement of the suprapatellar pouch and intercondylar notch is recommended. Elevation of the patellar tendon from the anterior aspect of the tibia proximal to the tibial tuberosity may be necessary as well as tibial tubercle repositioning.[4] Unfortunately, surgical intervention can inhibit quadriceps muscle function further because of postoperative knee joint effusion and pain.[45] Therefore, surgical intervention must be used with caution; only after active quadriceps function has been achieved should surgical treatment be considered. Performing surgical procedures around the knee in these situations before the development of adequate quadriceps muscle function is ill-advised. Worsening of the quadriceps condition by further inhibition of the extensor mechanism and decreasing the tensile forces applied to the patellar tendon allows the patella to remain in the inferior, hazardous position.

Despite difficulties in explaining why some patients develop the rapid sequence of problems demonstrated in these four patients, we believe that certain empirical precautions are prudent after injury and/or surgery about the knee. These include: (1) avoiding immobilization whenever possible after injury and/or surgery, (2) mobilizing the peripatellar soft tissues as soon as possible, through (3) range of motion exercises for the tibial femoral joint and patellar mobilization in the medial-lateral and superior-inferior planes, (4) encouraging active quadriceps contraction within 3 days of injury or operation, and (5) early lateral radiographic assessment of the knee in 30° to 60° of knee flexion for these patients to document patellar position to detect the possible rapid contraction of soft tissue.

References

1. Blazina ME, Fox JM, Carlson GJ, et al: Abstract: Patella baja: A technical consideration in evaluating results of tibial tubercle transplantation. *J Bone Joint Surg* 1975;57A:1027.
2. Caton J, Deschamps G, Chambat P, et al: Patella infera: A propos of 128 cases. *Rev Chir Orthop Reparatrice Appar Mot* 1982;68:317–325.
3. Linclau L, Dokter G: Iatrogenic patella "baja". *Acta Orthop Belg* 1984;50:75–80.
4. Noyes FR, Wojtys EM, Marshall MT: The early diagnosis and treatment of developmental patella infera syndrome. *Clin Orthop* 1991;265:241–252.
5. Paulos LE, Rosenberg TD, Drawbert J, et al: Infrapatellar contracture syndrome: An unrecognized cause of knee stiffness with patella entrapment and patella infera. *Am J Sports Med* 1987;15:331–341.
6. Wojtys EM, Noyes FR, Gikas P: Patella baja syndrome. Proceedings of the American Academy of Orthopaedic Surgeons 53rd Annual Meeting, New Orleans, LA. Park Ridge, IL, American Academy of Orthopaedic Surgeons, 1986, p 118.
7. Booth FW, Gould EW: Effects of training and disuse on connective tissue. *Excer Sports Sci Rev* 1975;3:83–112.
8. Brickley-Parsons D, Glimcher MJ, Smith RJ, et al: Biochemical changes in the collagen of the palmar fascia in patients with Dupuytren's disease. *J Bone Joint Surg* 1981;63A:787–797.
9. Buck RC: Regeneration of tendon. *J Pathol Bacteriol* 1953; 66:1–18.
10. Butler DL, Grood ES, Noyes FR: Biomechanics of ligaments and tendons. *Exerc Sport Sci Rev* 1978;6:125–181.
11. Dahners LE, Banes AJ, Burridge KW: The relationship of actin to ligament contraction. *Clin Orthop* 1986;210: 246–251.
12. Flint MH; Lyons MF, Meaney MF, et al: The Masson staining of collagen: An explanation of an apparent paradox. *Histochem J* 1975;7:529–546.
13. Gabbiani G, Majno G: Dupuytren's contracture: Fibroblast contraction? An ultrastructural study. *Am J Pathol* 1972;66:131–146.
14. Gelberman RH, Amiel D, Rudolph RM, et al: Dupuytren's contracture: An electron microscopic, biochemical, and clinical correlative study. *J Bone Joint Surg* 1980;62A:425–432.
15. Gillard GC, Reilly HC, Bell-Booth PG, et al: The influence of mechanical forces on the glycosaminoglycan content of the rabbit flexor digitorum profundus tendon. *Connect Tissue Res* 1979;7:37–46.
16. Postacchini F, De Martino C: Regeneration of rabbit calcaneal tendon maturation of collagen and elastic fibers following partial tenotomy. *Connect Tissue Res* 1980;8:41–47.
17. Woo SL, Ritter MA, Amiel D, et al: The biomechanical and biochemical properties of swine tendons: Long term effects of exercise on digital extensors. *Connect Tissue Res* 1980;7:177–183.
18. Flint M: Interrelationships of mucopolysaccharide and collagen in connective tissue remodelling. *J Embryol Exp Morph* 1972; 27:481–495.
19. Noyes FR, Wojtys EM: The early recognition, diagnosis, and treatment of patella infera syndrome, in Tullos H (ed): *Instructional Course Lectures XL*. Park Ridge, IL, American Academy of Orthopaedic Surgeons 1991, pp 233–247.
20. van Eijden TM, Kouwenhoven E, Weijs WA: Mechanics of the patellar articulation: Effects of patellar ligament length studied with a mathematical model. *Acta Orthop Scand* 1987;58:560–566.
21. Tardieu C, Blanchard O, Tabary JC, et al: Tendon adaptation to bone shortening. *Connect Tissue Res* 1983;11:35–44.
22. Tipton CM, Matthes RD, Maynard JA, et al: The influence of physical activity on ligaments and tendons. *Med Sci Sports* 1975;7:165–175.
23. Burks RT, Haut RC, Lancaster RL: Biomechanical and histological observations of the dog patellar tendon after removal of its central one-third. *Am J Sports Med* 1990;18:146–153.
24. Piper TL, Whiteside LA: Early mobilization after knee ligament repair in dogs: An experimental study. *Clin Orthop* 1980; 150:277–282.
25. Vailas AC, Tipton CM, Matthes RD, et al: Physical activity and its influence on the repair process of medial collateral ligaments. *Connect Tissue Res* 1981;9:25–31.
26. Ohno K, Yasuda K, Yamamoto N, et al: Effects of stress shielding on the mechanical properties of normal and in situ frozen patellar tendon. *Trans Orthop Res Soc* 1991;16:134.
27. Vailas AC, Deluna DM, Lewis LL, et al: Adaptation of bone and tendon to prolonged hindlimb suspension in rats. *J Appl Physiol* 1988;65:373–376.
28. Oakes BW, Parker AW, Norman J: Changes in collagen fibre populations in young rat cruciate ligaments in response to an

intensive one month's exercise program, in Russo P (ed): *Human Adaption: A Workshop.* Sydney, Australia, Cumberland College of Health Sciences, 1981, pp 223–230.

29. Ito S, Karnovsky MJ: Abstract: Formaldehyde-glutaraldehyde fixatives containing trinitro compounds. *J Cell Biol* 1968; 39(suppl 168A):1689–1699.
30. Parker AW: Changes in the strength of bone and ligament in response to training, in Russo P (ed): *Human Adaption: A Workshop.* Sydney, Australia, Cumberland College of Health Sciences, 1981, pp 209–221.
31. Parry DA, Craig AS, Barnes GR: Tendon and ligament from the horse: An ultrastructural study of collagen fibrils and elastic fibres as a function of age. *Proc R Soc Lond B Biol Sci* 1978;203:293–303.
32. Parry DA, Craig AS: Collagen fibrils during development and maturation and their contribution to the mechanical attributes of connective tissue, in Nimni ME (ed): *Collagen.* Boca Raton, Florida, CRC Press, 1988, vol 2, pp 1–23.
33. Parry DA, Craig AS: Growth and development of collagen fibrils in connective tissue, in Ruggeri A, Motta PM (eds): *The Ultrastructure of the Connective Tissue Matrix.* Boston, MA, Martinus Nijhoff, 1984, pp 34–64.
34. Frank C, Woo S, Andriacchi T, et al: Normal ligament: Structure, function, and compositions, in Woo SL-Y, Buckwalter J (eds): *Injury and Repair of the Musculoskeletal Soft Tissues.* Park Ridge, IL, American Academy of Orthopaedic Surgeons, 1988, pp 45–101.
35. Outerbridge RE: Further studies on the etiology of chondromalacia patellae. *J Bone Joint Surg* 1964;46B:179–190.
36. Shino K, Oakes BW, Inoue M, et al: Human ACL allograft: Collagen fibril populations studied as a function of age of the graft. *Trans Orthop Res Soc* 1990;15:520.
37. Kleiner JB, Amiel D, Harwood FL, et al: Early histologic, metabolic, and vascular assessment of anterior cruciate ligament autografts. *J Orthop Res* 1989;7:235–242.
38. Oakes BW, Bialkower B: Biomechanical and ultrastructural studies on the elastic wing tendon of the domestic fowl. *J Anat* 1977;123:369–387.
39. James DW, Taylor JF: The stress developed by sheets of chick fibroblasts in vitro. *Exp Cell Res* 1969;54:107–110.
40. Hay ED: Extracellular matrix, cell skeletons, and embryonic development. *Am J Med Genet* 1989;34:14–29.
41. Ippolito E, Natali PG, Postacchini F, et al: Ultrastructural and immunochemical evidence of actin in the tendon cells. *Clin Orthop* 1977;126:282–284.
42. Shadwick RE: Elastic energy storage in tendons: Mechanical differences related to function and age. *J Appl Physiol* 1990; 68:1033–1040.
43. Oakes BW: Connective tissue adaptation to loading: Fibroblasts, fibres, fibrils and free grafts. *Proc First Int Olympic Com World Cong Sports Sci* 1989:156–160.
44. Ogata K, Whiteside LA, Andersen DA: The intra-articular effect of various postoperative managements following knee ligament repair: An experimental study in dogs. *Clin Orthop* 1980; 150:271–276.
45. deAndrade JR, Grant C, Dixon A-St J: Joint distention and reflex muscle inhibition in the knee. *J Bone Joint Surg* 1965;47A: 313–322.

CHAPTER 25

Reflex Sympathetic Dystrophy, Patella Infera Contracture Syndrome, and Loss of Motion Following Anterior Cruciate Ligament Surgery

Bernard R. Bach, Jr, MD
Edward M. Wojtys, MD
Thomas N. Lindenfeld, MD

The complications of reflex sympathetic dystrophy, patella infera contracture syndrome, or arthrofibrosis following reconstructive surgery can be devastating. Of these three major complications, loss of motion secondary to arthrofibrosis (Figs. 1 and 2) is the most easily treated. The purpose of this chapter is to discuss (1) the timing of anterior cruciate ligament (ACL) surgery, (2) methods to minimize the complication of arthrofibrosis, (3) operative factors that may contribute to reduced knee motion, (4) treatment for the patient who presents with a stiff knee following ACL surgical treatment, and (5) the results in the literature concerning arthrofibrosis.

When considering the timing of ACL reconstructive surgery, three questions arise. (1) Why intervene surgically on an acute basis? (2) Can we intervene safely on an acute basis? (3) Should we intervene surgically on an acute basis? Biologic considerations, such as posttraumatic or postsurgical inflammation, associated collateral ligament injury, and a potentially repairable meniscal tear, are important factors that govern decisions regarding early surgical reconstruction. The disadvantage of acute ACL surgical reconstruction is that often the knee is inflamed, particularly in individuals who have sustained "loading" injuries while playing sports such as football, basketball, volleyball, or rugby. These patients frequently come to the office with a large hemarthrosis and decreased motion. These symptoms are in contrast to those seen in many individuals who sustain acute ski-related injuries, which are generally "unloading" injuries with different mechanisms of injury and a reduced incidence of meniscal tears. Patients may present to the physician's office within several days after an acute ski injury with nearly normal motion. In the acute setting, it may be difficult for the physician to accurately assess the patient's expectations regarding their injured knee. Conversely, the patient who has sustained an acute injury has not experienced the potential disability associated with a chronic ACL-deficient knee. The individual with a chronic ACL-deficient knee who has experienced episodes of instability and knows the unpredictability of the knee may have expectations entirely different from those of the acute patient subgroup. Although the patient's perceptions regarding ACL surgical treatment, reduced perioperative morbidity, and markedly improved results have changed, there remains a role for conservative treatment of the ACL-deficient knee. In the patient with an acutely injured ACL it can be difficult to predict who will benefit optimally from surgical treatment.

The advantages of acute ACL surgical reconstruction include the potential for less articular surface

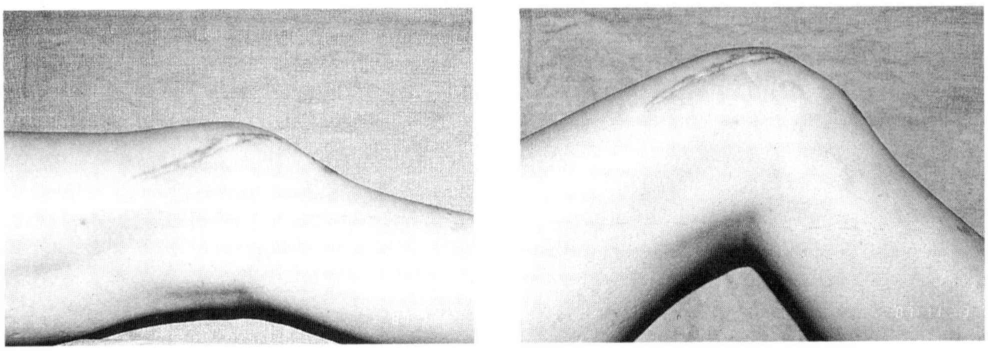

Fig. 1 Left, Knee flexion contracture following arthrotomy, acute repair and reconstruction of a combined grade 3 ski-related injury to the medial collateral and anterior cruciate ligaments initially seen in our office at 4 months postoperatively. Subsequent arthroscopic debridement of intercondylar notch, fat pad, and adhesions within the medial and lateral gutters and manipulation under anesthesia resulted in recovery of symmetric extension and flexion. **Right,** Knee extension contracture in aforementioned patient when examined under anesthesia prior to arthroscopic debridement and manipulation.

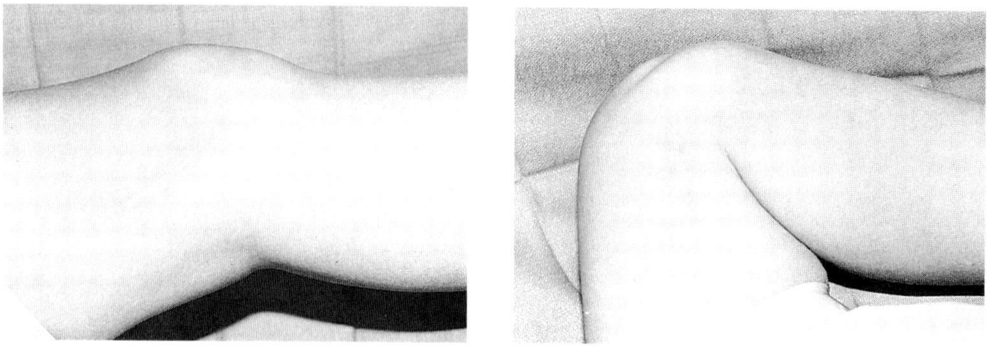

Fig. 2 Preoperative flexion, **left,** and extension, **right,** contractures demonstrated a combined 40-cm (40°) asymmetry at 18 months postoperatively when this patient presented to our office following arthroscopically assisted anterior cruciate ligament reconstruction with patellar tendon autograft for chronic anterior cruciate ligament deficiency. Following arthroscopic debridement, expansion notchplasty, and manipulation, the patient made dramatic gains in motion recovery with an ultimate asymmetry in extension and flexion of only 6 cm.

injury and reduced incidence and severity of meniscal pathology. In the acute setting, the lateral meniscus is more frequently injured than the medial meniscus. In the chronic setting, the medial meniscus is more frequently injured. In individuals who sustain peripheral longitudinal meniscal tears that are amenable to meniscal repair, the medial meniscus predominates in a 4:1 ratio. For these reasons, many ligament surgeons prefer subacute surgical treatment in appropriately selected individuals.

When considering acute or subacute ACL reconstructive surgery, the tissues most commonly used include patellar tendon autograft or medial hamstrings. The hamstrings may be used as doubled, tripled, or quadrupled length grafts. Primary repair of the ACL tissue with semitendinosus augmentation is performed less frequently today. Some surgeons prefer patellar tendon allograft as an alternative graft source. Overall, the use of the hamstring tendons is a more forgiving procedure, and knee stiffness after acute reconstruction is less likely than with patellar tendon autogenous tissue.

The timing of surgical intervention in the acute phase remains controversial. Urgent surgical intervention has evolved to a concept of subacute surgical treatment for patients who are considered reconstruction candidates. In the era of arthrotomy, primary and acute ACL repair with augmentation within 2 to 3 weeks was frequently performed so that ACL ligamentous tissue could be incorporated into the repair, but this is rarely done today. Several authors have recommended a minimal time for surgical intervention to minimize knee motion problems. The studies of Shelbourne and associates,[1-3] Mohtadi and associates,[4] and Cosgarea and associates,[5] demonstrated that motion problems are reduced if subacute reconstruction is deferred until after 3 weeks from the index injury, whereas the study of Harner and associates[6] suggested a 4-week delay.

The development of arthrofibrosis has been attributed to a myriad of factors, including gender, associated meniscal repair, extra-articular repair, concomitant medial collateral ligament (MCL) injury, infection, reflex sympathetic dystrophy, preoperative range of motion, type of tissue used for reconstruction, postoperative immobilization, and the interval from index injury to reconstruction. Review of the literature sheds considerable insight into the problems of knee stiffness with ACL injuries.

Literature Review

Sachs and associates[7] prospectively reviewed 126 patients who between 1982 and 1986 underwent ACL reconstruction with intra-articular patellar tendon, hamstring, or iliotibial band tissues. Postoperatively, patients were casted in 30° of knee flexion for 3 weeks. Limited motion was then instituted with a 30° extension stop for another 3 to 5 weeks. Full weightbearing was delayed until between 6 and 8 weeks postoperatively. Terminal extension exercises were not used until 1 year postoperatively. In this study, the authors reported a high incidence (24%) of knee flexion contractures greater than 5° as measured by prone heel height differences. Quadriceps deficiency, as demonstrated by Cybex isokinetic testing at 60°/s, demonstrated deficits of greater than 20% in 65% of the patients. Patellar pain was present in 19% of their patients. The authors recommended that efforts be made to achieve full extension earlier and concluded that knee flexion contractures were frequently associated with patellar pain and quadriceps weakness.

In 1990, Jackson and Schaefer[8] reviewed the arthroscopic findings of 13 of 230 patients (6%) who required arthroscopic evaluation for symptomatic knee flexion contractures. They described a characteristic "cyclops" scar nodule (Fig. 3) near the base of the ACL insertion site in all patients. The nodule was noted to impinge within the intercondylar notch in extension. Routine

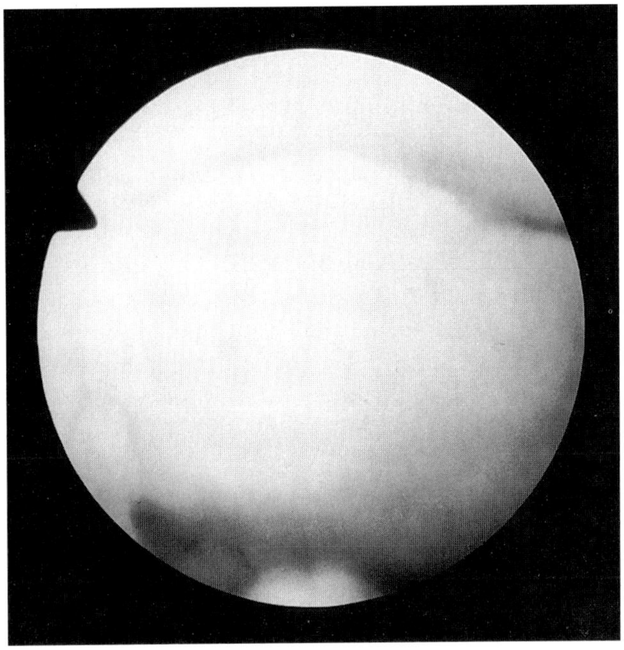

Fig. 3 This intraoperative arthroscopic photograph demonstrates a characteristic fibroproliferative scar nodule (cyclops lesion) which responded to arthroscopic debridement and notchplasty following anterior cruciate ligament reconstruction.

expansion notchplasty was not performed in these patients. They attributed the loss of extension and a characteristic audible clunk with terminal extension to this nodule. Surgical intervention was performed at an average of 16 weeks postoperatively (range 8 to 36 weeks). Prior to repeat arthroscopy, the mean knee flexion contracture was 16°. At final follow-up, the mean knee flexion contracture was 3.8° and all patients had greater than 130° of knee flexion. In these 13 patients, 11 had undergone reconstruction within 6 weeks of the index injury, although preoperative range of motion was not described. Four patients had an associated extra-articular reconstruction, and two had associated collateral ligament injuries. The nodules were examined histologically and described as dense fibrous tissue with a central area of granulation tissue with occasional osseous or cartilaginous tissue within the lesion.

Marzo and associates[9] retrospectively reviewed The Hospital for Special Surgery experience with arthrofibrosis between 1988 and 1991. Eighteen patients were personally evaluated by the authors. Thirteen had undergone either patellar tendon or hamstring reconstruction by the authors, whereas three patients transferred their care. During this period of time, 640 arthroscopically assisted ACL reconstructions were performed with a 2% reoperation rate for symptomatic knee flexion contractures. Nine patients had undergone index reconstruction acutely (< 2 weeks). Six patients had a medial and/or lateral meniscal repair, and two patients had an associated extra-articular reconstruction. Patients were reoperated at a mean of 11 months postreconstruction (range 3 to 21 months). The average knee flexion contracture was 11° (range 3° to 20°). Prone heel height differences were not mentioned. Intraoperative improvements in knee extension were readily observed, with a mean improvement of 8° (range 3° to 17°). At a mean follow-up of 16 months, the mean extension was 0° (range -7° to 5°). The authors characteristically observed a fibrous scar nodule within the intercondylar notch. Histologically, this nodule had the appearance of disorganized fibrous connective tissue, with a paucity of vascular ingrowth, no apparent inflammatory or granulation response, and a tendency toward chondroid metaplasia. It should be noted that this patient population underwent arthroscopic debridement much later than the patients in the study reported by Jackson. This interval to surgery, they postulated, might account for the lack of granulation tissue noted in the specimens that Jackson observed. Nevertheless, even at a mean intervention of 11 months, patients dramatically benefited from arthroscopic debridement.

Shelbourne and associates[2] reviewed 169 acute ACL injuries. The authors defined a knee flexion contracture as greater than or equal to 5°. They stratified their subgroups of surgical treatment (which was done with patellar tendon autograft via a mini-incision secured with buttons) as less than 1 week (Group I), 1 to 3 weeks (Group II), and greater than 3 weeks (Group III) as the surgical interval from index injury. The authors noted a statistically significant difference in the incidence of knee flexion contracture in the Group I and II patients versus patients treated after 3 weeks (Group III), which led them to defer surgical treatment until after 3 weeks from the index injury. In their report the authors did not specifically address a recommended range of motion that would minimize the likelihood of knee stiffness.

Harner and associates[6] retrospectively reviewed knee stiffness in 244 patients, 82 of whom were treated with patellar tendon autograft. Of the 244, 162 patients were treated with patellar tendon allograft in an arthroscopically assisted fashion. Associated extra-articular ligamentous repair was performed in 33% of the patients, and meniscal repair was performed in 25% of the patients. The authors defined arthrofibrosis as greater than a 10° knee flexion contracture or less than 125° of knee flexion. The authors observed that in those patients in whom surgical treatment was performed at less than 1 month from the initial injury, 37% met their definition of arthrofibrosis. In contrast, only 5.5% of their patients who underwent surgery at greater than 1 month developed arthrofibrosis. This observation was statistically significant ($p < .001$). The authors also noted that those individuals who underwent MCL repair, with or without posterior oblique repairs, had an arthrofibrosis incidence of 44% in contrast to only 7% in those without MCL repairs. There was also a gender difference, with males having a higher incidence of arthrofibrosis than females.

Fisher and Shelbourne[10] retrospectively reviewed 42 of 959 patients who developed a knee flexion contracture.[10] They reported that prior to 1987 there was a reoperation incidence of 10% for knee flexion contractures. They instituted an accelerated rehabilitation program that resulted in a reduced incidence of knee flexion contracture between 1987 and 1989, when they reported a 4% reoperation rate. They observed that in those individuals undergoing acute ACL reconstruction there was a twofold incidence of reoperation in those individuals whose surgery was done less than 3 weeks after the index injury.

Wasilewski and associates[11] retrospectively reviewed 87 patients in whom an arthroscopically assisted hamstring reconstruction procedure was performed.[11] The author defined arthrofibrosis as greater than 25° of combined flexion or extension deficit at 6 months postoperatively. A conservative early range of motion and weightbearing protocol was utilized and, in those patients undergoing meniscal repairs, immobilization was continued for up to 1 month. The authors noted an incidence of 15% arthrofibrosis in acute patients undergoing surgery at less than 1 month from the index injury, 0% in the subacute patients (1 to 6 months), and a 13% incidence in the chronic subgroup operated on greater than 6 months from the index injury.

Hardin and associates'[12] initial experience of 200 arthroscopically assisted ACL reconstructions using patellar tendon autograft without extra-articular augmentation was retrospectively reviewed and reported in 1993. Twelve patients (6%) required reoperation for symptomatic knee flexion contractures. An early range of motion (-10° to 90°) was the standard protocol until 1989. For individuals undergoing repeat surgery for scar excision, the mean interval to surgical treatment was 8 months postoperatively. Predebridement knee flexion contracture averaged 12° (5° to 20°). Following surgery, the mean knee flexion contracture was 3°, with all patients having significant improvements in range of motion. At the time of surgery, scar nodules were noted in ten of 12 patients. Eleven of 12 patients demonstrated intercondylar notch stenosis. At follow-up, all patients demonstrated stable knees by KT-1000 arthrometry and negative pivot shift testing. Nine of 12 had returned to sports, and six of 12 demonstrated some degree of patellofemoral crepitation.

Bach and associates[13] retrospectively reviewed their initial experience with arthroscopically assisted ACL reconstruction and in 1994 reported a retrospective review of 62 of 75 patients. There was no statistically significant difference in the range of motion in the acute versus chronic subgroup, no difference in the incidence of reoperation for the acute versus chronic subgroup, and no differences in the incidence of knee flexion contractures defined by prone heel height discrepancies in the acute and chronic subgroups. The author, however, has used preoperative motion as the criteria for surgical intervention.

In another study, Shelbourne and Johnson[1] reviewed nine patients with symptomatic knee flexion contracture greater than 15° compared to the opposite knee.[1] He noted that eight of the nine patients had undergone surgery at less than 2 weeks from the index injury. Five of these patients underwent open patellar tendon autograft reconstruction, and two of the nine had associated MCL repair.

Cosgarea and associates[14] retrospectively reviewed DeHaven's experience with arthrofibrosis. Between 1981 and 1990, 61 patients required arthroscopic debridement for stiff knees. Ligament surgery had been performed in 43 knees (37 patients). In 30 of the patients, surgical treatment included arthroscopic debridements, lysis of adhesions, lateral retinacular release, and notchplasty; six patients required mini-anterior arthrotomy and extra-articular scar resection, while one patient required a posteromedial arthrotomy, excision of posterior intra-articular adhesions, and posterior capsular release. Although marked improvements in range of motion were observed by the authors, with the mean knee flexion contracture improving from -14° to -3°, and flexion improving from 83% to 97% of the normal knee, only 62% of their patients achieved satisfactory functional results. Patella infera, soft-tissue calcification, and radiographic degenerative joint disease was noted in 9%, 51%, and 89%, respectively. They also noted that those patients who underwent arthroscopic debridement at less than 6 months from the time of index ligament surgery had improved results.

Hunter, in 1994, reported at the Arthroscopy Association of North America meeting a prospective study of 185 patients surgically reconstructed at a ski resort setting. The mean age of the predominantly skiing patient population was 34 years, which is older than the mean patient age for most reported studies. An arthroscopically assisted ACL reconstruction with patellar tendon autograft without extra-articular augmentation was performed on all patients. The authors stratified their patient subgroups from injury to surgical intervention as less than 2 days, 3 to 7 days, 1 to 3 weeks, and greater than 3 weeks. No statistically significant differences in range of motion, stability, or KT-1000 parameters were reported. Eleven reoperations were performed, all of them in patients who underwent ACL surgical treatment at less than 3 weeks from the initial injury. Hunter concluded that there was no advantage to immediate surgery. Although he also concluded that there was reason to wait to perform surgery, collective reoperation of 11 patients in those individuals at less than 3 weeks from the index injury might suggest otherwise.

A retrospective review of 373 patients was reported by Graf and associates.[15] In this mixed patient population, an arthrotomy was performed in 40% of patients who underwent intra-articular ligament reconstruction. The authors defined arthrofibrosis as a range of motion at less than 10° of knee extension and less than 125° of knee flexion. They stratified the patient subgroups as less than 1 week, 2 to 6 weeks, 6 weeks to 6 months, and greater than 6 months from the index injury. In this patient population, the periods of immobilization varied. Several factors were identified as high risk factors for the development of the stiff knee. Open surgery ($p < .0008$), surgery performed at less than 1 week from the index injury ($p < .04$), and motion delayed until the second day following surgery ($p < .04$) are three factors noted to be associated with arthrofibrosis. The authors also reported that an early motion protocol reduced the incidence of arthrofibrosis from 25% to 9%. They also observed that an early motion rehabilitation protocol reduced the likelihood of manipulation from 15% to 1.5%.

In another study, Cosgarea and associates[5] reported an arthrofibrosis incidence of 12% in a review of 188 patients who underwent ACL reconstruction. Group I patients (n = 64) were splinted postoperatively in 45° of knee flexion for 7 days prior to allowing passive extension. Group II patients (n = 49) were splinted at 45° for 48 hours. Group III patients (n = 75) were splinted in full extension, and active flexion and full passive extension were immediately allowed. A mini-arthrotomy technique was used in 101 patients (54%) and an arthroscopically assisted technique in 87 patients (46%). Overall, an arthrofibrosis incidence of 12% was noted, defined as a knee flexion contracture ≥ 10° and/or knee flexion of ≤ 125°. The authors noted that preoperative motion was an important criteria that was directly related to developing arthrofibrosis ($p < .05$). An arthrofibrosis incidence of 21% was reported in acute patients, reconstructed less than 3 weeks from index injury, representing a twofold factor greater than the chronic subgroup (9%). The incidence of arthrofibrosis was reported as 23%, 10%, and 3% for Groups I, II, and III, respectively ($p < .0005$). There were no statistical associations between patient age, gender, associated meniscal surgery, or type of immediate postoperative analgesic. Acute surgery, motion deficits, and postoperative immobilization in flexion were significant factors associated with the development of arthrofibrosis.

Patel and associates[16] have recently reported their 10-year experience with 72 patients between 1983 and 1993 who required repeat arthroscopy for arthrofibrosis. The authors described a classification based on four patterns of knee stiffness, which aided them in predicting which type of arthroscopic surgery would be required. Type I patients (n = 25) had normal flexion and < 10° of extension loss. Type II patients (n = 16) had > 10° extension loss and normal flexion. Type III patients (n = 15) had a combined knee flexion and extension contracture (> 10° flexion, > 25° flexion) and evidence of a peripatellar fibrosis. Type IV patients (n = 16) had > 10° of knee extension, < 120° of knee flexion, and evidence of a patellar infera contracture syndrome. The mean interval from initial ACL reconstruction and arthroscopic debridement was 12.5 months (range 2.4 to 60 months). The authors recommended arthroscopic debridement and notchplasty for the Type I patients. The Type II, III, and IV patients represent a progressively more severe spectrum of knee stiffness, requiring medial and lateral releases along with intercondylar scar debridement and expansion notchplasty. The authors described dense scar formation in the medial and lateral gutters and extrasynovial scar formation between the fat pad and patellar tendon in the Type III patients, and a similar but more severe involvement in the Type IV patients. All arthroscopic debridements were performed on an outpatient basis, and serial extension casts were used in Types II, III, and IV patients. The authors did not mention the use of open posterior capsular releases or continuous passive motion (CPM) machines in this population. Overall, at a mean follow-up of 35 months, full extension compared to the opposite knee was noted in 88%, 81%, 80%, and 60% of Types I, II, III, and IV, respectively. The authors reported significant improvements in knee flexion in the Type IV patients. The mean postoperative modified Noyes score was 92, 94, 93, and 86 for these groups, respectively.

Hutton and associates retrospectively reported, at the 1995 American Orthopaedic Society for Sports Medicine's Specialty Day Meeting, on Steadman's experience with the issue of arthrofibrosis in 160 patients undergoing arthroscopically assisted ACL reconstruction using a double-incision patellar tendon autograft without extra-articular augmentation (Hutton KS, Scheinberg RR, Burns T, Steadman JR, Sterrett W, unpublished data, 1995). The definition of arthrofibrosis was less than 10° of extension or less than 120° of knee flexion. The patient subgroups were stratified as less than 1 week, 1 to 3 weeks, and greater than 3 weeks from the index injury. The authors reported no statistically significant difference in the range of motion. Overall, a 6% reoperation rate was reported. The authors emphasized using a protocol of attaining near complete extension and 120° of knee range of motion prior to surgical treatment as a primary goal before surgery is contemplated. Using this concept of adequate preoperative range of motion, quadriceps control and near resolution of posttraumatic swelling, the authors questioned the "golden time period" as previously advocated by Shelbourne and associates[2] and Harner and associates.[6] It should be noted, however, that this patient population is almost exclusively a skiing patient population. It may not be possible to extrapolate these results to the athlete who sustains a loading injury or to the individual who has an associated MCL sprain.

Management

The management of arthrofibrosis can be divided into prevention, recognition, and treatment phases. As a generalization, it is safer to avoid acute ACL surgery. Motion should be regained prior to surgical reconstruction if early surgical reconstruction is warranted. Our protocol has been similar to that advocated by Steadman. Since the late 1980s we have avoided operating on patients who have had poor range of motion in the acute or subacute phase. Occasionally this may necessitate observing a patient for up to 6 to 8 weeks subsequent to their injury and prior to reconstruction. Associated MCL injury should heighten the awareness of the potential development of knee stiffness. The more proximal MCL injury has been reported to have a higher association with delayed motion recovery.[17] If the patient has a combined ACL-MCL injury and is noted to have localized tenderness over the adductor tubercle, the motion must be carefully monitored. Preoperative or postoperative casting can be abandoned with contemporary methods of ACL surgical treatment with either multistrand hamstring or patellar tendon auto- or allograft surgical reconstruction. Post injury or postoperatively, early complete extension should be the principal treatment. We no longer immobilize our ACL-MCL injuries at 30° and, in fact, allow complete extension prior to any consideration for ACL surgical treatment.[13,18] There has been controversy with regard to the combined ACL-MCL injury, particularly the grade 3 MCL injury. There are advocates of combined MCL repair with ACL reconstruction. We, however, advocate isolated ACL reconstruction rather than combined MCL repair with reconstruction. Shelbourne and others have also advocated ACL reconstruction rather than combined MCL repair with ACL reconstruction.[3,19]

Postoperatively, the accelerated rehabilitation protocol advocated by Shelbourne and associates is used.[2] Complete extension and full weightbearing with the knee in extension is allowed. Following an injury or reconstructive surgery, the patella should be mobilized to minimize the development of scar tissue. Because most patients will sleep with their knees flexed, night extension splinting is routinely used in our patients to reduce the likelihood of a knee flexion contracture. This technique has been particularly helpful at achieving complete extension. Although basic science literature suggests early strain on the ACL tissue in the terminal 30° of extension, clinical observations suggest that early quadriceps rehabilitation can be performed without resultant failure of the ACL graft. For this reason, early active extension and straight leg raising exercises following patellar tendon autograft reconstruction for ACL deficiency is allowed. If an ACL orthosis is being used, an extension block is avoided. In some patients who develop an early abnormal gait following ACL reconstructive surgery, the use of an ACL orthosis is abandoned.

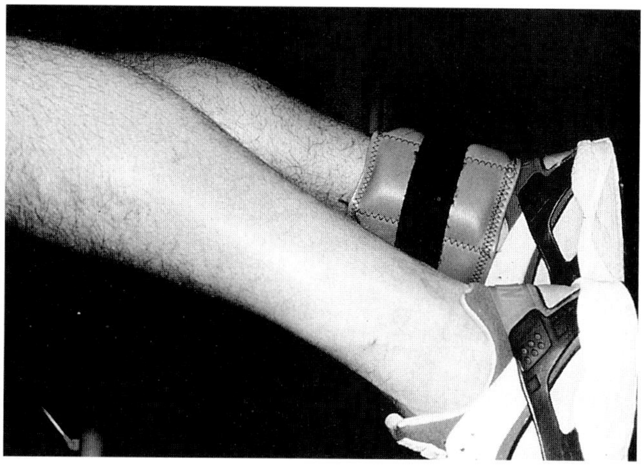

Fig. 4 Assessment of prone heel height asymmetries should be made on a regular basis postoperatively. Ankle weights may be necessary to achieve complete extension.

Careful monitoring of knee range of motion following ACL reconstructive surgery allows early recognition of the "problem" knee. One should monitor heel height discrepancies of extension and flexion with the patient in the prone position. A 5-cm asymmetry correlates with a 5° contracture.[7] Prone heel hangs postoperatively are initiated immediately after surgery (Fig. 4). In patients who have difficulty obtaining extension, ankle weights may be applied to the heel at anywhere from 2.5 to 20 pounds depending on the circumstances. If one assesses knee flexion both in the supine and prone position and there is a difference of more than 10°, this may imply that there is associated quadriceps contracture, which may necessitate aggressive stretching.

In the early postoperative course (eg, 2 weeks), our goal is to obtain 0° to 90° of knee motion. If the patient is having difficulty gaining extension in the first 2 weeks and has a prone heel height discrepancy greater than 5 cm, we will follow the patient weekly in the office. In contrast, if the patient is quickly gaining extension, we will routinely perform our second follow-up visit at 6 weeks postoperatively. Our decision to institute prone hangs with ankle weights depends on the sensation of the end point in "extension." If the patient demonstrates an abnormal knee flexion gait pattern at 6 weeks postoperatively, we will eliminate the ACL orthosis from our protocol to encourage a more normal heel-toe gait. We do not use an extension block when an orthosis is used.

Many surgeons continue to use the CPM machine to enhance early knee range of motion following ACL reconstruction. Surgeons should be cognizant that the CPM encourages flexion but does not promote extension. The literature clearly indicates that there is no advantage for a home CPM greater than 3 days postoperatively.[20]

This author (BRB) has not used CPM since early 1994. This change was based on our observations when a transition was made from the two-incision arthroscopically assisted technique to a single-incision technique. Between 1987 and 1991, we used a two-incision arthroscopically assisted technique with patellar tendon autograft, which required an average 2.9 days hospitalization.[21] CPM was used while the patients were hospitalized. In October of 1991 we made a prospective transition to a single-incision endoscopic technique.[18] We also began the use of Toradol (ketoralac tromethamine, Syntex Laboratories, Inc., Palo Alto, CA), Propofol (diprivan, Stuart Pharmaceuticals, Wilmington, DE), and ice cryotherapy units postoperatively. This resulted in a decreased hospitalization, so that by 1993 all patients were being discharged the day after surgery. Although we reduced hospitalization time by 2 days, our incidence of symptomatic knee flexion contractures and need for secondary arthroscopic scar resection were reduced. When we instituted our prospective outpatient endoscopic ACL reconstruction effort in May of 1994, we eliminated the use of the CPM in our postoperative protocol. At this time we have not seen any deleterious effect of abandoning CPM for our patient population.

Active flexion/extension must be monitored carefully, listening for an audible "clunk" in extension, which may suggest the development or presence of a fibroproliferative scar nodule, commonly referred to as a "cyclops" lesion.[8] If the patient has less than a 5-cm prone heel height discrepancy in extension at 3 months postoperatively without a "clunk," has a soft end point to extension, has appropriately placed tunnels, and does not have any significant patellofemoral pain symptoms, we continue to monitor the patient. One must recall that even up into the late 1980s it was common to limit extension purposely until 6 months postoperatively to "protect" the ACL reconstruction. Nevertheless, the majority of those patients regained complete extension. If a patient has between a 5- and 10-cm prone heel height discrepancy beyond 3 months and has an audible "clunk," has developed patellofemoral symptoms, or has pain referred in the retropatellar region with attempts to extend the knee, one should consider arthroscopic surgical treatment. If the patient has more than 10 cm of prone heel height discrepancy in extension beyond 3 months, surgery is a recommended treatment.

In most instances involving a symptomatic knee flexion contracture, surgical treatment can be performed arthroscopically on an outpatient basis.[1,7] Preoperatively, radiographs should be obtained to assess tunnel placement. A true lateral radiograph with the knee in extension may reveal an abnormal anterior tibial tunnel placement that results in impingement upon the intercondylar region.

Loss of knee motion may be attributable to intraoperative technical errors. Anterior tibial tunnel placement may result in graft impingement in extension (Fig. 5, *left*). Howell[22] has extensively studied and promoted the concept of intercondylar roof impingement of the ACL graft when it is placed too far anteriorly. MRI scanning has demonstrated characteristic signal changes in the impinged and nonimpinged graft (Fig. 5, *right*).[23] Anterior femoral tunnel placement may contribute to loss of knee flexion (Fig. 6). Excessive graft tensioning may overconstrain the knee. Bach has recommended fixation of the ACL graft in complete extension, in contrast to the concept of securing the graft at 30° of knee flexion and applying a posterior Lachman force to reduce the possibility of overconstraining the joint.[13,18]

Bilateral lateral radiographs to rule out patella infera contracture syndrome should be considered.[24,25] If the patient has disproportionate pain, one must consider reflex sympathetic dystrophy and begin an appropriate work-up, including a triple-phase bone scan, prior to surgical treatment. Recurrent effusions mandate a work-up for an occult infection.

Limitations to extension generally are secondary to pathology within the intercondylar notch region. In contrast, limitations to knee flexion generally are secondary to scar within the medial and/or lateral gutters or within the suprapatellar pouch region. At the time of arthroscopy, one may encounter considerable difficulty making a transition from the intercondylar notch region to the suprapatellar pouch. This difficulty, which is generally secondary to marked fat pad scarring, may necessitate transfer of the arthroscope to an inferomedial portal to allow initial debridement of the fat pad and scar tissue in the anterior intercondylar region or, on occasion, fat pad tissue that has filled the anterolateral joint line region. A fibroproliferative scar nodule, the "cyclops lesion," should be assessed at the anterior base of the ACL insertion.[8,9] As the knee is brought into extension, this scar nodule may be noted to slide into the patellotrochlear interval and make contact in this

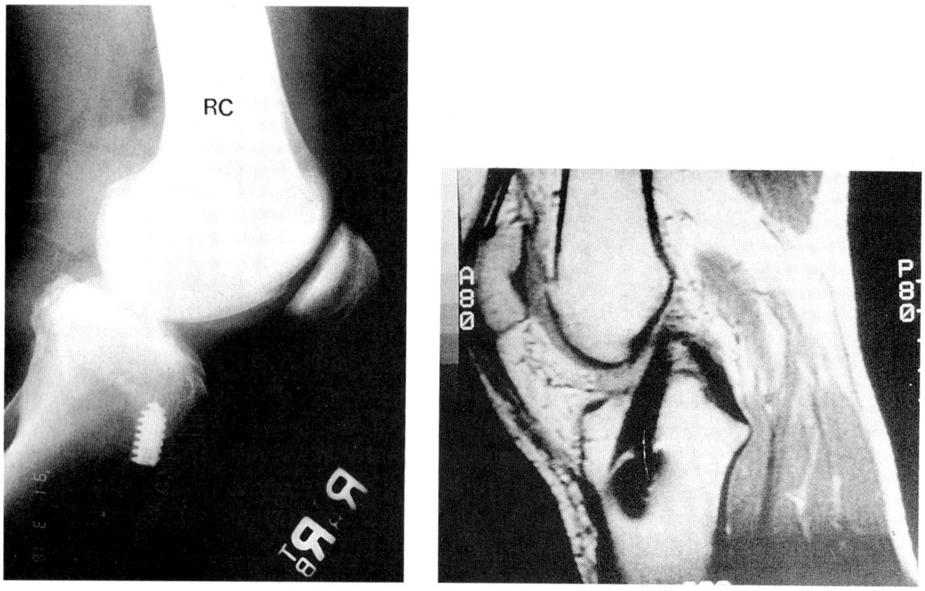

Fig. 5 **Left,** This lateral radiograph demonstrates anterior femoral tunnel placement using a two-incision outside-in technique. This revision procedure had been performed after a failed Andrews' mini extra-articular tenodesis. Anterior tibial tunnel placement resulted in graft failure of the revision procedure. **Right,** This postoperative MRI following ACL reconstruction demonstrates a normal signal within the ACL autograft. Impingement would demonstrate signal changes and edema within the graft.

region. Aggressive debridement should be performed, but one must avoid debriding the intermeniscal ligament. The intercondylar notch should be visualized from both inferolateral and inferomedial portals, because a surprising amount of scar tissue may be present in the anterolateral compartment, thus tethering the patella. Once this tissue is debrided, the patella becomes more mobile, allowing a transition from the suprapatellar pouch into the lateral gutter. Variations include a cord of tissue, which may partially obscure the most distal portion of the patella and extend directly down onto the anterior region of the tibial articular surface. If present, this tissue must be carefully debrided to avoid injuring the patellar tendon. Revision expansion notchplasty is performed with an arthroscopic shaver or burr. Care must be taken not to damage the ACL tissue, but hypertrophic synovium and scar overlying the ACL may require debridement. The ACL should be carefully assessed at this time. The assessment should include its tension, its orientation, synovialization and vascularity, any fraying of the ligament, and any torn portions of the ACL graft bundle. Improvement of knee extension must be confirmed intraoperatively. A sterile goniometer is used to measure the improvement in extension gained at surgery. At the conclusion of the procedure, manipulation may be performed to gain flexion. Manipulation in flexion is deferred until after intercondylar notch debridement has been performed. Prior to manipulation, scar may also be encountered in the medial or lateral gutter, and this can be lysed with the tip of the shaver. The ACL integrity should be documented with an examination under anesthesia at the beginning and conclusion of the procedure, and this information should be confirmed in the operative report. In some circumstances, graft malposition may contribute to lack of knee motion, which may require debridement of a portion of the graft.[9] Patients rarely develop unstable knees following debridement in this unusual situation. If patellar mobilization is significantly reduced, arthroscopic lateral and/or medial release should be considered.

Although hemovac drains are generally not used following ACL surgical reconstruction, a hemovac is placed into the knee joint and removed in the recovery room to minimize any hemarthrosis in the postarthroscopic resection patient. Marcaine is injected into the knee joint and Toradol (ketoralac tromethamine, Syntex Laboratories, Inc., Palo Alto, CA) is administered during anesthesia. Every effort should be made to minimize discomfort and swelling in the immediate postoperative phase. Complete extension is recommended using prone heel hangs beginning immediately on the day of surgery and supervised physical therapy during the first 1 to 2 weeks on a daily basis. Full weightbearing is allowed immediately. Consideration should be made for the use of CPM machine to assist with flexion. One may use CPM during the day and use night extension splinting to maintain extension. One must recognize that the CPM machine will not contribute to regaining extension. One may also consider a bivalved extension casting or a hyperextension "board" as popularized by Shelbourne.[1,10] Efforts should be directed toward patellar mobilization.

In summary, arthrofibrosis should be viewed as a spectrum of knee stiffness, which in its mildest form results in loss of extension. More extensive involvement is manifested by knee flexion and extension contractures with concomitant patellar entrapment. In its most severe form, patella infera contracture syndrome may occur. Reflex sympathetic dystrophy or occult infection

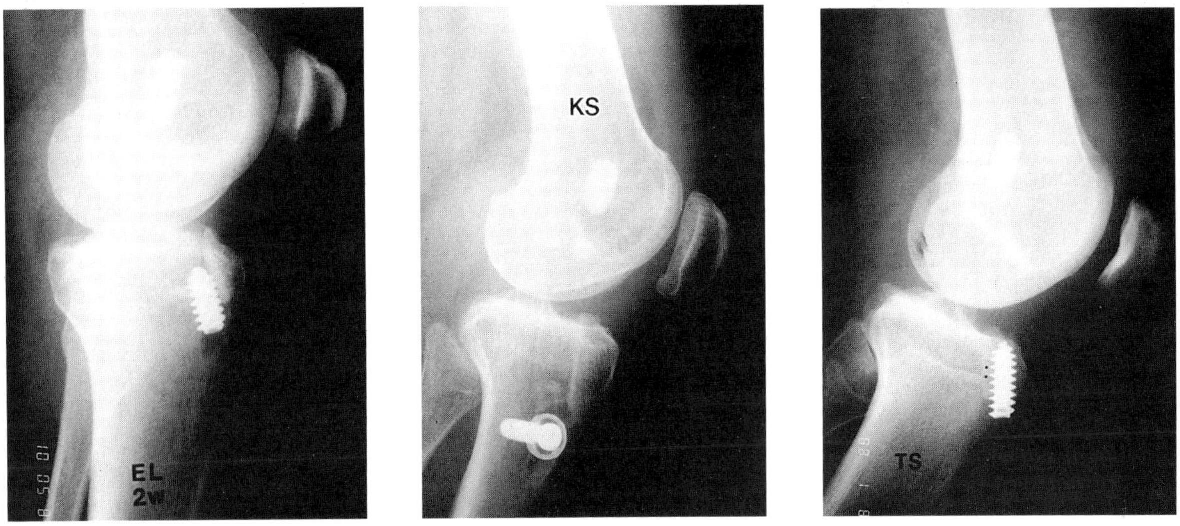

Fig. 6 **Left,** This lateral radiograph demonstrates anterior femoral and tibial tunnel placement using a double-incision endoscopic technique which contributed to loss of knee flexion and extension. **Center,** This patient underwent acute anterior cruciate ligament reconstruction with medial collateral ligament repair via an arthrotomy and was then casted. A significant knee flexion and extension contracture resulted. The femoral and tibial tunnels are anteriorly placed. **Right,** Another radiographic example of anterior tibial tunnel placement which can contribute to a knee flexion contracture or, ultimately, graft failure.

may be an underlying component to this complication. Knee stiffness may occur following injury or surgery. The literature suggests that careful monitoring of motion, an early rehabilitation program to regain quadriceps control, and delaying surgery following the index injury until the inflammatory phase has resolved will dramatically reduce the incidence of arthrofibrosis. Immediate postoperative extension, early range of motion, avoidance of casting, and early quadriceps usage are preventive factors. Loss of extension with an audible clunk in extension suggests the development of a fibroproliferative scar nodule, which is amenable to arthroscopic resection. Patients who have improperly placed tunnels are less likely to benefit from debridement and more likely to have ultimate graft failure. In general, patients who require arthroscopic debridement, notchplasty, scar resection, and manipulation predictably will have significant gains in motion.

References

1. Shelbourne KD, Johnson GE: Outpatient surgical management of arthrofibrosis after anterior cruciate ligament surgery. *Am J Sports Med* 1994;22:192–197.
2. Shelbourne KD, Wilckens JH, Mollabashy A, et al: Arthrofibrosis in acute anterior cruciate ligament reconstruction: The effect of timing of reconstruction and rehabilitation. *Am J Sports Med* 1991;19:332–336.
3. Shelbourne KD, Porter DA: Anterior cruciate ligament-medial collateral ligament injury: Nonoperative management of medial collateral ligament tears with anterior cruciate ligament reconstruction. A preliminary report. *Am J Sports Med* 1992;20: 283–286.
4. Mohtadi NG, Webster-Bogaert S, Fowler PJ: Limitation of motion following anterior cruciate ligament reconstruction: A case-control study. *Am J Sports Med* 1991;19:620–625.
5. Cosgarea AJ, Sebastianelli WJ, DeHaven KE: Prevention of arthrofibrosis after anterior cruciate ligament reconstruction using the central third patellar tendon autograft. *Am J Sports Med* 1995;23:87–92.
6. Harner CD, Irrgang JJ, Paul J, et al: Loss of motion after anterior cruciate ligament reconstruction. *Am J Sports Med* 1992;20: 499–506.
7. Sachs RA, Daniel DM, Stone ML, et al: Patellofemoral problems after anterior cruciate ligament reconstruction. *Am J Sports Med* 1989;17:760–765.
8. Jackson DW, Schaefer RK: Cyclops syndrome: Loss of extension following intra-articular anterior cruciate ligament reconstruction. *Arthroscopy* 1990;6:171–178.
9. Marzo JM, Bowen MK, Warren RF, et al: Intraarticular fibrous nodule as a cause of loss of extension following anterior cruciate ligament reconstruction. *Arthroscopy* 1992;8:10–18.
10. Fisher SE, Shelbourne KD: Arthroscopic treatment of symptomatic extension block complicating anterior cruciate ligament reconstruction. *Am J Sports Med* 1993;21:558–564.
11. Wasilewski SA, Covall DJ, Cohen S: Effect of surgical timing on recovery and associated injuries after anterior cruciate ligament reconstruction. *Am J Sports Med* 1993;21:338–342.
12. Hardin GT, Bach BR Jr, Bush-Joseph C: Extension loss following arthroscopic ACL reconstruction. *Orthop Intl* 1993;1:405–410.
13. Bach BR Jr, Jones GT, Sweet FA, et al: Arthroscopy-assisted anterior cruciate ligament reconstruction using patellar tendon substitution: Two- to four-year follow-up results. *Am J Sports Med* 1994;22:758–767.
14. Cosgarea AJ, DeHaven KE, Lovelock JE: The surgical treatment of arthrofibrosis of the knee. *Am J Sports Med* 1994;22:184–191.
15. Graf BK, Ott JW, Lange RH, et al: Risk factors for restricted motion after anterior cruciate reconstruction. *Orthopedics* 1994; 17:909–912.
16. Patel DV, Shelbourne DK, Martini DJ: Classification and man-

agement of arthrofibrosis of the knee following anterior cruciate ligament reconstruction. Proceedings of the American Academy of Orthopaedic Surgeons 63rd Annual Meeting, Atlanta, GA. Rosemont, IL, American Academy of Orthopaedic Surgeons, 1996.

17. Robins AJ, Newman AP, Burks RT: Postoperative return of motion in anterior cruciate ligament and medial collateral ligament injuries: The effect of medial collateral ligament rupture location. *Am J Sports Med* 1993;21:20–25.

18. Hardin GT, Bach BR Jr, Bush-Joseph CA, et al: Endoscopic single-incision anterior cruciate ligament reconstruction using patellar tendon autograft: Surgical technique. *Am J Knee Surg* 1992;5:144–155.

19. Aglietti P, Buzzi R, Zaccherotti G, et al: Operative treatment of acute complete lesions of the anterior cruciate and medial collateral ligaments: A 4- to 7-year follow-up study. *Am J Knee Surg* 1991;4:186–194.

20. Richmond JC, Gladstone J, MacGillivray J: Continuous passive motion after arthroscopically assisted anterior cruciate ligament reconstruction: Comparison of short-term versus long-term use. *Arthroscopy* 1991;7:39–44.

21. Nogalski MP, Bach BR Jr, Bush-Joseph CA, et al: Trends in decreased hospitalization for anterior cruciate ligament surgery: Double-incision versus single-incision reconstruction. *Arthroscopy* 1995;11:134–138.

22. Howell SM: Arthroscopic roofplasty: A method for correcting an extension deficit caused by roof impingement of an anterior cruciate ligament graft. *Arthroscopy* 1992;8:375–379.

23. Howell SM, Clark JA, Farley TE: Serial magnetic resonance study assessing the effects of impingement on the MR image of the patellar tendon graft. *Arthroscopy* 1992;8:350–358.

24. Paulos LE, Rosenberg TD, Drawbert J, et al: Infrapatellar contracture syndrome: An unrecognized cause of knee stiffness with patellar entrapment and patella infera. *Am J Sports Med* 1987;15:331–341.

25. Richmond JC, al Assal M: Arthroscopic management of arthrofibrosis of the knee, including infrapatellar contraction syndrome. *Arthroscopy* 1991;7:144–147.

CHAPTER 26

Reflex Sympathetic Dystrophy and Pain Dysfunction in the Lower Extremity

Thomas N. Lindenfeld, MD
Bernard R. Bach, Jr, MD
Edward M. Wojtys, MD

Most orthopaedic surgeons have faced the challenge of managing patients who have marked limitation of motion of the knee. Others have managed patients who have a disability because of sympathetically maintained pain (SMP)—that is, reflex sympathetic dystrophy. Both of these conditions can be difficult to treat. When SMP and severe contractures occur together in the knee, the problems of diagnosis and treatment are magnified. SMP can be disproportionately severe and associated with periarticular swelling as well as with muscle inhibition,[1,2] which may lead to a slow and painful course in physical therapy. The relative lack of progress in rehabilitation of the knee, as well as the SMP itself, frequently produce anxiety and depression in these patients, which can lead to poor compliance and worsening stiffness. Increasing stiffness in the knee often limits the ability of a patient to walk, kneel, climb, sit, work, or participate in sports activities and leads to additional emotional stress and upset. As the depression worsens, a vicious cycle results. Unless early and appropriate measures are taken to break the cycle, both the patient and the treating physician will be faced with anger, frustration, and ultimately, an unsatisfactory outcome.

Although hand surgeons have long dealt with SMP in the upper extremity,[3] the syndrome has not been as well recognized or treated as frequently in the lower extremity.[4-7] However, recent reports[1,8-13] have helped to delineate SMP in the lower extremity, and we now have a better understanding of the pathophysiology and treatment of the condition. The keystone of treatment for this type of stiff and painful knee is early recognition.[14] SMP, patella infera, and arthrofibrosis may be interrelated, and all are best treated early in their course, because they can progress quickly to the point where resolution becomes quite difficult.[3] Too often, early signs and symptoms of these processes are not recognized or are ignored, making treatment received later much more complicated.[15,16] Early treatment is important because of the difficulty in managing more chronic syndromes and because irreversible changes are more likely to occur when the condition persists untreated. Alterations in collagen crimp patterns and crosslinks result in permanent shortening of the periarticular soft tissues.[17] Furthermore, alterations in patellar height and in the mechanics of the tibiofemoral joint can ultimately lead to the breakdown of the articular surface. The pain and dysfunction caused by this chondral degeneration can make SMP even more difficult to treat and can lead to irreversible and painful conditions such as arthritis within the joint.

Successful management of a patient who has a stiff and painful knee requires an understanding of the basic mechanisms that cause SMP, arthrofibrosis, and patella infera. This basic understanding can lead to early recognition of this difficult problem, and treatment can be initiated as soon as possible, creating the best chance of success.

Sympathetic Nervous System Dysfunction

Most clinicians recognize the full-blown syndrome of reflex sympathetic dystrophy, which is characterized by a stiff, swollen extremity and pain that is out of proportion to the underlying mechanical problem.[3] Pain that is out of proportion to the inciting cause is the hallmark of the condition. The extremity usually shows changes in color, temperature (vasomotor changes), and sweating (sudomotor changes). Frequently, however, sympathetic dysfunction presents in a more subtle and limited way.[18] Only a localized area of the extremity may be painful, and there may be no sweating or changes in color. Unfortunately, even these milder forms of sympathetic dysfunction may be associated with substantial functional limitations. If not recognized, mild sympathetic dysfunction can progress to full-blown reflex sympathetic dystrophy. Recognition and treatment of sympathetic nervous system dysfunction in its earliest stages can prevent the pain and limited function from becoming worse.

Terminology

The terminology of sympathetic nervous system dysfunction has been confusing. Reflex sympathetic dystrophy, major and minor causalgia, reflex algodystrophy, mimo-causalgia (a causalgia-like syndrome without documented nerve injury[19]), and many other terms have been used to describe different clinical manifestations of sympathetic nervous system dysfunction.[1,20] The major reason for the many and often confusing terms is that the root cause of sympathetic nervous system dysfunction and its true pathophysiology have yet to be completely understood.[18] Recent work[9,12,21-27] in this area has improved the understanding of sympathetic dysfunction and has led to simplified terminology.

Sympathetic nervous system dysfunction is often part of a pain dysfunction syndrome. A pain dysfunction syndrome is a group of symptoms that are manifested by pain that appears to be excessive and nonanatomic and does not seem to match the underlying physical findings.[28] The dysfunction may be physical (swelling, stiffness, atrophy, weakness, or the inability to function) or mental (the patient may be withdrawn or depressed).

The three primary components of a pain dysfunction syndrome are a local trigger—that is, a painful organic condition—such as patellofemoral pain, a fracture, or a nerve injury; psychological factors (a personality disorder or particular social circumstances, perhaps reinforced by underlying secondary gain); and systemic factors (a generalized condition that causes or exacerbates pain, such as a peripheral neuropathy or arteritis). These three primary components of the pain dysfunction syndrome are not related to sympathetic nervous system dysfunction. Therefore, they are known as sympathetically independent pain.

A secondary component of the pain dysfunction syndrome is sympathetic nervous system dysfunction. It is secondary because it is initiated by an injury of nonsympathetic tissues. Examples include the development of reflex sympathetic dystrophy after traumatic injury of a limb and the development of shoulder-hand syndrome after myocardial infarction. This pain is, by definition, relieved by sympathetic blockade. In 1986, Roberts termed this type of pain SMP.[29] The terminology allows all painful sympathetic nervous system dysfunctions to be grouped under one heading, eliminating the need to describe these conditions by their confusing and often overlapping clinical signs and symptoms.

More recently, the International Association for the Study of Pain revised the taxonomy for disorders of the sympathetic system.[30] These disorders are now referred to as a complex regional pain syndrome. A complex regional pain syndrome is present when regional pain and sensory changes occur after a noxious event. The pain is associated with other findings of a sympathetic disorder, such as changes in skin color and temperature and abnormal swelling and sudomotor activity. These changes are greater than would be expected to result from the initiating noxious event. Complex regional pain syndrome is further categorized into type I and type II. Type I describes an area of sympathetic dysfunction that does not follow the course of a peripheral nerve. After a noxious event, ongoing pain and hyperalgesia develop. At some time in the course of the syndrome, typical sympathetic nervous system dysfunction—that is, edema and sudomotor or surface bloodflow changes—is noted. Classic reflex sympathetic dystrophy fits into this category. Type II complex regional pain syndrome has a similar constellation of clinical signs and symptoms; however, it is associated with a known nerve injury. The syndromes that were previously termed major and minor causalgia fit best into this category. Although it seems logical, this terminology is too new for us to judge its ultimate utility for describing the patterns of sympathetic nervous system dysfunction.

Sympathetic Nervous System

The sympathetic nervous system is the larger of the two divisions of the autonomic nervous system.[31,32] Although the sympathetic system is relatively primitive, it has connections to the neocortex of the brain and its function may be modified by many higher autonomic centers (the hypothalamus, the thalamus, and even the cerebral cortex). Although there are some afferent (peripheral-to-central) fibers, the sympathetic nervous system is mostly an efferent (central-to-peripheral) system. The two main ganglionic trunks are the cervical and lumbar trunks. However, there are many other ganglia throughout the paraspinal area, which form complex interconnections within the sympathetic nervous system and between it and the brain. The complexity of this system makes it difficult to disable the sympathetic system completely in any one anatomic region.

Preganglionic fibers arise from the cell bodies in the gray matter of the spine. They exit the spinal cord in the ventral roots of the spinal nerves, and either they reenter the spinal cord through the white rami communicans at the same or an adjacent level or they connect to a peripheral sympathetic ganglion. Postganglionic fibers may reenter the corresponding spinal nerve through the gray rami communicans to innervate viscera or to travel with blood vessels. They also may move to a higher or lower level and may cross the midline at multiple points.

The sympathetic nervous system innervates many peripheral structures and affects many bodily functions (Table 1). The easiest way to remember the potential of a stimulated sympathetic nervous system is to recall that it prepares one for fight or flight. The sympathetic nervous system has both alpha and beta receptors. Either of these receptors can be excitatory or inhibitory at the end organ. When stimulated, an alpha receptor tends to cause skin vasoconstriction, pilomotor contraction, cardiac acceleration, and intestinal relaxation. Stimulation of a beta receptor causes muscle vasodilation, bronchial relaxation, and cardiac acceleration.

Table 1
Effects of sympathetic stimulation mediated by alpha and beta receptors

Alpha Receptor	Beta Receptor
Vasoconstriction (skin)	Vasodilation (muscle)
Pilomotor contraction	Bronchial relaxation
Cardiac acceleration	Cardiac acceleration
Intestinal relaxation	

Pathophysiology

The confusion and complexity of the clinical terminology of sympathetic nervous system dysfunction are largely due to an incomplete understanding of its actions.[3] The following theories of the pathophysiology of these disorders have the most clinical and basic science support.

It has long been believed that sensitization of peripheral mechanoreceptors and nociceptors can be a cause of SMP.[22,25] The findings of recent studies[14,23,26,33,34] suggest that there is a sympathetic-afferent coupling at sensory nerve endings, mediated through sensitive alpha adrenergic receptors. Norepinephrine that is released from sympathetic terminals, as a result of increased sympathetic tone, can stimulate the peripheral sensory nerves of the afferent spinothalamic tract, which transmit intense pain and temperture signals to the neocortex.

Another mechanism may involve the formation of artificial synapses (ephapses) after nerve injury.[24] Ephapses can simply shunt impulses from efferent (sympathetic) to afferent (sensory) fibers.

Additionally, direct injury of a nerve may allow for an epileptic-type discharge of electrical energy in the area of the injured nerve.[35] This may either directly stimulate sensory nerves or allow for excessive neurotransmitter release, which in turn can stimulate pain fibers.

Finally, deafferentation may affect sympathetic output.[27] Simply stated, deafferentation is a substantial decrease in afferent signals to the spinal cord and to other neurologic centers. Constant and normal sensory input is thought to suppress sympathetic activity; this is known as the gate theory. When an extremity becomes painful, it is used less. In the case of SMP, skin sensitivity causes the patient to minimize contact, which eventually results in decreased afferent activity. This decreased afferent activity limits the normal inhibition of the sympathetic system, allowing increased sympathetic discharge. Such a mechanism can explain the positive clinical results seen with massage and desensitization of a body part affected by SMP.

Diagnosis

History

SMP is initiated by a noxious event. It may be surprising to those who do not treat this condition routinely that the inciting event may be a very small or even a trivial injury that normally would be expected to resolve quickly without any adverse sequelae.[36] A simple ankle sprain, a minor injury of a branch of the saphenous nerve, or a mild sprain of a collateral ligament during knee arthroscopy can initiate a pain dysfunction syndrome. If a patient has an unusual amount of pain immediately postoperatively or postinjury and healing does not progress as expected, sympathetic dysfunction should be suspected.

Signs and Symptoms

SMP has a variable presentation.[7] In the classic case, within the first 6 weeks or so after injury the sympathetic overreaction causes a swollen, immobile, and painful limb. The pain is in a nonanatomic distribution, that is, it does not follow the distribution of a single peripheral nerve, and it often is described as burning in nature. There is usually an increase in sweating, and often there are color changes (ranging from blue to dusky red) in the extremity. Frequently, there is allodynia, which is pain that is produced by a nonnoxious stimulus such as the light touch of a bedsheet. There also may be hyperpathia, which is an overreaction to a painful stimulus. These factors help to explain why forcing joint motion during physical therapy is not productive. Late in the course of the disease, there are trophic changes: dystrophic, smooth, shiny skin; osteoporosis; fast-growing and brittle nails; hypertrichosis; and muscular and subcutaneous atrophy. Patients who have chronic SMP may also have extra-articular swelling and joint contractures.

One of the earliest and most helpful signs of early sympathetic dysfunction is intolerance to cold.[34] Frequently, patients tell the physical therapist that they cannot stand an ice pack or they cannot tolerate winter weather.

Pain that is located specifically in the distribution of the saphenous nerve may represent a saphenous neuralgia, which is really a *forme fruste* of SMP.[37] This dysfunction previously was termed minor causalgia. With the increasing prevalence of meniscal repair, the saphenous nerve is at risk more frequently. Direct injury of this nerve during surgery can cause saphenous neuritis. This diagnosis can be made when a history of burning pain along the medial side of the knee is noted or when percussing the origin of the nerve at the adductor canal elicits a sensation of burning pain.

Diffuse pain and skin sensitivity about the joint after major surgery are also early signs of SMP. Although the clinician who treats musculoskeletal conditions about the knee should be able to recognize the early signs of this disorder, it is helpful for other health-care providers to suspect and report signs as well. In the weeks between follow-up visits, early SMP can develop and progress quickly into a severe and less treatable condition. Frequently, the patient does not progress as expected with physical therapy and may become intolerant of joint manipulation or of the application of wraps or braces. Therapists should refer such patients immediately to the physician for evaluation and treatment.

It should be remembered that SMP follows a nonanatomic distribution. The pain may not involve an entire extremity or even a large part of the extremity. For example, a 42-year-old female mail carrier was first seen by us after she had missed almost 6 months of work. She had had an excision of a Morton neuroma, but a 2-cm area of pain had developed postoperatively on the plantar aspect of the foot, in the area of the old incision. The neuroma appeared to have been adequately excised, but multiple attempts to treat the pain had been unsuccessful. When she was questioned, the patient reported that she had skin sensitivity and intolerance to cold in this discrete area of the foot. A series of lumbar sympathetic blocks were performed, and the pain completely resolved. Within 10 days after the initiation of treatment, the patient had returned to work full time and she had had no recurrence of symptoms.

Diagnostic Studies

Technetium-99m bone-scanning is a very sensitive but not very specific diagnostic tool. Holder and Mackinnon[38] reported that 22 of 23 patients who had reflex sympathetic dystrophy in the hands had a positive bone scan. Because of its lack of specificity, we do not recommend bone-scanning for the diagnosis of reflex sympathetic dystrophy. Bone-scanning may be helpful, however, for finding an occult lesion in a patient who has SMP that is resistant to treatment.

Sympathetic blockade is the best method for the diagnosis of SMP.[29] If a complete sympathetic blockade does not relieve the pain, the disorder most likely is not SMP. In our clinical experience, on occasion a patient with SMP has had incomplete pain relief even with complete sympathetic blockade. The reason for this remains unclear.

There are a variety of ways to achieve a sympathetic blockade, the easiest of which is intravenous administration of an alpha blocker such as phentolamine.[21,39] This creates a complete sympathetic blockade so the pain relief should correlate closely with the degree of SMP. The disadvantage of this method is that the blockade is of short duration and, as a result, does not help in the treatment of the condition.

There are several methods for spinal sympathetic blockade.[40] To be effective, they must deliver the anesthetic agent to the appropriate area, as documented by an increase of 2° to 3°C in the skin temperature of the involved extremity. Simple visual-analog pain scales should be used to measure the amount of pain relief achieved with the blockade. Our experience in the management of several hundred patients has led us to believe that a decrease in pain of at least 50% must be documented in order for the physician to be confident of a diagnosis of SMP.

Differential spinal blockade is achieved with use of a simple spinal puncture. This commonly used technique depends on the principle that myelin slows the rate of penetration of an anesthetic agent. Because motor fibers are the most heavily myelinated, sensory fibers are less myelinated, and sympathetic fibers are the least, a low concentration of an anesthetic agent (0.25% lidocaine), placed in the subarachnoid space, penetrates mainly unmyelinated sympathetic fibers. The advantage of this method is that it is a simple, commonly used way to provide a complete sympathetic blockade. Unfortunately, this method rarely achieves a purely sympathetic blockade. Most often, there is some blockade of the sensory system. Therefore, pain relief may be partially due to sensory blockade rather than entirely due to sympathetic blockade. This makes it difficult to establish a clear diagnosis of SMP.

Epidural sympathetic blockade has virtually all of the same strengths and weaknesses as spinal blockade. However, it has one added strength—it may be administered continuously for several days.

Paravertebral blockade is the best method of spinal blockade for SMP. With this method, a local anesthetic is delivered to the sympathetic chain in the paravertebral area. The advantage is that the anesthetic agent is delivered outside of the spinal column to the sympathetic ganglia, avoiding any blockade of the sensory or motor nerves. It may be done on an outpatient basis, and long-lasting anesthetic agents may be used. The disadvantage of this technique is that a skilled anesthesiologist is required to administer the anesthetic effectively.

Treatment

The treatment of SMP of the lower extremity involves three separate areas: lumbar sympathetic blockade, through either blocks or surgical interruption; pharmacologic treatment for both sympathetic and nonsympathetic symptoms; and physical therapy (Fig. 1).

When SMP is diagnosed in the early stages, repeated long-lasting paravertebral blocks can be an effective treatment,[41] as demonstrated in our patient who had postoperative pain in the foot. The results of paravertebral blocks should be monitored closely to assess their effect. The blocks may provide sympathetic pain relief for much longer than the duration of the pharmacologic effect of the anesthetic agent. Our clinical

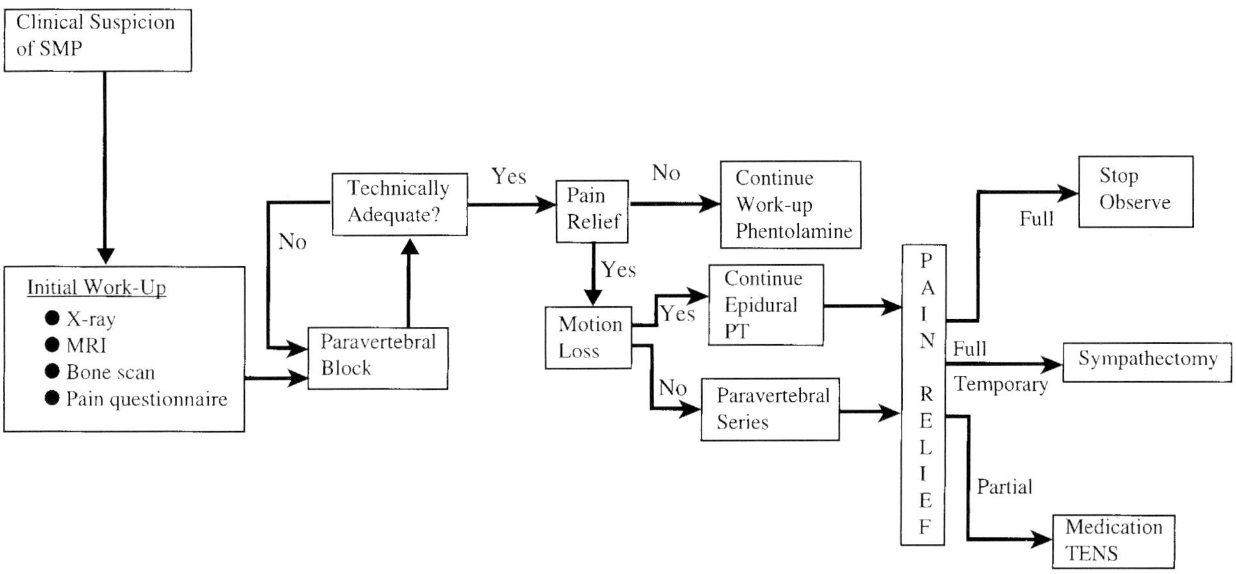

Fig. 1 The decision-making process in the diagnosis and treatment of sympathetically maintained pain.

experience indicates that the more complete and long-lasting the pain relief from a lumbar sympathetic block, the better the prognosis for recovery. Blocks may be used as frequently as every other day for 2 weeks to achieve a long-lasting effect.

Pharmacologic Therapy

Several drugs are useful in the treatment of SMP,[42] although they cannot be expected to take the place of early diagnosis and appropriate treatment with sympathetic blockade. In fact, they are used more commonly to control the symptoms associated with the chronic stages of this condition (Table 2).

Although not universally accepted as an effective treatment, orally administered corticosteroids may interrupt or reverse early SMP.[17,43] If used in the first week or two after injury, an orally administered steroid medication, tapered over 3 to 5 days, can be effective in relieving symptoms. We have had good results after administering commercially available drugs such as methylprednisolone to patients in our clinic who had early SMP. Nonsteroidal anti-inflammatory medications may have some benefit for patients who have SMP,[11] as these drugs are cyclooxgenase inhibitors and interfere with the production of prostanoids. They can, therefore, minimize inflammation facilitated by prostaglandins and decrease peripheral pain secondary to injury. They also may block spinal prostanoids, which facilitate transmission of substance P receptors and glutamate pain fiber in the spinal cord.

Some oral medications for SMP are safe and can be administered relatively easily by the practicing orthopaedist. However, other medications can be more difficult and dangerous to use. Multiple side effects and drug interactions can occur, and these probably are best monitored by a physician who is experienced in the use of the medication.

The use of narcotics and benzodiazepines, such as diazepam, chlordiazepoxide, and alprazolam, is not recommended for the treatment of SMP. These medications tend to lead to drug dependence, depression, and increased pain.[3] Frequently, however, patients who have SMP have already been managed with these drugs and, if they have become dependent on them, management is complicated. In order to prevent such abuse, it is best to insist early in the course of treatment that the patient obtain all drugs from one source. If physicians who previously managed a patient are informed that the patient is under the care of a new physician, the problem of multiple prescriptions for addictive drugs can be decreased.

Lumbar sympathectomy is used generally as a procedure of last resort.[44-48] It is used if anesthetic sympathetic blockade has provided good short-term but not good long-term relief. Although many patients have good early relief with lumbar sympathectomy, the symptoms of SMP tend to recur[45,47] and, after 5 years, many patients have a return to the pretreatment condition.[32,49] Thus, lumbar sympathectomy may be most helpful for patients who have a limited life expectancy. Sympathectomy for multiple extremities is not tolerated well because of problems with thermal regulation and control of the bowel, the bladder, or ejaculation. For an effective lumbar sympathectomy, a complete

Table 2
Pharmacologic treatment for sympathetically maintained pain

Drug	Dose	Mechanism of Action	Use	Side Effects
Alpha blockade				
Phenoxybenzamine (Dibenzyline; SmithKline Beechman, Philadelphia, PA)	10 mg every night, may increase to 10 mg 3 times a day	Blocks peripheral $alpha_1$ receptors, decreases sympathetic tone	Causalgias	Hypotension
Prazosin (Minipress; Pfizer, Parsippany, NJ)				Hypotension, tachycardia, decreased sexual function, nasal congestion
Terazosin (Hytrin; Abbott Laboratories, North Chicago, IL)				May have fewer side effects than other alpha blockers
Clonidine	Pain relief can be obtained with use of Clonidine patches	$Alpha_2$ agonist, blocks $alpha_1$ transmission both peripherally and centrally		Hypotension
Antidepressants				
Trazodone (Desyrel; Apothecon, Princeton, NJ)	50 mg 3 times a day	Blocks serotonin receptors, activates descending pain inhibitory fibers	Most chronic pain syndromes	Multiple side effects
Trycyclic antidepressants				
Desipramine (Norpramin; Marion Merrell Dow, Kansas City, MO)	100 to 200 mg a day			Myocardial ischemia, urinary retention
Doxepin (Sinequan; Roerig Division, Pfizer, New York, NY)	10 to 25 mg 3 times a day			
Amitriptyline (Elavil; Stuart Pharmaceuticals, Wilmington, DE)	25 mg 3 times a day			Orthostatic hypotension
Calcium channel blockers				
Nifedipine (Procardia; Pratt Pharmaceuticals, New York, NY)	10 to 30 mg 3 times a day	Relaxes smooth muscle, increases peripheral blood flow, decreases discharges from ephaptic scars	Peripheral nerve injury, especially in patients who have decreased blood flow	Headaches, hypotension
Diltiazem (Cardizem; Marion Merrell Dow, Kansas City, MO)	30 mg 4 times a day, increased to 60 to 90 mg 4 times a day			
Verapamil (Calan; G.D. Searle, Chicago, IL)				
Nicardipine (Cardene; Syntex, Palo Alto, CA)				
Anticonvulsants				
Carbamazepine (Tegretol; Basel, Summit, NJ)	100 mg by mouth twice a day, up to 800 mg a day	Supresses pathologic electrical discharges in central nervous system and in peripheral nervous system	Ephapses, burning pain, sharp discharges	Depression of central nervous system, drowsiness, multiple side effects
Clonazepam (Klonopin; Roche Laboratories, Nutley, NJ), tricyclic	0.5 mg twice a day to 3 times a day, may be increased			
Gabapentin (Neurontin, Parke-Davis, Morris Plains, NJ)				
Valproic acid				

ganglionectomy from at least the tenth thoracic vertebra to the fourth lumbar vertebra should be done.

One difficult area in the management of these patients is the differentiation of sympathetically independent pain from the SMP. Painful stimuli not only initiate SMP but also help to maintain it. It is important that the orthopaedist not miss the potentially painful lesion hidden in the morass of signs and symptoms of reflex sympathetic dystrophy. A workup for potentially painful lesions should be complete in order to provide the best prognosis for the patient. A painful chronic infection, a neuroma, an undiagnosed meniscal tear or chondral lesion, and a myriad of other conditions can provide a painful somatic focus for recurrent flare-ups of SMP, even with use of adequate repeated sympathetic blockade. If surgery is needed to correct a painful area, epidural anesthesia should be used and then maintained continuously for 3 to 4 days postoperatively to decrease the potential for a flare-up of the SMP.

Physical Therapy and Exercise

Physical therapy is an important part of the management of patients who have SMP.[33,50,51] Recovery from the muscle dysfunction, swelling, and joint stiffness requires appropriate exercise. Therapists must understand that a patient who has SMP cannot be managed with normal postoperative care.

These patients have a pain response to normally nonpainful stimuli (allodynia), such as light touch, and an excessive response to any stimulus that is painful (hyperpathia). These stimuli are encountered normally during physical therapy. When excessive pain is created, SMP may worsen. The therapist must have the patient progress slowly with strengthening and range-of-motion exercises and not force the pace too vigorously. Intolerance to cold obviates the use of cold packs and, in fact, moist heat is more effective for reducing pain and stiffness. Possibly the most important element for successful rehabilitation is the avoidance of personality confrontations. These patients are frequently withdrawn, depressed, angry, and unwilling to cooperate with therapy because of the pain and dysfunction.[15] It has been our experience that when SMP is treated successfully, the behavior of the patient may return to normal. Therefore, the personality defects should be assumed to be a part of the disease and not an integral part of the patient. The therapist must learn to ignore some of the unpleasant aspects of the personality of the patient that are created by this disease and focus patiently on muscle-strengthening and range-of-motion exercises.

In order to lessen pain during therapy, active and active-assisted range-of-motion exercises should be encouraged and passive-motion exercises should be discouraged. Transcutaneous electrical nerve stimulation may be helpful to control the pain. Swelling should be controlled with massage instead of ice. It is important for the therapist to listen to the patient, who knows what is working and what is not. Frequently, exercises that are appropriate for a patient who has SMP differ from those of the typical physical therapy routines.

Overview

SMP may affect the lower extremity more commonly than is currently recognized. When a patient is having unusual trouble with pain or stiffness in relation to the inciting injury, a diagnosis of SMP should be considered. Because this condition frequently does not manifest all of its possible symptoms, the clinician should be aware that other findings, such as intolerance to cold or allodynia, may be the only clinical signs of SMP. The key to successful management is early diagnosis and treatment. Lumbar sympathetic blockade can both confirm a diagnosis of SMP and provide an appropriate early treatment. Many other medications can be useful for treating the symptoms. The help of a practitioner who is experienced in the use of multiple-drug therapy may be necessary. The patient who has SMP presents a true clinical challenge. The patience, concern, and skill of the surgeon, anesthesiologist, physical therapist, and other health-care professionals, working as a team, are necessary for a successful outcome.

References

1. Inhofe PD, Garcia-Moral CA: Reflex sympathetic dystrophy: A review of the literature and a long-term outcome study. *Orthop Rev* 1994;23:655–661.
2. Schwartzman RJ, McLellan TL: Reflex sympathetic dystrophy: A review. *Arch Neurol* 1987;44:555–561.
3. Dzwierzynski WW, Sanger JR: Reflex sympathetic dystrophy. *Hand Clin* 1994;10:29–44.
4. Cameron HU, Park YS, Krestow M: Reflex sympathetic dystrophy following total knee replacement. *Contemp Orthop* 1994; 29:279–281.
5. Finsterbush A, Frankl U, Mann G, et al: Reflex sympathetic dystrophy of the patellofemoral joint. *Orthop Rev* 1991;20:877–885.
6. Luerssen TG, Campbell RL, Defalque RJ, et al: Spontaneous saphenous neuralgia. *Neurosurgery* 1983;13:238–241.
7. Poehling GG, Koman LA, Pollock FE Jr: Reflex sympathetic dystrophy of the knee, in Sprague NF III (ed): *Complications in Arthroscopy*. New York, NY, Raven Press, 1989, pp 53–72.
8. AbuRahma AF, Robinson PA, Powell M, et al: Sympathectomy for reflex sympathetic dystrophy: Factors affecting outcome. *Ann Vasc Surg* 1994;8:372–379.
9. Backonja MM: Reflex sympathetic dystrophy/sympathetically maintained pain/causalgia: The syndrome of neuropathic pain with dysautonomia. *Semin Neurol* 1994;14:263–271.
10. Chabal C, Jacobson L, Mariano A, et al: The use of oral mexiletine for the treatment of pain after peripheral nerve injury. *Anesthesiology* 1992;76:513–517.
11. Cooper DE, DeLee JC, Ramamurthy S: Reflex sympathetic dystrophy of the knee: Treatment using continuous epidural anesthesia. *J Bone Joint Surg* 1989;71A:365–369.
12. Harden RN, Duc TA, Williams TR, et al: Norepinephrine and epinephrine levels in affected versus unaffected limbs in sympathetically maintained pain. *Clin J Pain* 1994;10:324–330.

13. Jadad AR, Carroll D, Glynn CJ, et al: Intravenous regional sympathetic blockade for pain relief in reflex sympathetic dystrophy: A systematic review and a randomized, double-blind crossover study. *J Pain Symptom Manage* 1995;10:13–20.
14. Katz MM, Hungerford DS: Reflex sympathetic dystrophy affecting the knee. *J Bone Joint Surg* 1987;69B:797–803.
15. Geertzen JH, de Bruijn H, de Bruijn-Kofman AT, et al: Reflex sympathetic dystrophy: Early treatment and psychological aspects. *Arch Phys Med Rehabil* 1994;75:442–446.
16. Noyes FR, Wojtys EM, Marshall MT: The early diagnosis and treatment of developmental patella infera syndrome. *Clin Orthop* 1991;265:241–252.
17. Glick EN: Reflex dystrophy (algoneurodystrophy): Results of treatment by corticosteroids. *Rheum Phys Med* 1973;12:84–88.
18. Gragnani J: A review of reflex sympathetic dystrophy and related syndromes. *Mo Med* 1994;91:680–683.
19. Patman RD, Thompson JE, Persson AV: Management of posttraumatic pain syndromes: Report of 113 cases. *Ann Surg* 1973; 177:780–787.
20. O'Brien SJ, Ngeow J, Gibney MA, et al: Reflex sympathetic dystrophy of the knee: Causes, diagnosis, and treatment. *Am J Sports Med* 1995;23:655–659.
21. Arner S: Intravenous phentolamine test: Diagnostic and prognostic use in reflex sympathetic dystrophy. *Pain* 1991;46:17–22.
22. Barasi S, Lynn B: Effects of sympathetic stimulation on mechanoreceptor and nociceptor afferent units with small myelinated (A-delta) and unmyelinated (C) axons innervating the rabbit pinna. *J Physiol* 1983;341:51P.
23. Devor M, Janig W: Activation of myelinated afferents ending in a neuroma by stimulation of the sympathetic supply in the rat. *Neurosci Lett* 1981;24:43–47.
24. Jänig W: Causalgia and reflex sympathetic dystrophy: In which way is the sympathetic nervous system involved? *Trends Neurosci* 1985;8:471–477.
25. Roberts WJ, Elardo SM: Sympathetic activation of A-delta nociceptors. *Somatosens Res* 1985;3:33–44.
26. Scadding JW: Development of ongoing activity, mechanosensitivity, and adrenaline sensitivity in severed peripheral nerve axons. *Exp Neurol* 1981;73:345–364.
27. Wall PD, Devor M: The effect of peripheral nerve injury on dorsal root potentials and on transmission of afferent signals into the spinal cord. *Brain Res* 1981;209:95–111.
28. Amadio PC: Pain dysfunction syndromes. *J Bone Joint Surg* 1988;70A:944–949.
29. Roberts WJ: A hypothesis on the physiological basis for causalgia and related pains. *Pain* 1986;24:297–311.
30. Merskey H, Bogduk N (eds): *Classification of Chronic Pain: Descriptions of Chronic Pain Syndromes and Definitions of Pain Terms*, ed 2. Seattle, WA, IASP Press, 1994, pp 40–43.
31. Pick TP, Howden R (eds): *Anatomy: Descriptive and Surgical*, ed 15. New York, NY, Bounty Books, 1977.
32. Hooshmand H (ed): *Chronic Pain: Reflex Sympathetic Dystrophy. Prevention and Management.* Boca Raton, FL, CRC Press, 1993, pp 123–168.
33. Duncan KH, Lewis RC Jr, Racz G, et al: Treatment of upper extremity reflex sympathetic dystrophy with joint stiffness using sympatholytic Bier blocks and manipulation. *Orthopedics* 1988; 11:883–886.
34. Koman LA, Nunley JA, Goldner JL, et al: Isolated cold stress testing in the assessment of symptoms in the upper extremity: Preliminary communication. *J Hand Surg* 1984;9A:305–313.
35. Sunderland S (ed): *Nerves and Nerve Injuries*, ed 2. Edinburgh, Scotland, Churchill Livingstone, 1978, pp 343–480.
36. Neuschwander D, Drez D Jr, Heck S: Pain dysfunction syndrome of the knee. *Orthopedics* 1996;19:27–32.
37. Poehling GG, Pollock FE Jr, Koman LA: Reflex sympathetic dystrophy of the knee after sensory nerve injury. *Arthroscopy* 1988;4:31–35.
38. Holder LE, Mackinnon SE: Reflex sympathetic dystrophy in the hands: Clinical and scintigraphic criteria. *Radiology* 1984; 152:517–522.
39. Abram SE, Lightfoot RW: Treatment of long-standing causalgia with prazosin. *Reg Anesth* 1981;6:79–81.
40. Löfström JB, Cousins MJ: Sympathetic neural blockade of upper and lower extremity, in Cousins MJ, Bridenbaugh PO (eds): *Neural Blockade in Clinical Anesthesia and Management of Pain*, ed 2. Philadelphia, PA, JB Lippincott, 1988, pp 461–500.
41. Leipzig TJ, Mullan SF: Causalgic pain relieved by prolonged procaine amide sympathetic blockade. *J Neurosurg* 1984;60: 1095–1096.
42. Payne R: Neuropathic pain syndromes, with special reference to causalgia and reflex sympathetic dystrophy. *Clin J Pain* 1986;2: 59–73.
43. Rosen PS, Graham W: The shoulder-hand syndrome: Historical review with observations on seventy-three patients. *Can Med Assoc J* 1957;77:86–91.
44. Barnes R: The role of sympathectomy in the treatment of causalgia. *J Bone Joint Surg* 1953;35B:172–180.
45. Persson AV, Anderson LA, Padberg FT Jr: Selection of patients for lumbar sympathectomy. *Surg Clin North Am* 1985;65: 393–403.
46. Schutzer SF, Gossling HR: The treatment of reflex sympathetic dystrophy syndrome. *J Bone Joint Surg* 1984;66A:625–629.
47. Shumacker HB Jr: A personal overview of causalgia and other reflex dystrophies. *Ann Surg* 1985;201:278–289.
48. Shumacker HB Jr, Spiegel IJ, Upjohn RH: Causalgia: I. The role of sympathetic interruptions in treatment. *Surg Gynecol Obstet* 1948;86:76–86.
49. Bonica JJ: Causalgia and other reflex sympathetic dystrophies, in Bonica JJ, Liebeskind JC, Albe-Fessard DG, et al (eds): *Advances in Pain Research and Therapy*. New York, NY, Raven Press, 1979, vol 3, pp 141–166.
50. Kozin F: Reflex sympathetic dystrophy syndrome. *Bull Rheum Dis* 1986;36:1–8.
51. Lankford LL, Thompson JE: Reflex sympathetic dystrophy, upper and lower extremity: Diagnosis and management, in Wissinger HA (ed): American Academy of Orthopaedic Surgeons *Instructional Course Lectures XXVI*. St Louis, MO, CV Mosby, 1977, pp 163–178.

Tibial Fractures

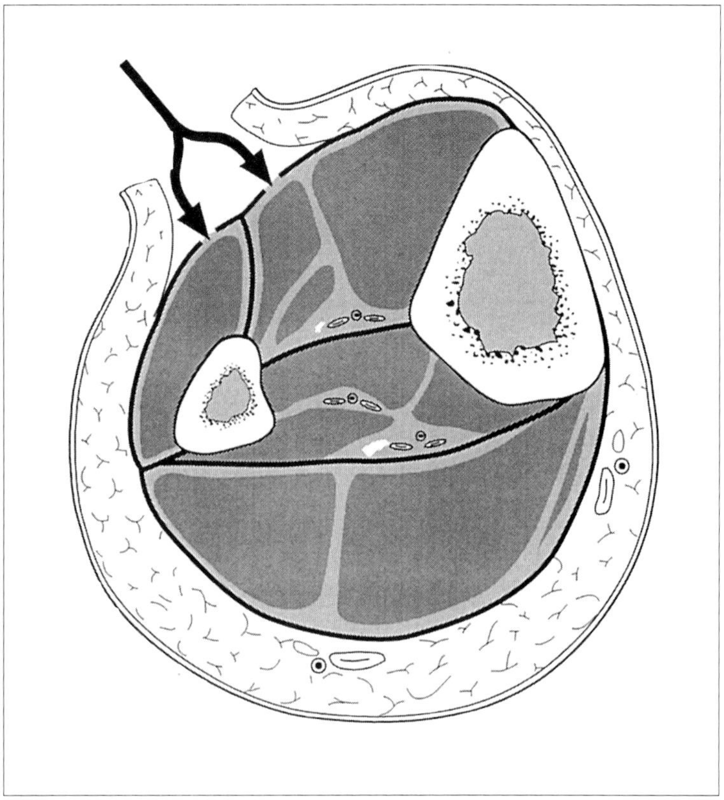

CHAPTER 27

Technical Considerations in the Surgical Management of Tibial Fractures

Paul Tornetta III, MD

Introduction

Tibial shaft fractures are common injuries. Isolated closed tibial fractures can usually be treated nonsurgically.[1] Surgical management is reserved for open fractures; closed fractures in multitrauma patients; fractures with severe soft-tissue injury, unstable patterns, and concomitant fractures; and for fractures treated with nonsurgical management that failed.

Nailing has become the preferred method of surgical stabilization of the tibia, because this procedure provides an early return to function and has a high rate of union. However, recent reports have raised questions about efficacy relating to several areas, including the use of unreamed nailing techniques and the nailing of proximal fractures.[2,3] This chapter will focus on several of the technical difficulties associated with the surgical management of acute tibial shaft fractures and will offer some possible solutions.

Setup

The standard setup for tibial nailing is on a fracture table in the 90°-90° position,[4] which provides enough knee flexion to allow nail placement without steric interference from the patella, and which allows relatively straightforward biplanar imaging. However, this position may make the leg more susceptible to compartment syndrome and requires significant setup time.[5,6] Alternative techniques in patient positioning are faster to set up and can provide the same degree of access to the proximal tibia. One method uses ceiling traction via a distal femoral pin (Fig. 1), which allows easy access for portal placement and does not require continuous traction. The reduction can be maintained manually during reaming (if chosen) and nail passage.

Alternatively, many surgeons now routinely perform tibial nailings without continuous traction on a radiolucent table.[7,8] The initial incision and location of the portal is done with the knee slightly flexed over a bolster. The leg is then flexed by an assistant, who holds the proximal fragment from anteriorly while the portal is completed and the nail is passed. This technique is most useful when an unreamed nailing technique is chosen. If the fracture is significantly short and cannot be held out to length, a femoral distractor or external fixator can be added temporarily to accomplish the reduction.[9] The distractor may be placed on either the medial or the lateral side of the leg, but use of the medial side is usually easier. The proximal pin is positioned in the posterior tibial metaphysis behind the tract that the nail will occupy (Fig. 2). Several options are available distally. For fractures in the proximal two thirds of the tibia, placement of the distal pin in the tibia just above the plafond is recommended. With this configuration the reduction force is directly in line with the tibia and does not exert any force across the joint. For distal fractures, a pin in the center of the talar body works well. The calcaneus is another option for pin placement, but the axis of distraction falls posterior to the tibia, forcing distal fractures into posterior angulation.

Portal Placement

Approach

The incision can be either transverse or vertical. A vertical incision is more forgiving and can be used for future procedures around the knee if required. Once the skin incision is made, access to the proximal tibia may be via a patellar tendon splitting or paratendinous exposure. Although the tendon splitting approach is more direct, the incidence of knee pain is significantly

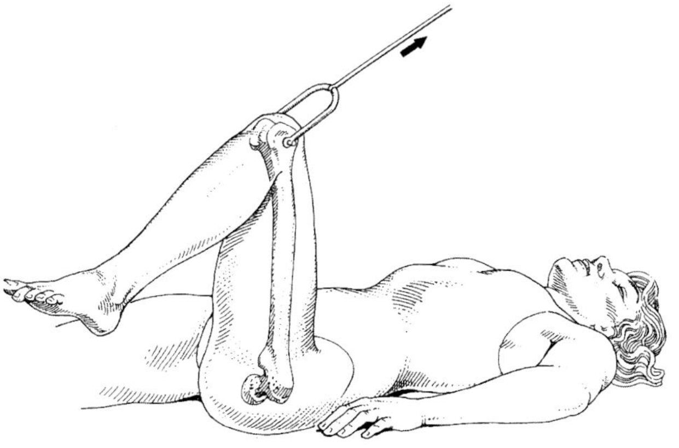

Fig. 1 Ceiling traction from a distal femoral pin allows for nailing without a fracture table when limited assistance is available.

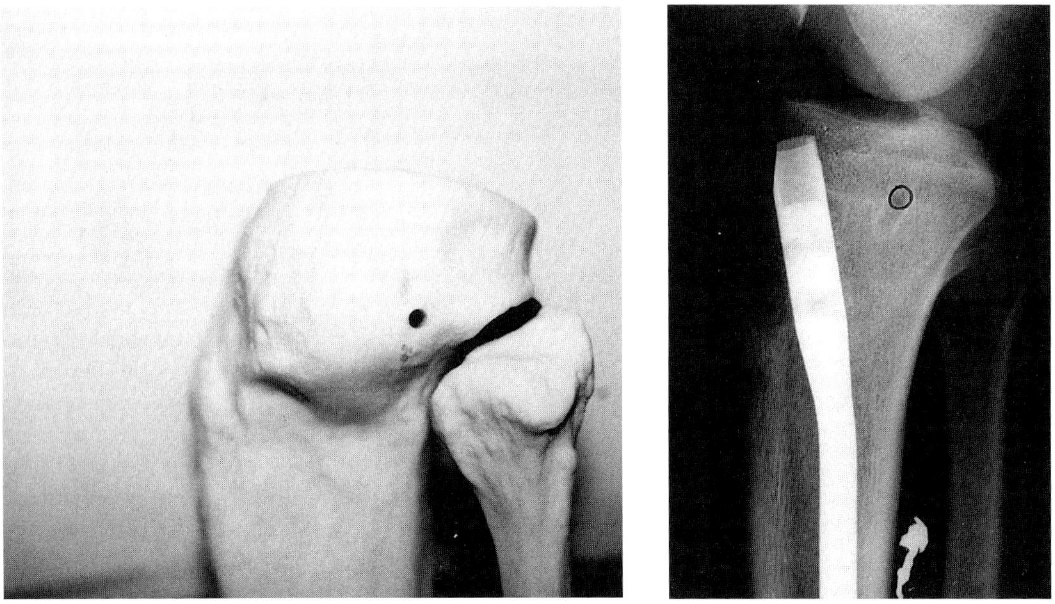

Fig. 2 The location of pin placement in the proximal tibia for use of the femoral distractor **(left)**. This position (circle) is posterior to the tract of the nail and does not hinder nail placement **(right)**.

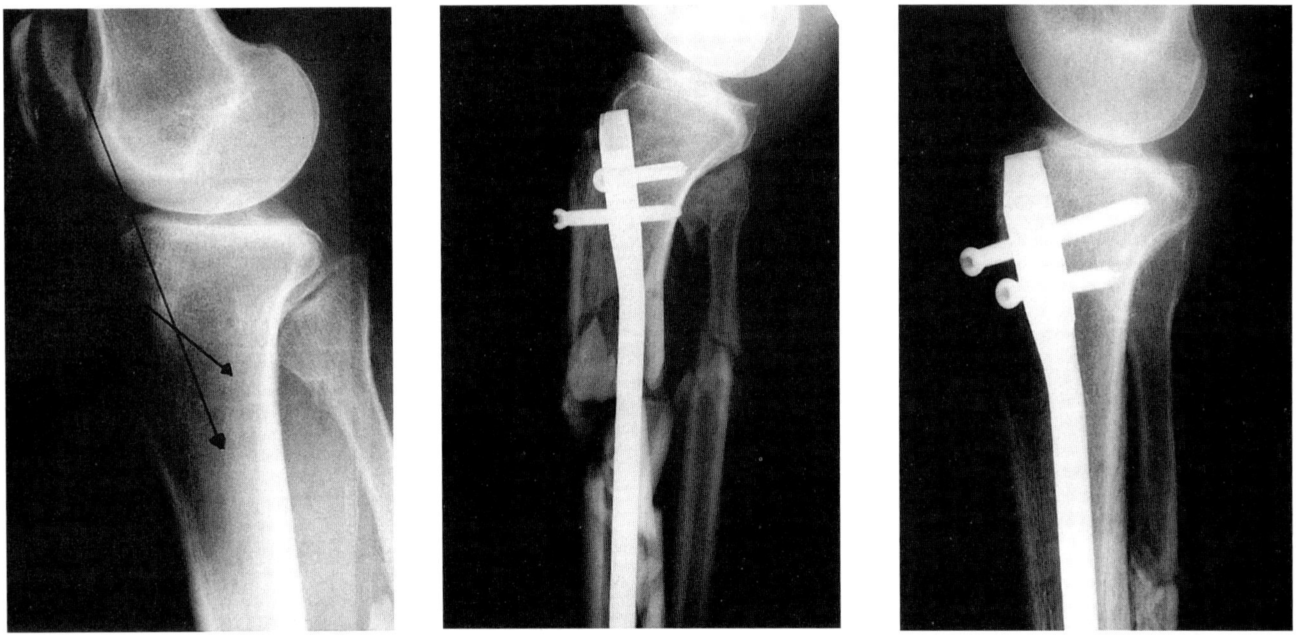

Fig. 3 The previously used portal is more distal than the currently used one. **Left** and **center,** When the oblique area just above the tubercle is used, the nail is directed posteriorly. **Left** and **right,** A more proximal portal introduces the nail closer to the intramedullary axis.

higher when this technique is used.[10] In addition, several cases of heterotopic ossification have been reported following tendon splitting approaches.[11,12] For these reasons an incision medial to the tendon is generally chosen.

Position

Earlier descriptions of tibial nailing recommended that the portal be placed on the oblique facet of the tibial metaphysis just cephalad to the tubercle.[8] This position is easily accessible, but is not in line with the tibial medullary canal. Placement of the nail through this location directs the nail toward the posterior cortex. In older patients and in those with comminuted or proximal fractures, posterior blowout can occur, which may be difficult to manage. A more proximal portal beginning approximately 3 to 4 mm back on the superior surface of the tibia is closer to the intramedullary axis and avoids these problems (Fig. 3). This position also creates less stress in the proximal tibia during nail placement.[13] When this portal is used, it should be noted that the original starting point of the awl will become the posterior aspect of the portal because of the relative strength of the subchondral bone and the force vector of the awl. The anterior cortex is preferentially opened by the awl. Thus, the starting point for the awl should be slightly posterior to the intended center of the portal.

Reaming

For open fractures, unreamed nails are advantageous compared to reamed nails, because they have a less deleterious effect on the endosteal blood supply, and have infection rates similar to external fixation.[14-17] Higher infection rates have been reported for reamed nailing, even if delayed.[18,19]

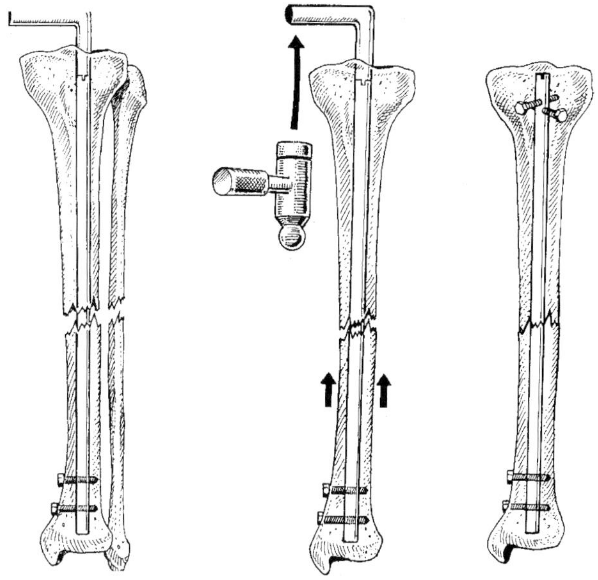

Fig. 4 Any distraction that occurs during nail passage must be corrected and cortical contact achieved. **Left,** The nail should be overseated by the amount of the distraction and distally locked. **Center,** Backtapping the jig will then reduce the distraction, allowing for proximal locking after cortical contact is achieved **(right)**.

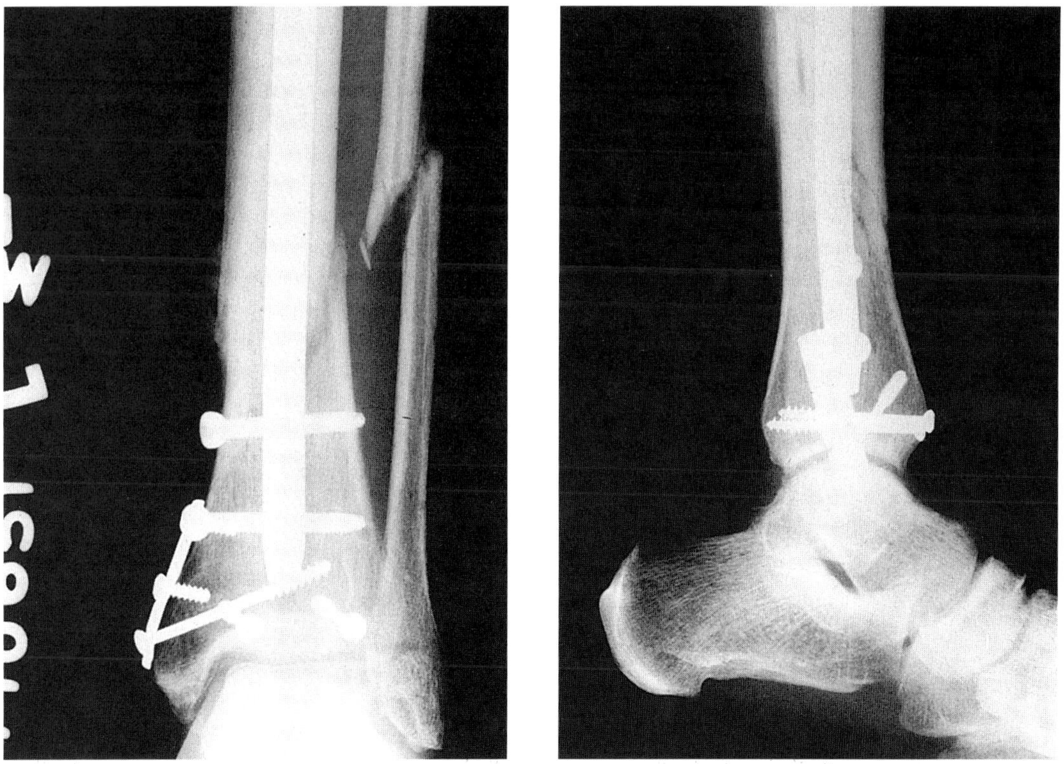

Fig. 5 A patient with an ipsilateral segmental tibia fracture and an indirect ankle fracture. The ankle was fixed with standard techniques and the tibial shaft fracture was treated with an intramedullary nail. The healed anteroposterior **(left)** and lateral **(right)** radiographs demonstrate the fixation.

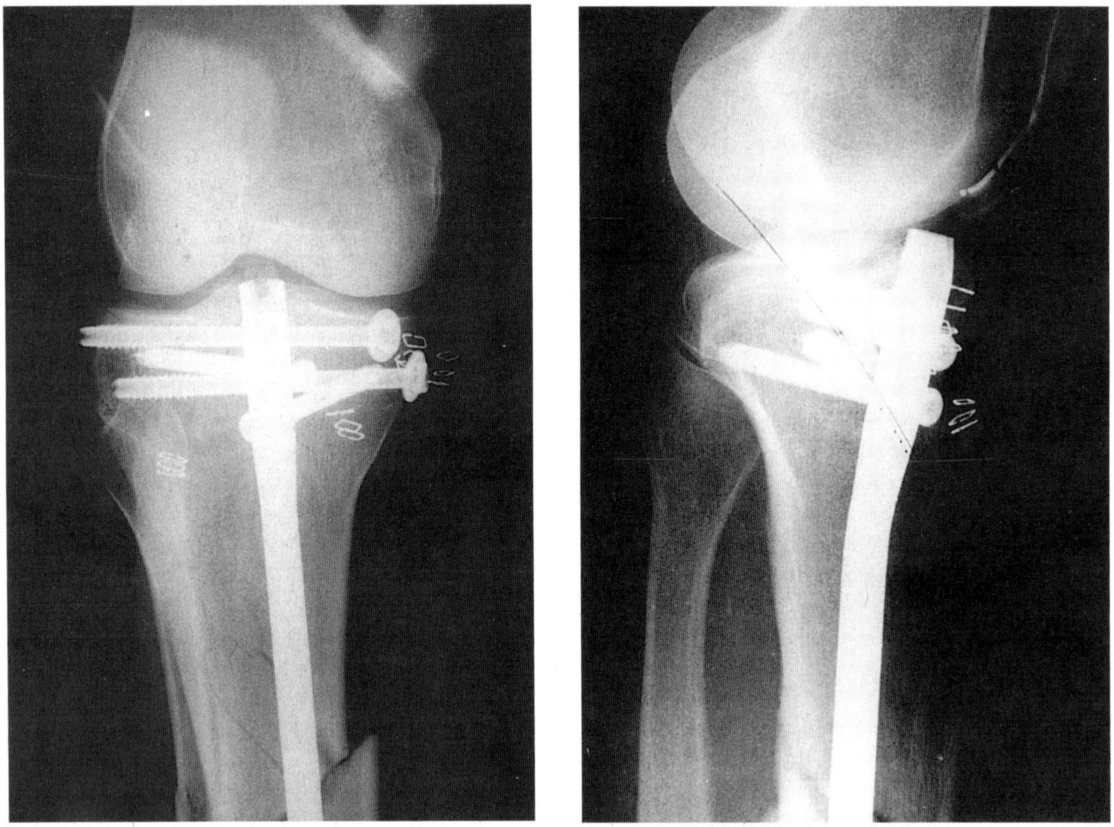

Fig. 6 A nondisplaced lateral plateau fracture was identified before nailing in the patient in Figure 5. This was stabilized with percutaneous lag screws before the nail was placed.

For closed fractures, however, the question of reaming is much more controversial. There are theoretical benefits to an unreamed technique, but reamed nails are stronger and more stable. Thus, each technique has advantages.

In addition to better endosteal blood flow, another benefit of unreamed nailing is that in a sheep model the time to maximal callus formation was found to be 33% faster.[20] The heat created during reaming may be a factor in delayed healing. In fact, hand reaming leads to earlier union than power reaming.[21] Thus, patients with significant soft-tissue injury associated with their fractures and patients with open fractures may both benefit from the omission of reaming. Excellent results in patients with soft-tissue injury have been reported with the use of unreamed nailing, although secondary procedures to obtain union are more common than in those with fractures without soft-tissue injury.[22-24]

Several studies have compared the results of reamed versus unreamed nailing for closed fractures. Court-Brown and associates[2] randomized 50 patients with closed fractures of the tibia without significant soft-tissue injury (Tscherne C1) to either a reamed or unreamed tibial nail. Compared to results of unreamed nailing, reamed nailing resulted in faster weightbearing and union with fewer secondary procedures. Ruchholtz and associates[25] studied 56 patients over a 3-year period and did not find any difference in time to union or functional results between reamed and unreamed nailing. However, the patients who underwent unreamed nailing began walking 3 weeks earlier than those with reamed nails. Mayr and associates[26] studied 70 patients evenly divided into two groups: reamed and unreamed. There were no differences in the groups with respect to soft-tissue injury. The patients treated with unreamed nails had a shorter hospital stay, began partial weightbearing sooner, and union was achieved faster than in those with a reamed nail. Also, more pseudarthroses occurred in the reamed group. McClellan and associates,[27] in a nonrandomized multicenter study, found that more secondary procedures were needed after reamed nailing than after unreamed nailing.

Some of the differences seen in various series may be related to technique. Placement of an unreamed nail results in the distribution of a relatively small amount of bone graft. For this reason, obtaining cortical contact in order to allow for early weightbearing is paramount. Bone and associates[28] and Riemer and associates[22] found that static locking of unreamed nails was

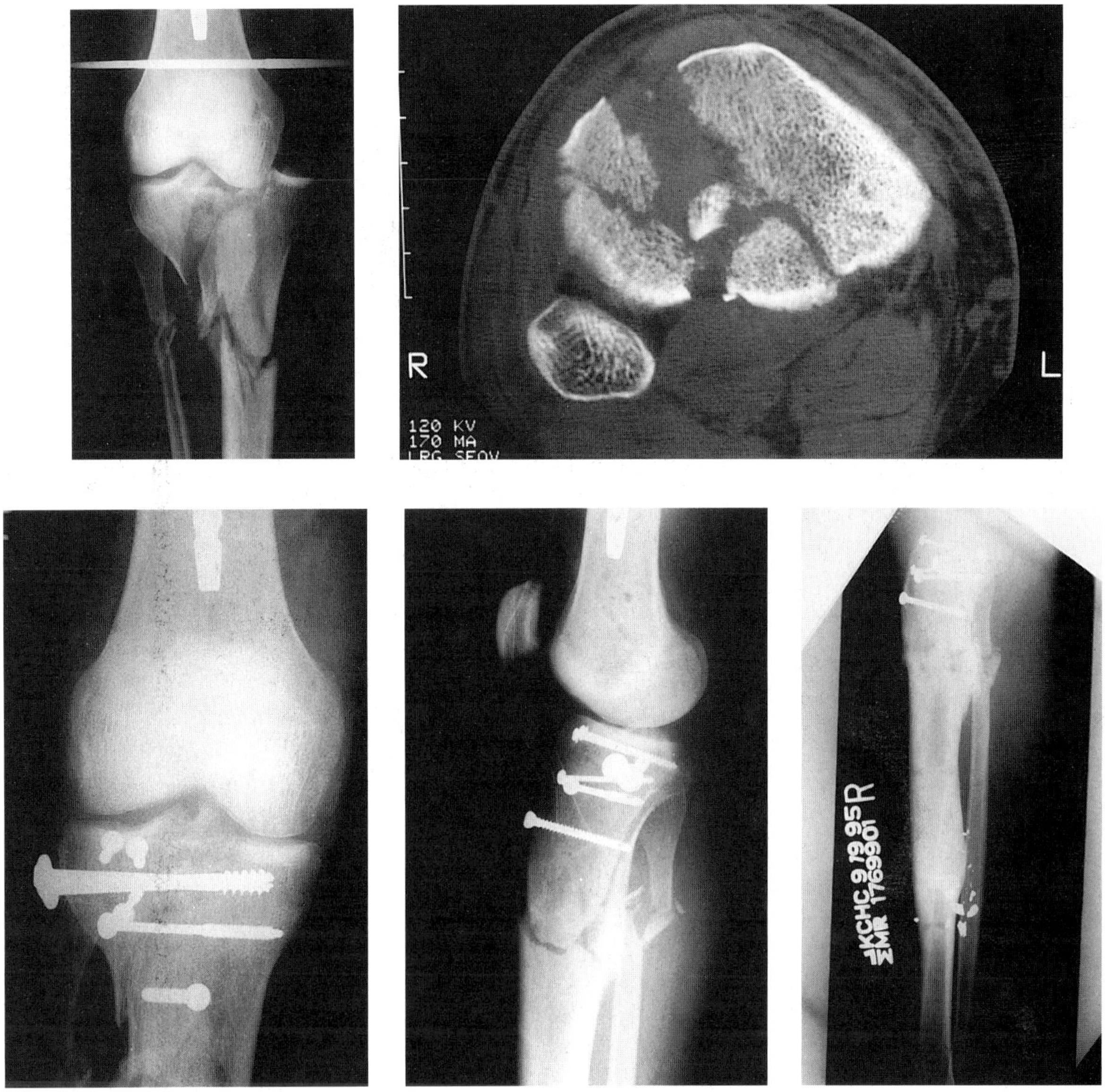

Fig. 7 A comminuted intra-articular fracture in combination with a shaft fracture **(top left** and **center)** is treated with formal open reduction of the joint **(top right, bottom left)** and external fixation. This patient went on to solid union in 5 months **(bottom right)**.

associated with delayed union and the requirement for secondary procedures. As a result, both groups recommended early intervention to dynamize or bone graft these fractures. This recommendation was most important in fractures that were nailed in distraction without cortical contact.

Other differences in reamed and unreamed nailing exist with regard to compartment syndromes and hardware failure. Reaming causes increased intramedullary pressure and has been linked to compartment syndromes of the leg.[29,30] Although a potential disadvantage of reamed nailing, monitoring of compartment pressures during nailing can help establish the diagnosis before permanent damage occurs.[31]

Unlike reamed nails, unreamed nails have a high rate of hardware failure,[23,32] which results partly from the small diameters of nails and screws required for this application. However, the materials and designs used also contribute to the rate of hardware failure. Small diameter titanium implants have a much lower failure rate than stainless steel, especially if the nails are solid.[22,33] Failure rates for these implants are approximately the same as those for reamed nails.[34]

The question of whether or not reamed nailing should be done with closed fractures may not have an answer. Different applications may be useful for specific situations. However, several recommendations can be made. The potential benefits of reaming include

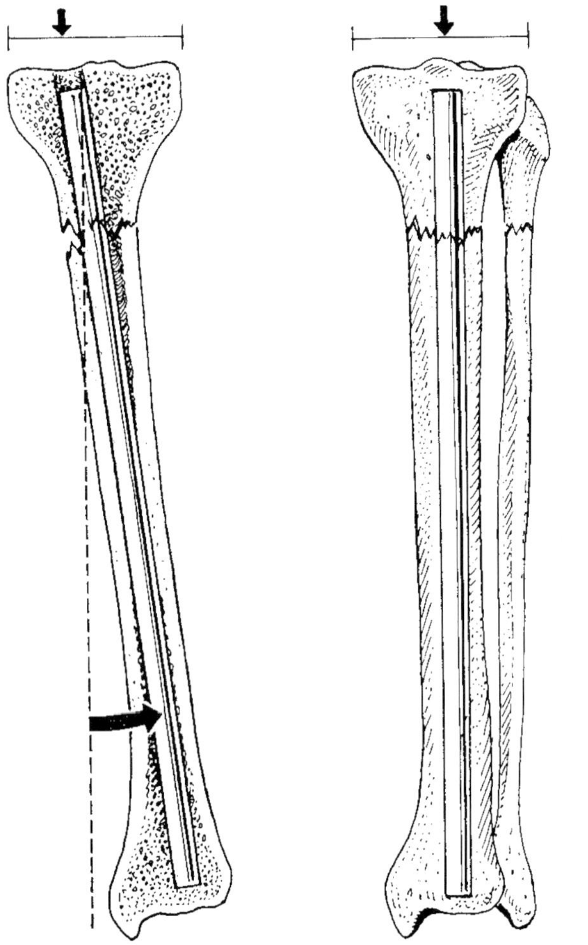

Fig. 8 If the portal for nail placement is medial then the nail will deflect off the inner cortex of the proximal fragment and result in a valgus position **(left)**. A central portal aids in proper coronal plane angulation **(right)**.

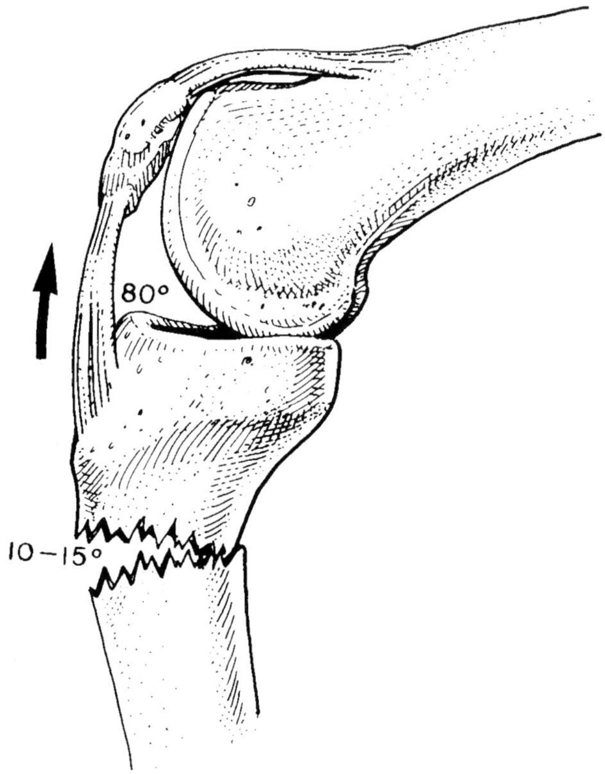

Fig. 9 In cases of proximal fracture, knee flexion leads to anterior angulation at the fracture site secondary to the pull of the quadriceps. (Reproduced with permission from Tornetta P III, Collins E: Semiextended position for intramedullary nailing of the proximal tibia. *Clin Orthop* 1996;328:185-189.)

bone grafting, increased stability from a larger implant, and a stronger implant. If unreamed nailing is chosen, attempts to equal the mechanical advantages of reaming must be made. First, and most important, cortical contact must be achieved. When passing an unreamed nail across a fracture site, the fracture is frequently distracted. Distraction of the fracture is not as common after reamed canal preparation because the nail is undersized compared to the canal. Efforts must be made to avoid or correct this distraction during unreamed nailing. Therefore, the surgeon should use a nail at least 1 mm narrower than the smallest measurement of the canal on the anteroposterior and lateral radiographs (usually the lateral) at the isthmus. With exceptions for very large patients, an 8-mm or 9-mm nail usually suffices. No attempt should be made to obtain a tight cortical fit for stability, because locking will maintain the reduction. Even using small diameter nails, the fracture must be carefully examined intraoperatively using fluoroscopy or plain films. If any distraction is present, it must be corrected. The best way to accomplish this is to overseat the nail by the amount of distraction present, lock the nail distally, and then backtap until cortical contact is achieved. The nail can then be locked proximally (Fig. 4). This technique is relatively simple and may help to avoid secondary procedures. Second, the use of a titanium implant will offset the small size of the nail and allow for early weightbearing with an acceptable hardware failure rate.

Last, walking should begin no later than 8 weeks postoperatively, because the stimulus of weightbearing promotes union.[35] If strong implants are used, weightbearing may begin as early as 2 weeks postoperatively.[33]

Special Fractures

Combined Injuries

Tibial shaft fractures may occur in conjunction with intra-articular fractures of the knee or ankle. The association of tibial shaft fractures with ipsilateral ankle fractures has recently been described by Lonner and

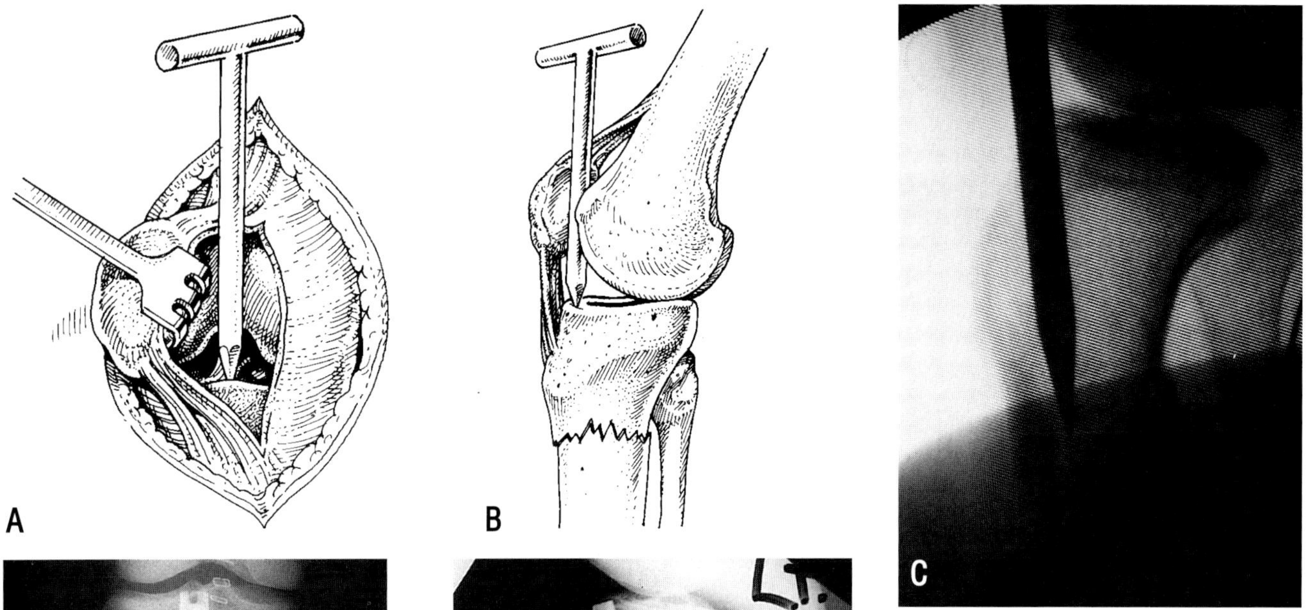

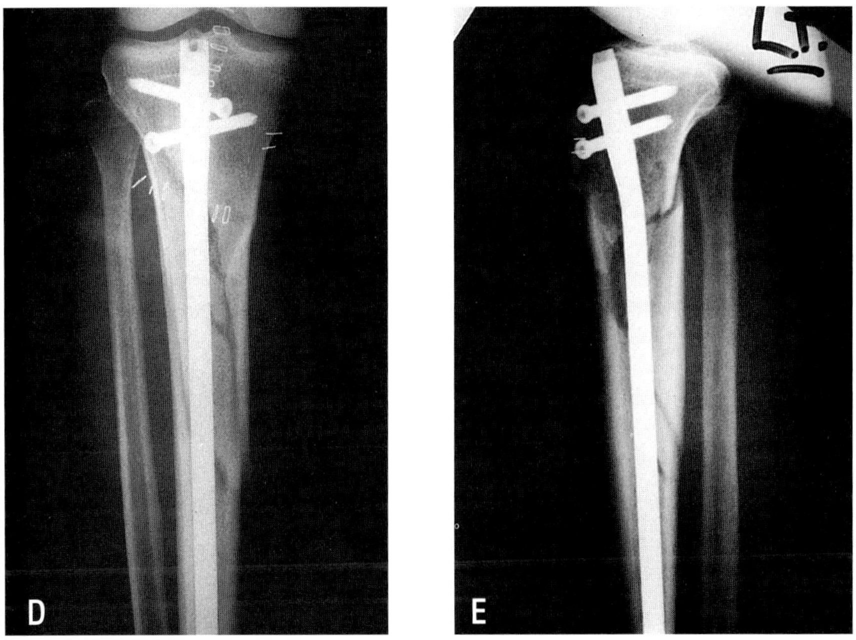

Fig. 10 Nailing in the semiextended position requires subluxation of the patella (**A**). This avails the trochlear groove as a conduit for straight awl and nail placement (**B**). Efforts must be made to direct the awl anteriorly as the nail will follow the tract set by the awl (**C**). Postoperative radiographs of a proximal segmental fracture treated with this technique (**D, E**). (Reproduced with permission from Tornetta P III, Collins E: Semiextended position for intramedullary nailing of the proximal tibia. *Clin Orthop* 1996;328:185-189.)

associates,[36] who along with Keating and associates[37] found that surgical treatment of both injuries led to better results than nonsurgical management.

The type of fixation used for these injuries depends on the type of ankle fracture. If the ankle fracture is rotational in nature (indirect), the ankle may be fixed using standard techniques with lag screws and plates and the shaft with an intramedullary device (Fig. 5). If the ankle injury is the result of impaction (direct) such as a pilon fracture, then both injuries can be managed with an external fixator that is placed following formal open reduction and limited internal fixation of the intra-articular component. The fixator is kept within the tibia if the fracture pattern and soft-tissue injury permit.[38] Extension across the joint may be required if there is a significant soft-tissue injury about the ankle or if comminution precludes adequate stability from a hybrid frame.

Likewise, the type of plateau fracture dictates treatment when it is associated with a shaft fracture. If the intra-articular component is simple, it can be fixed with lag screws and the shaft can be nailed. The lag screws are placed posterior to the location of the nail and, if needed, a buttress plate placed with unicortical screws in the tibial shaft may be added (Fig. 6). A nail with very proximal locking screws should be chosen to add to the fixation of the plateau. If, however, the intra-articular component of the injury is comminuted, then

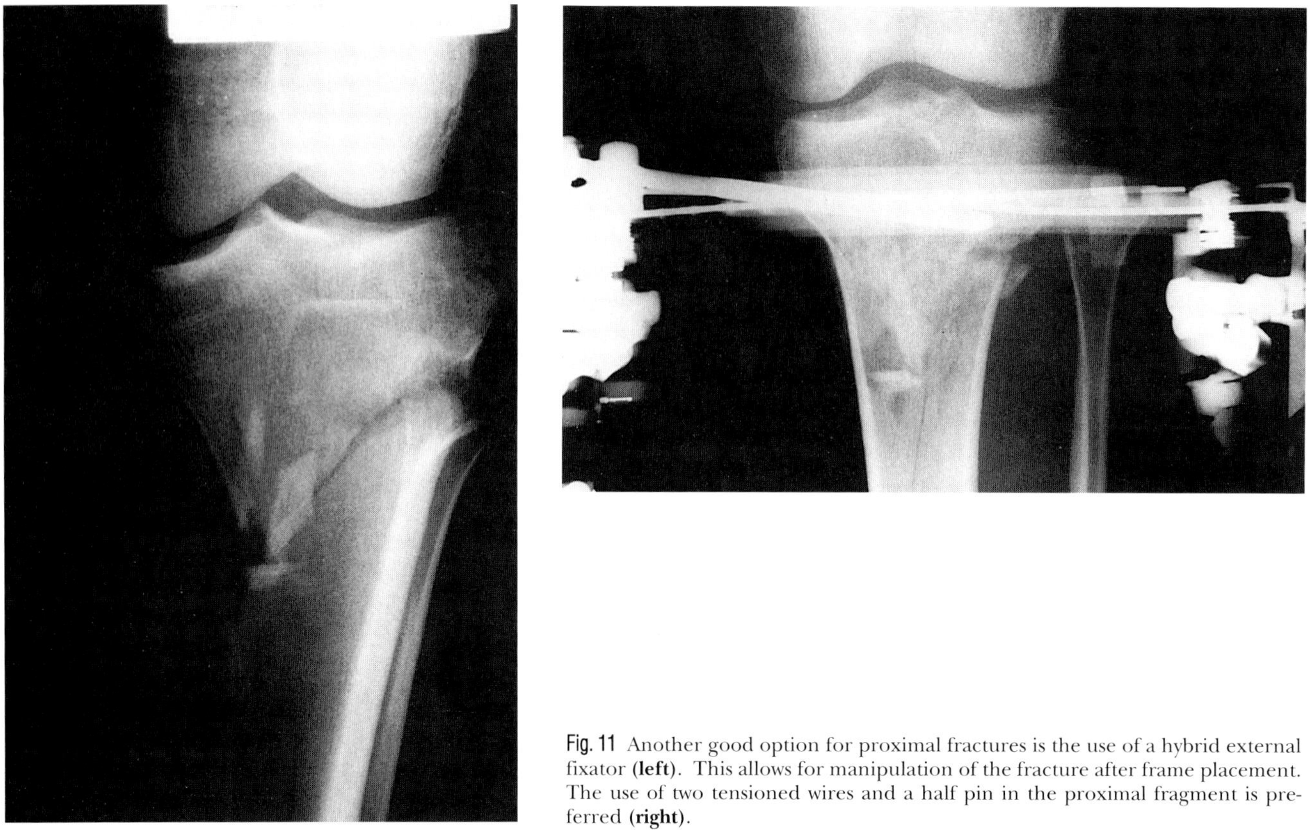

Fig. 11 Another good option for proximal fractures is the use of a hybrid external fixator **(left)**. This allows for manipulation of the fracture after frame placement. The use of two tensioned wires and a half pin in the proximal fragment is preferred **(right)**.

external fixation is the best option. Once again, the frame is placed after limited internal fixation of the joint and, if possible, should not span the knee (Fig. 7).

Weightbearing for these combined injuries is determined by the joint injury. For indirect ankle fractures, weightbearing usually begins at 6 to 8 weeks. For pilon or plateau fractures, it should be delayed for 10 to 12 weeks.

Proximal Fractures

The treatment of proximal tibial shaft fractures is an area of great controversy. Included in this discussion are fractures that extend into the proximal third of the tibia but remain distal to the tubercle. The anatomy of the proximal tibia makes nailing these fractures technically difficult. Lang and associates[3] reported malunions in 84% and loss of reduction in 25% of such fractures. Freedman and Johnson[39] reviewed 133 cases of tibial nailings. The rate of malalignment was 58%, 7%, and 8% for proximal, middle, and distal fractures, respectively. Both sets of authors found poor portal placement to be part of the problem.

However, specific techniques to address the problems encountered in nailing proximal fractures have been reported by others. Cole[40] had only three (5%) malunions in 57 cases. Tornetta and Collins[41] reported no cases of sagittal plane malalignment and two cases of 5° of coronal malalignment in 25 patients using a semiextended position for nailing.

Nailing of proximal fractures can result in two failure types: device or technical. Henley[42] demonstrated that if the bend at the top of a nail is at or below the level of the fracture, it will displace the fracture. Thus, nails used for proximal fractures should have their bend as high as possible. Technical failures are related to the anatomy of the proximal tibia and to the deforming forces on the fracture fragments. The proximal tibia is much wider than any nail that is placed. Thus, as opposed to fractures of the tibial shaft, simply passing the nail across the fracture site will not reduce the fracture.

The most common deformity is anterior angulation from the pull of the extensor mechanism. The origin of the anterior compartment musculature also creates a deformity by tethering the lateral side of the fracture, which leads to valgus malalignment. In addition to these deforming forces, placement of the portal in the center of the proximal fragment is difficult. Palpation of the center of the proximal fragment is rarely possible in very proximal fractures. Additionally, angulation at the fracture site is often present during portal placement. A central portal is extremely important. If the portal is placed eccentrically, the nail will deflect off the inner cortex and force coronal plane angulation (Fig.

8). This deformity can be avoided if a good anteroposterior (AP) image is available during the nailing.

Use of a semiextended position can help to solve most of these problems.[41] Maintaining the knee in approximately 20° of flexion on a bolster will eliminate the pull of the extensor mechanism (Fig. 9). Additionally, excellent AP and lateral images can be obtained. Nailing in this position is not possible unless the patella is subluxated. This is accomplished with a partial parapatellar incision. With the patella lateralized, a straight line entrance into the proximal tibia is available. The use of a straight awl eases creation of a tract in the anterior part of the tibia. The awl should be placed using biplanar image confirmation because the tract cut by the awl will be followed by the nail. It is important not to widen the portal excessively, because a snug fit between the nail and the subchondral bone adds to stability. This technique is depicted in Figure 10. The addition of blocking screws to decrease the available canal size during nailing may also be useful.[24,40] This technique is particularly helpful if anterior angulation is present after the nail has been placed. A percutaneous screw abuts the nail posteriorly while the tibia is held manually reduced. This screw prevents displacement of the proximal fragment. If varus or valgus deformity is present after nail placement, then a blocking screw may also be used to correct this. However, it is often simpler to rotate the nail within the tibia and reduce these malalignments with the proximal bend. After these corrections are made, the nail is then locked proximally.

Hybrid external fixation is another excellent option for very proximal fractures. If used, two tensioned wires may be insufficient. A third wire or preferably a single anteroposterior half pin should be added to counteract the pull of the extensor mechanism (Fig. 11).

Summary

The surgical treatment of tibial shaft fractures is generally successful. However, significant controversy exists regarding the indications for specific types of fixation and the techniques used to apply them. Advances to meet the technical challenges of tibial fracture fixation continue to be made, and orthopaedic surgeons should have these new techniques at their disposal for application to each individual patient's injury.

References

1. Sarmiento A, Sharpe FE, Ebramzadeh E, et al: Factors influencing the outcome of closed tibial fractures treated with functional bracing. *Clin Orthop* 1995;315:8–24.
2. Court-Brown CM, Will EM, McQueen MM, et al: Reamed or unreamed nailing in closed tibial fractures. *J Bone Joint Surg* 1996;78B:580–583.
3. Lang GJ, Cohen BE, Bosse MJ, et al: Proximal third tibial shaft fractures: Should they be nailed? *Clin Orthop* 1995;315:64–74.
4. Koval KJ, Clapper MF, Brumback RJ, et al: Complications of reamed intramedullary nailing of the tibia. *J Orthop Trauma* 1991;5:184–189.
5. Matsen FA III, Mayo KA, Krugmire RB Jr, et al: A model compartmental syndrome in man with particular reference to the quantification of nerve function. *J Bone Joint Surg* 1977; 59A:648–653.
6. Templeman D, Tornetta P III: Compartment syndrome and tibial shaft fractures, in Springfield DS (ed): *Instructional Course Lectures 46.* Rosemont, IL, American Academy of Orthopaedic Surgeons, 1997.
7. Tornetta P III, Bergman M, Watnik N, et al: Treatment of grade-IIIb open tibial fractures: A prospective randomised comparison of external fixation and non-reamed locked nailing. *J Bone Joint Surg* 1994;76B:13–19.
8. Hansen ST Jr, Veith RG: Closed Küntscher nailing of the tibia, in Browner BD, Edwards CC (eds): *The Science and Practice of Intramedullary Nailing.* Philadelphia, PA, Lea & Febiger, 1987, pp 267–279.
9. Moed BR, Watson JT: Intramedullary nailing of aseptic tibial nonunions without the use of the fracture table. *J Orthop Trauma* 1995;9:128–134.
10. Keating JF, Orfaly RM, O'Brien PJ: Knee pain following tibial nailing. *Orthop Trans,* in press.
11. Tornetta P III, Barbera C: Severe heterotopic bone formation in the knee after tibial intramedullary nailing. *J Orthop Trauma* 1992;6:113–115.
12. Gosselin RA, Belzer JP, Contreras DM: Heterotopic ossification of the patellar tendon following intramedullary nailing of the tibia: Report on two cases. *J Trauma* 1993; 34:161–163.
13. Carr J, Sobba D, Bear L: Abstract: Biomechanics of rigid tibial nail insertion sites. *J Orthop Trauma* 1991;5:238.
14. Schemitsch EH, Kowalski MJ, Swiontkowski MF, et al: Comparison of the effect of reamed and unreamed locked intramedullary nailing on blood flow in the callus and strength of union following fracture of the sheep tibia. *J Orthop Res* 1995;13:382–389.
15. Singer RW, Kellam JF: Open tibial diaphyseal fractures: Results of unreamed locked intramedullary nailing. *Clin Orthop* 1995;315:114–118.
16. Stegemann P, Lorio M, Soriano R, et al: Management protocol for unreamed interlocking tibial nails for open tibial fractures. *J Orthop Trauma* 1995;9:117–120.
17. Sanders R, Jersinovich I, Anglen J, et al: The treatment of open tibial shaft fractures using an interlocked intramedullary nail without reaming. *J Orthop Trauma* 1994;8:504–510.
18. Court-Brown CM, McQueen MM, Quaba AA, et al: Locked intramedullary nailing of open tibial fractures. *J Bone Joint Surg* 1991;73B:959–964.
19. MacKenzie DA, Martimbeau C, Mudge K, et al: Abstract: A prospective study of closed reamed locking intramedullary rods in the early management of open tibial fractures. *J Orthop Trauma* 1991;5:239–240.
20. Runkel M, Wenda K, Ritter G, et al: Bone healing after unreamed intramedullary nailing. *Unfallchirurg* 1994;97:1–7.
21. O'Dwyer KJ, Chakravarty RD, Esler CN: Intramedullary nailing technique and its effect on union rates of tibial shaft fractures. *Injury* 1994;25:461–464.
22. Riemer BL, DiChristina DG, Cooper A, et al: Nonreamed nailing of tibial diaphyseal fractures in blunt polytrauma patients. *J Orthop Trauma* 1995;9:66–75.
23. Gregory P, Sanders R: The treatment of closed, unstable tibial shaft fractures with unreamed interlocking nails. *Clin Orthop* 1995;315:48–55.
24. Krettek C, Schandelmaier P, Tscherne H: Nonreamed interlocking nailing of closed tibial fractures with severe soft tissue

injury. *Clin Orthop* 1995;315:34–47.
25. Ruchholtz S, Nast-Kolb D, Betz A, et al: Fracture healing after intramedullary nailing of simple tibial shaft fractures: A clinical comparison of reamed and unreamed procedures. *Unfallchirurg* 1995;98:369–375.
26. Mayr E, Barnikel C, Braun W, et al: Closed tibial fracture: Reamed or unreamed intramedullary nailing. A clinical study. *Zentralbl Chir* 1995;120:24–30.
27. McClellan RT, Comstock CP, Henry SL, et al: Intramedullary nailing of closed tibial shaft fractures. Proceedings of the American Academy of Orthopaedic Surgeons 63rd Annual Meeting, Atlanta, GA. Rosemont, IL, American Academy of Orthopaedic Surgeons, 1996, p 159.
28. Bone LB, Kassman S, Stegemann P, et al: Prospective study of union rate of open tibial fractures treated with locked, unreamed intramedullary nails. *J Orthop Trauma* 1994;8:45–49.
29. Tischenko GJ, Goodman SB: Compartment syndrome after intramedullary nailing of the tibia. *J Bone Joint Surg* 1990;72A:41–44.
30. Mawhinney IN, Maginn P, McCoy GF: Tibial compartment syndromes after tibial nailing. *J Orthop Trauma* 1994;8:212–214.
31. McQueen MM, Court-Brown CM: Compartment monitoring in tibial fractures: The pressure threshold for decompression. *J Bone Joint Surg* 1996;78B:99–104.
32. Whittle AP, Wester W, Russell TA: Fatigue failure in small diameter tibial nails. *Clin Orthop* 1995;315:119–128.
33. Weckbach A, Blattert TR, Kunz E: Differential indications for intramedullary nailing of the tibia with the reamed and unreamed technique. *Zentralbl Chir* 1994;119:556–563.
34. Tornetta P III, McClellan T, Comstock C, et al: Tibial nailing: A multicenter study. *Orthop Trans* 1995;19:483.
35. O'Sullivan ME, Bronk JT, Chao EY, et al: Experimental study of the effect of weight bearing on fracture healing in the canine tibia. *Clin Orthop* 1994;302:273–283.
36. Lonner JH, Jupiter JB, Healy WL: Ipsilateral tibia and ankle fractures. *J Orthop Trauma* 1993;7:130–137.
37. Keating JF, Kuo RS, Court-Brown CM: Bifocal fractures of the tibia and fibula: Incidence, classification and treatment. *J Bone Joint Surg* 1994;76B:395–400.
38. Tornetta P III, Weiner L, Bergman M, et al: Pilon fractures: Treatment with combined internal and external fixation. *J Orthop Trauma* 1993;7:489–496.
39. Freedman EL, Johnson EE: Radiographic analysis of tibial fracture malalignment following intramedullary nailing. *Clin Orthop* 1995;315:25–33.
40. Cole JD: Intramedullary nailing of proximal fourth tibia fractures. *Orthop Trans*, in press.
41. Tornetta P III, Collins E: Semiextended position for intramedullary nailing of the proximal tibia. *Clin Orthop* 1996;328:185–189.
42. Henley MB: Intramedullary devices for tibial fracture stabilization. *Clin Orthop* 1989; 240:87–96.

CHAPTER 28

Delayed Union and Nonunion of Tibial Shaft Fractures

James A. Goulet, MD
David Templeman, MD

Nonunion of the tibial shaft is a common problem that is severe and disabling. Failure of tibial fractures to unite can lead to multiple surgical procedures and prolonged hospitalization, with years of disability before a union is obtained or amputation is performed. Although in some series of tibial fractures high rates of union have been obtained with simple methods,[1-4] nonunion is seen by all practitioners treating tibial fractures. This chapter provides an overview of tibial nonunions and reviews the treatment options available for management of this diverse group of clinical problems. Finally, it makes recommendations for the treatment of tibial diaphyseal fractures that fail to unite after initial appropriate treatment. These nonunions occur relatively frequently and are treated by most orthopaedic surgeons.

The definitions of nonunion and malunion are arbitrary and, therefore, warrant careful attention by the reviewer of fracture literature trying to interpret results from previous series. Nonunion is defined as a condition in which, in the opinion of the surgeon, further nonsurgical management will fail to unite the fragments.[5] Müller's definition—failure to unite after 8 months of nonsurgical treatment—is the most widely used arbitrary criterion for nonunion of the tibia.[6] Delayed union is defined as the state in which the expected progression to union has not been observed at a specified time. Failure to see evidence of union on radiographs at various times ranging from 20 to 26 weeks has been the criterion used by several authors to define delayed union.[5-9] It is most useful to think of delayed union as the point at which alteration of treatment to achieve union should be considered. Although this determination is frequently made 20 weeks after the fracture, certain fractures, such as type III open tibial fractures, may benefit from earlier intervention.

Malunion of a tibial shaft fracture refers to healing of the fracture in a nonanatomic position. Functional malposition, rather than cosmetic deformity, constitutes an indication for surgical intervention. Although this chapter will not deal explicitly with tibial malunions, tibial nonunions may be shortened or angulated, and the same alignment and length criteria that apply to tibial malunions also apply to tibial nonunions. The most frequently encountered problem in malalignment is shortening. Shortening of less than 1 cm is acceptable. Shortening of greater than 15 mm may be symptomatic and necessitate a lift or leg length equalization procedure. Varus and valgus angulation should be limited to less than 10°. Recurvatum is functionally less well-tolerated than anterior bowing and should not exceed 10°. Anterior bowing of less than 10° is rarely of functional significance, but it can be cosmetically unacceptable. Rotatory malalignment is better tolerated than varus-valgus angulation. Internal rotation that exceeds 5° is noticeable; if it exceeds 10°, it is usually unacceptable. External rotation is better tolerated, but will become noticeable when it exceeds 10° and may become functionally significant when it exceeds 15°. Although some degree of malalignment is common following tibial fractures, osteotomy is rarely indicated. Close follow-up of patients with acute tibial fractures and early intervention in cases of developing angular deformity will prevent most unacceptable malunions and angulated nonunions.

Incidence and Etiology

The incidence of nonunion and delayed union are estimated from reports published in the literature. In historic series, including all types of tibial fractures, the incidence of nonunion has been between 2% and 3% and the incidence of delayed union between 4% and 5%.[1-4,8,10-26] Open fractures with gross contamination and extensive soft-tissue damage have a much higher incidence of nonunion and delayed union. In series of open tibial fractures, Clancy and associates[13] reported a 13% incidence of delayed union, Widenfalk and associates[4] reported a 31% incidence of delayed union, and Edwards and associates[27] reported that 41% of grade III fractures required bone grafting to achieve union. In type II and type III open tibial fractures, Velazco and associates[25] reported a 14% rate of nonunion. A higher incidence of tibial nonunions and malunions should be expected by orthopaedic surgeons in view of the increased incidence of high-energy trauma associated with motor vehicle accidents.

Many factors have been associated with delayed union or nonunion. The incidence of nonunion, and especially of infected nonunion, increases with the severity of open fractures. The presenting factors contributing to nonunion or delayed union include fracture displacement, bone loss, associated fibular fractures, comminution, and infection.[16-19,21,28-31] A direct correlation exists between the energy absorbed by the bone and soft tissues and the complications of wound healing, including delayed union, nonunion, infection, and skin slough.[32,33]

The common factor that determines healing of tibial fractures is the preservation of the tibial blood supply. The nutrient vessels provide the endosteal blood supply to the tibia, supplying as much as 90% of the inner cortex.[34] Destruction of the endosteal blood supply is most extensive when the fracture occurs in the middle one third of the tibia,[34] but the distribution of nonunions among proximal, middle, and distal thirds of the shaft appears to be equal.[5] The blood supply to the subcutaneous anteromedial periosteum is precarious and easily destroyed. The degree of periosteal stripping and the resultant amount of devascularized bone varies with the fracture type. Increased periosteal stripping, as seen in high-grade open fractures, contributes substantially to delayed union or nonunion.

Failure to manage tibial fractures properly has been shown to increase the incidence of nonunion. Distraction at the fracture site and failure to immobilize the fracture adequately are known to increase the time to union.[35] Adherence to the principles of open fracture management, including aggressive multiple debridements, administration of antibiotics, and stable immobilization of fracture fragments, has also been shown to substantially decrease the incidence of infection and nonunion.

Goals of Tibial Nonunion Treatment

The ultimate goal of a functional lower extremity should not be overlooked in attempts to achieve bone union. Amputation is a reasonable alternative to heroic efforts that pursue union in the face of major bone loss, infection, and posterior tibial nerve lesions. Patients frequently require 18 months of intensive orthopaedic care to achieve union, but a poor functional result. Optimal treatment seeks to avoid the muscle atrophy, muscle and tendon contractures, joint stiffness, and disuse osteoporosis that have been associated with prolonged cast immobilization.[1]

Assessment of Tibial Nonunion

Treatment of tibial nonunions requires critical analysis. The fracture configuration, location, extent of soft-tissue damage, and history of infection or previous external fixation are essential elements of the history. Physical examination determines the status of the soft tissue, the presence or absence of a draining sinus, and the neurovascular status of the foot. Initial and current fracture alignment should be radiographically assessed and note made of any significant bony defect that limits the choices for managing the nonunion.

The algorithm for surgical therapy of tibial nonunions is based on eliminating the factors responsible for development of the nonunion, correcting any deformity, gaining union, and controlling infection. Infection, soft-tissue defects, atrophic nonunions, and malalignment substantially alter treatment options in tibial nonunions.

Closed, uninfected nonunions with anatomic alignment require intervention only to achieve union. Atrophic nonunions require altering the local biology of the nonunion site, usually with bone grafting, in addition to providing mechanical stability at the fracture site. The methods by which bone defects are overcome include cancellous bone grafting, vascularized bone grafts, and distraction osteogenesis with application of Ilizarov-type devices.

Infection must be excluded before a treatment protocol for any tibial nonunion is begun. Routine assessment of tibial nonunions includes a complete blood count with differential and assessment of acute-phase reactants, including the erythrocyte sedimentation rate and C-reactive proteins. Routine radiographs should be studied for changes consistent with infection, including decreases in cortical density, increased radiolucency around implants, increased periosteal reaction, and the formation of sequestra and involucrum. The absence of these radiographic findings does not exclude infections, because these changes often occur late in the course of infection. In contrast, increased uptake on technetium and indium scans does not confirm the presence of infection, because these findings may be observed for several months or years following tibial fracture fixation. Aspiration at the site of maximum inflammation or maximum tenderness with Gram staining and culture of the fluid will establish or confirm the diagnosis of infection in most patients. The scope of treatment and types of decisions that need to be made for these patients differ substantially from the algorithms used for tibial nonunions without existing or previous infection. The management of infected tibial nonunions poses a substantial challenge, requiring adequate debridement and soft-tissue coverage in addition to other procedures. This topic exceeds the scope of this chapter; the reader is advised to consult other resources before treating infected nonunions.[2,26,32,36-38]

Treatment of Tibial Nonunion

A wide variety of tools and methods are used in the management of tibial nonunions. While some interventions are more universally accepted and more frequently successful than others, each of the methods discussed below is popular for the treatment of tibial nonunions. A brief overview is provided to place each technique in perspective.

Bone Grafting

Many methods of bone grafting for tibial defects have been described. These include many forms of sliding-onlay grafts,[39-41] inlay grafts,[42] nonvascularized fibular transplants,[43,44] and other techniques for creating tibiofibular synostosis.[45,46] The primary function of a bone graft is to alter the local biology of the nonunion site. Proposed alternatives to cancellous bone grafting include the use of percutaneous marrow injections,[47] human bone morphogenic protein,[48] and synthetic bone graft substitutes.[49] Although promising, these techniques are not currently available to practicing physicians, and the precise role of each of these alternatives has yet to be defined.

Cancellous bone grafting is the best method to alter the local biology of the nonunion site. Anteromedial bone grafting is preferable for proximal nonunions.[50] The posterolateral approach described by Harmon[51] is best in the distal two thirds of the tibia; it avoids the typical anteromedial open wound and places bone in the most vascular portion of the leg. In several large series, in which cancellous bone grafting was used for tibial nonunions, union rates of 87% to 100% have been reported.[7,17,52-58] Complications, which are uncommon, include stiffness, deformity, and loss of ankle motion. These complications have been ascribed to the initial injury, but may be aggravated by the prolonged immobilization associated with bone grafting. Paresthesia in the sole of the foot and delayed vascular impairment have been reported, but seem to be rare.[7,55] Formation of a synostosis has been associated with, but is not clearly the cause of, ankle pain.[9] Because these complications are uncommon and the union rate following posterolateral bone grafting is high, the posterolateral approach may be used in conjunction with other procedures for angulated or infected nonunions.

Anteromedial Bone Grafting For delayed unions or nonunions in the proximal third of the tibia, we prefer an anteromedial approach to a posterolateral approach. Due to difficulties in management trifurcation of the popliteal artery and the vascular supply to the entire lower extremity, the anteromedial approach is safer and easily accessible. Surgery is performed with the patient supine, and the anterior iliac crest provides enough bone graft for union to be achieved.

The anteromedial approach provides a smaller tissue envelope for massive amounts of cancellous bone than does the posterolateral approach. The incision is frequently dictated by the injury. However, in uninjured skin, a straight vertical incision is made just medial to the crest and straight to bone. Great care is taken in dissecting the soft tissues off the anterior tibia. The development of skin flaps compromises soft tissue, causes skin sloughs, and may necessitate skin grafting or rotational flaps as salvage procedures. Once the cancellous bone has been harvested, the hypertrophic nonunion is recontoured to recreate the normal shape of the bone, and bone is packed anteromedially and anterolaterally. No attempt is made to dissect deep into the anterior compartment along the lateral crest of the tibia, because to do so can injure the already compromised soft tissues and vascular structures.

Posterolateral Bone Grafting We prefer the posterolateral approach to the tibia with the patient prone. This allows a two-team approach; one surgeon can begin harvesting the bone graft from the posterior iliac crest while the other begins the approach to the tibia. This method decreases surgical operating time and provides maximum exposure to the posterior crest and tibia. Depending on the level of the nonunion, a generous skin incision is made 10 cm above and 10 cm below the level of nonunion. A longitudinal incision, medial to the palpable border of the fibula, is made between the gastrocnemius/soleus and flexor hallucis longus and the peroneal muscles. After the fascia of the soleus has been entered, the fixed palpable fascia on the anteromedial border of the fibula provides a landmark for the next level of dissection. The soleus and flexor hallucis longus muscles are reflected, using a periosteal elevator, and a periosteal elevator is passed against the fibula superficial to the posterior tibial muscle and neurovascular bundle to elevate the posterior compartment free from the fibula. Care is taken at this level to avoid inadvertent entry into the posterior tibial compartment, which could injure the posterior tibial neurovascular bundle. Dissection should always begin in areas of known anatomy far away from the fracture and nonunion site. Once the appropriate plane has been entered, carry the dissection to the nonunion site, which frequently is encased in a scar. At this point, lift the posterior tibial compartment off the interosseous membrane with a periosteal elevator. Hold the posterior compartment, neurovascular bundle, soleus, and gastrocnemius free with Bennett or Hohmann retractors. After the nonunion has been identified, petal the shaft from 5 cm above to 5 cm below with a sharp .5-inch osteotome. Copiously irrigate the wound and pack the harvested cancellous bone into this compartment. After the bone graft is in place, insert a suction drain, loosely close the soleus fascia to the peroneal fascia to hold the bone graft in position, and close the skin in the standard fashion. Finally, apply a long-leg Robert Jones dressing, which allows easy access to the wound and drain.

Defect Nonunion

Large segmental defects of the tibia are usually the result of severe open tibial fractures. In the past, the treatment of choice has frequently been amputation, which decreases the length of hospitalization and decreases the risk of adult respiratory distress syndrome associated with necrotic tissue during acute management.

Our approach to these large segmental defects had previously been initial surgical debridement, stable external fixation, and soft-tissue coverage with late massive posterolateral cancellous bone grafting. Using this approach, a synostosis can be created proximally and distally with internal fixation of the fibula to provide a strut for bone-grafting procedures. Achievement of a stable functional union may take 2 years, and multiple bone-grafting procedures are sometimes necessary. Intramedullary fixation and tibial plate fixation are associated with a higher risk of infection, and are therefore not used in this setting. Although the length of treatment is prolonged and requires multiple hospitalizations and bone grafting, massive posterolateral bone grafting appears to be a viable alternative in the treatment of patients with severe segmental bone loss. It is the only technique with an acceptable rate of success that does not require the use of specialized instrumentation and training.

Distraction Osteogenesis (Ilizarov Technique)

More recently, segmental defects have been treated effectively using the Ilizarov technique of corticotomy and bone transport. Available reports of results using this technique have been enthusiastic and promising,[59] and our initial experience has confirmed the utility of this technique in our own practice. To date, only small series have been reported from North America with sufficient follow-up to critically evaluate the outcome and complication rate associated with this technique. Because the Ilizarov technique differs substantially from other available techniques for treating segmental bone loss, a steep learning curve is likely to be encountered by the orthopaedist treating segmental bone loss with bone transport for the first time. Formal training in this technique is recommended before proceeding with any Ilizarov procedure. A relatively high rate of pin tract problems and other potentially more significant problems might be anticipated as this technique is initially applied, and a good ancillary medical support network is highly recommended.

Free Microvascular Bone Transfers

Free microvascular bone transfers may be useful for osseous reconstruction following extensive resections. First successfully reported by Taylor and associates[23] in 1978, the technique involves the isolation and transfer of a bone segment, most commonly the contralateral fibula. The technique has the advantages of a one-stage procedure, which is relatively independent of the recipient bed and other available procedures, has a fast union rate, and has the potential for graft hypertrophy. However, the procedure is long and demanding, necessitates a vascular sacrifice, may lead to graft fracture, and creates a donor bone defect that may result in instability of the contralateral foot, with restricted motion of the ankle and great toe.[60,61] The technique may be considered for defects greater than 6 cm. There is no role for this technique in infected nonunions until the infection is completely under control, adequate soft tissue coverage has been obtained, and drainage has been eliminated with the patient free of all antibiotics.

Treatment Protocols for Common Tibial Nonunions

External Fixation

Tibial nonunions have been treated with a variety of internal and external fixation devices. External fixation is the preferred method of stabilization in cases of previous infection with the risk of reactivation of quiescent sepsis, following grade II and grade III open fractures, and in the presence of thin secondary epithelium adherent to bone that might slough after surgical dissection.[62] Experimentally and clinically, the single-frame anterior fixator using 4.5-mm or 5.0-mm half pins has been shown to be the best device.[63-65] This form of external fixation provides free wound access, allows stabilization of bone fragments at a distance from the lesion, permits motion of adjacent joints, and encourages patient mobility. Pin tract drainage, reported to occur in 5% to 10% of all pins and responsible for removal or alteration of one out of 30 frames, may be minimized with compulsive local care.[66,67]

Ilizarov Technique

The Ilizarov technique has been used with increasing frequency to treat angulated malunions, and there is considerable early enthusiasm for this approach. Inconveniences associated with the need for frequent postoperative visits, as well as a relatively high rate of pin tract problems and overall complications, may temper enthusiasm for this technique in less complicated cases. The versatility of this method, however, may make it the salvage procedure of choice for some of the more difficult tibial malunion problems that would otherwise not be amenable to functional limb salvage. This technique may be especially useful when shortening or compromised soft tissue complicate the more readily approachable simple angular malunion.

Intramedullary Nailing

Intramedullary nailing has many applications in the treatment of the uninfected tibial nonunion. Nonreamed intramedullary nailing, as advocated by Lottes[68] for the treatment of nonunion, is a relatively simple procedure, especially if the tibia is well aligned. However, unreamed nails that are not interlocked do not provide adequate rotational control and function solely as a form of internal splint.

Reamed tibial nails have a wider application than nonreamed nails, but prohibitively high infection and reinfection rates preclude their use in infected or previously infected tibial nonunions.[69,70] Even recent reports advocating the use of reamed intramedullary nails in the setting of previous infection document a reinfection rate of 22% to 38% when union is achieved.[71,72] In the patient with a noninfected tibial nonunion, the procedure stimulates the fracture site with the autogenous graft provided by the reamer and provides greater stabilization than does nonreamed nailing. Union rates of 95% to 100% have been reported with reamed nailing in tibial nonunions and delayed unions with no prior history of infection.[13,73,74] Mean healing time with reamed nailing in this setting has ranged from 5 to 9 months.[13,74] Unlike compression plating, reamed intramedullary nailing offers the advantage of full function, including weightbearing, after treatment, in addition to allowing motion at the adjacent joints.

The surgeon using reamed tibial nails must adhere especially closely to the principles of management of tibial nonunions outlined earlier in this chapter. The tibial blood supply has usually been adequately reestablished from surrounding soft tissues by the time reamed nailing for nonunion is considered. Care must be taken to avoid interfering with associated soft tissues, and surgery at the fracture site must be limited to the minimum necessary to achieve alignment. In a previously nonsurgically treated tibial nonunion, a very limited open procedure may be necessary to remove fibrous tissue and bone to align the canal. If the tibia is malaligned, a small osteotomy of the malunited fibula near the tibial fracture is frequently necessary to achieve tibial alignment. Whenever possible, reamed tibial nailing should be done as a closed procedure.

Nonunion After Nailing Without Reaming

Treatments for delayed union and nonunion after intramedullary nailing of the tibia continue to evolve. The recent popularity of the use of interlocking nails without reaming to stabilize open tibial fractures has expanded the indications for intramedullary nailing of tibial shaft fractures.[75-78] Despite early aggressive care and the absence of initial complications, many fractures that are initially treated with interlocking nailing without reaming require additional procedures to achieve union (Figs. 1 and 2).

Delayed union and nonunion are common sequelae after high-energy tibial fractures, and have been referred to as the negative biology of tibial fractures. Although interlocking nailing without reaming addresses the mechanical demands of the fracture, the nails do not sufficiently alter the local biology of the fracture; additional procedures are frequently required to achieve union. Recent reports indicate that between 20% and 57% of fractures treated with nailing without reaming required at least one additional procedure to obtain union.[74,78,79]

After nailing without reaming, delayed union and nonunion are managed by observation, dynamization, exchange nailing, or bone grafting.[76,78,80-83] The indications for these different treatments are based upon the severity of the soft-tissue injury, the geometry and comminution of the fracture site, location of the fracture, bone loss, fracture-implant stability, and the specific patient. These factors that direct which form of treatment to use are likely to be refined with further experience. The indications described here should be considered to be relative indications rather than absolute indications for treatment.

At the time of the initial irrigation and debridement, the extent and anatomic location of bone loss should be documented. Bone loss of more than 30% of the cortex predisposes the fracture to nonunion. In separate studies Whittle, Templeman, and Sanders found that bone grafting is the most reliable method to promote union in the presence of bone loss. In addition to bone loss, open tibial fractures that require free or local tissue transfers do not predictably unite their fractures after intramedullary nailing.[78,82,84,87] Further experience is needed to develop protocols for the treatment of severe open tibial fractures that require tissue transfers.

When bone grafting is used to promote union, the grafting should be delayed for a minimum of 6 weeks after injury. After 6 weeks, the soft-tissue edema and erythema at the fracture site have usually resolved.[85,86] In series in which the bone graft was applied earlier, the bone grafts have been resorbed. This presumably happens because the bone graft was placed in the wound during the inflammatory stage of fracture healing, which results in resorption of the graft.

In the absence of bone loss, it becomes more difficult to determine the best procedure to promote union. Observation, dynamization (removal of interlocking bolts), exchange nailing and bone grafting are all advocated.[74,78,82,87] When the fracture is unstable (due to shortening, angulation, or rotation), the nail should not be dynamized. Fractures with segmental comminution, fractures located at the metaphyseal-diaphyseal junction, and spiral fractures may be unstable after the interlocking bolts are removed.[76,78,88] In these situations, either bone grafting or exchange nailing is performed.

Breakage of the interlocking bolts has been reported to be as high as 25%[89] after nailing without reaming. Avoiding distraction at the fracture site, dynamization at 6 weeks, and the use of titanium implants are all reported to decrease the incidence of implant failure. If the fracture site is stable and not distracted, many patients can be allowed to weightbear. These patients

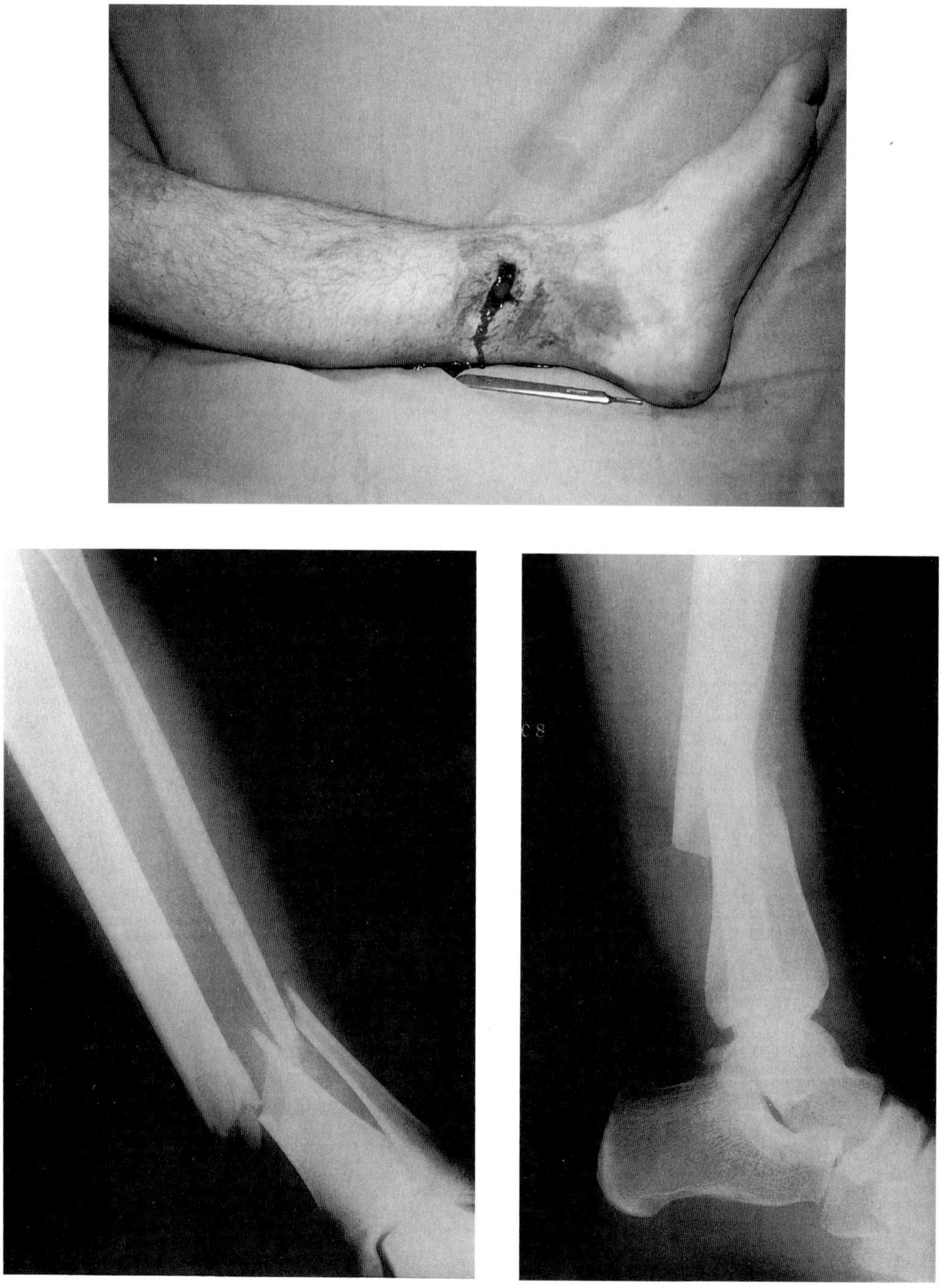

Fig. 1 A 19-year-old man sustained an open fracture of the distal tibia when he was run over by a truck.

are seen monthly to assess pain and to look for the development of callus on radiograms. Callus is usually first seen along the posterior cortex of the tibia. Sanders recommended at least 9 months of observation after the initial use of unreamed nailing techniques before performing a secondary procedure.

In our experience, the patient's level of comfort is a useful clue in assessing stability. Patients who are comfortable weightbearing can be observed for fracture healing. Continued pain is an indication that the nail-fracture construct is unstable and additional surgery is needed to promote healing.

To reduce the time to union, Stegemann and Bone recommend early intervention. Bone and Johnson[74] observed that unstable fractures that required the use of statically locked nails had a longer time to union and

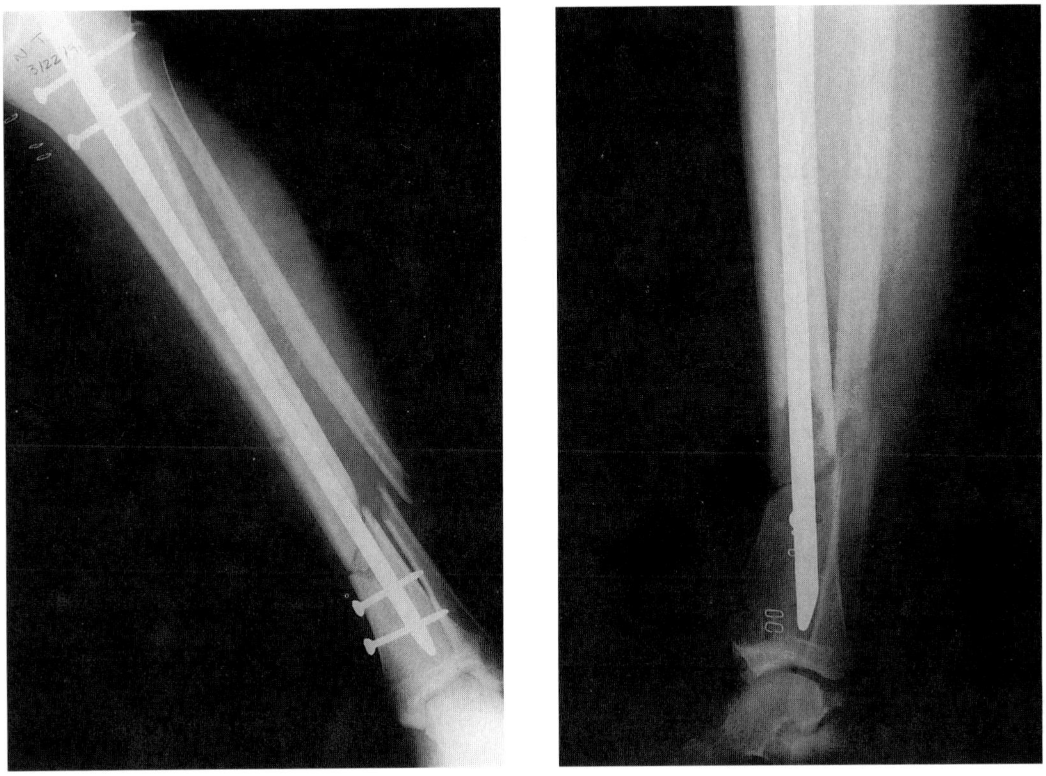

Fig. 2 Following emergent irrigation and debridement, the fracture was treated by insertion of interlocking nail without reaming.

required additional procedures to achieve union, as compared to stable fracture patterns that did not need static locking of the nails. To promote union and shorten healing times, patients with statically locked nails either have the nails dynamized, or bone grafting is performed within a 6- to 10-week period after the time of the injury. This protocol of early secondary surgery reduced the time to union from 37 to 24 weeks in a series of high-energy open tibial fractures.[90]

Exchange reamed intramedullary nailing after the initial use of nails without reaming is another method to promote union. The initial use of nails, as opposed to external fixators, avoids problems with pin tract infections and aligns the tibia for secondary nailing.[91-93]

The conversion of the small nails inserted without reaming to larger diameter nails promotes healing in several ways. Reaming may act as a physiologic stimulus to healing.[94,95] In some cases, the insertion of a larger nail with a snug fit in the intramedullary canal will improve the stability of the nail-fracture construct enough to allow weightbearing and loading of the fracture (Fig. 3).[96]

Despite the avoidance of pin tract problems, the infection rate after exchange nailing was 11% in one series.[82] Complications with exchange nailing, infection, and nonunion are higher in patients with Grade IIIB fractures or bone loss. Autogenous bone grafting appears to be a more predictable procedure for these injuries.

Exchange nailing is a relatively simple procedure with low morbidity. Reaming alone may provide an important stimulus to healing. Static locking of the larger nail is rarely needed and early weightbearing is possible. Exchange nailing is a safe and effective treatment for delayed union of closed and Grades I, II, and IIIA open tibial fractures (Fig. 4).[97]

Initial Treatment With External Fixation

Additional procedures are frequently required to promote union after the initial use of external fixation. This is because external fixators are frequently used to treat the most severe tibial fractures. These fractures are predisposed to delayed union and nonunion. However, union rates are high when autogenous bone grafting is performed in conjunction with external fixation. Blick and associates[85] and Behrens and associates[75] report union rates approximating 90% when bone grafting was used in combination with external fixation.

Many traumatologists believe that once external fixation is used, it should be continued until the fracture unites. This is an excellent protocol that maintains alignment, and autogenous bone graft provides the biologic stimulus for healing, while permitting motion

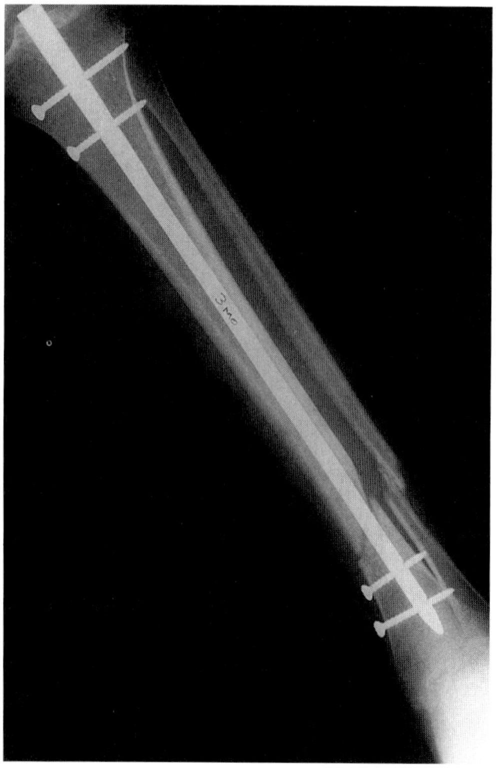

Fig. 3 (Same patient as in Figs. 1 and 2) Three months after the injury, there is no evidence of callus formation. Exchange nailing was performed within the next month; a large diameter nail with reaming was used.

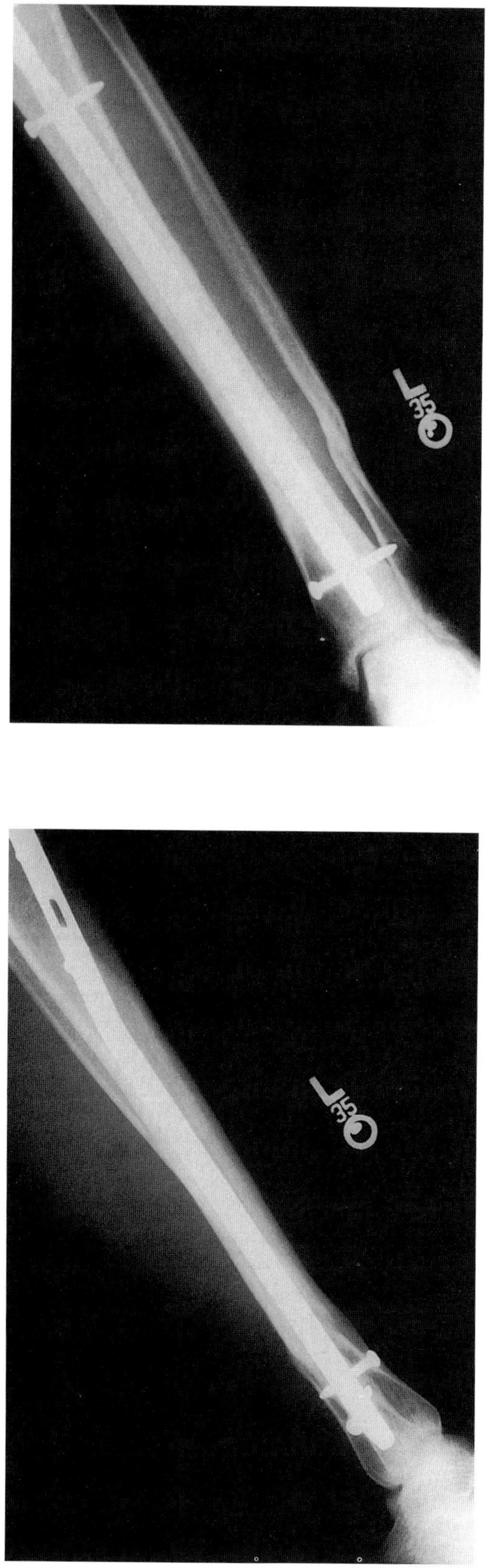

Fig. 4 (Same patient) One year after the injury, the fracture has remodeled.

of the knee and ankle.[75] Additional procedures, such as removal and/or replacement of infected pins, are performed as needed. Removal of external fixators before union of the fracture frequently results in the development of malalignment because secure fixation of the fracture is lost.

Open reduction and plate fixation for aseptic nonunion of the tibia is a reliable treatment. Müller and Thomas[98] achieved union in 21 of 23 tibial nonunions; Rosen[99] reported union in 31 of 33 cases; and Weber and Brunner[100] secured union in 126 of 127 cases.

Wiss[96] addressed the use of compression plating after the initial use of external fixation in 50 patients. Initially, 46 of the 50 fractures were open fractures. Compression plating was performed at an average of 8 months after the initial injury. In this series, 72% of the nonunions were classified as atrophic; autogenous bone grafting was used for 78% of the fractures treated. Union was achieved for 92% of the fractures after plate fixation; the infection rate was 6%. Compared to the experience with the use of reamed intramedullary nailing of the tibia, Wiss recommends the use of external fixation for the treatment of tibial nonunions initially treated by external fixation.

Plating also avoids problems with malalignment, which requires soft-tissue stripping to realign the fracture. This last point addresses the blood supply of the fracture site. When extraperiosteal stripping is needed to realign the tibia, it should not be followed with intramedullary nailing, which further compromises the intramedullary blood supply. In this setting, plating causes less vascular damage than intramedullary nailing.

References

1. Brown PW, Urban JG: Early weight-bearing treatment of open fractures of the tibia: An end–result study of sixty-three cases. *J Bone Joint Surg* 1969;51A:59–75.
2. Dehne E, Metz CW, Deffer PA, et al: Nonoperative treatment of the fractured tibia by immediate weight bearing. *J Trauma* 1961;1:514–535.
3. Sarmiento A, Sobol PA, Sew Hoy AL, et al: Prefabricated functional braces for the treatment of fractures of the tibial diaphysis. *J Bone Joint Surg* 1984;66A:1328–1339.
4. Widenfalk B, Ponten B, Karlström G: Open fractures of the shaft of the tibia: Analysis of wound and fracture treatment. *Injury* 1979;11:136–143.
5. Nicoll EA: Fractures of the tibial shaft: A survey of 705 cases. *J Bone Joint Surg* 1964;46B:373–387.
6. Muller ME, Allgöwer M, Schneider R, et al (eds): *Manual of Internal Fixation: Techniques Recommended by the AO Group*, ed 2. Berlin, Germany, Springer–Verlag, 1979.
7. Jones KG: Treatment of infected nonunion of the tibia through the posterolateral approach. *Clin Orthop* 1965;43:103–109.
8. Rosenthal RE, MacPhail JA, Oritz JE: Non-union in open tibial fractures: Analysis of reasons for failure of treatment. *J Bone Joint Surg* 1977;59A:244–248.
9. Skelley JW, Hardy AE: Results of bone grafts in the treatment of tibial fractures. *Clin Orthop* 1981;158:108–110.
10. Anderson LD, Hutchins WC, Wright PE, et al: Fractures of the tibia and fibula treated by casts and transfixing pins. *Clin Orthop* 1974;105:179–191.
11. D'Aubigne RM, Maurer P, Zucman J, et al: Blind intramedullary nailing for tibial fractures. *Clin Orthop* 1974;105:267–275.
12. Christensen NO: Küntscher intramedullary reaming and nail fixation for non–union of fracture of the femur and the tibia. *J Bone Joint Surg* 1973;55B:312–318.
13. Clancey GJ, Winquist RA, Hansen ST Jr: Nonunion of the tibia treated with Küntscher intramedullary nailing. *Clin Orthop* 1982;167:191–196.
14. Donald G, Seligson D: Treatment of tibial shaft fractures by percutaneous Küntscher nailing: Technical difficulties and a review of 50 consecutive cases. *Clin Orthop* 1983;178:64–73.
15. Gershuni DH, Halma G: The A-O external skeletal fixator in the treatment of severe tibia fractures. *J Trauma* 1983;23:986–990.
16. Karlstrom G, Olerud S: Fractures of the tibial shaft: A critical evaluation of treatment alternatives. *Clin Orthop* 1974;105: 82–115.
17. Lamb RH: Posterolateral bone graft for nonunion of the tibia. *Clin Orthop* 1969;64:114–120.
18. Mayer L, Werbie T, Schwab JP, et al: The use of Ender nails in fractures of the tibial shaft. *J Bone Joint Surg* 1985;67A:446–455.
19. Nicoll EA: Closed and open management of tibial fractures. *Clin Orthop* 1974;105:144–153.
20. Pankovich AM, Tarabishy IE, Yelda S: Flexible intramedullary nailing of tibial-shaft fractures. *Clin Orthop* 1981;160:185–195.
21. Sakellarides HT, Freeman PA, Grant BD: Delayed union and non-union of tibial-shaft fractures: A review of 100 cases. *J Bone Joint Surg* 1964;46A:557–569.
22. Sedlin ED, Zitner DT: The Lottes nail in the closed treatment of tibial fractures. *Clin Orthop* 1985;192:185–192.
23. Taylor GI, Miller GD, Ham FJ: The free vascularized bone graft: A clinical extension of microvascular techniques. *Plast Reconstr Surg* 1975;55:533–544.
24. Velazco A, Fleming LL: Open fractures of the tibia treated by the Hoffmann external fixator. *Clin Orthop* 1983;180:125–132.
25. Velazco A, Whitesides TE Jr, Fleming LL: Open fractures of the tibia treated with the Lottes nail. *J Bone Joint Surg* 1983; 65A:879–885.
26. Witschi TH, Omer GE Jr: The treatment of open tibial shaft fractures from the Vietnam War. *J Trauma* 1970;10:105–111.
27. Edwards CC, Jaworski MF: Hoffman external fixation in open tibial fractures with tissue loss. *Orthop Trans* 1979;3:261–262.
28. Boyd HB, Lipinski SW: Causes and treatment of non-union of the shafts of the long bones, with a review of 741 patients, in Reynolds FC (ed): American Academy of Orthopaedic Surgeons *Instructional Course Lectures XVII.* St. Louis, MO, CV Mosby, 1960, pp 165–182.
29. Ellis H: *A Study of Some Factors Affecting Prognosis Following Tibial Shaft Fractures.* Oxford, England, Bodlein Library, 1956. Thesis.
30. Urist MR, Mazet R Jr, McLean FC: The pathogenesis and treatment of delayed union and non–union: A survey of eighty-five ununited fractures of the shaft of the tibia and one hundred control cases with similar injuries. *J Bone Joint Surg* 1954; 36A:931–968.
31. Watson–Jones R, Coltart WD: Slow union of fractures: With a study of 804 fractures of the shafts of the tibia and femur. *Br J Surg* 1943;30:260–276.
32. Cierny G III, Byrd HS, Jones RE: Primary versus delayed soft tissue coverage for severe open tibial fractures: A comparison of results. *Clin Orthop* 1983;178:54–63.
33. Hoaglund FT, States JD: Factors influencing the rate of healing in tibial shaft fractures. *Surg Gynecol Obstet* 1967;124:71–76.
34. Macnab I: Blood supply of the tibia. *J Bone Joint Surg* 1957;39B:799.
35. Connolly JF: Common avoidable problems in nonunions. *Clin Orthop* 1985;194:226–235.
36. Ger R: Muscle transposition for treatment and prevention of chronic post-traumatic osteomyelitis of the tibia. *J Bone Joint Surg* 1977;59A:784–791.
37. Weiland AJ, Moore JR, Daniel RK: The efficacy of free tissue transfer in the treatment of osteomyelitis. *J Bone Joint Surg* 1984;66A:181–193.
38. Weiland AJ, Moore JR, Hotchkiss RN: Soft tissue procedures for reconstruction of tibial shaft fractures. *Clin Orthop* 1983;178: 42–53.
39. Boyd HB: The treatment of difficult and unusual non-unions: With special reference to the bridging of defects. *J Bone Joint Surg* 1943;25:535–552.
40. Flanagan JJ, Burem HS: Reconstruction of defects of the tibia and femur with apposing massive grafts from the affected bone. *J Bone Joint Surg* 1947;29:587–597.
41. Milch H: Tibiofibular synostosis for non-union of the tibia. *Surgery* 1950;27:770–779.
42. Wagner JH: Anterolateral approach in bone grafting for ununited fractures of tibia. *Am J Surg* 1947;73:282–299.
43. Carnesale PL, Guerrieri AG: Fibular transplant for loss of substance of tibia: Report of a case. *J Bone Joint Surg* 1955; 37A:204–206.
44. Davis AG: Fibular substitution for tibial defects. *J Bone Joint Surg* 1944;26:229–237.
45. Campanacci M, Zanoli S: Double tibiofibular synostosis (fibula pro tibia) for non–union and delayed union of the tibia: End-

result review of one hundred seventy–one cases. *J Bone Joint Surg* 1966;48A:44–56.
46. Hand FM: Crisscross tibiofibular graft for nonunion of the tibia. *Clin Orthop* 1953;1:154–160.
47. Connolly JF, Guse R, Tiedeman J, et al: Autologous marrow injection for delayed unions of the tibia: A preliminary report. *J Orthop Trauma* 1989;3:276–282.
48. Johnson EE, Urist MR, Finerman GA: Distal metaphyseal tibial nonunion: Deformity and bone loss treated by open reduction, internal fixation, and human bone morphogenetic protein (hBMP). *Clin Orthop* 1990;250:234–240.
49. McAndrew MP, Gorman PW, Lange TA: Tricalcium phosphate as a bone graft substitute in trauma: Preliminary report. *J Orthop Trauma* 1988;2:333–339.
50. Behrens F: Bone grafting: General principles and use in open fractures, in Murray DG (ed): American Academy of Orthopaedic Surgeons *Instructional Course Lectures XXX.* St. Louis, MO, CV Mosby, 1981, pp 152–156.
51. Harmon PH: A simplified surgical approach to the posterior tibia for bone-grafting and fibular transference. *J Bone Joint Surg* 1945;27:496–498.
52. Freeland AE, Mutz SB: Posterior bone–grafting for infected ununited fracture of the tibia. *J Bone Joint Surg* 1976; 58A:653–657.
53. Hanson LW, Eppright RH: Posterior bone-grafting of the tibia for non–union: A review of twenty-four cases. *J Bone Joint Surg* 1966;48A:27–43.
54. Harkins HN, Phemister DB: Simplified technique of onlay grafts for all ununited fractures in acceptable position. *JAMA* 1937;109:1501–1506.
55. Jones KG, Barnett HC: Cancellous-bone grafting for non-union of the tibia through the posterolateral approach. *J Bone Joint Surg* 1955;37A:1250–1260.
56. McCarroll HR: The surgical management of ununited fractures of the tibia. *JAMA* 1961;175:578–583.
57. Simon JP, Hoogmartens M: The value of posterolateral bone-grafting for non-union of the tibia. *Acta Orthop Belg* 1984; 50:557–564.
58. Souter WA: Autogenous cancellous strip grafts in the treatment of delayed union of long bone fractures. *J Bone Joint Surg* 1969;51B:63–75.
59. Paley D: Treatment of tibial nonunion and bone loss with the Ilizarov technique, in Greene WB (ed): *Instructional Course Lectures XXXIX.* Park Ridge, IL, American Academy of Orthopaedic Surgeons, 1990, pp 185–197.
60. Ito T, Kohno T, Kojima T: Free vascularized fibular graft. *J Trauma* 1984;24:756–760.
61. Osterman AL, Bora FW: Free vascularized bone grafting for large-gap nonunion of long bones. *Orthop Clin North Am* 1984;15:131–142.
62. Green SA, Garland DE, Moore TJ, et al: External fixation for the uninfected angulated nonunion of the tibia. *Clin Orthop* 1984; 190:204–211.
63. Behrens F: External skeletal fixation: Basic concepts and applications in open tibial fractures, in Murray JA (ed): American Academy of Orthopaedic Surgeons *Instructional Course Lectures XXXIII.* St. Louis, MO, CV Mosby, 1984, pp 124–130.
64. Behrens F, Johnson WD, Koch TW, et al: Bending stiffness of unilateral and bilateral fixator frames. *Clin Orthop* 1983; 178:103–110.
65. Wu JJ, Shyr HS, Chao EY, et al: Comparison of osteotomy healing under external fixation devices with different stiffness characteristics. *J Bone Joint Surg* 1984;66A:1258–1264.
66. Behrens F: Introduction to external skeletal fixation, in Murray DG (ed): American Academy of Orthopaedic Surgeons *Instructional Course Lectures XXX.* St. Louis, MO, CV Mosby, 1981, pp 112–118.
67. Green SA: Complications of external skeletal fixation. *Clin Orthop* 1983;180:109–116.
68. Lottes JO: Treatment of delayed or nonunion fractures of the tibia by a medullary nail. *Clin Orthop* 1965;43:111–128.
69. Laurent LE, Langenskiöld A: Osteosynthesis with a thick medullary nail in non-union of long bones. *Acta Orthop Scand* 1967;38:341–358.
70. Lidgren L, Onnerfält R: Infected non-union of the tibial shaft treated by Küntscher intramedullary reaming and nail fixation: A report of four cases. *Acta Orthop Scand* 1982;53:669–674.
71. Miller ME, Ada JR, Webb LX: Treatment of infected nonunion and delayed union of tibia fractures with locking intramedullary nails. *Clin Orthop* 1989;245:233–238.
72. Sledge SL, Johnson KD, Henley MB, et al: Intramedullary nailing with reaming to treat non-union of the tibia. *J Bone Joint Surg* 1989;71A:1004–1019.
73. Böhler J: Treatment of nonunion of the tibia with closed and semiclosed intramedullary nailing. *Clin Orthop* 1965;43:93–101.
74. Bone LB, Johnson KD: Treatment of tibial fractures by reaming and intramedullary nailing. *J Bone Joint Surg* 1986;68A:877–887.
75. Behrens F, Comfort TH, Searls K, et al: Unilateral external fixation for severe open tibial fractures: Preliminary report of a prospective study. *Clin Orthop* 1983;178:111–120.
76. Bone LB, Kassman S, Stegemann P, et al: Prospective study of union rate of open tibial fractures treated with locked, unreamed intramedullary nails. *J Orthop Trauma* 1994;8:45–49.
77. Rubinstein RA Jr, Green JM, Duweilus PJ: Intramedullary interlocked tibial nailing: A new technique (preliminary report). *J Orthop Trauma* 1992;6:90–95.
78. Whittle AP, Russell TA, Taylor JC, et al: Treatment of open fractures of the tibial shaft with the use of interlocking nailing without reaming. *J Bone Joint Surg* 1992;74A:1162–1171.
79. Duwelius PJ, Schmidt AH, Rubenstein RA, et al: Nonreamed interlocked intramedullary tibial nailing: One community's experience. *Clin Orthop* 1995;315:104–113.
80. Olerud S, Karlstrom G: Secondary intramedullary nailing of tibial fractures. *J Bone Joint Surg* 1972;54A:1419–1428.
81. Siebenrock KA, Schillig B, Jakob RP: Treatment of complex tibial shaft fractures: Arguments for early secondary intramedullary nailing. *Clin Orthop* 1993;290:267–274.
82. Templeman D, Thomas M, Varecka T, et al: Exchange reamed intramedullary nailing for delayed union and nonunion of the tibia. *Clin Orthop* 1995;315:169–175.
83. Webb LX, Winquist RA, Hansen ST: Intramedullary nailing and reaming for delayed union or nonunion of the femoral shaft: A report of 105 consecutive cases. *Clin Orthop* 1986;212:133–141.
84. Blachut PA, Meek RN, O'Brien PJ: External fixation and delayed intramedullary nailing of open fractures of the tibial shaft: A sequential protocol. *J Bone Joint Surg* 1990;72A:729–735.
85. Blick SS, Brumback RJ, Lakatos R, et al: Early prophylactic bone grafting of high-energy tibial fractures. *Clin Orthop* 1989; 240:21–41.
86. Gustilo RB, Mendoza RM, Williams DN: Problems in the management of Type III (severe) open fractures: A new classification of Type III open fractures. *J Trauma* 1984;24:742–746.
87. Sanders R, Jersinovich I, Anglen J, et al: The treatment of open tibial shaft fractures using an interlocked intramedullary nail without reaming. *J Orthop Trauma* 1994;8:504–510.
88. Templeman DC, Larson C, Varecka TF, et al: Decision-making errors in the use of interlocking tibial nails. *Orthop Trans* 1995; 19:142.
89. Riemer BL, DiChristina DG, Cooper A, et al: Nonreamed nailing of tibial diaphyseal fractures in blunt polytrauma patients. *J Orthop Trauma* 1995;9:66–75.
90. Stegemann P, Lorio M, Soriano R, et al: Management protocol for unreamed interlocking tibial nails for open tibial fractures. *J Orthop Trauma* 1995;9:117–120.

91. Maurer DJ, Merkow RL, Gustilo RB: Infection after intramedullary nailing of severe open tibial fractures initially treated with external fixation. *J Bone Joint Surg* 1989;71A: 835–838.
92. McGraw JM, Lim EV: Treatment of open tibial–shaft fractures: External fixation and secondary intramedullary nailing. *J Bone Joint Surg* 1988;70A:900–911.
93. Törnqvist H: Tibia nonunions treated by interlocked nailing: Increased risk of infection after previous external fixation. *J Orthop Trauma* 1990;4:109–114.
94. Johnson EE, Marder RA: Open intramedullary nailing and bone-grafting for non-union of tibial diaphyseal fracture. *J Bone Joint Surg* 1987;69A:375–380.
95. Kessler SB, Hallfeldt KK, Perren SM, et al: The effects of reaming and intramedullary nailing on fracture healing. *Clin Orthop* 1986;212:18–25.
96. Wiss DA: Flexible medullary nailing of acute tibial shaft fractures. *Clin Orthop* 1986;212:122–132.
97. Court-Brown CM, Gustilo T, Christie J, et al: Exchange tibial nailing for aseptic non-union. *Orthop Trans* 1995;19:146.
98. Müller ME, Thomas RJ: Treatment of non-union in fractures of long bones. *Clin Orthop* 1979;138:141–153.
99. Rosen H: Compression treatment of long bone pseudarthroses. *Clin Orthop* 1979;138:154–166.
100. Weber BG, Brunner C: The treatment of nonunions without electrical stimulation. *Clin Orthop* 1981;161:24–32.

CHAPTER 29

Open Fractures of the Tibial Shaft

Steven A. Olson, MD

The tibial shaft is one of the most common sites of an open fracture,[1] a fracture that involves a break in the skin with soft tissues communicating with the fracture or its hematoma, or both. The specific methods of skeletal stabilization and soft-tissue treatment of open and closed fractures continue to be topics of debate in orthopaedic traumatology. The type of treatment selected for open tibial fractures depends on the individual characteristics of the fracture and the concomitant soft-tissue injury, making experience and clinical judgment an important part of the overall treatment.[2,3] Most orthopaedists treat only a few of these injuries each year; however, there are increasing expectations for surgeons to understand and apply the techniques of treatment of open fractures, such as the use of flap coverage and bone transplant techniques, to help patients to obtain an optimum functional outcome.[2]

Treatment in the Emergency Room

In the emergency room, initial attention should be given to resuscitation and assessment of the patient according to the guidelines of *Advanced Trauma Life Support*.[4] Specific assessment of the extremities other than to control active hemorrhage should be part of a secondary survey. The orthopaedist must be aware of other injuries, because severe pulmonary, intra-abdominal, or head injuries may limit the extent of intial debridement and stabilization that can be performed acutely for the open tibial fracture.[1] Concomitant fractures of the long bones and unstable fractures of the posterior part of the pelvic ring associated with hemodynamic instability should be stabilized within the first 24 hours after the injury whenever possible.

The physical examination should include a thorough inspection and palpation of the extremities.[1] Occult open fractures may be missed if the examining physician does not elevate the extremity and inspect it circumferentially. The initial evaluation should include assessment of the neurovascular status, the soft-tissue injury, and the osseous deformity. The vascular status can be documented by palpation of pulses, examination for capillary refill, and notation of the color of the limb and the presence of bleeding from open wounds. Any osseous deformity should be evaluated. Legs that have a gross rotational deformity or angular deformity, or both, at the site of a tibial fracture should be realigned promptly in an anatomic position.[1,4] Associated deformities of the foot, ankle, knee, or femur should also be noted. Pulses should be documented before and after alignment. The pulses often improve with realignment; persistently diminished pulses may indicate a vascular injury and the need for arteriographic evaluation. Gross motor function and sensibility of the foot and leg should be documented whenever possible. The presence or absence of plantar sensation can be an important factor in determining whether a limb-salvage procedure is the best treatment for a severe injury.[1,5]

Often, soft-tissue injuries can be assessed only superficially in the emergency room. Knowledge of the history of the injury and its location is often helpful when determining the extent of soft-tissue damage and the level of contamination. Blistering, contusions, crushed areas of skin, and burns reflect the transfer of a large amount of energy to the limb.[6] Gross contamination with soil, grass, or other foreign material should be noted. The dimensions and location of all open wounds should be recorded. A photograph of the open wound helps to document its characteristics. Extensive or contaminated wounds should be lavaged with a liter of sterile saline solution. Superficial foreign bodies, such as leaves and grass, that are immediately accessible should be removed from the wound before it is sealed. The surgeon should take care to use a sterile technique so as not to increase the contamination of the wound during the initial inspection phase. A clean sterile dressing should be applied to the wound and should not be removed until the patient is taken to the operating room.[1,6] The limb should be placed in a well-padded plaster splint in grossly normal alignment.

Early intravenous administration of antibiotics is associated with a decreased rate of infection[7] and thus should be begun in the emergency room.[1,2,6,7] Coverage for gram-positive organisms with cefazolin (1 g every 8 hours) should be routine for all open fractures. Coverage for gram-negative organisms, typically with an aminoglycoside, is used for open fractures with more extensive soft-tissue injury or extensive contamination, or both.[1,6] Coverage for anaerobic organisms, typically with penicillin, should be used whenever there is the possibility of infection with *Clostridium perfringens*, such as from contamination with soil (particularly with injuries that occur on a farm) or public waters such as rivers or lakes.[1,8] Antibiotic therapy should be continued for 48 to 72 hours after the initial debridement for type-I and type-II open fractures, as classified by Gustilo and Anderson.[9] Antibiotics should be given for as long as 120 hours after debridement of a type-III open fracture.[1,2,6,7]

Prophylaxis against tetanus should also be considered with any open fracture. Patients who were immunized in the last 5 years before the injury do not need prophylaxis. Those who were immunized more than 5 years before the injury should receive a tetanus booster. Patients for whom the time of the last immunization is unknown or who have never been immunized should receive a tetanus immunization booster as well as tetanus immune globulin.[4]

Classification

Classification of an open fracture facilitates the description of the severity of the injury among physicians, and it can provide useful guidance for treatment as well. The classification of an open fracture is based on a number of factors, including the mechanism of injury, the vascular status of the extremity, the size of soft-tissue defects and lacerations of the extremity, the extent of soft-tissue crush or loss, the extent of comminution, the amount of bone loss, the degree of periosteal stripping, and the degree of bacterial contamination.[2,9] The final classification of an open fracture should be delayed until the time of the initial surgical debridement, as many of these factors cannot be assessed fully before that time.[6]

The most common classification system for open fractures used in the United States is that of Gustilo and associates.[9,10] As originally described by Gustilo and Anderson[9] in 1976, this classification divided fractures into types I, II, and III. With its revision in 1984,[10] the classification subdivided type-III injuries into types IIIA, IIIB, and IIIC.

A type-I fracture is a low-energy injury with minimum soft-tissue damage and a small (less than 1 cm) wound; the fracture typically occurs as an inside-to-out puncture from an underlying spike of bone. Typically, there is slight comminution of the bone.[9]

A type-II fracture represents a transition between the low-energy type-I and the high-energy type-III fracture. Type-II fractures may have associated soft-tissue lacerations 1 to 10 cm long, slight or moderate comminution, and no or slight periosteal stripping of the bone fragments.[9]

The most severe pattern of open fractures is type III. Gustilo and associates[10] defined type-IIIA open fractures as those having adequate coverage with soft tissue despite extensive soft-tissue lacerations or flaps or injuries reflecting high-energy trauma, such as extensive osseous comminution, a segmental fracture pattern, or extensive soft-tissue injury (irrespective of the size of the wound), or a combination of any of these. Open fractures that occur in an environment that predisposes to extensive bacterial contamination, such as a barnyard setting or a public waterway, are also classified as type IIIA.

Type-IIIB fractures were originally defined as fractures with extensive soft-tissue injury, periosteal stripping, and exposed bone.[10] This definition has led to debate as to whether a fracture with areas of periosteal stripping but adequate muscle coverage of the bone should be classified as type IIIA or type IIIB. We prefer to define type-IIIB open fractures as those that necessitate local or distant flap coverage of areas of exposed bone.[1] These fractures are commonly associated with extensive periosteal stripping.

A type-IIIC fracture is associated with a vascular injury that requires repair for survival of the limb.[10] A tibial fracture with only an isolated injury of the anterior or posterior tibial artery should not be considered type IIIC.

The introduction of the classification of Gustilo and associates[9,10] for open fractures was a major step forward in the treatment of these complex injuries. Recently, Brumback and Jones[11] surveyed a group of orthopaedic surgeons interested in the treatment of open fractures, in order to assess the interobserver reliability associated with this classification system. The surgeons viewed video presentations of the history, physical examination, radiographs, and operative debridement of the wound for 13 open fractures. The average overall interobserver agreement for classification was 60% (range, 42% to 94%). The average agreement was 59% (range, 33% to 94%) for residents and fellows and 66% (range, 39% to 100%) for trauma-fellowship-trained, academic orthopaedic surgeons who treated more than 12 open tibial fractures a year.[11] These low levels of interobserver agreement emphasize that the classification of open fractures is subjective.

Other classification systems for open fractures are available. The AO/ASIF classification for soft-tissue injuries uses a combination of the alpha-numeric fracture classification system and an IMN system wherein the injury to the integument (I), muscle (M), and nerve (N) is each judged independently. This classification system has several potential benefits for clinical research; however, it is cumbersome in clinical situations. The Hannover open-fracture classification, developed by Südkamp and associates,[12] is based on a point-scale system for bone injury, soft-tissue injury, vascular injury, and contamination. Open fractures are classified as types I through IV. This system has not been widely used in North America.

Initial Surgical Treatment

An open tibial fracture is a surgical emergency. The primary treatment is early surgical debridement and stabilization of the bone. Debridement of an open tibial fracture involves surgical exploration of the wound or wounds to define the zone of injury, removal of devitalized tissue, and use of pulsed lavage to achieve additional mechanical debridement of the wound.[1,2,6] Experience and judgment are required to determine the appropriate extent of debridement. The wound should be extended with the use of sharp dissection until healthy tissue is seen at each end. The wound should then be explored systematically to ensure complete debridement of all contaminants and devitalized tissue.

Debridement should begin with the skin. After surgical extension, the edges of the skin should be inspected carefully about the entire wound. Evidence of skin and subcutaneous tissue that has been avulsed from underlying fascial structures should be noted, because this is an indicator of high-energy trauma and may be indicative of underlying muscle injury.[1,13] The debridement should continue in a methodical way with careful inspection of the subcutaneous tissue, muscle, and finally bone to avoid overlooking any devitalized tissue. The skin and subcutaneous tissue are inspected throughout the entire extent of the wound. Any obviously nonviable or crushed skin should be excised. Skin with questionable viability can be retained until a later debridement. This is especially important in the area of the subcutaneous border of the tibia, where injudicious removal of skin may necessitate later use of a local or distant flap to cover the bone.[1,13]

Muscle should be inspected carefully for signs of viability, which can be assessed with the so-called four C's: color, consistency, contractility, and capacity to bleed.[1] Of these four, the latter two, particularly contractility, are the more sensitive indicators of viable muscle. Clearly nonviable muscle should be debrided. Muscle that is weakly contractile and appears contused can be left and reinspected in 24 to 48 hours. Attempts should be made to maintain the integrity of musculotendinous units whenever possible without compromising the debridement. It must be remembered that the presence of an open fracture does not preclude the development of a compartment syndrome,[1,14] and fasciotomy of the compartment or compartments containing structures that may have been damaged by the injury through the open fracture wound should be performed routinely as part of the initial debridement.[1] However, fasciotomy of all four compartments should be reserved for injuries with extensive soft-tissue swelling and increased intracompartmental pressures (to within 20 to 30 mm of mercury of the diastolic blood pressure).[15,16] The more extensive use of fasciotomy may be warranted for patients who have moderate swelling of the leg (intracompartmental pressures of 25 to 35 mm of mercury), for those who have sustained systemic hypotension (diastolic blood pressure of approximately 55 mm of mercury or less), for those with severe polytrauma in whom an accurate clinical examination may be difficult postoperatively, or after revascularization for salvage of the limb.[1]

Bone that is stripped of all soft-tissue attachments is necrotic and can act as a substrate for organisms that cause infection.[1,6,17] Small-to-moderate avascular segments of bone should be removed. The decision to debride large portions of devascularized diaphyseal or metaphyseal bone, or both, is often a difficult one. Major articular segments of the tibial plateau and the tibial plafond should be retained, even when there is extensive stripping, if the surgeon believes that salvage of the involved joint is possible.[1] Areas of bone that have been stripped of periosteum but that are in continuity with a vascularized portion of the tibia can be retained if there is adequate soft-tissue coverage to allow early revascularization. Debridement of free segments of devascularized diaphyseal bone has been reported to result in a decreased prevalence of infection.[17] In the first part of their series, Edwards and associates[17] reported deep infection associated with 18 of 85 tibial fractures in which visually clean necrotic bone had been retained. In the second half of the series, the prevalence of deep infection decreased to eight of 86 fractures with debridement of all necrotic bone. The retention of completely free segments of devascularized diaphyseal or metaphyseal bone should be considered only rarely. The surgeon should be aware that the risk of postoperative infection is higher when necrotic bone remains in the wound.[6,13,17]

After thorough surgical debridement of the wound, mechanical debridement is performed with pulsed lavage irrigation.[18,19] Pulsed lavage with use of several different types of irrigation solution resulted in decreased bacterial counts compared with those associated with standard irrigation with use of a bulb syringe.[20] Recently, investigators found that antiseptic solutions of hydrogen peroxide, Betadine (povidone-iodine) solution, and Betadine scrub are toxic to osteoblasts in culture at concentrations used clinically, while bacitracin in normal saline solution had no similar toxic effects.[21]

Stabilization of Open Fractures

After the initial irrigation and debridement, the next step is stabilization of the osseous injury. Controlling instability of the bone provides several benefits: continued damage to the surrounding soft tissue by displaced bone fragments is decreased, care of the soft-tissue injuries is facilitated, and the patient's comfort is increased. Options for stabilization include immobilization in a cast, external fixation, internal fixation with plates and screws, and intramedullary nailing. Immobilization of open fractures in a cast is associated with an increased prevalence of nonunion and delayed union (ten of 205 to 45 of 112 fractures in reported series) as well as late osseous deformity (17 of 33 fractures in reported series).[22-25] Sarmiento and associates[26] reported that the average time to union in a series of 34 grade-III open tibial fractures was 26 weeks. Prolonged immobilization in a cast or orthosis may increase stiffness, muscle atrophy, and dysfunction of the limb.[27] Type-I and some type-II open fractures with minimum soft-tissue injuries and slight-to-moderate displacement of the bone can be treated with immobilization in a cast. However, such treatment precludes access for wound care for fractures with more extensive soft-tissue injury.[1] Hooper and associates[24] performed a prospective randomized trial comparing the results of immobilization in a cast with those of intramedullary nailing of closed and type-I open fractures of the tibial shaft and demonstrated a significantly ($p < 0.05$) higher prevalence of varus or valgus malalignment and shortening with the former treatment. Seventeen of the 33 fractures that were treated in a cast had a malunion, as defined by more than 5° of varus or valgus angulation, at least 10° of anteroposterior angulation, and at least 1 cm of shortening. One of the 29 fractures treated with intramedullary nailing had a malunion.[24]

External fixation offers several advantages in the treatment of open tibial fractures.[17,28-30] Most modern external fixation frames provide acceptable stability for such fractures.[31] Generally, there is good access to the soft tissues, and most forms of external fixation do not substantially impair the range of motion of the knee or ankle. External fixation is typically applied as a static form of immobilization to maintain skeletal alignment. Newer forms of external fixation allow compression of the fracture site with weightbearing.[32,33]

External fixation has also been associated with some difficulties. Irritation of the pin track with inflammation of the skin at the interface between the bone and the pin is a common problem[34] that can present in a variety of ways, ranging from mild erythema about the pin to a frank pin-track infection. Pin-track infections are associated with thermal necrosis of bone at the time of insertion of the pin. Green and Ripley[35] reported 14 cases of osteomyelitis that occurred in the tracks of pins that had been placed entirely in cortical bone. Infection can be avoided by predrilling pin tracks and by not placing the pin entirely through cortical bone.[35,36] External fixator pins have a limited life span and typically loosen between 3 to 6 months after application of the fixator, necessitating either revision of the fixator or conversion to another form of treatment. Iliac-crest bone-grafting early (within the first 6 weeks) after the injury frequently is recommended to accelerate union of the fracture before the fixator becomes loose.[37] Delayed conversion from an external fixator to an intramedullary nail has been associated with an increased prevalence of infection.[38] Wiss and Stetson[38] reported on a series in which 33 nonunions of open fractures of the tibia were treated with intramedullary nailing. An infection developed at the sites of five of the fractures, all of which had been treated initially with external fixation, with the removal of the fixator at least 11 weeks before the intramedullary nailing. McGraw and Lim[3] found an infection around seven of 16 open fractures of the tibial shaft that had been treated with external fixation followed by intramedullary nailing. In a study of two groups of comparable open fractures of the tibial shaft treated with external fixation followed by delayed intramedullary nailing, Maurer and associates[39] observed that the rate of infection was much higher (five of seven compared with one of 17) when a pin-track infection had developed before the intramedullary nailing. In fact, those authors found that a pin-track infection during the course of external fixation was the most sensitive predictor of infection after intramedullary nailing. Fractures that have been treated with external fixation for more than 21 days and are being considered for treatment with delayed intramedullary nailing should be assessed carefully for any history of drainage around or infection of the pin track to evaluate the risk of deep infection. However, good results have been reported with intramedullary nailing following short-term (ten- to 18-day) use of external fixation to facilitate initial soft-tissue treatment.[40]

Edwards and associates[17] reported on 171 type-III open fractures that had been treated with external fixation. They reported complications related to the pin track following treatment of 50 fractures and only four cases of pin-induced local osteomyelitis. The prevalence of drainage associated with anteromedial half-pins in the tibial diaphysis was noted to be approximately one third that associated with comparably placed transfixion pins.[17] Marsh and associates[32] reported 39 pin-track complications after the treatment of 101 open tibial fractures with the dynamic axial fixator. Ten of the complications necessitated removal or reinsertion of the screw or some other change in the treatment of the fracture. The overall prevalence of deep infection at the site of the fracture was 6%.[32]

Fixation with a plate typically is reserved for the treatment of open periarticular fractures of the tibial plateau and selected fractures of the tibial plafond.[1,6,13] Rhinelander[41] demonstrated that the normal pattern of bone circulation (from the medullary artery to the periosteum) is reversed following a fracture. A transient increase in periosteal blood flow supplies most of the circulation in the first weeks after a fracture.[41,42] The application of a plate requires extensive dissection, which devitalizes soft tissue and bone and may lead to more frequent complications.[43,44] Rüedi and associates[45] reported a prevalence of infection of 12% after fixation of open fractures of the tibial shaft with a plate. In a prospective, randomized study, Bach and Hansen[43] compared the use of external fixation with that of open reduction and internal fixation with plates and screws for type-II and type-III open fractures of the tibial shaft. They found a prevalence of infection of 35% and a prevalence of osteomyelitis of 19% after fixation with plates and screws, compared with prevalences of 13% and 3% after external fixation. The prevalence of malunion was slightly lower (4%) after fixation with a plate than after external fixation (10%).

Stabilization with an intramedullary nail has become increasingly popular for the treatment of fractures of the tibial shaft.[46-54] One study demonstrated a decreased prevalence of deep infection with use of Ender nails (two of 29) compared with the prevalence with use of external nails (four of 28), and there were no pin-track infections associated with the Ender nails.[49] Similar findings were noted in a comparison of external fixation with Lottes nails.[55,56] However, the use of Ender or Lottes nails for axially unstable fractures often results in malunion and creates the need for prolonged immobilization in a cast.[49-51,53,57] The development of the interlocking technique has greatly enhanced the use of tibial nailing in the treatment of more extensively comminuted fractures (Fig. 1).

Nailing without reaming has been advocated for open tibial fractures to minimize the injury to the endosteal circulation caused by reaming.[1,6,13] Several authors have reported on the use of locking nails without reaming for the treatment of open fractures of the tibial shaft (Table 1).[58-64] Overall, the prevalence of both deep infection and nonunion in association with type-I, -II, and -IIIA open fractures treated with intramedullary nailing without reaming has been lower than that associated with similar fractures treated with other fixation devices.

The role of interlocking tibial nailing without reaming in the treatment of type-IIIB fractures remains controversial. The early results reported with this technique have been promising.[58-64] Because such extensive soft-tissue injuries to the leg are relatively uncommon, multicenter studies may be needed to address this issue fully.

Chapman and associates[60] and Tornetta and associates[65] performed prospective randomized studies comparing the use of external fixation with interlocking tibial nailing without reaming. Chapman and associates[60] reported the results of 174 type-II, -IIIA, and -IIIB open fractures of the tibial shaft and found that the prevalence of deep traumatic wound infections after intramedullary nailing was 7% and the prevalence of such infections after external fixation was 11%. There was no difference in the time to union between the two groups. Tornetta and associates[65] reported on 29 type-IIIB open fractures of the tibial shaft that had been randomized alternatively to treatment with external fixation or with interlocking nailing. There was one deep infection in each group and no difference in the time to union between the two groups.

The use of reaming in the treatment of open fractures continues to be a source of controversy.[1,2,6,48] A small, prospective, randomized series in which tibial nailing of open fractures with reaming was compared with that without reaming demonstrated no detectable differences between the techniques; an infection developed at the site of two of 49 fractures treated with intramedullary nailing with reaming compared with none of 38 fractures treated without reaming. (P O'Brien, R Meek, P Blachet, personal communication, 1993). However, Bone and Johnson[66] reported an infection at the site of two of eight type-II or type-III open fractures of the tibial shaft that had been treated with intramedullary nailing with reaming, compared with two of 68 closed or type-I open fractures that had been treated with primary intramedullary nailing with reaming. Furthermore, in a laser Doppler flowmetry study of cortical circulation after intramedullary nailing with and without reaming in a sheep tibial-fracture model, revascularization occurred 6 weeks after nailing without reaming but not until 12 weeks after nailing with reaming; this finding suggests an advantage of nailing without reaming in the treatment of severe open tibial fractures.[67]

The transition from a 9-mm-diameter nail to a 10-mm-diameter nail in most current tibial nailing systems includes the use of larger-diameter cross-locking screws that increase the stability of the fixation. Thus, the debate regarding reaming versus nonreaming techniques centers on fractures with a small-diameter canal. In this case, it is not clear whether the benefits of minimum reaming to allow a 10-mm nail to be used outweigh the risks of increased vascular injury from the reaming. I believe that tibial nailing without reaming is still preferable and that reaming to accommodate nail sizes of 11 mm or larger is contraindicated for open fractures of the tibia.

I prefer interlocking intramedullary nailing without reaming for skeletal stabilization of type-I, -II, and -IIIA open fractures of the tibial shaft with a nailable fracture pattern (fractures involving the middle three fifths of the tibial shaft). For type-IIIB fractures, the results with interlocking intramedullary nailing without reaming are equivalent to, but not better than, those with external fixation.[60,65] Intramedullary nailing offers several advantages in the treatment of these severe soft-tissue injuries. No external fixation pins or circumferential plaster dressing is needed, facilitating free-tissue transfer or local rotational flap coverage. An early range of motion of the knee and ankle is also facilitated with intramedullary fixation. Intramedullary nailing offers many of the advantages of external fixation; moreover, several of the drawbacks associated with external fixation, such as loosening of the pins and loss of fixation,

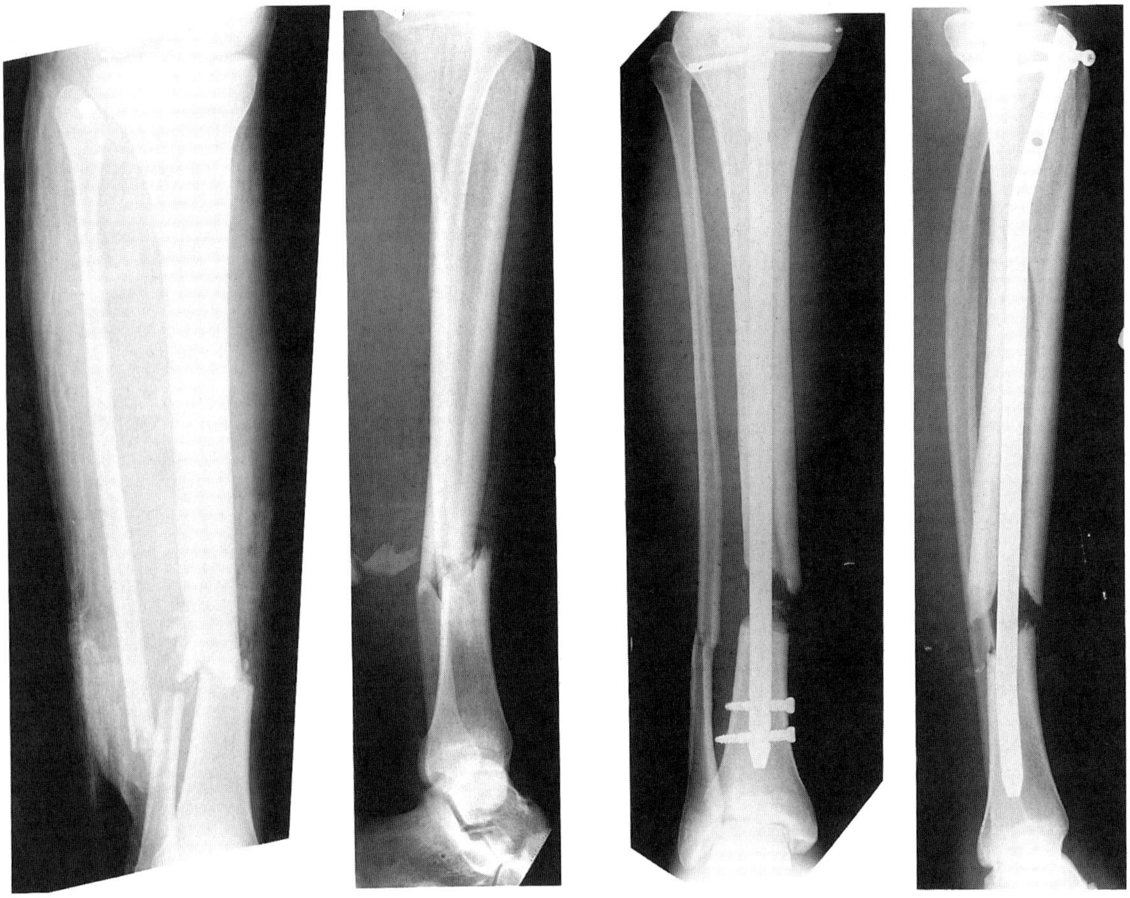

Fig. 1 A type-IIIA open fracture of the distal third of the tibial shaft. **Left,** Anteroposterior and lateral radiographs showing initial shortening of the tibia through the region of the fracture. **Right,** Anteroposterior and lateral radiographs made after debridement and stabilization with a static locking tibial nail. There is segmental loss of the distal third of the tibial shaft.

are avoided.[58-64] It should be appreciated that both external fixation and intramedullary nailing of open tibial fractures require technical expertise to obtain acceptable reduction and stable fixation.[2,17,32,6]

Treatment of the Wound

After the initial irrigation and debridement and stabilization of the bone, the surgeon must treat the traumatic wounds. Surgical extensions of the initial wound may be sutured primarily.[1] The initial traumatic wound should be left open. Early intensive repeated debridement is a fundamental principle of treatment of severe soft-tissue injuries. Patients who have a type-III injury with extensive soft-tissue damage should be returned to the operating room within 24 to 48 hours for reinspection and additional debridement of the soft tissues.[1,6,13] The goal of repeated debridement is to remove all necrotic tissue from the wound so as to remove the substrate for infection. Repeated debridement every 24 to 48 hours may be necessary to achieve this goal. When the soft-tissue bed is stable and no necrotic tissue is evident, delayed closure or coverage of the fracture can be performed. Gustilo and Anderson[9] originally recommended delayed primary closure of open-fracture wounds 5 days after the initial debridement. In general, delayed primary closure or split-thickness skin-grafting can be performed when there is a healthy soft-tissue envelope with adequate muscle coverage over the fracture. Ideally, this objective is achieved within 5 to 7 days after the initial debridement.

Polymethylmethacrylate beads impregnated with antibiotics can be used in severe soft-tissue injuries[68] to deliver locally high concentrations of antibiotics without serious systemic effects other than the possibility of an allergic reaction. An occlusive dressing must be placed over the wound to form a bead pouch, which allows the antibiotics to remain in the local environment. The bead-pouch technique is an excellent way to

Table 1
Reported rates of deep infection, malunion, delayed union, and nonunion following fixation with interlocking nailing without reaming

Study	Total No. of Fractures	Rate of Infection*					No. of Malunions†	No. of Delayed Unions†	No. of Persistent Nonunions
		Type I	Type II	Type IIIA	Type IIIB	Type IIIC			
Bonatus et al[58]	72	0/27	1/22	1/11	1/12	0/0	7	13	0
Helfet et al[59]	37	0/8	0/14	2/11	0/2	0/2	0	2	2
Henley et al[60]	104	0/0	2/52	4/40	1/12	0/0	8	13	9
Sanders et al[61]	64	0/10	0/16	1/17	5/21	0/0	0	17	1
Singer and Kellam[62]	43	0/6	1/11	1/16	2/9	0/1	20	NR	1
Stegemann et al[63]	41	0/15	1/12	1/14	0/0	0/0	NR	2	0
Whittle et al[64]	50	0/3	0/13	1/22	3/12	0/0	0	25	2

*Number of fractures associated with a deep infection/total number of fractures of that type[9,10]
†NR = not reported

deal with dead space and to prevent desiccation of exposed bone in open wounds before soft-tissue coverage.[1] Ostermann and associates[68] reported a significant decrease ($p < 0.05$) in the rate of infection with the combined use of systemic antibiotics administered intravenously and antibiotic beads for type-IIIB open fractures (an infection developed in ten of 144 fractures treated with antibiotic beads and systemic antibiotics, compared with 11 of 27 fractures treated with systemic antibiotics alone) and type-IIIC open fractures (an infection developed in two of 40 fractures treated with antibiotic beads and systemic antibiotics, compared with eight of 32 fractures treated with systemic antibiotics alone).

Exposed tendon and bone without peritenon or periosteal coverage necessitates flap coverage.[1,6,13] Ideally, if rotational or free-flap coverage of the fracture is needed, it should be done within the first 7 days after the injury.[69,70] Delay beyond this time has been associated with an increased prevalence of late infection.[69] Flap coverage can be performed with a local rotational muscle flap, a free vascularized muscle flap, or a local fasciocutaneous flap. Muscle flaps have been shown to aid revascularization of underlying exposed bone,[1,6] and they are superior to fasciocutaneous flaps in the treatment of dead space caused by a loss of bone or soft tissue.[1,6,13] In general, tissue defects in the proximal third of the tibia are covered with a gastrocnemius rotational flap. A soleus rotational flap is recommended for defects in the middle third of the tibial shaft, and a free vascularized muscle flap typically is needed for those in the distal third of the tibia.[1] However, the success of a local muscle rotational flap may be compromised if the muscle to be mobilized—that is, the gastrocnemius or the soleus—was involved in the zone of injury,[1,6,13] and severe muscle contusion precludes the local rotation of the muscle for flap coverage. In these cases, free vascularized flaps may be necessary.

With fasciocutaneous flap coverage, a segment of the skin, the underlying subcutaneous tissue, and fascia are mobilized to cover the exposed bone or tendon, or both.[71] Fasciocutaneous flaps are based on circulation from the posterior tibial or peroneal systems. With careful planning, a flap with as high as a 3:1 length-to-width ratio can be created safely, while a 1:1 ratio is necessary for random flaps.[71] Recently, good results have been reported following treatment of open tibial fractures with fasciocutaneous flaps.[47] Rotational or free flap coverage of the fracture is best done within the first 7 days, because delay beyond that has been associated with an increased incidence of late infection.

Bone-Grafting

Early iliac-crest bone-grafting is recommended for fractures with extensive soft-tissue stripping, especially those treated with external fixation, as well as fractures with a loss of more than 50% of the circumference of the bone or areas of segmental loss.[1,37] The bone-grafting should be performed after soft-tissue coverage has been achieved (Fig. 2). Fischer and associates[70] reported that bone-grafting of type-IIIA and -IIIB fractures before a healed soft-tissue envelope was present led to an infection in four of 15 patients, whereas delayed bone-grafting performed after a well vascularized soft-tissue envelope was present (6 to 8 weeks after the fracture) did not lead to an infection in any of the 16 patients who were managed in this fashion. Bone-grafting should be considered for type-IIIB fractures that are not associated with a loss of bone if there is no callus 3 months after the injury.[1]

Rehabilitation

Early functional rehabilitation should be a key part of the treatment of open fractures of the tibial shaft.

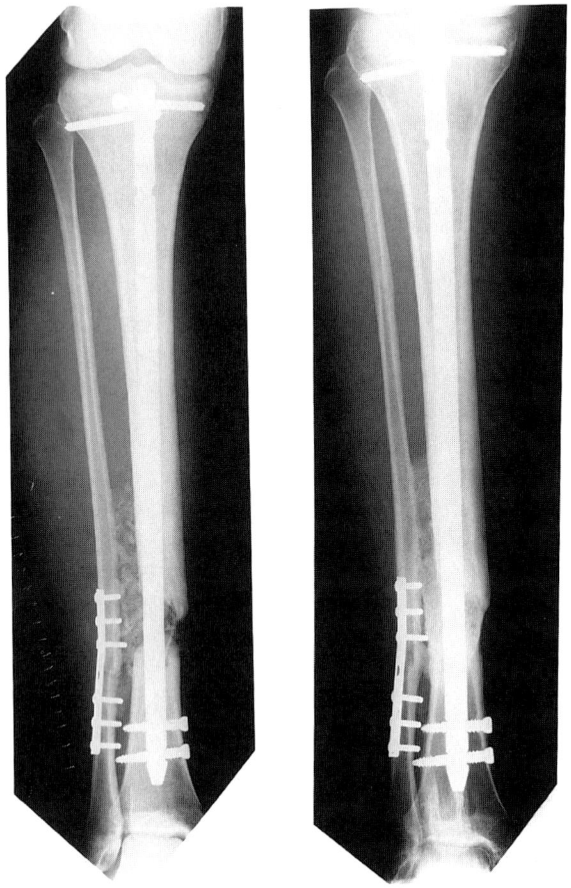

Fig. 2 Same patient as Fig. 1. **Left,** This anteroposterior radiograph was made 8 weeks after the initial injury. A posterolateral iliac-crest bone graft was inserted and internal fixation of the fibula was performed. **Right,** Anteroposterior radiograph made 10 months after the initial injury. The fracture united, with good incorporation of the bone graft.

Physical therapy programs to emphasize the range of motion of the knee and ankle are critical in the first few weeks after the injury.[1,6] The patient should be encouraged to maintain good muscle tone, even if no weightbearing or only toe-touch weightbearing is allowed. Patients who have an axially stable fracture pattern can begin bearing weight immediately,[1,72] whereas those who have an axially unstable fracture pattern should delay weightbearing until the first callus is seen. Patients who have a fracture with segmental bone loss should not be allowed to bear weight on the affected extremity until there are radiographic signs of incorporation of the bone graft (callus).[1]

Overview

In summary, open fractures of the tibial shaft represent a limb-threatening, and potentially life-threatening, emergency. Optimum treatment involves appropriate initial evaluation and administration of antibiotics; urgent operative debridement and skeletal stabilization; repeated soft-tissue debridements; and early soft-tissue closure or flap coverage, or both. This intensive treatment allows early functional rehabilitation and an improved clinical outcome for patients who have an open fracture of the tibial shaft.

References

1. Chapman MW, Olson SA: Open fractures, in Rockwood CA Jr, Green DP, Bucholz RW, et al (eds): *Fractures in Adults*, ed 4. Philadelphia, PA, Lippincott-Raven, 1996, vol 1, pp 305–352.
2. Brumback RJ: Open tibial fractures: Current orthopaedic management, in Eilert RE (ed): *Instructional Course Lectures XLI*. Park Ridge, IL, American Academy of Orthopaedic Surgeons, 1992, pp 101–117.
3. McGraw JM, Lim EV: Treatment of open tibial-shaft fractures: External fixation and secondary intramedullary nailing. *J Bone Joint Surg* 1988;70A:900–911.
4. American College of Surgeons, Committee on Trauma: *Advanced Trauma Life Support*, ed 5. Chicago, IL, American College of Surgeons, 1993.
5. Hansen ST Jr: Overview of the severely traumatized lower limb: Reconstruction versus amputation. *Clin Orthop* 1989;243:17–19.
6. Behrens F: Fractures with soft tissue injuries, in Browner BD, Jupiter JB, Levine AM, et al (eds): *Skeletal Trauma: Fractures, Dislocations, Ligamentous Injuries*. Philadelphia, PA, WB Saunders, 1992, vol 1, pp 311–336.
7. Patzakis MJ, Harvey JP Jr, Ivler D: The role of antibiotics in the management of open fractures. *J Bone Joint Surg* 1974;56A: 532–541.
8. Patzakis MJ, Dorr LD, Hammond W, et al: The effect of antibiotics, primary and secondary closure on clostridial contaminated open fracture wounds in rats. *J Trauma* 1978;18:34–37.
9. Gustilo RB, Anderson JT: Prevention of infection in the treatment of one thousand and twenty-five open fractures of long bones: Retrospective and prospective analyses. *J Bone Joint Surg* 1976;58A:453–458.
10. Gustilo RB, Mendoza RM, Williams DN: Problems in the management of type III (severe) open fractures: A new classification of type III open fractures. *J Trauma* 1984;24:742–746.
11. Brumback RJ, Jones AL: Interobserver agreement in the classification of open fractures of the tibia: The results of a survey of two hundred and forty-five orthopaedic surgeons. *J Bone Joint Surg* 1994;76A:1162–1166.
12. Südkamp NP, Haas NP, Sinnig M, et al: Incidence of pseudarthroses in open fractures: Analysis of 948 open fractures. *Aktuelle Traumatol* 1993;23:59–67.
13. Sanders R, Swiontkowski M, Nunley J, et al: The management of fractures with soft-tissue disruptions. *J Bone Joint Surg* 1993;75A: 778–789.
14. Heckman MM, Whitesides TE Jr, Grewe SR, et al: Compartment pressure in association with closed tibial fractures: The relationship between tissue pressure, compartment, and the distance from the site of the fracture. *J Bone Joint Surg* 1994;76A: 1285–1292.
15. Heckman MM, Whitesides TE Jr, Grewe SR, et al: Histologic determination of the ischemic threshold of muscle in the canine compartment syndrome model. *J Orthop Trauma* 1993;7:199–210.
16. McQueen MM, Christie J, Court-Brown CM: Compartment pressure monitoring in tibial fractures. *Orthop Trans* 1995;19:142.
17. Edwards CC, Simmons SC, Browner BD, et al: Severe open tibial fractures: Results treating 202 injuries with external fixation.

Clin Orthop 1988;230:98–115.
18. Benjamin JB, Volz RG: Efficacy of a topical antibiotic irrigant in decreasing or eliminating bacterial contamination in surgical wounds. *Clin Orthop* 1984;184:114–117.
19. Gross A, Cutright DE, Bhaskar SN: Effectiveness of pulsating water jet lavage in treatment of contaminated crushed wounds. *Am J Surg* 1972;12:373–377.
20. Anglen JO, Apostoles S, Christensen G, et al: The efficacy of various irrigation solutions in removing slime-producing Staphylococcus. *J Orthop Trauma* 1994;8:390–396.
21. Kaysinger KK, Nicholson NC, Ramp WK, et al: Toxic effects of wound irrigation solutions on cultured tibiae and osteoblasts. *J Orthop Trauma* 1995;9:303–311.
22. Anderson LD, Hutchins WC, Wright PE, et al: Fractures of the tibia and fibula treated by casts and transfixing pins. *Clin Orthop* 1974;105:179–191.
23. Brown PW, Urban JG: Early weight-bearing treatment of open fractures of the tibia: An end-result study of sixty-three cases. *J Bone Joint Surg* 1969;51A:59–75.
24. Hooper GJ, Keddell RG, Penny ID: Conservative management or closed nailing for tibial shaft fractures: A randomised prospective trial. *J Bone Joint Surg* 1991;73B:83–85.
25. Nicoll EA: Fractures of the tibial shaft: A survey of 705 cases. *J Bone Joint Surg* 1964;46B:373–387.
26. Sarmiento A, Gersten LM, Sobol PA, et al: Tibial shaft fractures treated with functional braces: Experience with 780 fractures. *J Bone Joint Surg* 1989;71B:602–609.
27. Müller, ME, Allgöwer M, Schneider R, et al (eds): *Manual of Internal Fixation: Techniques Recommended by the AO-ASIF Group*, ed 3. Berlin, Germany, Springer-Verlag, 1991.
28. Caudle RJ, Stern PJ: Severe open fractures of the tibia. *J Bone Joint Surg* 1987;69A:801–807.
29. Gershuni DH, Halma G: The A-O external skeletal fixator in the treatment of severe tibia fractures. *J Trauma* 1983;23:986–990.
30. Kimmel RB: Results of treatment using the Hoffmann external fixator for fractures of the tibial diaphysis. *J Trauma* 1982; 22:960–965.
31. Behrens F, Searls K: External fixation of the tibia: Basic concepts and prospective evaluation. *J Bone Joint Surg* 1986;68B:246–254.
32. Marsh JL, Nepola JV, Wuest TK, et al: Unilateral external fixation until healing with the dynamic axial fixator for severe open tibial fractures. *J Orthop Trauma* 1991;5:341–348.
33. Melendez EM, Colon C: Treatment of open tibial fractures with the Orthofix fixator. *Clin Orthop* 1989;241:224–230.
34. Green SA: *Complications of External Skeletal Fixation: Causes, Prevention and Treatment.* Springfield, IL, Charles C Thomas, 1981.
35. Green SA, Ripley MJ: Chronic osteomyelitis in pin tracks. *J Bone Joint Surg* 1984;66A:1092–1098.
36. Matthews LS, Green CA, Goldstein SA: The thermal effects of skeletal fixation-pin insertion in bone. *J Bone Joint Surg* 1984; 66A:1077–1083.
37. Blick SS, Brumback RJ, Lakatos R, et al: Early prophylactic bone grafting of high-energy tibial fractures. *Clin Orthop* 1989; 240:21–41.
38. Wiss DA, Stetson WB: Nonunion of the tibia treated with a reamed intramedullary nail. *J Orthop Trauma* 1994;8:189–194.
39. Maurer DJ, Merkow RL, Gustilo RB: Infection after intramedullary nailing of severe open tibial fractures initially treated with external fixation. *J Bone Joint Surg* 1989;71A:835–838.
40. Blachut PA, Meek RN, O'Brien PJ: External fixation and delayed intramedullary nailing of open fractures of the tibial shaft: A sequential protocol. *J Bone Joint Surg* 1990;72A:729–735.
41. Rhinelander FW: The normal microcirculation of diaphyseal cortex and its response to fracture. *J Bone Joint Surg* 1968; 50A:784–800.
42. Rhinelander FW: Tibial blood supply in relation to fracture healing. *Clin Orthop* 1974;105:34–81.
43. Bach AW, Hansen ST Jr: Plates versus external fixation in severe open tibial shaft fractures: A randomized trial. *Clin Orthop* 1989;241:89–94.
44. Burwell HN: Plate fixation of tibial shaft fractures: A survey of 181 injuries. *J Bone Joint Surg* 1971;53B:258–271.
45. Rüedi T, Webb JK, Allgöwer M: Experience with the dynamic compression plate (DCP) in 418 recent fractures of the tibial shaft. *Injury* 1976;7:252–257.
46. Chapman MW: The role of intramedullary fixation in open fractures. *Clin Orthop* 1986;212:26–34.
47. Cole JD, Ansel LJ, Schwartzberg R: A sequential protocol for management of severe open tibial fractures. *Clin Orthop* 1995; 315:84–103.
48. Court-Brown CM, McQueen MM, Quaba AA, et al: Locked intramedullary nailing of open tibial fractures. *J Bone Joint Surg* 1991;73B:959–964.
49. Holbrook JL, Swiontkowski MF, Sanders R: Treatment of open fractures of the tibial shaft: Ender nailing versus external fixation. A randomized, prospective comparison. *J Bone Joint Surg* 1989;71A:1231–1238.
50. Lottes JO: Medullary nailing of the tibia with the triflange nail. *Clin Orthop* 1974;105:53–66.
51. Mayer L, Werbie T, Schwab JP, et al: The use of Ender nails in fractures of the tibial shaft. *J Bone Joint Surg* 1985;67A:446–455.
52. Merianos P, Cambouridis P, Smyrnis P: The treatment of 143 tibial shaft fractures by Ender's nailing and early weight-bearing. *J Bone Joint Surg* 1985;67B:576–580.
53. Velazco A, Whitesides TE Jr, Fleming LL: Open fractures of the tibia treated with the Lottes nail. *J Bone Joint Surg* 1983;65A: 879–885.
54. Wiss DA: Flexible medullary nailing of acute tibial shaft fractures. *Clin Orthop* 1986;212:122–132.
55. Spiegel J, Bray T, Chapman M, et al: The Lottes nail vs. AO external fixation in open tibia fractures. *Orthop Trans* 1988; 12:656.
56. Swanson TV, Spiegel JD, Sutherland TB, et al: A prospective, comparative study of the Lottes nail versus external fixation in 100 open tibia fractures. *Orthop Trans* 1990;14:716–717.
57. Howard MW, Zinar DM, Stryker WS: The use of the Lottes nail in the treatment of closed and open tibial shaft fractures. *Clin Orthop* 1992;279:246–253.
58. Bonatus T, Olson SA, Lee S, et al: Non-reamed locking intramedullary nailing for open fractures of the tibia. *Clin Orthop*, in press.
59. Helfet DL, Howey T, Dipasquale T, et al: The treatment of open and/or unstable tibial fractures with an unreamed double-locked tibial nail. *Orthop Rev* 1994;23(suppl):9–17.
60. Chapman JR, Henley MB, Agel J, et al: Comparison of unreamed tibial nails and external fixateurs in the treatment of grade II and III open tibial shaft fractures. *Orthop Trans* 1995; 19:143–144.
61. Sanders R, Jersinovich I, Anglen J, et al: The treatment of open tibial shaft fractures using an interlocked intramedullary nail without reaming. *J Orthop Trauma* 1994;8:504–510.
62. Singer RW, Kellam JF: Open tibial diaphyseal fractures: Results of unreamed locked intramedullary nailing. *Clin Orthop* 1995;315:114–118.
63. Stegemann P, Lorio M, Soriano R, et al: Management protocol for unreamed interlocking tibial nails for open tibial fractures. *J Orthop Trauma* 1995;9:117–120.
64. Whittle AP, Russell TA, Taylor JC, et al: Treatment of open fractures of the tibial shaft with the use of interlocking nailing without reaming. *J Bone Joint Surg* 1992;74A:1162–1171.
65. Tornetta P III, Bergman M, Watnik N, et al: Treatment of grade-IIIB open tibial fractures: A prospective randomised comparison of external fixation and non-reamed locked nailing. *J Bone*

Joint Surg 1994;76B:13–19.
66. Bone LB, Johnson KD: Treatment of tibial fractures by reaming and intramedullary nailing. *J Bone Joint Surg* 1986;68A:877–887.
67. Schemitsch EH, Kowalski MJ, Swiontkowski MF, et al: Cortical bone blood flow in reamed and unreamed locked intramedullary nailing: A fractured tibia model in sheep. *J Orthop Trauma* 1994;8:373–382.
68. Ostermann PA, Seligson D, Henry SL: Local antibiotic therapy for severe open fractures: A review of 1085 consecutive cases. *J Bone Joint Surg* 1995;77B:93–97.
69. Cierny G III, Byrd HS, Jones RE: Primary versus delayed soft tissue coverage for severe open tibial fractures: A comparison of results. *Clin Orthop* 1983;178:54–63.
70. Fischer MD, Gustilo RB, Varecka TF: The timing of flap coverage, bone-grafting, and intramedullary nailing in patients who have a fracture of the tibial shaft with extensive soft-tissue injury. *J Bone Joint Surg* 1991;73A:1316–1322.
71. Louton RB, Harley RA, Hagerty RC: A fasciocutaneous transposition flap for coverage of defects of the lower extremity. *J Bone Joint Surg* 1989;71A:988–994.
72. Winquist RA, Hansen ST Jr, Clawson DK: Closed intramedullary nailing of femoral fractures: A report of five hundred and twenty cases. *J Bone Joint Surg* 1984;66A:529–539.

CHAPTER 30

Compartment Syndrome Associated with Tibial Fracture

Paul Tornetta III, MD
David Templeman, MD

Compartment syndrome is a well-recognized complication of a fracture of the tibial shaft.[1-5] Despite attempts to document the pathophysiology of compartment syndrome, the clinical recognition of this disorder is frequently difficult. If left untreated, compartment syndrome not only results in the loss of nerve and muscle function but also can lead to infection, myoglobinuria and renal failure, and even amputation.

A closed tibial fracture is one of the conditions most frequently associated with the development of compartment syndrome. Compartment syndrome occurs after both closed and open tibial fractures; the prevalence has ranged from five of 411 fractures to 18 of 198 fractures.[1] The range probably reflects the varying percentage of high-velocity injuries seen at different medical centers.[5]

The Clinical Problem

Despite an increased sensitivity of clinicians to the diagnosis of compartment syndrome, few criteria are available to serve as guidelines for making the diagnosis. The subjective criteria include pain, sensory changes, motor function, and turgor, but the sole objective criterion is the measurement of intracompartmental pressures. However, even the definition of abnormal tissue pressure is difficult, as anatomic compartments are not homogeneous and an equilibrium of pressure cannot be expected.[6] Heckman and associates[7] measured intracompartmental pressures at multiple sites in patients who had a tibial fracture. They documented localized areas of increased tissue pressure within single compartments. These differences were significant ($p < 0.0005$) at distances of as little as 5 cm from the site of the fracture. In 24 of the 25 patients, the highest pressures were found in the anterior and posterior compartments. Those authors recommended the measurement of pressure at multiple sites, especially at the level of the fracture, and the careful assessment of all compartments.[7]

For the clinician, the fundamental problem is the inability to identify the pressure at which nerve and muscle become ischemic. There is no reliable objective method to determine when a fasciotomy is required. Despite the development of various techniques for the measurement of intracompartmental pressure, it is not appropriate to rely on this measurement only; the diagnosis of a compartment syndrome is made from a constellation of clinical findings. The clinician should consider several key points when evaluating a patient for the development of compartment syndrome: (1) intracompartmental pressures are not a measure of muscle and nerve ischemia; (2) the development of muscle ischemia depends on the magnitude and duration of the elevated pressure; and (3) the tolerance of muscle to ischemia may vary among patients because of associated conditions such as shock, compensatory hypertension, or altered tone of the resistance vessels.

Many researchers have tried to identify a critical value for intracompartmental pressure that will lead to the development of tissue necrosis if no treatment is given. Probably because of the variable factors just mentioned, different critical values have been identified by various authors.[1,4,8-12] There have been two approaches to the problem of a critical value. Some investigators have tried to identify an absolute tissue pressure above which the risk of tissue necrosis is great enough that a fasciotomy should be performed. This value has been determined to be 30[1,8,11] or 45[10] mm of mercury. Others have suggested that the critical value must reflect a decrease in tissue perfusion, which occurs when the intracompartmental pressure approaches the perfusion pressure, as reflected by some measurement of the systemic blood pressure.[9,13,14] This critical difference between blood pressure and compartmental pressure, differential pressure (DP), has been suggested to be 30[4,9,12] to 40[9] mm of mercury.

Diagnosis

The mechanism of injury is the first indication that a patient may be at risk for a compartment syndrome. Chapman[2] estimated the amount of energy associated with various mechanisms of tibial fracture: a fall was associated with 100 foot-pounds (136 N·m) of energy, whereas an injury caused by the bumper of a motor vehicle striking a pedestrian was associated with as much as 100,000 foot-pounds (135,600 N·m) of energy. According to Tscherne and Gotzen,[5] the more severe the initial soft-tissue injury, the greater the probability that soft-tissue complications, including compartment syndrome, will develop. Because the development of a compartment syndrome is unpredictable, close observation is required until the acute swelling begins to subside. A single examination of a patient who has a tibial fracture may not reveal a compartment syndrome, which may develop hours or days after the initial injury.

Severe or increasing pain, tightness in the leg, and

sensory changes are frequently the first symptoms. All complaints should be thoroughly investigated. A careful physical examination is necessary and should include testing of muscle strength in the leg and foot as well as sensory testing of the superficial and deep peroneal nerves and the tibial nerve. Because nerve tissue is very sensitive to ischemia, sensory changes frequently herald the onset of decreased tissue perfusion.

Matsen[6] created a model to explain the development of compartment syndrome. This model was based on the premise that when local blood flow is unable to meet the metabolic demands of the tissue, ischemia begins. When tissue pressure increases, the intraluminal venous pressures within the compartment increase. This increase reduces the magnitude of the arteriovenous pressure gradient, which in turn reduces the blood flow to the tissues of the compartment. Both the magnitude and the duration of increased tissue pressure adversely affect the perfusion of the compartment. For example, it takes longer for a lower tissue pressure to adversely affect perfusion than it does for a higher tissue pressure, which quickly reduces the amount of blood flowing into the compartment.

Although the measurement of intracompartmental pressure is a critical step in the evaluation of a patient who is suspected of having a compartment syndrome, the interpretation of the results raises several points of controversy. As already discussed, either an absolute value of intracompartmental pressure or the difference between the diastolic blood pressure and the intracompartmental pressure (which is used to identify a perfusion pressure) has been used by some as an indication to perform a fasciotomy.[1,4,8-12] McQueen and associates[4,15] recently reported on the use of a differential pressure of less than 30 mm of mercury as the threshold for a fasciotomy. With use of this criterion, three of 116 patients with a tibial fracture had a fasciotomy and none of the 116 patients were observed to have sequelae.[4] Several patients had an absolute intracompartmental pressure of greater than 40 mm of mercury but were simply observed because the differential pressure was more than 30 mm of mercury. The authors concluded that simple observation was safe, even when the absolute compartmental pressure was high, if the diastolic pressure remained high enough to perfuse the compartment.[4,15]

Compartment Syndrome and Tibial Nailing

In 1971, Hamza and associates[3] reported on 50 patients who had nailing with reaming because of a tibial fracture; there were five neuromuscular complications that, in retrospect, seem to have been the consequences of a compartment syndrome. Two patients had clawing of the toes, two had a transient peroneal nerve palsy, and one had an equinus contracture. More recently, Koval and associates[16] retrospectively reviewed the records concerning 60 acute fractures of the tibia that had been treated with nailing and reaming with the limb in the 90°/90° position on a fracture table. The purpose of that report was to delineate clearly the complications associated with tibial nailing with reaming. The average time from the injury to the operation was 10 days. The authors found that 18 of the 60 fractures were associated with neurologic complications, which included paresthesias in the distribution of the peroneal nerve (11 lower extremities), foot drop (three lower extremities), and combined sensory and motor deficits (four lower extremities). Sixteen of the 18 neurologic manifestations were transient; the foot drop persisted in one patient and the peroneal paresthesias persisted in another. The specific cause of these neurologic problems could not be determined, and many probably were multifactorial. The authors implicated several factors: the presence of soft-tissue swelling, bleeding into the compartment as a result of reaming, and the use of calcaneal traction over a popliteal post. In such acute fractures, all of these factors can lead to increased intracompartmental pressures and possible neurologic damage. Alternatively, this nerve damage may have resulted from traction or a compression injury to the nerve during the procedure.

Several other investigators have specifically addressed the possible association between tibial nailing and the development of compartment syndrome. Tischenko and Goodman[17] reported on three patients in whom a compartment syndrome developed immediately after tibial nailing with reaming. They prospectively studied an additional seven patients who had continuous monitoring of the pressure in the deep posterior compartment during nailing with reaming. Two peak pressures were seen: one during reduction of the fracture and the other during reaming. On the basis of these findings, they recommended that intracompartmental pressure should be monitored in patients for whom prolonged traction is needed intraoperatively. Compartment syndrome developed after nailing with reaming in three patients of Mawhinney and associates[18] and in two patients of Ho and Lau.[19] The common factors in these case reports were the use of reaming and the use of a posterior thigh bar for positioning of the limb for longitudinal traction.

McQueen and associates[20] conducted a prospective study of intracompartmental pressures during and after tibial nailing with reaming. The pressure in the anterior compartment was continuously monitored before, during, and for 24 to 36 hours after the operation in 66 patients (67 fractures). In general, the pressure was seen to increase during the surgical procedure and then to dissipate during the postoperative period. Peak pressures of more than 30 mm of mercury were seen during traction and during reaming. The pressure decreased to a mean of 23 mm of mercury within 24 to 36 hours after the procedure. The actual pressures were not reported, nor were the blood pressures of the patients. A compartment syndrome developed in one patient postoperatively. The authors found no significant difference between the intracompartmental pressures that were measured during acute nailing procedures and those that were measured during delayed nailing procedures. There also were no significant differences among the intracompartmental pressures that were associated with the various types of fractures (as classified according to the system of Tscherne and Gotzen[5]). McQueen and associates[15] later reported that a compartment syndrome had developed in 22 (6.4%) of 342 patients who were 35 years old or less. Most of the patients in the second report had isolated injuries and may not have been considered for intramedullary nailing. Thus, it is clear that patient selection may play a role in the percentage of patients who develop a compartment syndrome after reamed nailing.

Because of the seemingly contradictory evidence in these clinical series, objective data must be evaluated. The development of compartment syndrome in two patients managed with nailing with reaming prompted Moed and Strom[21] to study the pressures in the anterior and deep posterior compartments in dogs during and after nailing with reaming. Intracompartmental pressures increased during nailing with reaming and then returned to normal after fasciotomy in two of the ten dogs in the study group, whereas the intracompartmental pressures did not increase in any of the ten dogs in the control group (dogs that had a fracture but did not have nailing). The mean pressure was significantly higher ($p < 0.05$) in the anterolateral compartment of the dogs that had had intramedullary nailing. This difference persisted for 3 hours postoperatively. No traction devices were used during the nailing procedures, which more strongly implicates reaming as the cause of the high intracompartmental pressures.

In contrast, Tornetta and French (personal communication, 1996) studied intracompartmental pressures during tibial nailing without reaming and without the use of continuous traction. They continuously monitored the pressure in the anterior compartment in 30 patients and found that the peak intracompartmental pressures occurred during manual reduction and during insertion of the nail. The pressure exceeded 40 mm of mercury in 12 of the 30 patients and was within 30 mm of mercury of the diastolic blood pressure in 15. All of the increased pressures returned to baseline levels immediately after the nail had been inserted, and there were no residual neurologic abnormalities in any of the 56 patients who had had no clinical signs of compartment syndrome when they were first seen.

After evaluation of these studies, several conclusions can be made. First, acute compartment syndrome is seen after tibial nailing with reaming. Second, efforts should be made to avoid mechanical factors that may potentiate compartment syndrome. The most important factors that increase the intracompartmental pressure seem to be longitudinal traction, reaming, and the position of the lower limb. Shakespeare and Henderson[22] showed that, in patients who had an acute tibial fracture, the pressure in the deep posterior compartment increased 5.7% per kilogram of weight applied for calcaneal traction. Wozasek and associates[23] in an experimental study in sheep, reported that the intramedullary pressure increased as much as tenfold during reaming. This increased pressure may cause extrusion of blood and marrow products through the fracture into the compartments. The position of the limb also must be considered. The standard 90°/90° position requires countertraction with the use of a posterior thigh bar. The use of this bar can decrease arterial flow and venous return and contribute to ischemia of the leg. Matsen and associates[24] showed that, in three normal human subjects, elevation of the limb to the 90°/90° position decreased the tolerance to external pressure by 35 mm of mercury. Lastly, hemorrhagic shock decreases the mean arterial pressure and can be an important factor in the development of a compartment syndrome, particularly in a multiply injured patient. For these same reasons, a tourniquet should not be used for a patient who has a tibial fracture and is at risk for a compartment syndrome.[25]

These considerations should be understood by any surgeon who is planning a tibial nailing. When a compartment syndrome is clinically suspected, monitoring of the pressure in the anterior compartment near the site of the fracture may be helpful during and even after the nailing procedure. The indication for fasciotomy should be a pressure that is persistently 30 mm of mercury of the diastolic blood pressure, as recommended by McQueen and Court-Brown.[4] Use of this guideline will allow the surgeon to avoid many unnecessary fasciotomies that would be done on the basis of a raw measurement of pressure alone. Transient elevations should not be considered evidence of compartment syndrome, as they are common and are not associated with sequelae.[15,20,22]

Surgical Technique for Fasciotomy

To perform an adequate fasciotomy, we use extensive incisions that approximate the proximal-to-distal length of the compartment to be decompressed. A long fasciotomy is required for reliable decompression of an acute compartment syndrome.[26] We do not recommend the use of a short incision that does not span the length of the compartment. Adequate decompression of the four fascial compartments of the leg can be achieved with either one or two incisions.

Regardless of the approach used, all four compartments of the leg must be thoroughly decompressed. We recommend that all of the compartments be decompressed at the time of the initial fasciotomy because, after one compartment has been released, hyperemia may precipitate increased pressures in adjacent compartments. If the anterior tibial artery was injured at the time of the tibial fracture, the anterior skin bridge created by the two-incision technique survives only as a fasciocutaneous flap. Because the acceptable length-to-width ratio for this type of flap may be exceeded, the skin bridge, particularly if injured, may be placed at risk when the two-incision technique is used.

Matsen and associates[10] modified the single lateral incision advocated by Kelly and Whitesides,[27] who performed decompression by fibulectomy. (We do not believe that the fibula should be removed during the treatment of a tibial fracture.) With this modified method,[10] the incision is made from the fibular neck to the lateral malleolus. The skin is then retracted to expose and decompress the anterior, peroneal, and superficial posterior compartments. The deep posterior compartment is exposed by retraction of the peroneal compartment anteriorly and releasing the soleus from the fibula, which exposes the fascia of the deep posterior compartment.

In most instances, the two-incision technique affords better exposure of the four compartments, and release of the soleus from the fibula is not required. A lateral incision is made over the intermuscular septum between the anterior and lateral compartments to release these two compartments. The medial incision is made 2 cm from the medial crest of the tibial shaft. The superficial posterior compartment is exposed by retracting the skin. After the superficial posterior compartment has been released, the deep posterior compartment is exposed by retracting the superficial compartment posteriorly. The interval between the superficial and deep compartments is best identified in the distal third of the leg where the gastrocnemius-soleus unit becomes tendinous. The deep posterior compartment should be released throughout its entire length.

After the fasciotomy, a bulky compression dressing and a splint are applied. The foot should be placed in slight dorsiflexion to prevent an equinus contracture. The incision for the fasciotomy usually can be closed after 3 to 5 days. When two incisions have been made and it is not possible to close both, delayed primary closure of the medial wound should be performed. On the lateral side, where there is good muscle coverage over the bone, the wound may be closed by one of several methods involving the use of split-thickness skin grafts, relaxing incisions, or skin-stretching devices. Regardless of the method, excessive skin tension must be avoided with closure.

It is important to understand the course of the superficial nerves, especially the divisions of the peroneal nerve, in relation to the techniques of fasciotomy, because these nerves can be damaged when the lateral incision is made. The common peroneal nerve originates from the sciatic nerve in the thigh. It enters the leg by passing anteriorly around the fibular head under the proximal portion of the peroneus longus muscle.[28] It then divides into the superficial and deep branches between the peroneus longus and the fibular neck. The deep peroneal nerve courses distally in the anterior compartment and supplies the muscles therein. The superficial peroneal nerve passes through the lateral compartment and supplies the peroneus brevis and longus muscles before it pierces the fascia in the distal third of the leg and terminates as the medial and intermediate dorsal cutaneous nerves of the foot.

Recent attention has been given to the variations in the course of the superficial peroneal nerve and its cutaneous branches. Adkison and associates[29] studied the nerve in 85 legs from cadavera. In only 62 legs (73%) did the nerve remain in the lateral compartment from its origin to its exit through the deep fascia, 3 to 18 cm proximal to the lateral malleolus. In 22 legs (26%), the nerve or one of its branches passed through the anterior compartment. In one leg, the nerve coursed directly beneath the deep fascia and superficial to the peroneus brevis and longus muscles.

Great variation has also been found in the course of the cutaneous branches of the superficial peroneal nerve. Blair and Botte[30] recently reported that the most common pattern was a single nerve that exited the crural fascia at an average of 12 cm proximal to the ankle joint and then divided into its terminal branches approximately 4 cm proximal to the ankle joint. In the other patterns, the medial and intermediate dorsal cutaneous nerves arose independently from the superficial peroneal nerve and pierced the fascia separately; the intermediate dorsal cutaneous nerve penetrated the fascia more distally than did the medial dorsal cutaneous nerve (usually within about 6 cm proximal to the ankle joint). The intermediate dorsal cutaneous nerve may be located anterior or posterior to the lateral malleolus and may remain in close proximity to it.

The locations of the muscular branches of the peroneal nerve also have been more clearly delineated recently.[31,32] In addition to its recurrent, deep, and superficial branches, the common peroneal nerve was found to give off several muscular branches near the fibular neck. Most of these branches supplied the peroneus longus and extensor digitorum muscles. This leash of nerve fibers was located in the anterior compartment, 2 to 5 cm distal to the head of the fibula.

An important implication of these recent anatomic studies relates to the technique used for the release of the anterior and lateral compartments. This can be done either by dividing the deep fascia of one compartment and then dividing the intermuscular septum for the release of the other compartment (Fig. 1) or by the individual release of each compartment through its outer fascia (Fig. 2). Because of the variable location of the superficial peroneal nerve within and crossing the anterior compartment, the second technique is safer. However, it must be remembered that the nerve may lie immediately beneath the fascia and therefore may be vulnerable to injury when this method is used.

The terminal cutaneous branches of the superficial peroneal nerve are at risk at the distal end of the fasciotomy after they pierce the crural fascia, most commonly at the junction of the middle and distal thirds of the leg, approximately 12 cm proximal to the ankle. The intermediate dorsal cutaneous nerve is at particular risk if it crosses the fibula or lies too close to it. Likewise, care must be taken in the proximal region of the leg to avoid damage to the branches of the common peroneal nerve.

Outcome of Compartment Syndrome

When the diagnosis of a compartment syndrome is made early and a fasciotomy is performed promptly, most patients have few sequelae. Rorabeck and Macnab[33] documented that patients who had a release within 6 hours of the diagnosis had a full recovery, whereas those who had a release after 6 hours (mean time to operation, 18 hours) had sequelae. In a study of the malpractice costs associated with a missed diagnosis of compartment syndrome in eight patients,[34] the average indemnity was nearly $280,000. The sequelae included amputation and complete loss of function of the lower extremity. The costs were high because the patients were young (average age, 16 years), with an average work-life expectancy of 30 years; thus, the loss of productivity in these patients was severe. Two factors were found to contribute to the missed diagnosis. First, intracompartmental pressure had not been measured in any of the patients. This points to the need for early diagnosis of a compartment syndrome and the timely measurement of intracompartmental pressure. Second, some patients had been evaluated by more than one physician as the syndrome evolved over a period of time. This demonstrates the need for improved communication between health-care providers in the assessment and observation of patients who are at risk for the development of a compartment syndrome.

Overview

A compartment syndrome of the leg may be a devastating complication of a tibial fracture. Meticulous and repeated examinations of the patient who has such a

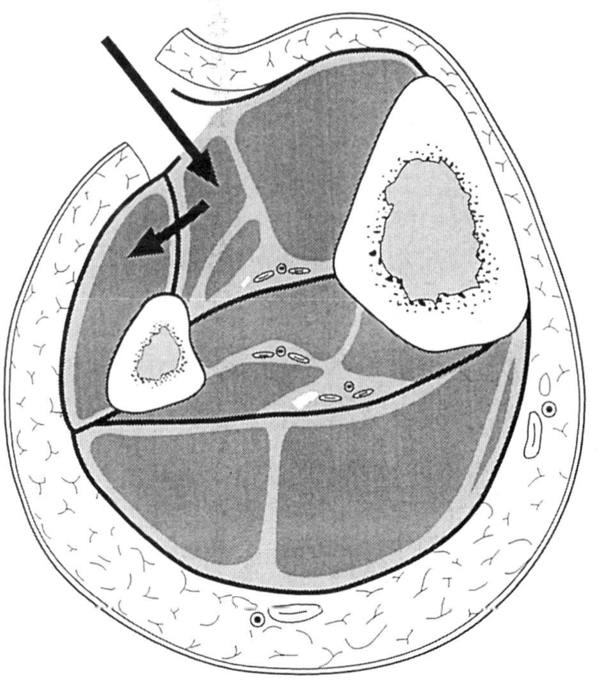

Fig. 1 Release of the compartments by dividing the deep fascia of the anterior compartment first and then dividing the intermuscular septum to release the lateral compartment.

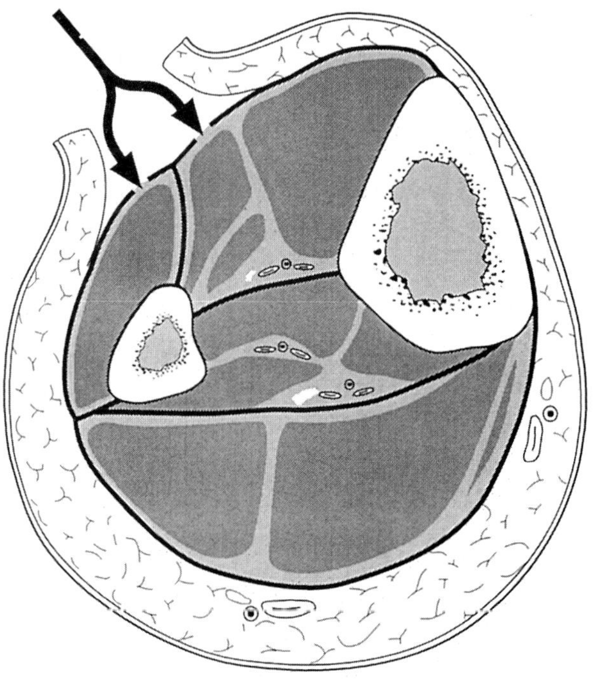

Fig. 2 The preferred technique, individual release of each compartment through its outer fascia.

fracture are needed to ensure that the diagnosis is not missed. In patients who are conscious, sensory changes usually occur before motor changes. Pain on passive stretching of the muscles in a given compartment may be the earliest clinical indicator.[33] In patients who are obtunded or anesthetized, objective criteria must be used to make the diagnosis. Intracompartmental pressure is the sole objective measurement and constitutes an indirect measurement of muscle and nerve ischemia. We believe that the most reliable measurement is the difference between the diastolic blood pressure and the intracompartmental pressure, and we consider a differential pressure of less than 30 mm of mercury to be indicative of compartment syndrome. Patients managed with tibial nailing are at particular risk, especially if reamers and prolonged traction are used.[17,21] In these situations, monitoring of the pressure in the anterior compartment is a judicious step. If the nail is inserted without continuous traction or reaming, incidental but short-lived increases in pressure will occur, but continuous monitoring is not needed. Once a compartment syndrome has been diagnosed, emergent fasciotomy is needed to avoid permanent neurologic sequelae.[33] Many techniques are available, but regardless of the method chosen, all four compartments must be released throughout their entire extent. A delay of more than 6 hours in the diagnosis or the fasciotomy usually leads to permanent weakness. The surgeon must have a high index of suspicion for compartment syndrome for all patients who have a tibial fracture.

References

1. Blick SS, Brumback RJ, Poka A, et al: Compartment syndrome in open tibial fractures. *J Bone Joint Surg* 1986;68A:1348–1353.
2. Chapman MW: Fractures of the tibial and fibular shafts, in Evarts CM (ed): *Surgery of the Musculoskeletal System.* New York, NY, Churchill Livingstone, 1983, vol 3, pp 8:5–8:62.
3. Hamza KN, Dunkerley GE, Murray CM: Fractures of the tibia: A report on fifty patients treated by intramedullary nailing. *J Bone Joint Surg* 1971;53B:696–700.
4. McQueen MM, Court-Brown CM: Compartment monitoring in tibial fractures: The pressure threshold for decompression. *J Bone Joint Surg* 1996;78B:99–104.
5. Tscherne H, Gotzen L (eds): *Fractures with Soft Tissue Injuries.* Berlin, Germany, Springer-Verlag, 1984.
6. Matsen FA III: Compartment syndromes: Part A. Pathophysiology of compartment syndromes, in Barr JS Jr (ed): *Instructional Course Lectures XXXVIII.* Park Ridge, IL, American Academy of Orthopaedic Surgeons, 1989, pp 463–466.
7. Heckman MM, Whitesides TE Jr, Grewe SR, et al: Compartment pressure in association with closed tibial fractures: The relationship between tissue pressure, compartment, and the distance from the site of the fracture. *J Bone Joint Surg* 1994;76A:1285–1292.
8. Hargens AR, Romine JS, Sipe JC, et al: Peripheral nerve-conduction block by high muscle-compartment pressure. *J Bone Joint Surg* 1979;61A:192–200.
9. Heppenstall RB, Sapega AA, Scott R, et al: The compartment syndrome: An experimental and clinical study of muscular energy metabolism using phosphorus nuclear magnetic resonance spectroscopy. *Clin Orthop* 1988;226:138–155.
10. Matsen FA III, Winquist RA, Krugmire RB Jr: Diagnosis and management of compartmental syndromes. *J Bone Joint Surg* 1980;62A:286–291.
11. Mubarak SJ, Owen CA, Hargens AR, et al: Acute compartment syndromes: Diagnosis and treatment with the aid of the wick catheter. *J Bone Joint Surg* 1978;60A:1091–1095.
12. Whitesides TE Jr, Haney TC, Morimoto K, et al: Tissue pressure measurements as a determinant for the need of fasciotomy. *Clin Orthop* 1975;113:43–51.
13. Heckman MM, Whitesides TE Jr, Grewe SR, et al: Histologic determination of the ischemic threshold of muscle in the canine compartment syndrome model. *J Orthop Trauma* 1993;7:199–210.
14. Heppenstall RB, Scott R, Sapega A, et al: A comparative study of the tolerance of skeletal muscle to ischemia: Tourniquet application compared with acute compartment syndrome. *J Bone Joint Surg* 1986;68A:820–828.
15. McQueen MM, Christie J, Court-Brown CM: Acute compartment syndrome in tibial diaphyseal fractures. *J Bone Joint Surg* 1996;78B:95–98.
16. Koval KJ, Clapper MF, Brumback RJ, et al: Complications of reamed intramedullary nailing of the tibia. *J Orthop Trauma* 1991;5:184–189.
17. Tischenko GJ, Goodman SB: Compartment syndrome after intramedullary nailing of the tibia. *J Bone Joint Surg* 1990;72A:41–44.
18. Mawhinney IN, Maginn P, McCoy GF: Tibial compartment syndromes after tibial nailing. *J Orthop Trauma* 1994;8:212–214.
19. Ho YK, Lau PY: Compartment syndrome after intramedullary interlocking nailing of a tibial fracture. *Injury* 1991;22:490–491.
20. McQueen MM, Christie J, Court-Brown CM: Compartment pressures after intramedullary nailing of the tibia. *J Bone Joint Surg* 1990;72B:395–397.
21. Moed BR, Strom DE: Compartment syndrome after closed intramedullary nailing of the tibia: a canine model and report of two cases. *J Orthop Trauma* 1991;5:71–77.
22. Shakespeare DT, Henderson NJ: Compartmental pressure changes during calcaneal traction in tibial fractures. *J Bone Joint Surg* 1982;64B:498–499.
23. Wozasek GE, Simon P, Redl H, et al: Intramedullary pressure changes and fat intravasation during intramedullary nailing: An experimental study in sheep. *J Trauma* 1994;36:202–207.
24. Matsen FA III, Mayo KA, Krugmire RB Jr, et al: A model compartmental syndrome in man with particular reference to the quantification of nerve function. *J Bone Joint Surg* 1977;59A:648–653.
25. Zweifach SS, Hargens AR, Evans KL, et al: Skeletal muscle necrosis in pressurized compartments associated with hemorrhagic hypotension. *J Trauma* 1980;20:941–947.
26. Gaspard DJ, Kohl RD Jr: Compartmental syndromes in which the skin is the limiting boundary. *Clin Orthop* 1975;113:65–68.
27. Kelly RP, Whitesides TE Jr: Abstract: Transfibular route for fasciotomy of the leg. *J Bone Joint Surg* 1967;49A:1022–1023.
28. Woodburne RT (ed): *Essentials of Human Anatomy,* ed 7. New York, NY, Oxford University Press, 1983, pp 523–604.
29. Adkison DP, Bosse MJ, Gaccione DR, et al: Anatomical variations in the course of the superficial peroneal nerve. *J Bone Joint Surg* 1991;73A:112–114.
30. Blair JM, Botte MJ: Surgical anatomy of the superficial peroneal nerve in the ankle and foot. *Clin Orthop* 1994;305:229–238.
31. Soejima O, Ogata K, Ishinishi T, et al: Anatomic considerations of the peroneal nerve for division of the fibula during high tibial osteotomy. *Orthop Rev* 1994;23:244–247.
32. Stitgen SH, Cairns ER, Ebraheim NA, et al: Anatomic considerations of pin placement in the proximal tibia and its relationship to the peroneal nerve. *Clin Orthop* 1992;278:134–137.
33. Rorabeck CH, Macnab I: The pathophysiology of the anterior tibial compartmental syndrome. *Clin Orthop* 1975;113:52–57.
34. Templeman DC, Schmidt RD, Varecka TF: Economic costs of missed compartment syndromes. Proceedings of the American Academy of Orthopaedic Surgeons 60th Annual Meeting, San Francisco, CA. Rosemont, IL, American Academy of Orthopaedic Surgeons, 1993, p 157.

Foot and Ankle

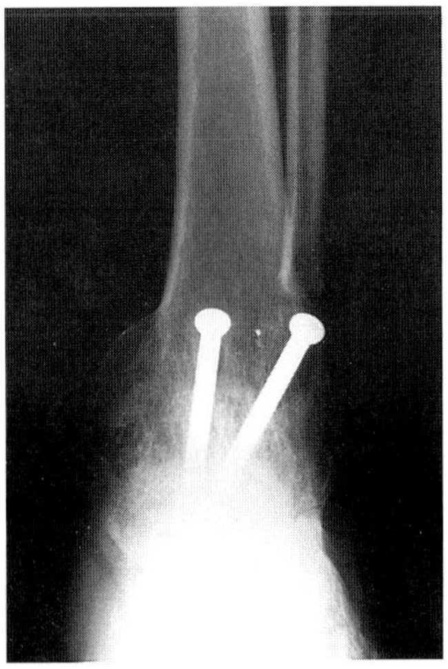

CHAPTER 31

Fractures of the Ankle and the Distal Part of the Tibia

Robert Vander Griend, MD
James D. Michelson, MD
Lawrence B. Bone, MD

Ankle Fractures

Ankle fractures are the most common types of fractures treated by orthopaedic surgeons.[1,2] There has been an increased prevalence of such fractures over the last two decades both in young, active patients and in the elderly.[1,2] There also seems to have been an increased prevalence of complex injuries of the ankle and foot as a result of the increased use of automobile safety devices, such as seat belts and air bags, which decrease mortality and protect the trunk but not necessarily the lower extremities.

As a result of a better understanding of the biomechanics of the ankle, improvements in fixation techniques, and findings of outcome studies, there has been a gradual evolution in the effective strategies for the treatment of ankle fractures. The goals of treatment continue to be both a healed fracture and an ankle that moves and functions normally without pain. The development of strategies for the treatment of various patterns of ankle injuries revolves around whether these goals can be achieved more predictably with surgical or nonsurgical means.

Surgical treatment is indicated when congruity of the joint cannot be restored with closed methods. With intra-articular fractures of the distal tibia, such as pilon fractures, there often is major incongruity of the weightbearing articular surface that must be corrected. With ankle fractures, the primary concern is residual instability of the joint, because malalignment or residual displacement can adversely affect the biomechanical behavior of the ankle and result in loss of function. Certain injury patterns have a better outcome after surgical treatment, while other patterns are better managed without surgery.

The treatment of ankle fractures involves both a risk-benefit and a cost-benefit analysis. The primary risk associated with closed treatment is inadequate restoration of the biomechanics of the ankle, which can lead to a poor outcome. Conversely, while open reduction and internal fixation is an excellent method for the restoration of the normal anatomy of the joint, it is accompanied by the costs and risks of surgery.

Anatomy and Biomechanics

An understanding of the anatomy and biomechanics of the ankle is essential before one can evaluate and treat injuries involving that joint. The ankle consists of the articulating surfaces of the talus, tibia, and fibula as well as their interconnecting ligaments and the joint capsule. The ankle often is divided into medial, lateral, and syndesmotic complexes to help the physician to understand the mechanism of injury better and to devise a treatment plan. The medial complex consists of the medial malleolus, the medial facet of the talus, and the superficial and deep components of the deltoid ligament; the lateral complex consists of the distal fibula, the lateral talus, and the lateral collateral ligaments of the ankle and subtalar joints; and the syndesmotic complex consists of the articulation between the tibia and the fibula as well as the interconnecting ligaments of the syndesmosis and the interosseous membrane.

While the ankle previously was considered to be a simple hinge joint, studies have shown clearly that the biomechanics of the ankle are quite complex.[3-6] The contributions of the articular surfaces, the ligaments, and the capsular and musculotendinous structures to the stability and function of the ankle are influenced by changes in loading characteristics and joint position and are altered in response to injury. These biomechanical studies have shown that as the ankle moves in the sagittal plane the talus both slides and rotates underneath the tibial plafond.[3,4,7] In addition, motion of the ankle in the sagittal plane induces coupled motions in both the coronal and the axial plane. Plantarflexion of the ankle results in internal rotation of the talus, while dorsiflexion results in external rotation (Fig. 1).[3,6,8] Dorsiflexion also results in posterolateral translation and external rotation, but in minimum vertical motion, of the fibula.[9-11]

It is now well recognized that the injury patterns associated with ankle fractures are more complex than simple lateral displacement of the talus in the injured mortise. It is difficult to assess displacement, which occurs in multiple planes, with use of two-dimensional radiographs. For example, what appears on plain radiographs to be direct lateral translation of the talus is actually anterolateral rotation of the talus within the mortise.[5,12-14] Failure to appreciate this fact can lead to a misunderstanding of the actual biomechanical changes that occur, can result in the design of inaccurate experimental models, and can contribute to confusion with regard to clinical treatment. Experimental models of ankle fractures that involve only direct later-

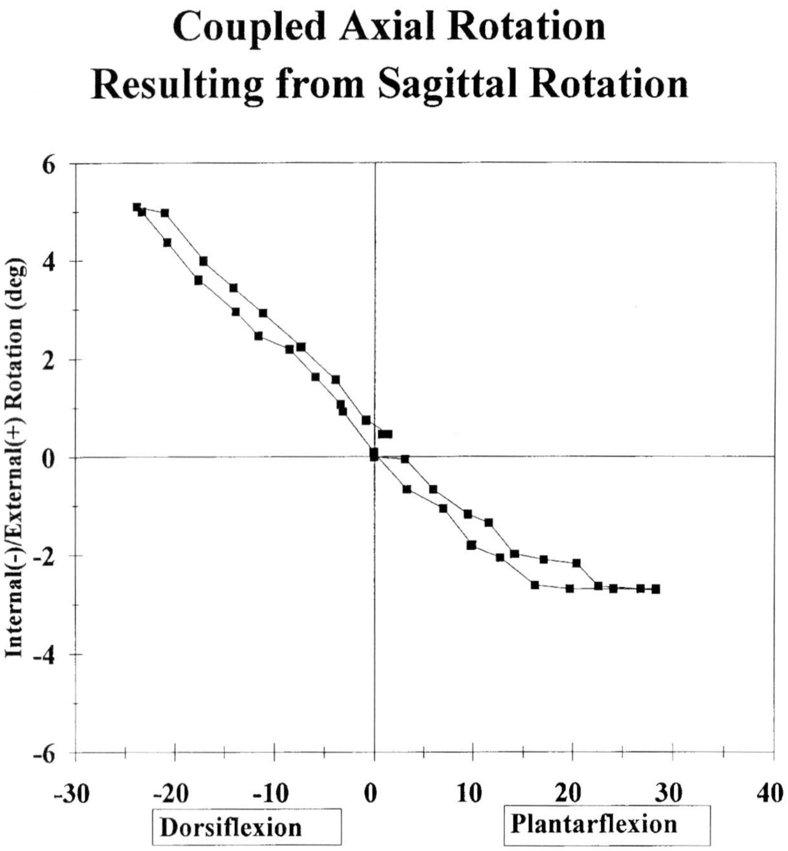

Fig. 1 Illustration of the coupled motion that occurs when the ankle is moved into dorsiflexion and plantarflexion. The talus rotates externally when the ankle is dorsiflexed and internally when the ankle is plantarflexed.

al translation of the talus do not accurately represent the consequences of the injury.

Historically, the primary goal of surgical treatment of ankle fractures was to stabilize the medial side. Later, the lateral side was considered to be more important.[15] More recent studies[4,7,15] have suggested that both sides are important, with the medial side (specifically, the deep component of the deltoid ligament) holding the talus in place and keeping it from displacing laterally and from rotating externally while the lateral side acts as a buttress. The biomechanical consequences of injury must be considered for both sides of the ankle when treatment is being planned.

Radiographic Evaluation

Fractures of the ankle are evaluated primarily with the use of plain radiographs. Instability is assessed by means of an analysis of the displacements of various parts of the ankle and the association of these displacements with their perceived biomechanical consequences. The measurements that typically can be obtained are the medial clear space, the tibiofibular clear space, the tibiofibular overlap, the talar tilt, and the talocrural angle (Fig. 2).

The utility of a radiographic examination of an ankle fracture is limited, as all of the measurements are subject to interobserver variability. In addition, the measurements vary depending on whether the radiographs are made during weightbearing or nonweightbearing, and the degree of magnification is uncalibrated and varies from patient to patient. Finally, there are differences in the literature with regard to what is normal, abnormal, or acceptable, and there is a limited understanding of the biomechanical consequences of small amounts of displacement.[15-19] Reevaluation of these measurements with newer techniques, such as computed tomography (CT), also has called into question the validity of some previously accepted concepts. For example, fibular length commonly has been estimated with use of the talocrural angle. Although it has been stated that a change in the talocrural angle of as little as 2° compared with the angle on the normal side reflects fibular shortening, examinations of fractures with use of three-dimensional CT scans have not supported this contention.[17,18,20,21]

Classification

The treatment of ankle fractures is based almost entirely on the radiographic findings. Currently, there are two widely used classification systems.

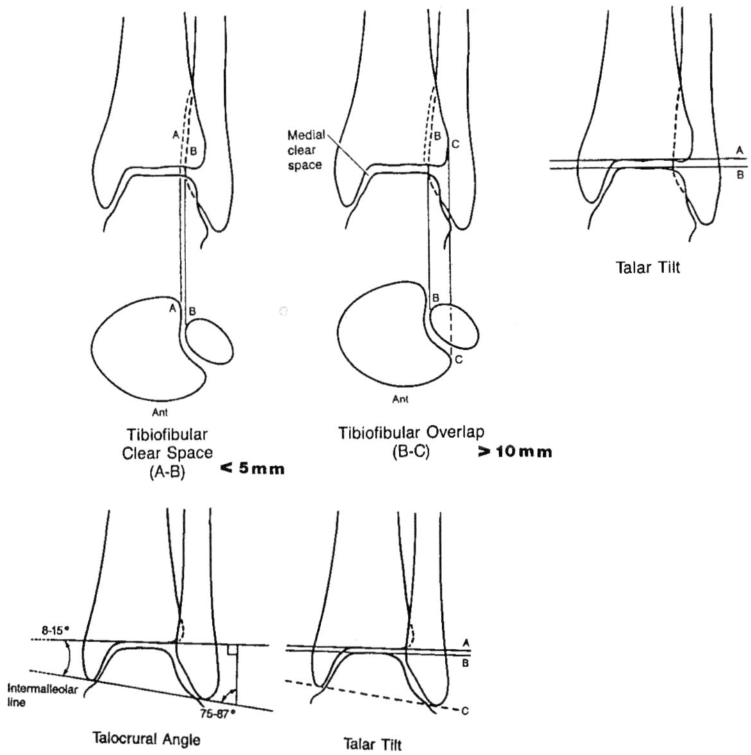

Fig. 2 Illustration of the measurements, made on plain radiographs, that are used to determine the displacement associated with an ankle fracture. The width of the syndesmosis is measured 1 cm proximal to the tibial plafond. (Adapted with permission from Vander Griend RA, Savoie FH, Hughes JL: Fractures of the ankle, in Rockwood CA Jr, Green DP, Bucholz RW (eds): *Fractures in Adults*, ed 3. Philadelphia, PA, JB Lippincott, 1991, vol 2, p 2003.)

Lauge-Hansen[22] apparently devised the first modern classification system that was based specifically on the mechanism of injury. This is a two-part system in which the first word of the classification denotes the position of the foot at the time of the injury and the second word indicates the direction of the deforming force. The initial position of the foot is important because it determines which structures are tight and therefore are most likely to be injured first. (For example, with the foot supinated, the medial structures are loose and the lateral structures are tight; the lateral structures, therefore, are injured first.) The severity of the injury then is defined as stage 1, 2, 3, or 4, depending on the particular pattern. The two most common injury patterns are the supination-external rotation and pronation-external rotation types. The supination-external rotation injury begins at the anterolateral corner of the ankle. The structures that are damaged are, in order, the anterior tibiofibular ligament (stage 1), the lateral malleolus (stage 2), the posterolateral aspect of the capsule or the posterior malleolus (stage 3), and the medial malleolus or the deltoid ligament (stage 4). The pronation-external rotation injury begins on the medial side of the ankle with an injury of the deltoid ligament or the medial malleolus (stage 1) and then progresses around the ankle to the anterolateral ligaments (stage 2), the lateral malleolus or the proximal part of the fibula (stage 3), and the posterolateral ligaments or the posterior malleolus (stage 4). Other, less common injury patterns include the supination-adduction and pronation-abduction types.

As the Lauge-Hansen classification system is based on the mechanism of injury, its primary advantage in the past was that it could be used as a guide for the closed reduction of ankle injuries. Although this system remains useful for describing the mechanism of injury, it is complicated and, regardless of the experience of those interpreting the radiographs, its clinical usefulness is limited by variable interobserver reliability.[23,24]

The Weber classification system is based on the level of the fibular fracture: type-A fractures occur distal to the level of the tibial plafond, type-B fractures start at the level of the plafond and frequently spiral proximally, and type-C fractures originate proximal to the level of the plafond and are associated with a variable amount of syndesmotic injury.[25] While this system is easy to use and provides information about the lateral fracture, it does not discriminate adequately between fractures that are quite distinct biomechanically.[26] For example, with use of this system, fibular fractures with a medial injury are indistinguishable from those without such an injury.

The AO classification system is a modification of the Weber system in which the A, B, and C fracture types are subdivided on the basis of the presence of medial or posterior injury.[27] Familiarity with both the Lauge-

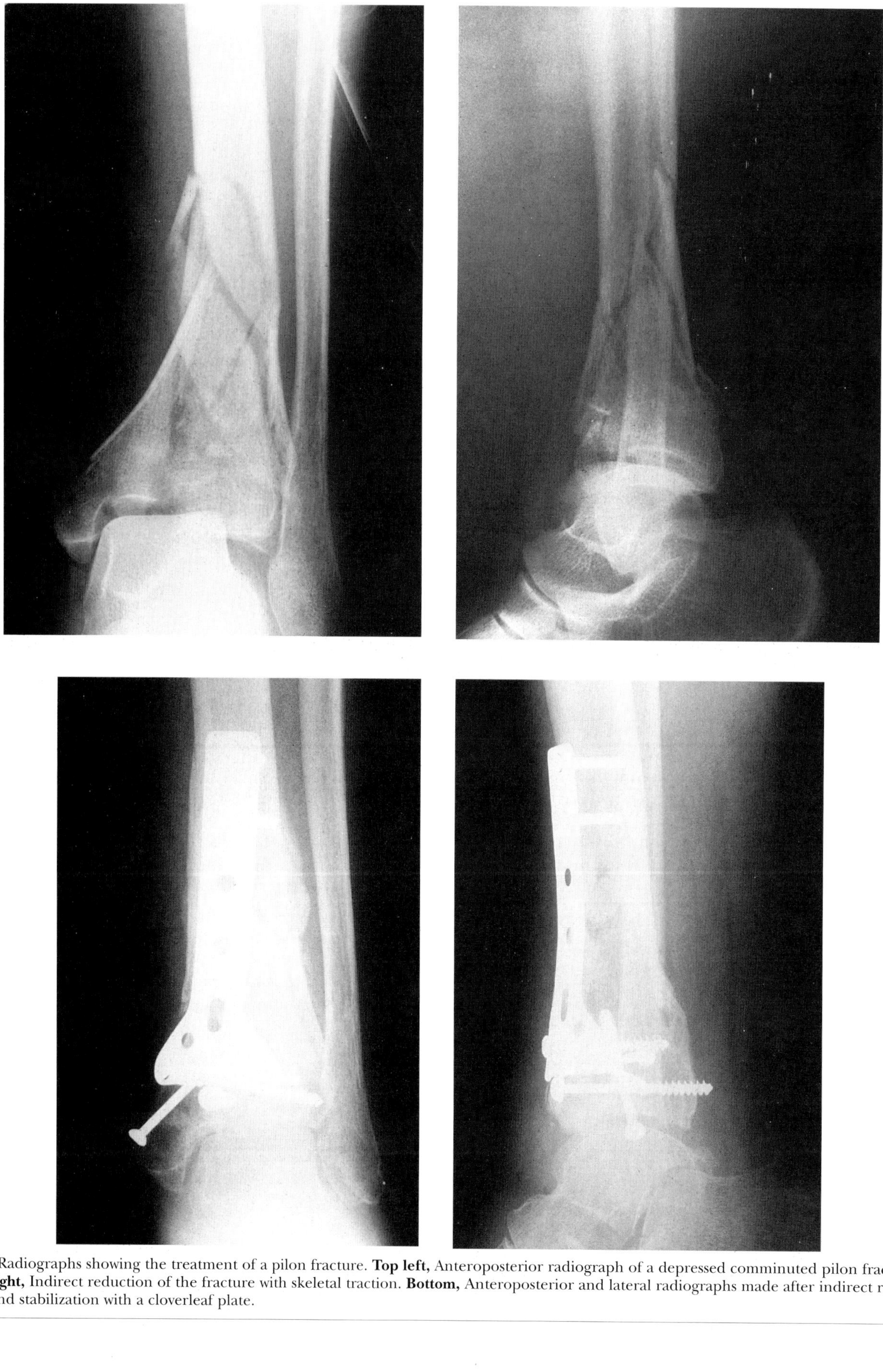

Fig. 3 Radiographs showing the treatment of a pilon fracture. **Top left,** Anteroposterior radiograph of a depressed comminuted pilon fracture. **Top right,** Indirect reduction of the fracture with skeletal traction. **Bottom,** Anteroposterior and lateral radiographs made after indirect reduction and stabilization with a cloverleaf plate.

Hansen and the AO-Weber system enables the surgeon to appreciate the mechanism of injury and yet still use the simpler, and now more comprehensive, AO system.

Current Issues in the Treatment of Ankle Fractures

Although the evolution of internal fixation techniques has settled much of the controversy regarding the treatment of ankle fractures, some aspects of treatment remain subject to debate.

As noted earlier, there have been several recent studies of the biomechanics of ankle motion. Of particular importance is the recognition that instability of the ankle results from external rotation of the talus.[5,12-14] The medial structures provide the primary restraint to this pattern of instability, while the lateral structures contribute relatively little to stability.[5,28] As this concept has become more widely recognized, surgical indications based strictly on the characteristics of the lateral injury pattern have been called into question. In pre-vious reports, the amount of acceptable fibular displacement has ranged from zero to as much as 5 mm.[1,17,21,29,30] This wide range supports the notion that apparent fibular displacement does not provide a satisfactory indication of ankle instability and does not define treatment requirements.

Isolated Lateral Malleolar Fractures

Isolated fractures of the lateral malleolus are the most common fractures of the ankle. By definition, this type of fracture is associated with no appreciable medial injury of either the deltoid ligament or the medial malleolus.

In recent years, there has been a trend toward treating this type of fracture with anatomical open reduction and internal fixation. This approach has been based, in part, on the finding that displacement of the talus follows displacement of the lateral malleolus[14] and on the experimental work of Ramsey and Hamilton,[31] who found that 1 mm of lateral talar shift reduces the ankle contact area by 42%. However, in that study,[31] the lateral talar shift was achieved by placing shims between the talus and the medial malleolus and loading the ankle in the neutral position only. That study reflected the then-current thought that a fracture causes the talus to shift laterally rather than to rotate anterolaterally, as is actually the case. In that study, ankle motion was constrained by the testing apparatus. Subsequent studies have shown that it is important for the models used for biomechanical testing to account for the normal complex coupled motions of the ankle.[4,5,32]

A number of recent studies have re-examined the biomechanics of lateral malleolar fractures. These studies have included measurements of the contact area through a full range of motion,[28] measurements of intra-articular pressure with use of a quasidynamic methodology,[33] and direct measurements of three-dimensional motion of the ankle.[4,5] None of these laboratory investigations demonstrated any change in the loading characteristics or the motion of the ankle as a result of an isolated lateral malleolar fracture.

CT studies have indicated that the amount of displacement of the distal fibular fragment with respect to the proximal portion of the fibular shaft is overestimated on plain radiographs.[20] The classic description of a lateral malleolar fracture is that of a fracture in which the distal fibular fragment is externally rotated; however, CT scans showed that such external rotation rarely occurs.[20] The typical deformity actually is characterized by internal rotation of the proximal portion of the fibular shaft relative to the tibia and no substantial rotation of the distal part of the fibula with respect to either the tibia or the talus. This internal rotation of the proximal portion of the fibular shaft most likely is a result of the muscular and syndesmotic attachments to that part of the bone. The talofibular articulation remains unchanged because of the preservation of the ligamentous and articular constraints. On the basis of these findings, it would be expected that the results of nonsurgical treatment of isolated lateral malleolar fractures would be as good as those of surgical treatment. This was, in fact, demonstrated in two studies,[16,34] in which 75 of 82 patients had a good clinical result—despite as much as 3 mm of apparent fibular displacement—at least 20 years after the closed treatment of a stage-2 supination-external rotation fracture. Furthermore, in three other studies, the outcome after anatomic open reduction and internal fixation was not found to be substantially different from that after nonsurgical treatment.[29,35,36] The findings of these studies[16,29,34-36] suggest that as much as 3 mm of residual displacement is well tolerated after an isolated fracture of the lateral malleolus.

Deltoid Ligament Injuries

A lateral malleolar fracture that is associated with a complete injury of the deltoid ligament is biomechanically equivalent to a bimalleolar fracture.[7,33,37] The diagnosis of a complete rupture of the deltoid ligament is based on the presence of medial tenderness as well as evidence of a talar shift as determined by more than 4 mm of widening of the medial clear space as seen on the post-injury radiographs.[17,38] The clinical situation is not as clear when there is medial tenderness without any discernible talar shift. Stress radiographs may be considered and close radiographic follow-up is necessary, especially when nonsurgical treatment is selected.

A fibular fracture with associated disruption of the deltoid ligament should be treated with surgical stabilization of the fibula. Unless an interposed deltoid ligament or other soft tissue blocks reduction of the talus, a medial arthrotomy and repair of the deep component of the deltoid ligament is not necessary to achieve a good outcome.[14,17,39] Postoperatively, the ankle should be immobilized in slight dorsiflexion for about 3 weeks. This minimizes the rotational forces on the talus that accompany normal dorsiflexion and plantarflexion of the ankle. Although some authors[38,39] have described the use of an above-the-knee cast, we have not found this to be necessary.[15,19]

Posterior Malleolar Fractures

A fracture of the posterior malleolus can occur in association with either external-rotation or abduction injuries of the ankle. The mechanism of injury is usually an avulsion force acting through the posterior syndesmotic ligaments on the posterolateral part of the tibia. Less commonly, the mechanism is impaction of the externally rotating talus on the posterior lip of the tibia. The primary issues regarding the treatment of a posterior malleolar fracture have been the effect of the size of the fragment on posterior stability of the ankle and what criteria should be used to determine when internal fixation is needed. Harper,[40] in an experimental study, showed that posterior malleolar fractures involving as much as 50% of the articular margin (as seen on the lateral radiograph) were not associated with posterior talar subluxation, provided that the lateral supporting structures were intact. Harper and Hardin,[41] in a clinical study, reported similar results when posterior malleolar fractures involving approximately 25% of the articular surface were treated with and without internal fixation, provided that the lateral and, if present, the medial fractures were anatomically reduced and stabilized.

Clinically, the posterior malleolar fragment often reduces with reduction of the fibula. Most current texts recommend internal fixation of the posterior malleolus if the reduced fragment comprises more than one fourth to one third of the articular surface.[15,19] An additional indication for open (or percutaneous) reduction and fixation is persistent intra-articular displacement of the posterior malleolar fragment after reduction of the lateral and, if present, the medial malleolar fractures. A step-off or gap of more than 2 to 3 mm should be reduced and fixed, especially if there is associated posterior subluxation of the talus. Residual posterior subluxation of the talus should not be accepted as it will lead to rapid destruction of the ankle joint. Fixation can be achieved with use of screws placed either posterior-to-anterior or anterior-to-posterior, depending on the size of the posterior fragment.[15] All of the fractures (those involving the medial malleolus, the lateral malleolus, the posterior malleolus, or any combination of the three) should be either reducible or reduced and provisionally stabilized with Kirschner wires or a malleolar clamp before definitive fixation is done.

Syndesmotic Injuries

There continues to be some controversy regarding the evaluation and treatment of syndesmotic injuries. The primary issues include determination of when the injured syndesmosis is unstable, when and what type of syndesmotic fixation is needed, and how the patient should be managed postoperatively.

Injuries of the syndesmotic ligaments occur as a result of abduction or external rotation of the talus within the ankle mortise. This mechanism most com-monly occurs in association with pronation-external rotation, pronation-abduction, and occasionally supination-external rotation injuries[22] (type-C and some type-B injuries).[25]

In abduction injuries, the medial side is injured first and then the syndesmotic ligaments are torn or avulsed along with their osseous attachments. The proximal extent of the injury of the interosseous membrane and the level of the fibular fracture depend on the loading forces. In external-rotation injuries, the anterior syndesmosis is disrupted. The interosseous membrane and the posterior tibiofibular ligament may or may not remain intact as the fibula rotates externally and subsequently fractures.

Stability of the ankle results from contributions of the medial complex (the medial malleolus and the deltoid ligament), the lateral complex (the lateral malleolus and the lateral ligament complex), and the syndesmotic complex. Usually, at least two of these complexes must be injured for the ankle to become unstable. Burns and associates,[33] in an in vitro biomechanical study, showed that the loading characteristics of the ankle did not change substantially when only the syndesmotic ligaments were cut; however, when both the syndesmotic and the medial ligaments were cut, there was an increase in both talar shift and joint-contact pressure as well as a 39% decrease in joint-contact area.

In another study,[37] the relationship between medial injury and the level of syndesmotic injury was studied. When there was no medial injury (that is, when the deep component of the deltoid ligament and the medial malleolus were intact), there was minimum widening of the syndesmosis, regardless of the proximal extent of the syndesmotic injury. When a medial injury was combined with a disruption of the syndesmosis that extended more than 4.5 cm proximal to the joint, there was widening of the syndesmosis and changes in the loading characteristics of the ankle. No changes in the loading characteristics were seen when the syndesmosis was disrupted for a distance of less than 3.0 cm proximal to the joint.

In the past, fixation of the syndesmosis was recommended routinely for patients who had a fracture of the fibula proximal to the level of the ankle joint. More recent reports have suggested that the need for trans-syndesmotic fixation may be less than was previously assumed.[15] Recent biomechanical testing and clinical outcome studies[7,37,42-45] have led to the following conclusions. (1) If the medial and lateral complexes are intact or can be restored anatomically and stabilized with internal fixation, the syndesmosis usually will be stable regardless of the degree of injury. (2) If the syndesmotic injury occurs as an osseous avulsion of the ligament or ligaments, reduction of these osseous fragments with or without fixation usually restores stability to the syndesmosis, especially if the medial and lateral complexes also are anatomically restored. (3) Internal fixation of the syndesmosis may be needed if there is a fracture of the fibula that extends more than 3 to 4 cm proximal to the joint line and an associated medial-side injury that cannot be fixed or repaired (even if the fibular fracture has been fixed anatomically). (4) Internal fixation of the syndesmosis may be needed if there is a fibular fracture proximal to the level of the ankle joint for which fixation is not planned and there also is a medial-side injury that cannot be fixed in a stable position.

Instability of the syndesmosis is identified primarily on the basis of the mechanism of injury and the fracture pattern. Clinical tests such as the squeeze test (manual medial-lateral compression across the syndesmosis) and the external-rotation stress test can elicit pain, but the findings may not be reliable in the acute setting. Radiographic parameters are helpful. A tibiofibular clear space (Fig. 2) of less than 5 mm and widening of the medial clear space of more than 4 mm are strong indications of a syndesmotic injury. Intraoperatively, the fibula can be manipulated to determine if there is excessive lateral displacement indicative of a syndesmotic injury. This is accomplished using the hook test, in which the fibula is grasped with bone forceps or a bone hook and is pulled laterally. While this test may demonstrate gross instability, this finding usually is already apparent on the preoperative radiographs. The sensitivity of this test for subtle instability is not known.

An external-rotation or abduction stress radiograph should be made when there is any remaining uncertainty with regard to the stability of the syndesmosis. The medial clear space normally widens by 2 to 3 mm with external-rotation or abduction stress. Widening of more than 4 mm indicates an injury of the syndesmotic and deltoid ligaments.

Apparent widening of the medial clear space may be observed if radiographs are made with the ankle in plantarflexion, especially if there is associated medial capsular or ligamentous injury. The reason for this apparent widening is that, with the ankle in plantarflexion, the narrowest part of the talus is within the mortise. With associated medial ligamentous injury, the talus can rotate externally, especially with plantarflexion and an anterior drawer effect from pressure on the posterior aspect of the heel; this situation also contributes to the appearance of medial widening. Radiographs made with the ankle in neutral prevent this misinterpretation.

If the syndesmosis is unstable, trans-syndesmotic fixation is recommended. Anatomic reduction of the syndesmosis is necessary, and the talus must be reduced in the mortise. If the fibula is fractured, its length, rotation, and alignment are restored first, and then the bone is reduced in the tibial notch. If the medial malleolus is fractured, it should be reduced and fixed as well. Reduction of the tibiofibular joint must be maintained during placement of any type of trans-syndesmotic fixation. Although many methods of fixation, including suture and use of synthetic grafts, have been reported,[15] fixation with screws is the most common technique.

The fixation screw is a positioning screw; its function is to hold the syndesmosis in the reduced position. The screw can be used independently or in conjunction with a plate, depending on the type and location of the fibular injury. The screw is inserted at the top of the fibular sulcus in the tibia, usually about 3 to 4 cm proximal and parallel to the ankle joint, and is angled approximately 30° anteriorly so that it is perpendicular to the tibiofibular joint and will not miss the tibia. Screws that are placed too far proximally may deform the fibula and widen the mortise. Screws that are not parallel to the ankle joint or perpendicular to the tibiofibular joint can cause the fibula to shift proximally or laterally.

If the fibular fracture is proximal, as it is in a Maisonneuve injury, and fixation of the fibula is not planned, accurate reduction of the fibula is essential. Determination of when the fibula is reduced can be difficult, especially if the fracture is comminuted. Guides to reduction include realignment of the articular surface of the fibula with the lateral facet of the talus, intraoperative measurement of the talocrural angle, and comparison with radiographs of the contralateral ankle. Alignment of the trans-syndesmotic screw is particularly important, as a misplaced screw can cause the fibula to shift and then can hold it in a malreduced position. In some situations (for example, when the patient is large or when compliance with nonweightbearing is in doubt), two syndesmotic screws may be used.

It has been recommended that fixation of the syndesmosis be performed with the ankle in full dorsiflexion to avoid overtightening of the mortise and loss of dorsiflexion postoperatively. However, in this fully dorsiflexed configuration, the mortise is in its widest position and the fibula is shifted laterally and rotated externally. There is concern that fixation of the syndesmosis in this position can result in persistent widening and predispose to instability, especially in plantarflexion and particularly if the screw is left in place or if ossification of the syndesmosis occurs.[46] We have found that placement of the screw with the ankle in 5° of dorsiflexion leads to a satisfactory result.

The type of screw that should be used and the number of cortices that should be fixed continue to be debated. Opinions have varied as to whether screws should be used in only the lateral tibial cortex or in both the lateral and the medial tibial cortex. If screw removal is planned, probably neither the screw size nor the number of tibial cortices fixed is crucial, provided that the syndesmosis is reduced and stabilized properly. If screw removal is not planned, fixation through the lateral cortex only provides adequate fixation, and later, with weightbearing, this unicortical screw will loosen rather than break, thereby allowing for the restoration of syndesmotic motion.

After fixation of the unstable syndesmosis, nonweightbearing in a cast or a fracture brace for 6 to 8 weeks generally is recommended. However, the time needed for healing of the syndesmotic complex is unknown. A very controversial topic is whether the syndesmotic screw should be removed before weightbearing is resumed. Those who advocate removal of the screw emphasize that motion of the fibula with respect to the tibia, which is an important part of the normal motion and function of the ankle, will be altered if the syndesmotic screw is left in place.[46] The goal is to avoid a fixed and nonresponsive syndesmosis caused by the replacement of the elastic ligaments with a stiff syndesmotic screw. Those who advocate leaving the screw in place note that there is no objective clinical evidence that this screw causes problems.[7] The screw usually loosens or breaks, permitting syndesmotic motion, and an additional surgical procedure is avoided. The optimum time for removal of the screw is unknown. We are aware of several instances in which displacement of the fibula occurred after a syndesmotic screw was removed at 6 to 8 weeks. The recommendations in the literature have ranged from 6 to 12 weeks;[15,19,46] it is probably better to leave the screw in place for the longer period of time. Our observation that, in some patients, symptoms seem to decrease after removal, loosening, or breakage of the syndesmotic screw suggests there may be individual differences in the ability of the ankle to tolerate a stiff syndesmosis.

Postoperative and Post-Injury Management

Early motion has been advocated after surgical treatment of an ankle fracture.[47,48] Theoretically, early motion reduces intra-articular adhesions and improves long-term function. However, in a study of the results 3 months after internal fixation, no difference in motion or function was found between patients managed with early motion and those managed with several weeks of immobilization.[49-52] Stuart and associates[48] reported that nonsurgical treatment of isolated fractures of the lateral malleolus with early motion in an air splint resulted in a greater range of motion and decreased time to rehabilitation compared with immobilization in a cast. There was no difference in the time to union. There is often concern that early weightbearing after an ankle fracture could lead to a loss of reduction. This has not been observed after isolated lateral malleolar fractures or other stable injuries.[53] Similarly, when stable internal fixation has been achieved, early weightbearing has not resulted in either late displacement of the fracture or a delay in healing.[49,51,52,54] Obviously, the decision as to whether stable fixation has been achieved and, thus, when weightbearing can begin is affected by many variables, such as the degree of comminution and the quality of the bone, and must be made by the treating surgeon on a patient-by-patient basis.

Pilon Fractures

Its name derived from the French word for pestle or rammer, a pilon fracture involves the tibial articular surface. Rüedi[55] and Rüedi and Allgöwer[56] reported the results of open reduction and early fixation of pilon fractures. Their basic treatment concepts included anatomic reduction and stabilization of the fibula, anatomic reduction of the articular surface of the distal part of the tibia, bone grafting of the metaphyseal defect, buttress plating of the tibia, and early mobilization of the ankle. They reported excellent results; however, most of their patients had sustained relatively low-energy injuries. Application of these techniques to high-energy injuries, both open and closed, resulted in a high rate of complications, most commonly soft-tissue problems and infection.[15,57] As a result, a number of modifications of the original technique have been introduced in an attempt to reduce the complications associated with the treatment of high-energy and open pilon fractures.[57-60]

Classification

The classification system described by Rüedi and Allgöwer,[56,61] which is commonly used today, includes three types of fractures: type I is an undisplaced, T-shaped fracture of the distal end of the tibia that extends into the joint; type II is the same as type I but with displacement of the intra-articular components; and type III is a complex, intra-articular, multifragmental fracture. Ovadia and Beals[57] added types IV and V to include fractures that extend into the metaphyseal and diaphyseal regions with more severe comminution, which is characteristic of many high-energy injuries.[60,62] The classification system of the AO/Orthopaedic Trauma Association is even more comprehensive and includes subdivisions that are based on the amount of comminution.[61] This system is very useful for research studies as it permits a more exact description of the injury and therefore allows better comparisons between studies.

As with any fracture, a thorough preoperative evaluation is essential for the effective treatment of a pilon fracture. It is important to understand the mechanism of injury, because these factors determine the amount and type of energy imparted to the bone as well as to the soft tissues. The fracture pattern is dictated by the position of the foot and the talus at the time of impact. A straight axial load creates a more central depression with circumferential splitting of the distal part of the tibia. An inverted or everted position of the ankle at the time of impact creates a split, or often a split-depression, fracture with comminution and compression of the distal metaphysis.

The pattern and extent of the injury of the bone, the articular surfaces, and the soft tissues determine the techniques of fixation that should be used. The options range from nonsurgical treatment to the traditional open reduction and internal fixation as described by Rüedi and Allgöwer.[56] It must be remembered that the soft-tissue envelope around the distal part of the tibia is the limiting factor in the treatment of these injuries. The soft-tissue injury must be evaluated carefully, as postoperative problems with soft-tissue healing or coverage are associated with a substantial increase in the morbidity associated with this injury.

Anteroposterior, lateral, and oblique radiographs should be made. A traction radiograph of the injured extremity is helpful, as traction and ligamentotaxis often cause the displaced fragments to be pulled back into position, which allows for a better definition and understanding of the fracture pattern (Fig. 3). When the injury pattern is not clearly visible on plain radiographs, a computed tomographic scan can be made to allow for a better, three-dimensional evaluation of the injury. Precise preoperative planning and drawings, using the uninjured ankle as a template, are helpful to ensure that the needed equipment and instruments are available. Careful planning also reduces the need for extensive soft-tissue dissection to allow the surgeon to see the fracture, reduces the time required, and facilitates each step of surgery.[63]

If more than a few hours have elapsed between the injury and the evaluation, the soft-tissue swelling will, as a rule, be too great to allow for an immediate open reduction and internal fixation. In this situation, skeletal traction, either with placement of the pin through the calcaneus or the application of an external fixator, should be used because soft-tissue recovery may take days or weeks and it is important to prevent skeletal shortening. Furthermore, indirect reduction with traction helps to realign the fracture surfaces, which makes subsequent internal fixation easier to accomplish.

The method that we commonly use to treat high-energy fractures involves the initial placement of an external fixation device with indirect reduction of the fracture. The fibula may or may not be fixed at the same time. After soft-tissue recovery has occurred, a limited open reduction and stabilization of the articular component is done with screws alone or with screws and a small buttress plate. The location of the incisions and the steps in reduction of the articular surface and the fracture fragments are based on the preoperative plan. Soft-tissue dissection should be minimized and, whenever possible, fragments should remain attached to the periosteum and the joint capsule.

The articular surface generally is reassembled from lateral to medial and from posterior to anterior. The anterolateral portion of the tubercle of Chaput usually is still attached to the anterior syndesmotic ligaments and is brought down into position at the time of fibular reduction. The anterolateral corner of this reduced fragment can be used as a guide for the restoration of tibial length. Any posterolateral or posterior fragments then are reduced to the anterolateral fragment. The remaining fragments, including any central depressed fragments, then are realigned. When necessary, the split medial malleolar fragment can be retracted posteriorly to allow for better visualization of the reduction of the articular surface. Temporary fixation is obtained with Kirschner wires, and the reduction is confirmed radiographically. Bone grafting of any structurally deficient areas in the cortical or cancellous bone of the metaphysis then should be done. Autogenous bone grafts commonly are used. While allograft and synthetic bone materials have been used, the efficacy of these grafts in the treatment of pilon fractures has not been reported.

When plate fixation is planned, an anterior or anteromedial buttress plate is used, depending on the fracture configuration. Large spoon and T-plates no longer are recommended because they are too bulky and their use can lead to compromise of the overlying soft tissues. A 3.5-mm cloverleaf plate has a much smaller profile than the large-fragment-system plates but still has adequate strength to maintain reduction and can be bent and contoured relatively easily for positioning on the tibia (Fig. 3). Cannulated screws can be placed independent of the plate, either through the wound or percutaneously, to secure isolated fragments. The importance of meticulous care of the soft tissues, including a tension-free closure, cannot be overemphasized.

The external fixator, if used, may be left in place for as long as is needed to achieve the specific goals of its use, such as soft-tissue stabilization, temporary buttressing, or definitive fixation. Weightbearing should be delayed until there is radiographic evidence of bone healing.

Open pilon fractures present an additional challenge. These injuries, like all open fractures, necessitate emergency debridement, irrigation, and stabilization. The typical wound associated with an open pilon fracture is a transverse distal anteromedial laceration. The proximal skin flap is contused, and use of the usual anteromedial incision may compromise its blood supply. When treating such an injury, it may be necessary to apply an external fixator, obtain indirect reduction, stabilize the fibula, and then perform the reconstruction of the articular surface through the open wound with use of cannulated screws for stabilization. This technique has been found to be less traumatic to the already injured soft tissues than the traditional extensile exposure.[59,64] Cancellous bone grafting and even internal fixation can, if necessary, be delayed until 4 to 6 weeks later, when the soft tissues have stabilized and the risk of soft-tissue slough and infection is reduced.

Complications

Pilon fractures, especially those caused by high-energy trauma, have been associated with a high rate of complications.[57-62,64] Early postoperative problems have included skin necrosis, superficial and deep infection, and loss of fixation. Complications with fracture healing have included delayed union or nonunion of the metaphyseal-diaphyseal junction, varus or valgus malunion of the distal part of the tibia, and nonanatomic reduction or postoperative loss of reduction of the articular surface.[57-59,61] Stabilization of the anterolateral fragment and bone grafting of the lateral border of the distal part of the tibia promote union and reduce the prevalence of both valgus malunion and nonunion of this fracture. The prevalence of postoperative skin and wound problems has been reduced substantially through the use of indirect reduction with external fixation and reconstruction of the articular surface with small plates and/or screws.[58,61,63-66]

Post-traumatic osteoarthrosis may occur as a result of damage of the articular cartilage at the time of the injury and also has been associated with fractures in which a congruous articular surface was not restored or maintained.[58,61,64] Primary arthrodesis of the ankle rarely is indicated because the long-term outcome is not easy to predict. Although some patients may need an arthrodesis of the ankle because of symptomatic osteoarthrosis, others do fairly well despite radiographic signs of posttraumatic osteoarthrosis.

Overview

The primary goal in the treatment of fractures of the ankle is to obtain union of the fracture and to restore normal function. Ankle fractures constitute a wide spectrum of injuries, ranging from undisplaced or minimally displaced stable fractures that can be treated nonsurgically to displaced unstable fractures that require surgical intervention. While some controversies remain, the general principles and techniques used for the surgical treatment of ankle fractures are well established.

References

1. Bauer M, Bengner U, Johnell O, et al: Supination-eversion fractures of the ankle joint: Changes in incidence over 30 years. *Foot Ankle* 1987;8:26–28.
2. Praemer A, Furner S, Rice DP (eds): *Musculoskeletal Conditions in the United States.* Park Ridge, IL, American Academy of Orthopaedic Surgeons, 1992.
3. Lundberg A, Goldie I, Kalin B, et al: Kinematics of the ankle/foot complex: Plantarflexion and dorsiflexion. *Foot Ankle* 1989;9:194–200.
4. Michelson JD, Helgemo SL Jr: Kinematics of the axially loaded ankle. *Foot Ankle Int* 1995;16:577–582.
5. Michelson JD, Helgemo SL, Ahn UM: Dynamic biomechanics of the normal and fractured ankle. *Trans Orthop Res Soc* 1994; 20:253.
6. Parlasca R, Shoji H, D'Ambrosia RD: Effects of ligamentous injury on ankle and subtalar joints: A kinematic study. *Clin Orthop* 1979;140:266–272.
7. Michelson JD: Fractures about the ankle. *J Bone Joint Surg* 1995; 77A:142–152.
8. Siegler S, Wang D, Plasha E, et al: Technique for in vivo measurement of the three-dimensional kinematics and laxity characteristics of the ankle joint complex. *J Orthop Res* 1994; 12:421–431.
9. Close JR: Some applications of the functional anatomy of the ankle joint. *J Bone Joint Surg* 1956;38A:761–781.
10. Lundberg A: Kinematics of the ankle and foot: In vivo roentgen stereophotogrammetry. *Acta Orthop Scand* 1989;233(suppl): 1–24.
11. Peter RE, Harrington RM, Tencer A, et al: Effect of implants on the motion of the distal tibio-fibular syndesmotic joint: Comparison of screw versus K-wire fixation of Weber type "C" injuries. *Orthop Trans* 1992;16:459–460.
12. Harper MC: An anatomic study of the short oblique fracture of the distal fibula and ankle stability. *Foot Ankle* 1983;4:23–29.
13. McCullough CJ, Burge PD: Rotatory stability of the load-bearing ankle: An experimental study. *J Bone Joint Surg* 1980;62B: 460–464.
14. Yablon IG, Heller FG, Shouse L: The key role of the lateral malleolus in displaced fractures of the ankle. *J Bone Joint Surg* 1977;59A:169–173.
15. Vander Griend RA, Savoie FH, Hughes JL: Fractures of the ankle, in Rockwood CA Jr, Green DP, Bucholz RW (eds): *Fractures in Adults,* ed 3. Philadelphia, PA, JB Lippincott, 1991, vol 2, pp 1983–2039.
16. Bauer M, Jonsson K, Nilsson B: Thirty-year follow-up of ankle fractures. *Acta Orthop Scand* 1985;56:103–106.
17. de Souza LJ, Gustilo RB, Meyer TJ: Results of operative treatment of displaced external rotation-abduction fractures of the ankle. *J Bone Joint Surg* 1985;67A:1066–1074.
18. Sarkisian JS, Cody GW: Closed treatment of ankle fractures: A new criterion for evaluation. A review of 250 cases. *J Trauma* 1976;16:323–326.
19. Trafton PG, Bray TJ, Simpson LA: Fractures and soft tissue injuries of the ankle, in Browner BD, Jupiter JB, Levine AM, et al (eds): *Skeletal Trauma: Fractures, Dislocations, Ligamentous Injuries.* Philadelphia, PA, WB Saunders, 1992, vol 2, pp 1871–1957.

20. Michelson JD, Magid D, Ney DR, et al: Examination of the pathologic anatomy of ankle fractures. *J Trauma* 1992;32:65–70.
21. Phillips WA, Schwartz HS, Keller CS, et al: A prospective, randomized study of the management of severe ankle fractures. *J Bone Joint Surg* 1985;67A:67–78.
22. Lauge-Hansen N: Fractures of the ankle: II. Combined experimental-surgical and experimental-roentgenologic investigations. *Arch Surg* 1950;60:957–985.
23. Nielsen JO, Dons-Jensen H, Sorensen HT: Lauge-Hansen classification of malleolar fractures: An assessment of the reproducibility in 118 cases. *Acta Orthop Scand* 1990;61:385–387.
24. Rasmussen S, Madsen PV, Bennicke K: Observer variation in the Lauge-Hansen classification of ankle fractures: Precision improved by instruction. *Acta Orthop Scand* 1993;64:693–694.
25. Müller ME, Allgöwer M, Schneider R, et al: *Manual of Internal Fixation: Techniques Recommended by the AO-Group*, ed 2. Berlin, Germany, Springer-Verlag, 1979.
26. Lindsjö U: Classification of ankle fractures: The Lauge-Hansen or AO system? *Clin Orthop* 1985;199:12–16.
27. Muller ME, Nazarian S, Koch P (eds): *The AO Classification of Fractures.* Berlin, Germany, Springer-Verlag, 1988.
28. Clarke HJ, Michelson JD, Cox QG, et al: Tibio-talar stability in bimalleolar ankle fractures: A dynamic in-vitro contact area study. *Foot Ankle* 1991;11:222–227.
29. Bauer M, Bergström B, Hemborg A, et al: Malleolar fractures: Nonoperative versus operative treatment. A controlled study. *Clin Orthop* 1985;199:17–27.
30. Joy G, Patzakis MJ, Harvey JP Jr: Precise evaluation of the reduction of severe ankle fractures. *J Bone Joint Surg* 1974;56A:979–993.
31. Ramsey PL, Hamilton W: Changes in tibiotalar area of contact caused by lateral talar shift. *J Bone Joint Surg* 1976;58A:356–357.
32. Cass JR, Settles H: Ankle instability: In vitro kinematics in response to axial load. *Foot Ankle Int* 1994;15:134–140.
33. Burns WC II, Prakash K, Adelaar R, et al: Tibiotalar joint dynamics: Indications for the syndesmotic screw. A cadaver study. *Foot Ankle* 1993;14:153–158.
34. Kristensen KD, Hansen T: Closed treatment of ankle fractures: Stage II supination-eversion fractures followed for 20 years. *Acta Orthop Scand* 1985;56:107–109.
35. Tunturi T, Kemppainen K, Pätiälä H, et al: Importance of anatomical reduction for subjective recovery after ankle fracture. *Acta Orthop Scand* 1983;54:641–647.
36. Yde J, Kristensen KD: Ankle fractures: Supination-eversion fractures of Stage IV. Primary and late results of operative and nonoperative treatment. *Acta Orthop Scand* 1980;51:981–990.
37. Boden SD, Labropoulos PA, McCowin P, et al: Mechanical considerations for the syndesmosis screw: A cadaver study. *J Bone Joint Surg* 1989;71A:1548–1555.
38. Harper MC: The deltoid ligament: An evaluation of need for surgical repair. *Clin Orthop* 1988;226:156–168.
39. Baird RA, Jackson ST: Fractures of the distal part of the fibula with associated disruption of the deltoid ligament: Treatment without repair of the deltoid ligament. *J Bone Joint Surg* 1987;69A:1346–1352.
40. Harper MC: Posterior instability of the talus: An anatomic evaluation. *Foot Ankle* 1989;10:36–39.
41. Harper MC, Hardin G: Posterior malleolar fractures of the ankle associated with external rotation-abduction injuries: Results with and without internal fixation. *J Bone Joint Surg* 1988;70A:1348–1356.
42. Amendola A: Controversies in diagnosis and management of syndesmosis injuries of the ankle. *Foot Ankle* 1992;13:44–50.
43. Pankovich AM: Maisonneuve fracture of the fibula. *J Bone Joint Surg* 1976;58A:337–342.
44. Pankovich AM: Fractures of the fibula proximal to the distal tibiofibular syndesmosis. *J Bone Joint Surg* 1978;60A:221–229.
45. Yamaguchi K, Martin CH, Boden SD, et al: Operative treatment of syndesmotic disruptions without use of a syndesmotic screw: A prospective clinical study. *Foot Ankle Int* 1994;15:407–414.
46. Needleman RL, Skrade DA, Stiehl JB: Effect of the syndesmotic screw on ankle motion. *Foot Ankle* 1989;10:17–24.
47. Segal D, Wiss DA, Whitelaw GP: Functional bracing and rehabilitation of ankle fractures. *Clin Orthop* 1985;199:39–45.
48. Stuart PR, Brumby C, Smith SR: Comparative study of functional bracing and plaster cast treatment of stable lateral malleolar fractures. *Injury* 1989;20:323–326.
49. Ahl T, Dalen N, Selvik G: Mobilization after operation of ankle fractures: Good results of early motion and weight bearing. *Acta Orthop Scand* 1988;59:302–306.
50. Cimino W, Ichtertz D, Slabaugh P: Early mobilization of ankle fractures after open reduction and internal fixation. *Clin Orthop* 1991;267:152–156.
51. Finsen V, Saetermo R, Kibsgaard L, et al: Early postoperative weight-bearing and muscle activity in patients who have a fracture of the ankle. *J Bone Joint Surg* 1989;71A:23–27.
52. Hedstrom M, Ahl T, Dalen N: Early postoperative ankle exercise: A study of postoperative lateral malleolar fractures. *Clin Orthop* 1994;300:193–196.
53. Ahl T, Dalen N, Selvik G: Ankle fractures: A clinical and roentgenographic stereophotogrammetric study. *Clin Orthop* 1989;245:246–255.
54. Ahl T, Dalen N, Lundberg A, et al: Early mobilization of operated on ankle fractures: Prospective, controlled study of 40 bimalleolar cases. *Acta Orthop Scand* 1993;64:95–99.
55. Rüedi T: Fractures of the lower end of the tibia into the ankle joint: Results 9 years after open reduction and internal fixation. *Injury* 1973;5:130–134.
56. Rüedi TP, Allgöwer M: The operative treatment of intra-articular fractures of the lower end of the tibia. *Clin Orthop* 1979;138:105–110.
57. Ovadia DN, Beals RK: Fractures of the tibial plafond. *J Bone Joint Surg* 1986;68A:543–551.
58. Bone LB: Fractures of the tibial plafond: The pilon fracture. *Orthop Clin North Am* 1987;18:95–104.
59. Bourne RB: Pylon fractures of the distal tibia. *Clin Orthop* 1989;240:42–46.
60. Pierce RO Jr, Heinrich JH: Comminuted intra-articular fractures of the distal tibia. *J Trauma* 1979;19:828–832.
61. Heim U (ed): *The Pilon-Tibial Fracture.* Philadelphia, PA, WB Saunders, 1995.
62. Tscherne H, Schatzker J: *Major Fractures of the Pilon, the Talus, and the Calcaneus: Current Concepts of Treatment.* Berlin, Germany, Springer-Verlag, 1993.
63. Mast J, Jakob R, Ganz R (eds): *Planning and Reduction Technique in Fracture Surgery.* Berlin, Germany, Springer-Verlag, 1989.
64. Bone L, Stegemann P, McNamara K, et al: External fixation of severely comminuted and open tibial pilon fractures. *Clin Orthop* 1993;292:101–107.
65. Kellam JF, Waddell JP: Fractures of the distal tibial metaphysis with intra-articular extension: The distal tibial explosion fracture. *J Trauma* 1979;19:593–601.
66. Tile M: Fractures of the distal tibial metaphysis involving the ankle joint: The pilon fracture, in Schatzker J, Tile M (eds): *The Rationale of Operative Fracture Care.* Berlin, Germany, Springer-Verlag, 1987, pp 343–369.

CHAPTER 32

Complex Fractures of the Talus

Robert S. Adelaar, MD

Introduction

The management of talus injuries has always been a challenge, because these injuries occur relatively infrequently, the fact that the talus is hidden by its anatomic location makes approaches difficult, and the blood supply to the talus is precarious. In this chapter, I will attempt to give you the approach to this injury at the Medical College of Virginia and compare it to current treatment protocols. I will emphasize the surgical management of talar neck fractures, which make up over 50% of all talar injuries.

History of Talar Injuries

The word talus has an interesting derivation. Roman soldiers originally made their dice from the heel bones of horses, which became known as the taxillus. Taxillus was eventually shortened to talus. The Greeks made dice from the second vertebrae of sheep and called the bone astragalus. Both words with gambling origin came to be applied to the same bone in the foot.[1] The first account of an accident to the talus was made in 1608 by Fabricius of Hilden who wrote about a man who dislocated his talus.[1-3] Many isolated cases have been reported since then, but the first to collect and classify a series of cases were H. G. Anderson and associates.[4] In 1919, Anderson, a consulting surgeon to the Royal Flying Corps of England, described 18 cases of fractures and dislocations of the talus associated with aircraft accidents (aviator astragalus). Coltart,[5] in a review of Royal Air Force studies between 1940 and 1945, reported that of 25,000 fractures and dislocations, 228 were fractures of the talus. Aviator injuries occurred with the foot positioned on the rudder bar in extreme plantarflexion.

Since then, many investigators[6-16] have reported series of talar injuries, drawing attention to the problems involved. Modern incidence of talus injuries has been detailed in a report by the Hanover Medical School,[17] in which there were 120 talar fractures out of approximately 1,500 injuries. There also were more than 1,200 ankle injuries and 200 calcaneal injuries in their series of complex foot and ankle trauma. With the advent of mandatory seat belts and more air bags, more of the people involved in high-speed crashes survive, which increases the number of injuries to the distal extremities that require treatment. Almost one half of talus injuries are secondary to motor vehicle accidents.

Anatomy

The talus has several anatomic features that predispose it to complex injury (Fig. 1). Because approximately 60% of the talar surface is cartilage, there often are problems with circulation. The talus has seven articular surfaces and is wider anteriorly than it is posteriorly; therefore, dorsiflexion increases stability. However, the talus is weakest at the neck where the bone is recessed to allow for dorsiflexion. The talar neck deviates medially and is shortened on the medial aspect. The orientation of the talar neck differs from that of the body of the talus in both the horizontal and sagittal planes. In the horizontal plane, the neck shifts medially with a deviation that can range from 10° to

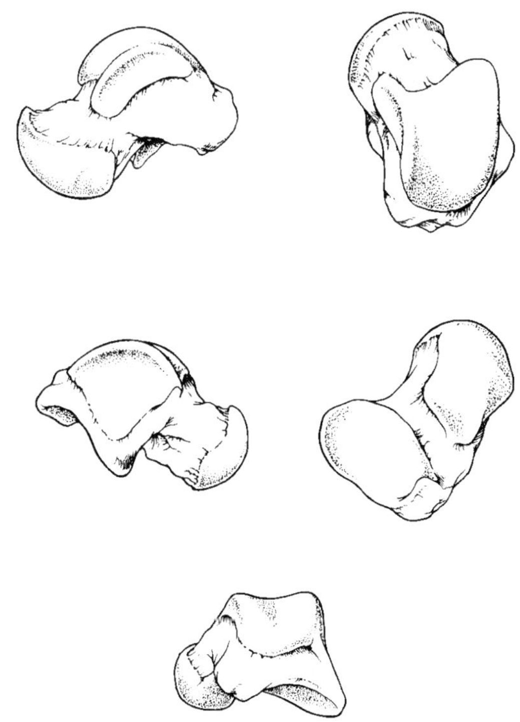

Fig. 1 Important anatomic features of the talus. (Reproduced with permission from Adelaar RS: Fractures of the talus, in Greene WB (ed): *Instructional Course Lectures XXXIX*. Park Ridge, IL, American Academy of Orthopaedic Surgeons, 1990, pp 147-156.)

Parts of this chapter were reproduced with permission from Adelaar RS: Surgical treatment of fractures of the talus, in Gould JS (ed): *Operative Foot Surgery*. Philadelphia, PA, WB Saunders, 1994, pp 377-398.

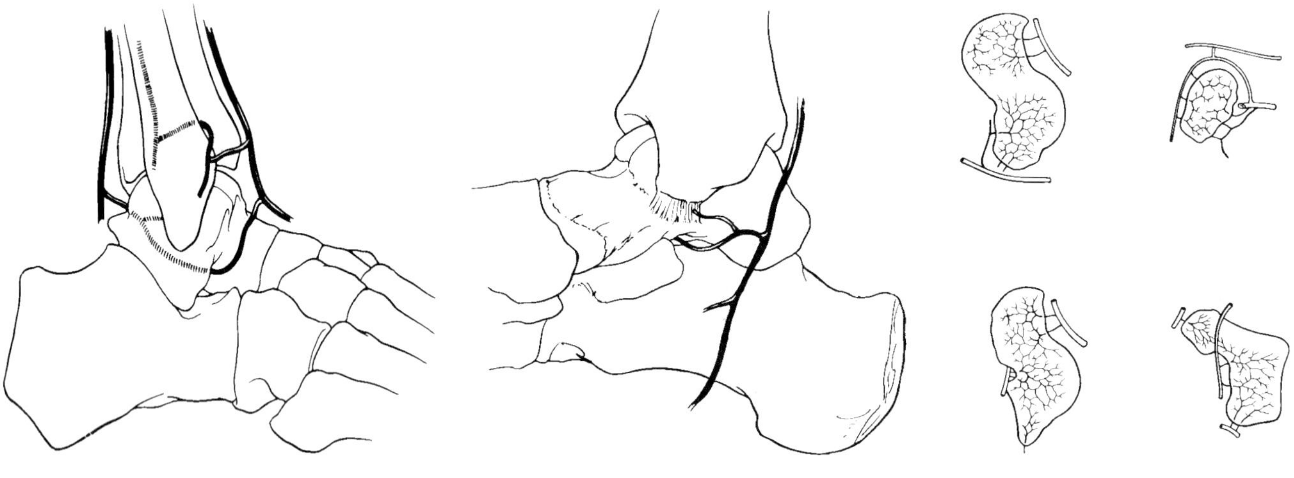

Fig. 2 **Left,** The vascular anatomy of the talus from three major vessels. (Reproduced with permission from Adelaar RS: Fractures of the talus, in Greene WB (ed): *Instructional Course Lectures XXXIX.* Park Ridge, IL, American Academy of Orthopaedic Surgeons, 1990, pp 147-156.) **Center,** The deltoid artery branch to the body of the talus from tarsal canal artery. **Right,** The regional blood supply to the talus.

44°, with an average of 24°. In the sagittal plane, the neck deviates downward with a range of 5° to 50° and an average of 24°.[18] Therefore, it is difficult to interpret radiographs with respect to accuracy of reduction. In addition, the alignment of the lateral talus axis with the first metatarsal affects attempts at screw fixation from the anterior medial approach. Screw fixation is difficult without damaging the navicular, and the short length and the direction of the screw may not give adequate fixation.

When the ankle is plantarflexed, there is increased mobility and anterior instability. In this position, rotational forces may cause subluxation and dislocation. The talar neck is the only extra-articular portion of the talus, and it forms a bridge between the posterior and anterior middle facets of the talus. The talocalcaneal ligament is important in stabilizing the talar neck and the distal fragment of talar neck fractures. Dorsal subluxation and varus displacement can occur if this ligament is ruptured. The posterior talocalcaneal ligament usually is the last supporting structure ruptured before the body of the talus is completely dislocated from the mortise.

The inferior portion of the talus articulates with the posterior calcaneal articular facet, which keeps the body of the talus in an upright position. The interosseous talocalcaneal ligament plays an important part in reduction of talar neck fractures. The medial and lateral posterior tubercles form a roof over the flexor hallucis longus. The os trigonum is a congenital nonunion of the lateral posterior process and is symptomatic in dancers. The lateral tubercle articulates with the fibula and tibial portion of the mortise; therefore, lateral tubercle injuries can involve articular surfaces. The lateral process also has strong anterior talofibular and posterior talocalcaneal ligamentous attachments.[19-21] The lateral process can act as a wedge to disrupt the angle of Gissane, which is the lateral angle of the subtalar joint, or the lateral strut of the calcaneus in calcaneal fractures.

Circulation of the Talus

Osteonecrosis is the most harmful complication of talar injuries, and, to avoid iatrogenic vascular injury, the surgeon must be very knowledgeable regarding the circulation of the talus. The blood supply to the talus comes mainly from the extraosseous and the intraosseous circulation. The extraosseous circulation, with contributions from the anterior tibial, posterior tibial, and peroneal vasculature, forms a vascular extraosseous ring, described by Wildenaur, around the talar neck and sinus tarsi.[22-26] The tarsal sinus artery forms from branches of the anterior tibial artery and the peroneal artery. The tarsal canal artery arises from the posterior tibial artery within the deltoid ligament below the medial malleolus (Fig. 2), and it branches to form the deltoid artery, which is an important source of extraosseous circulation to the body of the talus. Preservation of the deltoid artery is critical during stabilization or reduction of the talar neck and body.

A complete intraosseous anastomosis between all regions of the talus (Fig. 2, *right*) has been found in 60% of talar anatomic specimens. The vascular supply varies among the regional sections of the talus. The talar head has an abundant vasculature, which is supplied primarily by the anterior tibial artery. Multiple vascular foramina are seen in the superior and anterior portions of the talar head. The deltoid artery contributes significantly to the interosseous circulation in

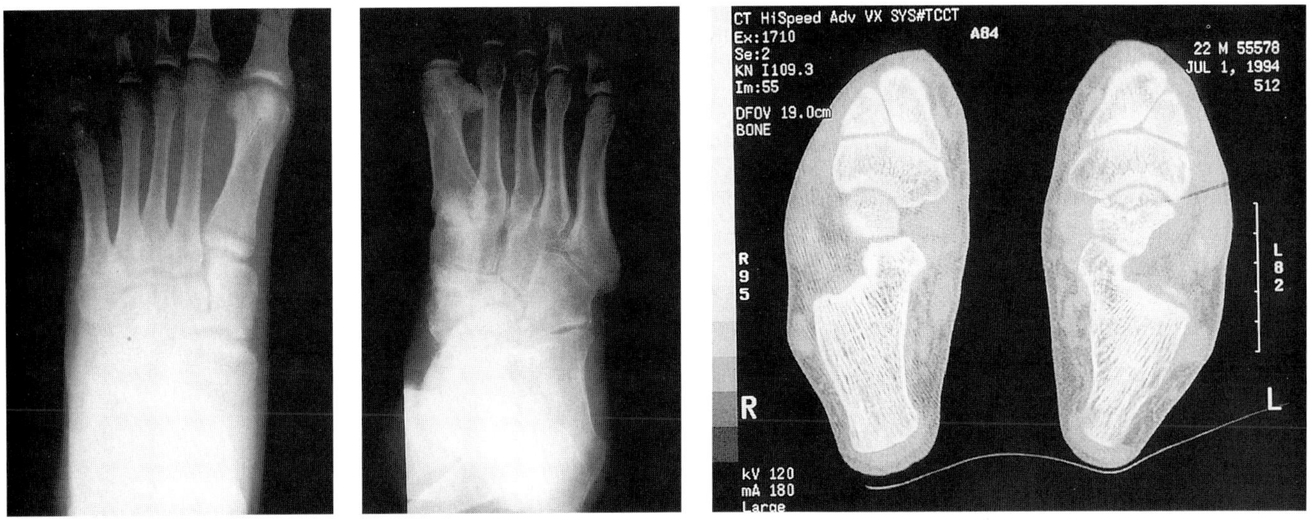

Fig. 3 **Left,** Radiographic view of the talar head fracture demonstrating an unstable midtarsal joint. **Center,** A Canale view of talar head fracture. **Right,** A computed tomography scan of talar head fractures.

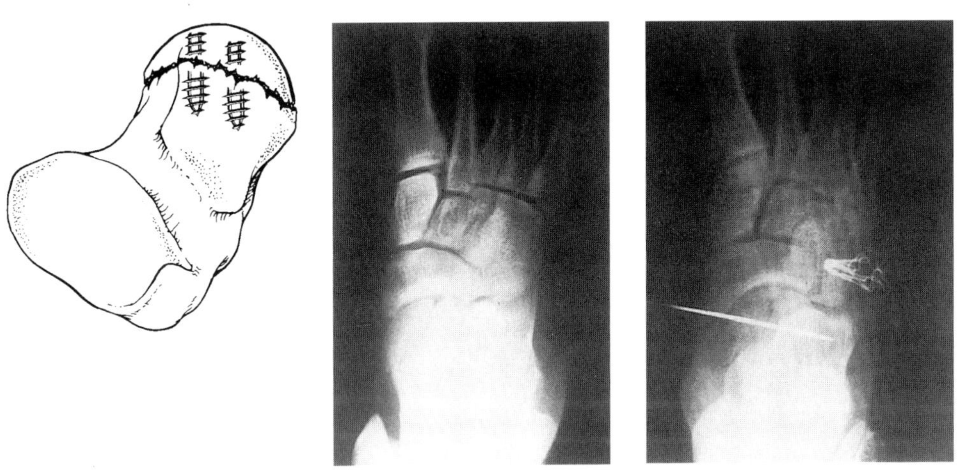

Fig. 4 **Left,** A talar head fracture can be stabilized with subarticular screws. **Right,** The radiographs show reduction of a talar head fracture with 0.062 Kirschner wires.

the medial and proximal portions of the body of the talus. However, the anterolateral surface of the talar body and the posterior tubercles of the talus are relatively avascular.

Talar Head Injuries

Talar head fractures constitute 5% to 10% of all talar injuries. The mechanism of injury is usually compressive forces secondary to hyperdorsiflexion. Because the talar head is well vascularized, the incidence of osteonecrosis is low. The key problem with this injury is recognition. Midtarsal instability and future arthrosis can occur from improper reduction. During physical examination, tenderness and possible instability in the talonavicular area are often present. Instability of the talonavicular joint can be caused by a fracture fragment of greater than 50% (Fig. 3, *left*). It is often necessary to obtain special oblique radiographs or Canale views in order to define the talar neck (Fig. 3, *center*).[12] Computed tomography (CT) also is used to define accurately the extent and location of injuries. CT is quite helpful in planning for reduction and fixation (Fig. 3, *right*).

Unstable talar head fractures, especially those that involve more than 50% of the talar head, require rigid fixation (Fig. 4). The surgeon should use a medial approach, taking care not to disturb the posterior tibial tendon attachment to the navicular or spring ligament. A portion of the medial and anterior talonavicular capsule needs to be released. The goal of reduction is rigid fixation in order to allow early motion after soft-tissue

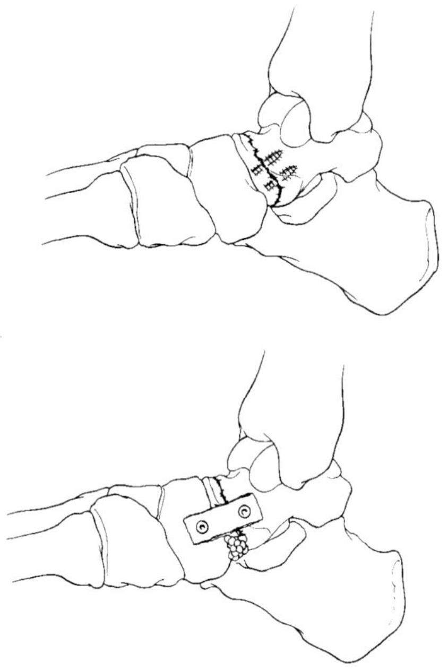

Fig. 5 A talonavicular fusion can be performed for articular pain after talar head fracture. A wedge graft is taken from the top of the iliac crest, and fixation is with one or two lag screws.

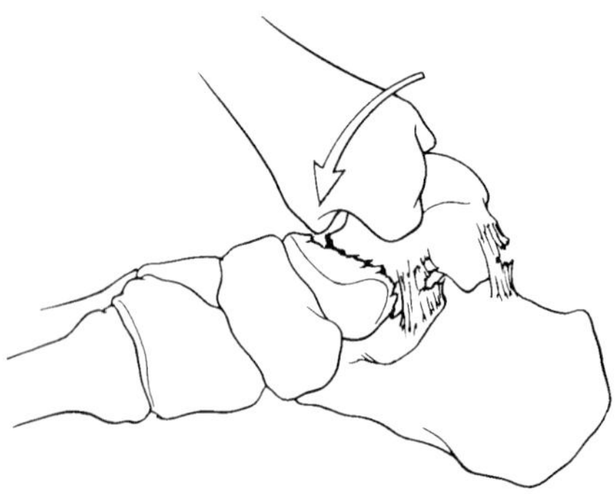

Fig. 6 The mechanism of injury for most talar neck fractures is hyperdorsiflexion with an axial load. After impingement of the trochlea (the talar neck) on the tibia, the posterior capsule is put under stretch and supination occurs, thereby stabilizing the subtalar joint.

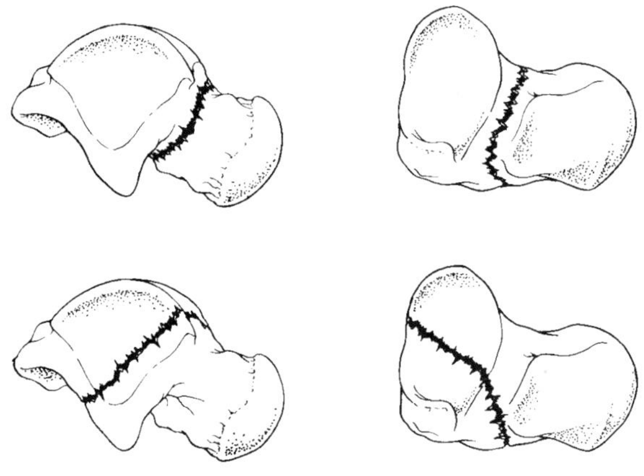

Fig. 7 The difference between talar neck and body fractures depends on whether the fracture exists in the posterior articular joint.

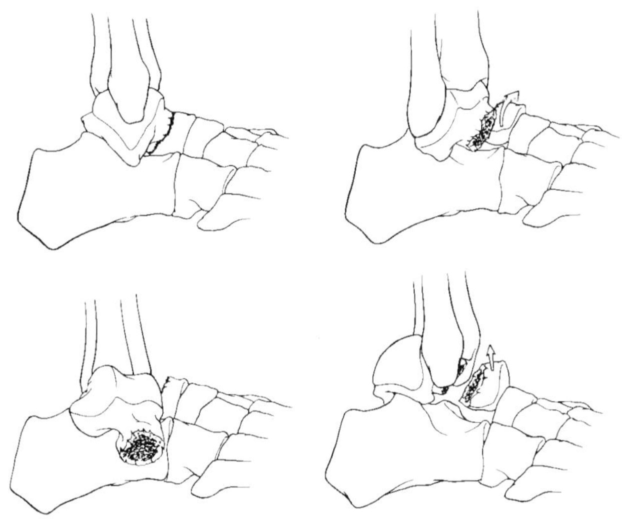

Fig. 8 Hawkins-type classification of talar neck injuries. **Top left,** Nondisplaced. **Top right,** Neck fracture with displacement. **Bottom left,** Displaced neck with subtalar ankle dislocation. **Bottom right,** Type II or III with talonavicular subluxation.

healing. Long-term problems with arthrosis depend on anatomic articular fixation. Subarticular cancellous lag screws (Fig. 4, *left*) are appropriate. Percutaneous Kirschner wires (K-wires) do not provide a stable reduction, and they cause soft-tissue problems (Fig. 4, *right*).

Complications that can occur with talar head fractures include instability from nonunion, missed fractures that do not unite, arthrosis of the talonavicular joint as a result of poor articular reduction, and, rarely, osteonecrosis. If complications occur and the fragment cannot be securely fixed, a talonavicular fusion should be considered. The fusion technique that we use at the Medical College of Virginia is screw fixation through the navicular with slotting of a corticocancellous wedge graft from the iliac crest into the talonavicular joint (Fig. 5). In addition, cancellous bone graft is packed into any spaces before screw fixation. When attempting a fusion or fracture reduction, it is important not to strip the blood supply entirely from the talar head and to approach the talar head only from the anteromedial aspect. The normal dimensions of the bones should be maintained.

Nondisplaced talar-head fractures should be treated nonsurgically. A nonweightbearing short leg cast is worn for approximately 8 to 12 weeks until healing can be confirmed radiographically. If a displaced fracture

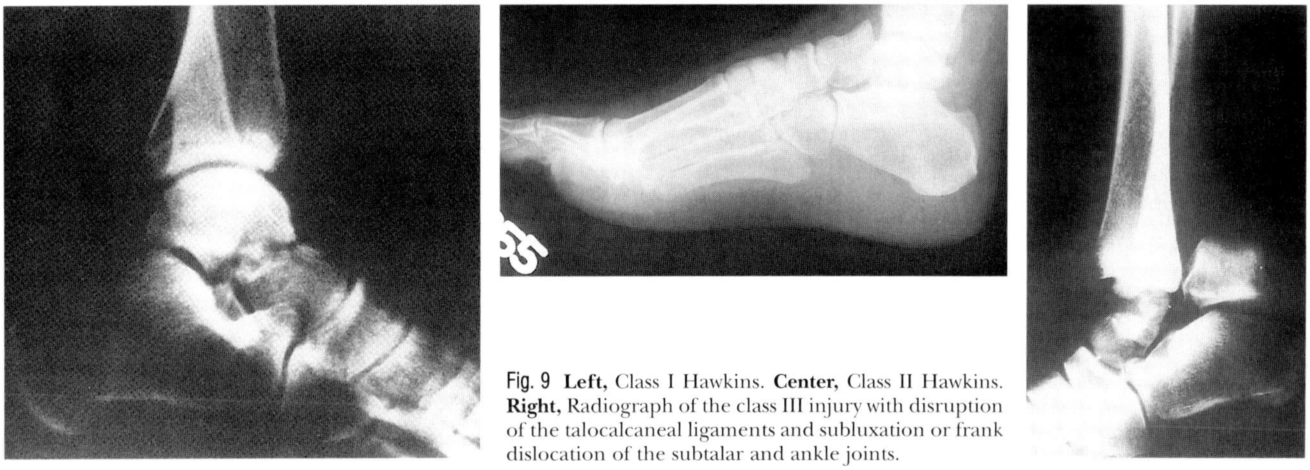

Fig. 9 **Left,** Class I Hawkins. **Center,** Class II Hawkins. **Right,** Radiograph of the class III injury with disruption of the talocalcaneal ligaments and subluxation or frank dislocation of the subtalar and ankle joints.

involves more than 50% of the talar head, it usually requires internal fixation. If it involves less than 50% with no instability of the talonavicular joint, excision of the displaced fragments can be considered.

Talar Neck Fractures

Talar neck fractures represent 50% of all talar injuries. The principles that apply to the treatment of talar neck injuries also apply to treatment of talar body fractures, with some modifications in exposure. The mechanism of injury has been described as a dorsiflexion of the foot against a stationary tibia, with impingement of the talar neck, or trochlea, which is the weakest area on the tibial dome (Figs. 6 and 7). As this force continues, there usually is medial and dorsal comminution of the talus, disruption of the talocalcaneal ligament, and disruption of the posterior and subtalar capsule. Supination of the ankle with impingement of the talar neck against the medial malleolus will cause subluxation of the subtalar joint and comminution of the medial neck.[18] This usually occurs in class II or III injuries (Fig. 8).[13] When the talar body dislocates, it usually is found at the posteromedial aspect of the Achilles tendon, where it can compress the adjacent neurovascular structures. Talar neck fractures can also occur from direct blows.

In laboratory experiments, it was difficult to produce talar neck fractures by wedging the talus against the tibial dome in dorsiflexion. These fractures could not be produced unless the ankle was in a neutral position and ankle motion was eliminated by compressing the calcaneus against the overlying talus and tibia.[18,27] Peterson and associates[27] felt that these forces could be reproduced in an extended leg if the triceps surae was contracted. Supination forces are more commonly associated with higher classes of Hawkins injuries because they produce fracture dislocation patterns and often cause a direct push-off injury to the medial malleolus. Fractures of the medial malleolus and lumbar spine injuries have been found in association with talar neck injuries.

Classification

The Medical College of Virginia uses a modified Hawkins classification (Fig. 8).[13] A class I injury is a nondisplaced vertical neck fracture with no subluxation; a class II injury has mild dorsal displacement of the distal talar neck fragment with subluxation of the subtalar joint; and a class III injury involves displacement of the talar body with associated subtalar subluxation and talar neck displacement (Fig. 9). As the displacement of the talar neck increases, the incidence of malunion, osteoarthritis, and osteonecrosis increases.[9,11,18,28,29] The talocalcaneal ligament is ruptured when dorsal displacement of the distal fragment is present. With rupture of this ligament, it is difficult to control talar neck fractures by closed means because of the supination deformity or varus and comminution that occur. Open techniques are recommended when it is not possible to achieve anatomic reduction and when there is at least 3 mm of dorsal displacement and 5° of varus rotation. Another type of talar neck fracture has been observed by Canale and Kelly,[12] who noted that a talonavicular dislocation could accompany a Hawkins class I or III injury. This has been called a Hawkins class IV (Fig. 8).

Talar Neck Malalignments

When reducing talar neck fractures, it is very important to maintain alignment of the talar neck; this often is difficult because of the comminution normally found on the medial side. The lateral portion of the talus is thought to have less comminution because the higher grades of injury are associated with a supination mechanism that impacts the talar neck against the medial

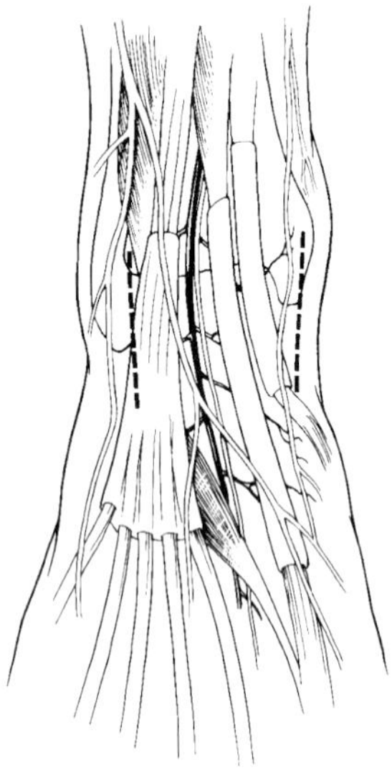

Fig. 10 An anteromedial approach to the talar neck fracture through the interval between the anterior tibial and extensor hallucis longus tendons, avoiding neurovascular bundles. Care should be taken not to do a great deal of stripping on the talar neck.

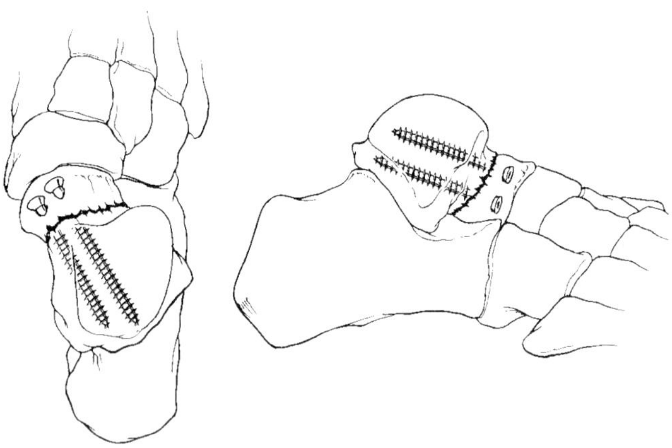

Fig. 11 **Left,** Fixation of a talar neck fracture with cannulated screw from the anteromedial approach. **Right,** An anterolateral approach to the talar neck.

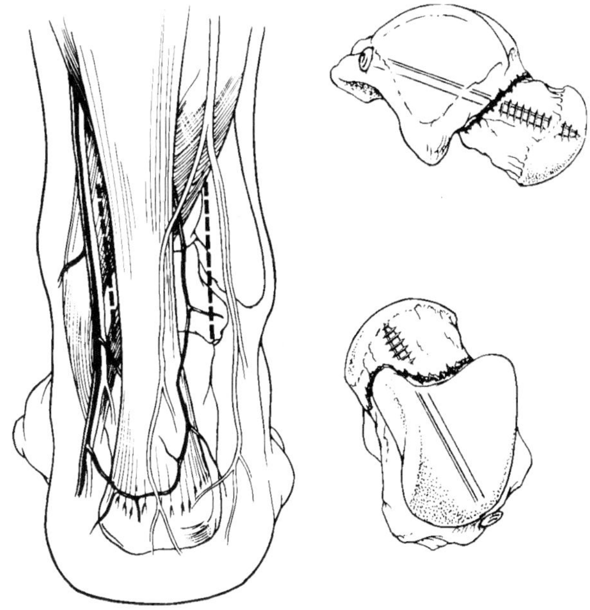

Fig. 12 **Left,** A posterolateral approach to the talus. A lateral approach adjacent to the Achilles tendon is carried out down to the posterolateral tubercle after reflection of the flexor hallucis longus. **Right,** Cannulated screws can be placed to this area at a biomechanical advantage for fracture fixation.

malleolus and causes comminution on the medial side.[18,30] Because the talus articulates with three facets of the calcaneus, a malalignment may alter the mechanical relationships and lead to future degeneration. Alterations in alignment may be responsible for delayed degenerative arthrosis in the subtalar joint and ankle.

To avoid these complications, we advocate use of anterolateral and anteromedial incisions to address the neck comminution and rotational malalignment. Because supination often plays a role in the higher grades of injury, rotation of the neck will occur. Subtalar instability also occurs and needs to be addressed in the reduction. When using a posterior lateral approach, an anteromedial or anterolateral approach also is necessary to achieve temporary reduction and to check alignment. The Canale view provides the best check for neck malalignment; it often is difficult to judge small degrees of malrotation using the image intensifier or routine radiograph. The importance of good talar neck alignment was brought out by a recent laboratory study in which certain degrees of malalignment were fixed into the talar neck reduction and contact stress areas were evaluated. It was found that there was a change in the weightbearing load pathway and in the contact stresses and peak pressures of the subtalar joint with talar neck malalignment.[30]

Treatment

Class I Injury Class I injuries occur when there is a minimal displacement of the distal fracture fragment (Fig. 9). These injuries can usually be treated by closed means with an anatomic reduction that includes correction of the minimal dorsal displacement and talar neck supination. The incidence of osteonecrosis is low (10%) because the circulation is usually intact.[2,3] If an anatomic reduction is obtained, as confirmed by appropriate radiographs, a cast can be used for treatment until trabeculation is demonstrated. Weightbearing is allowed only after trabeculation occurs across the talar neck because of the problem of shear forces with weightbearing before trabeculation, particularly without rigid fixation. If anatomic reduction cannot be obtained, or if there is significant comminution, open

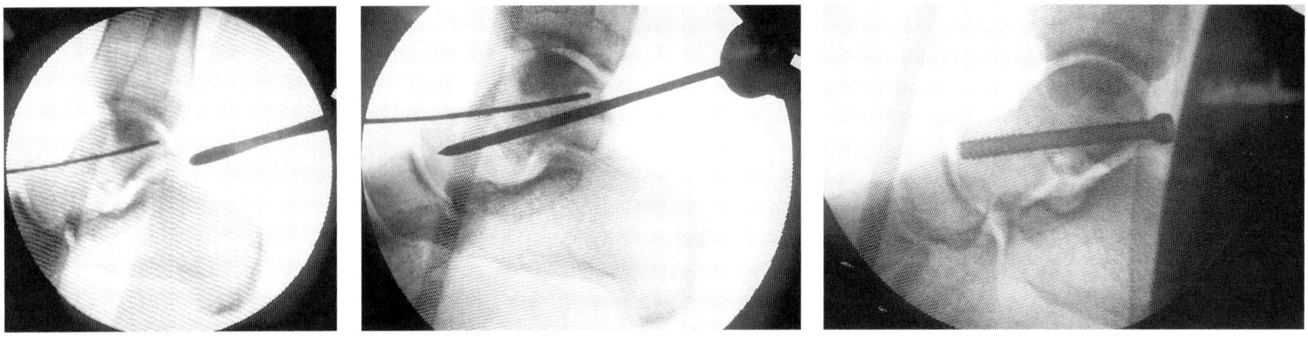

Fig. 13 **Left and center,** Fixation from the posterolateral approach provides the best biomechanical fixation for fractures of the talar neck and body. The screws are usually firmly fixed in the talar head at an angle between 90° and 45°. **Right,** The posterolateral approach with use of image intensifier and fixation with large titanium cannulated screws.

or percutaneous reduction with screws can be used. An anteromedial or anterolateral approach should be used to achieve provisional K-wire reduction, and it can be combined with a posterolateral approach for screw insertion for improved fracture mechanics.

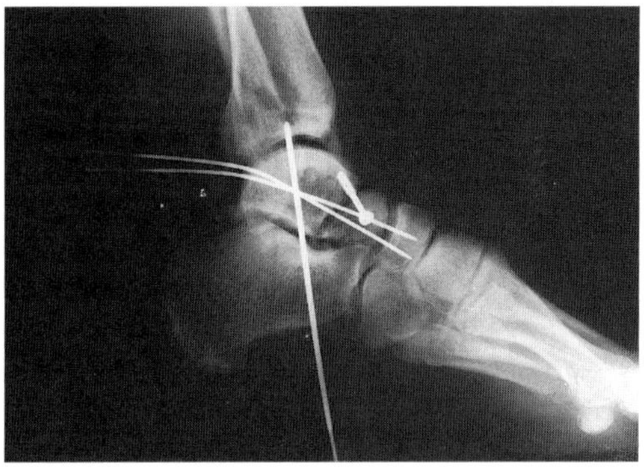

Fig. 14 Retrograde K-wires can be used from anterior medial approach.

The classic approach to the talar neck fracture has been the anteromedial approach (Fig. 10). There is a safe interval adjacent to the anterior tibial tendon. The incision may need to be extended to the ankle joint, and care should be taken to avoid any periosteal stripping. The problem with this approach is the difficulty in obtaining good biomechanical fixation at the fracture site because the talar neck is deviated and shortened in a medial direction. The threads of the screws usually exit the lateral cortex just proximal to the fracture and do not give adequate compression in an axis perpendicular to the fracture site. Although I do not believe that there is any place for K-wire fixation alone in open treatment, K-wires (0.062) often can be used in combination with an appropriate threaded screw to supply some rotational stability (Fig. 11). At our institution, 4.5- or 6.5-mm titanium cannulated screws have been very helpful. Other centers have felt that fully threaded screws were much stronger, but we have had no problem with breakage. It is important to restate that lateral, anterior, and oblique radiographs with Canale view should be obtained for each patient at the conclusion of treatment because the image intensifier often may fail to give an accurate picture of the reduction.

The anterolateral approach is a better approach for fixation of the fracture (Fig. 11, *right*). This approach is preferred in higher grades of injury, when the medial neck often is comminuted and the lateral aspect is not. When there is subtalar injury, the sinus tarsi may have bone fragmentation that needs debridement. The problem with this approach is the risk of causing damage to the anterior tibial perforating vessels and the superficial branch of the peroneal nerve. The anterolateral approach is appropriate for higher grades of injury, particularly when there is medial comminution or sinus tarsi debris.

A posterolateral approach, which was described by Trillat and associates[31] has been used in combination with an anteromedial open or closed manipulation of the fracture site.[32,33] In the posterolateral approach (Fig. 12, *left*) using an image intensifier, the patient is placed in the prone or lateral position, and the incision is made lateral to the heel cord. The enlarged lateral posterior process of the talus adjacent to the flexor hallucis muscle mass is identified. After fracture reduction with an anteromedial or anterolateral incision and provisional K-wire fixation, titanium cannulated screws are used (Figs. 12, *right*, and 13).

Another technique used is opening the fracture and, with the patient in the lateral position and using the anteromedial approach, passing K-wires retrograde across the proximal fracture and out the posterolateral aspect. The problem with this approach is that the cannulated K-wires often are not directed out the appropriate posterolateral tubercle (Fig. 14).

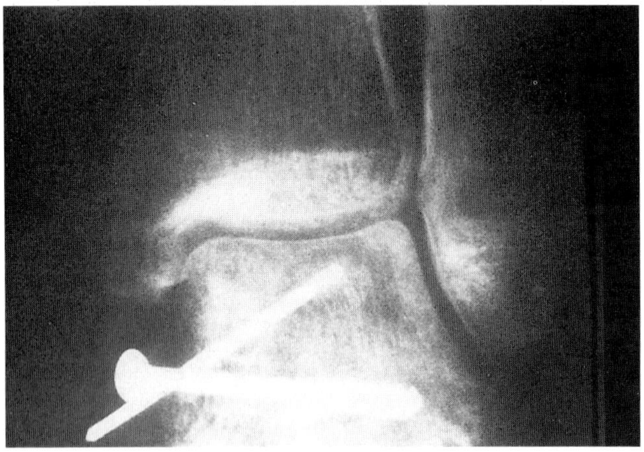

Fig. 15 A mortise view of the ankle between 6 and 10 weeks after injury can show evidence of some resorption, which indicates revascularization of the body of the talus (Hawkins sign).

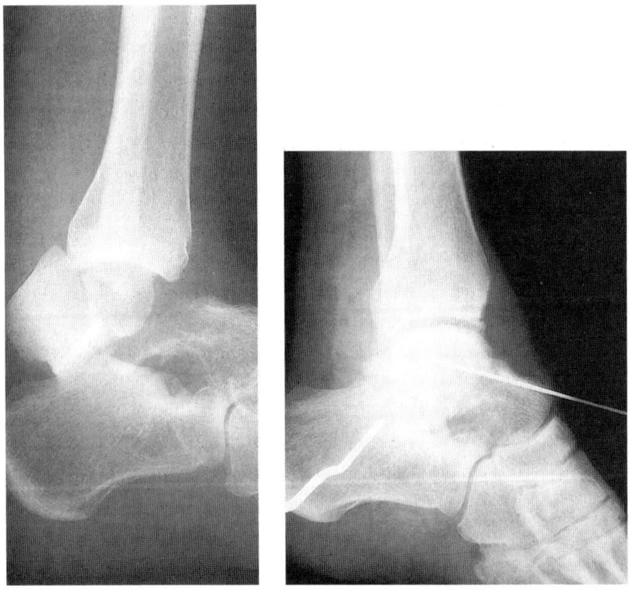

Fig. 16 **Left,** Closed reduction techniques are used for initial reduction of a class III injury in which the talus has been dislocated, usually in the medial direction. **Right,** Traction usually is applied with a pin through the os calcis in combination with equinus positioning and rotation to allow the talar body to be relocated in the subtalar joint. Getting the body over the posterior articular process is sometimes difficult, and a femoral distractor may be necessary.

We have found that it is difficult to obtain a good closed reduction. Therefore, a combined anteromedial or anterolateral approach should be used to open the fracture and anatomically hold it. We believe that no important blood supply is violated by either the anteromedial or the posterolateral approach. Once again, it is important to obtain good radiographs at the conclusion of treatment, particularly an oblique film as

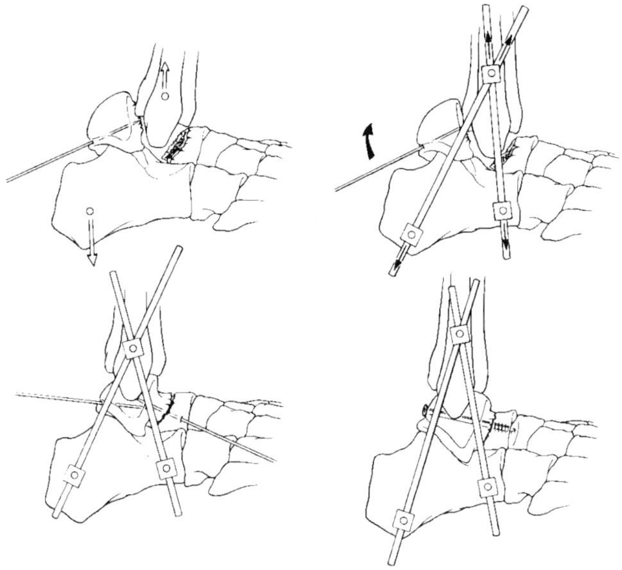

Fig. 17 A femoral distractor is used for difficult class III injuries to hold the anatomic height of the hindfoot. It can be used whether or not the talar body is available for reinsertion into the mortise.

described by Canale and Kelly,[12] before accepting a closed or open reduction.

In summary, closed reduction should never be done in displaced injuries. We do not use K-wires as a sole means of fixation because they have been found to be much weaker than screws. Histomorphic analysis has shown that bone density is greatest in the lateral portion of the head and inferior lateral portion of the body.[34] Screws inserted from the posterior to anterior provide better biomechanical fixation than those inserted from anterior to posterior.[34] We recommend the use of titanium screws, particularly in unstable fractures in which osteonecrosis is a possibility and magnetic resonance imaging (MRI) may be necessary, because MRI can be used with titanium screws.[35] The approach depends on the location of the comminution and the fracture type. We feel that a posterolateral approach gives the best biomechanical fixation. An anteromedial or anterolateral approach should accompany this approach to ensure an accurate reduction.

Class II Injury The disruption of the talocalcaneal ligament in class II injuries makes it difficult to obtain a closed anatomic reduction (Fig. 9, *center*). Open reduction is indicated in the presence of 3 mm of dorsal displacement or any rotational deformity that will impede the ability to obtain an accurate closed anatomic reduction. The anteromedial or anterolateral approach is combined with a posterolateral approach for screw fixation. It is critical to obtain an anatomic reduction and to ensure that the subtalar joint has been reduced.

The postoperative care of patients with class

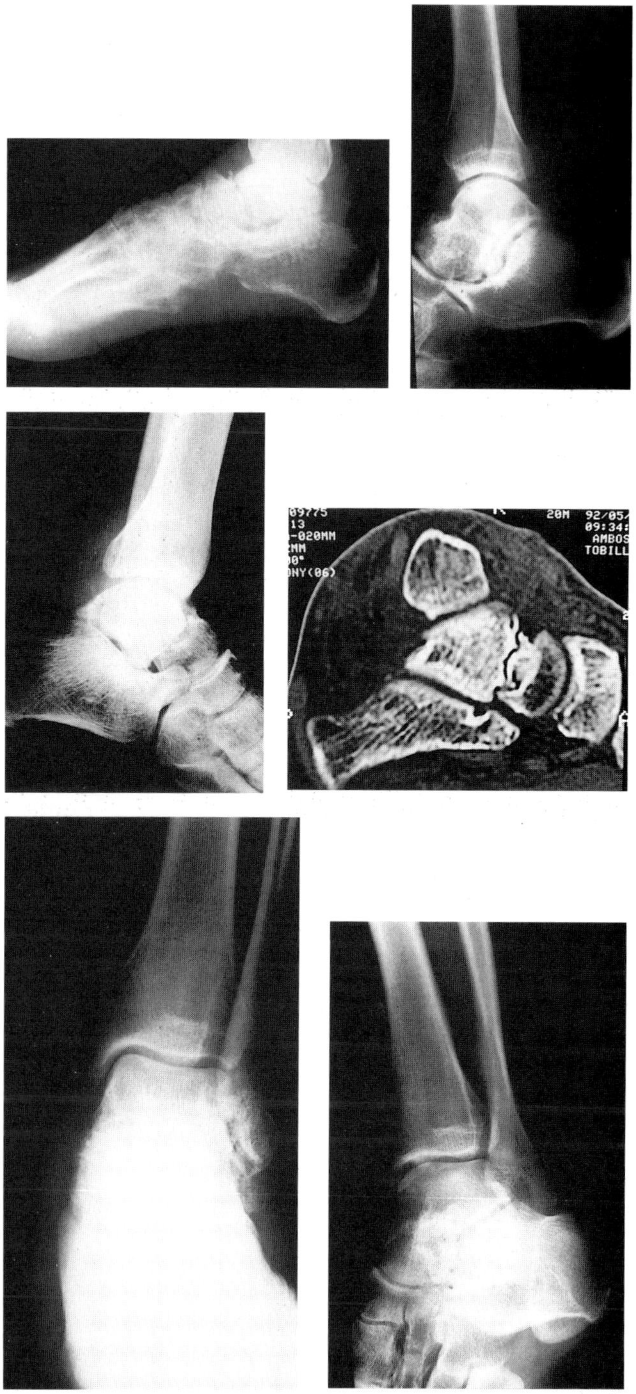

Fig. 18 **Top,** Malunion of talar neck. **Center,** Nonunion of talar neck. **Bottom,** Subtalar arthritis from fracture or sinus tarsi debris.

II injuries is directly related to the biomechanical rigidity of fixation. With rigid fixation, the patient should be encouraged to start early motion, but then a short leg cast should be used. It is important that no weightbearing be allowed for at least 3 months or until trabeculation is demonstrated to avoid shear forces. At 8 weeks, the orthopaedic surgeon should evaluate an anteroposterior (AP) or mortise view to determine signs of vascularization (Hawkins Sign)[13] (Fig. 15).

Class III Injury In class III talar neck fractures, the talar body and subtalar joint subluxate or dislocate (Fig. 9, *right,* and 16). A large percentage of these injuries are open (50%), and the incidence of osteonecrosis has been reported to be greater than 50%.[2,3,7] The body of the talus should be reduced by open reduction as soon as possible to decrease the stress on the medial neurovascular bundle. It is important not to injure the deltoid vessels. Manipulation requires the use of an os calcis traction pin and external fixator or femoral distraction (Figs. 16, *right,* and 17). This reduction can be difficult, requiring traction, equinus, and rotation. The associated soft-tissue injuries usually are debrided and left open if they do not violate a joint space or tendons. If the talar body cannot be relocated from its displaced position by closed manipulation, a posterior medial incision is required. The neurovascular bundle is retracted, and direct manipulation of the body of the talus is attempted. K-wires can be used to hold the body of the talus in the mortise temporarily and as a joy stick to reduce it. A femoral distractor is also helpful in cases that resist closed attempts (Fig. 17).

Complications

The complications that occur with talar neck fractures are delayed union, nonunion, malunion, subtalar and ankle arthritis, and osteonecrosis (Figs. 18 and 19). Reports of long-term complications from this injury[9,15,16,18,28,29,35] indicate that osteonecrosis occurred in only 10% of nondisplaced fracture cases but approached 70% when there was significant displacement. Delayed unions occurred primarily in class II and class III injuries, and the incidence of subtalar arthritis also became higher as the grade of injury increased. The major morbid complication of a talar neck fracture is osteonecrosis.

Osteonecrosis

Osteonecrosis has been shown to increase with severity of injury.[9,29] The Hawkins sign has been described as evidence of revascularization and is felt to be a specific, reliable early indicator of vascular viability with few false negatives. This sign of patchy subchondral osteoporosis usually occurs in 6 to 8 weeks and can be visualized radiographically on the AP or mortise view but not on the lateral view, because it is obscured by the fibula (Figs. 15 and 19).[13,36] MRI has been used to diagnose and quantify the degree of osteonecrosis. We usually recommend waiting at least 3 months until bone healing is present before doing an MRI. MRI has been very sensitive and few false negative reports have been published. In trabecular bone, the marrow elements are predominately fat cells. The fat cells are responsible for the strong T1-weighted MRI

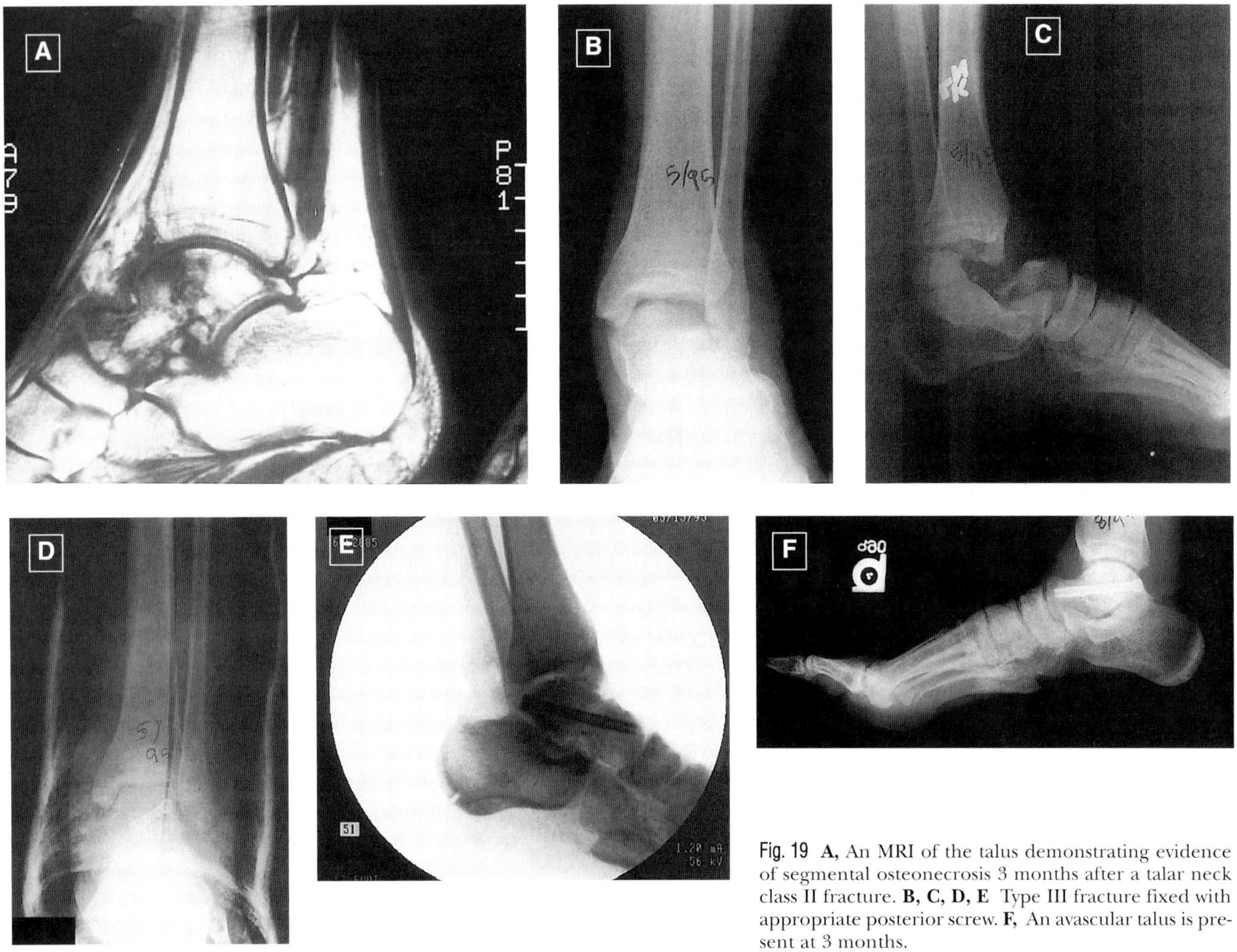

Fig. 19 **A,** An MRI of the talus demonstrating evidence of segmental osteonecrosis 3 months after a talar neck class II fracture. **B, C, D, E** Type III fracture fixed with appropriate posterior screw. **F,** An avascular talus is present at 3 months.

images and the MRI is sensitive to altered fat cell signals because marrow necrosis is an early part of osteonecrosis (Fig. 19).[37]

The determination of when to put weight on the talus is made from radiographic evidence of bone healing or trabeculation. The method of weightbearing, whether it is foot flat, associated with a patella tendon brace, or associated with some type of ankle orthosis to hold the ankle in equinus, is determined by the extent of osteonecrosis. Osteonecrosis may take up to 2 years to heal. There have been no outcome studies done on osteonecrosis of the talus and it is surprising how well patients do in the face of an avascular talus. We have counseled them as to their disease process and recommend that they not do running athletic events until there is evidence of healing. We do not believe that there is any clear evidence that revascularization procedures, subtalar arthrodesis, or core decompressions are of any long-term benefit. It has been recommended that displaced talar fractures or class II and III Hawkins fractures be treated with titanium screws in order to allow use of MRI in the event of osteonecrosis. Titanium has nonmagnetic properties and creates a signal void, which is only slightly larger than the actual implant. Stainless steel implants, however, have ferromagnetic properties, which cause significant distortion on the MRI.[35]

Talar Body Fractures

Fractures of the talar body are less common than talar neck fractures, and they are classified into five groups. These fractures constitute about 20% of all talar fractures (Fig. 20). The most common talar body fractures are located in the posterior process and lateral tubercle.[2,3] Talar fractures have been classified into group I, osteochondral fractures; group II, fractures of the body of the talus, including coronal, sagittal, horizontal, and shear fractures; group III, posterior process fractures of both the medial and the posterior tubercle; group IV, lateral tubercle fractures; and group V, crush or compression injuries of the talar body. The group II

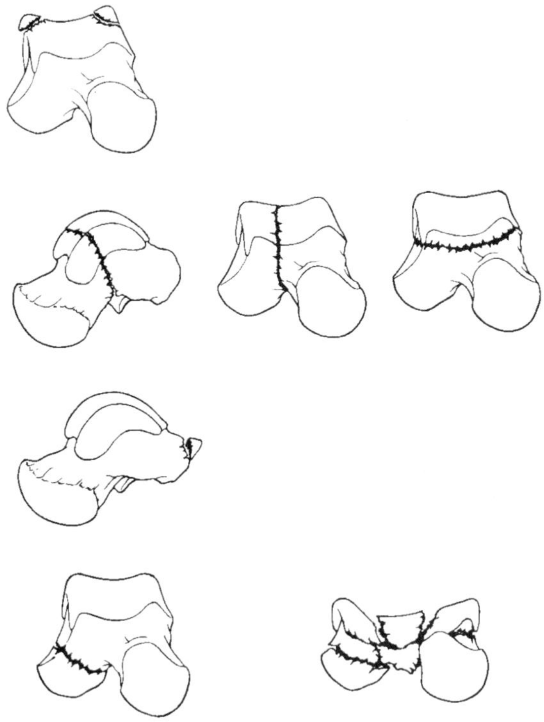

Fig. 20 Classification of talar body fractures. **Top,** Osteochondral fracture (class I). **Top center,** Sagittal, vertical, and horizontal talar body injuries (class II). **Bottom center,** Posterior process fracture (class III). **Bottom left,** Lateral tubercle fracture (class IV). **Bottom right,** Crush injury (class V).

and V fractures of the body of the talus have an osteonecrosis incidence of 25% when no dislocations occur. With dislocation, they have a greater than 50% incidence of osteonecrosis and take an average of 3 to 4 months for bone union. Nonunion and subtalar ankle osteoarthritis are common with these injuries. Group II fractures are body fractures without significant comminution. They are classified with respect to the direction of the fracture: vertical, horizontal, or coronal (Fig. 20).[38,39] It often is necessary to use CT to define the fracture pattern and plan surgical strategy (Fig. 21). Because these fractures occur underneath the ankle mortise, exposure is required to perform medial or lateral malleolar osteotomy or to retract the fractures (Fig. 22).[40]

Fixation of talar body fractures involves temporary fixation with K-wires, debridement of small articular fractures that cannot be fixed, and the use of 4.0-mm titanium cannulated lag screws or subarticular fixation. The small head subarticular 3.0-mm screws will not be removed. The critical factor is the best possible reconstruction of the body's articular surface. The articular gaps will fill in with fibrous tissue (Fig. 23).

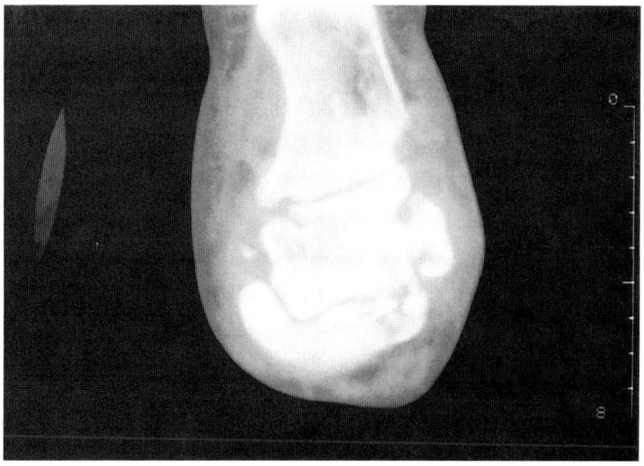

Fig. 21 A computed tomographic scan of a crushed or comminuted body of the talus (fracture class V).

Talar Salvage Problems

It is important to discuss the severely traumatized avascular or completely detached body of the talus. The goal is to preserve the body of the talus whenever it can be safely reimplanted into the mortise. The body of the talus is used to maintain the hindfoot architecture until soft-tissue healing will allow the best reconstructive procedure for the future. We use femoral distractors and external fixators to preserve hindfoot length and achieve soft-tissue healing or coverage (Fig. 24).

If the talus is missing or cannot be salvaged, then the best reconstructive procedure is a delayed Blair fusion (Fig. 25) or a tibiocalcaneal arthrodesis with iliac crest distraction grafts.[41,42] The Blair procedure is a good reconstructive procedure, but it is difficult to obtain union into the vascularized remaining portion of the talar head. With this procedure, the tibia is fused to the live portion of the talar neck after excision of the body of the talus. An attempt is made to leave the subtalar joint free to allow some minimal hindfoot motion in the area. It is difficult to obtain good fixation and not to alter the talonavicular articulation.

The tibiocalcaneal arthrodesis is done with the use of large corticocancellous iliac or bank bone grafts, which are implanted in place of the osteonecrotic body of the talus and are secured with cannulated screws from the heel to the tibia (Fig. 26). The use of good fixation screws with appropriate bone graft can maintain the anatomic hindfoot architecture; the rigidity of the fixation is important to allow revascularization. A talectomy is the last choice for a salvage procedure. A talectomy gives a severely unstable and uncosmetic shortened hindfoot, which is not tolerated well by the neurologically intact adult patient.

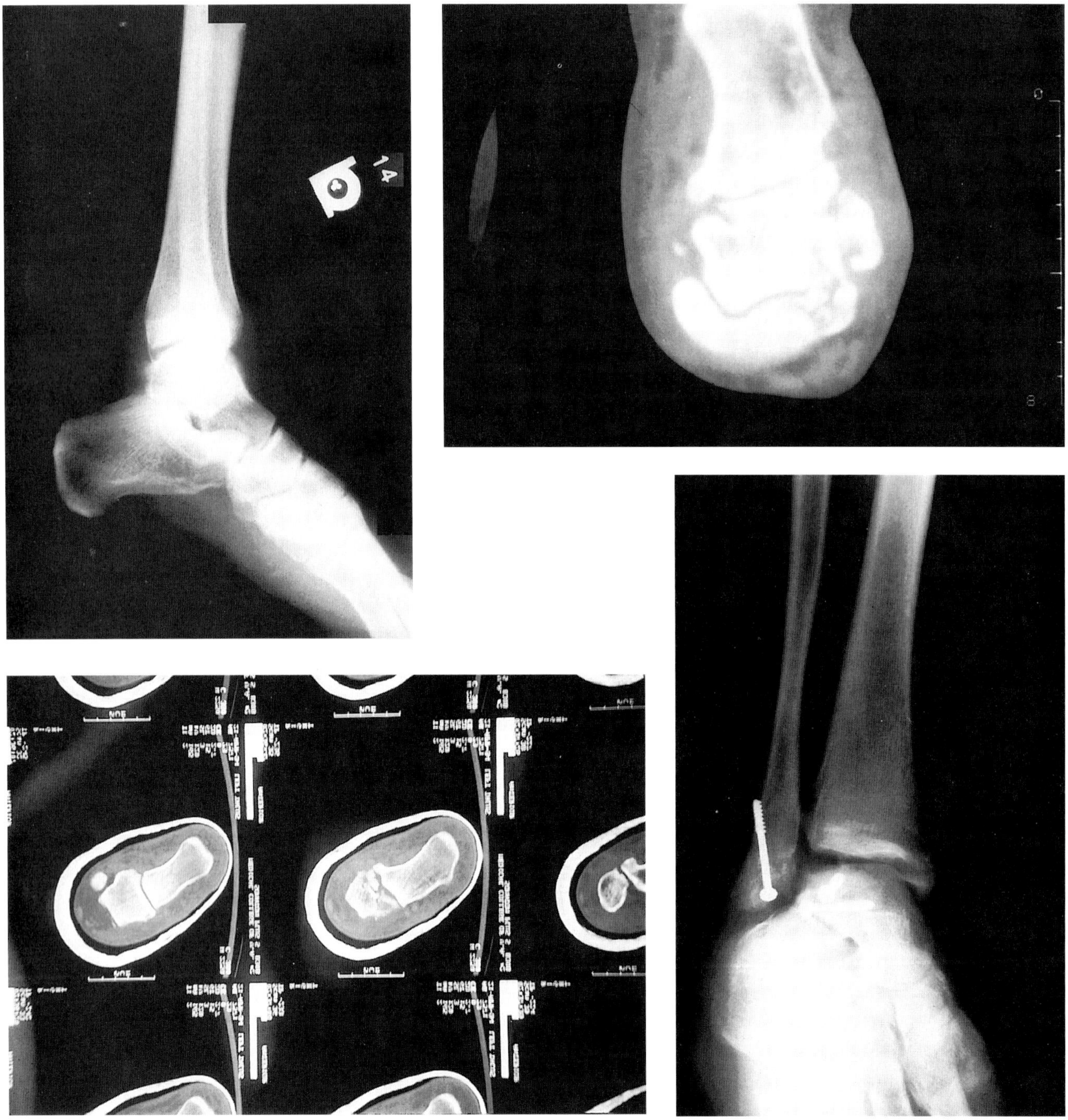

Fig. 22 Osteotomy of the lateral malleolus is often needed to treat comminuted fractures of the body of the talus. Care should be taken not to destroy the deltoid ligament.

Open Fractures of the Talus

Up to 50% of class III Hawkins injuries are open injuries of the talus. These injuries often involve marked fracture displacement, disrupted blood supply, severe soft-tissue damage, and contamination. The functional outcome of open injuries has recently been evaluated by Marsh and associates.[43] An infection rate of 38% for previously open injuries of the talus is quite high, and it appears higher than that associated with other open lower extremity injuries such as that to the tibia. The high infection rate associated with these open talar injuries was attributed to more skin damage, a larger dead space, and disruption of bone blood supply. The extruded talus has a particularly high inci-

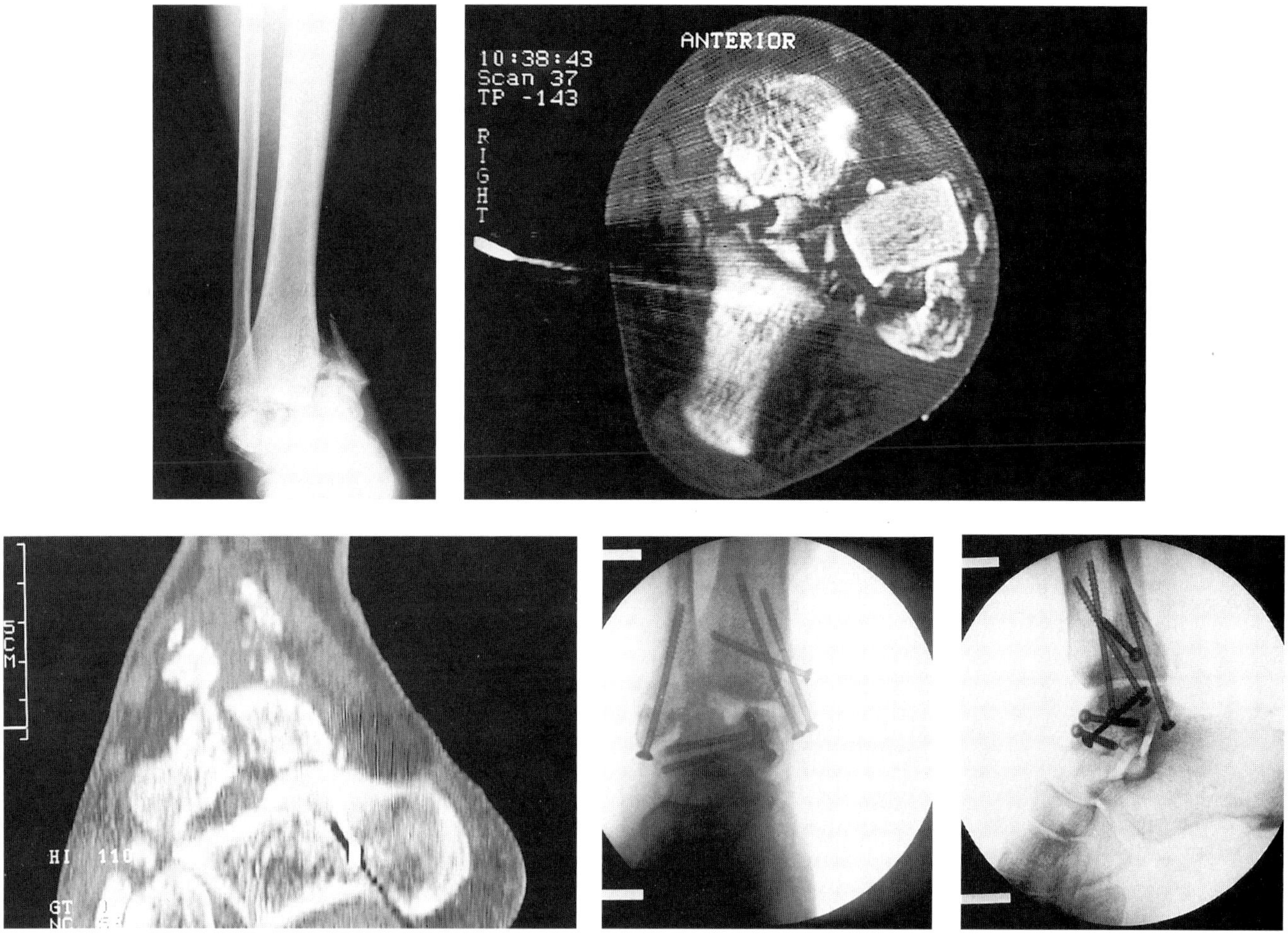

Fig. 23 A severely comminuted talar body can still be salvaged with fixation of larger fragments and debridement of smaller fragments.

dence of infection, which has a negative impact on outcome, with many requiring late partial to complete talar body excisions.[43] Therefore, if an open injury is associated with an extruded talus and there is significant contamination, it may be more appropriate to maintain hindfoot architecture with an external fixator and perform a late Blair fusion or tibiocalcaneal arthrodesis. This will always remain a judgment call, but I feel that it is appropriate to report that there is a higher incidence of late infections with open talar injuries.

Outcome of Talus Fractures

Recent literature has provided evidence of the outcome of talus fractures. The incidence of malunion is related to whether the fracture is opened appropriately for reduction. It is more difficult to determine the accuracy of the reduction in fractures treated closed. Canale views obtained after reduction of talar fractures have revealed incidences of malunion as high as 27%, with varus malunion being the most common deformity.[18,28,29,44] The degree of malunion decreases if the fractures were treated with open reduction. A malunion is much less of a problem if two incisions are made to fix an exposed lesion. Appropriate views in the operating room can be taken by image intensifier or by standard radiograph using the Canale technique. Dorsal malunions are usually taken care of by excision of the beak. Varus malunions are more difficult to control, and results of biomechanical studies indicate that they create problems in load transference to the foot.[30]

The incidence of posttraumatic arthritis differs depending on whether the injury was to the tibiotalar or the talocalcaneal joint. Subtalar arthrosis depends on degree of injury, with the more severe injuries having increased rates of postinjury arthrosis.[18,28,44] In a recent series of 108 patients with a 5-month follow-up,[28] the range of motion of the tibiotalar joint was restricted to about half of normal and inversion/eversion of the subtalar joint also was restricted by 50%. The incidence of arthrosis reached 50% in the highest Hawkins

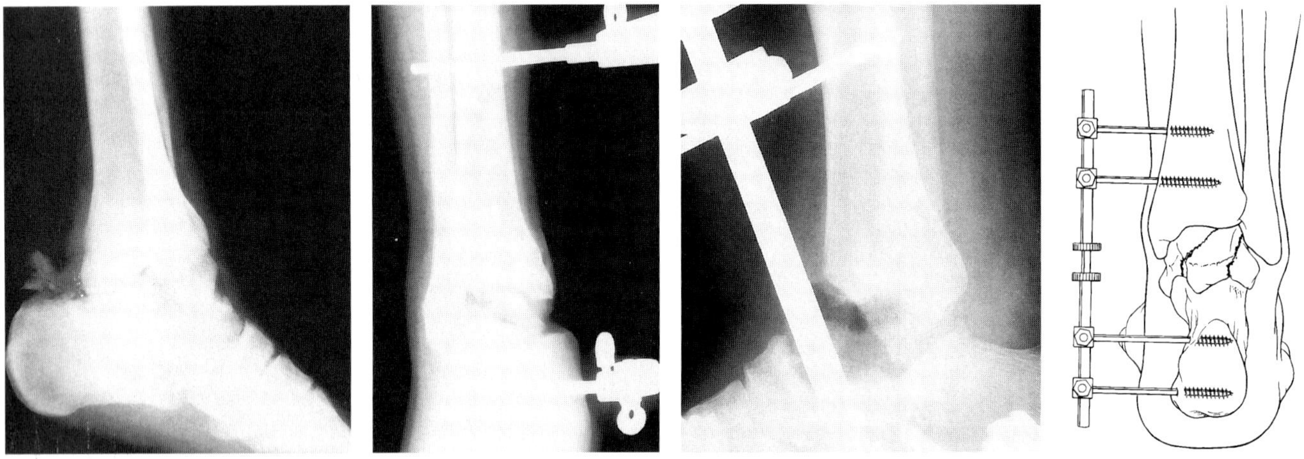

Fig. 24 A femoral distractor for an external fixator can maintain the height of the heel in the absence of the body of the talus until a secondary reconstructive procedure can be done (usually 6 to 8 weeks after injury) unless there is a severe soft-tissue compromise.

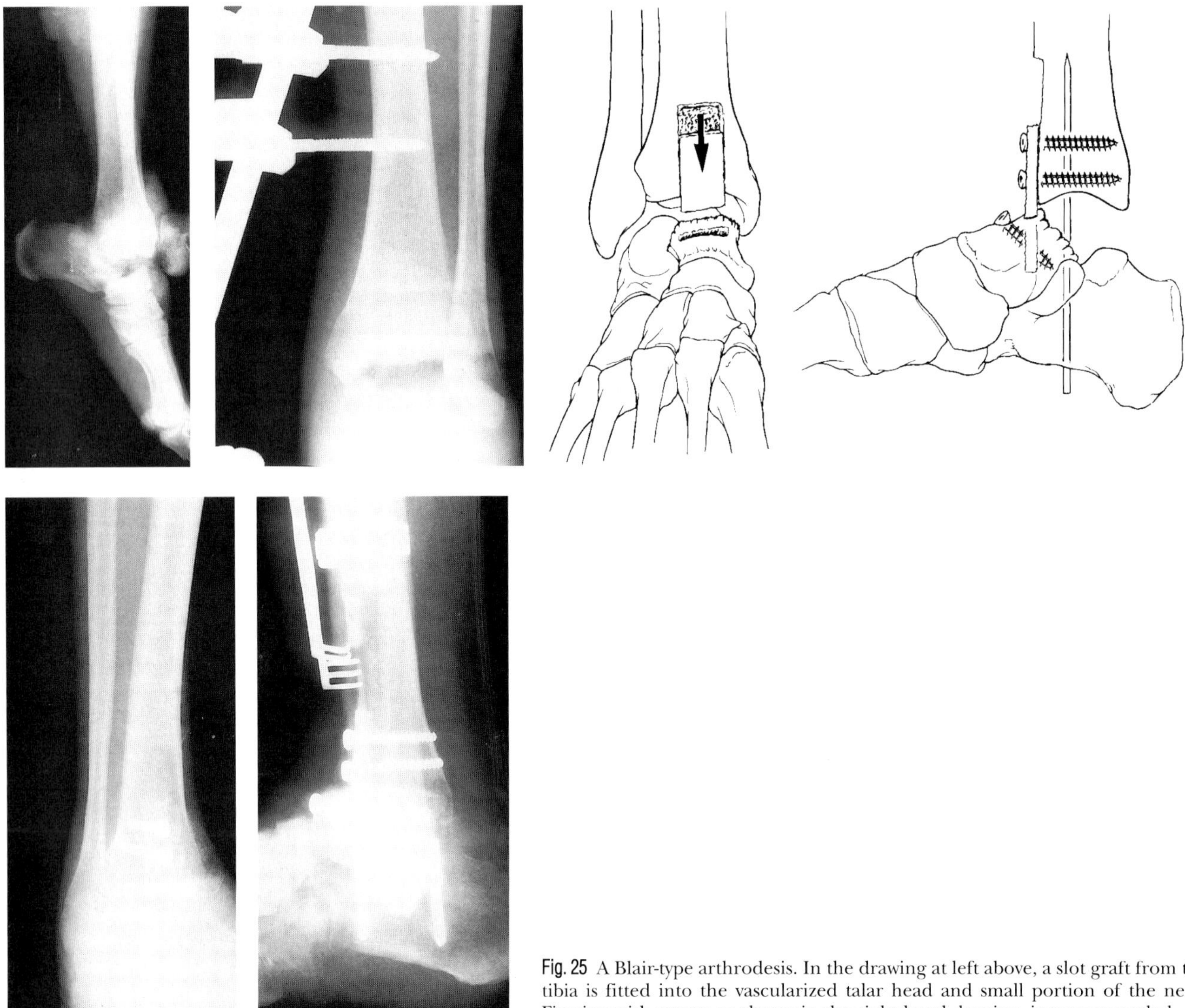

Fig. 25 A Blair-type arthrodesis. In the drawing at left above, a slot graft from the tibia is fitted into the vascularized talar head and small portion of the neck. Fixation with screws, as shown in the right hand drawing, is recommended.

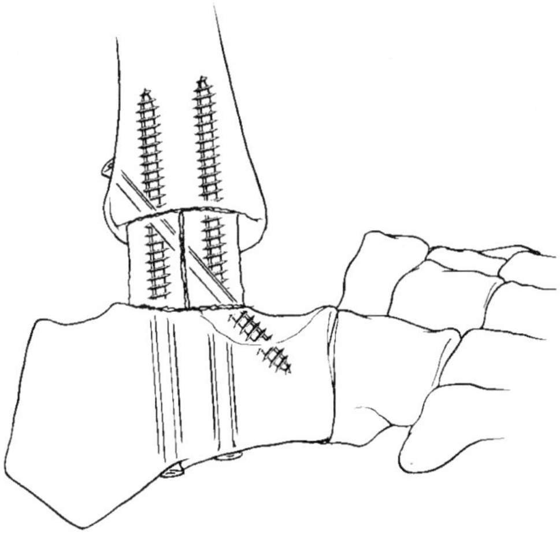

Fig. 26 Reconstruction for loss of the body of the talus. When there is insufficient talar head for a Blair fusion, a tibiocalcaneal fusion with a corticocancellous iliac slot graft and cancellous screw fixation from heel to tibia are done.

type III fractures. The results in this study paralleled the expected degree of injury. Tibiotalar joint arthrosis does not appear to parallel the degree of injury and stays fairly constant. Some have thought that prolonged periods of immobilization may play a role in the restricted range of motion and arthrosis. The use of more appropriate and early passive ranges of motion after surgery is being stressed to improve the degrees of arthrosis and restriction.

The incidence of osteonecrosis has certainly paralleled the degree of injury, but early appropriate reductions and rigid fixation should help reduce the degree of severity of the osteonecrosis in the talar body. It is much safer to walk on a partially osteonecrotic talus than on a completely osteonecrotic talus. The incidence of osteonecrosis cannot be prevented but the degree of osteonecrosis may depend on treatment. The morbidity of the osteonecrosis will also depend on the postoperative regimen and clear diagnosis using MRI when appropriate. Decreasing the amount of varus and valgus stresses and loads through the ankle should help decrease the morbidity from osteonecrosis. A higher percentage of excellent and good results has been found in those series in which weightbearing was delayed until there was evidence of bone healing.

Summary

Injuries of the talus make up a significant proportion of complex foot and ankle injuries. The severity of these injuries is increasing because the availability and use of better safety equipment has allowed more people to survive serious accidents. Early rigid and accurate anatomic fixation lead to the best possible outcome for each category of talar injury. If osteonecrosis is suspected, titanium screws should be used for fixation to allow better postoperative follow-up. Treatment of osteonecrosis of the talus still depends mainly on clinical judgment, with the MRI providing more clinical data. The outcome of the osteonecrotic talus has not been established at this point.

The approach to the talus depends on the judgment and skill of the surgeon; two approaches usually are indicated for more severe injuries. A CT scan is quite helpful for fractures of the talar body; preoperative planning and the judicious use of malleolar osteotomy with preservation of the deltoid artery are advocated. Tibiotalar and talocalcaneal motion have been altered as a result of talar fractures. Arthrosis of the subtalar joint depends on the degree of injury.

References

1. Bonnin JG: Dislocations and fracture-dislocations of the talus. *Br J Surg* 1940;28:88–100.
2. DeLee JC: Fractures and dislocations of the foot, in Mann RA (ed): *Surgery of the Foot,* ed 5. St Louis, MO, CV Mosby, 1986, pp 592–808.
3. Heckman JD: Fractures and dislocations of the foot, in Rockwood CA Jr, Green DP (eds): *Fractures in Adults.* Philadelphia, PA, JB Lippincott, 1984, vol 2, pp 1703–1832.
4. Anderson HG, Flack MW, Gotch OH (eds): *The Medical and Surgical Aspects of Aviation.* London, England, H Frowde, 1919.
5. Coltart WD: "Aviator's astragalus." *J Bone Joint Surg* 1952;34B:545–566.
6. Pennal GF: Fractures of the talus. *Clin Orthop* 1963;30:53–63.
7. Dunn AR, Jacobs B, Campbell RD Jr: Fractures of the talus. *J Trauma* 1966;6:443–468.
8. Penny JN, Davis LA: Fractures and fracture-dislocations of the neck of the talus. *J Trauma* 1980;20:1029–1037.
9. Gilquist J, Oretop N, Stenstrom A, et al: Late results after vertical fracture of the talus. *Injury* 1974;6:173–179.
10. Mindell ER, Cisek EE, Kartalian G, et al: Late results of injuries to the talus: Analysis of forty cases. *J Bone Joint Surg* 1963;45A:221–245.
11. Kenwright J, Taylor RG: Major injuries of the talus. *J Bone Joint Surg* 1970;52B:36–48.
12. Canale ST, Kelly FB Jr: Fractures of the neck of the talus: Long-term evaluation of seventy-one cases. *J Bone Joint Surg* 1978;60A:143–156.
13. Hawkins LG: Fractures of the neck of the talus. *J Bone Joint Surg* 1970;52A:991–1002.
14. Kleiger B: Fractures of the talus. *J Bone Joint Surg* 1948;30A:735–744.
15. Lorentzen JE, Christensen SB, Krogsoe O, et al: Fractures of the neck of the talus. *Acta Orthop Scand* 1977;48:115–120.
16. Pantazopoulos T, Galanos P, Vayanos E, et al: Fractures of the neck of the talus. *Acta Orthop Scand* 1974;45:296–306.
17. Zwipp H: Severe foot trauma in combination with talar injuries, in Tscherne H, Schatzker J (eds): *Major Fractures of the Pilon, the Talus, and the Calcaneus: Current Concepts of Treatment.* Berlin, Germany, Springer-Verlag, 1993, pp 123–135.
18. Daniels TR, Smith JW: Talar neck fractures. *Foot Ankle* 1993;14:225–234.
19. Hawkins LG: Fracture of the lateral process of the talus: A review of thirteen cases. *J Bone Joint Surg* 1965;47A:1170–1175.20. Heckman JD, McLean MR: Fractures of the lateral process of the talus. *Clin Orthop* 1985;199:108–113.

20. Heckman JD, McLean MR: Fractures of the lateral process of the talus. *Clin Orthop* 1985;199:108–113.
21. Mukherjee SK, Pringle RM, Baxter AD: Fracture of the lateral process of the talus: A report of thirteen cases. *J Bone Joint Surg* 1974;56B:263–273.
22. Haliburton RA, Sullivan CR, Kelly PJ, et al: The extra-osseous and intra-osseous blood supply of the talus. *J Bone Joint Surg* 1958;40A:1115–1120.
23. Kelly PJ, Sullivan CR: Blood supply of the talus. *Clin Orthop* 1963;30:37–44.
24. Mulfinger GL, Trueta J: The blood supply of the talus. *J Bone Joint Surg* 1970;52B:160–167.
25. Wildenauer E: Die Blutversorgung des Talus. *Z Anat Entwicklungsgesch* 1950;115:32–36.
26. Larson RL, Sullivan CR, Janes JM: Trauma, surgery, and circulation of the talus: What are the risks of avascular necrosis? *J Trauma* 1961;1:13–21.
27. Peterson L, Romanus B, Dahlberg E: Fracture of the collum tali: An experimental study. *J Biomech* 1976;9:277–279.
28. Szyszkowitz R, Seggl W, Wildburger R: Late results of fractures and fracture-dislocation after ORIF, in Tscherne H, Schatzker J (eds): *Major Fractures of the Pilon, the Talus, and the Calcaneus: Current Concepts of Treatment.* Berlin, Germany, Springer–Verlag, 1993, pp 105–112.
29. Behrens F: Long-term results of displaced talar neck fractures, in Tscherne H, Schatzker J (eds): *Major Fractures of the Pilon, the Talus, and the Calcaneus: Current Concepts of Treatment.* Berlin, Germany, Springer–Verlag, 1993, pp 113–121.
30. Sangeorzan BJ, Wagner UA, Harrington RM, et al: Contact characteristics of the subtalar joint: The effect of talar neck misalignment. *J Orthop Res* 1992;10:544–551.
31. Trillat A, Bousquet G, Lapeyre B: Displacerd fractures of the neck or of the body of the talus: Value of screwing by posterior surgical approach. *Rev Chir Orthop Reparatrice Appar Mot* 1970;56:529–536.
32. Gatellier J: The juxtoretroperoneal route in the operative treatment of fracture of the malleolus with posterior marginal fragment. *Surg Gynecol Obstet* 1931;52:67–70.
33. Lemaire RG, Bustin W: Screw fixation of fractures of the neck of the talus using a posterior approach. *J Trauma* 1980;20:669–673.
34. Swanson T, Bray T: Talar neck fractures: A mechanical and histomorphometric study of fixation. *Orthop Trans* 1989;13:762.
35. Comfort TH, Behrens F, Gaither DW, et al: Long-term results of displaced talar neck fractures. *Clin Orthop* 1985;199:81–87.
36. Henderson RC: Posttraumatic necrosis of the talus: The Hawkins sign versus magnetic resonance imaging. *J Orthop Trauma* 1991;5:96–99.
37. Bobechko WP, Harris WR: The radiographic density of avascular bone. *J Bone Joint Surg* 1960;42B:626–632.
38. Alexander AH, Lichtman DM: Surgical treatment of transchondral talar-dome fractures (osteochondritis dissecans): Long-term follow-up. *J Bone Joint Surg* 1980;62A:646–652.
39. Sneppen O, Christensen SB, Krogsoe O, et al: Fracture of the body of the talus. *Acta Orthop Scand* 1977;48:317–324.
40. Deyerle WM, Burkhardt B, Comfort T, et al: Displaced fractures of the talus: An agressive approach. *Orthop Trans* 1981;5:465.
41. Dennis MD, Tullos HS: Blair tibiotalar arthrodesis for injuries to the talus. *J Bone Joint Surg* 1980;62A:103–107.
42. Ries M, Healy WA Jr: Total dislocation of the talus: Case report with a 13-year follow up and review of the literature. *Orthop Rev* 1988;17:76–80.
43. Marsh JL, Iverson M, Shapiro D, et al: Major open injuries of the talus. *Orthop Trans* 1994;18:720–721.
44. Jensen I, Wester JU, Rasmussen F, et al: Prognosis of fracture of the talus in children: 21 (7–34) –year follow–up of 14 cases. *Acta Orthop Scand* 1994;65:398–400.

CHAPTER 33

Salvage Procedures for Calcaneus Fractures

Bruce J. Sangeorzan, MD

Introduction

A fracture of the calcaneus will heal reliably, although not anatomically, with closed treatment.[1,2] However, salvage or secondary reconstruction may be required when symptoms persist and are severe.[1,3-5] Patients may experience pain (subtalar, plantar heel, and ankle most often), stiffness, deformity, difficulty finding appropriately fitting shoewear, and difficulty walking without shoes. Many of these symptoms are directly attributable to known mechanical alterations that occur in the foot at the time of injury.[1,6-10] From a practical standpoint, the soft-tissue problems are often managed by nonsurgical means while some specific bony problems many be amenable to surgical management.

Initial Management

The most common sites of pain are the lateral subfibular area, the heel pad, and the ankle, in addition to generalized pain accompanied by stiffness and swelling. Heel pad pain, the second most common site of pain after calcaneus fracture regardless of fracture pattern or treatment,[1,7] normally occurs with weightbearing activity. In general, treatment is geared toward padding the heel externally. A simple soft heel cup, made of silicone or soft rubber and inserted in the shoe, is effective if the alignment is otherwise normal. It may be helpful to encourage the patient to wear a soft shoe with slight elevation of the heel.

The horizontal talus may abut the distal tibia anteriorly (see below).[3] Elevating the heel in a soft rubber insert or single axis cushioned heel (SACH) modification places the hindfoot into a slightly plantarflexed position in addition to providing a cushioning effect. Elevating the hind foot with an internal heel lift moves the malleoli away from the edges of the shoe so that they are not so easily irritated. Elevation also allows the hindfoot to plantarflex and corrects the dorsiflexed position of the talus within the tibiotalar joint (see below), which relieves the tibial abutment. Because the insert material is compressible, it provides additional padding beneath the heel that may compensate for the lost shock absorption of the subtalar joint. A soft heel cup allows the heel to tolerate pressure while it builds scar tissue to compensate for the loss of fat and fibrous septa. Additional modifications of the orthosis, such as adding medial or lateral post or stress relief areas, can be made to unload painful areas. An ankle lacer may be helpful when the patient is experiencing pain on uneven surfaces or to provide additional support.

Toe contractures occur for a number of reasons. Edema in the foot may lead to intrinsic contracture. These deformities are usually mild but static. The flexor digitorum longus (FDL) may be entrapped in the fracture or the fracture callous on the medial side of the heel. The FDL may also become entrapped above the ankle. In the latter case, the toes may be passively correctable with the foot fully plantarflexed. However, as the examiner dorsiflexes the ankle, the toe flexion becomes more severe and fixed. Release of the FDL or transfer into the extensor hood is usually sufficient to correct the deformity. The extra room needed for contracted toes can also be found in extra depth shoes. Toe contracture may also result from intrinsic damage from compartmental pressure.

Lindsay and Dewar[1] demonstrated a correlation between prolonged immobilization and edema. Generalized stiffness secondary to edema and prolonged immobilization is best treated by prevention. Patients whose treatment included prolonged cast treatment tend to have swelling and stiffness that is harmful to the outcome after calcaneus fracture. Whatever initial treatment is selected, it should be geared toward early mobilization and anti-edema measures to prevent severe soft-tissue contracture.

Bony Changes

The bony changes include a displaced joint surface leading to subtalar or transverse tarsal arthrosis; a wide heel with a laterally displaced but varus position; a flattened hindfoot with loss of height sufficient to restrict ankle dorsiflexion and cause the malleoli to impact on the shoe (diminished Böhler's angle with horizontal talus); and buckling of the lateral wall, causing subfibular impingement or displacing the peroneal tendons.[1,9-12] These changes can be visualized more readily when one considers the pathologic anatomy of displaced fracture.

The displacement in a typical calcaneus fracture portends the problems that occur in the unreduced but healed calcaneus fracture. The bony architecture of the calcaneus deforms into two general fracture patterns—tongue type and joint depression (Fig. 1).[9,10]

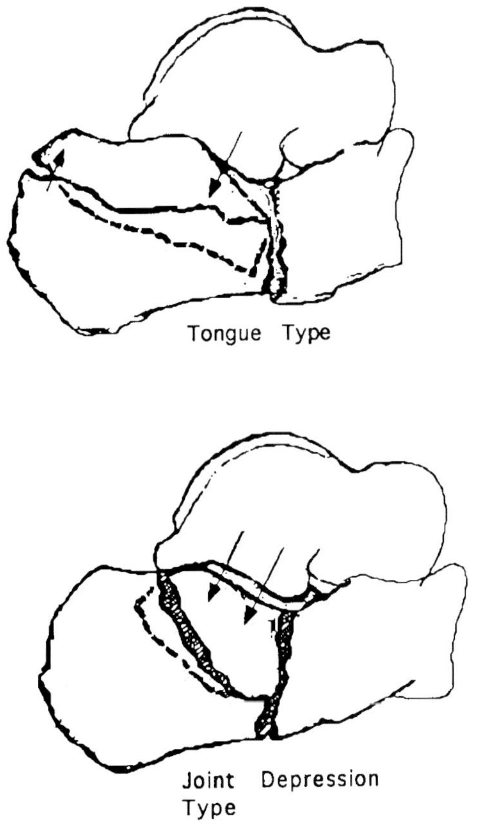

Fig. 1 Two general fracture patterns include joint depression and tongue type. In the joint-depression injury, the tuberosity breaks off along the primary fracture line and displaces laterally, anteriorly, and superiorly. The posterior facet that is attached to the tuberosity is broken off and depressed. In the tongue-type fracture, there is pure rotation of the posterior facet downward into the body of the calcaneus and upward rotation of the dorsal part of the tuberosity. With this pattern, there is less widening.

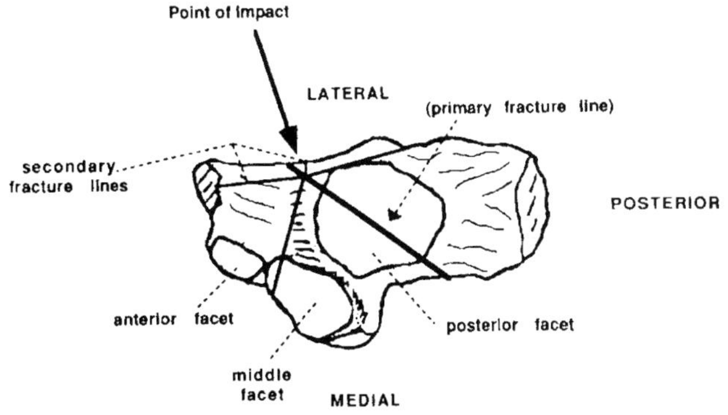

Fig. 2 The primary fracture line begins somewhere in the sinus tarsi, near the lateral wall. It passes posteriorly and medially through the posterior facet and exits medially. It separates the lateral part of the posterior facet and the tuberosity from the medial part of the posterior facet, sustentaculum tali, and the anterior and middle facet.

The fracture is most commonly caused by an axial load. In a joint depression fracture, the calcaneus is driven upward against the talus by the impact. In addition, there may be tension on the Achilles tendon acting specifically on the tuberosity. The lateral process of the talus acts as a fulcrum across which the calcaneus fractures. A fracture line is created that begins in the sinus tarsi near the lateral wall and propagates obliquely across the posterior facet to the medial wall. This fracture line, known as the primary fracture line or separation fracture, is common to most intra-articular fractures of the calcaneus (Fig. 2). The primary fracture line is less like a slice through the bone than it is like a reproducible part of a stellate fracture pattern centered in the sinus tarsi. Although its position can vary, it generally proceeds from anterolateral to posteromedial across the posterior facet and out the medial wall posterior to the sustentaculum. It divides the tuberosity and lateral wall, along with a variable part of the posterior facet, from the sustentacular fragment with the middle and anterior facet and some part of the posterior facet. In addition to this primary fracture line, many secondary fracture lines may occur. The location and number of these lines presumably is determined by the direction and force of impact, the quality of bone, and the position of the foot. Common secondary fracture lines include an anterior extension, which divides the anterior process, and a medial extension, which divides the middle facet from the posterior facet. The lateral edge of the posterior facet may be sheared off with the lateral wall.

Because the tuberosity is driven anteriorly and laterally along the oblique primary fracture line, it assumes a lateral and anterior position beneath the fibula. This leaves the heel widened and shortened. Because the fracture line is oblique, the tuberosity continues upward toward the tip of the fibula, and laterally and anteriorly. The net final position of the tuberosity is toward the underside of the fibula.

Because the posterior facet is no longer under the talus, the talus settles into a position parallel to the ground. As the tuberosity is moved laterally, it displaces further from the weightbearing axis of the limb. It may impinge on or dislocate the peroneal tendons. When the fracture heals and the individual begins bearing weight again, this relative change in the calcaneus results in a so-called horizontal talus (Fig. 3). The talus is parallel to the floor, often nearly fully dorsiflexed, even though the foot is only in a neutral position. Any attempt to dorsiflex the foot will cause the talar neck to impinge on the anterior aspect of the tibia.

The heel is wide and short for the same reasons. The fracture line is oblique, and the lateral and anterior movement leaves the heel relatively more short and wide. The subtalar joint incongruity comes from the

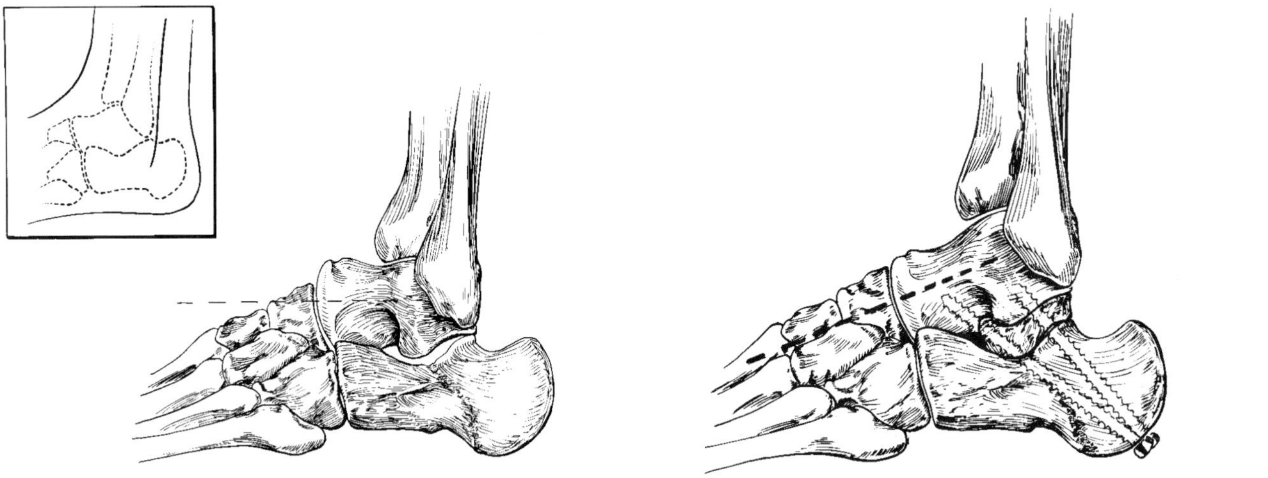

Fig. 3 **Left**, This is a schematic representation of the position the talus assumes after significant compression of the calcaneus. The axis of the talus, as seen on the lateral radiograph (dashed line), is nearly parallel to the floor when in the standing position. This is called a horizontal talus. The tibia is almost abutting the dorsum of the talus. There is no clear space to allow dorsiflexion. **Right**, This is a schematic representation of the corrected position the talus after a bone block distraction arthrodesis. Note that the axis now is properly plantarflexed and is approximately parallel to the first metatarsal. There is room for the talus to dorsiflex before impinging on the distal tibia.

obvious—the fracture displaces through the joint and it heals in that position. This constellation of changes in the subtalar joint also affects the transverse tarsal joint. Because the relative positions of the calcaneus at the cuboid (neutral) and the talus at the navicular (dorsiflexed) are different, this has the net effect of locking the transverse tarsal joint.

The so-called tongue-type fracture occurs by a similar mechanism but has less lateral translation. It may be pure downward rotation. In this pattern, there is less potential for subfibular impingement, and no alteration in the weightbearing axis. The talus is still in a horizontal position, and the ankle and transverse tarsal joints are still affected.

Simply stated, the surgically treatable anatomic problems are a wide, short heel; subfibular impingement; a horizontal talus; subtalar arthrosis; and Chopart arthrosis. Surgical techniques include ostectomy, osteotomy, arthrodeses, and structural bone grafting.

Treatment

The treatment algorithm for surgically treatable disorders includes ostectomy, osteotomy, arthrodesis, and a combination of all three. Selecting the appropriate treatment depends on history and physical examination and an understanding of the bony anatomy. Preoperative imaging includes weightbearing anteroposterior (AP) and lateral radiographs of the foot as well as an axial (Harris) view. If there is significant hindfoot deformity, ie, varus or valgus, an AP radiograph of the ankle may be helpful to determine whether there is tibiotalar arthrosis. Computed tomography (CT) is performed, when needed, in the semicoronal plane at 1.5 mm intervals. Intervals greater than 1.5 mm make reconstructions that are of poor quality. To achieve the semicoronal plane, flex both the hip and knee of the supine patient and tilt the gantry toward the patient's head. The images may be reconstructed in the sagittal or transverse plane or into 3-D format for planning an osteotomy. In addition, the degree of involvement of the joint surfaces may be evaluated best by CT.

In addition to physical examination and imaging, differential injection of local anesthetic may be a helpful diagnostic tool. The subfibular area is a common site of pain after calcaneus fracture.[1] Pain in this region may be from the subtalar joint, from the peroneal tendons, or from direct pressure between the calcaneus and fibula (Fig. 4). The altered anatomy may make injection difficult. An arthrogram done simultaneously will demonstrate irregularitites as well as confirm the anatomic placement of local anesthetic. If an injection in the subtalar joint relieves the patient's pain, it is likely a fusion will be helpful. If there is minimal pain relief, other causes of pain should be sought.

Simple Ostectomy

Simple ostectomy is used for extra-articular fractures or for those fractures in which the intra-articular component of the fracture line is limited. These might include peroneal tendon or subfibular impingement secondary to lateral wall displacement. The lateral wall may be intact but buckled outward, or the lateral wall

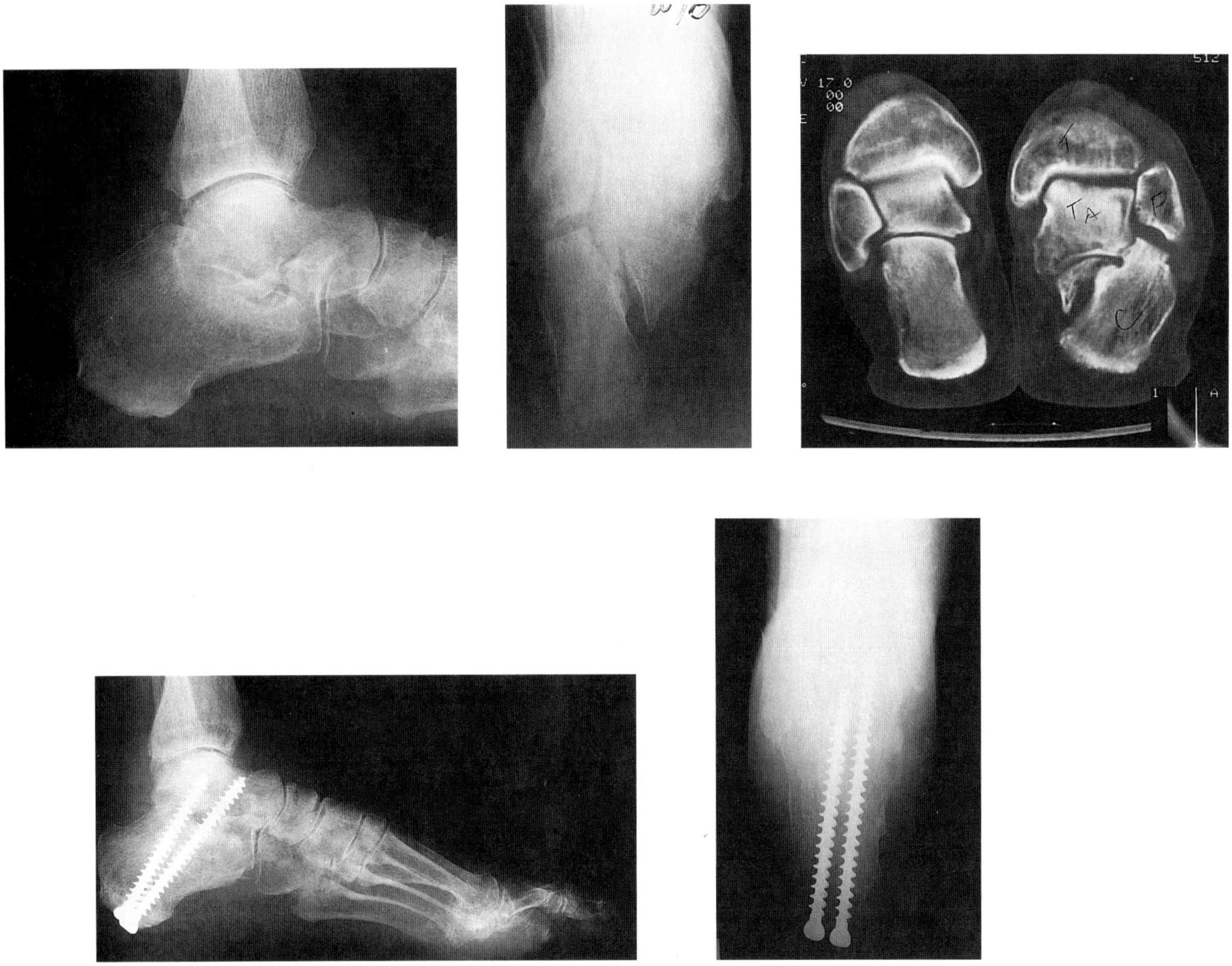

Fig. 4 **Top left,** shows a lateral radiograph of a 77-year-old female 1 year following an injury treated in a closed fashion. The lateral radiograph is suspicious for dislocation of the calcaneus, as the dorsum of the calcaneus is superior to the inferior aspect of the talus. **Top center,** This axial, or Harris, view shows that the primary fracture line has healed, but that the posterior facet is directly beneath the fibula, completely displacing the peroneal tendons. **Top right,** This computed tomographic scan through the hindfoot shows the calcaneus, again with the entire tuberosity and most of the posterior facet displaced laterally. More anterior cuts of the computed tomographic scan showed that the fracture had healed. **Bottom left,** This is a postoperative lateral view with the calcaneus reduced beneath the talus and the overall hindfoot alignment restored. Osteotomy was performed through the original fracture line before the tuberosity and body could be reduced. **Bottom right,** An axial view of the same patient shows the calcaneus now directly beneath the weightbearing axis of the talus. The patient went on to uneventful healing and full weightbearing within 3 months.

and lateral margin of the posterior facet may have been sheared off and never reduced. If symptoms are localized and the remaining joint surface is congruent, simple excision of the prominent bone may be adequate. Clues that impingement is causing the pain include a displaced or buckled lateral wall that narrows or eradicates the space deep to the fibula or at the lateral wall of the talus, swelling and pain in the peroneal tendons, pain with resisted eversion, and increased pain when weightbearing on a laterally inclined surface. Selective injection with local anesthetic may be inconclusive because the joint and subfibular space communicate.

For a simple subfibular ostectomy, the patient is placed in a lateral position. A curved incision is performed posterior to the peroneal tendons, taking care to avoid the sural nerve. The flap is raised subperiosteally, leaving the calcaneofibular ligament intact in the flap in order to help maintain the reduced position of the peroneal tendons. A curved periosteal elevator, or cob, is used to expose the prominent segment. A curved osteotome is placed at the anterior margin of the bone to be excised, and a small indentation is made to limit the anterior extension of the ostectomy. The saw is placed parallel to the lateral wall of the calcaneus and the prominent bone is removed. The margins should then be smoothed with a rongeur. The calcaneofibular ligament is then brought back to its native position, which helps to maintain the reduction of the peroneal tendons. The wound is closed and a padded dressing is applied. The dressing is created to apply light pressure to the flap by taking sponges and creating a defect in the sponge for the fibula. In doing so, slightly more pressure is held on the flap than on the fibula itself. An elastic wrap is then used to cover this dressing for 4 weeks. The patient is allowed partial weightbearing with crutch protection for 2 to 4 weeks.

Simple Osteotomy

Some extra-articular fractures may respond to osteotomy. This is particularly true when the tuberosity has displaced medially, laterally, or dorsally. When the tuberosity displaces, it may cause a disruption of the position of the plantar fascia and heel pad, which can be compensated for by the use of an orthosis. When not corrected by nonsurgical measures, an extra-articular osteotomy may be used to restore alignment. The goal of this osteotomy should be to realign the normal mechanics. This simple osteotomy is not commonly needed. More complex osteotomy may also be done in combination with arthrodesis.

A Dwyer-type osteotomy can be performed to move the tuberosity into appropriate position. The patient is placed in the lateral position. A curved incision is performed posterior to the peroneal tendons, taking care to avoid the sural nerve as well as the calcaneal branch of the sural nerve. The osteotomy should be performed behind the peroneal tendons, but should include the attachment of the origin of the plantar fascia. Make the osteotomy as close as possible to the original fracture line. When the osteotomy is completed, place a 1-inch osteotome into the cut and use it to lever the medial side open. Place a laminar spreader in the osteotomy to open it and use a blunt dissection technique to free the soft tissue from the bone. When there has been adequate medial soft-tissue release, move the bone into the desired position. Secure the position with two large screws directed upward and anteriorly from the heel.

When the osteotomy is intra-articular, it is slightly more complex. This technique is discussed below.

Arthrodesis

There are times when arthrodesis of the subtalar joint alone is adequate. In situ fusion is performed when the fracture displacement has caused subtalar arthrosis but has not disrupted the overall alignment of the hindfoot. This situation typically occurs in a person with soft bone who has had an impacting type fracture of the subtalar joint. Arthrodesis in situ may also be helpful in treatment of a patient whose calcaneus fracture has been reduced, but who has posttraumatic arthrosis. Meary's line should be intact on the lateral radiograph. A preoperative injection of the subtalar joint with local anesthesia relieves the pain in most cases when the pain is from the joint. Arthrodesis is performed in a routine way. The joint surfaces are debrided, and two screws are directed from the tuberosity upward into the talus. The two screws begin at the plantar side of the tuberosity and extend upward. The more lateral screw is directed into the dome of the talus, and the more medial one into the talar neck. Care should be taken to center these screws toward the midline of the tuberosity, not to the lateral side, because the slight lateral displacement may allow the screw to end up in the talofibular articulation. Use of two screws prevents rotation of the joint during healing.

Arthrodesis With Osteotomy

More commonly, before an arthrodesis can be performed, mechanical alignment of the hindfoot needs to be reestablished. The osteotomy used to accomplish the realignment must be tailored to the deformity. In general, the osteotomy allows the surgeon to undo the misalignment that occurred at the time of injury, ie, the translation along the primary fracture line. The osteotomy should therefore mimic the primary fracture line. By doing this osteotomy, it is possible to restore some height and narrow the heel simultaneously.

A lateral approach is used. Whether the incision is longitudinal or an oblique sinus tarsi incision depends on distal extension of the fracture malunion. If the fracture through the joint can be visualized, the osteotomy can follow that fracture line. The osteotomy should start just anterior to the sinus tarsi and should be directed laterally and obliquely into a plantar direction. The osteotomy is directed from lateral to medial and from dorsal to plantar. A Schanz pin is placed in the tuberosity before completion of the osteotomy to assist in upward rotation and medial translation of the tuberosity. The pin is directed axially from the plantar to dorsal. As the tuberosity is rotated counterclockwise for the right foot or clockwise for the left, it slides medially along this oblique line. This movement allows it to rotate the posterior facet upward, restoring height of the hindfoot. As it slides obliquely, it will also decompress the subfibular space and allow restoration of the position of peroneal tendons. The tuberosity can then be transfixed with lag screws, or with a small anti-glide plate placed laterally and combined with axially directed screws. The ideal configuration is to place two screws across the osteotomy and two screws from the tuberosity upward into the talus to complete the arthrodesis (Fig. 5).

Medial translation may be difficult to accomplish. Medial soft-tissue release may be helpful. When the osteotomy is completed, it should be opened up with a 1-inch osteotome. A laminar spreader is then placed and opened until the medial soft tissues are visualized. The medial soft tissues are bluntly dissected from the bone to allow the bone to move. The bone is then levered with small periosteal elevators until its native position is restored, and it is then transfixed with Kirschner wires. Implants can then be inserted.

If additional subfibular decompression is required, it can be done with a rongeur. Postoperatively, the patient is kept nonweightbearing for 8 to 12 weeks. The patient may, however, perform active range of motion of the ankle joints as soon after surgery as is comfortable.

A second type of osteotomy that is intra-articular is done after a tongue-type fracture. Tongue-type fractures are typically not as wide, but they do need an increase in the height. The planned procedure is to allow the tuberosity to be rotated upward until the height of the foot is restored. Although conceptually this should allow the height to be restored (by rotating the posterior facet upward toward the talus), it is often not possible to restore height completely when the soft tissues have been contracted for substantial amount of time.

A lateral approach is used. Whether the incision is longitudinal or an oblique sinus tarsi incision depends on distal extension of the fracture malunion. If the fracture through the joint can be visualized, the osteotomy can follow that fracture line. The osteotomy is directed from lateral to medial. A Schanz pin is placed in the tuberosity before completion of the osteotomy to assist in upward rotation of the tuberosity. When the orientation of the tuberosity is such that the posterior facet is reduced, it can be transfixed with axial lag screws. At times, a small anti-glide plate placed laterally may be needed as a tension band.

Arthrodesis Without Osteotomy: Subtalar Bone Block Distraction

When there is minimal misalignment in the coronal plane, but significant impaction, the talus comes to lie parallel to the floor. This so-called horizontal talus creates two problems. First, when the foot is in a neutral position, the talus is dorsiflexed because the body is more plantar than the head and neck. If the foot attempts to dorsiflex, the neck of the talus impinges on the anterior part of the tibia. Secondly, because the talus is dorsiflexed and the anterior part of the calcaneus is not, the transverse tarsal joint is incongruous. The goal of surgery is to restore the lost height and unlock the transverse tarsal joint. A compressed tongue-type fracture is another circumstance in which the height must be restored by elevation, although this may be accomplished without interposition of structural bone graft.

This technique was previously described by Carr and associates.[13] The patient is placed in the prone position, which allows easy access to the hindfoot and to the posterior iliac crest for donation of the autogenous graft. The surgical incision is made just posterior to the sural nerve and is carried sharply through the skin and subcutaneous tissue. The retinaculum is divided and the flexor hallucis muscle belly is identified. The muscle belly is then bluntly retracted medially, which protects the neurovascular bundle. The posterior aspect of the ankle and subtalar joint are easily identified. When the tuberosity is displaced upward, identification is less straightforward and fluoroscopy may be helpful. A

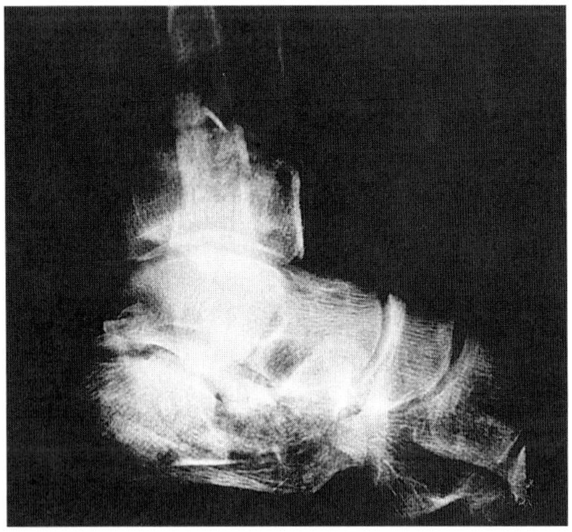

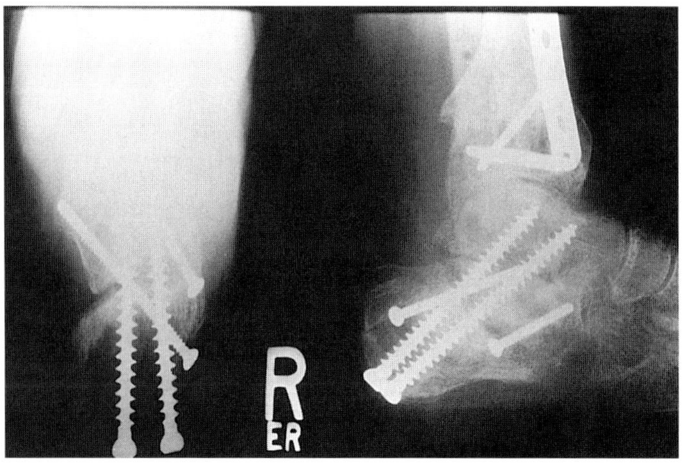

Fig. 5 Left, This preoperative radiograph shows a lateral view of a highly comminuted calcaneus fracture. The axial view, which was too dark to reproduce, demonstrated a grossly widened heel with abutment of the calcaneus in the subfibular area. **Right**, The postoperative axial and lateral view. Note that in sliding the calcaneus along this oblique osteotomy, the heel was narrowed and the hindfoot was elevated. Two screws crossed the fracture line and the osteotomy line, and another two screws were placed across the subtalar joint. Note that on the medial side of the reduced calcaneus, there is abundant bone, which shows the amount of displacement necessary to restore hindfoot alignment.

curved narrow osteotome is then placed into the joint and used to distract the talus and the calcaneus. A lamina spreader is placed in the posterior aspect of the joint, and debridement of scar tissue, articular cartilage, and bone fragments is performed. A femoral distractor is applied, a Schanz pin is placed into the tibia and into the calcaneus, and the two are distracted. The lamina spreader, which is placed slightly to the lateral side of the incision, balances the femoral distractor on the medial side. By continuing to increase the distraction with these instruments, a normal relationship between the talus and the calcaneus can be restored (Fig. 6). In essence this restores Böhler's angle. When the calcaneus and talus are distracted and the posterior and middle facets are denuded of cartilage, it is possible to measure the distance between the talus and calcaneus, which may be as much as 2 cm. The posterior iliac crest is identified, and a graft 1 mm to 2 mm larger than the gap is selected. If the crest is narrow, two pieces of graft may be selected. An osteotome is then used to petal the underside of the talus and the dorsum of the calcaneus, and multiple drill holes are placed in each. Cancellous graft is packed anteriorly in the area of the middle and anterior facet. Drill bits (4.5 mm) are used to drill from the calcaneus upward through what was once the posterior facet, directed toward the talus. A fully threaded 7-mm screw is then placed all the way up into the talus and is then backed out, so it is just visible at the level of the calcaneus. This procedure helps to ensure that screws will be directed appropriately after the graft is in place. The fully threaded screws act to buttress the gap filled by the bone graft. The structural cortical cancellous grafts are then oriented so that the cancellous surface is directed toward the calcaneus and talus, and the cortical surface is aligned superiorly and inferiorly (Fig. 5). The grafts are then placed into the gap between the talus and calcaneus, using a bone impactor, until they are flush with the posterior aspect of the talus. Care should be taken not to allow the grafts to be prominent at the posterior part of the talus, as they could potentially obstruct plantarflexion. With the impactor holding these grafts in place, the 7-mm screws are then repositioned into the talus, lateral and axial radiographs are obtained to confirm the connection, and a mortise view of the ankle is obtained to confirm that the screws are safely within the talus.

A posterior splint is applied for 2 weeks, after which the sutures are removed. The patient can then begin gentle ankle range of motion, wearing a clam shell or similar removable brace. At 6 weeks the patient is allowed to place approximately 50 pounds of weight on the limb, and at 12 weeks, if radiographs confirm consolidation, full weightbearing can be reinstituted.

Summary

Salvage procedures reverse the anatomic factors that cause widening and mechanical misalignment of the hindfoot. Posttraumatic arthrosis of the subtalar joint is treated by arthrodesis, using techniques that improve alignment. The easily measured goal is to restore the normal plantar alignment of the talus (Meary's line) and return the calcaneal tuberosity to the weightbearing line beneath the talus. The subtalar joint is the joint most often treated by arthrodesis, although a triple arthrodesis is sometimes required when Chopart's joint is involved.

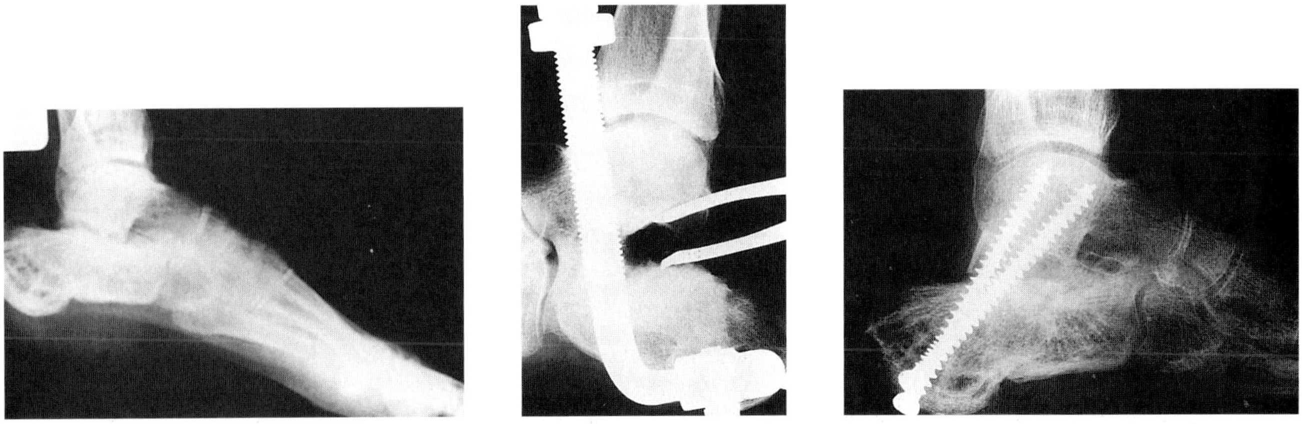

Fig. 6 **Left**, This is the preoperative, nonweightbearing radiograph of a patient 2 years following a tongue-type calcaneus fracture treated closed. He had minimal widening, but significant joint depression causing a horizontal talus and subtalar pain. He was unable to dorsiflex his foot or walk uphill. **Center**, In this intraoperative radiograph, the subtalar joint has been distracted until the talus follows a normal axis down the first metatarsal. A laminar spreader is within the subtalar joint and a femoral distractor is distracting from the calcaneus to the tibia. **Right**, The postoperative healed position of this same patient with the normal hindfoot axis restored. Note the use of the fully threaded screws across the subtalar joint to prevent collapse during healing.

References

1. Lindsay WRN, Dewar FP: Fractures of the calcaneus. *Am J Surg* 1958;95:555–576.
2. Pozo SL, Kirwan EO'G, Jackson AM: The long term results of conservative management of severely displaced fractures of the calcaneus. *J Bone Joint Surg* 1984;66B:386–390.
3. Carr JB, Hamilton JJ, Bear LS: Experimental intra-articular calcaneal fractures: Anatomic basis for a new classification. *Foot Ankle* 1989;10:81–87.
4. Gallie WE: Subastragalar arthrodesis in fractures of the os calcis. *J Bone Joint Surg* 1943;25:731–736.
5. Kalamchi A, Evans JG: Posterior subtalar fusion: A preliminary report on a modified Gallie's procedure. *J Bone Joint Surg* 1977;59B:287–289.
6. Bohler L: Diagnosis, pathology, and treatment of fractures of the calcaneus. *J Bone Joint Surg* 1931;13:75–89.
7. Cave EF: Fracture of the os calcus: The problem in general. *Clin Orthop* 1963;30:64–66.
8. Kitaoka HB, Schaap EJ, Chao EY, et al: Displaced intraarticular fractures of the calcaneus treated nonoperatively: Clinical results and ground reaction forces. *J Bone Joint Surg* 1994;76A:1531–1540.
9. Essex-Lopresti P: Results of reduction in fractures of the calcaneum. *J Bone Joint Surg* 1951;33B:284.
10. Essex-Lopresti P: The mechanism, reduction technique and results in fractures of the os calcuis. *Br J Surg* 1952;39:395–419.
11. Sangeorzan BJ, Benirschke SK, Carr JB: Surgical management of fractures of the os calcis, in Jackson D (ed): *Instructional Course Lectures 44.* Rosemont, IL, American Academy of Orthopaedic Surgeons, 1995, pp 359–370.
12. Benirschke SK, Sangeorzan BJ: Intraarticular fractures of the foot: Surgical management of calcaneal fractures. *Clin Orthop* 1993;292:128–134.
13. Carr JB, Hansen ST, Benirschke SK: Subtalar distraction bone block fusion for late complications of os calcis fractures. *Foot Ankle* 1988;9:81–86.

CHAPTER 34

Technical Factors in Hindfoot Arthrodesis

Arthur Manoli II, MD
Timothy C. Beals, MD
Sigvard T. Hansen, Jr, MD

Introduction

The purpose of this chapter is to review the basic principles of hindfoot arthrodesis and to emphasize those technical aspects of the procedures that will enhance the likelihood of clinical success. The general principles of hindfoot fusion techniques are addressed initially and are followed by a discussion of specific fusion operations with a recommended technique for arthrodesis. Finally, special circumstances affecting the recommended techniques for arthrodesis and management are reviewed.

Basic Principles

The goal of all hindfoot arthrodesis procedures is the ablation of articular surfaces with the subsequent development of a solid bony union with the hindfoot in a functional position. The most consistent way to achieve this is by adhering to several fundamental principles. First, it is necessary to recognize that well-performed arthrodesis procedures are primarily soft-tissue procedures. Approaches must respect the vascular supply to each bony surface that is to be fused.

Once the joint is visualized, the remaining cartilage must be carefully removed without destroying the subchondral bone that supports the bony architecture. The subchondral bone should be perforated in multiple locations to encourage union between surfaces, and the hindfoot must be held rigidly in a correct position with internal fixation. All joints that are to undergo fusion should be bone grafted in a manner that encourages early union.

Specifically, the use of 6.5-mm cancellous screws is recommended for hindfoot arthrodesis. These screws allow rigid internal fixation without the soft-tissue stripping and associated devascularization of plating techniques. Large screws also allow the maintenance of the desired position for fusion. It should be noted that rigid internal fixation is particularly important in a patient population with impaired healing potential, because it provides a solid scaffold that supports soft-tissue healing.

There are essentially three types of 6.5-mm cancellous screws. The three types are short-threaded screws, in which the terminal 16 mm are threaded; long-threaded screws, in which the terminal 32 mm are threaded; and fully-threaded screws. The two types of partially threaded screws are used when compression is desired. The fully-threaded screws are used when the goal is maintenance of a corrected position, as illustrated by the subtalar distraction bone block fusion technique. The AO technique manual recommends a 3.2-mm drill for the placement of 6.5-mm screws.[1] However, in dense bones, such as are found in the hindfoot, a combination of 4.5- and 3.5-mm drills is employed to avoid incarceration of the screw or difficulty initiating penetration of the screw into the drill hole. Our standard technique for compression screw placement is to drill with a 4.5-mm drill in the part of the bone that will engage the screw head and to drill the terminal portion of the screw hole with a 3.5-mm drill. This overdrilling allows the screws to be placed much more easily.

In the placement of all screws, the surgeon should avoid leaving screw threads across the fusion site. Short-threaded screws should be used if there is uncertainty about how closely the threads will abut subchondral surfaces. However, when more threads engage the distal bone stock, the screw has greater pull-out strength. Washers should be considered if the bone quality is poor in terms of density but only if the screw does not enter the bone at too great an angle. Using a washer with a sharply angled screw will create a stress riser effect beneath a portion of the washer.

An important technical aspect to the placement of screws is the "notch technique." This technique should be used whenever screws are inserted into bone at an angle. Angled screws are necessary during most joint fusions, and notch placement is essential to avoid splitting bone bridges near joints. The notch technique is distinct from countersinking. The notch technique creates a pathway for the head of the screw so that no part of the screw head engages the bone until its entire surface area is seated. This technique allows for maximum compression when tightening screws without the typical concerns of breaking the bone on the near surface of the site for fusion or altering the joint position due to sheer forces created by tightening the screw.[2]

The notch is made with a high speed burr and is half as deep as the diameter of the screw head. The deepest portion of the notch is toward the arthrodesis site, and it tapers away from that surface at the angle of the proposed screw placement. Thus, a path is created that allows the head of the screw to engage bone only when fully seated. The most important aspect of the notch technique is to ensure that the gliding hole is drilled with the drill bit starting not in the base of the notch, but rather near the cortical surface where the notch begins (Fig. 1). If the head of the screw engages either soft tissue or bone before fully seating, the screw head will be lifted away from the bone, which can result in a fracture of the near cortex or distort the position of the arthrodesis surface.

The preparation of bone surfaces for fusion and the grafting of those surfaces deserves special emphasis. For the removal of cartilage, we advocate techniques that preserve the subchondral bone. Osteotomes must be used with great care to avoid fracture of the joint surfaces and inadvertent deep penetration of soft bone. The use of ring curettes can be helpful in this regard. If the site of fusion is a joint surface, the subchondral bone is typically drilled with a 2.0-mm drill in multiple sites to enhance vascular penetration of the fusion surface (Fig. 2). This technique maintains the congruent surfaces of the joint, and these can then be optimally positioned and compressed to encourage rapid fusion. Techniques such as "petalling" can yield an undulating surface with increased "dead space" after compression fixation and less surface area for primary bone healing.

Grafting of all joint surfaces should be performed routinely. The source of graft bone can be the iliac crest or proximal tibia. Small grafts can be taken from local sites. We advocate the use of autologous bone for the best results with arthrodesis. One important technique that is used regardless of the site of fusion is the preparation of a shear-strain-relieved bone graft site.[3] In this technique, cancellous bone graft is packed into a small area that is created across the fusion site. The shear-strain-relieved bone graft site is created by placing a high speed burr at the fusion site, making a hole 4 to 5 mm deep, and packing this area with cancellous graft. This technique allows a portion of the arthrodesis surface to heal devoid of shear. We believe this site serves as a "spot weld" and encourages early fusion across the bony surface undergoing arthrodesis.

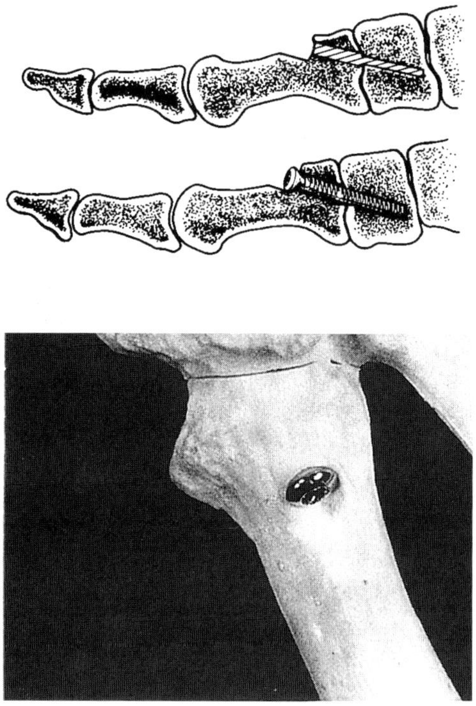

Fig. 1 **Top,** Graphic illustration of the correct location of the gliding drill hole and screw relative to the notch in the notch technique. **Bottom,** Demonstration of a screw placed using the notch technique.

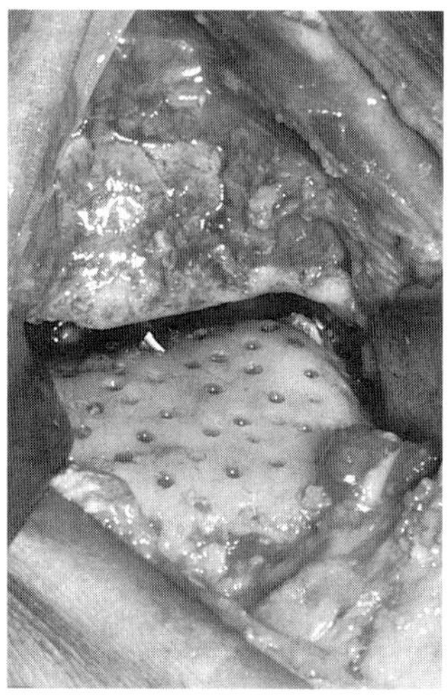

Fig. 2 Bone surface after cartilage debridement and placement of multiple 2.0-mm drill holes.

Ankle Arthrodesis

Ankle arthrodesis is undertaken for end-stage degenerative disease of the tibiotalar joint. It has been shown to be a reliable procedure for pain relief but a number of patients have less than optimal results due to technical errors in the course of arthrodesis.[4-9] In determining candidates for ankle arthrodesis, particular consideration should be given to patients who smoke, because the risk of non-union is significantly higher in such patients. We do not recommend major hindfoot arthrodesis in patients who smoke, and we specifically require 3 months of abstinence from smoking and nicotine products before a patient can be a candidate for this procedure.

Ankle arthrodesis can be performed with various techniques.[10-14] Different fixation constructs may require three, four, or five screws. The goal is to obtain screws that cross at right angles to each other in the hindfoot, compress surfaces effectively, and have solid purchase.

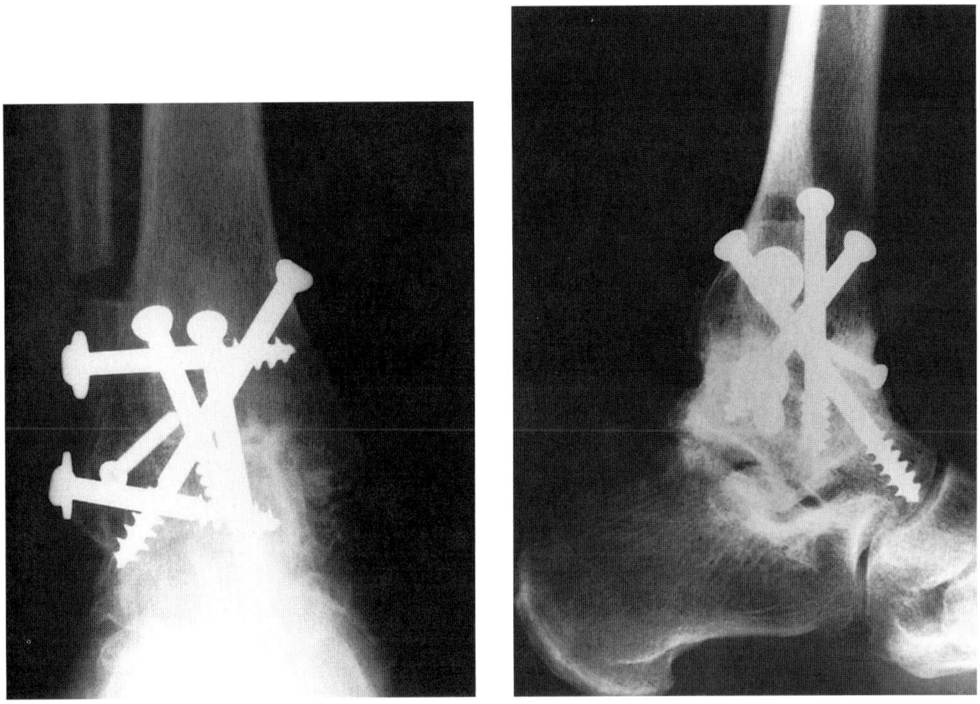

Fig. 3 **Left,** Anteroposterior view of an ankle fusion with 6.5-mm screws compressing the ankle joint and 6.5-mm screws with washers compressing the fibula as a vascularized bone graft. **Right,** Lateral view of an ankle arthrodesis demonstrating a 6.5-mm screw into the talar neck from the posterolateral aspect of the distal tibia.

The lateral approach is most commonly used for ankle arthrodesis. It is particularly appropriate if hardware removal is required, if anterior soft tissues are poor, or if the talus is extruded anteriorly from the mortise. The lateral approach allows for a transfibular osteotomy to be performed, which exposes the mortise by reflecting the fibula posteriorly on its soft-tissue attachments and associated blood supply.[12] The transverse fibular osteotomy is performed approximately 5 cm above the mortise. A 0.5-cm segment of the fibula is removed to prevent a painful nonunion from developing, and the removed fibular bone segment is retained as bone graft.

Once the ankle joint is visualized, the joint surfaces are debrided of cartilage. The dome and lateral side of the talus are visualized directly. The medial side of the talus is debrided of cartilage with the use of curved curettes and by gently tilting the ankle into varus. The medial malleolus can be visualized directly through the ankle joint with the lateral approach. The tibial plafond is also carefully scraped to remove remaining cartilage. Regular and ring curettes as well as a curved osteotome are used to remove the cartilage. Multiple 2.0-mm drill holes are made in all surfaces to be fused.

A series of decisions are then made that relate to achieving the optimum position for ankle fusion. It is not uncommon to see patients with unsatisfactory ankle fusions in which the talus is fixed too anteriorly relative to the tibia. This creates a "longer" foot, which makes it difficult for patients to "roll over" the hindfoot during single leg stance without excessively externally rotating the limb. To achieve a satisfactory position, it is occasionally necessary to remove bone at the back of the plafond in order to translate the talus posteriorly into the mortise. Usually, the heelcord is lengthened to achieve proper position. Heelcord lengthening is performed percutaneously with three incisions of half of the transverse width of the Achilles tendon spaced approximately 3 cm apart.[15] The heelcord is lengthened until the ankle dorsiflexes to between neutral and 5° of dorsiflexion with the talus pushed posteriorly into the mortise.

The first screw to be placed is a 6.5-mm cancellous screw from the posterior aspect of the tibia to the middle of the neck of the talus. A 4.5-mm drill hole that exits 1 cm posterior to the anterior aspect of the plafond is made. It should be noted that anterior osteophytes need to be removed to properly judge the location for this drilling or the drill hole may be made too far anteriorly. The drill hole should be 45° from the long axis of the tibia and should exit just medial to the midline of the tibia. An "ACL type" drill guide can be helpful to properly position this drill hole.[16] A small incision is necessary to pass the drills and screw just lateral to the heelcord. The ankle is then postioned for fusion. The position for arthrodesis is between neutral and 5° of dorsiflexion and neutral in terms of varus and valgus. The talus must be translated posteriorly

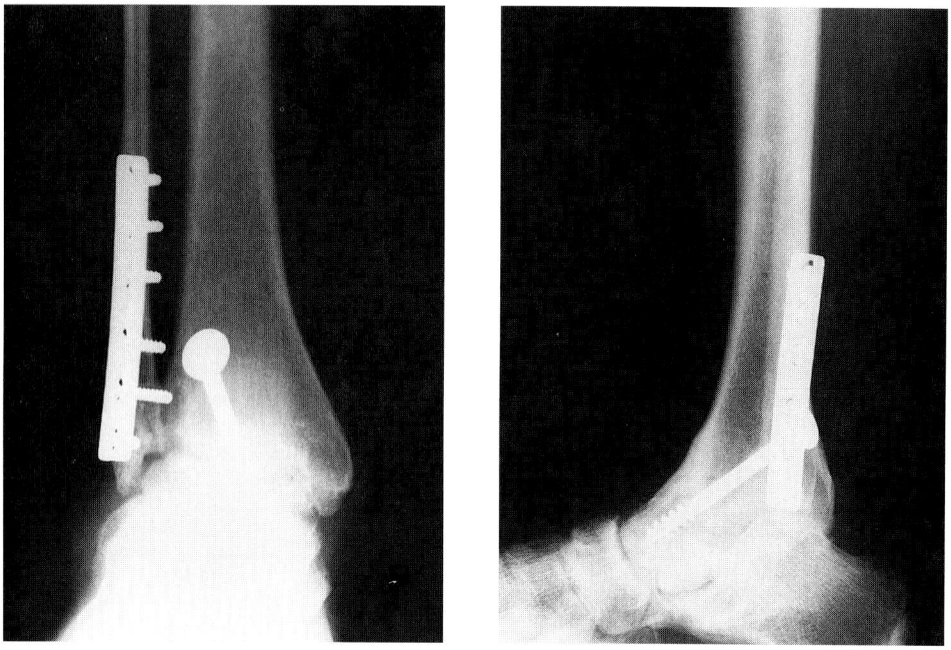

Fig. 4 **Left,** Anteroposterior view shows a single 6.5-mm cancellous screw placed into the talus to secure the position of a modified Blair fusion. **Right,** Lateral view of a modified Blair fusion demonstrating proper positioning of the screw into the head and neck of the talus.

into the mortise. A 3.5-mm hole is made into the neck of the talus. Typically, a short-threaded screw, 75 to 80 mm in length, is used.

Radiographs are taken after initial screw placement to verify that an appropriate position has been achieved. Three views are routinely done; they are a lateral hindfoot, an anteroposterior (AP) hindfoot, and an AP ankle. These films should determine the position of the fusion and that the location of the screw is in the talar neck. If the position is unacceptable, the screw is removed and appropriate adjustments are made.

Once the initially placed screw is in an acceptable position, a short-threaded 6.5-mm screw is placed through a stab wound over the medial malleolus into the middle of the body of the talus. The medial half of the distal fibula is removed with an oscillating saw or an osteotome. The fibula is held carefully with two towel clips so that its posterior blood supply is maintained. Resection of the medial fibula during the initial approach is not recommended, because the fibula is more prone to fracture from retraction once the medial portion has been removed. The medial fibular bone is kept for graft material and often is of adequate volume to make formal bone graft harvest unnecessary. The distal fibula is transfixed with two 6.5-mm screws. A cephalad screw is placed into the tibia. A second screw is placed approximately 2 cm from the distal end of the fibula into the lateral talar body. This technique of using the distal fibula as a plate enhances fixation and provides an additional vascularized bone surface for healing.

A final screw is placed from the anterior tibia into the body of the talus. Final radiographs are taken. The AP hindfoot view is not necessary at this time, because none of the subsequently placed screws are directed into the neck of the talus and the previously taken films illustrate the position of the initial screw. The AP ankle and lateral hindfoot views allow visualization and assessment of all screws placed except the first screw that entered the talar neck. Screws may be shortened if necessary. The surgeon must be critical in the assessment of screw placement to ensure that no screw enters or limits the function of the subtalar joint (Fig. 3).

Bone grafting is performed as described previously. Shear-strain-relieved bone grafting can be performed on all surfaces except that between the medial talus and the medial malleolus. If a bone defect is present, a block of bone can be placed in the location of the tubercle of Chaput and transfixed with a 3.5-mm screw. If additional bone graft is necessary, we typically harvest graft from the ipsilateral anterior iliac crest.

Postoperative management consists of a nonweight-bearing cast for 6 weeks and a walking cast or cast brace for an additional 4 weeks.

Modified Blair Arthrodesis

A modified Blair arthrodesis has few and specific indications.[17,18] Osteonecrosis of the talar body, traumatic bone loss of the talar body, and infection are three indications. The technique for arthrodesis is similar to the previously described technique for ankle arthrodesis. A lateral transfibular approach is used. Particularly with this procedure, the fibula must be

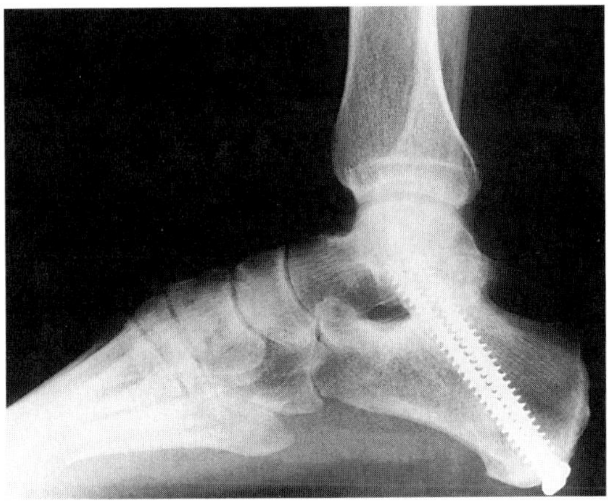

Fig. 5 Lateral view of a subtalar distraction bone block fusion with two fully-threaded 6.5-mm screws crossing the subtalar joint.

shortened to avoid heel varus from body impingement laterally.

The body of the talus is removed and the talar neck and head are positioned onto the anterior aspect of the tibial plafond. The back-to-front screw is placed from the tibia into the talar head and neck. The tibial drill hole for the screw exits just above the anterior margin of the tibia rather than 1 cm posteriorly as described for ankle fusion. A bone bridge is maintained below the screw. The screw is otherwise placed as described for the initial screw in ankle arthrodesis (Fig. 4).

Shear-strain-relieved bone graft sites are created between the talar neck and the tibia. The postoperative management is the same as described for ankle arthrodesis. If well positioned, a good approximation of subtalar motion can be obtained with this procedure but it should be recognized that mild equinus may also result to make up for the necessary shortening. A 1-cm heel lift may be helpful postoperatively.

Subtalar Arthrodesis

Indications for subtalar arthrodesis include degenerative arthritis of the subtalar joint and posttraumatic dysfunction after calcaneal fracture.[19-21] In the cases of degenerative arthritis and calcaneal fractures, the hindfoot architecture is abnormal, with shortening of the hindfoot and tipping of the talus into a more horizontal position.[19] If a posterior bone block is placed at the time of subtalar fusion, it prevents anterior impingement of the ankle and recreates the normal hindfoot height. The height of the bone block depends on the degree and etiology of the shortening. When used for subtalar arthritis, bone blocks are typically 5 to 8 mm in height. For shortening associated with old calcaneal fractures, bone blocks are 10 to 15 mm in height.

Patients are placed in a lateral position. A straight posterolateral incision is made and the subtalar joint entered. Care must be taken to avoid entering the ankle joint, because the two joints are adjacent when viewed from this approach, particularly with the foot in a plantarflexed position. The subtalar joint is opened and the posterior facet scraped of residual cartilage. Lamina spreaders are essential to assist in visualization. Another important technique for exposure and for the determination of correct hindfoot position is a medially placed femoral distractor. Pins are placed into the middle of the tibia and the calcaneous through stab wounds. The fixator allows for removal of the lamina spreader and enhances visualization. Additionally, it is easier to place the blocks into the subtalar joint with the hindfoot secured by the fixator. The most important function of the femoral distractor is to assist positioning of the hindfoot so that heel varus is avoided.

Tricortical blocks are harvested from the posterior iliac crest and are placed into the subtalar joint with a tamp. The "upper" cortical surface of the graft is placed posteriorly, and the blocks are shaped into wedges with the longest dimension facing posteriorly. Prior to placing the blocks, an "ACL type" drill guide can be helpful to position two 4.5-mm drill holes through the calcaneus.[16] Drilling and screw placement are performed percutaneously through the heel. A lateral hindfoot screw is relatively vertically positioned so that it enters the talar body. A more medial screw is placed into the talar neck. Both screws are fully threaded and serve as an internal distractor. Once the 4.5-mm drill holes are made through the calcaneus, the blocks are positioned and a 3.5-mm drill is used to complete the screw holes for the two fully threaded 6.5-mm screws. Screws are usually 75 to 80 mm in length (Fig. 5).

Once the screws are placed, intraoperative radiographs are taken to assure that the screws do not engage the ankle joint and are positioned well into the talus. If the radiographic appearance is satisfactory, as much cancellous graft as can be accommodated is packed into the subtalar region, and the wound is closed. The femoral distractor is removed after radiographs are taken. Subsequently, the subtalar region is tested manually for rigidity. The patient is kept nonweightbearing for 12 weeks in a short limb cast.

Triple Arthrodesis

There are a number of indications for a triple hindfoot fusion.[4,22,23] Commonly encountered pathology leading to a fixed deformity of the hindfoot includes posterior tibial tendon insufficiency, tarsal coalitions, and degenerative arthritis. The goal of a triple arthrodesis is to fuse the subtalar, talonavicular, and calcaneocuboid jonts in a position of mild (5°) hind-foot valgus with an associated correction of any midfoot or forefoot deformity through proper positioning.

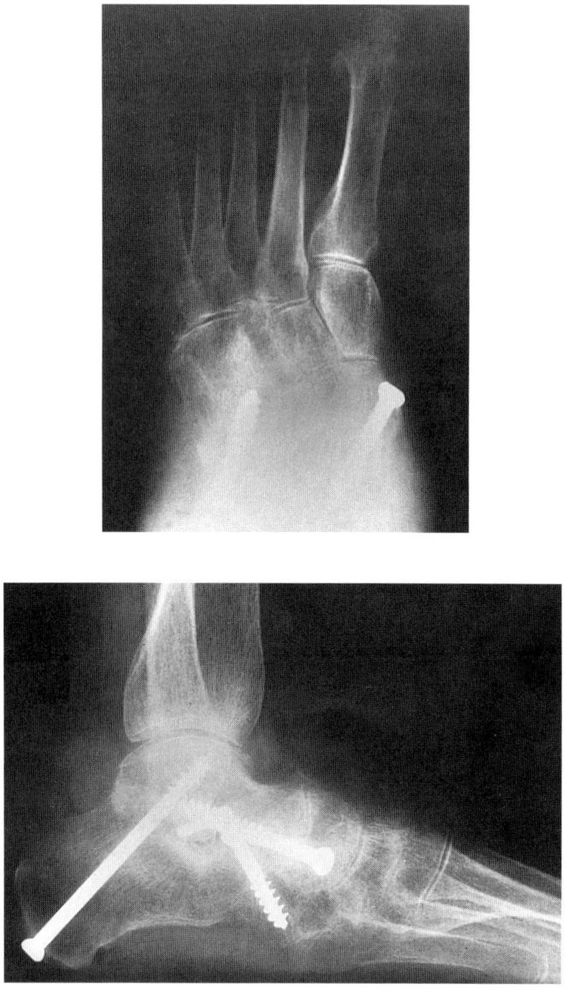

Fig. 6 **Top,** Anteroposterior view of a triple arthrodesis with screws compressing the talonavicular and calcaneocuboid joints. **Bottom,** Lateral view of a triple arthrodesis fixed with 6.5-mm cancellous screws.

Two incisions are used to expose the articulations of the hindfoot. An extensile medial incision that follows the course of the posterior tibial tendon is used to debride the talonavicular joint of remnant cartilage. The lateral incision as described by Ollier allows access to the posterior and middle facets of the subtalar joint and the calcaneocuboid joint. During the lateral approach, an exposure is created between the long extensor tendons and the peroneal tendons. Care is taken to identify and protect the sural nerve as it travels adjacent to the peroneal tendons. The extensor digitorum brevis muscle is reflected distally as a subperiosteal flap, which exposes both the calcaneocuboid and subtalar joints.

The cartilage is scraped off the exposed joints and multiple 2.0-mm drill holes are made in the subchondral bone surfaces to be fused. Lamina spreaders are extremely helpful to allow full visualization of the posterior and middle facets of the subtalar joint. We typically drill the surfaces of a particular joint as soon as it is debrided. Doing so minimizes soft-tissue manipulation and operative time, because exposure only needs to be achieved once.

The foot must be carefully positioned in an anatomic configuration. This almost always requires a heelcord lengthening. Once the hindfoot is reduced, a plantarflexion deformity is typically apparent. This is most obvious in the planovalgus foot with hindfoot equinus. A percutaneous, triple-cut heelcord lengthening is performed.[15]

The subtalar joint is rigidly fixed after positioning the hindfoot in 5° of valgus. Through a 1-cm incision made just off the plantar surface in the center of the heel, a 4.5-mm drill is used to make a gliding hole in the calcaneus. The hole should pass through the mid-

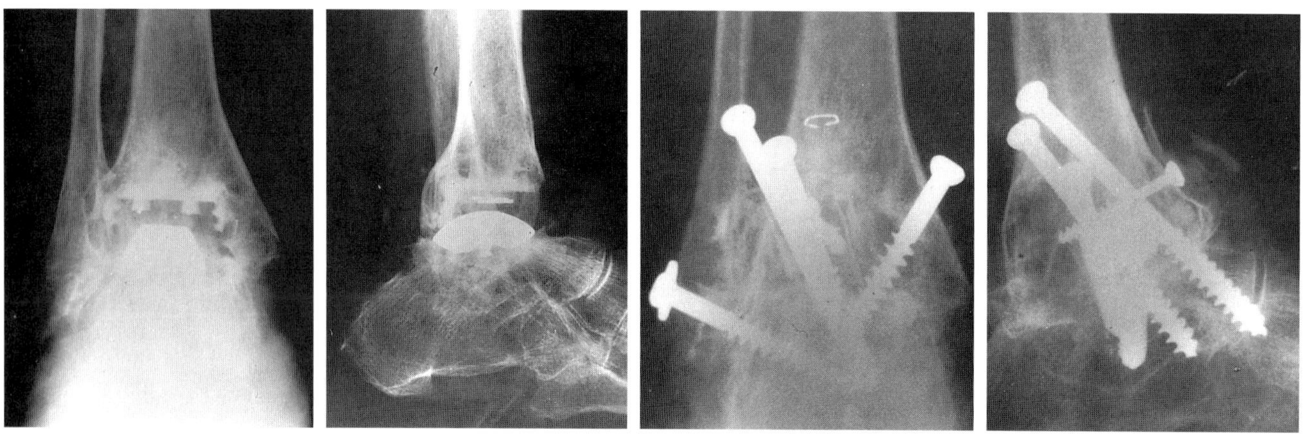

Fig. 7 **Left,** Anteroposterior view of a loose total ankle arthroplasty. **Center left,** Lateral view of a total ankle arthroplasty with cystic bone changes. **Center right,** Construct of ankle fusion stabilization after removal of ankle arthroplasty components and placement of tricortical pelvic grafts. **Right,** Lateral view of ankle fusion after "Crawford Campbell" bone graft.

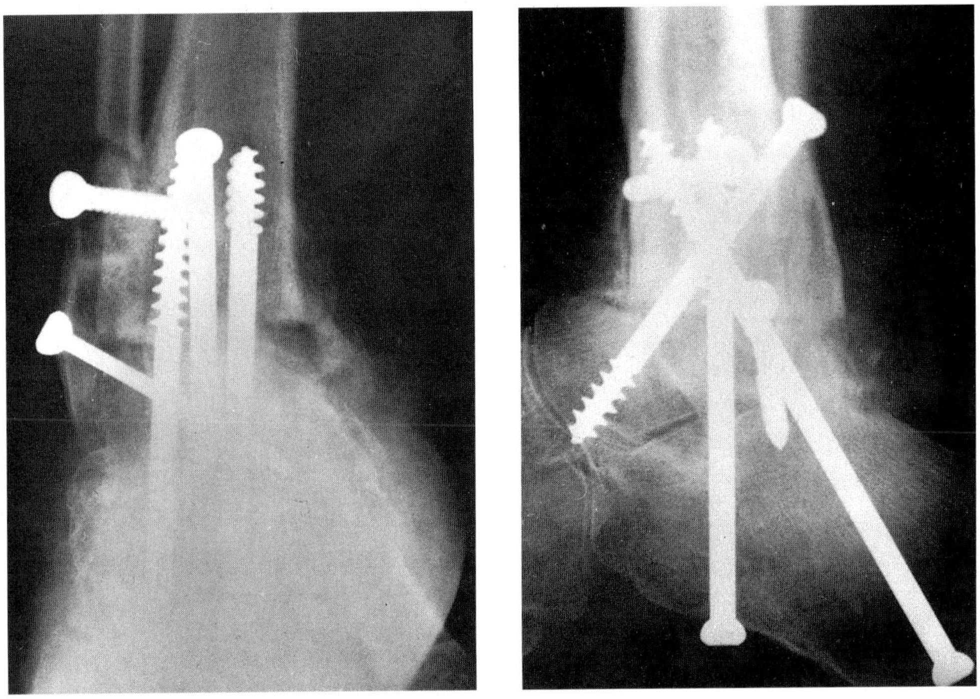

Fig. 8 Left, Anteroposterior view of a pantalar arthrodesis showing large cancellous screws. **Right,** Lateral view of pantalar arthrodesis demonstrating a well-positioned talus relative to the tibia.

dle of the posterior facet of the subtalar joint. An "ACL type" drill guide can be helpful to consistently achieve the proper location of the gliding hole.[16] The talus is then drilled with a 3.5-mm drill. A 6.5-mm short-threaded cancellous screw 75 to 80 mm in length is typically used.

There are a number of advantages to using a "bottom up" screw to fix the subtalar joint as compared to a screw placed from the dorsal side of the hindfoot. The screw is easier to aim and a drill guide can be used to assist in positioning. This technique avoids the deep peroneal nerve, the dorsalis pedis artery, and the blood supply of the talar neck. The screw is more perpendicular to the posterior facet and the screw head does not impinge on the tibia with dorsiflexion of the ankle. A potential stress riser is also avoided on the talar neck. Occasionally, the screw head of the "bottom up" can be bothersome. This screw can be removed under local block after fusion is complete. Another risk of the "bottom up" screw is that it can impinge on the fibula if it is directed too far laterally.

Once the hindfoot is fixed with the subtalar joint screw, the talonavicular joint must be positioned to properly align the midfoot and forefoot to the hindfoot. In a planovalgus deformity, the forefoot is supinated relative to the hindfoot so that the first ray must be "turned down" through the positioning of the talonavicular and calcaneocuboid joints. In a cavus foot, the forefoot is pronated and the first ray must be "turned up" through the talonavicular and calcaneocuboid joints. Once the triple arthrodesis is completed, careful inspection of the attitude of the foot is essential. A plantarflexing modified Lapidus fusion in the planovalgus foot or a first metatarsal dorsiflexion osteotomy in the cavus foot may be necessary to improve alignment if the deformity cannot be fully corrected through the transverse tarsal joints.

The talonavicular joint is fixed with a 6.5-mm long-threaded cancellous screw after drilling with 4.5-mm and 3.5-mm drills respectively. Screw length is usually 55 mm. The notch technique is essential to avoid breaking the bone bridge in the region of the navicular tuberosity. We typically expose the navicular back to the naviculocuneiform joint to maximize the thickness of the bone bridge. The screw must be directed superiorly and laterally to avoid passing into the subtalar joint area.

The calcaneocuboid joint is fixed with a short-threaded 6.5-mm cancellous screw, which averages 35 to 40 mm in length. The notch technique is applied to the anterior process of the calcaneus. When aiming this screw, a common error is to direct it too vertically and medially. The drill should be juxtaposed to the fibula to ensure adequate purchase of this screw (Fig. 6).

Radiographs should be taken to evaluate hindfoot correction and proper placement of screws. A mortise view of the ankle ensures that no undetected penetra-

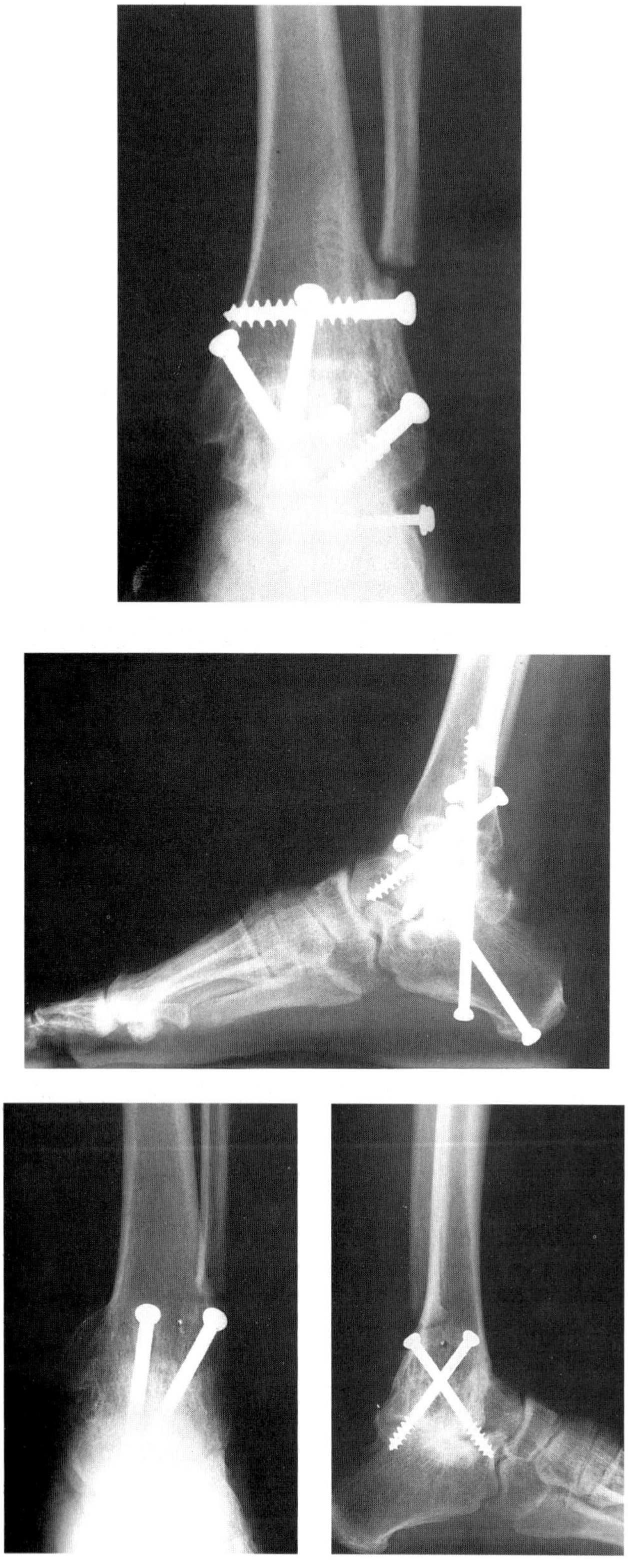

Fig. 9 **Top,** Anteroposterior (AP) view of a healed pantalar fusion. **Center,** Lateral view shows excessive plantarflexion of pantalar arthrodesis. **Bottom left,** AP ankle view showing two 6.5-mm screws securing a revision ankle level osteotomy. **Bottom right,** Crossed screws used to fix revision closing wedge osteotomy of pantalar arthrodesis.

tion of the ankle joint occurs. A lateral hindfoot radiograph allows an assessment of the position of each of the screws. The AP hindfoot view allows visualization of the navicular bone bridge and an assessment of the relationship between the hindfoot and forefoot.

Shear-strain-relieved bone grafts are routinely performed on all three joints. A corticocancellous bone block is occasionally fixed into the sinus tarsi with a 3.5-mm screw. The amount of graft necessary is best obtained from the iliac crest. Few absorbable sutures are placed in the deep soft tissues and the skin is closed with staples. A short limb cast is applied and the patient is kept nonweightbearing for 4 weeks with an additional 4 weeks in a walking cast.

Special Circumstances

Ankle Fusion With Bone Loss

The loss of bone stock presents an additional challenge for surgeons performing ankle arthrodesis. In the case of arthrodesis after a failed ankle arthroplasty or a healed pilon fracture with severe anterior bone loss, the surgeon must be prepared to replenish bone stock with large corticocancellous pelvic bone grafts. A technique referred to as the "Crawford Campbell" bone graft has been found to be effective.[6] This technique involves harvesting iliac crest bone in tricortical segments that are cut and stacked like books on a shelf. The graft segments must be placed so that they are stable, and screw fixation can augment their stability.

In situations with abnormal bone stock, it is particularly important that the proper position for fusion be attained. The talus should be placed as posteriorly as possible, because this is the region where the bone stock typically is best preserved. A heelcord lengthening should be considered if any element of equinus is present, because the equinus would place undue stress on the fusion site. Multiple 6.5-mm cancellous screws will be necessary to ensure proper fixation (Fig. 7).

Pantalar Arthrodesis

In rare cases, a pantalar arthrodesis will be necessary to address the complaints of a patient. Although a true pantalar arthrodesis involves fusion of the ankle, subtalar, talonavicular, and calcaneocuboid joints, we attempt in most cases to fuse only the ankle and subtalar joints if possible. The additional Chopart fusion adds considerable stiffness and should be avoided unless the talonavicular and calcaneocuboid joints are arthritic and painful.

The technique for pantalar arthrodesis is a combination of the ankle and subtalar fusion techniques described previously. A supplementary 6.5-mm "bottom-up" screw is placed from the calcaneus to the tibia. Typically a short-threaded screw, 110 to 120 mm in length, is used (Fig. 8).

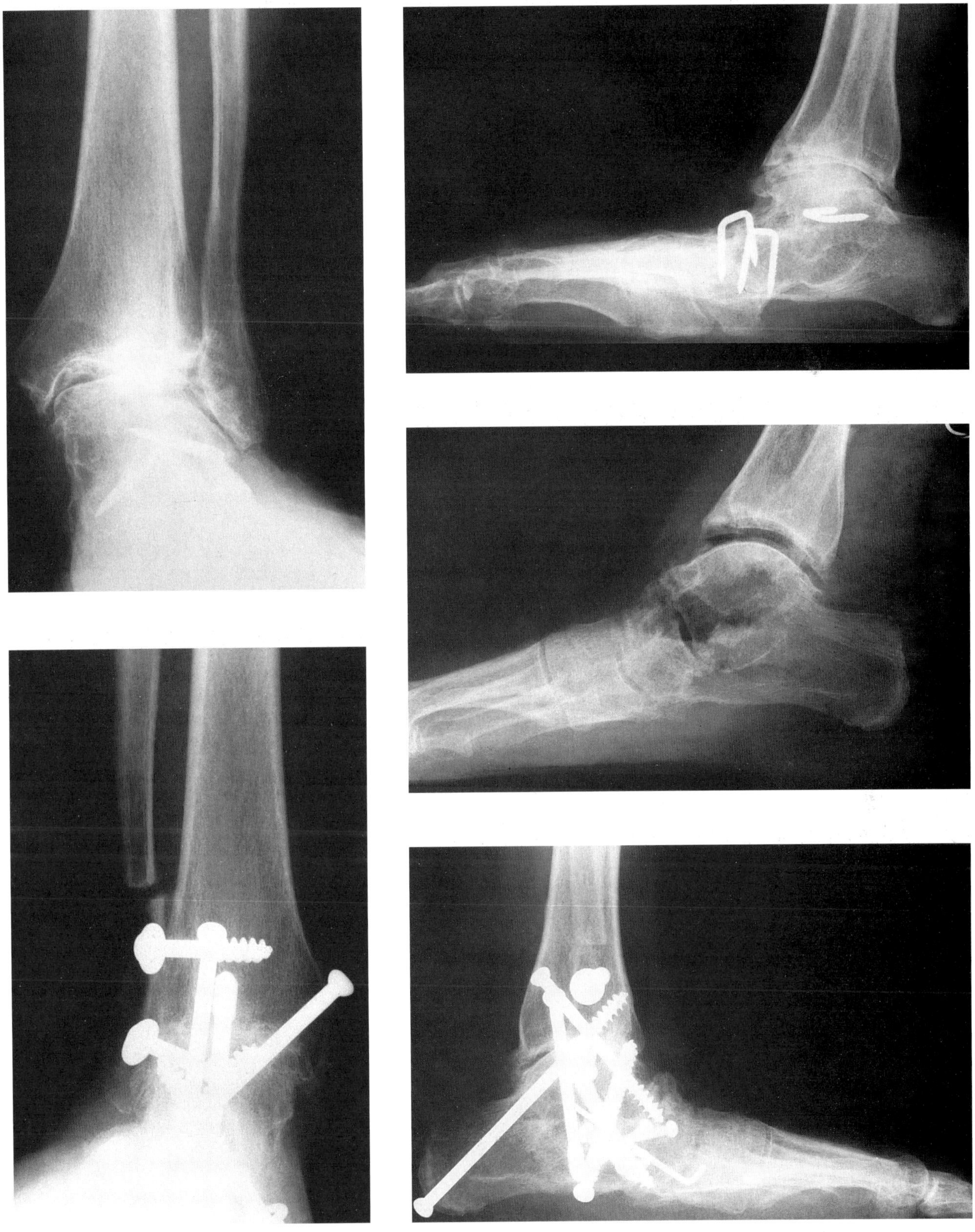

Fig. 10 **Top left,** Anteroposterior (AP) view showing severe ankle degenerative disease above triple arthrodesis. **Top right,** Lateral view showing ankle arthrosis and poorly positioned triple arthrodesis. **Center right,** Intraoperative film demonstrating osteotomies through talonavicular and subtalar regions for repositioning of hindfoot arthrodesis. **Bottom left,** AP view demonstrating construct for ankle arthrodesis. **Bottom right,** Lateral view demonstrating fixation for revision triple arthrodesis in conjunction with ankle fusion.

Charcot Joints

Each of the described fusions can be performed in patients with neuropathic joints. The fundamental principles of achieving good position and fixation must be emphasized. Multiple large screws with excellent purchase on both sides of the site of fusion should be used. No bending moments should be created by the position, and the construct must be biomechanically sound. Bone grafting is essential. Postoperative immobilization should continue until solid fusion is evident radiographically. Due to the associated neuropathy, the ability of neuropathic patients to discern the pain of an ununited arthrodesis is impaired.

Osteotomy Through A Previous Ankle Fusion

Despite the best efforts to properly position a patient for an arthrodesis of the ankle, some patients are left with an unacceptable position. One must attempt to modify shoe wear before considering osteotomy, but some deformities are too severe for compensatory arrangements with orthotics. Additionally, one must consider if there are deformities of the forefoot or midfoot that contribute to the disability. For example, if a patient has an excessively plantarflexed first ray, a dorsiflexion osteotomy of the first metatarsal should be considered instead of or in addition to an ankle osteotomy.

The most common deformity of an ankle fusion is equinus. This can be corrected with an anterior closing wedge osteotomy. Either the anterior or lateral approach can be used. Crossed 6.5-mm cancellous compression screws are effective. Crossed anterior to posterior and posterior to anterior screws are preferred (Fig. 9).

Osteotomy Through A Triple Arthrodesis

Residual heel varus from an old clubfoot deformity or undercorrection of hindfoot valgus secondary to posterior tibial tendon dysfunction are two common causes of unacceptable hindfoot deformity after triple arthrodesis. Revision osteotomy is performed with medial and lateral approaches as described for an initial triple arthrodesis. An initial osteotomy is made through the talonavicular and subtalar joint areas (Fig. 10).

The hindfoot must be rigidly fixed in the proper position. Optimal positioning may require an additional calcaneocubiod osteotomy to align the forefoot with the hindfoot. Again, one must consider the need for a plantarflexing Lapidus procedure to "desupinate" the forefoot when correcting heel valgus or a first metatarsal dorsiflexion osteotomy to correct forefoot pronation when correcting hindfoot varus.

References

1. Müller ME, Allgöwer M, Schneider R, et al (eds): *Manual of Internal Fixation: Techniques Recommended by the AO-ASIF Group*, ed 3. Berlin, Germany, Springer-Verlag, 1991.
2. Manoli A II, Hansen ST Jr: Screw hole preparation in foot surgery. *Foot Ankle* 1990;11:105–106.
3. Perren SM: The biomechanics and biology of internal fixation using plates and nails. *Orthopedics* 1989;12:21–34.
4. Alexander IJ: Osteoarthritis and static deformities of the midfoot and hindfoot, in Sammarco GJ (ed): *Foot and Ankle Manual*. Philadelphia, PA, Lea & Febiger, 1991, pp 145–162.
5. Buck P, Morrey BF, Chao EY: The optimum position of arthrodesis of the ankle: A gait study of the knee and ankle. *J Bone Joint Surg* 1987;69A:1052–1062.
6. Campbell CJ, Rinehart WT, Kalenak A: Arthrodesis of the ankle: Deep autogenous inlay grafts with maximum cancellous-bone apposition. *J Bone Joint Surg* 1974;56A:63–70.
7. Hefti FL, Baumann JU, Morscher EW: Ankle joint fusion: Determination of optimal position by gait analysis. *Arch Orthop Trauma Surg* 1980;96:187–195.
8. Mazur JM, Schwartz E, Simon SR: Ankle arthrodesis: Long-term follow-up with gait analysis. *J Bone Joint Surg* 1979;61A:964–975.
9. Morrey BF, Wiedeman GP Jr: Complications and long-term results of ankle arthrodeses following trauma. *J Bone Joint Surg* 1980;62A:777–784.
10. Charnley J: Compression arthrodesis of the ankle and shoulder. *J Bone Joint Surg* 1951;33B:180–191.
11. Holt ES, Hansen ST, Mayo KA, et al: Ankle arthrodesis using internal screw fixation. *Clin Orthop* 1991;268:21–28.
12. Mead NC: Fusion of the ankle joint: A description of a simple, effective surgical technic. *Clin Orthop* 1953;2:211–215.
13. Verhelst MP, Mulier JC, Hoogmartens MJ, et al: Arthrodesis of the ankle joint with complete removal of the distal part of the fibula: Experience with the transfibular approach and three different types of fixation. *Clin Orthop* 1976;118:93–99.
14. White AA III: A precision posterior ankle fusion. *Clin Orthop* 1974;98:239–250.
15. Hatt RN, Lamphier TA: Triple hemisection: A simplified procedure for lengthening the Achilles tendon. *N Engl J Med* 1947;236:166–169.
16. Gable ST, Bohay DR, Manoli A II: Technique tip: Aiming guide for accurate placement of subtalar joint screws. *Foot Ankle Int* 1995;16:238–239.
17. Lionberger DR, Bishop JO, Tullos HS: The modified Blair fusion. *Foot Ankle* 1982;3:60–62.
18. Morris HD, Hand WL, Dunn AW: The modified Blair fusion for fractures of the talus. *J Bone Joint Surg* 1971;53A:1289–1297.
19. Carr JB, Hansen ST, Benirschke SK: Subtalar distraction bone block fusion for late complications of os calcis fractures. *Foot Ankle* 1988;9:81–86.
20. Hansen ST Jr: Foot injuries, in Browner BD, Jupiter JB, Levine AM, et al (eds): *Skeletal Trauma: Fractures, Dislocations, Ligamentous Injuries*. Philadelphia, PA, WB Saunders, 1992, vol 2, pp 1959–1991.
21. Sanders R, Hansen ST Jr, McReynolds IS: Trauma to the calcaneus and its tendon: Fractures of the calcaneus, in Jahss MH (ed): *Disorders of the Foot and Ankle: Medical and Surgical Management*, ed 2. Philadelphia, PA, WB Saunders, 1991, vol 3, pp 2326–2354.
22. Sangeorzan BJ, Hansen ST Jr: Early and late posttraumatic foot reconstruction. *Clin Orthop* 1989;243:86–91.
23. Sangeorzan BJ, Smith DG, Veith RG, et al: Triple arthrodesis using internal fixation in treatment of adult foot disorders. *Clin Orthop* 1993;294:299–307.

CHAPTER 35

Hallux Valgus

Michael J. Coughlin, MD

Hallux valgus occurs with lateral deviation of the great toe and medial deviation of the first metatarsal. Commonly, the deformity is characterized by progressive subluxation of the first metatarsophalangeal (MTP) joint (Fig. 1). Occasionally, there is a static deformity due to valgus angulation of the distal articular surface of the first metatarsal or the proximal phalangeal articular surface (Fig. 2).

Hallux valgus occurs almost exclusively in shoe-wearing societies.[1] Coughlin and Thompson,[2] noting the extremely high prevalence of bunions in American women in the fourth, fifth, or sixth decade of life, implicated constricting footwear as a cause of hallux valgus. This notion is supported by a study from China, where the prevalence of hallux valgus was 15 times higher in people who wore shoes than in those who did not.[3] Likewise, in Japan, Kato and Watanabe[4] noted that the prevalence of hallux valgus in women increased dramatically following the introduction of high-fashion footwear after World War II.

While constricting footwear appears to be the major extrinsic cause of hallux valgus, intrinsic factors play a role as well. Inman[5] and Hohmann[6] both suggested pronation of the hindfoot as a major cause of bunion formation, while Mann and Coughlin[7] as well as others[8,9] reported that pes planus plays a minor role in this process. An increased angle between the first and second metatarsals (metatarsus primus varus) is often associated with a hallux valgus deformity. Hardy and Clapham[10] reported an association between the magnitude of the hallux valgus angle and the first-second intermetatarsal angle and stated that metatarsus primus varus is secondary to an increased hallux valgus angle. Other intrinsic causes of hallux valgus may include contracture of the Achilles tendon, generalized joint laxity, hypermobility of the first metatarsocuneiform joint, and neuromuscular disorders (including cerebral palsy and stroke).[11] Heredity is thought to influence the development of hallux valgus in many individuals. Hardy and Clapham noted that 63% of the

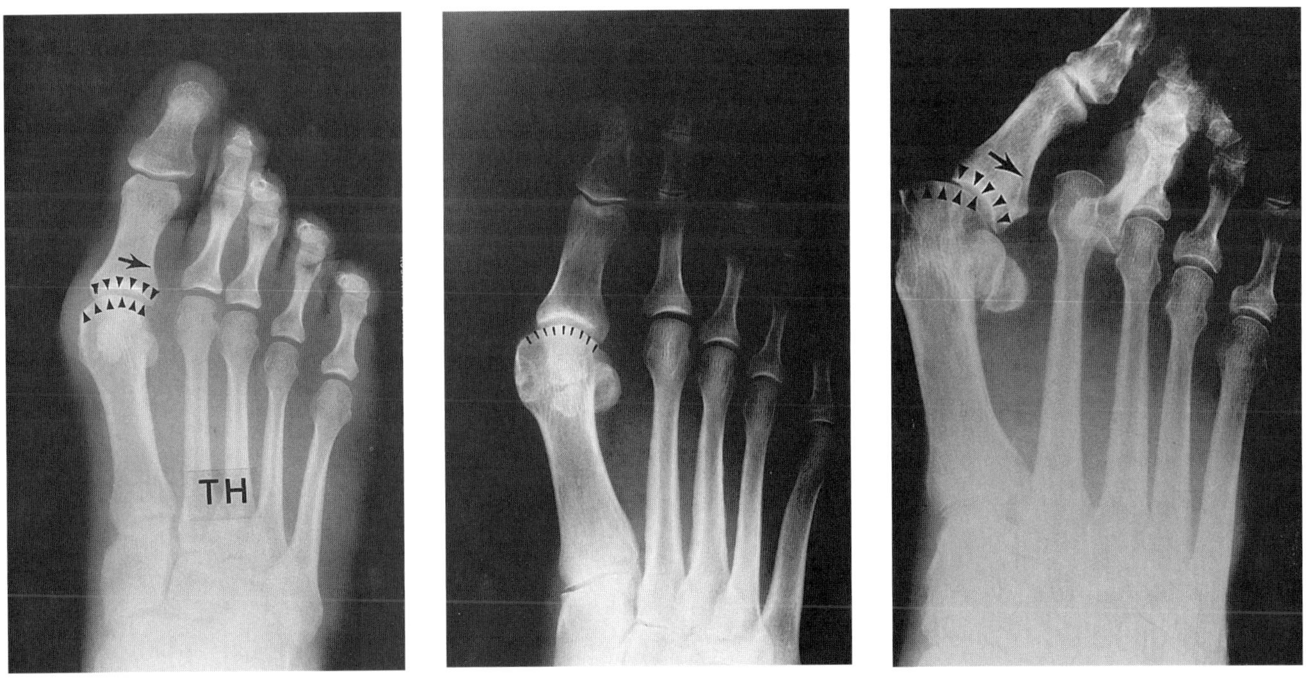

Fig. 1 Radiographs demonstrating the different degrees of a hallux valgus deformity. The arrows indicate the direction of the subluxation, and the arrowheads indicate the extent of the joint surface. **Left,** A mild hallux valgus deformity with subluxation of the first metatarsophalangeal joint. The hallux valgus angle is 19°, the first-second intermetatarsal angle is 10°, and there is less than 50% (mild) subluxation of the sesamoids. **Center,** A moderate hallux valgus deformity with subluxation of the first metatarsophalangeal joint. The hallux valgus angle is 30°, the first-second intermetatarsal angle is 14°, and there is 50% to 75% (moderate) subluxation of the sesamoids. **Right,** A severe, recurrent hallux valgus deformity with severe subluxation of the first metatarsophalangeal joint. The hallux valgus angle is 50°, the first-second intermetatarsal angle is 17°, and there is more than 75% (severe) subluxation of the sesamoids. The second metatarsophalangeal joint is dislocated.

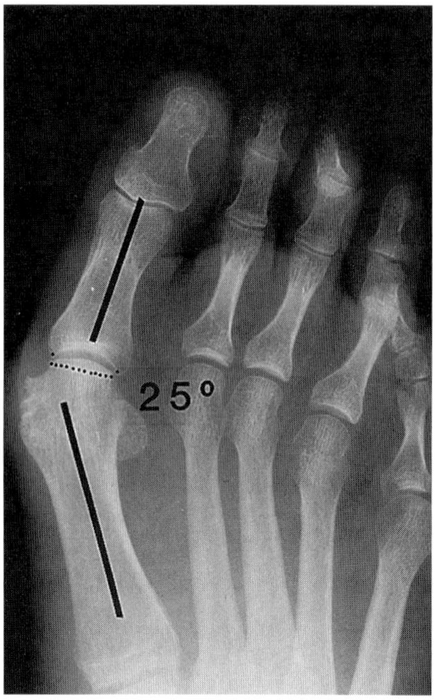

Fig. 2 Radiograph of a foot with a moderate hallux valgus deformity without subluxation of the first metatarsophalangeal joint. The hallux valgus is due mainly to 25° of valgus angulation of the distal articular surface of the metatarsal. A sagittal groove (or sulcus) has developed medial to the articular surface. There is a prominent medial eminence. The dotted line indicates the medial and lateral extent of the distal articular surface of the metatarsal.

91 patients in their series had a parent who had hallux valgus, and I[8] reported that a bunion was identified in 94% of 31 mothers of children who had hallux valgus.

Anatomy

The MTP joint of the great toe is different from that of the lesser toes because it has a sesamoid mechanism and a set of intrinsic muscles that stabilize the joint and provide motor strength to the first ray.[12] The muscles and tendons that control the great toe are divided into four groups that encircle the first MTP joint (Fig. 3, *top*). On the dorsal aspect of the great toe, the extensor hallucis longus and brevis pass centrally, inserting into the distal and proximal phalanges, respectively. The extensor hallucis longus is anchored by the hood ligaments,[13] a fibrous band that interdigitates medially and laterally with the collateral and sesamoid ligaments, forming the capsule of the MTP joint. The short and long flexor tendons pass on the plantar surface, with the tendons of the medial and lateral heads of the flexor hallucis brevis inserting into the medial and lateral sesamoids (Fig. 3, *center*). Distally, the sesamoids are attached to the base of the proximal phalanx by the plantar plate (Fig. 3, *bottom*). The flexor hallucis longus tendon is located plantar to the sesamoid complex,

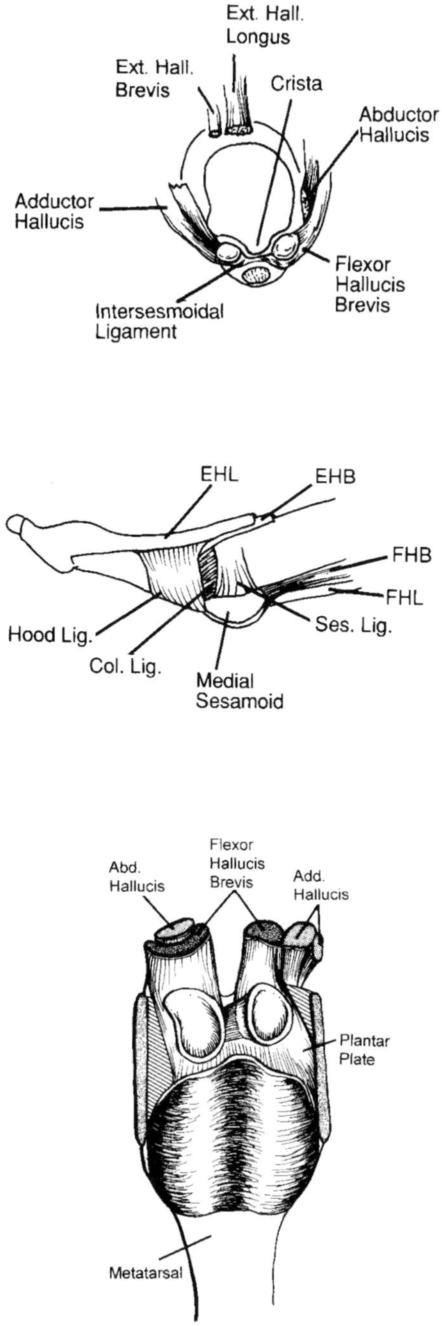

Fig. 3 Drawings illustrating the anatomy of the foot. **Top,** A transverse section through the first ray at the level of the first metatarsal head. The long and short extensors are the major tendinous structures on the dorsal aspect of the first metatarsophalangeal joint. **Center,** The hood ligament interdigitates with the extensor hallucis longus (EHL). The flexors pass on the plantar aspect, with the flexor hallucis brevis (FHB) inserting into the sesamoids. EHB = extensor hallucis brevis, FHL = flexor hallucis longus, Ses. Lig. = sesamoid ligament, Col. Lig. = collateral ligament, and Medial Ses. = medial sesamoid. **Bottom,** The plantar aspect of the first metatarsophalangeal joint. The sesamoid complex has been reflected distally to reveal the plantar plate. The plantar plate connects the sesamoids and the flexor hallucis brevis to the base of the proximal phalanx plantarly.

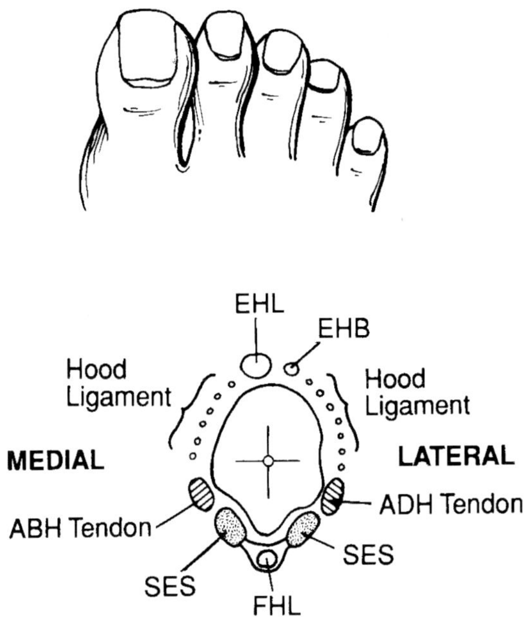

Fig. 4 Illustration of the anatomy of a foot with the great toe in normal alignment. The sesamoids (Ses.) and intrinsic muscles stabilize the plantar aspect of the first metatarsal head. The hood ligaments make up much of the dorsal aspect of the capsule. EHL = extensor hallucis longus, EHB = extensor hallucis brevis, ADH = adductor hallucis, FHL = flexor hallucis longus, and ABH = abductor hallucis.

passing within a tendon sheath to insert into the base of the distal phalanx.

The abductor and adductor hallucis tendons are located on the plantar-medial and plantar-lateral aspects, respectively, of the MTP joint and insert into the base of the proximal phalanx and the adjacent sesamoids (Fig. 4). The plantar half of the MTP joint capsule is reinforced by the tendons of the abductor hallucis and adductor hallucis, while the dorsal half of the MTP capsule is comparatively thin, without tendinous constraints. With the development of hallux valgus (Fig. 5), the abductor hallucis tendon is displaced plantarward, leaving only the thinner and weaker dorsal half of the capsule as the major restraining force on the medial aspect.[14]

In its normal position, the abductor hallucis provides major support to the well-aligned great toe.[12] On the lateral aspect, the adductor hallucis provides stability as well; however, its insertion into the plantar-lateral aspect of the base of the proximal phalanx and lateral sesamoid becomes a deforming force as the hallux valgus deformity increases. Because it arises from the shafts of the lesser metatarsals, the adductor hallucis tends to tether the sesamoids and proximal phalanx as the first metatarsal deviates medially. Because it inserts on the plantar aspect of the proximal phalanx, the adductor hallucis also exerts a rotational force on the great toe, pronating it as the phalanx deviates laterally (Fig. 6). With continued lateral movement, the imbalance progresses and the intrinsic plantar cuff (the

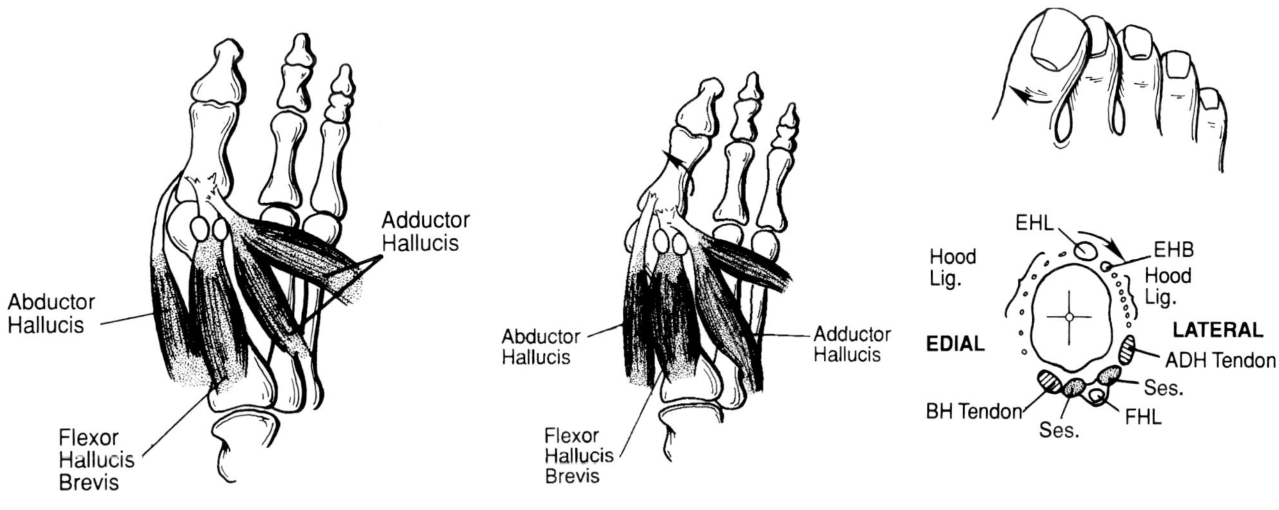

Fig. 5, **Left** and **center,** Drawings of the plantar aspect of a foot with hallux valgus. **Left,** The great toe deviates laterally. **Center,** The great toe pronates (arrow) as it rotates on the axis of the conjoined adductor hallucis tendon. **Right,** Dorsal aspect of the toes of a foot with hallux valgus and a cross section through the first metatarsal head. The crista (intersesamoid ridge) is diminished in height as the sesamoids (Ses.) assume a more lateral orientation and the abductor hallucis (ABH) tendon migrates plantarward (arrows), leaving the thin extensor hood ligament as the major soft-tissue constraint against progressive hallux valgus. EHL = extensor hallucis longus, EHB = extensor hallucis brevis, ADH = adductor hallucis, and FHL = flexor hallucis longus.

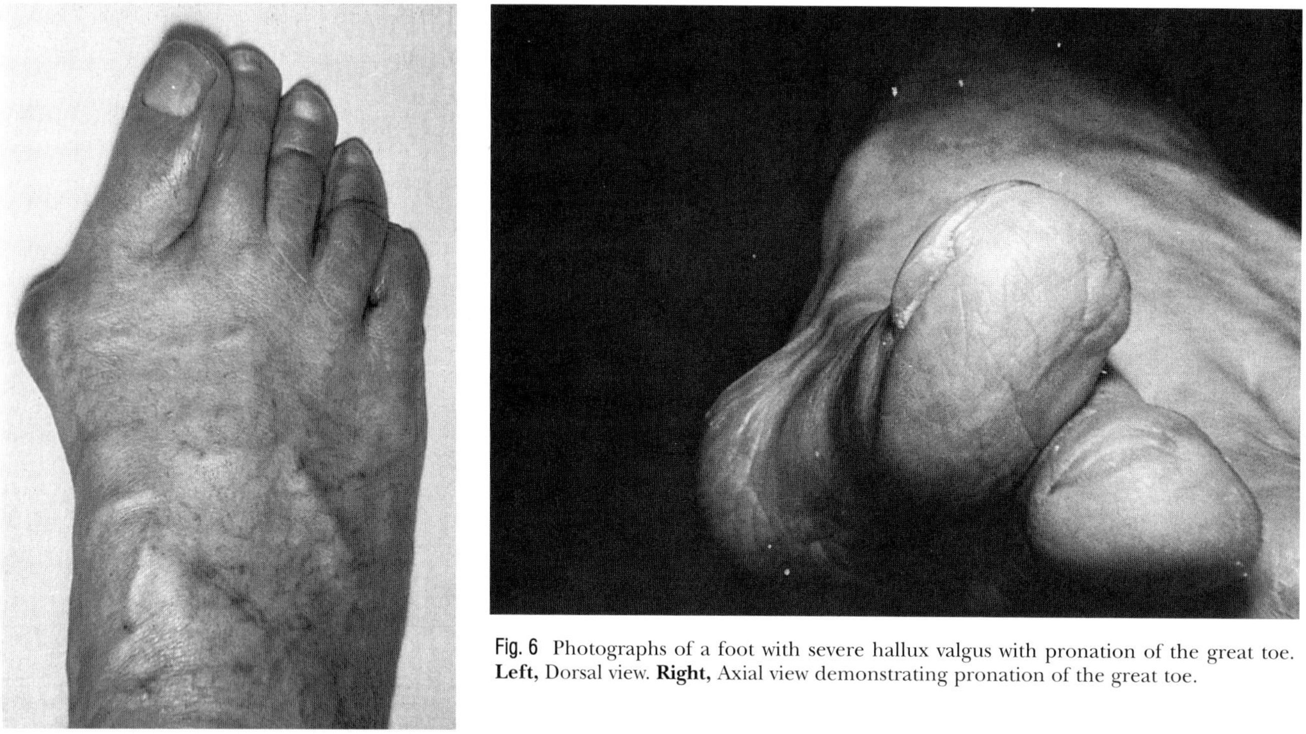

Fig. 6 Photographs of a foot with severe hallux valgus with pronation of the great toe. **Left,** Dorsal view. **Right,** Axial view demonstrating pronation of the great toe.

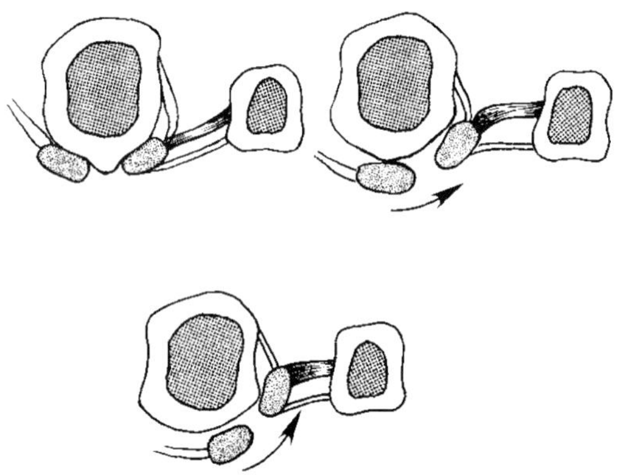

Fig. 7 Normal alignment and subluxation of the sesamoids. **Top Left,** Normal alignment of the sesamoids. **Top right,** As the first metatarsal migrates medially, the crista is eroded and the medial sesamoid assumes a more central location (arrow). **Bottom,** With a severe deformity, the lateral sesamoid comes to lie vertically dorsal to the medial sesamoid (arrow), and a lateral soft-tissue contracture occurs.

adductor hallucis, flexor hallucis brevis, and abductor hallucis) rotates in a lateral direction (in relation to the head of the first metatarsal), leaving the thin dorsal half of the capsule that is at risk for additional deformation.[12] As the hallux valgus deformity progresses, the extensor hallucis longus displaces into the first interspace and becomes an adduction force on the great toe.

Continuing lateral rotation of the intrinsic plantar cuff leads to displacement or subluxation of the medial and lateral sesamoids in relation to the plantar surface of the first metatarsal (Fig. 7). While this phenomenon has been described as subluxation of the sesamoids, it is actually the first metatarsal that deviates medially away from the sesamoid complex.

The plantar surface of the first metatarsal is characterized by a crista, or intersesamoid ridge, that articulates with the medial and lateral sesamoids (Fig. 8, *left*). As displacement occurs, this ridge is gradually smoothed out until it offers no additional resistance to displacement of the sesamoid,[15] as can be demonstrated on an axial radiograph (Fig. 8, *center*). On an anteroposterior (AP) radiograph of a joint with moderate subluxation, the lateral sesamoid is uncovered 50% to 75% within the first intermetatarsal space and the medial sesamoid is located in a central position plantar to the first metatarsal head (Fig. 8, *center*). With a severe hallux valgus deformity, the lateral sesamoid migrates to the lateral aspect of the first metatarsal head and lies vertically dorsal to the medial sesamoid (Fig. 8, *right*).[13]

It is important to recognize the magnitude of subluxation of the sesamoids because this will guide the choice of the method of surgical reconstruction. A surgical correction that does not reduce this subluxation by relocating the first metatarsal head to a normal articulation with both the medial and the lateral sesamoid is at risk for recurrent deformity. As the hallux valgus deformity increases in magnitude, there is a corre-

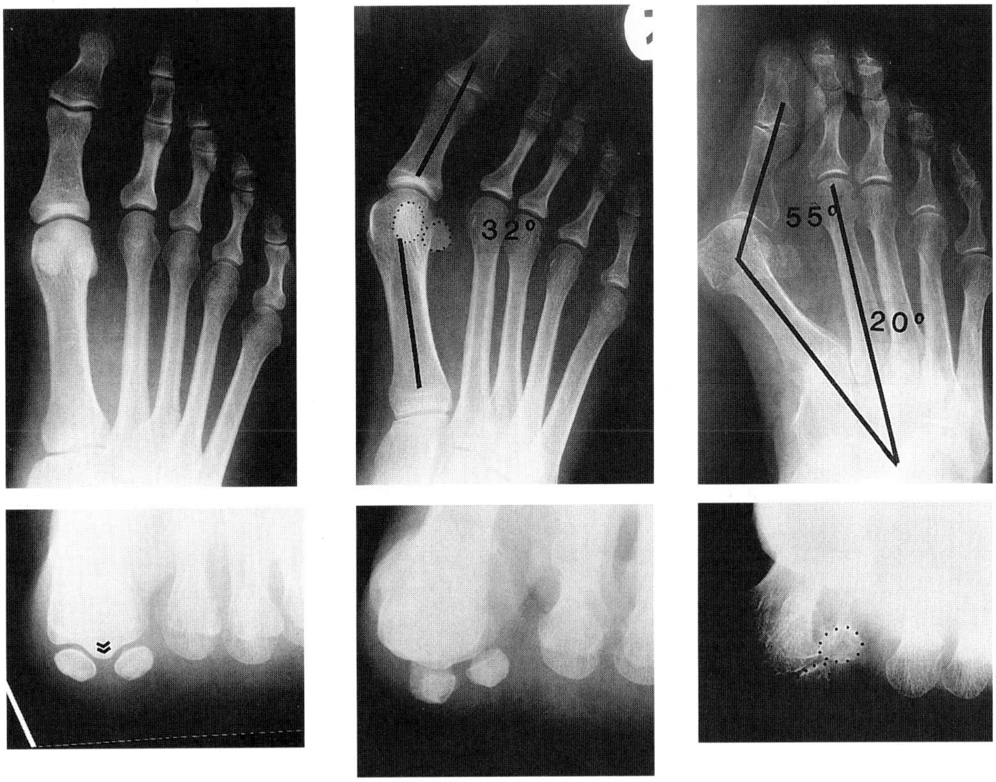

Fig. 8 Radiographs showing normal alignment and subluxation of the sesamoids. **Left,** Anteroposterior, **top,** and axial, **bottom,** radiographs, made with the patient standing, demonstrating the normal alignment of the sesamoids with a straight great toe. Note the crista (double chevrons). **Center,** Anteroposterior and axial radiographs, made with the patient standing, showing a moderate hallux valgus deformity. The hallux valgus angle is 32°, and there is 75% subluxation of the sesamoids (dotted outlines). **Right,** Anteroposterior and axial radiographs, made with the patient standing, showing a severe hallux valgus deformity. The hallux valgus angle is 55°, with vertical orientation of the lateral sesamoid dorsal to the medial sesamoid (dotted outlines).

sponding increase in both the subluxation of the sesamoids and the pronation of the great toe. Surgical techniques for correction may vary considerably, depending on the magnitude of both of these deformities.

Angular measurements on radiographs made with the patient standing are helpful to define the magnitude of the hallux valgus deformity (Fig. 9). The hallux valgus angle is formed by the intersection of the longitudinal axes of the proximal phalanx and the first metatarsal. A hallux valgus angle of less than 15° is considered normal.[10] The first-second intermetatarsal angle is formed by the intersection of the longitudinal axes of the first and second metatarsals, and an angle of less than 9° is considered normal.[11] With the use of these two measurements, a general classification scheme for hallux valgus was developed. It is helpful to define mild, moderate, and severe deformities, both to standardize their description and to assist in preoperative planning.[11] A mild hallux valgus deformity is characterized by a hallux valgus angle of less than 20° and a first-second intermetatarsal angle of 11° or less (Fig. 1, *left*). Subluxation of the lateral sesamoid, as measured on an AP radiograph, is less than 50%. A moderate deformity is characterized by a hallux valgus angle of 20° to 40°, a first-second intermetatarsal angle of less than 16°, and 50% to 75% subluxation of the lateral sesamoid (Figs. 1, *center* and 8, *center*). A severe deformity is characterized by a hallux valgus angle of more than 40°, a first-second intermetatarsal angle of 16° or more, and more than 75% subluxation of the lateral sesamoid (Figs. 1, *right* and 8, *right*).

There is significant variation in the shape of the distal articular surface of the first metatarsal. A rounded surface is most common (Fig. 10, *top left*), and it is more prone to subluxation and to the development of a progressive hallux valgus deformity. A flattened or chevron-shaped MTP articulation is more stable and tends to resist subluxation (Fig. 10, *top right*).[11] The term congruity describes the relationship of the metatarsal and phalangeal articular surfaces. When the surfaces are aligned, the joint is said to be congruous (Fig. 10, *bottom*).[16] When they are not aligned, the articulation is non-congruous (subluxation of the MTP

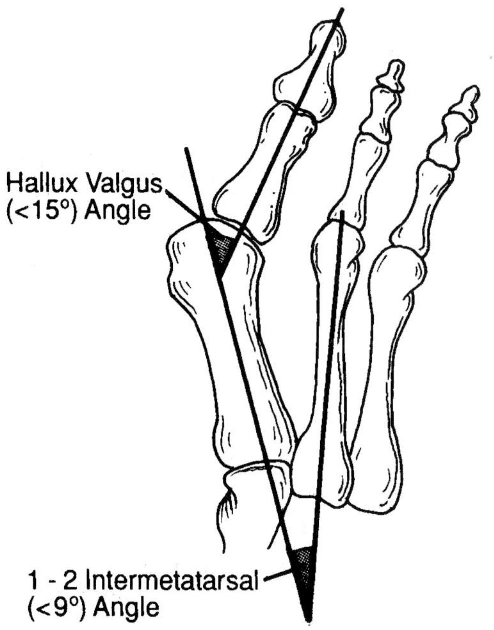

Fig. 9 Illustration demonstrating the radiographic measurements in the assessment of hallux valgus. The hallux valgus angle is formed by the intersection of the longitudinal axes of the first metatarsal and the proximal phalanx. A normal angle is less than 15°. The first-second intermetatarsal angle is formed by the intersection of the longitudinal axes of the first and second metatarsals. A normal angle is less than 9°.

joint) (Fig. 1). The distal metatarsal articular surface forms an angle with the longitudinal axis of the first metatarsal (the distal metatarsal articular angle, or DMAA). The proximal articular surface of the proximal phalanx forms a similar angle with the longitudinal axis of the proximal phalanx (the proximal phalangeal articular angle, or PPAA). These two angles reflect the basic inclination of the MTP joint. Normally, the great toe is in slight valgus angulation (0° to 15°) as a result of the lateral inclination or sloping of the distal metatarsal articular surface.[8,16,17] This angulation is also known as the metatarsal articular orientation or the proximal articular set angle; however, the term DMAA describes more clearly the inclination of the metatarsal articular surface. The PPAA has also been called the phalangeal articular orientation and the distal articular set angle. Although substantial angulation of the phalangeal articular surface in relation to the shaft of the phalanx is uncommon (two of 65 feet in one series[8]), when it is present a hallux valgus interphalangeus deformity is created (Fig. 11). Angulation of the phalangeal articular surface can occur in the presence of an increased DMAA or subluxation of the MTP joint, or both. A normal MTP articulation occurs with a hallux valgus angle of less than 15°. Angulation of the MTP joint may be created by mild subluxation of that joint, by a lateral sloping of the distal metatarsal articular surface, by increased lateral sloping of the proximal phalangeal articular surface, or by a combination of these.

Piggott,[16] in an analysis of congruous and noncongruous MTP joints with hallux valgus, determined that a congruous joint was less likely to have progression of the hallux valgus deformity. A noncongruous joint was likely to subluxate further with time. Twenty (9%) of 215 adult feet with hallux valgus in the series reviewed by Piggott had a congruous joint, and 28 (47%) of 60 juvenile feet with hallux valgus reported on by me had a congruous joint. It is important to distinguish a congruous MTP joint from a noncongruous one when treating hallux valgus, as the choice of a specific surgical approach depends on the pathologic elements present. An intra-articular realignment (such as a McBride procedure or another distal soft-tissue reconstruction) achieves correction by rotating the articular surface of the phalanx across the articular surface of the metatarsal to reduce the hallux valgus angle. In contrast, an extra-articular correction (an Akin, Reverdin, chevron, or Mitchell osteotomy; proximal metatarsal osteotomy; or cuneiform osteotomy) achieves correction through periarticular osteotomies, which do not change the articular orientation or congruency of the MTP joint. Realignment of a congruous hallux valgus deformity with an intra-articular procedure may be complicated postoperatively either by recurrence of the deformity or by restricted motion of the MTP joint.[11]

The medial eminence, or bunion, is often the most visible component of a hallux valgus deformity. Often preoperative pain is centered in this region because of irritation of the dorsal cutaneous nerve of the great toe or an inflamed or thickened bursa overlying the medial eminence. Occasionally the medial eminence is hypertrophied, but frequently it is not much enlarged. An increase in the first-second intermetatarsal angle with lateral deviation of the great toe leaves the medial eminence prominent and easily irritated by constricting footwear. As the proximal phalanx deviates laterally, the head of the metatarsal is pushed medially. The lateral soft-tissue structures contract as the medial soft-tissue constraints become attenuated. The medial deviation of the first metatarsal gradually uncovers the lateral sesamoid. The intrinsic muscles, which normally act to stabilize the MTP joint, become deforming forces. There are no muscle insertions into the first metatarsal head; thus, its position is influenced to a great extent by the position of the proximal phalanx. With progressive MTP subluxation, a groove (or sagittal sulcus) develops at the medial border of the metatarsal articular surface. The magnitude of the

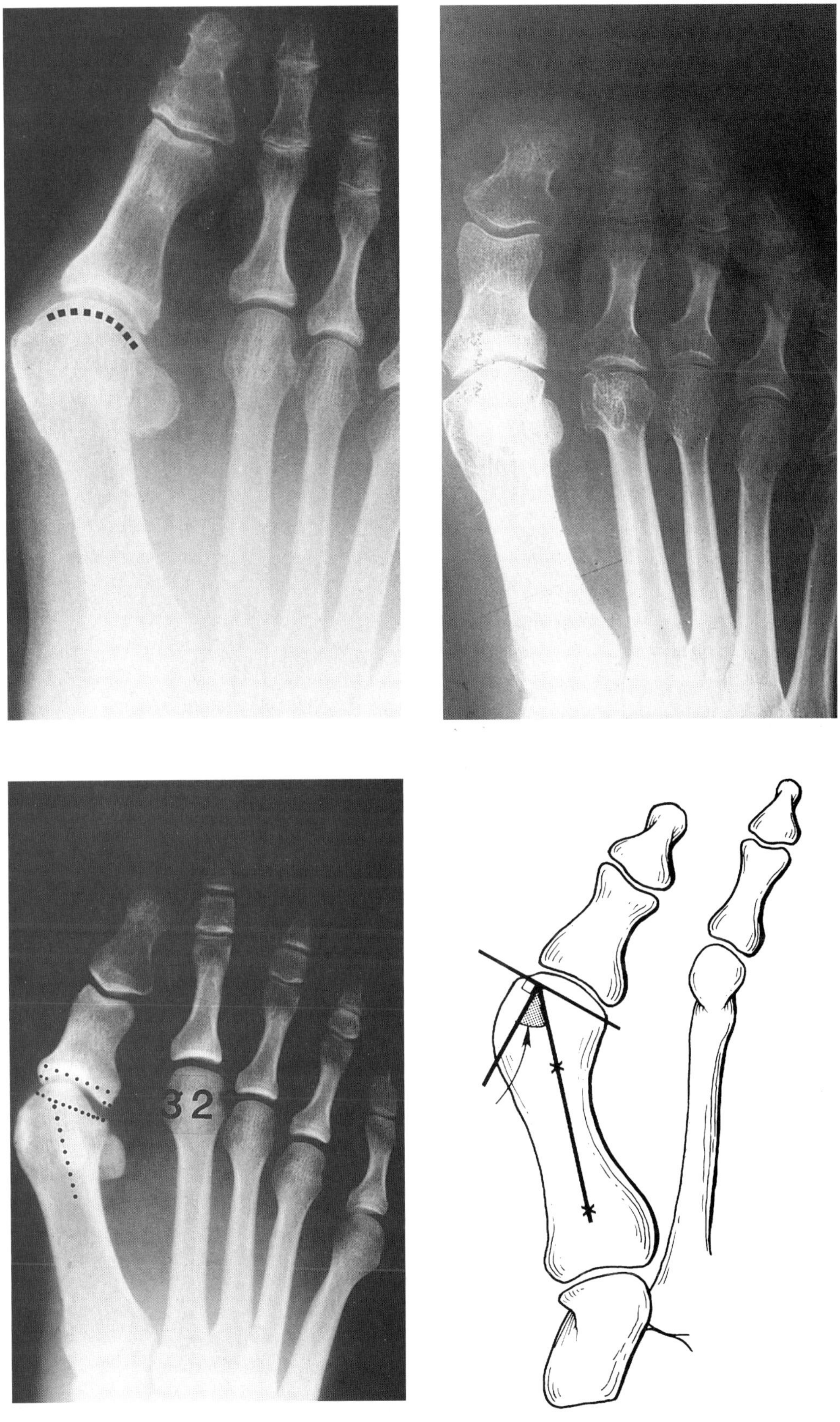

Fig. 10 Anteroposterior radiographs and a drawing demonstrating the shapes of the metatarsophalangeal articular surfaces. **Top left,** A rounded articular surface (dotted line) is more prone to subluxation of the metatarsophalangeal joint. **Top right,** The joint is congruous without subluxation. A flattened or chevron-shaped metatarsophalangeal joint tends to resist subluxation. **Bottom left,** A hallux valgus deformity with a congruous metatarsophalangeal joint (dotted lines). **Bottom right,** This drawing illustrates how the distal metatarsal articular angle measures the lateral slope of the articular surface of the metatarsal. The distal metatarsal articular angle is the angle subtended by a line drawn perpendicular to the metatarsal articular surface and the longitudinal axis of the first metatarsal. With increasing lateral angulation of the articular surface, the angle increases.

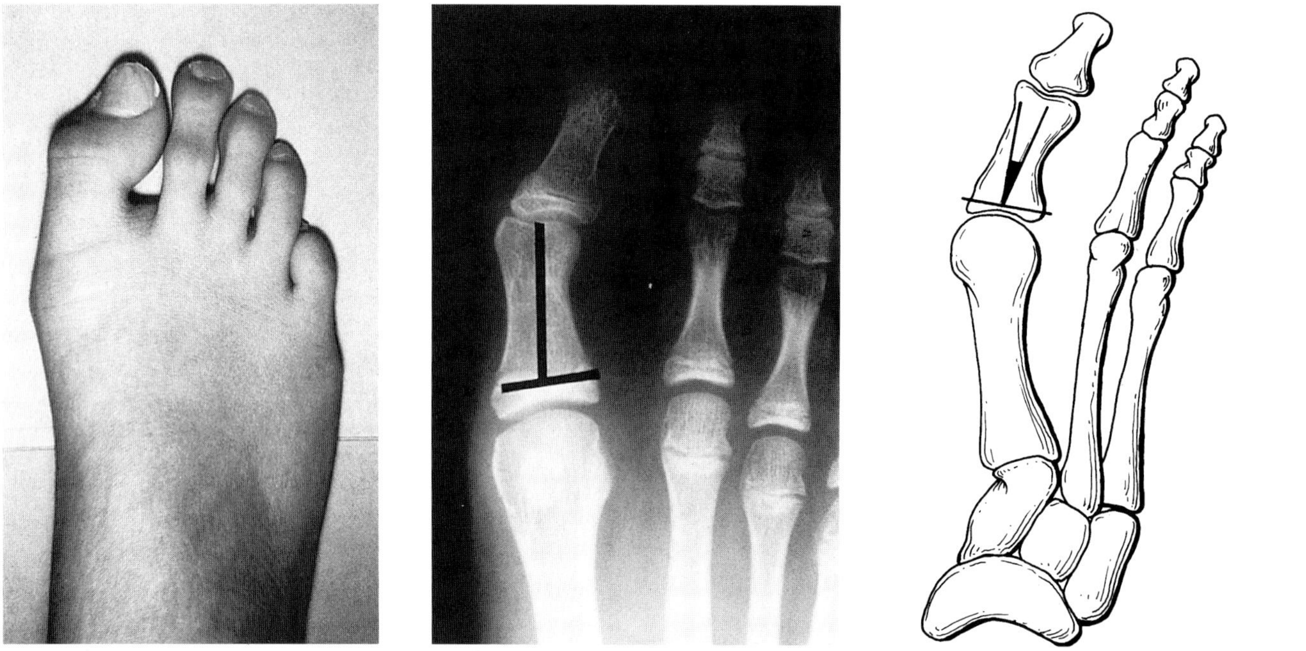

Fig. 11 **Left** and **center,** Photograph and radiograph of a foot with hallux valgus interphalangeus. **Right,** The drawing illustrates how the proximal phalangeal articular angle increases with hallux valgus interphalangeus. The proximal phalangeal articular angle is the angle subtended by a line drawn perpendicular to the phalangeal articular surface and the longitudinal axis of the proximal phalanx.

hallux valgus deformity determines the presence and location of the sagittal sulcus. While this groove does delineate the border of the articular surface, it is an unreliable landmark for the planning of a medial exostectomy. The sagittal sulcus may be located in the center of the metatarsal head when the deformity is severe, and it may be located more medially when the deformity is mild or moderate.[13] It is important not to rely on the sagittal sulcus as the guide for resection of the medial eminence because, with a severe deformity, doing so may lead to excessive bone resection.

The shape and orientation of the metatarsocuneiform joint are variable factors that influence the magnitude of medial inclination of the first metatarsal. Normally the first metatarsocuneiform joint is inclined medially, but occasionally there is marked medial obliquity, which is believed by some to result in instability of the metatarsocuneiform joint.[18,19] Radiographically, the metatarsocuneiform joint may appear to be flat, curved, or oblique, and the appearance can vary dramatically depending on the plane of the weightbearing radiograph.[18] Undoubtedly, there is a certain amount of flexibility in the metatarsocuneiform joint,[20] and this is demonstrated by the decrease in the size of the first-second intermetatarsal angle following a distal soft-tissue reconstruction. Excessive flexibility at this joint may be inferred from a radiograph, but it is best ascertained by physical examination.[18,19]

History and Physical Examination

The primary symptom of hallux valgus is pain over the medial eminence. Pressure from footwear is the most frequent cause of this discomfort. Bursal inflammation, irritation of the skin, and even breakdown of the skin may be noted.

The physical examination of a hallux valgus deformity must be performed with the patient sitting and standing. The deformity is often accentuated with weightbearing. The foot is examined for a pes planus deformity and for contracture of the Achilles tendon, both of which may affect the choice and success of the surgical technique. The magnitude of the hallux valgus deformity is noted, as is any pronation of the great toe. The passive and active range of motion of the MTP joint is measured.[21] Pain or crepitus, or both, with motion of the MTP joint is often indicative of degenerative osteoarthrosis and often alters the choice of the surgical procedure. To check the metatarsocuneiform joint for hypermobility, the examiner grasps the first metatarsal with the thumb and index finger and pushes it in a plantar lateral-to-dorsomedial direction.[19] Mobility of more than 9 mm represents hypermobility,[19] which, according to Mann and Coughlin,[11] is present in less than 5% of patients. The neurovascular status of the foot must also be assessed. Doppler studies may be performed if there is a question regarding the adequacy of circulation. The foot is inspected for deformities of the lesser toes that may cause discomfort as well. Other frequent symptoms are hammer-toe deformities of the second toe or metatarsalgia of the lesser MTP joints. The plantar surface of the foot should be inspected for intractable plantar keratoses or callosities.

An attempt should be made to reduce the first MTP joint by passive correction of the hallux valgus def-ormity. This may be difficult if there is a soft-tissue contracture. This maneuver helps the examiner to assess the congruency of the MTP joint. Passive attempts to alter the alignment of a congruous MTP joint frequently limit its passive range of motion.

An interview with the patient is important not only to evaluate the major symptoms associated with the hallux valgus deformity but also to educate the patient with regard to the problem, the alternatives for treatment, and the risks and complications when surgery is indicated. A patient's preoperative expectations play a major role in his or her postoperative satisfaction. Relief of pain is frequently the major objective, but an improved appearance of the foot and the ability to wear smaller or narrower shoes are frequent (and often unstated) goals as well. Mann and associates[22] reported that, while 59% of patients were able to wear their choice of shoes after repair of a hallux valgus deformity, 41% were not. It is important to educate the patient regarding the likely result of surgery as well as its limitations.

Radiographic Examination

Weightbearing AP, lateral, and axial (sesamoid) radiographs should be made. Evaluation of the radiographs includes measurement of the hallux valgus angle and the first-second intermetatarsal angle. The first MTP joint is evaluated for osteoarthrosis and congruity, and the DMAA and the PPAA are measured. The size of the medial eminence and the magnitude of sesamoid subluxation are assessed. The forefoot alignment is evaluated for metatarsus adductus, and the hindfoot is inspected for pes planus or pes cavus.

Decision-Making for Treatment

Conservative care is always the first option for a patient with hallux valgus deformity. Often, pain, blistering, and bursal inflammation can be relieved by eliminating friction over the medial eminence. Evaluation of the patient's footwear may prove helpful for making recommendations for modifications or a change in the size or style of the shoes. A wider toe box may reduce symptoms substantially.[2] Stretching of areas of the shoe that cause increased pressure can result in complete relief of the symptoms overlying a painful bunion. A patient who has pes planus can be managed with an orthosis. A contracture of the Achilles tendon may be treated with stretching exercises or, sometimes, with lengthening of the Achilles tendon. Severe pes planus not only may be a factor in the etiology of hallux valgus but also may lead to recurrent deformity. On rare occasions, stabilization or realignment of the hindfoot may be necessary in conjunction with a bunion operation.

Despite conservative measures, some patients eventually need surgical intervention. The patient should be counseled regarding the risks, complications, and expectations of the surgery. Various magnitudes of deformity, different pathologic elements, and anatomic abnormalities make it important for the surgeon to have several techniques of hallux valgus repair available. The selection of the specific procedure is often based on the severity of the hallux valgus deformity and the magnitude of the first-second intermetatarsal angle but may vary from surgeon to surgeon. Angular measurements provide only some of the indications for a particular procedure. The chosen surgical technique must correct all elements of the problem: prominence of the medial eminence, increased valgus angulation of the proximal phalanx, an increased first-second intermetatarsal angle, congruency of the MTP joint, subluxation of the sesamoids, and pronation of the great toe. When surgical treatment is planned, association of the main symptom with the physical findings as well as the radiographic information helps the surgeon to select the best procedure for correction of a hallux valgus deformity.

Surgical Correction

The goal of hallux valgus surgery is to correct all pathologic elements and yet maintain a biomechanically functional forefoot. The vast number of surgical techniques that have been described indicates that no one procedure is universally applicable for all deformities and that many procedures have serious shortcomings. The history and physical examination provide information regarding postural deformities, tendon contractures, neurologic and vascular abnormalities, and the alignment and range of motion of the first ray. Radiographic evaluation demonstrates the congruency of the MTP joint, the magnitudes of the hallux valgus and first-second intermetatarsal angles, and the degree of any osteoarthrosis of the joint. If correction is to be successful, the choice of surgical technique must depend on the anatomic and pathologic abnormalities that are present. Options include MTP soft-tissue reconstruction, distal or proximal metatarsal osteotomy, cuneiform osteotomy, arthrodesis of the MTP joint, and excisional arthroplasty.

Joint implants are not considered in this discussion, as I believe that they are rarely indicated in the treatment of hallux valgus, although some surgeons may consider them when there is concomitant hallux rigidus. If a joint replacement is performed in a patient who has osteoarthrosis of the MTP joint as well as hallux valgus, the first-second intermetatarsal and hallux valgus angles must be corrected adequately at the time of the arthroplasty.[23] I believe that any attempt to use an implant to achieve angular realignment is associated with a high risk of postoperative failure. A combination of procedures may occasionally be necessary to obtain a successful result. The surgeon should be aware that any of these procedures may fail and that a reasonable method of salvage should be possible after a failed hallux valgus reconstruction. It is not the purpose of this review to discuss the surgical technique of every bunion procedure but rather to present an approach to surgical intervention that involves several different techniques.

A mild hallux valgus deformity,[11] with or without a congruous MTP joint, can be satisfactorily corrected with a chevron or Mitchell osteotomy. A distal soft-tissue reconstruction may be considered, in addition to these procedures, for a mild hallux valgus deformity with subluxation of the metatarsophalangeal joint. However, a distal soft-tissue reconstruction cannot be used to correct a hallux valgus deformity with a congruous metatarsophalangeal joint, as an intra-articular realignment may create a noncongruous joint that is at risk for recurrence of the deformity or the development of degenerative osteoarthrosis.[15,24]

For a moderate hallux valgus deformity[11] with subluxation of the MTP joint, a Mitchell osteotomy may be considered; however, a distal soft-tissue reconstruction combined with an osteotomy of the proximal end of the metatarsal is more commonly performed. For a moderate hallux valgus deformity with degenerative changes of the MTP joint, an excisional arthroplasty or arthrodesis should be done. A moderate hallux valgus deformity with a congruous MTP joint is not common; however, when one is present, satisfactory correction may necessitate a Mitchell osteotomy or a double or triple osteotomy (an Akin osteotomy of the proximal phalanx combined with an osteotomy of the metatarsal and, on occasion, an additional cuneiform osteotomy).[8]

A severe hallux valgus deformity[11] most commonly includes subluxation of the metatarsophalangeal joint. A distal soft-tissue reconstruction with a proximal metatarsal osteotomy is frequently used to achieve correction. In the presence of hypermobility of the metatarsocuneiform joint, which typically is associated with subluxation of the MTP joint, a distal soft-tissue reconstruction should be combined with arthrodesis of the metatarsocuneiform joint. With osteoarthrosis of the MTP joint, an arthrodesis may be considered. A severe hallux valgus deformity with a congruous MTP joint is uncommon; however, when one is present, a double or triple osteotomy is the procedure of choice.

Proximal Phalangeal Osteotomy (Akin Procedure)

The Akin procedure[25-29] achieves correction of a hallux valgus deformity with a medial eminence resection and medial capsular reefing, combined with a medial closing-wedge phalangeal osteotomy. An increased first-second intermetatarsal angle is not corrected with this procedure. The indications for the Akin procedure include hallux valgus interphalangeus, mild hallux valgus without metatarsus primus varus, and mild hallux valgus with an enlarged medial eminence. In the presence of a congruous MTP joint with hallux valgus, a phalangeal osteotomy can be combined with a metatarsal osteotomy[26,30] in order to create an extra-articular realignment.

Technique With the Akin technique,[25-29] a longitudinal incision is centered over the medial eminence and extends from the interphalangeal joint to just proximal to the distal metaphysis of the metatarsal. Care is taken to protect the plantar and dorsal digital nerves within the skin flap. An L-shaped capsular flap is developed by reflecting the capsule from the medial eminence (Fig. 12, *top*).[27] The weakest capsular attachments on the dorsal and proximal aspects are released, and the stout plantar and distal attachments are left intact to provide a secure flap that can later be reattached. The medial eminence is resected with an oscillating saw along a line parallel with the medial border of the first metatarsal (Fig. 12, *center left*). Usually, the resection is carried out just medial to the sagittal sulcus. If any portion of the sagittal sulcus remains, it should be beveled with a rongeur. The capsule is then repaired with interrupted absorbable sutures. A drill-hole may be placed in the medial aspect of the metatarsal metaphysis to anchor the capsular flap. An osteotomy is performed in the proximal metaphyseal region of the proximal phalanx. Care must be taken to protect the distal insertion of the MTP capsular attachment and to avoid penetration of the interphalangeal or MTP joint with the saw blade.[30] Subperiosteal dissection is used to reflect tissue in the metaphyseal region dorsally, medially, and plantarly, but extensive soft-tissue dissection is avoided. An oscillating saw is used to remove a medially based wedge of bone from the metaphysis. The lateral cortex is left intact. The size of the medial wedge depends on the magnitude of either the PPAA or the hallux valgus angle. An adequate wedge is removed to achieve correction of the deformity; typically, the wedge measures 0.125 to 0.188 in (0.318 to 0.478 cm) at its base. The osteotomy site is closed by cracking the remaining lateral cortex and is stabilized with two 0.062-in (0.157-cm) Kirschner wires placed in an oblique fashion (Fig.

12, *center right* and *bottom*). Pronation of the great toe may be corrected at the time of the osteotomy by derotation of the toe.[26]

Postoperative Care A compression dressing is applied at surgery and is changed weekly for 6 weeks. The patient is allowed to walk while wearing a postoperative shoe. The fixation pins are removed after 4 to 6 weeks. Walking is encouraged, and range-of-motion exercises of the MTP and interphalangeal joints are initiated 6 weeks after the operation, after use of the compression dressing has been discontinued.

Results and Complications The Akin procedure achieves slight, if any, correction of the first-second intermetatarsal angle (Fig. 13, *left*).[28,31] Plattner and Van Manen,[28] in a series of 22 patients, initially found an average correction of the hallux valgus angle of 13°. However, after long-term follow-up, at 4.5 years, the hallux valgus angle was decreased only 6° compared with the preoperative measurement. Seelenfreund and Fried[32] reported recurrence in eight (16%) of 50 patients, and Goldberg and associates[31] reported recurrence in 75 (21%) of 351 patients (Fig. 13, *right*).

The use of internal fixation to stabilize the site of the osteotomy usually prevents malunion. Nonunion is uncommon.[32] Although Colloff and Weitz[33] recommended the use of a lateral MTP capsular and adductor release, I do not advise this because of the increased chance of devascularization of the proximal phalangeal fragment. Other complications that can occur when the Akin procedure is used as a primary procedure include poor cosmetic appearance[31] and a high rate of postoperative dissatisfaction.[28,31] Goldberg and associates[31] concluded that isolated phalangeal osteotomy as treatment for a hallux valgus deformity "does not have a sound biomechanical basis and should not be performed as an isolated . . . procedure." Plattner and Van Manen[28] concluded that the major indication for the Akin procedure is hallux valgus interphalangeus and that the technique is not indicated for hallux valgus with subluxation of the MTP joint. Colloff and Weitz[33] as well as Mitchell and Baxter[30] suggested that a phalangeal osteotomy may be used in combination with a more proximal osteotomy to align a congruous MTP joint in the presence of hallux valgus and an increased first-second intermetatarsal angle.

Distal Soft-Tissue Reconstruction

The technique of distal soft-tissue reconstruction for correction of a hallux valgus deformity has been advocated by many authors;[7,14,34-37] however, it was Silver[38] who popularized it by performing a medial capsulorrhaphy, a medial exostectomy, and a lateral capsular and adductor release. This technique was later modified by McBride,[14,35,36] who advocated removal of the lateral sesamoid and transfer of the adductor tendon to

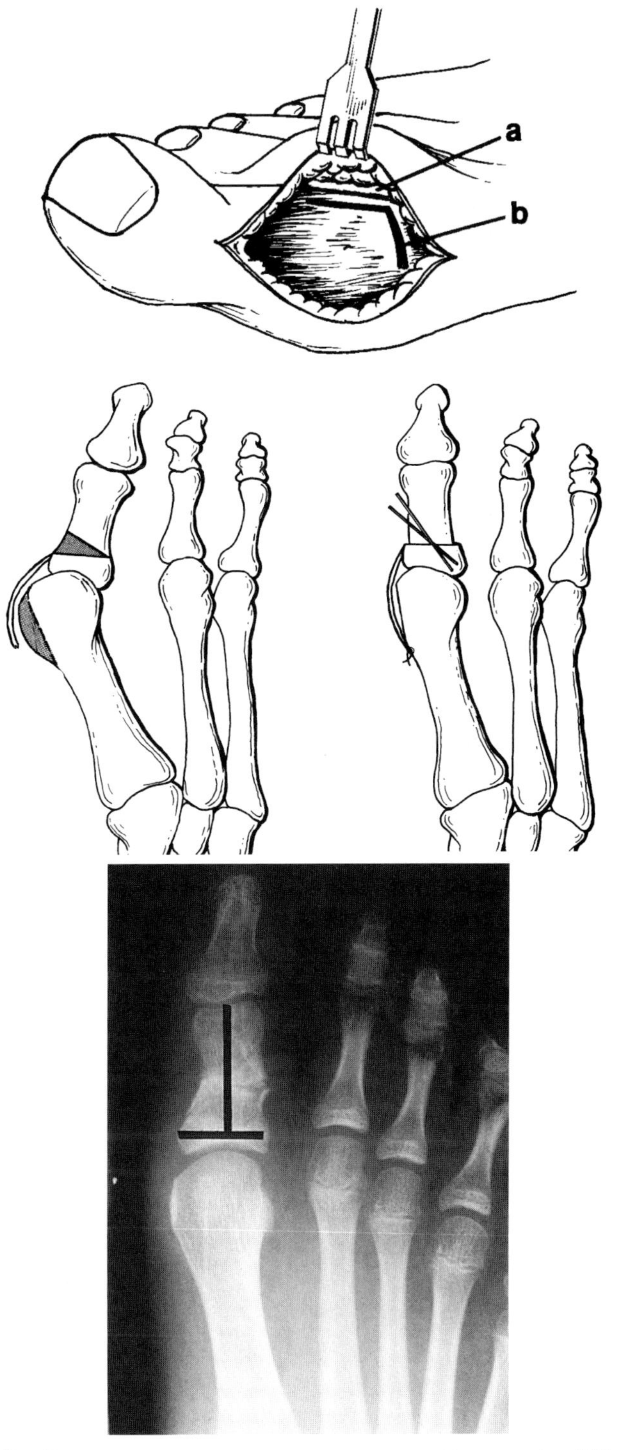

Fig. 12 The proximal phalangeal osteotomy (Akin procedure[25-29]). **Top,** An L-shaped capsulotomy releases the dorsal and proximal attachments of the metatarsophalangeal capsule. a = dorsal neurovascular bundle and b = capsular incision. **Left center,** The medial eminence is excised in line with the medial aspect of the first metatarsal (lower shaded area). The medial-based osteotomy is located in the proximal phalangeal metaphysis (upper shaded area). **Right center,** The osteotomy is approximated and fixed internally with K-wires. The capsule is secured through a drill-hole in the metaphysis. **Bottom,** Radiograph after correction of the hallux valgus interphalangeus deformity with the Akin procedure.

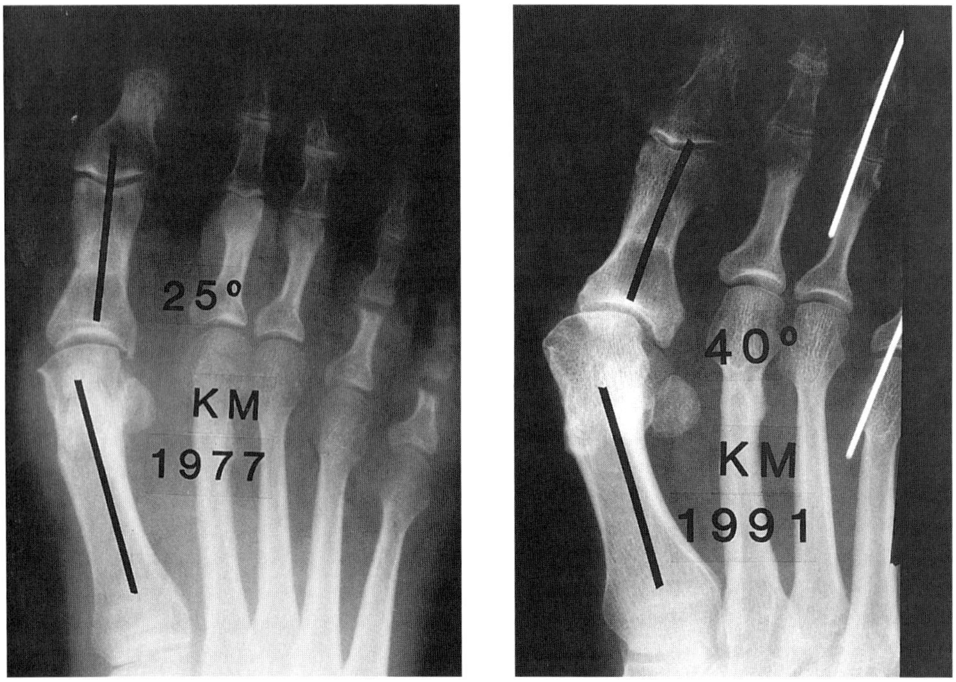

Fig. 13 Radiographs made after the performance of an Akin procedure in a foot with a moderate hallux valgus deformity. **Left,** Postoperatively, there is no correction of the first-second intermetatarsal angle and little correction of the hallux valgus angle. **Right,** 14 years postoperatively, there is recurrent deformity with increased subluxation of the sesamoids.

the lateral aspect of the first metatarsal head. DuVries[34] and others[7,15,24,27,39] have modified the procedure so that the eponym McBride is no longer appropriate. Mann and Coughlin[7] and later Mann and Pfeffinger[39] reviewed the results of this procedure and recommended preservation of the fibular sesamoid because of the high rate of postoperative hallux varus when it was excised.

The indication for a distal soft-tissue reconstruction is a noncongruous hallux valgus deformity (a subluxated MTP joint) of less than 30° and a first-second intermetatarsal angle of less than 15°. A fixed intermetatarsal angle prevents the achievement of a long-lasting distal correction and, therefore, the first metatarsocuneiform joint must have adequate mobility so that the first-second intermetatarsal angle can decrease after the surgery.

Technique This technique[7,34,39] involves a 3-cm dorsal longitudinal incision centered over the first intermetatarsal space to expose the conjoined adductor tendon. The tendon is dissected from the lateral sesamoid. The distal part of the tendon is left attached to its insertion on the base of the proximal phalanx and the tendon is severed approximately 1.5 cm proximal to the musculotendinous junction, allowing the adductor hallucis muscle to retract (Fig. 14). The distal stump of the tendon is later sutured into the lateral aspect of the metatarsal capsule. The lateral sesamoid is freed of any lateral soft-tissue attachments, and the transverse intermetatarsal ligament is released. Care must be taken not to injure the common digital nerve directly beneath this ligament. Several stab wounds are made in the lateral aspect of the capsule with a number-11 knife blade to release it, and the remaining lateral part of the capsule is torn by abduction of the great toe. The purpose of this tearing technique is to leave some lateral capsular tissue that will heal to stabilize the MTP joint and to minimize the chance of a postoperative hallux varus deformity. Three interrupted absorbable 2-0 sutures are placed in the lateral aspect of the capsule of the MTP joint and the medial aspect of the capsule of the second MTP joint within the first intermetatarsal space. They are tied later to approximate the first and second MTP capsules.

A longitudinal incision is then centered over the medial eminence, and the dissection is deepened to the MTP joint capsule. Care is taken to protect the dorsal and plantar digital nerves, which are contained in the skin flaps. An L-shaped capsular release (Fig. 12, *top*) detaches the dorsal and proximal attachments, exposing the medial eminence. The medial eminence is resected in a line parallel with the medial diaphyseal cortex of the first metatarsal (Fig. 15). The cut is made without reference to the sagittal sulcus, although frequently (with mild and moderate deformities) it is approximately 1 to 2 mm medial to the sulcus. A drill-hole is then made in the medial aspect of the metaphysis of the first metatarsal, and the medial aspect of the capsule is secured with an absorbable suture. The distal stump of the adductor tendon is sutured into the later-

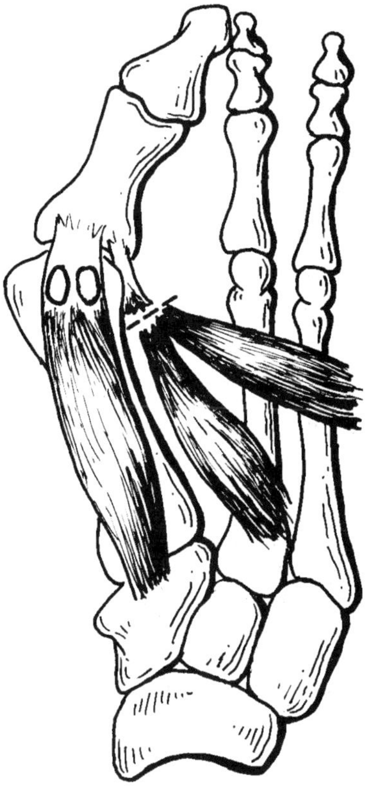

Fig. 14 A distal soft-tissue reconstruction. The conjoined adductor tendon is released, leaving a 1.5-cm stump of tendon, which is secured to the lateral aspect of the metatarsal capsule at the conclusion of the procedure.

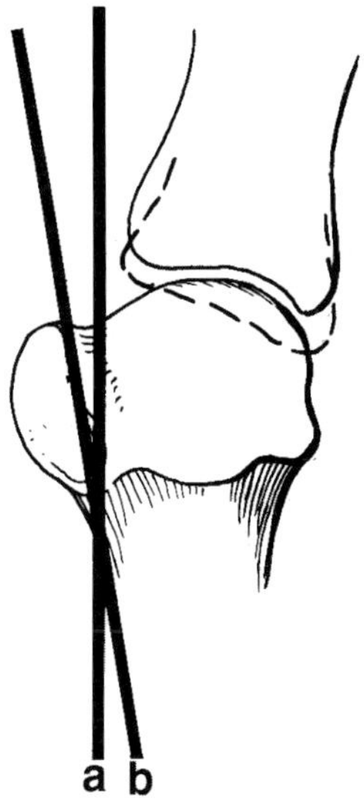

Fig. 15 This drawing compares the resection of the medial eminence for the distal soft-tissue reconstruction with that for the chevron osteotomy. For the distal soft-tissue reconstruction, the excision of the medial eminence (line b) is in line with the medial diaphyseal cortex of the first metatarsal. However, for the chevron osteotomy, the osteotomy (line a) is in line with the medial border of the foot.

al aspect of the capsule, and the three sutures that were previously placed in the first web space are tied to approximate the first and second MTP capsules. Several sutures are placed medially in the proximal aspect of the capsule, incorporating the abductor hallucis tendon. The dorsal capsular incision is repaired with interrupted suture as well, and the skin is closed in a routine fashion.

Postoperative Care A gauze-and-tape compression dressing is applied at surgery and is changed weekly for 8 weeks. The patient is allowed to walk in a postoperative wooden-soled shoe, with weightbearing as tolerated. Passive and active range-of-motion exercises are initiated 6 weeks after the operation.

Results and Complications Although Silver[38] advocated resection of the medial eminence and lateral soft-tissue release, he did not report the results of this procedure. Kitaoka and associates,[40] in a review of the results of simple bunionectomy and medial capsulorrhaphy with or without lateral capsulotomy in 33 patients (49 feet), found that at 4.8 years the average hallux valgus angle had increased 4.8° from the preoperative deformity and the first-second intermetatarsal angle had increased 1.7°. Twenty-nine percent of the feet that had had the bunionectomy without the lateral capsulotomy had had a reoperation at 5 years. The rate of failure was 24%.[40]

Bonney and Macnab[41] reported generally poor results after simple exostectomy (Fig. 16). Twenty-five (37%) of their 68 patients needed additional treatment, and the authors concluded that the only indication for a simple exostectomy is a large medial eminence that is the sole cause of symptoms in a patient whose general medical condition contraindicates an extensive procedure and to whom postoperative appearance is not important.

Johnson and associates[42] and Meyer and associates[37] reported a high degree of clinical success in the treatment of mild-to-moderate hallux valgus with the modified McBride procedure. Mann and Coughlin,[7] in a review of the results of 100 McBride procedures, found an average correction of the hallux valgus angle of 14.8° and an average correction of the first-second intermetatarsal angle of 5.2°. However, they recommended that if more than 20° of correction of the hallux valgus angle is needed, this procedure should be combined with an osteotomy of the first metatarsal.[7] Hallux varus is a serious complication of the McBride procedure. Mann and Coughlin[7] reported this complication in 11 of their 100 patients, although it was severe in only four. Mann and Pfeffinger[39] noted that the prevalence of hallux varus is higher after attempted correction of more severe deformities. They also reported that 43 (91%) of their 47 patients were satisfied with the result of the modified McBride procedure and there was no postoperative progression of the hallux valgus deformity at an average of 4 years.

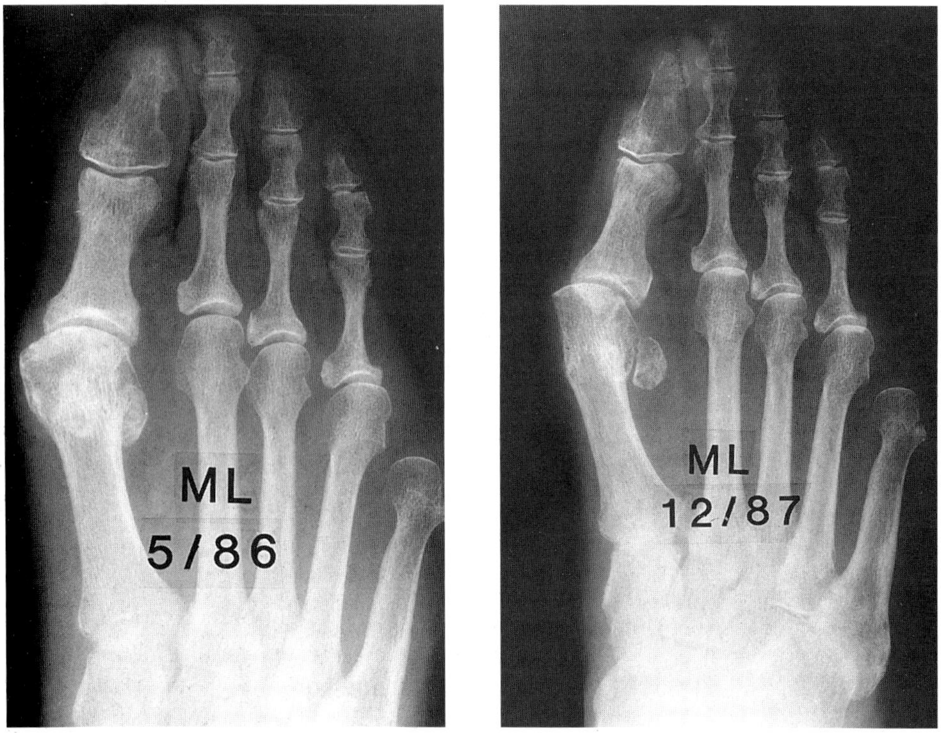

Fig. 16 Radiographs made before and after exostectomy in a foot with a moderate hallux valgus deformity. **Left,** Preoperatively, the lateral sesamoid is displaced 50%. The fifth toe had been amputated previously as a result of trauma. **Right,** After the surgery, the hallux valgus recurred, with progression of the deformity. The hallux valgus is now characterized by severe subluxation of the metatarsophalangeal joint and progression of the sesamoid displacement.

The limitations of an isolated distal soft-tissue reconstruction are substantial. Mann and Pfeffinger[39] concluded that a severe hallux valgus deformity was not well corrected by a distal soft-tissue reconstruction, as only approximately 50% of the hallux valgus angle was corrected in such deformities. Therefore, I believe that the indications for a distal soft-tissue reconstruction are a hallux valgus angle of less than 30° (with MTP subluxation) and an intermetatarsal angle of less than 15° (Fig. 17).

Chevron Osteotomy

The chevron procedure (a distal metatarsal osteotomy) is indicated for mild and some moderate hallux valgus deformities (a hallux valgus angle of less than 30° and a first-second intermetatarsal angle of less than 13°) with subluxation of the MTP joint.[43-45] Because the chevron osteotomy achieves an extra-articular correction, it may also be considered for the treatment of a hallux valgus deformity with a congruous MTP joint if the DMAA is not severe (15° or less). With this procedure, a medial eminence resection, a distal metatarsal osteotomy, and a medial capsulorrhaphy are used to realign the great toe. A chevron osteotomy does not correct pronation of the great toe and only partially corrects subluxation of the sesamoids. This procedure is contraindicated for a severe hallux valgus deformity, for hallux valgus associated with degenerative osteoarthrosis, in the presence of a congruous MTP joint with a DMAA of more than 15°, and for patients who are more than 60 years old.[46] The indications for this procedure when it is combined with a phalangeal osteotomy[47] include a hallux valgus deformity with a congruous MTP joint (a distal metatarsal articular angle of less than 20°) and with pronation of the great toe. If residual valgus angulation of the great toe remains after a chevron osteotomy, an additional phalangeal osteotomy may help to improve alignment.

Technique This technique[43,48] is done through a longitudinal incision centered over the medial eminence that is extended from the mid-portion of the proximal phalanx to a point proximal to the metaphysis of the first metatarsal. Care is taken to protect the dorsal and plantar cutaneous nerves in the skin flaps. The incision is carried directly down to the MTP capsule. An inverted L-shaped plantar and distally based capsular flap is developed to expose the medial eminence (Fig. 12, *top*).[43] The medial eminence is resected with an oscillating saw at a point just medial to the sagittal sulcus, in line with the medial border of the foot (Fig. 15). The location of the sagittal sulcus may vary, depending on the size of the hallus valgus deformity. Because the chevron osteotomy is typically performed on hallux valgus deformities of 30° or less, the use of the sagittal sulcus as a marker for the distal point of the medial emi-

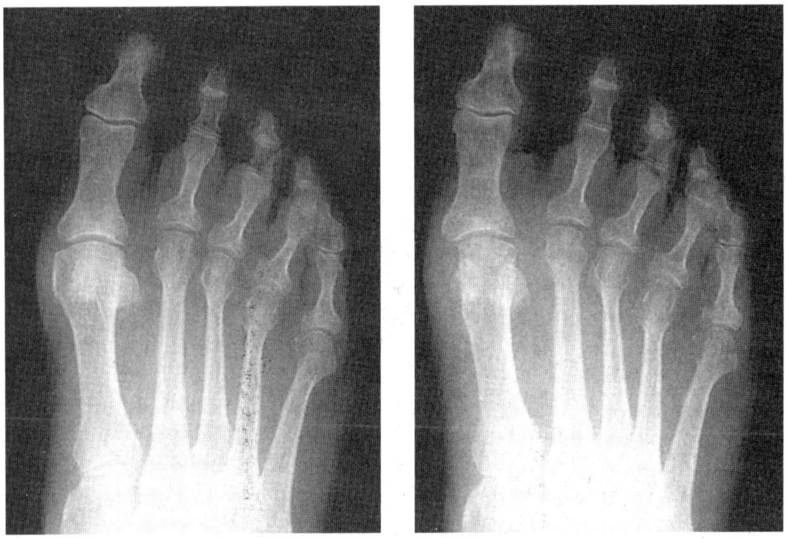

Fig. 17 Radiographs made before and after a distal soft-tissue reconstruction in a foot with a mild hallux valgus deformity, subluxation of the metatarsophalangeal joint, and 50% subluxation of the lateral sesamoid. **Left,** Preoperatively, the hallux valgus angle is 17°, and the first-second intermetatarsal angle is 10°. **Right,** Postoperatively, the hallux valgus and first-second intermetatarsal angles have been corrected. The hallux valgus angle is 9°, and the first-second intermetatarsal angle is 5°.

nence resection is more reliable. With a more severe deformity, the sulcus shifts lateral-ward, and its use as a guide may lead to excessive medial eminence resection. A transverse medial-to-lateral drill-hole is made in the center of the metatarsal head to mark the apex of the chevron osteotomy. An oscillating saw blade with very fine in-line teeth (number 2296-3-414 or 2296-3-115; Stryker, Kalamazoo, MI) to minimize shortening is used to create a V-shaped osteotomy in the coronal plane (Fig. 18). Excessive dorsal or lateral penetration of the saw blade or excessive soft-tissue dissection may disrupt critical soft-tissue attachments and devascularize the metatarsal head. For this reason, a lateral soft-tissue release is discouraged (Fig. 19),[44,48-53] although Hetherington and associates[54] and others[55-59] have performed lateral releases without complications. The metatarsal shaft is then grasped with a bone clamp, and the capital fragment is translated approximately 4 to 5 mm in a lateral direction (Fig. 20, *left*).[44,50] If additional medial angulation of the osteotomy is desired (to accommodate an increased DMAA), more metaphyseal bone is resected medially, allowing the capital fragment to incline medially. The metatarsal head is then impacted on the proximal fragment and stabilized with a 0.062-in (0.157-cm) Kirschner wire (Fig. 20, *right*). Care is taken to avoid penetration of the sesamoid mechanism plantarly by the Kirschner wire. The prominent metaphyseal flare created by displacement at the site of the osteotomy is then beveled with the oscillating saw. A drill-hole is made in the metaphysis, and the medial aspect of the capsule is anchored through this hole. Several interrupted absorbable sutures are used to complete the capsulorrhaphy. The skin is approximated in a routine fashion.

Postoperative Care A gauze-and-tape compression dressing is applied at surgery and is changed weekly for 6 weeks. The Kirschner wire is removed 3 to 4 weeks following surgery, and passive range-of-motion exercises are initiated at this time. Weightbearing is allowed on the heel and the lateral aspect of the foot. At 4 weeks, plantigrade walking is allowed while the patient is wearing a wooden-soled postoperative shoe. If the site of the osteotomy is unstable, a below-the-knee weightbearing cast is applied for 3 weeks or until adequate bone-healing has been documented radiographically.

Results and Complications Johnson and associates[48] and others[44,46,56,58] have reported excellent results with this procedure. After a chevron osteotomy, the average correction of the hallux valgus angle has been reported to be 12° to 13°, and the average correction of

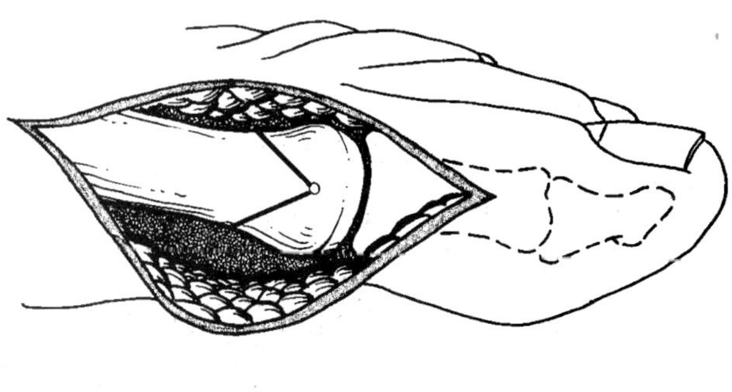

Fig. 18 Illustration of the chevron osteotomy. A drill-hole in the center of the metatarsal head marks the apex of the osteotomy. The angle of the osteotomy cut is 60° to 90°, providing a large, stable surface area.

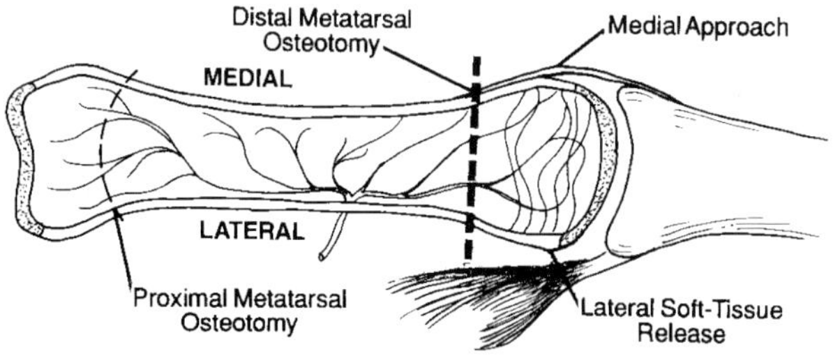

Fig. 19 A dorsal view of the first metatarsal. The vascular supply to the head of the first metatarsal is through the medial and lateral soft-tissue structures and medullary vessels. A proximal metatarsal osteotomy does not interrupt the intramedullary supply. A distal metatarsal osteotomy, when combined with an extensive lateral soft-tissue release, may compromise the vascularity of the capital fragment.

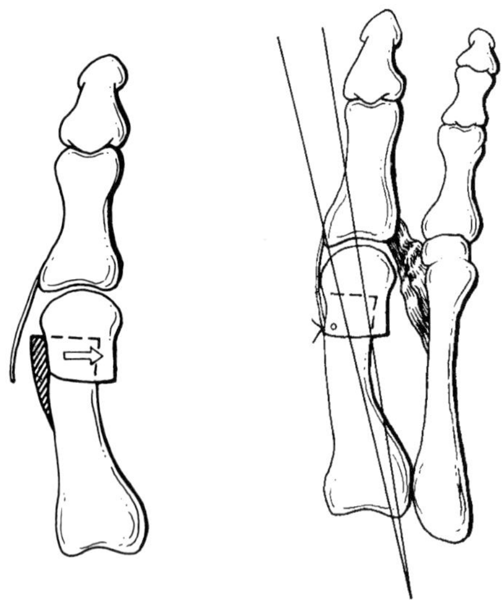

Fig. 20 The chevron osteotomy. **Left,** The capital fragment is translated laterally (arrow). **Right,** The osteotomy is stabilized with a K-wire, and the capsule is anchored with a suture through the metaphysis.

the first-second intermetatarsal angle has been 4° to 5°.[44,46,48,54,56-58] Because of the limited correction of the hallux valgus, the chevron procedure is reserved for mild and some moderate deformities. Expansion of the indications for this procedure to more severe deformities appears to increase the risk of complications and patient dissatisfaction. Meier and Kenzora,[45] in a series of 50 patients (72 feet) who had had an osteotomy of the distal end of the metatarsal, noted a rate of satisfaction of 74% when the preoperative first-second intermetatarsal angle had been more than 12° and a rate of 94% when the intermetatarsal angle had been 12° or less.

The most frequent complications associated with this procedure are recurrence or undercorrection of the deformity (four of 29 feet, 14%;[57] eight of 78 feet, 10%;[44] and 30 of 300 feet, 10%[55]). Hallux valgus may recur when the indications for the chevron procedure are expanded to include more severe deformities. Loss of correction (overcorrection or undercorrection) can be caused by slippage at the site of the osteotomy.[44,45] Although internal fixation was not advocated originally by Austin and Leventen[55] or by others,[53,56,60] its use decreases the possibility of postoperative displacement of the capital fragment (Fig. 21).[48,58] Shortening may occur as a result of excessive bone loss,[44,45,51,55] and Klosok and associates[61] reported a postoperative transfer lesion in five (12%) of 43 feet and postoperative metatarsalgia in ten (43%) of 23 patients.

The most serious complication following this procedure is osteonecrosis of the first metatarsal head (Fig. 22). Meier and Kenzora[45] reported that osteonecrosis developed in 20% (12) of 60 feet after a chevron osteotomy, and this rate increased to four of ten feet when the osteotomy had been combined with an adductor tenotomy. Horne and associates[62] reported osteonecrosis in 12% (nine) of 76 feet, and Mann[51] as well as others[63,64] reported several isolated cases of partial and whole-head osteonecrosis after osteotomy of the distal end of the metatarsal. In contrast, Johnson and associates[48] and others[55,58,61] reported no evidence of osteonecrosis after osteotomy. Hattrup and Johnson[46] as well as Shereff and associates[52] cautioned that lateral release increases the risk of osteonecrosis. Release of the lateral structures may enable greater correction, but I believe that the risk of osteonecrosis is indeed increased.[45,53,56,63]

Distal Metatarsal Osteotomy (Mitchell or Wilson Osteotomy)

Correction of a hallux valgus deformity with a distal first metatarsal osteotomy was reported first by Reverdin,[65] in 1881, and later by Hohmann[47] and by Peabody,[66] who described variations in the technique. It was Mitchell who popularized the technique of biplanar distal metatarsal osteotomy,[67,68] which achieves lateral and plantar displacement as well as shortening of the first metatarsal. Wilson[69] and others[70-73] have described an oblique metaphyseal osteotomy in this same region. Variations in the technique have included changes in the capsulorrhaphy,[71,72,74,75] the metaphyseal osteotomy,[69,71-73,75-77] the use of internal fixation,[71,72,74,76-79] and the postoperative care.[71,74,79] These many changes make the eponym Mitchell inadequate to describe the procedure as performed in many series.

Indications for a transverse or oblique osteotomy of the distal end of the metatarsal include moderate

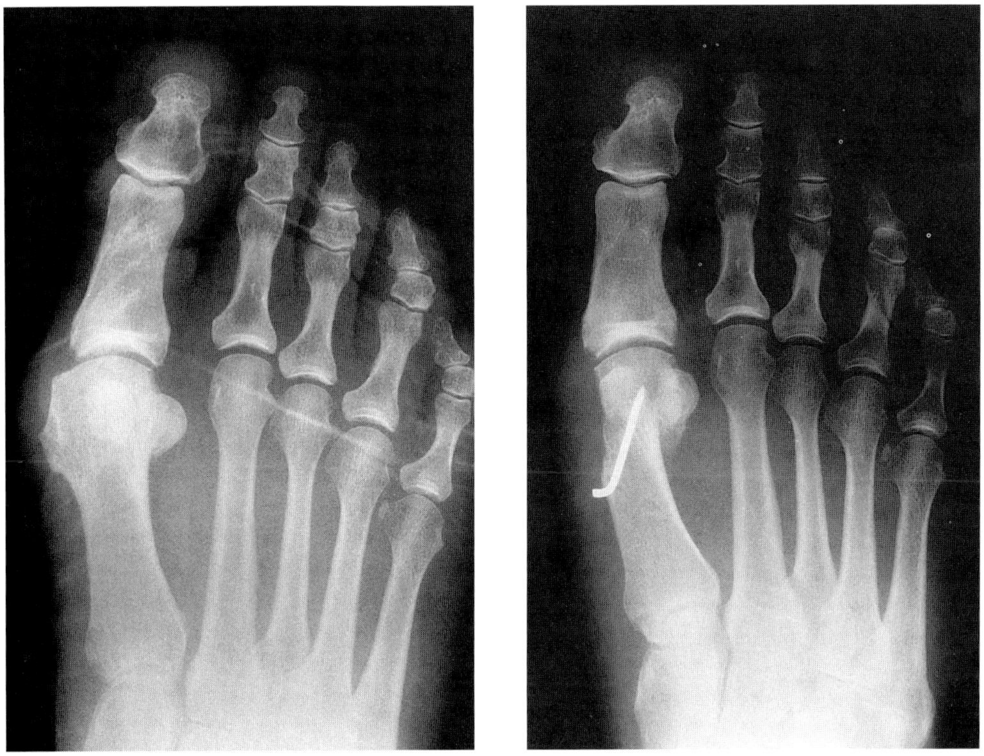

Fig. 21 Radiographs made before and after a chevron osteotomy in a foot with a moderate hallux valgus deformity and subluxation of the metatarsophalangeal joint. **Left,** Preoperative appearance. **Right,** Postoperatively, satisfactory correction has been achieved. Note the internal fixation with a K-wire.

hallux valgus with subluxation of the MTP joint; however, if the DMAA is not severe (if it is less than 15°), this distal metatarsal osteotomy is still indicated. The upper limits for deformity are a hallux valgus angle of 35° and a first-second intermetatarsal angle of 15°. Contraindications include a hallux valgus deformity with concurrent degenerative osteoarthrosis, a short first metatarsal, lateral metatarsalgia, and a congruous MTP joint with a DMAA of more than 15°.

Technique A longitudinal skin incision is centered over the dorsomedial aspect of the first MTP joint and extends from the mid-portion of the proximal phalanx to the mid-portion of the first metatarsal. A distally based capsular flap[74] or a V-Y capsular flap[68] is created over the medial aspect of the MTP joint. The adductor tendon and lateral capsular attachments are not disturbed, in order to protect the vascularity of the metatarsal head.[45] The medial eminence is exposed and osteotomized in line with the shaft of the first metatarsal. Two dorsal-to-plantar drill-holes are made in the distal end of the metatarsal. The first hole, 1.5 cm proximal to the articular surface, is made near the medial cortex, and the second hole, 2.5 cm proximal to the articular surface, is made nearer to the lateral cortex. The drill-holes are positioned so that they will line up as the capital fragment is shifted laterally. An incomplete osteotomy is performed 2 cm proximal to the articular surface of the metatarsal, midway between the two drill-holes (Fig. 23, *left*). The distal cut is made partway through the shaft, with the depth depending on the desired width of the lateral shelf. The second osteotomy cut is made completely through the metatarsal, approximately 2 mm proximal to the initial cut and diverging plantarward, with removal of approximately 1 to 2 mm more bone on the plantar aspect (Fig. 23, *top right*).

The magnitude of the deformity (the first-second intermetatarsal angle) determines both the amount of longitudinal shortening to be achieved at the site of the osteotomy and the width of the incomplete osteotomy. With a moderate deformity, a lateral shelf one sixth the width of the shaft is left on the distal fragment. With a severe deformity, a lateral shelf one third the width of the shaft should remain.

The capital fragment is then displaced 4 to 5 mm laterally until the lateral shelf locks over the lateral aspect of the proximal part of the shaft (Fig. 23, *bottom left*). Care is taken to ensure that the capital fragment either is angulated plantarward approximately 10° or is displaced plantarward 2 to 3 mm. With lateral sloping of the DMAA, more bone can be resected medially (Fig. 23, *bottom right*) to rotate the articular surface perpendicular to the long axis of the first metatarsal. The osteotomy site is stabilized with a circumferential suture placed through the now-parallel drill-holes and tied dorsally[67,68,76,77] or is fixed with Kirschner

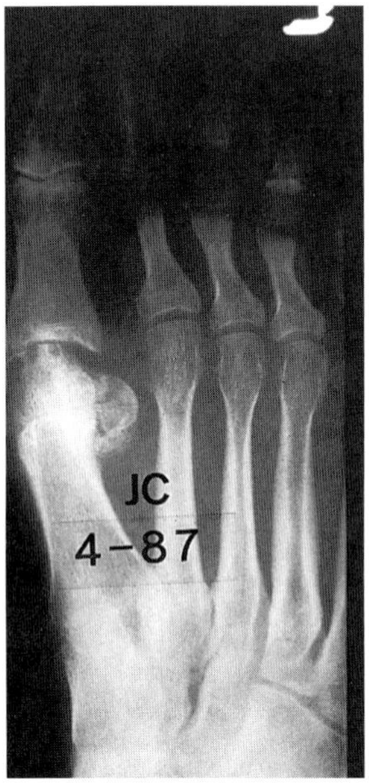

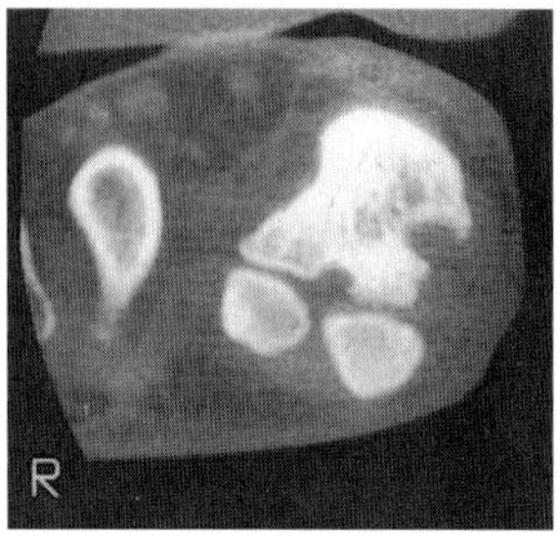

Fig. 22 Anteroposterior and axial (sesamoid) radiographs showing osteonecrosis after a chevron osteotomy combined with a lateral release.

wires,[71,78,79] staples,[74] or screws.[76,77] The remaining medial metaphyseal flare created by lateral displacement of the capital fragment is removed with a power saw, and the metaphyseal capsule is plicated with interrupted sutures. The skin is closed in a routine fashion.

Postoperative Care A gauze-and-tape compression dressing is applied at surgery.[74] A nonweightbearing cast typically is applied a week after surgery. Most surgeons prefer a 4-week course of nonweightbearing, after which walking is permitted with the foot immobilized in a below-the-knee cast until the site of the osteotomy has healed at 8 to 10 weeks postoperatively.

Results and Complications Overall, distal metatarsal osteotomies have resulted in satisfactory correction of the hallux valgus deformity in 82% to 97% of feet (Fig. 24).[49,67,68,76,77,80,81] In the two larger series, 185 (91%) of 204 patients[80] and 182 (97%) of 188 patients[67] were satisfied with the result of the procedure. The average reported correction of the hallux valgus deformity has ranged from 10° to 25°[49,74,76,77,80,82] and the average correction of the first-second intermetatarsal angle, from 5° to 10°.[49,67,74,76,77,80,82] These results are consistent with those of Jahss and associates,[50] who estimated that an average of 4.3° of correction of the intermetatarsal angle could be achieved with a distal metatarsal osteotomy.

Shortening of the first metatarsal is an important part of this procedure as it helps to correct the deformity. However, excessive shortening is a frequent complication, which is undesirable as it may lead to transfer metatarsalgia.[67] Merkel and associates[78] reported an average shortening of 7 mm in their series; however, patients who had more than 10 mm of shortening had a higher degree of dissatisfaction and an increased frequency of metatarsalgia. Lateral metatarsalgia and callus formation, the most frequently recognized complications, have been reported in almost all series in which distal osteotomy has been performed.[49,67-69,72,75,81,82] Rates of 20% to 40% have been reported,[67,68,82] with a 31% rate (59 of 188 feet) in the largest series.[67] While some calluses are asymptomatic, they may become painful in time. Plantar displacement, as advocated by Mitchell and associates[68] and by others,[49,67,81] and plantar angulation, as recommended by Wu[76,77] and by Merkel and associates,[78] have both been proposed to diminish the ill effects of shortening of the first metatarsal. Glynn and associates[49] stressed that failure to depress the capital fragment eventually predisposes to metatarsalgia. Dorsal angulation[74,76-78] is associated with patient dissatisfaction as it magnifies the effects of shortening of the first metatarsal.

Undercorrection and recurrence of the deformity are also recognized as common complications following this osteotomy. Such complications have been reported in approximately 10% of patients,[49,67,68,75-77,80] with six of the series including at least 100 patients. The use of a distal metatarsal osteotomy for more severe deformities increases the risk of undercorrection or recurrence.

Mitchell and associates[68] and others[45,51,63,70,72,81] have reported osteonecrosis after distal metatarsal osteotomy. Wu[76,77] mentioned the occasional use of lateral capsular and adductor release in combination with such an osteotomy, but Carr and Boyd[81] as well as others[67,68,73] recommended avoidance of a lateral capsular release to minimize this problem.

The nature of this transverse osteotomy makes it relatively unstable, and loss of correction,[14,82] malunion,[74,76,77] delayed union,[68,75,78] and nonunion[78] have all been reported. The technique is demanding[76,77] and this may be one reason for the high prevalence of complications, which has led to less frequent use of this procedure in favor of others.

Distal Soft-Tissue Reconstruction with Osteotomy of the First Metatarsal

The primary indication for a distal soft-tissue reconstruction combined with a proximal osteotomy of the first metatarsal is a moderate or severe hallux valgus deformity (a hallux valgus angle of at least 35° and an intermetatarsal angle of at least 13°) with subluxation of the MTP joint.[11,27] Techniques of proximal osteotomy of the first metatarsal include an opening-wedge,[41,83-85] closing-wedge,[84,86,87] proximal chevron,[88] and crescentic osteotomy.[8,11,22,23,89-91] Although an opening or closing-wedge osteotomy may be performed, substantial lengthening or shortening of the first ray is usually not necessary. In a study of more than 7,000

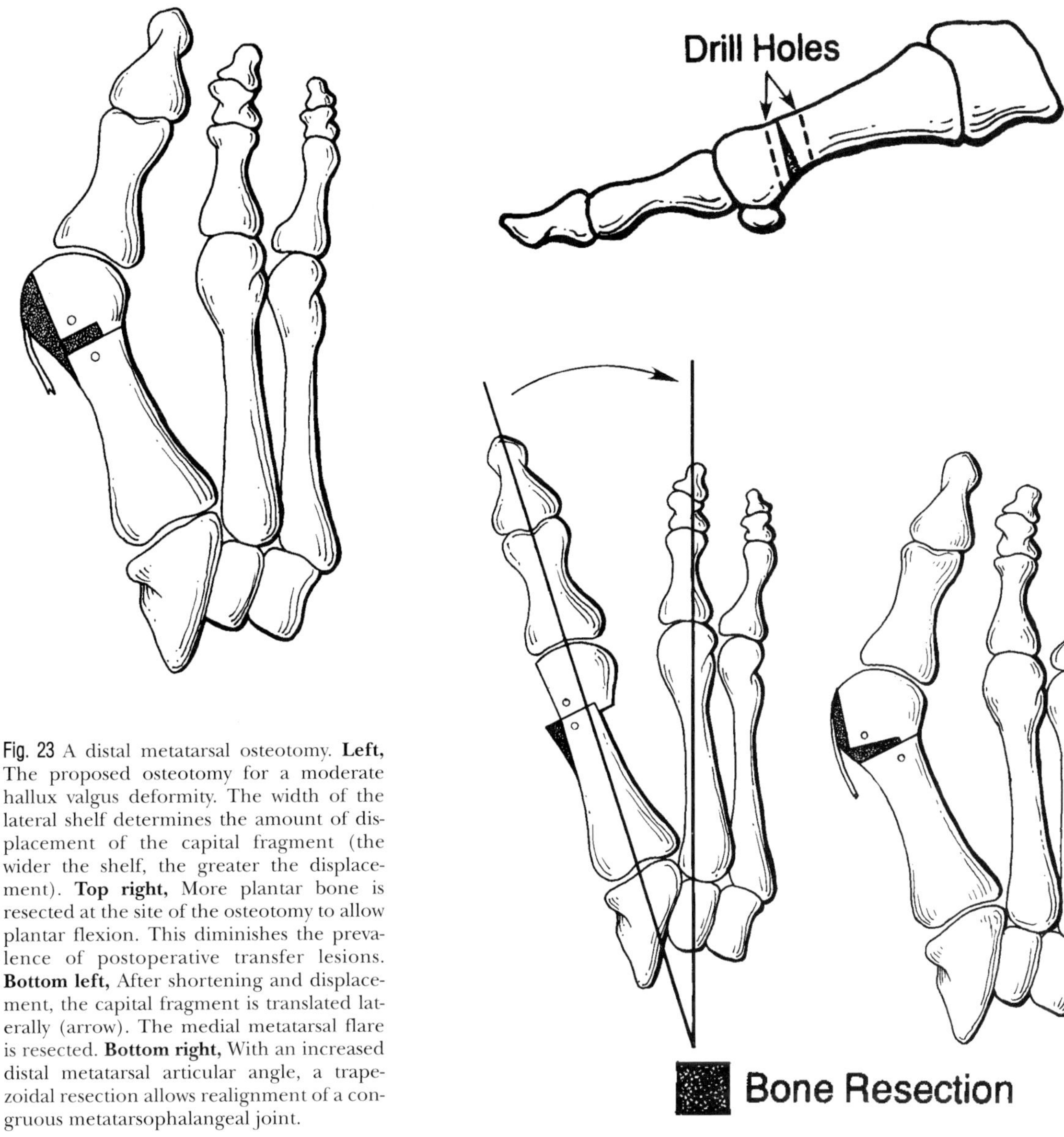

Fig. 23 A distal metatarsal osteotomy. **Left,** The proposed osteotomy for a moderate hallux valgus deformity. The width of the lateral shelf determines the amount of displacement of the capital fragment (the wider the shelf, the greater the displacement). **Top right,** More plantar bone is resected at the site of the osteotomy to allow plantar flexion. This diminishes the prevalence of postoperative transfer lesions. **Bottom left,** After shortening and displacement, the capital fragment is translated laterally (arrow). The medial metatarsal flare is resected. **Bottom right,** With an increased distal metatarsal articular angle, a trapezoidal resection allows realignment of a congruous metatarsophalangeal joint.

feet, Harris and Beath[92] reported that, in most feet, the lengths of the first and second metatarsals were either equal or within a few millimeters of one another. Thus, I usually prefer a proximal crescentic osteotomy. Contraindications to this procedure include a congruous MTP joint (a distal metatarsal articular angle of more than 15°),[83,89,91] degenerative osteoarthrosis of the first MTP joint,[89,91] and severe metatarsus adductus.[89]

Technique With this technique,[22,83,89] a 3-cm dorsal longitudinal incision is centered over the proximal part of the first metatarsal medial to the extensor hallucis longus tendon and is deepened to the shaft of the first metatarsal. The metatarsocuneiform (MC) joint is identified. The crescentic osteotomy is performed 1.0 to 1.3 cm distal to the MC joint with a curved saw blade (number 5053-176; Zimmer, Warsaw, IN, or number 2296-31-41657 or 277-31-41651; Stryker). The osteotomy is directed in a dorsal-to-plantar direction at a 120° angle with the shaft of the first metatarsal (Fig. 25). Care is taken to avoid either medial or lateral deviation of the saw blade, which could lead to plantarflexion or dorsiflexion at the site of the osteotomy.[90] The orientation of the osteotomy may be concave distal[89,93] or concave proximal.[22] The proximal fragment is rotated medially and the distal fragment is rotated laterally for approximately 2 to 3 mm, decreasing the first-second intermetatarsal angle. Care must be taken not to overcorrect the deformity. The osteotomy is fixed with both a 0.062-in (0.157-cm) Kirschner wire and a small-fragment compression screw to provide compression as well as rotational stability (Fig. 26). A

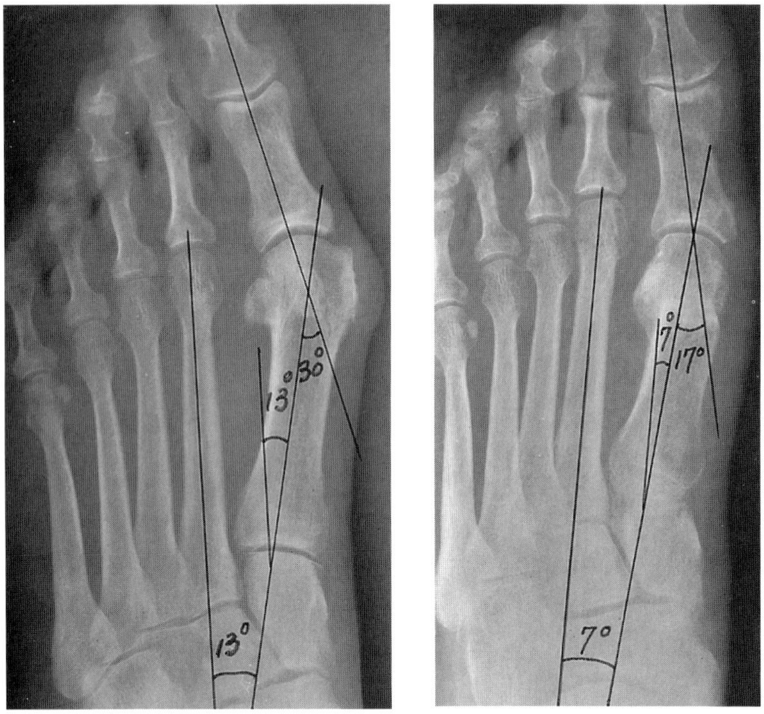

Fig. 24 Radiographs made before and after a distal metatarsal osteotomy in a foot with a moderate hallux valgus deformity and subluxation of the metatarsophalangeal joint. (Radiographs courtesy of Kent K. Wu, MD) **Left,** Preoperative appearance. **Right,** Postoperatively, there is satisfactory correction.

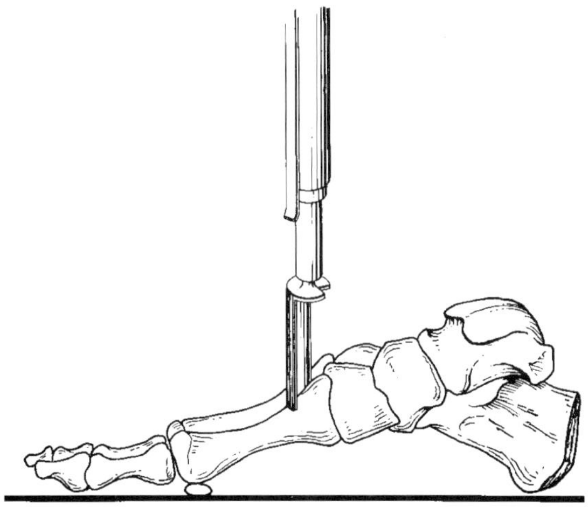

Fig. 25 Orientation of the saw blade at a 120° angle to the shaft of the first metatarsal during a distal soft-tissue reconstruction with a proximal osteotomy of the first metatarsal.

distal soft-tissue reconstruction is then performed as described previously. Intraoperative radiographs are made to evaluate the correction of the first-second intermetatarsal angle, the placement of the internal fixation, and the alignment of the metatarsophalangeal joint (Fig. 27).

Postoperative Care The foot is placed in a gauze-and-tape compression dressing at surgery, and the dressing is changed weekly. Weightbearing on the heel and lateral aspect of the foot is initially allowed with the patient wearing a wooden-soled postoperative shoe. The foot is rarely immobilized in a cast. MTP range-of-motion exercises are initiated 3 to 4 weeks following surgery, while the foot is still maintained in the dressing. The internal fixation hardware is routinely removed 6 weeks following surgery in an outpatient or office setting with the patient under local anesthesia. An intensive walking program is begun at 7 to 8 weeks.

Results and Complications The reported rate of patient satisfaction with this combined procedure[22,85,86,88,91,94] has ranged from 78%[88] to 93%,[91] with a 92% rate in the largest series.[22] The average correction of the hallux valgus angle has been consistently reported to be 23° or 24°.[8,22,91,93] The degree of improvement is directly proportional to the severity of the preoperative deformity, and Mann[23] noted that, for more severe deformities (a hallux valgus angle of more than 40°), the average correction was 30°. The correction of the first-second intermetatarsal angle has averaged 8° to 11°[8,22,91,93] after a crescentic osteotomy, 3° to 6°[84,86,87] after a closing-wedge proximal metatarsal osteotomy, and 7°[83,85] after an opening-wedge osteotomy. Wanivenhaus and Feldner-Busztin[87] reported an average shortening of the first metatarsal of 3.6 mm

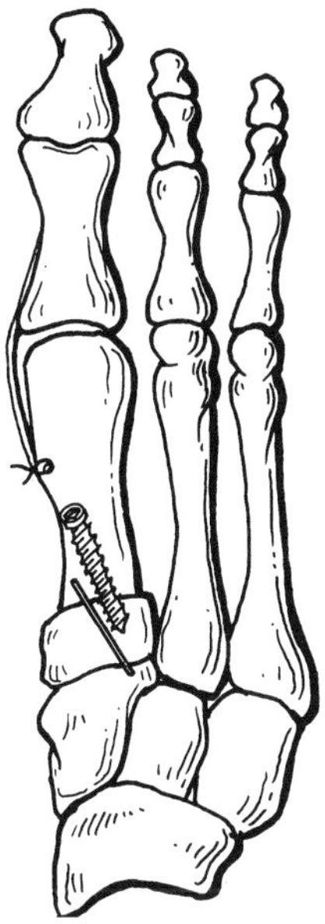

Fig. 26 A foot after distal soft-tissue reconstruction with a proximal osteotomy of the first metatarsal and internal fixation with a compression screw and a K-wire.

after a closing-wedge osteotomy, and shortening of the first metatarsal has been reported by other authors as well.[84,86,87,94] Shortening or dorsiflexion as the site of the osteotomy is closed predisposes to the development of lateral metatarsalgia.[23,86]

I prefer a crescentic osteotomy because it results in minimum shortening.[11,93] Lengthening of the first metatarsal through an opening-wedge osteotomy[3,41,83,84] may lead to instability as well as malunion at the site of the osteotomy. An opening-wedge osteotomy also lengthens the adjacent soft tissues, which may increase tension on an already tight MTP joint and lead to recurrence.[23,84]

Complications with this procedure include recurrence or undercorrection of the deformity,[8,84,85,88,89] overcorrection (hallux varus),[8,22,89,91] inadequacy or failure of the internal fixation,[22,89] shortening,[22,86] metatarsalgia,[22,91] delayed union,[88,89] and malunion[88,90,91] (Fig. 28). Overcorrection frequently has been associated with lateral sesamoidectomy. Simmonds and Menelaus[85] and later Mann and Coughlin[7] cautioned that the sesamoid should rarely, if ever, be removed. Retention of the sesamoid when possible decreased the prevalence of hallux varus in one series from 11 of 100 patients[7] to six of 72 patients.[22] Many postoperative hallux varus deformities of less than 10° are asymptomatic and do not preclude a satisfactory result.[91]

The deformity may recur for a variety of reasons.

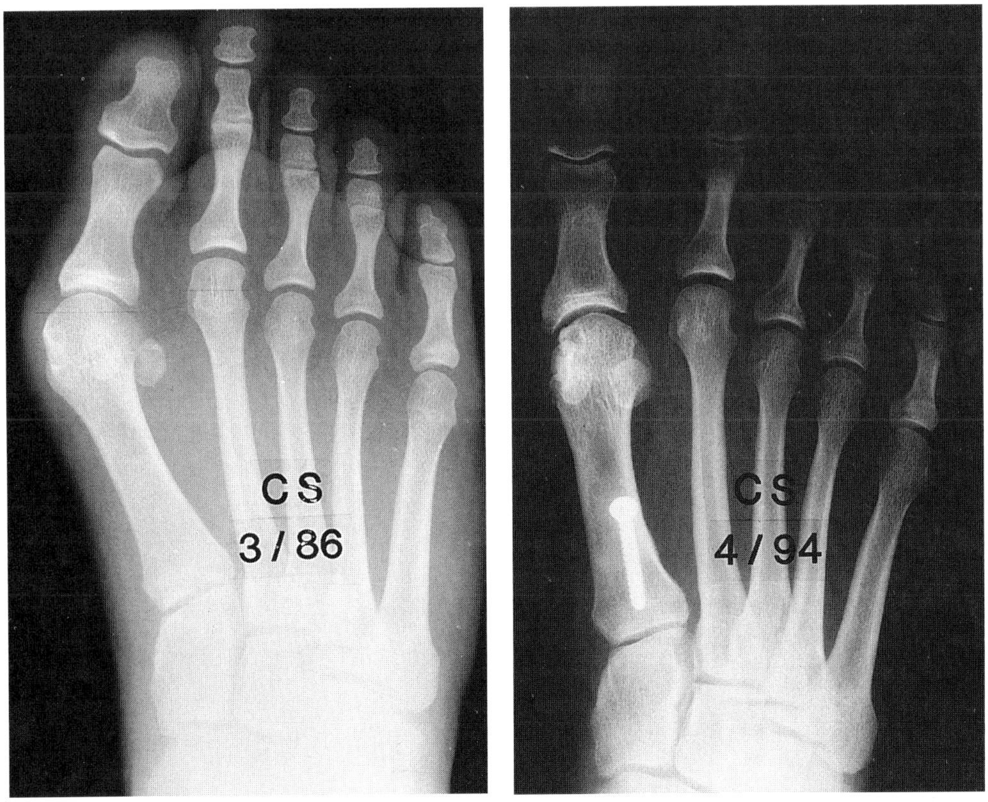

Fig. 27 Radiographs made before and after a proximal osteotomy of the first metatarsal in a foot with a hallux valgus deformity. **Left,** Preoperatively, the hallux valgus angle is 45° and the first-second intermetatarsal angle is 13°. **Right,** Eight years later, the hallux valgus angle is 15° and the first-second intermetatarsal angle is 6°.

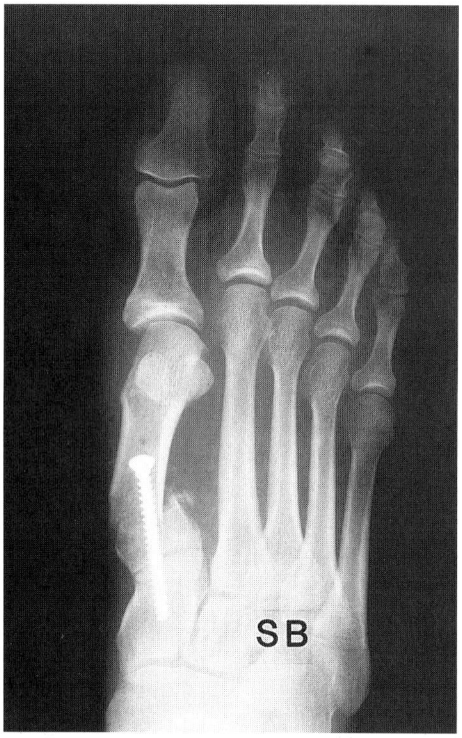

Fig. 28 Radiograph of a foot with overcorrection (negative first-second intermetatarsal angle) and malunion at the site of the proximal osteotomy, which leads to an increased risk of hallux varus.

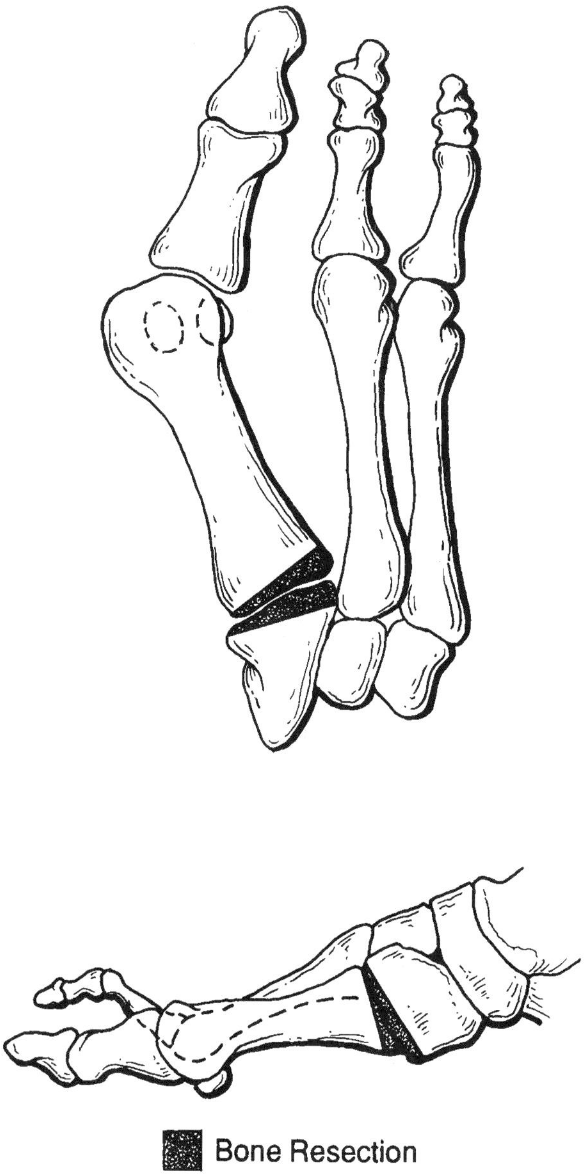

Fig. 29 Arthrodesis of the first metatarsocuneiform joint. **Top,** Minimum resection of the articular surface and subchondral bone decreases the first-second intermetatarsal angle. **Bottom,** Slightly more bone is resected on the plantar surface to achieve plantarflexion at the site of the arthrodesis.

A distal soft-tissue reconstruction should be avoided in the presence of a congruous MTP joint because it will probably lead to recurrence. Meticulous attention to surgical technique may reduce the prevalence of malunion. Lippert and McDermott[90] stressed the importance of correct positioning of the saw blade to avoid a dorsiflexion malunion (with medial rotation of the saw blade) or a plantarflexion and supination malunion (with lateral rotation of the saw blade). Thordarson and Leventen[91] emphasized that adequate internal fixation is the most important factor in the avoidance of a dorsiflexion malunion and the lateral metatarsalgia that accompanies it. Mann and associates[22] noted dorsiflexion at the site of the osteotomy in 30 of 109 feet, but they had used a single Steinmann pin for internal fixation. The use of screws[91] or screws and Kirschner wires[89] appears to increase the stability of the osteotomy site, and Thordarson and Leventen[91] documented less shortening with a more stable construct. Malunion can be extremely difficult to treat and may necessitate a complex and extensive salvage procedure that involves a corrective osteotomy and a distal soft-tissue realignment. Use of intraoperative radiographs may help to diminish malalignment.

A proximal metatarsal osteotomy combined with a distal soft-tissue reconstruction is technically demanding. In the treatment of moderate and severe hallux valgus deformities with MTP subluxation, meticulous attention to surgical technique, coupled with careful preoperative planning, can minimize postoperative complications.

Arthrodesis of the Metatarsocuneiform Joint (Modified Lapidus Procedure)

Arthrodesis of the first metatarsocuneiform (MC) joint can be combined with a distal soft-tissue realignment at the MTP joint to correct a hallux valgus deformity. On occasion, with a congruous MTP joint, a phalangeal osteotomy may be combined with the arthrodesis to achieve an extra-articular correction.[95] The major indication for this procedure is a moderate or severe hallux valgus deformity (a hallux valgus angle of at least 30° and an intermetatarsal angle of at least 16°[95]) with MTP subluxation associated with MC hypermobility[96] or generalized ligamentous laxity.[95] It is also used as a salvage procedure after a failed repair of hallux valgus.[95,96] Contraindications include a short first ray, juvenile hallux valgus with an open epiphysis, a moderate hallux valgus deformity without excessive MC hypermobility, and MTP degenerative osteoarthrosis.[97]

Technique A distal soft-tissue reconstruction, as described earlier, is routinely performed in conjunction with MC arthrodesis. The joint is then exposed through a 3-cm dorsal longitudinal incision just medial to the extensor hallucis longus tendon. A biplanar joint resection is performed to lateralize the first metatarsal, decrease the first-second intermetatarsal angle, and flex the first ray plantarly to diminish the prevalence of lateral metatarsalgia (Fig. 29). Meticulous preparation is necessary to ensure a successful arthrodesis. Excessive resection of bone is avoided as it may destabilize the MC joint, increasing the chance of malunion. The metatarsal should be aligned in neutral rotation in relation to the first cuneiform. A cancellous-bone graft[96] obtained from the distal tibial metaphysis, the iliac crest, or the calcaneus is added to the site of the arthrodesis to promote healing.

Internal fixation is an important aspect of the arthrodesis. Lapidus[98] recommended a heavy suture to secure the site of the arthrodesis; however, compression of the arthrodesis site with 3.5-mm fully threaded lag screws or 4.0-mm cancellous-bone screws is preferred. The first screw is introduced from the dorsal aspect of the base of the first metatarsal, 1.5 cm distal to the site of the arthrodesis, and is directed at a 45° angle into the first cuneiform. Care must be taken not to fracture the dorsal medial cortex or to depress the shaft of the first metatarsal excessively as the screw is tightened. A second screw is directed from the dorsal aspect of the first cuneiform distally into the first metatarsal. An optional third screw may be placed across the base of the first metatarsal into the second metatarsal. After adequate stabilization and alignment of the MC joint is confirmed with intraoperative radiographs or fluoroscopy, the wound is closed in a routine fashion.

Postoperative Care A gauze-and-tape compression dressing is applied at surgery and is changed 24 hours later, at which point a below-the-knee nonweightbearing cast is applied. At 4 weeks, the cast is changed and weightbearing is permitted.[96] Immobilization in a cast is continued until radiographic confirmation of fusion has been obtained. The hardware may be removed at 12 to 16 weeks after the arthrodesis, when radiographs show that fusion has occurred (Fig. 30).

Results and Complications In 1934, Lapidus[98] described a first and second MC arthrodesis combined with a distal soft-tissue reconstruction for the treatment of hallux valgus. Neither that report nor a follow-up report[99] contained any analysis of the results of the procedure. Mauldin and associates[100] as well as others[95,96] modified this procedure so that the second metatarsal is no

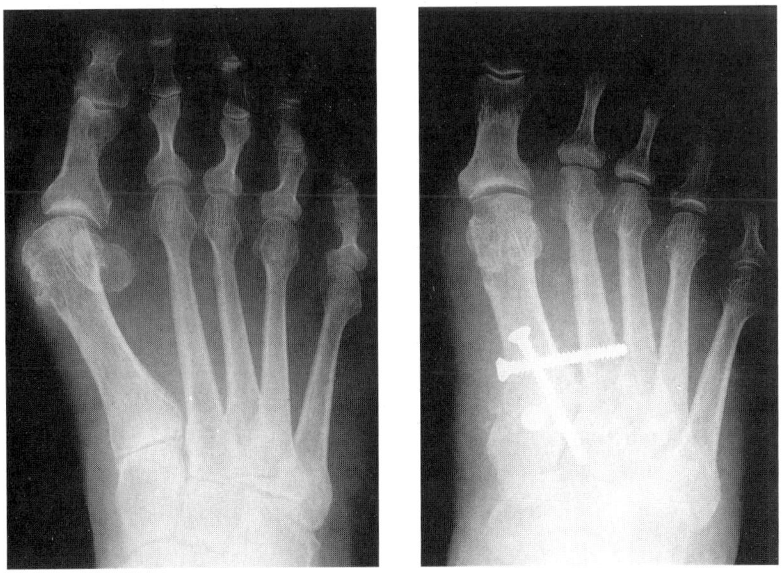

Fig. 30 Radiographs made before and after a distal soft-tissue repair and arthrodesis of the metatarsocuneiform joint in a foot with a moderate hallux valgus deformity and subluxation of the metatarsophalangeal joint. On preoperative examination, the patient had hypermobility of the metatarsocuneiform joint. **Left,** Preoperative appearance. **Right,** Postoperatively, correction has been achieved. Internal fixation is routinely removed at 12 to 16 weeks after a successful arthrodesis, to avoid breakage of the intermetatarsal screw.

longer included in the arthrodesis.

Mauldin and associates,[100] Myerson,[95] and Sangeorzan and Hansen[96] reported rates of patient satisfaction with the result of this procedure ranging from 75%[96] to 90%.[100] These authors reported an average correction of the hallux valgus angle of 18°[95,100] and an average correction of the first-second intermetatarsal angle of 6° to 8°.[95,96,100]

Sangeorzan and Hansen[96] as well as Myerson[95] observed prolonged swelling and a lengthy convalescent period after this procedure, compared with the findings after other bunion operations. Sangeorzan and Hansen also reported that only 12 of 28 feet were pain-free at the time of long-term follow-up. High rates of nonunion (10% and 12%) at the site of the arthrodesis have been reported,[95,96] and Mauldin and associates[100] confirmed fusion radiographically in only 13 of 51 feet. Rigid internal fixation and bone-grafting appear to reduce the prevalence of complications. Fixation with screws, as observed by Sangeorzan and Hansen, maintains position but is "quite unforgiving [and the] metatarsal must be positioned exactly at the time of surgery."

Inadequate preparation of the joint surfaces or inadequate internal fixation may lead to malposition at the site of the arthrodesis. Sangeorzan and Hansen[96] reported that five of 40 feet required surgical revision. The overall rate of failure in their study was 20%.

Excessive plantarflexion may lead to an intractable plantar keratosis beneath the first metatarsal, and excessive dorsiflexion may lead to lateral metatarsalgia. If a hallux valgus deformity is associated with shortening of the first ray or if the arthrodesis creates shortening without compensatory plantarflexion of the first ray, lateral metatarsalgia may be a serious problem. Myerson[95] noted that six of 62 metatarsals were fused in dorsiflexion, and three of these resulted in a transfer lesion or lateral metatarsalgia. Undercorrection may lead to recurrent hallux valgus, while overcorrection may actually create a negative intermetatarsal angle with subsequent hallux varus.[101] Postoperative hallux varus was reported in eight of 51 feet by Mauldin and associates,[100] a rate similar to that reported by Mann and Coughlin[7] after distal soft-tissue reconstruction alone.

Sangeorzan and Hansen[96] believed that the frequent failures of this procedure can be attributed to its technical complexity, and they concluded that the procedure should be reserved for hallux valgus deformities with hypermobility of the first ray[11,19,20,95] and recurrent deformity in young adults or adolescents.

Arthrodesis of the First Metatarsophalangeal Joint

Arthrodesis of the first MTP joint is recommended as a salvage procedure for various conditions, including severe hallux valgus,[102-104] recurrent hallux valgus,[103,105] rheumatoid arthritis,[102,104,106-109] hallux rigidus,[103,105,108,110-113] previous infection,[113] traumatic osteoarthrosis,[112] and hallux valgus associated with a neuromuscular disorder.[103-105] This arthrodesis was initially described by Clutton,[114] and various approaches, techniques for preparing the joint, and methods of internal fixation have been performed in an effort to improve the success rate of the procedure. Flat surfaces have been advocated because of the simplicity of preparation;[104,106,107,111,115,116] however, creation of a flat surface requires precision to achieve the desired alignment in all planes. Attempts to vary alignment in one plane intraoperatively may simultaneously affect alignment in another, creating an undesirable effect. The difficulty in achieving acceptable triplanar alignment at the site of the arthrodesis led Lipscomb[102] and others[86,108,109,113,115,117-121] to curve and contour the surfaces of the bone to enable adjustment of the alignment before placement of the internal fixation device. Later, cannulated cup-shaped power reamers were introduced to create congruous arthrodesis surfaces.[122-124] Both flat[104,106,107,111,115,116] and curved surfaces[86,109,117,119,120,125] have yielded relatively high rates of fusion. Various internal fixation devices have been used, including compression screws,[102,109,112,115,117,119,120] Steinmann pins,[103,104,107,126] Kirschner wires,[118] staples,[106] and compression plates,[108,122-124]

Contraindications to MTP fusion include active infection, substantial interphalangeal joint osteoarthrosis,[108,112,117,127] and severe osteoporosis.[86]

Technique With this technique,[49,122-124] a dorsal longitudinal incision is centered over the first MTP joint on the medial aspect of the extensor hallucis longus tendon. When necessary, the tendon is divided to aid exposure. The dissection is deepened to the MTP joint, and the capsular structures are released. An oscillating saw is used to resect the medial eminence and the articular surfaces of the base of the proximal phalanx and the first metatarsal head (Fig. 31). The amount of bone resected determines the eventual length of the ray. Preparation of the joint surfaces for arthrodesis is critical to achieve proper alignment.[122] I prefer to use cup-shaped power reamers for this purpose. The concave female reamer shapes the metatarsal head into a convex hemisphere (Fig. 32, *left*), and the phalangeal reamer is used to excavate the base of the proximal phalanx (Fig. 32, *center*). (Numbers 6514-7-216, 6514-7-316, and 6514-7-416 reamers [Howmedica, East Rutherford, NJ] are used.) After preparation, the surfaces are coapted (Fig. 32, *right*) in the desired alignment (15° to 20° of valgus, 20° to 30° of dorsiflexion, and neutral rotation) and are temporarily stabilized with a Kirschner wire. A small or mini-fragment plate is bent to the desired angle of dorsiflexion, positioned on the dorsal aspect of the

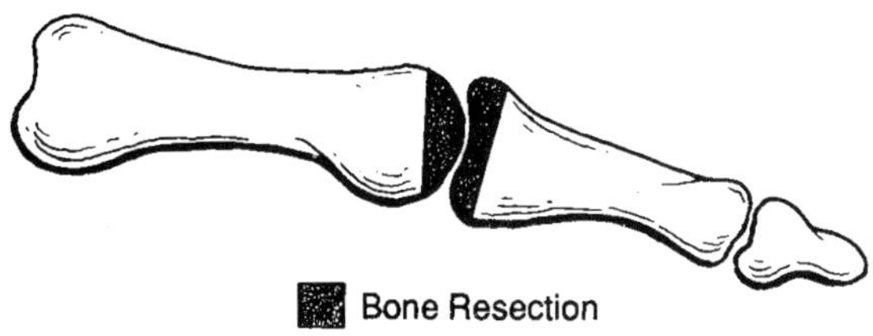

Fig. 31 Illustration demonstrating how the two articular surfaces are resected in preparation for arthrodesis of the first metatarsophalangeal joint.

phalanx and metatarsal, and secured with bicortical screws (Fig. 33). The K-wire is then removed, an oblique screw is introduced at the base of the proximal phalanx, and the screw is driven in a proximal-lateral direction across the site of the arthrodesis. The position of the arthrodesis should be confirmed with intraoperative radiographs. The extensor hallucis longus is repaired if necessary, and a routine capsular and skin closure is performed.

Postoperative Care A gauze-and-tape compression dressing is applied at surgery and is changed weekly. Walking is initiated with the patient wearing a postoperative shoe, with weightbearing on the heel and lateral aspect of the foot. Alternatively, the foot may be immobilized in a cast. The first ray is protected until adequate union is demonstrated radiographically, usually at 8 to 12 weeks postoperatively.

Results and Complications The rate of fusion varies substantially depending on surgical technique, the method of internal fixation, and the preoperative diagnosis. The reported prevalences of success have ranged from 77% to 100%,[104,105,107-109,111,112,116-121,125,126,128,129] with an average rate of 90%.[122] The rate of success in the largest series[125] was 91%. With use of a dorsal compression plate, the reported rate of successful fusion[108,123,124,130] has ranged from 92%[130] to 100%.[123] Coughlin and Abdo[124] reported a 93% subjective good or excellent result. While inadequate fixation is the most frequent cause of nonunion,[86,116,118] failure of the internal fixation is uncommon[125] and an unsuccessful arthrodesis or a pseudarthrosis may still lead to a painless and acceptable result (Fig. 34).[132]

The achievement of good alignment at the site of the arthrodesis is critically important for ultimate patient satisfaction. Recommendations for alignment in the frontal plane have ranged from 5° to 30° of valgus,[101,107,110,120,125-128] with an average of 15°.[104,122-124] After arthrodesis of the MTP joint, a widened first-second intermetatarsal angle associated with a severe hallux valgus deformity is usually reduced (Fig. 35),[102,103,115,119,120,125,129] and only rarely is an additional metatarsal osteotomy necessary.[103,111,129] Fitzgerald[128] cautioned that arthrodesis in less than 20° of valgus is associated with a threefold increase in the prevalence of interphalangeal joint osteoarthrosis. Recommendations for alignment in the sagittal plane have ranged from 10° to 40° of dorsiflex-ion[104,107,108,112,113,115,116,120,124-127] (in relation to the shaft of the first metatarsal), with 20° to 25° being the most commonly recommended position.[122] Excessive plantarflexion leads to pressure beneath the tip of the toe while excessive dorsiflexion frequently leads to an intractable plantar keratosis

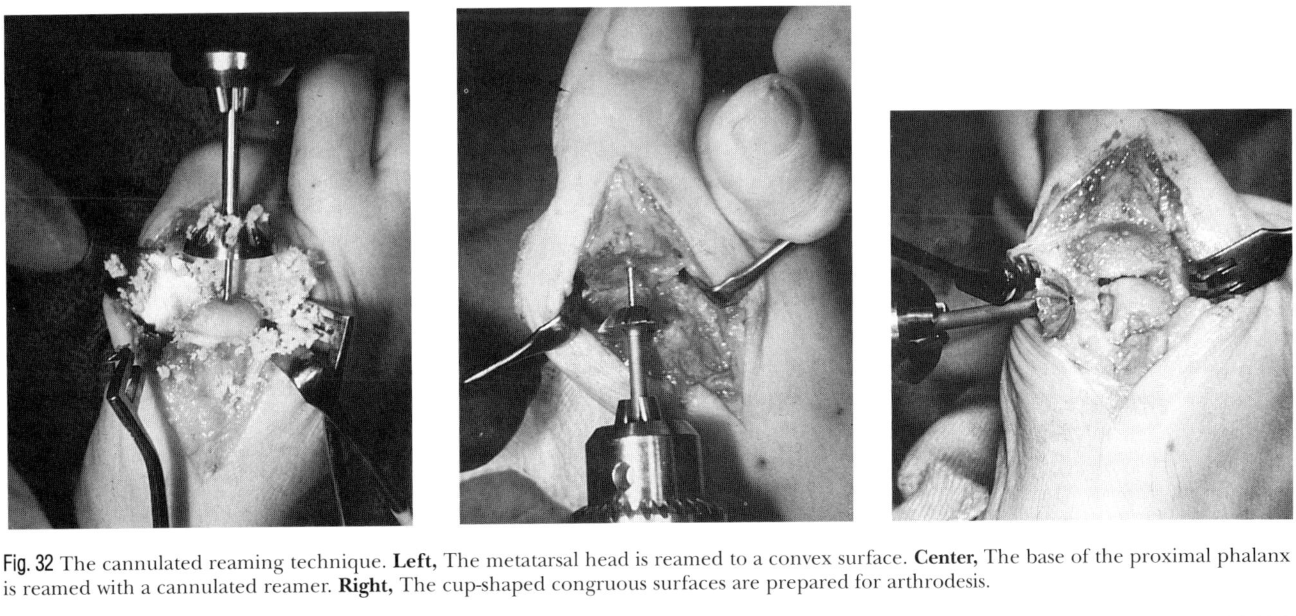

Fig. 32 The cannulated reaming technique. **Left,** The metatarsal head is reamed to a convex surface. **Center,** The base of the proximal phalanx is reamed with a cannulated reamer. **Right,** The cup-shaped congruous surfaces are prepared for arthrodesis.

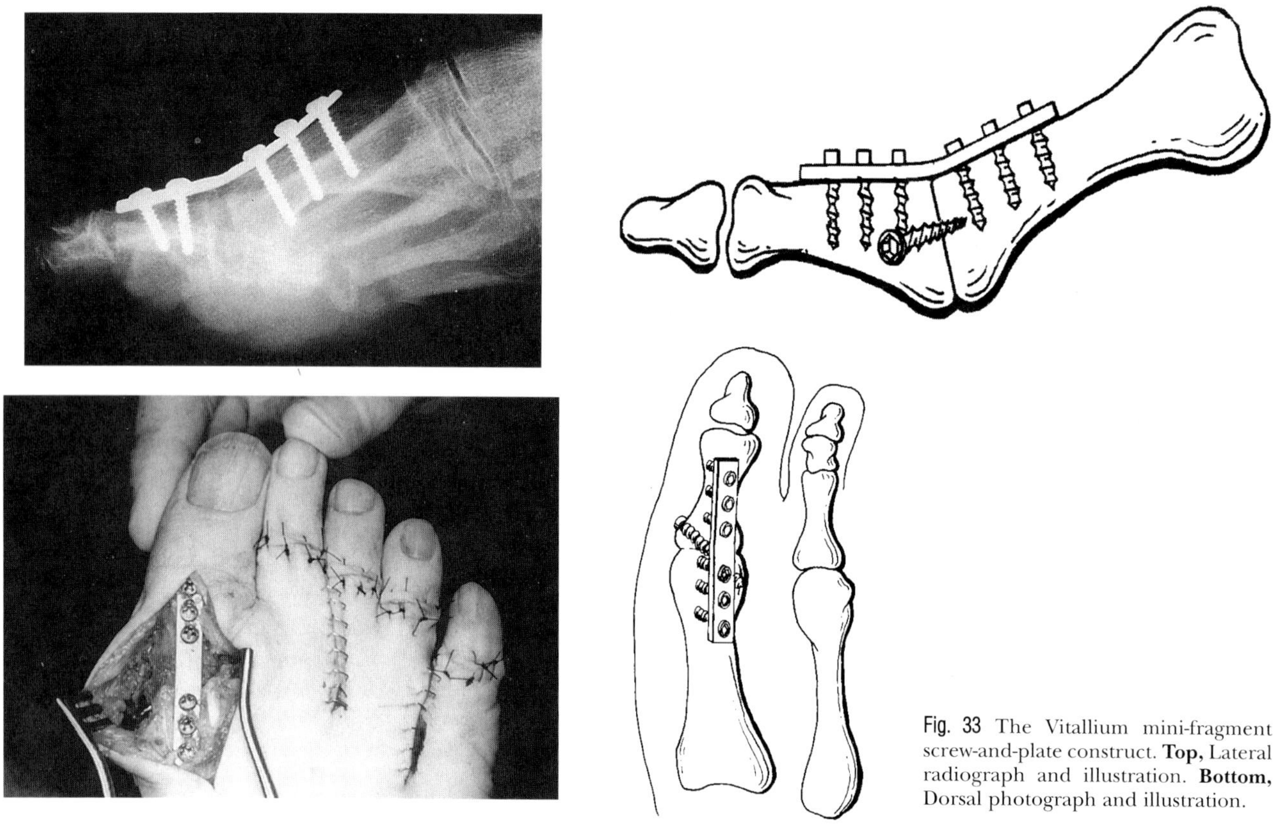

Fig. 33 The Vitallium mini-fragment screw-and-plate construct. **Top,** Lateral radiograph and illustration. **Bottom,** Dorsal photograph and illustration.

beneath the sesamoids. Malunion in any plane, however, is poorly tolerated and underscores the necessity of meticulous attention to the final position of the arthrodesis. No bunion procedure requires a technique that is more exacting and unforgiving than that required in arthrodesis of the first MTP joint.

When an arthrodesis is combined with MTP joint resection arthroplasties of the lesser toes, shortening of the first ray is not a problem. When only the first ray is operated on, slight shortening is of little consequence; however, marked shortening may be unacceptable, particularly from a cosmetic standpoint.[104,124]

The use of a dorsal compression plate is relatively easy and is associated with high rates of fusion and patient satisfaction. One major concern is that the plate, from a mechanical standpoint, is on the compression surface rather than the tension surface. I have not found this to be a problem. While bulky mini-fragment stainless-steel plates usually have to be removed,[108,123,130] the low-profile Vitallium plate that I currently use usually does not.[124] Alternatively, others have found that fixation with compression screws also offers a reliable means of internal fixation with a high degree of patient satisfaction.[112]

The surgical technique should be easy to perform and should achieve a predictable result. The shaping of congruous cancellous surfaces that allow easy adjustment to the desired position (varus and valgus angulation, dorsiflexion and plantarflexion, and rotation) and the use of rigid internal fixation are both important factors in achieving and maintaining position while attaining a high rate of osseous fusion. However, as McKeever[119] stated: "It is the [fusion] and its position that is important and not the method by which it is produced."

Excisional Arthroplasty

The Keller excisional arthroplasty is indicated for moderate hallux valgus deformities (a hallux valgus angle of less than 30°) associated with degenerative osteoarthrosis of the MTP joint in older, more sedentary patients who have limited expectations with regard to walking.[131] The procedure is contraindicated in young, active individuals,[132] older patients in whom function of the first MTP joint should be preserved; and patients who have a severe deformity and who consider subtotal correction unacceptable. With this technique, a resection of the medial eminence, partial proximal phalangectomy, and medial capsular plication are used to realign the great toe.[27,133-135] Often considered a salvage procedure, the technique involves resection of as much as one third of the proximal aspect of the proximal phalanx to decompress the metatarsophalangeal joint.[131,136]

Technique With this technique,[27,134,135,137] a medial longitudinal skin incision is centered over the MTP joint

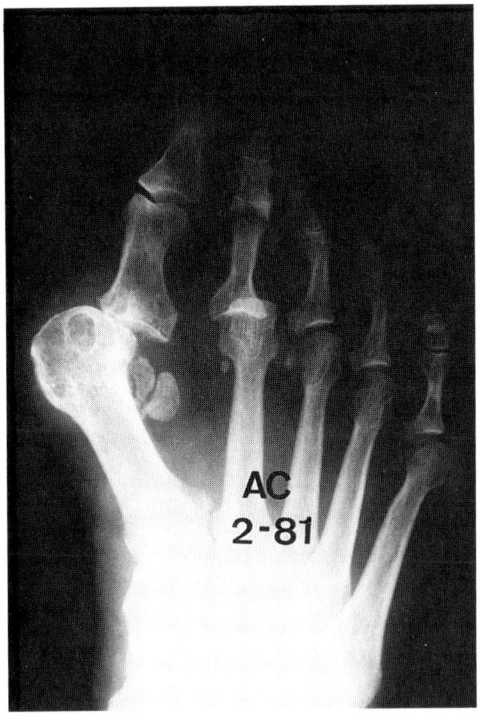

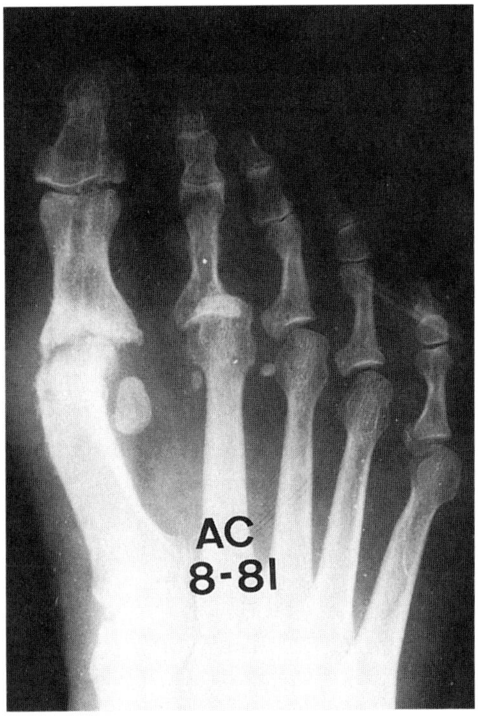

Fig. 34 Radiographs made before and after arthrodesis of the first metatarsophalangeal joint in a patient who had rheumatoid arthritis and a severe hallux valgus deformity. **Left,** Preoperative appearance. **Right,** Six months postoperatively, there is a painless fibrous union and the deformity is much less severe.

and extends from the interphalangeal joint to a point proximal to the medial eminence. A proximally based capsular flap is developed by detaching it from the base of the proximal phalanx, exposing the medial eminence. The base of the proximal phalanx is exposed by a subperiosteal dissection. The medial eminence is excised with a power saw in line with the medial border of the foot. Any remaining osteophytes in the area of the sagittal sulcus are removed with a rongeur. The proximal fourth of the proximal phalanx is then osteotomized at the level of the metaphyseal flare with an oscillating saw, is carefully released from the plantar plate, and is removed (Fig. 36, *left* and *center*).[134] Two drill-holes are made plantarly in the diaphyseal portion of the remaining proximal phalangeal segment, and the plantar plate with the attached sesamoids and intrinsic muscles is sutured to the base of the phalanx with interrupted non-absorbable sutures (Fig. 36, *right*).[135] The joint is then stabilized with one or two 0.062-in (0.157-cm) K-wires[131,134,138] introduced at the joint, drilled distally, and then drilled in a retrograde direction into the metatarsal head. The pins are bent at the tip of the toe to prevent proximal migration. The medial part of the capsule is then reattached to the proximal phalanx with interrupted absorbable sutures. The wound is closed in a routine fashion.

Postoperative Care The foot is placed in a gauze-and-tape compression dressing, which is changed weekly for 6 weeks. Walking with weightbearing is permitted with the patient wearing a wooden-soled shoe. The K-wires are removed 4 weeks following surgery, at which point MTP range-of-motion and plantarflexion exercises are initiated.[134]

Results and Complications After excisional arthroplasty, the hallux valgus angle is usually reduced approximately 50% or less,[73,131,139] and the intermetatarsal angle is not changed much at all (Fig. 37).[73,140] Satisfactory results occur more often when the hallux valgus angle is less than 30°, because correction can be obtained with removal of less than one-third of the proximal phalanx. Pain is reduced with decompression of the osteoarthrotic joint. Pain from a prominent medial eminence is reduced as well, and frequently this allows the patient to wear more comfortable shoes. Reported rates of subjective satisfaction,[131,132,136,141] as judged mainly on the basis of relief of bunion-related pain and not on the basis of the absence of metatarsalgia, have ranged from 72%[136] to 96%.[141] Bonney and Macnab[41] observed that functional results may deteriorate with time. Rogers and Joplin[140] reported generally poor results with this procedure, noting marked objective improvement in five of 55 feet, no change in 39 feet, and postoperative deterioration in 11 feet.

Henry and associates[142] documented that the inability of the great toe to bear weight postoperatively is associated with metatarsalgia. Coughlin and Mann[126] as well as others[73,133,134,136,140-142] reported postoperative

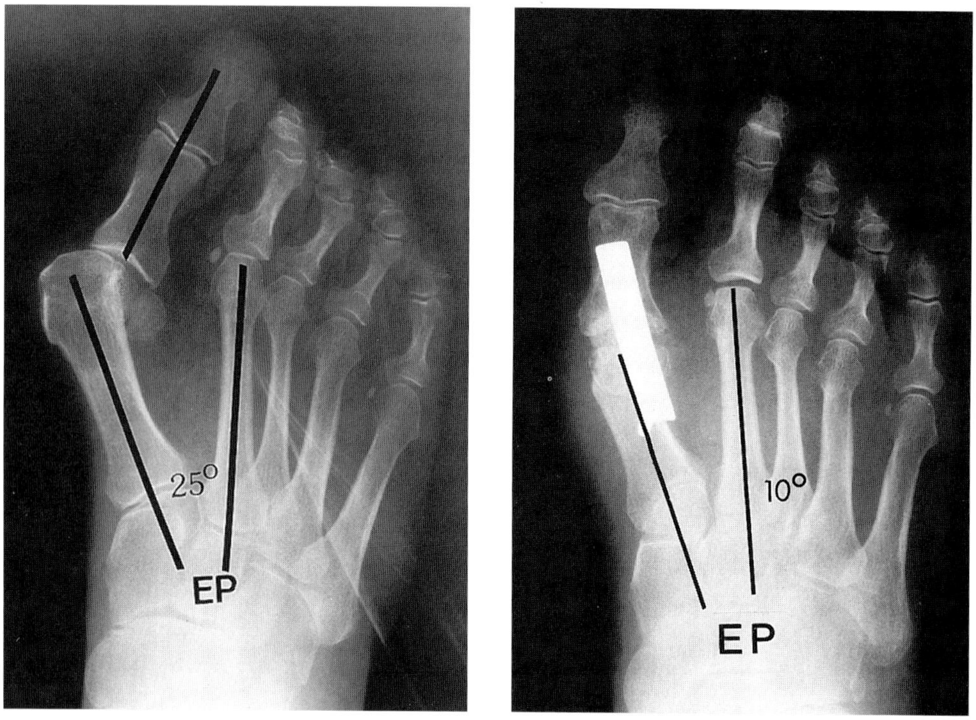

Fig. 35 Radiographs made before and after arthrodesis of the metatarsophalangeal joint in a foot with a severe hallux valgus deformity and widening of the first-second intermetatarsal angle to 25°. **Left,** Preoperative appearance. **Right,** Postoperatively, the first-second intermetatarsal angle decreased to 10° as the hallux valgus angle was corrected.

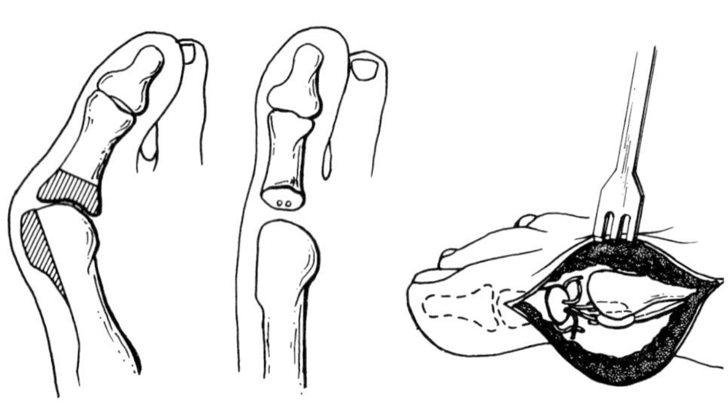

Fig. 36 An excisional arthroplasty. **Left,** Proposed resection of the medial eminence and the proximal quarter of the proximal phalanx. **Center,** After resection of the bone. **Right,** The plantar plate is reapproximated to the residual proximal phalanx.

metatarsalgia as a frequent complication following a Keller procedure. While excision of at least one half of the phalanx has been recommended,[41,133,141] Vallier and associates[131] and Wrighton[136] reported that limited phalangeal resection is associated with a higher rate of postoperative satisfaction. Henry and associates noted an association between an increased phalangeal resection and increased weightbearing on the lateral part of the forefoot as well as increased lateral metatarsalgia. Weightbearing on the great toe was noted in 24 of the 33 feet from which one third or less of the proximal phalanx had been resected, while it was noted in only nine of the 47 feet from which more than one third of the proximal phalanx had been resected.[45] With more severe deformities, there is a tendency to resect a larger amount of the proximal phalanx in order to correct the hallux valgus. Vallier and associates stressed that this tendency may lead to a short, flail, functionless great toe.

Besides postoperative metatarsalgia, which has been reported in almost all series,[31,46,131,134,136,140,141,143] other complications include a cock-up deformity of the great toe (Fig. 38);[73,126,132,139,140] stiffness of the interphalangeal joint;[126,142] and marked shortening,[126,142] impaired control and function,[126,136,142] and diminished flexor strength[73,126,131,139,143] of the great toe.

Because of the high frequency of incomplete correction and associated postoperative metatarsalgia, excisional arthroplasty of the first MTP joint is recommended for elderly, low-demand patients who have osteoarthrotic changes of that joint in the absence of lateral metatarsalgia.[139] As Henry and associates[142] observed: "Any operation for hallux valgus should attempt to restore (or at least not destroy) the ability of the big toe to bear weight."

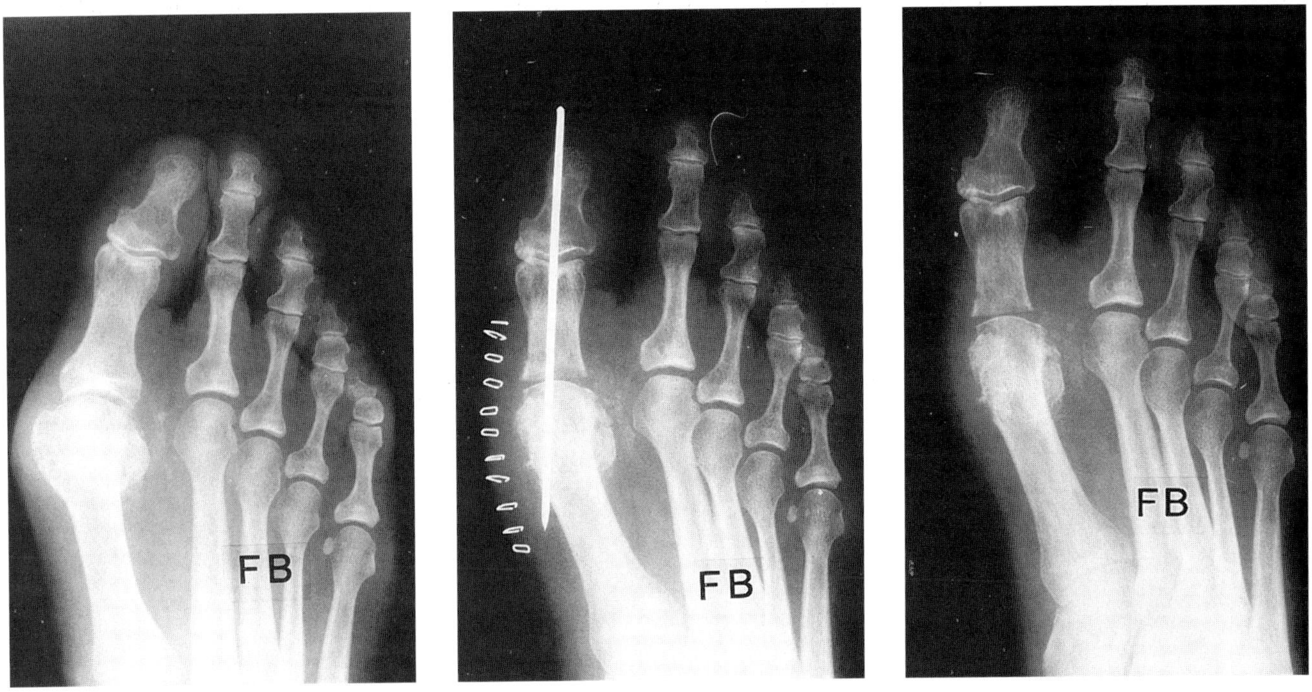

Fig. 37 Radiographs made before and after excisisonal arthroplasty in an 80-year-old woman who had a moderate hallux valgus deformity as well as osteoarthrosis of the metatarsophalangeal joint. **Left,** Preoperative appearance. **Center,** Postoperatively, intramedullaray fixation with one K-wire is seen. **Right,** One year after surgery, there is continued good alignment.

Multiple Osteotomies

An intra-articular or soft-tissue reconstruction is contraindicated for the surgical treatment of hallux valgus in the presence of a congruous MTP joint (a distal metatarsal articular angle of greater than 15°).[8] In this situation, an extra-articular correction may be achieved with either a double or a triple osteotomy. An Akin phalangeal osteotomy[8,24,144,145] can decrease phalangeal angulation due to an increased PPAA; a proximal first metatarsal osteotomy[146,147] or a cuneiform osteotmy[24,148] can diminish an increased intermetatarsal angle; and, in some cases, an increase in the DMAA necessitates a medial closing-wedge osteotomy of the distal end of the metatarsal.[47,65,66,149] Mitchell and Baxter[30] recommended combining a chevron osteotomy with a phalangeal osteotomy. In general, the magnitude of the DMAA determines the need for multiple osteotomies of the first ray. Richardson and associates[17] found that, on anatomic and radiographic analysis, the average DMAA in 100 normal feet was 6° or 7°. As this angle increases, the magnitude of the hallux valgus angle increases.[8] As previously mentioned, Piggott[16] noted that 9% of adults who have hallux valgus have congruous MTP joints, and I[8] found congruous joints in 28 of 60 children who had hallux valgus. It is in these patients who have a congruous joint and a large DMAA that a double or triple osteotomy has the best capacity to correct a hallux valgus deformity.

Technique Distal metatarsal osteotomy: With use of this technique,[65,66,146,147,149] a medial longitudinal incision is centered over the MTP joint. The dissection is deepened to the capsule. The medial part of the capsule is released on the dorsal and proximal aspect with an L-shaped distally based capsular flap. At a point approximately 1.5 cm proximal to the surface of the MTP joint, a medial closing-wedge osteotomy of the proximal metatarsal metaphysis is performed (Fig. 39). The magnitude of the medial closing wedge depends on the magnitude of the lateral slope of the DMAA. Usually, the wedge is 6 to 10 mm wide at its base. Care must be taken to avoid injury of the sesamoid complex on the plantar aspect with this closing-wedge osteotomy. Loretz and associates[150] and Kramer and associates[151] both described a Z-shaped osteotomy of the distal end of the metatarsal that protects the sesamoid mechanism. Once the wedge has been removed, the osteotomy is closed and fixed with two oblique 0.062-in (0.157-cm) K-wires. The medial eminence is then resected with an oscillating saw. The medial part of the capsule is approximated and secured to the first metatarsal with a suture placed through a metaphyseal drill-hole. The capsular repair is completed with interrupted

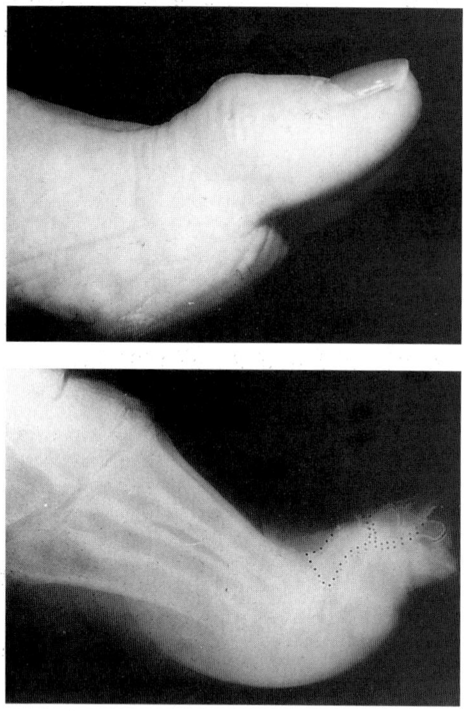

Fig. 38 Photograph and radiograph of a cock-up deformity of the great toe after an excisional arthroplasty.

absorbable sutures. After completion of this osteotomy, the great toe may appear to be in slight varus because the toe now more closely parallels the long axis of the shaft of the metatarsal. This situation creates the need for a proximal osteotomy of the first ray to diminish the first-second intermetatarsal angle. A proximal osteotomy of the first metatarsal may be considered but should be approached with caution as extensive soft-tissue stripping of the first metatarsal may devascularize it. An alternative osteotomy, therefore, is an opening-wedge first cuneiform osteotomy.[24]

Osteotomy of the first cuneiform: This technique[24] involves a medial longitudinal incision centered over the first cuneiform. Care is taken to identify the naviculocuneiform and metatarsocuneiform joints, exposing the entire medial aspect of the first cuneiform, which is approximately 3 cm high and 2 cm long (Fig. 39). A vertical osteotomy is made in the center of the bone, and the osteotomy site is opened medially. Once the osteotomy site has been distracted, a triangular bicortical iliac-crest bone graft is impacted into place and stabilized with two 0.062-in (0.157-cm) K-wires. Bone removed from the metatarsal head or the medial eminence usually is insufficient to serve as a graft. The incision is closed in a routine fashion.

Postoperative Care The foot is placed in a gauze-and-tape compression dressing at surgery, and a nonweightbear-

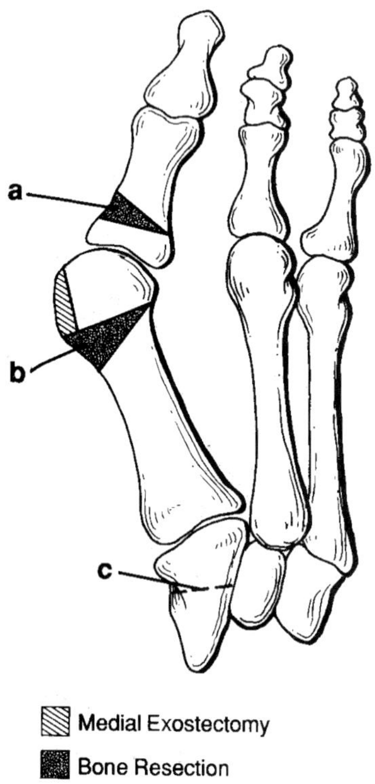

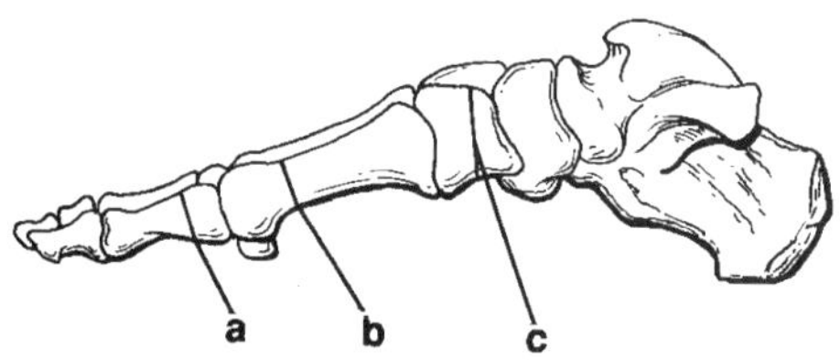

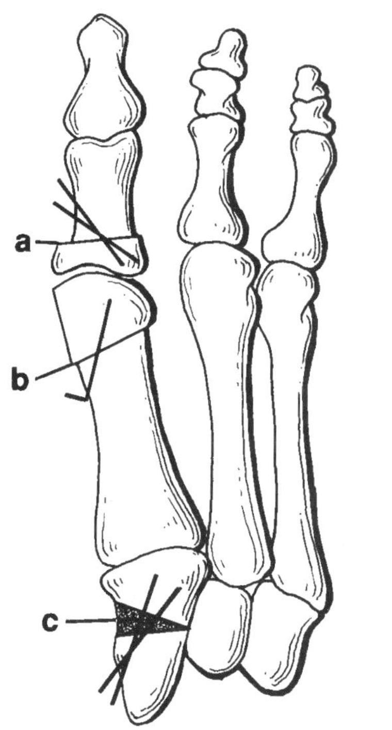

Fig. 39 Illustrations demonstrating how multiple osteotomies can be performed to achieve extra-articular correction of a hallux valgus deformity, especially when the distal metatarsal articular angle is increased. **Left,** A closing-wedge phalangeal osteotomy (a), a closing-wedge osteotomy of the distal end of the metatarsal with exostectomy of the medial eminence (b), and an opening-wedge osteotomy of the first cuneiform (c). **Center,** Lateral view showing the locations of the osteotomies. **Right,** Appearance of a foot after a triple osteotomy. There is overall improved alignment of the first ray and the first metatarsophalangeal joint.

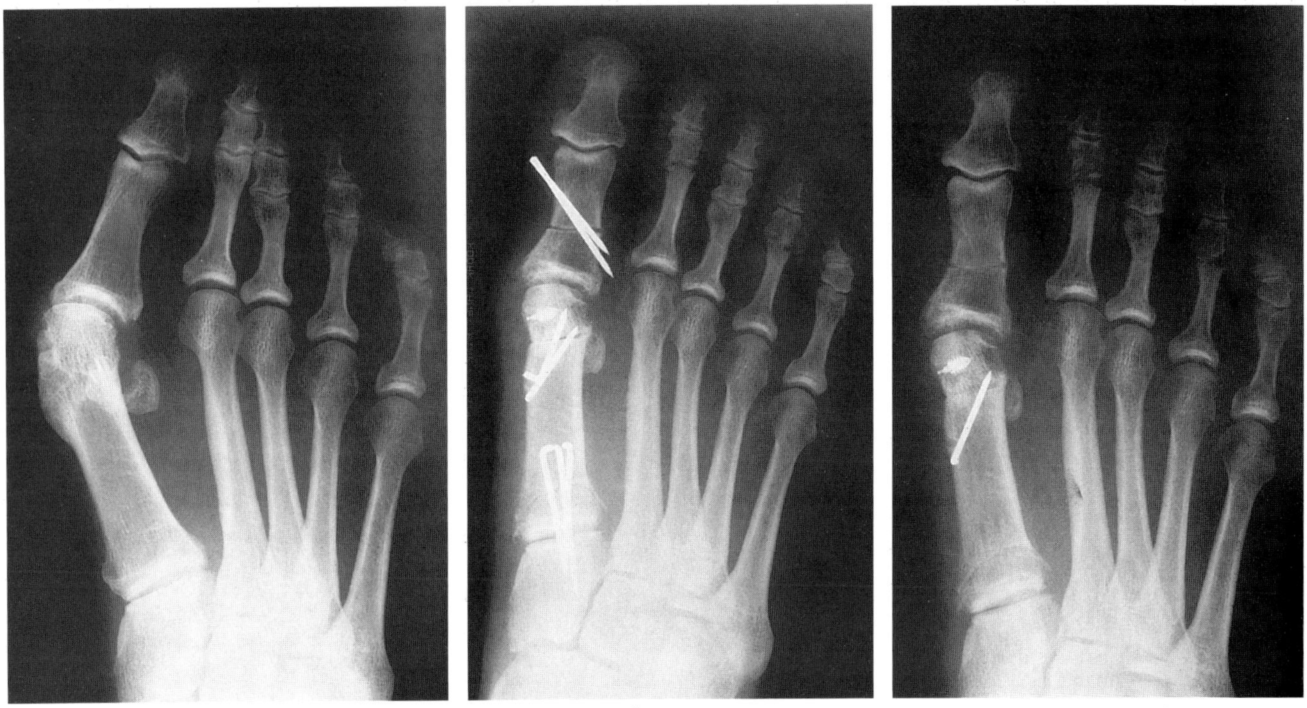

Fig. 40 Radiographs made before and after a closing-wedge phalangeal osteotomy, a crescentic osteotomy of the proximal end of the metatarsal, and a closing-wedge osteotomy of the distal end of the metatarsal in a foot that had recurrent hallux valgus after a McBride procedure. **Left,** Preoperatively, the hallus valgus angle is 40° and the distal metatarsal articular angle is 30°. **Center,** Immediate postoperative appearance. **Right,** Six months mostoperatively, there has been excellent correction. The hallux valgue angle is 11°, andf the distal metatarsal articular angle is 2°.

ing below-the-knee cast is applied. At 4 weeks, the cast is changed and weightbearing is allowed. Usually, the sites of the osteotomies heal in 6 to 8 weeks. The cast is removed after radiographic confirmation of healing, and range-of-motion exercises are initiated.

Results and Complications While Funk and Wells,[149] Peabody,[66] Hohmann,[47] and Reverdin[65] reported success with distal osteotomies of the first metatarsal, and Durman[146] as well as Goldner and Gaines[145] reported success with double osteotomies, very few investigators have reported quantitative results of these procedures.

Kramer and associates[151] reported an average 15° correction of the DMAA with a distal Z-type rotational osteotomy, and Loretz and associates[150] reported a similar improvement in this angle. Funk and Wells[149] reported an average 7.2° correction of the intermetatarsal angle with a distal closing-wedge osteotomy of the metatarsal. A variety of double osteotomies have been advocated, including phalangeal with metatarsal osteotomy,[8,144,145] double metatarsal osteotomies,[8,146] phalangeal with chevron osteotomy,[30] and phalangeal with cuneiform osteotomy[24,148] (Fig. 40).

Reporting on the use of double and triple osteotomies for the treatment of adolescent hallux valgus with congruous metatarsophalangeal joints, I noted an average hallux valgus correction of 22.9° and an average correction of the first-second intermetatarsal angle of 8.3° in seven patients. This correction was in the presence of an average DMAA of 18.9°. These results are similar to those obtained by Peterson and Newman,[147] who reported on ten adolescent patients who had an average correction of the hallux valgus angle of 24° and an average correction of the first-second intermetatarsal angle of 8.2° after double osteotomies. A high rate of subjective satisfaction was reported in both series.

Complications with multiple metatarsal osteotomies include loss of fixation, loss of correction,[24] malunion,[24] osteonecrosis,[63] intra-articular extension of the osteotomy,[30] and degenerative osteoarthrosis of the interphalangeal or MTP joint. These techniques are difficult and should be reserved for the occasional case of a hallux valgus deformity with a congruous joint associated with an increased DMAA of more than 15°.

Overview

The process of deciding which procedure to perform for a patient who has a bunion or bunions requires a careful preoperative physical evaluation and radiographic assessment to determine the specific pathologic elements that need surgical correction. All elements of the deformity, including an increased hallux valgus angle, increased first-second intermetatarsal angle, pronation of the great toe, increased DMAA, enlarged medial eminence, and subluxation of the sesamoids, must be corrected. Failure to correct any of these components places the foot at substantial risk of recurrent deformity.

The large number of procedures that are available testifies to the fact that no one method sufficiently corrects all bunion deformities. While it is not uncommon for a surgeon to be comfortable with one specific procedure and to use it to correct most hallux valgus deformities, different deformities have various pathologic components and magnitudes and may require distinctly different surgical approaches if consistently good results are to be achieved. Likewise, the upper limits of deformities that can be corrected successfully on a routine basis vary from surgeon to surgeon and may depend in part on the familiarity with the procedure, the surgical technique used, and the frequency with which it is used. Surgical versatility is important, and several types of operations should be at the disposal of the surgeon in order to address the different anatomic abnormalities.

Some surgical procedures have very limited indications. Choosing a procedure that has the capacity to correct a hallux valgus deformity easily is preferable to stretching the indications of a less intensive procedure, as doing so invites postoperative complications. In selecting a specific surgical technique, the surgeon must attempt to maintain a flexible first MTP joint, preserve the normal weightbearing pattern of the forefoot, and retain a reasonable means of salvage should a complication occur.

References

1. Coughlin MJ: Hallux valgus: Causes, evaluation, and treatment. *Postgrad Med* 1984;75:174–187.
2. Coughlin MJ, Thompson FM: The high price of high-fashion footwear, in Jackson DW (ed): *Instructional Course Lectures 44.* Rosemont, IL, American Academy of Orthopaedic Surgeons, 1995, pp 371–377.
3. Sim Fook L, Hodgson AR: A comparison of foot forms among the non-shoe and shoe-wearing Chinese population. *J Bone Joint Surg* 1958;40A:1058–1062.
4. Kato T, Watanabe S: The etiology of hallux valgus in Japan. *Clin Orthop* 1981;157:78–81.
5. Inman VT: Hallux valgus: A review of etiologic factors. *Orthop Clin North Am* 1974;5:59–66.
6. Hohmann G: Der hallux valgus und die ubrigen Zehenverkrummungen Ergebn. *Chir Orthop* 1925;18:308–376.
7. Mann RA, Coughlin MJ: Hallux valgus: Etiology, anatomy, treatment and surgical considerations. *Clin Orthop* 1981; 157:31–41.
8. Coughlin MJ: Juvenile hallux valgus: Etiology and treatment. *Foot Ankle Int* 1995;16:692–697.
9. Kilmartin TE, Wallace WA: The significance of pes planus in juvenile hallux valgus. *Foot Ankle* 1992;13:53–56.
10. Hardy RH, Clapham JCR: Observations on hallux valgus: Based on a controlled series. *J Bone Joint Surg* 1951;33B: 376–391.
11. Mann RA, Coughlin MJ: Adult hallux valgus, in Mann RA, Coughlin MJ (eds): *Surgery of the Foot and Ankle,* ed 6. St. Louis, MO, Mosby-Year book, 1993, pp 167–296.
12. Stein HC: Hallux valgus. *Surg Gynecol Obstet* 1938;66:889–898.
13. Haines RW, McDougall A: The anatomy of hallux valgus. *J Bone Joint Surg* 1954;36B:272–293.
14. McBride ED: A conservative operation for bunions. *J Bone Joint Surg* 1928;10:735–739.
15. Coughlin MJ, Mann RA: The pathophysiology of the juvenile bunion, in Griffin PP (ed): *Instructional Course Lectures XXXVI.* Park Ridge, IL, American Academy of Orthopaedic Surgeons, 1987, pp 123–136.
16. Piggott H: The natural history of hallux valgus in adolescence and early adult life. *J Bone Joint Surg* 1960;42B:749–760.
17. Richardson EG, Graves SC, McClure JT, et al: First metatarsal head-shaft angle: A method of determination. *Foot Ankle* 1993;14:181–185.
18. Brage ME, Holmes JR, Sangeorzan BJ: The influence of x-ray orientation on the first metatarsocuneiform joint angle. *Foot Ankle Int* 1994;15:495–497.
19. Klaue K, Hansen ST, Masquelet AC: Clinical, quantitative assessment of first tarsometatarsal mobility in the sagittal plane and its relation to hallux valgus deformity. *Foot Ankle Int* 1994;15:9–13.
20. Wanivenhaus A, Pretterklieber M: First tarsometatarsal joint: Anatomical, biomechanical study. *Foot Ankle* 1989;9:153–157.
21. Smith RW, Reynolds JC, Stewart MJ: Hallux valgus assessment: Report of research committee of American Orthopaedic Foot and Ankle Society. *Foot Ankle* 1984;5:92–103.
22. Mann RA, Rudicel S, Graves SC: Repair of hallux valgus with a distal soft-tissue procedure and proximal metatarsal osteotomy: A long-term follow-up. *J Bone Joint Surg* 1992;74A:124–129.
23. Mann RA: Decision-making in bunion surgery, in Greene WB (ed): *Instructional Course Lectures XXXIX.* Park Ridge, IL, American Academy of Orthopaedic Surgeons, 1990, pp 3–13.
24. Coughlin MJ: Juvenile bunions, in Mann RA, Coughlin MJ (eds): *Surgery of the Foot and Ankle,* ed 6. St. Louis, MO, Mosby-Year Book, 1993, vol 1, pp 297–339.
25. Akin OF: The treatment of hallux valgus: A new operative procedure and its results. *Medical Sentinel* 1925;33:678–679.
26. Brahms MA: Hallux valgus: The Akin procedure. *Clin Orthop* 1981;157:47–49.
27. Mann RA, Coughlin MJ: *Video Textbook of Foot and Ankle Surgery.* St. Louis, MO, Medical Video Productions, 1991, pp 146–184.
28. Plattner PF, Van Manen JW: Results of Akin type proximal phalangeal osteotomy for correction of hallux valgus deformity. *Orthopedics* 1990;13:989–996.
29. Silberman FS: Proximal phalangeal osteotomy for the correction of hallux valgus. *Clin Orthop* 1972;85:98–100.
30. Mitchell LA, Baxter DE: A Chevron-Akin double osteotomy for correction of hallux valgus. *Foot Ankle* 1991;12:7–14.
31. Goldberg I, Bahar A, Yosipovitch Z: Late results after correction of hallux valgus deformity by basilar phalangeal osteotomy. *J Bone Joint Surg* 1987;69A:64–67.
32. Seelenfreund M, Fried A, Tikva P: Correction of hallux valgus deformity by basal phalanx osteotomy of the big toe. *J Bone Joint Surg* 1973;55A:1411–1415.
33. Colloff B, Weitz EM: Proximal phalangeal osteotomy in hallux valgus. *Clin Orthop* 1967;54:105–113.
34. DuVries HL (ed): *Surgery of the Foot.* St. Louis, MO, CV Mosby, 1959, pp 381–388.
35. McBride ED: The conservative operation for "bunions": End results and refinements of technic. *JAMA* 1935;105:1164–1168.
36. McBride ED: The McBride bunion hallux valgus operation: Refinements in the successive surgical steps of the operation. *J Bone Joint Surg* 1967;49A:1675–1683.

37. Meyer JM, Hoffmeyer P, Borst F: The treatment of hallux valgus in runners using a modified McBride procedure. *Int Orthop* 1987;11:197–200.
38. Silver D: The operative treatment of hallux valgus. *J Bone Joint Surg* 1923;5:225–232.
39. Mann RA, Pfeffinger L: Hallux valgus repair: DuVries modified McBride procedure. *Clin Orthop* 1991;272:213–218.
40. Kitaoka HB, Franco MG, Weaver AL, et al: Simple bunionectomy with medial capsulorrhaphy. *Foot Ankle* 1991;12:86–91.
41. Bonney G, Macnab I: Hallux valgus and hallux rigidus: A critical survey of operative results. *J Bone Joint Surg* 1952;34B: 366–385.
42. Johnson JE, Clanton TO, Baxter DE, et al: Comparison of Chevron osteotomy and modified McBride bunionectomy for correction of mild to moderate hallux valgus deformity. *Foot Ankle* 1991;12:61–68.
43. Coughlin MJ: Chevron procedure. *Contemp Orthop* 1991;23: 45–49.
44. Hirvensalo E, Böstman O, Törmälä P, et al: Chevron osteotomy fixed with absorbable polyglycolide pins. *Foot Ankle* 1991; 1:212–218.
45. Meier PJ, Kenzora JE: The risks and benefits of distal first metatarsal osteotomies. *Foot Ankle* 1985;6:7–17.
46. Hattrup SJ, Johnson KA: Chevron osteotomy: Analysis of factors in patients' dissatisfaction. *Foot Ankle* 1985;5:327–332.
47. Hohmann G (ed): *Fuss und Bein, ihre Erkrankungen und deren Behandlung, ein Lehrbuch*, ed 4. Munchen, Germany, JF Bergmann, 1948, p 167.
48. Johnson KA, Cofield RH, Morrey BF: Chevron osteotomy for hallux valgus. *Clin Orthop* 1979;142:44–47.
49. Glynn MK, Dunlop JB, Fitzpatrick D: The Mitchell distal metatarsal osteotomy for hallux valgus. *J Bone Joint Surg* 1980; 62B:188–191.
50. Jahss MH, Troy AI, Kummer F: Roentgenographic and mathematical analysis of first metatarsal osteotomies for metatarsus primus varus: A comparative study. *Foot Ankle* 1985;5:280–321.
51. Mann RA: Complications associated with the Chevron osteotomy. *Foot Ankle* 1982;3:125–129.
52. Shereff MJ, Yang QM, Kummer FJ: Extraosseous and intraosseous arterial supply to the first metatarsal and metatarsophalangeal joint. *Foot Ankle* 1987;8:81–93.
53. Williams WW, Barrett DS, Copeland SA: Avascular necrosis following Chevron distal metatarsal osteotomy: A significant risk? *J Foot Surg* 1989;28:414–416.
54. Hetherington VJ, Steinbock G, LaPorta D, et al: The Austin bunionectomy: A follow-up study. *J Foot Ankle Surg* 1993; 32:162–166.
55. Austin DW, Leventen EO: A new osteotomy for hallux valgus: A horizontally directed "V" displacement osteotomy of the metatarsal head for hallux valgus and primus varus. *Clin Orthop* 1981;157:25–30.
56. Leventen EO: The Chevron procedure. *Orthopedics* 1990; 13:973–976.
57. Lewis RJ, Feffer HL: Modified Chevron osteotomy of the first metatarsal. *Clin Orthop* 1981;157:105–109.
58. Pochatko DJ, Schlehr FJ, Murphey MD, et al: Distal Chevron osteotomy with lateral release for treatment of hallux valgus deformity. *Foot Ankle Int* 1994;15:457–461.
59. Resch S, Stenström A, Gustafson T: Circulatory disturbance of the first metatarsal head after Chevron osteotomy as shown by bone scintigraphy. *Foot Ankle* 1992;13:137–142.
60. Corless JR: Abstract: A modification of the Mitchell procedure. *J Bone Joint Surg* 1976;58B:138.
61. Klosok JK, Pring DJ, Jessop JH, et al: Chevron or Wilson metatarsal osteotomy for hallux valgus: A prospective randomised trial. *J Bone Joint Surg* 1993;75B:825–829.
62. Horne G, Tanzer T, Ford M: Chevron osteotomy for the treatment of hallux valgus. *Clin Orthop* 1984;183:32–36.
63. Jahss MH: Editorial: Hallux valgus: Further considerations. The first metatarsal head. *Foot Ankle* 1981;2:1–4.
64. Wilkinson SV, Jones RO, Sisk LE, et al: Austin bunionectomy: Postoperative MRI evaluation for avascular necrosis. *J Foot Surg* 1992;31:469–477.
65. Reverdin J: De la déviation en dehors du gros orteil (hallux valgus, vulg, "aignon," "bunions," "Ballen") et de son traitement chirurgical. *Trans Int Med Congress* 1881;2:408–412.
66. Peabody CW: The surgical cure of hallux valgus. *J Bone Joint Surg* 1931;13:273–282.
67. Hawkins FB, Mitchell CL, Hedrick DW: Correction of hallux valgus by metatarsal osteotomy. *J Bone Joint Surg* 1945;27: 387–394.
68. Mitchell CL, Fleming JL, Allen R, et al: Osteotomy-bunionectomy for hallux valgus. *J Bone Joint Surg* 1958;40A:41–60.
69. Wilson JN: Oblique displacement osteotomy for hallux valgus. *J Bone Joint Surg* 1963;45B:552–556.
70. Grace D, Hughes J, Klenerman L: A comparison of Wilson and Hohmann osteotomies in the treatment of hallux valgus. *J Bone Joint Surg* 1988;70B:236–241.
71. Mizuno K, Hashimura M, Kimura M, et al: Treatment of hallux valgus by oblique osteotomy of the first metatarsal. *Foot Ankle* 1992;13:447–452.
72. Schemitsch E, Horne G: Wilson's osteotomy for the treatment of hallux valgus. *Clin Orthop* 1989;240:221–225.
73. Turnbull T, Grange W: A comparison of Keller's arthroplasty and distal metatarsal osteotomy in the treatment of adult hallux valgus. *J Bone Joint Surg* 1986;68B:132–137.
74. Briggs TW, Smith P, McAuliffe TB: Mitchell's osteotomy using internal fixation and early mobilisation. *J Bone Joint Surg* 1992; 74B:137–139.
75. Miller JW: Distal first metatarsal displacement osteotomy: Its place in the schema of bunion surgery. *J Bone Joint Surg* 1974; 56A:923–931.
76. Wu KK: Mitchell's bunionectomy and Wu's bunionectomy: A comparison of 100 cases of each procedure. *Orthopedics* 1990; 13:1001–1007.
77. Wu KK: Wu's bunionectomy: A clinical analysis of 150 personal cases. *J Foot Surg* 1992;31:288–297.
78. Merkel KD, Katoh Y, Johnson EW Jr, et al: Mitchell osteotomy for hallux valgus: Long-term follow-up and gait analysis. *Foot Ankle* 1983;3:189–196.
79. Szaboky GT, Raghaven VC: Modification of Mitchell's lateral displacement angulation osteotomy. *J Bone Joint Surg* 1969; 51A:1430–1431.
80. Blum JL: The modified Mitchell osteotomy-bunionectomy: Indications and technical considerations. *Foot Ankle Int* 1994; 15:103–106.
81. Carr CR, Boyd BM: Correctional osteotomy for metatarsus primus varus and hallux valgus. *J Bone Joint Surg* 1968;50A: 1353–1367.
82. Kinnard P, Gordon D: A comparison between Chevron and Mitchell osteotomies for hallux valgus. *Foot Ankle* 1984;4: 241–243.
83. Limbird TJ, DaSilva RM, Green NE: Osteotomy of the first metatarsal base for metatarsus primus varus. *Foot Ankle* 1989; 9:158–162.
84. Scranton PE Jr, Zuckerman JD: Bunion surgery in adolescents: Results of surgical treatment. *J Pediatr Orthop* 1984;4:39–43.
85. Simmonds FA, Menelaus MB: Hallux valgus in adolescents. *J Bone Joint Surg* 1960;42B:761–768.
86. Resch S, Stenström A, Egund N: Proximal closing wedge osteotomy and adductor tenotomy for treatment of hallux valgus. *Foot Ankle* 1989;9:272–280.
87. Wanivenhaus AH, Feldner-Busztin H: Basal osteotomy of the first metatarsal for the correction of metatarsus primus

varus associated with hallux valgus. *Foot Ankle* 1988;8:337–343.

88. Sammarco GJ, Brainard BJ, Sammarco VJ: Bunion correction using proximal Chevron osteotomy. *Foot Ankle* 1993;14:8–14.
89. Coughlin MJ: Proximal first metatarsal osteotomy, in Johnson KA (ed): *The Foot and Ankle.* New York, NY, Raven Press, 1994, pp 85–105.
90. Lippert FG III, McDermott JE: Crescentic osteotomy for hallux valgus: A biomechanical study of variables affecting the final position of the first metatarsal. *Foot Ankle* 1991;11:204–207.
91. Thordarson DB, Leventen EO: Hallux valgus correction with proximal metatarsal osteotomy: Two-year follow-up. *Foot Ankle* 1992;13:321–326.
92. Harris RI, Beath T: The short first metatarsal: Its incidence and clinical significance. *J Bone Joint Surg* 1949;31A:553–565.
93. Mann RA: Hallux valgus, in Anderson LD (ed): American Academy of Orthopaedic Surgeons *Instructional Course Lectures XXXV.* St. Louis, MO, CV Mosby, 1986, pp 339–353.
94. Cedell CA, Aström M: Proximal metatarsal osteotomy in hallux valgus. *Acta Orthop Scand* 1982;53:1013–1018.
95. Myerson M: Metatarsocuneiform arthrodesis for treatment of hallux valgus and metatarsus primus varus. *Orthopedics* 1990;13:1025–1031.
96. Sangeorzan BJ, Hansen ST Jr: Modified Lapidus procedure for hallux valgus. *Foot Ankle* 1989;9:262–266.
97. Maguire WB: The Lapidus procedure for hallux valgus. *J Bone Joint Surg* 1973;55B:221.
98. Lapidus PW: Operative correction of the metatarsus varus primus in hallux valgus. *Surg Gynecol Obstet* 1934;58:183–191.
99. Lapidus PW: The author's bunion operation from 1931 to 1959. *Clin Orthop* 1960;16:119–135.
100. Mauldin DM, Sanders M, Whitmer WW: Correction of hallux valgus with metatarsocuneiform stabilization. *Foot Ankle* 1990;11:59–66.
101. Butson AR: A modification of the Lapidus operation for hallux valgus. *J Bone Joint Surg* 1980;62B:350–352.
102. Lipscomb PR: Arthrodesis of the first metatarsophalangeal joint for severe bunions and hallux rigidus. *Clin Orthop* 1979;142:48–54.
103. Mann RA, Katcherian DA: Relationship of metatarsophalangeal joint fusion on the intermetatarsal angle. *Foot Ankle* 1989;10:8–11.
104. Mann RA, Oates JC: Arthrodesis of the first metatarsophalangeal joint. *Foot Ankle* 1980;1:159–166.
105. Tupman S: Abstract: Arthrodesis of first metatarsophalangeal joint. *J Bone Joint Surg* 1958;40B:826.
106. Mann RA, Coughlin MJ: The rheumatoid foot: Review of literature and method of treatment. *Orthop Rev* 1979;8:105–112.
107. Mann RA, Thompson FM: Arthrodesis of the first metatarsophalangeal joint for hallux valgus in rheumatoid arthritis. *J Bone Joint Surg* 1984;66A:687–692.
108. von Salis-Soglio G, Thomas W: Arthrodesis of the metatarsophalangeal joint of the great toe. *Arch Orthop Trauma Surg* 1979;95:7–12.
109. Wilkinson J: Cone arthrodesis of the first metatarsophalangeal joint. *Acta Orthop Scand* 1978;49:627–630.
110. Fitzgerald JA, Wilkinson JM: Arthrodesis of the metatarsophalangeal joint of the great toe. *Clin Orthop* 1981;157:70–77.
111. Harrison MHM, Harvey FJ: Arthrodesis of the first metatarsophalangeal joint for hallux valgus and rigidus. *J Bone Joint Surg* 1963;45A:471–480.
112. Johansson JE, Barrington TW: Cone arthrodesis of the first metatarsophalangeal joint. *Foot Ankle* 1984;4:244–248.
113. Thompson FR, McElvenny RT: Arthrodesis of the first metatarsophalangeal joint. *J Bone Joint Surg* 1940;22:555–558.
114. Clutton HH: The treatment of hallux valgus. *St. Thomas Hosp Rep* 1894;22:1–12.
115. Moynihan FJ: Arthrodesis of the metatarsophalangeal joint of the great toe. *J Bone Joint Surg* 1967;49B:544–551.
116. Turan I, Lindgren U: Compression-screw arthrodesis of the first metatarsophalangeal joint of the foot. *Clin Orthop* 1987;221:292–295.
117. Bingold AC: Arthrodesis of the great toe. *Proc R Soc Med* 1958;51:435–437.
118. Gimple K, Amspacher JC, Kopta JA: Metatarsophalangeal joint fusion of the great toe. *Orthopedics* 1978;1:462–467.
119. McKeever DC: Arthrodesis of the first metatarsophalangeal joint for hallux valgus, hallux rigidus, and metatarsus primus varus. *J Bone Joint Surg* 1952;34A:129–134.
120. Raymakers R, Waugh W: The treatment of metatarsalgia with hallux valgus. *J Bone Joint Surg* 1971;53B:684–687.
121. Wilson JN: Cone arthrodesis of the first metatarsophalangeal joint. *J Bone Joint Surg* 1967;49B:98–101.
122. Coughlin MJ: Arthrodesis of the first metatarsophalangeal joint. *Orthop Rev* 1990;19:177–186.
123. Coughlin MJ: Arthrodesis of the first metatarsophalangeal joint with mini-fragment plate fixation. *Orthopedics* 1990;13:1037–1044.
124. Coughlin MJ, Abdo RV: Arthrodesis of the first metatarsophalangeal joint with Vitallium plate fixation. *Foot Ankle Int* 1994;15:18–28.
125. Riggs SA Jr, Johnson EW Jr: McKeever arthrodesis for the painful hallux. *Foot Ankle* 1983;3:248–253.
126. Coughlin MJ, Mann RA: Arthrodesis of the first metatarsophalangeal joint as salvage for the failed Keller procedure. *J Bone Joint Surg* 1987;69A:68–75.
127. Marin GA: Arthrodesis of the metatarsophalangeal joint of the big toe for hallux valgus and hallux rigidus: A new method. *Int Surg* 1968;50:175–180.
128. Fitzgerald JA: A review of long-term results of arthrodesis of the first metatarso-phalangeal joint. *J Bone Joint Surg* 1969;51B:488–493.
129. Humbert JL, Bourbonniere C, Laurin CA: Metatarsophalangeal fusion for hallux valgus: Indications and effect on the first metatarsal ray. *Can Med Assoc J* 1979;120:937–941.
130. Mankey MG, Mann RA: Arthrodesis of the first metatarsophalangeal joint utilizing a dorsal plate. *Orthop Trans* 1992;16:782–783.
131. Vallier GT, Petersen SA, LaGrone MO: The Keller resection arthroplasty: A 13-year experience. *Foot Ankle* 1991;11:187–194.
132. Love TR, Whynot AS, Farine I, et al: Keller arthroplasty: A prospective review. *Foot Ankle* 1987;8:46–54.
133. Jordan HH, Brodsky AE: Keller operation for hallux valgus and hallux rigidus: An end result study. *Arch Surg* 1951;62:586–596.
134. Richardson EG: Keller resection arthroplasty. *Orthopedics* 1990;13:1049–1053.
135. Wagner FW Jr: Technique & rationale: Bunion surgery. *Contemp Orthop* 1981;3:1040–1053.
136. Wrighton JD: A ten-year review of Keller's operation: Review of Keller's operation at the Princess Elizabeth Orthopaedic Hospital, Exeter. *Clin Orthop* 1972;89:207–214.
137. Keller WL: The surgical treatment of bunions and hallux valgus. *New York Med J* 1904;80:741–742.
138. Thomas FB: Keller's arthroplasty modified: A technique to ensure post-operative distraction of the toe. *J Bone Joint Surg* 1962;44B:356–365.
139. Majkowski RS, Galloway S: Excision arthroplasty for hallux valgus in the elderly: A comparison between the Keller and modified Mayo operations. *Foot Ankle* 1992;13:317–320.
140. Rogers WA, Joplin RJ: Hallux valgus, weak foot and the Keller operation: An end-result study. *Surg Clin North Am* 1947;27:1295–1302.

141. Cleveland M, Winant EM: An end-result study of the Keller operation. *J Bone Joint Surg* 1950;32A:163–175.
142. Henry AP, Waugh W, Wood H: The use of footprints in assessing the results of operations for hallux valgus: A comparison of Keller's operation and arthrodesis. *J Bone Joint Surg* 1975;57B: 478–481.
143. Sherman KP, Douglas DL, Benson MK: Keller's arthroplasty: Is distraction useful? A prospective trial. *J Bone Joint Surg* 1984; 66B:765–769.
144. Amarnek DL, Jacobs AM, Oloff LM: Adolescent hallux valgus: Its etiology and surgical management. *J Foot Surg* 1985;24:54–61.
145. Goldner JL, Gaines RW: Adult and juvenile hallux valgus: Analysis and treatment. *Orthop Clin North Am* 1976;7:863–887.
146. Durman DC: Metatarsus primus varus and hallux valgus. *Arch Surg* 1957;74:128–135.
147. Peterson HA, Newman SR: Adolescent bunion deformity treated with double osteotomy and longitudinal pin fixation of the first ray. *J Pediatr Orthop* 1993;13:80–84.
148. Hara B, Beck JC, Woo RA: First cuneiform closing abductory osteotomy for reduction of metatarsus primus adductus. *J Foot Surg* 1992;31:434–439.
149. Funk FJ Jr, Wells RE: Bunionectomy: With distal osteotomy. *Clin Orthop* 1972;85:71–74.
150. Loretz L, DeValentine S, Yamaguchi K: The first metatarsal bicorrectional head osteotomy (distal "L"/Reverdin-Laird procedure) for correction of hallux abducto valgus: A retrospective study. *J Foot Ankle Surg* 1993;32:554–568.
151. Kramer J, Barry LD, Helfman DN, et al: The modified Scarf bunionectomy. *J Foot Surg* 1992;31:360–367.

CHAPTER 36

Adult Acquired Flatfoot Deformity: Treatment of Dysfunction of the Posterior Tibial Tendon

Mark S. Myerson, MD

Acquired flatfoot deformity caused by dysfunction of the posterior tibial tendon (PTT) is a common clinical problem. Treatment, which depends on the severity of the symptoms and the stage of the disease, includes nonsurgical options, such as rest, administration of anti-inflammatory medication, and immobilization, as well as surgical options, such as tendon transfer, calcaneal osteotomy, and several methods of arthrodesis.

Anatomy and Pathophysiology

The posterior tibial muscle forms part of the deep posterior compartment of the calf. It originates from the proximal third of the tibia and the interosseous membrane and passes immediately posterior to the medial malleolus, where it changes direction acutely.[1] A groove in the posteromedial aspect of the distal part of the tibia holds the PTT but is not deep enough to keep the tendon from bow-stringing or dislocating after an injury.[2] The flexor retinaculum, which is adjacent to the medial malleolus, tethers the PTT and keeps it in the groove, preventing dislocation. Distally, this retinaculum blends with the sheath of the PTT and the superficial deltoid ligament. The PTT does not have a mesotendon, and there is an area of relative hypovascularity immediately distal to the medial malleolus that may contribute to degenerative changes of the tendon.[3] The PTT divides anterior to the tuberosity of the navicular. An anterior slip, which is in direct continuity with the main tendon, inserts onto the tuberosity of the navicular, the inferior aspect of the capsule of the medial naviculocuneiform joint, and the inferior surface of the medial cuneiform. A second slip attaches to the plantar surfaces of the middle and lateral cuneiforms and the cuboid as well as to the bases of the corresponding metatarsals.[4]

The PTT passes posterior to the axis of the ankle and medial to the axis of the subtalar joint. Because of its insertion on the navicular and the plantar aspect of the mid-part of the tarsus, the PTT acts to plantarflex as well as to invert the middle part of the foot with an action that occurs primarily across the transverse tarsal joint (the talonavicular and calcaneocuboid joints). The PTT therefore functions predominantly to invert the midfoot and to elevate the medial longitudinal arch rather than having a specific effect on the hindfoot. However, the tendon does support the calcaneus and the rest of the hindfoot indirectly by means of its action within the pulley posterior to the medial malleolus as well as its relationship with the deep deltoid ligament, the talonavicular capsule, and the spring (calcaneonavicular) ligament.[1]

With dysfunction of the PTT, the medial longitudinal arch collapses, the subtalar joint everts, the heel assumes a valgus position, and the foot abducts at the talonavicular joint. This excessive movement around the talus suggests that the loss of function occurs as a result of dysfunction of the PTT at the site of its insertion on the navicular or through secondary stretching of the spring ligament.[5] The valgus angulation of the heel is probably a result of the loss of secondary soft-tissue supportive structures, including the deltoid ligament, the talonavicular capsule, and the spring ligament. Once the heel assumes a more valgus position, the Achilles tendon begins to act as an evertor of the calcaneus as it is then lateral to the axis of rotation of the subtalar joint.

Dysfunction of the PTT therefore results in a reversal of its primary actions, with relative internal rotation of the tibia and talus and flattening of the medial longitudinal arch. Secondary changes that may develop over time include an equinus deformity of the ankle, a more horizontal orientation of the subtalar joint, and valgus angulation of the heel. The associated contracture of the Achilles tendon causes more sagittal-plane motion to occur at the subtalar joint rather than at the tibiotalar joint. As the deformity progresses, this change eventually causes the calcaneus to impinge against the fibula, creating pain in the lateral part of the foot and ankle.

The clinical deformity associated with dysfunction of the PTT reflects the loss of support from the spring, deltoid, and talocalcaneal interosseous ligaments as well as from the talonavicular capsule and the plantar fascia. Normally, the deltoid ligament has a substantial stabilizing effect on the tibiotalocalcaneal joint complex.[6-10] As the deformity progresses, the deltoid ligament becomes attenuated and the talus begins to tilt in the ankle joint, leading to valgus deformity of the tibiotalar joint.[6,9,11] Deland and associates[11] demonstrated, in a cadaveric model, that no abnormality can be seen radiographically when there is dysfunction of the PTT alone and that a static deformity occurs only when there is also associated ligamentous damage. Although one cannot extrapolate these data directly to the clinical situation, it is important to recognize that dysfunction of the PTT usually is associated with changes in the ligamentous support of the hindfoot.

Etiology

The etiology of dysfunction of the PTT is varied, ranging from inflammatory synovitis to degenerative rupture and, occasionally, to acute trauma. A number of investigators have identified an increased prevalence of rupture of the PTT in middle-aged obese women.[12-15] Holmes and Mann[16] reported that 40 (60%) of 67 patients who had a rupture of the PTT had a history of hypertension, obesity, diabetes, prior surgery or trauma about the medial aspect of the foot, or treatment with steroids. Although acute trauma rarely plays a substantial role in ruptures of the PTT and although only a few patients can recall a specific history of a sprain or another injury about the foot and ankle, the tendon is at risk of injury because of its close proximity to the medial malleolar sulcus. For example, an acute rupture of the PTT occasionally has occurred in association with a closed fracture or dislocation of the ankle.[17]

There appears to be an association between dysfunction of the PTT and the injection of steroids. Jahss[1] reported that three of ten patients who had a rupture of the PTT had received multiple injections of corticosteroids around the medial aspect of the foot months to years earlier. Holmes and Mann[16] reported that the injection of corticosteroids about the PTT or the oral intake of corticosteroids increased the likelihood of rupture of the PTT.

It is likely that most ruptures of the PTT are due to an intrinsic abnormality or a failure of the tendon rather than to extrinsic trauma. A rupture may result from the acute angulation of the tendon as it passes posterior to the medial malleolus, from the relative hypovascularity of the tendon just distal to the medial malleolus, or from degeneration associated with an inflammatory disorder. Neither the flexor digitorum longus nor the flexor hallucis longus angulates as acutely behind the medial malleolus as does the PTT, and the former two tendons rarely rupture.[1] Frey and associates[3] showed that the PTT has a zone of hypovascularity that begins 1 to 1.5 cm distal to the medial malleolus and extends 1 cm farther distally. It is in this area where degenerative changes and ruptures most often are found. Dysfunction of the PTT also has been linked to seronegative inflammatory disorders, such as ankylosing spondylitis, Reiter syndrome, and psoriasis. Myerson and associates[18] reported on a group of 76 patients, 47 of whom had inflammation or rupture, or both, of the PTT in association with a seronegative inflammatory disorder and manifestations of enthesopathy. Whereas Anzel and associates[19] suggested that ruptures of the PTT are common in patients who have rheumatoid arthritis, other authors have found no strong relationship between rheumatoid arthritis and PTT ruptures.[12,16,18] It is my impression that flatfoot deformity associated with rheumatoid arthritis is more likely to be caused by synovitis of the talonavicular and subtalar joints.[20]

Diagnosis

History

In the early stages of dysfunction of the PTT, most of the discomfort is located medially along the course of the tendon and the patient reports fatigue and aching on the plantar-medial aspect of the foot and ankle. Swelling is common if the dysfunction is associated with tenosynovitis. As dysfunction of the tendon progresses, maximum pain occurs laterally in the sinus tarsi because of impingement of the fibula against the calcaneus. With increasing deformity, patients report that the shape of the foot changes and that it becomes increasingly difficult to wear shoes. Many patients no longer report pain in the medial part of the foot and ankle after a complete rupture of the PTT has occurred; instead, the pain is located laterally. If a fixed deformity has not occurred, the patient may report that standing or walking with the hindfoot slightly inverted alleviates the lateral impingement and relieves the pain in the lateral part of the foot.

Examination of the Patient

First, both feet should be examined with the patient standing and the entire lower extremity visible. The foot should be inspected from above as well as from behind the patient, as valgus angulation of the hindfoot is best appreciated when the foot is viewed from behind. Johnson[13] described the so-called more-toes sign: with more advanced deformity and abduction of the forefoot, more of the lateral toes become visible when the foot is viewed from behind. The single-limb heel-rise test is an excellent determinant of the function of the PTT. The patient is asked to attempt to rise onto the ball of one foot while the other foot is suspended off the floor. Under normal circumstances, the posterior tibial muscle, which inverts and stabilizes the hindfoot, is activated as the patient begins to rise onto the forefoot. The gastrocnemius-soleus muscle group then elevates the calcaneus, and the heel-rise is accomplished. With dysfunction of the PTT, however, inversion of the heel is weak, and either the heel remains in valgus or the patient is unable to rise onto the forefoot. If the patient can do a single-limb heel-rise, the limb may be stressed further by asking the patient to perform this maneuver repetitively.

With the patient seated, the strength of the posterior tibial muscle is evaluated by asking the patient to plantarflex and invert the foot against resistance. During the test, the examiner should hold the hindfoot of the patient in plantarflexion and eversion and the forefoot in abduction. This eliminates the synergistic action of the anterior tibial muscle and allows the strength of the posterior tibial muscle to be quantified more accurately.

The integrity of the tendon and the location of maximum tenderness are established with palpation. Occasionally, an acquired flatfoot deformity is due not to a rupture of the PTT but to a tear of the spring or deltoid ligament.[15] Therefore, the integrity of the tendon should be assessed with palpation while the patient attempts to invert the foot against resistance.

After the sites of tenderness have been located, the subtalar and ankle joints are assessed for mobility and the presence of any contracture of the Achilles tendon. With increased valgus angulation of the heel, the Achilles tendon assumes a position lateral to the axis of the subtalar joint and the gastrocnemius-soleus muscle group shortens over time. If the subtalar joint is mobile, the examiner should assess dorsiflexion of the ankle while passively correcting any heel valgus to be sure that the dorsiflexion that is present is occurring through the ankle and not through the transverse tarsal joint. The position of the forefoot is assessed with the heel held in neutral. In the early stages of flatfoot deformity, the forefoot remains plantigrade when the subtalar joint is placed in the neutral position. As the deformity worsens, however, a fixed supination deformity of the forefoot occurs and can be identified by holding the subtalar joint reduced in a neutral position. It is important to identify any fixed supination deformity of the forefoot because such a deformity will have an effect on treatment. With more advanced dysfunction of the PTT, rigidity of the subtalar joint may be present and may make it impossible to reduce the valgus deformity.

Radiography

Anteroposterior and lateral weightbearing radiographs of both feet and mortise radiographs of both ankles are recommended for the evaluation of flatfoot deformity.[20] If the deformity is present, the anteroposterior radiograph shows abduction of the forefoot at the transverse tarsal joint, with the navicular sliding laterally on the talar head. The lateral radiograph shows a decrease in the talometatarsal angle (normal angle, 0° to 10°) and in the distance of the medial cuneiform from the floor (normal distance, 15 to 25 mm) when the involved foot is compared with the contralateral foot. In patients who have an advanced deformity, subluxation or dislocation of the talonavicular joint may occur in association with degenerative osteoarthrosis of the posterior facet of the subtalar joint.[1]

It should be emphasized that the diagnosis of PTT dysfunction is based on a thorough examination of the foot as well as plain radiographs, which confirm the extent of the deformity and the presence of osteoarthrosis. Magnetic resonance imaging (MRI) is not required to make the diagnosis and does not assist in the planning of treatment. Although some authors have suggested that MRI is a useful diagnostic tool in the evaluation of PTT dysfunction,[21-23] other authors have asserted that it is used far too frequently in clinical practice and that its clinical usefulness is questionable at best.[15,16]

Classification

There is a continuum of PTT dysfunction, ranging from tenosynovitis to fixed deformity. Any grading or staging system of this dysfunction is therefore somewhat arbitrary. It is useful, however, to describe the dysfunction in stages in order to present treatment alternatives in a more logical manner. Johnson and Strom,[24] in 1989, described three clinical stages of PTT dysfunction. Stage I is characterized by pain and swelling of the medial aspect of the foot and ankle. The length of the tendon is normal, and tendinitis may be associated with mild degeneration. Mild weakness and minimum deformity are present. In stage II, the tendon is torn, the limb is weak, and the patient is unable to stand on tiptoe on the affected side. Secondary deformity is present as the midfoot pronates and the forefoot abducts at the transverse tarsal joint. The subtalar joint, however, remains flexible. In stage III, degeneration of the tendon is present, the deformity is more severe, and the hindfoot is rigid. Stage IV, which was not described by Johnson and Strom, is characterized by valgus angulation of the talus and early degeneration of the ankle joint.

Treatment

Nonsurgical management should be attempted for most symptomatic patients who have PTT dysfunction. Most patients who have tenosynovitis or stage-I disease respond to nonsurgical management. Patients who have more advanced (stage-II or -III) disease also benefit from nonsurgical management, but the risk of progressive deformity must be considered when planning treatment.

Nonsurgical Treatment

A patient who has acute tenosynovitis has pain and swelling along the medial aspect of the ankle. The patient is able to perform a single-limb heel-rise test but has pain when doing so. Inversion of the foot

Table 1
Treatment of dysfunction of the posterior tibial tendon

Stage	Characteristics	Treatment	
		Nonsurgical	Surgical
Tenosynovitis	Acute medial pain and swelling, can perform heel-rise, seronegative inflammation, extensive tearing	Anti-inflammatory medication, immobilization for 6 to 8 weeks; if symptoms improve, ankle stirrup-brace; if symptoms do not improve, surgical treatment	Tenosynovectomy, tenosynovectomy + calcaneal osteotomy, or tenosynovectomy + tenodesis of flexor digitorum longus to posterior tibial tendon
Rupture			
Stage I	Medial pain and swelling, hindfoot flexible, can perform heel-rise	Medial heel-and-sole shoe wedge, hinged ankle-foot orthosis, orthotic arch-supports	Debridement of posterior tibial tendon, flexor digitorum longus transfer, or flexor digitorum longus transfer + calcaneal osteotomy
Stage II	Valgus angulation of heel, lateral pain, hindfoot flexible, cannot perform heel-rise	Medial heel-and-sole shoe wedge, stiff orthotic support, hinged ankle-foot orthosis, injection of steroids into the sinus tarsi	Flexor digitorum longus transfer + calcaneal osteotomy or flexor digitorum longus transfer + bone-block arthrodesis at calcaneocuboid joint
Stage III	Valgus angulation of heel, lateral pain, hindfoot rigid, cannot perform heel-rise	Rigid ankle-foot orthosis	Triple arthrodesis
Stage IV	Hindfoot rigid, valgus angulation of talus	Rigid ankle-foot orthosis	Tibiotalocalcaneal arthrodesis

against resistance is painful but still strong. The patient should be managed with rest, the administration of appropriate anti-inflammatory medication, and immobilization. The injection of corticosteroids is not recommended. Immobilization with either a rigid below-the-knee cast or a removable cast or boot may be used to prevent overuse and subsequent rupture of the tendon. A removable stirrup-brace is not initially sufficient as it does not limit motion in the sagittal plane, a component of the pathologic process. Patients are allowed to walk in the cast or boot during the 6- to 8-week period of immobilization. At the end of that time, a decision must be made regarding the need for additional treatment. If there has been marked improvement, the patient may begin wearing a stiff-soled shoe with a medial heel-and-sole wedge to invert the hindfoot. If there has been only mild or moderate improvement, a longer period in the cast or boot may be tried.

Chao and associates[25] demonstrated that when the flatfoot deformity is caused by a nonfunctioning PTT, the deformity usually is progressive. However, they showed that a molded ankle-foot orthosis or a rigid orthotic support can control the deformity and alleviate symptoms in many elderly patients who have a relatively sedentary lifestyle. They concluded, therefore, that surgical treatment should be considered only for patients for whom an adequate trial of bracing has failed.

Surgical Treatment

Many surgical options are available for the treatment of PTT dysfunction after a thorough program of nonsurgical treatment has failed. The type of surgery selected is determined by the patient's age, weight, level of activity, and the extent of the deformity. The clinical stages outlined previously are a useful guide to surgical care (Table 1). In general, the clinician should perform the least invasive procedure that will decrease pain and improve function. One should consider the effects of each procedure, particularly those of arthrodesis, on the function of the rest of the foot and ankle.

Pathologic Findings The pathologic findings vary according to the underlying etiology of the PTT dysfunction. Myerson and associates[18] demonstrated that patients who have a seronegative inflammatory disorder have a proliferative synovial membrane that adheres to the tendon. In these patients, the tendon often is found to be attenuated and to contain longitudinal fissures, and a chronic nonspecific inflammatory infiltrate is noted histologically. In contrast, in patients who have degenerative tendinosis, the tendon sheath is edematous and thickened. Fibrous adhesions usually are present and often extend posteriorly from the inner (medial) aspect of the tendon. If a degenerative tear is present, it commonly is located 1 to 2 cm distal to the medial malleolus. Partial or complete rupture of the tendon occurs approximately 2 cm proximal to the tubercle of the navicular. In most instances, the scarred tendon is adherent to the tendon sheath. Longitudinal fissures commonly are found in the posterior aspect of the tendon that lies in proximity to the deeper soft tissues and tendon sheath.[1,18]

I have noted that the extent of clinical and radiographic deformity does not always correspond with the degree of degeneration of the PTT, and I have encountered patients who have had severe unilateral flatfoot deformity in association with an intact and grossly normal PTT.[15] Such patients have a rupture of the spring ligament, the talonavicular capsule, or the deltoid ligament.

Tenosynovectomy Patients who have tenosynovitis have an acute onset of pain and swelling along the medial aspect of the foot immediately inferior to the medial malleolus. This finding is associated with aching of the foot and an inability to stand for a long time or to walk for a long distance. The area directly over the tendon is tender to palpation. Inversion of the foot against resistance is strong, and the patient is able to perform single or even repetitive heel-rises, albeit with pain. Tenosynovectomy should be considered if the patient shows no improvement after 6 to 8 weeks of nonsurgical care. This intensive approach is particularly important in younger patients in whom tenosynovitis may have developed in association with a seronegative inflammatory disorder. This type of tenosynovitis appears to be particularly aggressive and is associated with an inflammatory infiltrate into the tendon that leads to rupture of the tendon unless treated expeditiously.[18]

A tenosynovectomy may be performed with ankle-block anesthesia.[26] A posteromedial incision is made from the musculotendinous junction to the insertion of the PTT. It is useful to preserve a 1-cm strip of the flexor retinaculum adjacent to the medial malleolus to prevent subsequent dislocation of the PTT, which may occur if the flexor retinaculum is not preserved or repaired after having been opened completely.[2,27]

Once the tendon sheath is opened, the tendon is inspected. When tenosynovitis is associated with a seronegative inflammatory disorder, the synovial membrane adheres to and infiltrates both the sheath and the tendon; this inflammatory tissue should be debrided thoroughly. Tenosynovitis associated with stage-I degenerative tendinosis has a less florid appearance, and bulbous swelling of the tendon associated with longitudinal fissuring (particularly on the posterior surface) typically is present. These fissures should be debrided, and the tendon splits should be repaired with 4-0 non-absorbable sutures. Any bulbous degenerated area of the tendon should be excised, and the tendon should be thinned so that it easily passes posterior to the malleolus. After the debridement, the retinaculum immediately posterior to the medial malleolus is repaired if it was detached completely, but otherwise the tendon sheath is left open to minimize the subsequent formation of adhesions.

It is unlikely that young patients who have tenosynovitis in association with a seronegative inflammatory disorder will need further surgery.[18] Tenosynovectomy usually is sufficient unless attritional tearing of the tendon already has occurred. This approach was substantiated by Teasdall and Johnson,[27] who recommended that stage-I PTT dysfunction be treated with synovectomy and debridement of the torn tendon. In the study, 16 of the 19 patients reported subjective improvement, with a return of the function of the PTT.

In contrast, in older patients who have stage-I disease but in whom the degeneration of the tendon is more advanced than the symptoms suggested, it is important to consider another procedure in addition to tenosynovectomy to support the diseased tendon. If one assumes that the tenosynovitis is a manifestation of early degeneration of the tendon, then the underlying pathologic process may continue to worsen after a simple tenosynovectomy. Some authors have suggested that such patients should be managed with a side-to-side tenodesis of the flexor digitorum longus tendon to the PTT[1,21] or a calcaneal osteotomy[28] in addition to tenosynovectomy.

Calcaneal Osteotomy The use of a calcaneal osteotomy to treat valgus angulation of the heel shifts the calcaneus medially and alters the mechanical axis of the lower limb, thereby reducing the valgus thrust on the hindfoot.[29,30] The medial displacement of the calcaneus redirects the pull of the gastrocnemius-soleus muscle group slightly medial to the axis of the subtalar joint,[29,30] increasing its varus pull on the hindfoot. Calcaneal osteotomy was performed first by Gleich[31] in 1893, in an attempt to displace the posterior calcaneal tuberosity both medially and inferiorly in order to restore the calcaneal pitch angle. Subsequent authors have reported on the treatment of flatfoot deformity with calcaneal osteotomy.[30,32-34] In the osteotomy described by Rose,[29] a triangular portion of bone is resected from the posteroinferior fragment, to create a medial ridge that passes medial to the inner side of the proximal fragment and locks the osteotomy in a stable configuration. This osteotomy creates both varus angulation and medial displacement of the calcaneus.[29,33]

The osteotomy recommended by Myerson and associates,[28] Saxby and Myerson,[34] Fairbank and associates,[6] and Koutsogiannis[35] is a simpler medial displacement osteotomy of the posterior part of the calcaneus. This procedure is indicated in combination with tenosynovectomy for patients who have advanced stage-I dysfunction of the PTT and in conjunction with a flexor tendon transfer for those who have stage-II disease. The patient is placed in the lateral decubitus position, and an incision is made inferior and parallel to the peroneal tendons and posterior to the sural nerve. The incision extends from the superior border of the calcaneal tuberosity anterior to the retrocalcaneal space to the inferior border of the calcaneus superficial to the plantar fascia. The incision is deepened to the periosteum, and the soft tissues are retracted with a self-retaining retractor. The periosteum is reflected. A transverse osteotomy is made in the calcaneus in line with the incision in the skin with use of an oscillating saw. The cut is made at a right angle to the lateral border of the calcaneus and is inclined posteriorly at an angle of approximately 45° to the plane of the sole of the foot. No wedge is removed from the calcaneus, and no attempt is made to tilt the tuberosity into varus angulation.[15] A lamina spreader is inserted into the site of the osteotomy, and the medial soft-tissue attachments onto the calcaneus are released by spreading the device open. The lamina spreader then is withdrawn, and the posterior fragment of the calcaneal tuberosity is translated medially 10 mm and secured with a cannulated cancellous-bone lag screw (Fig. 1).

Another procedure, which involves lengthening the lateral column of the foot by means of an osteotomy of the neck of the calcaneus and the interposition of a tricortical bone graft, recently has gained popularity (K Bandani, MD, A Gabriel, MD, HW Wagner Jr, MD, unpublished data, 1995). Evans[36] recommended that the osteotomy be done 1.5 cm proximal to the calcaneocuboid joint. Other authors[37,38] have reported good results with this procedure. Sangeorzan and associates[39] investigated the effect of calcaneal lengthening on the osseous relationships of the hindfoot, midfoot, and forefoot and noted improvement in the flatfoot deformity with respect to the lateral talocalcaneal angle, the lateral talometatarsal angle, the anteroposterior talometatarsal angle, the calcaneal pitch angle, and the talonavicular coverage angle. The results of in vitro studies have suggested that this procedure is a good option because it allows maintenance of motion of the talonavicular joint and, to some extent, that of the subtalar joint (American Orthopaedic Foot and Ankle Society Annual Meeting, unpublished data, 1995). This may have a positive effect on adjacent joints, including the ankle, by decreasing stress and thereby indirectly reducing the prevalence of osteoarthrosis. However, there have been reports that this procedure is associated with an increased prevalence of symptoms in the calcaneocuboid joint in adults (PS Cooper, MD, M Nowack, MD, J Schear, MD, unpublished data, 1995). When lengthening of the lateral column is performed in an adult who has acquired flatfoot deformity, I think that it probably should be done through the calcaneocuboid joint itself, with use of a tricortical bone graft for arthrodesis of the joint. I believe that this procedure is indicated for a patient who has stage-II dysfunction with pain in the lateral part of the foot, a mobile subtalar joint, and no fixed supination deformity of the forefoot when the heel is held in a neutral position. Lengthening of the lateral aspect of the hindfoot, whether through a calcaneal osteotomy or through the calcaneocuboid joint by arthrodesis, is an excellent option because in vitro studies have documented that motion of the talonavicular joint, and to some extent that of the subtalar joint, is still maintained. This may therefore have a positive effect on stress of adjacent joints, thereby indirectly reducing the incidence of adjacent arthrosis, including the ankle.

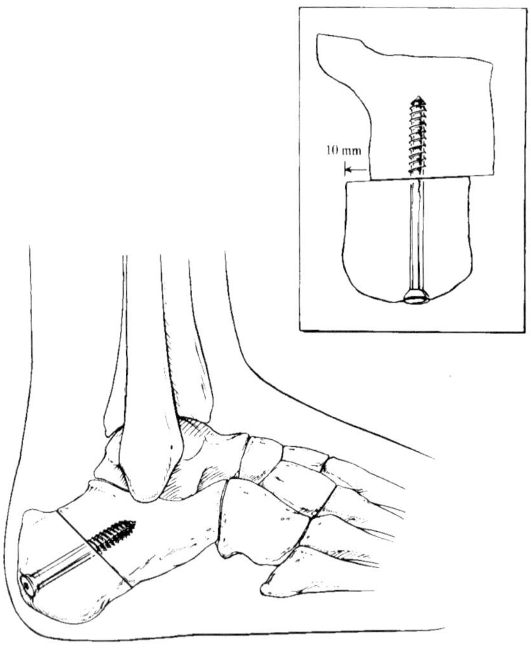

Fig. 1 Drawing of a calcaneal osteotomy. The calcaneus is shifted 10 mm medially and is secured with a cannulated screw. (Reproduced with permission from Myerson MS, Corrigan AJ, Schon L, et al: Tendon transfer combined with calcaneal osteotomy for treatment of posterior tibial tendon insufficiency: A radiological investigation. *Foot Ankle Int* 1995;16:712-718.)

Flexor Tendon Transfer Flexor tendon transfer is performed for patients who have stage-I or -II PTT dysfunction in association with weakness, valgus angulation of the hindfoot, pain in the medial part of the foot, and a mobile subtalar joint. A number of authors have recommended use of the flexor digitorum longus (FDL) tendon to substitute for the ruptured posterior tibial tendon.[12-14,40] Goldner and associates[5] recommended use of the flexor hallucis longus (FHL) for the reconstruction. With that procedure, however, the dissection is more complicated, the neurovascular bundle is in closer proximity to the FHL, and the deficit at the donor site is more substantial. Although the FHL muscle is markedly stronger than the FDL, the proximity of the PTT to the FDL makes the latter a more suitable

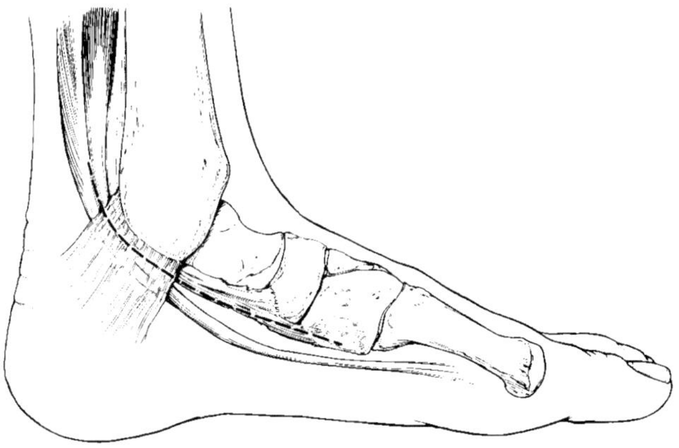

Fig. 2 Figures 2 through 6 are drawings of the various steps of a flexor tendon transfer. In this figure, the dashed line indicates the posteromedial incision used for the tendon transfer. (Reproduced with permission from Myerson MS, Corrigan AJ, Schon L, et al: Tendon transfer combined with calcaneal osteotomy for treatment of posterior tibial tendon insufficiency: A radiological investigation. *Foot Ankle Int* 1995;16:712-718.)

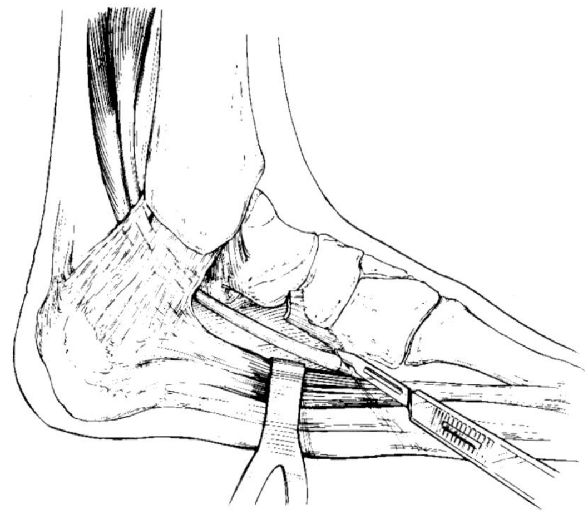

Fig. 3 The flexor digitorum longus tendon is cut as far distally as possible under direct vision. (Reproduced with permission from Myerson M: Posterior tibial tendon insufficiency, in Myerson M (ed): *Current Therapy in Foot and Ankle Surgery*. St. Louis, MO, Mosby-Year Book, 1993, pp 123-135.)

tendon for transfer. The transfer involves cutting the FDL tendon distally and rerouting it through the undersurface of the navicular through a drill hole. The incision is made along the entire length of the PTT from the musculotendinous junction distally beyond the navicular in line with the first metatarsal (Fig. 2). The sheath of the PTT is opened, and the tendon is inspected and cut transversely adjacent to the medial malleolus, leaving a 1-cm stump attached to the navicular distally.

Chronic rupture of the PTT may be associated with atrophy and fibrosis of the muscle. If the posterior tibial muscle is healthy, however, the tendon should be sutured to the FDL tendon at the level of the medial malleolus. When the proximal stump of the tendon is pulled in a distal direction, its normal excursion is approximately 1 cm. If there is no excursion of the musculotendinous unit when it is pulled in a distal direction, the muscle is either scarred or fibrotic, and a tenodesis to the FDL should not be performed.

The sheath of the FDL tendon is identified posterior to the PTT and is opened longitudinally and distally. The plane of dissection should be deep to the abductor hallucis and flexor digitorum brevis muscles. Distal dissection should allow identification of both the FHL and the FDL tendon. The FDL tendon should be cut as far distally as possible under direct vision (Fig. 3). It is not necessary to perform a tenodesis of the FHL to the stump of the FDL as there are multiple interconnections between the two.[41]

The periosteum over the navicular then is dissected, and a 4.5-mm drill hole is made in the tuberosity from dorsal to plantar (Fig. 4). The tendon is passed through the drill hole from plantar to dorsal. Before

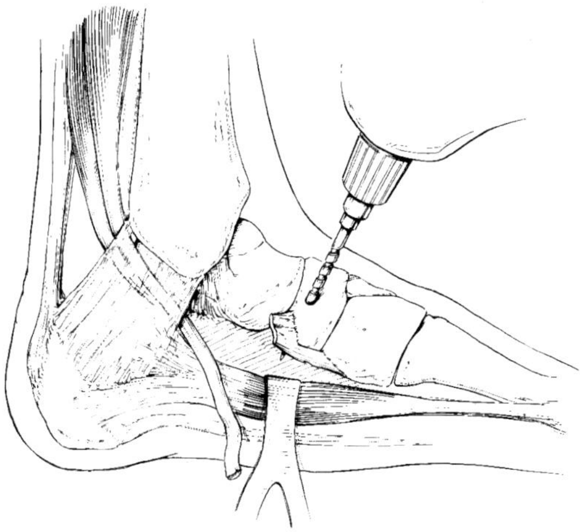

Fig. 4 A 4.5-mm drill hole is made in the navicular from dorsal to plantar. (Reproduced with permission from Myerson M: Posterior tibial tendon insufficiency, in Myerson M (ed): *Current Therapy in Foot and Ankle Surgery*. St. Louis, MO, Mosby-Year Book, 1993, pp 123-135.)

the FDL tendon is sutured, a vertical ellipse is removed from the talonavicular capsule. The ellipse should be approximately 8 mm wide and extend inferiorly from the dorsal aspect of the joint toward the spring ligament (Fig. 5). Once the FDL tendon has been transferred and attached, it is secured under moderate tension, and, finally, the shortened capsule is closed. To avoid overstretching the FDL muscle, the tension on its tendon is set halfway between maximum tension and complete relaxation (Fig. 6).[15]

At the completion of the reconstruction, the foot should rest in a slight equinovarus position. If a tourni-

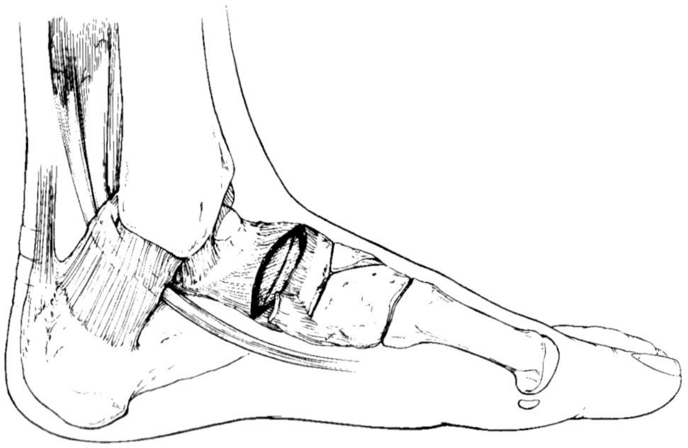

Fig. 5 A vertical ellipse over the talonavicular capsule is excised before the flexor digitorum longus tendon is sutured.

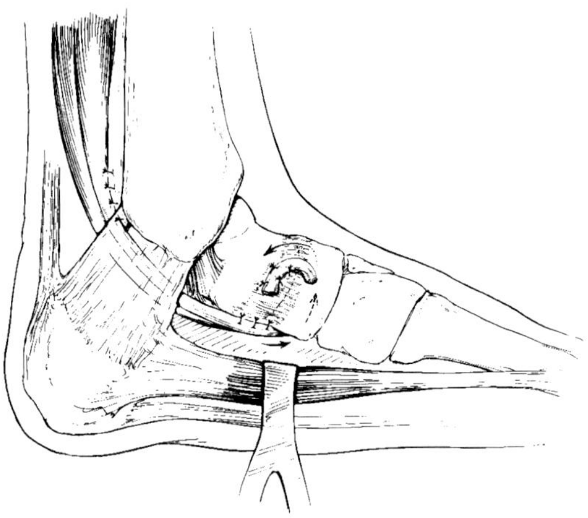

Fig. 6 The flexor digitorum longus tendon is sutured under tension to the stump of the posterior tibial tendon or to the periosteum overlying the navicular. A tenodesis of the proximal stump of the flexor digitorum longus tendon to the cut posterior tibial tendon is performed. (Reproduced with permission from Myerson MS, Corrigan J, Thompson F, et al: Tendon transfer combined with calcaneal osteotomy for treatment of posterior tibial tendon insufficiency: A radiological investigation. *Foot Ankle Int* 1995;16:712-718.)

quet was used, a suction drain should be inserted and left in place for 24 hours. No weightbearing is permitted for 4 weeks, after which partial weightbearing is permitted while wearing either a below-the-knee cast or a hinged range-of-motion walker boot for an additional 4 weeks. By 8 weeks, the patient begins walking with full weightbearing while wearing a shoe that has an ankle stirrup-brace, and physical therapy is started to strengthen the muscles of the leg (Fig. 7).

Arthrodesis An arthrodesis is indicated for a patient who has PTT dysfunction as well as pain in the lateral part of the foot, a rigid (stage-III) valgus deformity of the hindfoot, or a valgus deformity of the hindfoot that, when corrected to neutral, is associated with a fixed supination deformity of the forefoot. Numerous procedures have been described, including isolated talonavicular,[42-44] talonavicular and calcaneocuboid,[45] subtalar,[46] and triple arthrodesis.[47-50] According to Johnson and Lester,[46] it does not make much difference which procedure is performed, because fusion of any one of the joints of the hindfoot effectively blocks motion of the hindfoot. They noted that it is important not to disturb the position of the calcaneocuboid and talonavicular joints when performing a subtalar arthrodesis; however, this is not always possible, particularly if the deformity is rigid and a fixed supination deformity of the midfoot and forefoot occurs when the subtalar joint is reduced into a neutral position. In their technique, a morcelized bone graft obtained from the anterior part of the iliac crest is inserted into the anterior aspect of the subtalar joint. Temporary fixation is achieved with a Steinmann pin introduced percutaneously from the neck of the talus dorsally into the calcaneus.

Although triple arthrodesis has a long history of success for the treatment of neuromuscular deformities in children, fewer reports are available on its effectiveness in adults, particularly with respect to the treatment of planovalgus deformity of the hindfoot. A triple arthrodesis is indicated for a patient who has a fixed hindfoot deformity that is associated with pain in the lateral part of the foot. The goals of the triple arthrodesis are to realign the hindfoot; to establish a plantigrade weightbearing surface; to maintain the integrity of the adjacent joints, particularly the ankle; and to avoid incisional neuromas.

The technique of triple arthrodesis should be meticulous. The use of a single incision on the lateral aspect of the foot places both the sural nerve and the lateral cutaneous branch of the superficial peroneal nerve at risk for incisional neuromas, and it does not allow visualization of most of the talonavicular joint.[51] Therefore, two incisions should be used. The first incision parallels the inferior surface of the peroneal tendons from the tip of the fibula over the sinus tarsi; the second incision lies medial to the anterior tibial tendon and extends from the tibiotalar joint to the naviculocuneiform joint. Laterally, the contents of the sinus tarsi are excised and the joints are denuded of articular cartilage with the use of a sharp osteotome or chisel. The correction is achieved by adequate subtalar and talonavicular rotation, not by the resection of bone wedges.

It is particularly important to identify the recess between the navicular and the cuboid, at which point all four bones (the talus, the navicular, the calcaneus, and the cuboid) may come into contact with each other. If osseous bridging can be obtained in this loca-

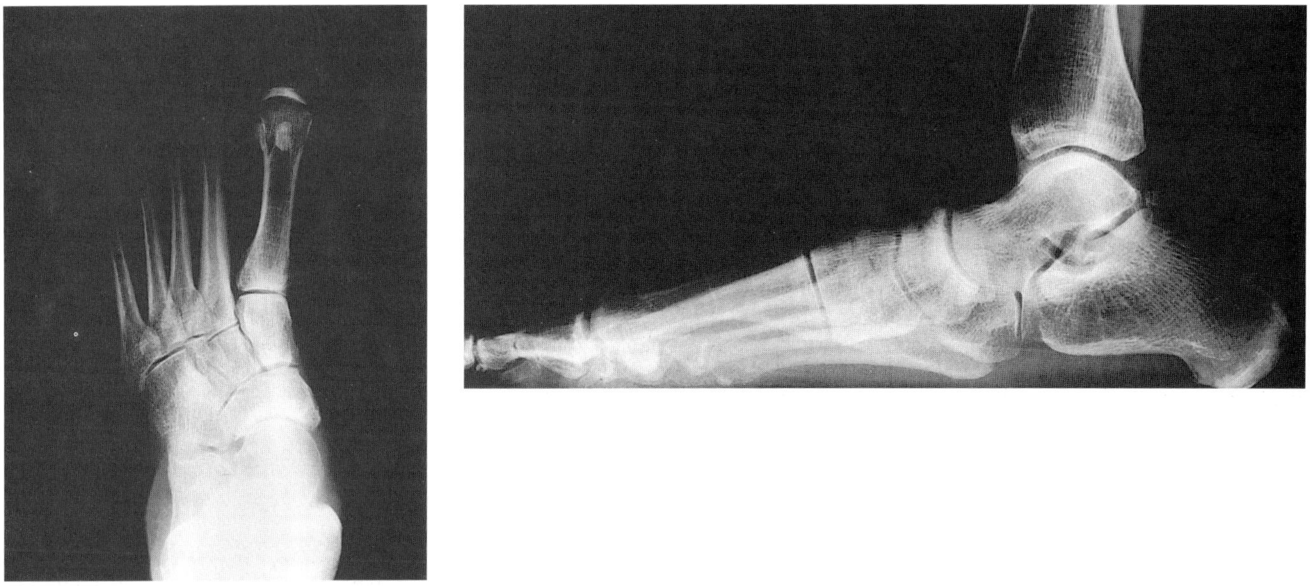

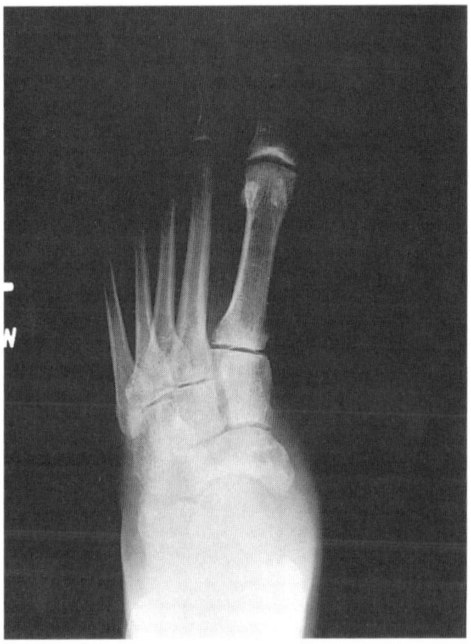

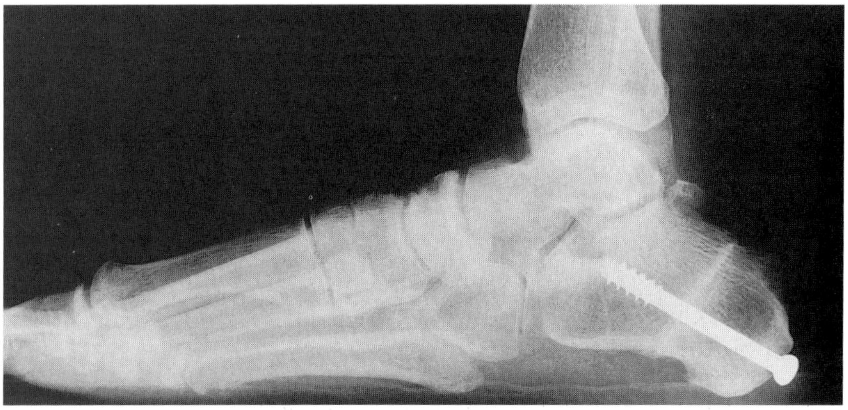

Fig. 7 A 46-year-old woman who was managed with calcaneal osteotomy and transfer of the flexor digitorum longus because of dysfunction of the posterior tibial tendon. **Top,** Preoperative radiographs. Note the uncovering of the talar head and the increased talometatarsal angle on the anteroposterior radiograph, **top left,** and the decreased distance between the medial cuneiform and the floor on the lateral radiograph, **top right. Bottom,** The postoperative radiographs show a decrease in the deformities.

tion, the foot will be stable even if there are radiographic signs of nonunion of one of the triple joints. Jahss and associates[52] called this concept a quadruple arthrodesis. Although they described this procedure with the use of cancellous bone graft, no internal fixation was used. Bone graft is not necessary if rigid internal fixation is used to stabilize the arthrodesis.

I prefer to achieve internal fixation with compression screws and have found it unnecessary to use bone graft. I have found the prevalence of nonunion associated with this technique to be negligible, provided that broad surfaces of bleeding bone are present and that rigid compression fixation is achieved (Fig. 8). In a recent institutional review of 143 triple arthrodeses performed between 1986 and 1994, my colleagues and I found that only one nonunion of the talonavicular joint had occurred (unpublished data).

Some clinicians advocate fixing the talonavicular joint first;[15] others believe that the subtalar joint should be stabilized first. It is my belief that realigning the medial column at the talonavicular joint is the key to aligning the rest of the foot. The forefoot is adducted and plantarflexed across the talonavicular joint, and that joint is held secure with a guide pin for a cannulated screw. Talonavicular correction should result in passive correction of the subtalar joint, which ideally should be aligned and stabilized in slight valgus. When stabilizing the calcaneocuboid joint, it is very important to elevate the cuboid forcefully to prevent any inferior sag that later may create pain along the lateral surface

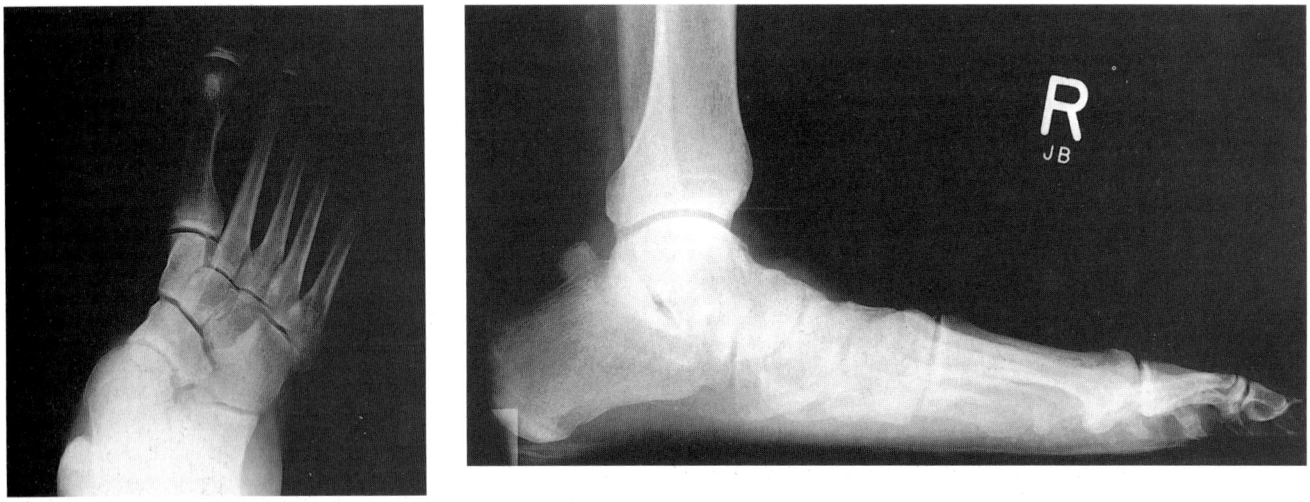

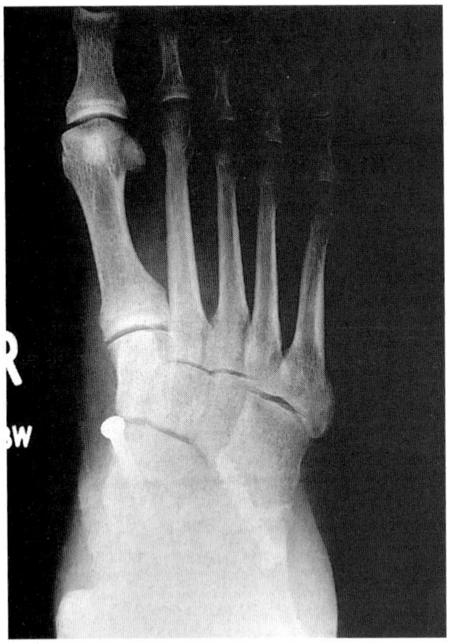

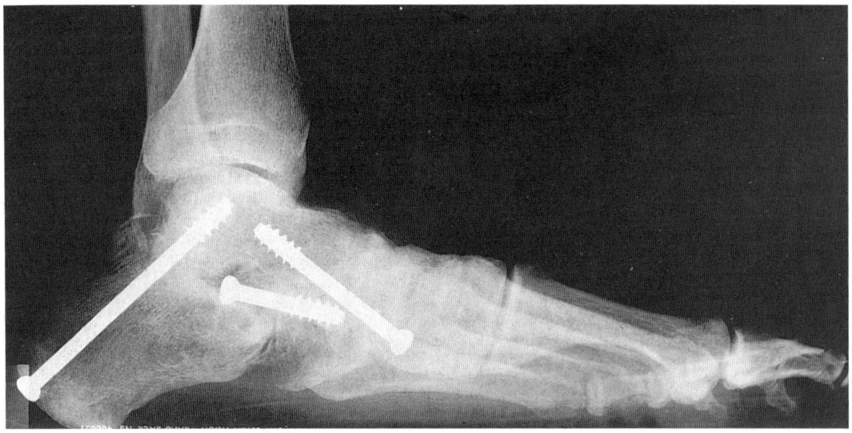

Fig. 8 A 62-year-old woman who was managed with a triple arthrodesis because of a stage-III flatfoot deformity. **Top,** Preoperative radiographs. Note the marked abduction of the forefoot and the decrease in talonavicular coverage on the anteroposterior radiograph, **top left,** as well as the complete loss of the medial longitudinal arch on the lateral radiograph, **top right. Bottom,** Postoperative radiographs showing correction of the deformities.

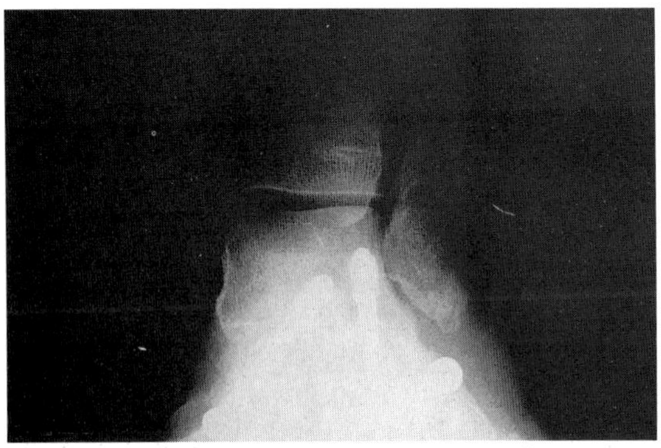

Fig. 9 Radiograph of a 63-year-old woman, made 28 months after a triple arthrodesis, showing valgus angulation of the talus.

of the foot with weightbearing.

It is far preferable to leave the foot in slight valgus than in neutral or varus, despite the possibility that impingement may occur between the fibula and the calcaneus in some patients who have more advanced deformity. One must be careful not to overcorrect the foot by internally rotating the subtalar joint and adducting the forefoot severely at the transverse tarsal joint. In contrast, an in situ arthrodesis that leaves the calcaneus in marked valgus will place undue stress on the tibiotalar joint. On the basis of these findings, Jahss (MH Jahss, MD, unpublished data, 1994) recommended adding a medial displacement osteotomy of the calcaneus to a triple arthrodesis in the presence of a fixed deformity of the hindfoot. Such a medial displacement osteotomy may normalize the weightbearing

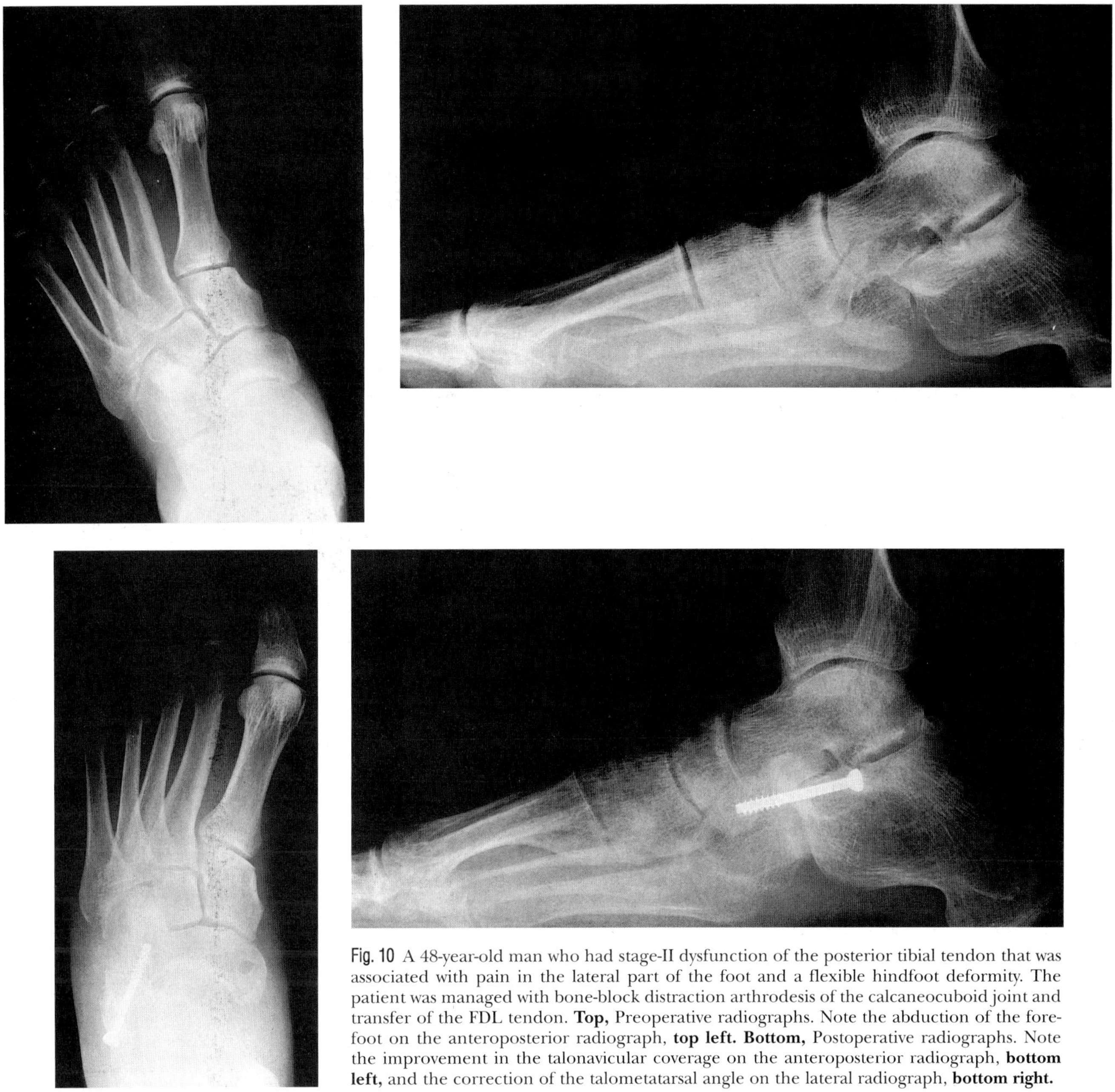

Fig. 10 A 48-year-old man who had stage-II dysfunction of the posterior tibial tendon that was associated with pain in the lateral part of the foot and a flexible hindfoot deformity. The patient was managed with bone-block distraction arthrodesis of the calcaneocuboid joint and transfer of the FDL tendon. **Top,** Preoperative radiographs. Note the abduction of the forefoot on the anteroposterior radiograph, **top left. Bottom,** Postoperative radiographs. Note the improvement in the talonavicular coverage on the anteroposterior radiograph, **bottom left,** and the correction of the talometatarsal angle on the lateral radiograph, **bottom right.**

surface of the hindfoot and improve the distribution of weightbearing forces across the medial part of the ankle, thereby reducing the stress on the tibiotalar joint and the deltoid ligament.[6,9,28,30] This is certainly an option for the treatment of a fixed valgus deformity that is associated with valgus tilting of the ankle, but every effort should be made to reduce the hindfoot deformity intraoperatively.

Unfortunately, the results of triple arthrodesis in older adults who have flatfoot deformity are disappointing, as many of these patients have later problems with the ankle joint. Graves and associates[47] found that triple arthrodesis in older patients eliminated or decreased the pain, but they cautioned that this procedure should be used only in a salvage attempt for fixed deformity because of the high rate of postoperative complications. With severe deformity, the hindfoot may become rigidly fixed in valgus and the talus may begin to tilt into valgus in the tibiotalar joint, perhaps as a result of attritional changes in the deltoid ligament. Triple arthrodesis fails in many of these patients (Fig. 9). Johnson and Lester[46] were perhaps the first to recognize this fact, and they recommended a primary tibiotalocalcaneal arthrodesis to address the problem.

The use of an arthrodesis to lengthen the lateral column has been successful for the treatment of severe planovalgus deformity of the foot, with excellent results and long-term maintenance of correction.[36,53] This procedure is indicated for a patient who has a valgus deformity that is not fixed (stage-II disease) (A Sands, L Grujic, B Sangeorzan, unpublished data, 1995). Options for bone graft include autogenous graft from the iliac crest and allograft. While the use of allograft is far easier and involves less morbidity, it is important to advise patients of its greater potential for nonunion (WC McGarvey, WG Braly, unpublished data, 1995). I prefer to use a femoral-head allograft, contouring a trapezoidal block of bone in two planes. The trapezoid is fashioned so that it is wider (12 mm) dorsally and laterally and narrower medially and inferiorly. On the plantar surface, the trapezoid tapers to 8 mm on both sides to achieve adduction of the midfoot and plantarflexion of the hindfoot (Fig. 10). The lengthening arthrodesis of the calcaneocuboid joint is facilitated with use of a smooth lamina spreader (without teeth), which can be removed smoothly from the joint as the bone graft is tamped into place. Although securing the bone graft may not be necessary as it is inserted under compression, I prefer to use either a cannulated screw or a percutaneous Kirschner wire to hold it in place.

Conclusion

The options for nonsurgical and surgical treatment of acquired flatfoot deformity in adults are numerous. Although each classification or treatment regimen has its flaws, the steps described should help the clinician to make an appropriate treatment decision.

References

1. Jahss MH: Spontaneous rupture of the tibialis posterior tendon: Clinical findings, tenographic studies, and a new technique of repair. *Foot Ankle* 1982;3:158–166.
2. Ouzounian TJ, Myerson MS: Dislocation of the posterior tibial tendon. *Foot Ankle* 1992;13:215–219.
3. Frey C, Shereff M, Greenidge N: Vascularity of the posterior tibial tendon. *J Bone Joint Surg* 1990;72A:884–888.
4. Sarrafian SK (ed): *Anatomy of the Foot and Ankle: Descriptive, Topographic, Functional,* ed 2. Philadelphia, PA, JB Lippincott, 1993.
5. Goldner JL, Keats PK, Bassett FH III, et al: Progressive talipes equinovalgus due to trauma or degeneration of the posterior tibial tendon and medial plantar ligaments. *Orthop Clin North Am* 1974;5:39–51.
6. Fairbank A, Myerson MS, Fortin P, et al: The effect of calcaneal osteotomy on contact characteristics of the tibiotalar joint. *Foot* 1995;5:137–142.
7. Harper MC: Deltoid ligament: An anatomical evaluation of function. *Foot Ankle* 1987;8:19–22.
8. Kjærsgaard-Andersen P, Wethelund J-O, Helmig P, et al: Stabilizing effect of the tibiocalcaneal fascicle of the deltoid ligament on hindfoot joint movements: An experimental study. *Foot Ankle* 1989;10:30–35.
9. Resnick RB, Jahss MH, Choueka J, et al: Deltoid ligament forces after tibialis posterior tendon rupture: Effects of triple arthrodesis and calcaneal displacement osteotomies. *Foot Ankle* 1995;16:14–20.
10. Stormont DM, Morrey BF, An KN, et al: Stability of the loaded ankle: Relation between articular restraint and primary and secondary static restraints. *Am J Sports Med* 1985;13:295–300.
11. Deland JT, Arnoczky SP, Thompson FM: Adult acquired flatfoot deformity at the talonavicular joint: Reconstruction of the spring ligament in an in vitro model. *Foot Ankle* 1992; 13:327–332.
12. Funk DA, Cass JR, Johnson KA: Acquired adult flat foot secondary to posterior tibial-tendon pathology. *J Bone Joint Surg* 1986;68A:95–102.
13. Johnson KA: Tibialis posterior tendon rupture. *Clin Orthop* 1983;177:140–147.
14. Mann RA, Thompson FM: Rupture of the posterior tibial tendon causing flat foot: Surgical treatment. *J Bone Joint Surg* 1985;67A:556–561.
15. Myerson M: Posterior tibial tendon insufficiency, in Myerson M (ed): *Current Therapy in Foot and Ankle Surgery.* St. Louis, MO, Mosby-Year Book, 1993, pp 123–135.
16. Holmes GB Jr, Mann RA: Possible epidemiological factors associated with rupture of the posterior tibial tendon. *Foot Ankle* 1992;13:70–79.
17. Monto RR, Moorman CT III, Mallon WJ, et al: Rupture of the posterior tibial tendon associated with closed ankle fracture. *Foot Ankle* 1991;11:400–403.
18. Myerson M, Solomon G, Shereff M: Posterior tibial tendon dysfunction: Its association with seronegative inflammatory disease. *Foot Ankle* 1989;9:219–225.
19. Anzel SH, Covey KW, Weiner AD, et al: Disruption of muscles and tendons: An analysis of 1,014 cases. *Surgery* 1959;45:406-414.
20. Myerson MS: Acquired flatfoot in the adult. *Adv Orthop Surg* 1989;12:155–165.
21. Conti S, Michelson J, Jahss M: Clinical significance of magnetic resonance imaging in preoperative planning for reconstruction of posterior tibial tendon ruptures. *Foot Ankle* 1992;13:208–214.
22. Rosenberg ZS, Cheung Y, Jahss MH, et al: Rupture of posterior tibial tendon: CT and MR imaging with surgical correlation. *Radiology* 1988;169:229–235.
23. Rosenberg ZS, Jahss MH, Noto AM, et al: Rupture of the posterior tibial tendon: CT and surgical findings. *Radiology* 1988;167:489–493.
24. Johnson KA, Strom DE: Tibialis posterior tendon dysfunction. *Clin Orthop* 1989;239:196–206.
25. Chao W, Lee TH, Hecht PJ, et al: Conservative management of posterior tibial tendon rupture. *Orthop Trans* 1994;18:1030.
26. Myerson MS, Ruland CM, Allon SM: Regional anesthesia for foot and ankle surgery. *Foot Ankle* 1992;13:282–288.
27. Teasdall RD, Johnson KA: Surgical treatment of stage I posterior tibial tendon dysfunction. *Foot Ankle Int* 1994;15:646–648.
28. Myerson MS, Corrigan AJ, Schon L, et al: Tendon transfer combined with calcaneal osteotomy for treatment of posterior tibial tendon insufficiency: A radiological investigation. *Foot Ankle Int* 1995;16:712–718.
29. Rose GK: Pes planus, in Jahss MH (ed): *Disorders of the Foot and Ankle: Medical and Surgical Management,* ed 2. Philadelphia, PA, WB Saunders, 1991, pp 892–920.
30. Welton EA, Rose GK: Posterior tibial tendon pathology: The foot at risk and its treatment by os calcis osteotomy. *Foot* 1993;3:168–174.
31. Gleich A: Beitrag zur operativen Plattfussbehandlung. *Arch Klin Chir* 1893;46:358–362.
32. Lord JP: Correction of extreme flatfoot: Value of osteotomy of

os calcis and inward displacement of posterior fragment (Gleich operation). *JAMA* 1923;81:1502–1507.
33. Nayak RK, Cotterill CP: Osteotomy of the calcaneum for symptomatic idiopathic valgus heel. *Foot* 1992;2:111–116.
34. Saxby T, Myerson M: Calcaneus osteotomy, in Myerson M (ed): *Current Therapy in Foot and Ankle Surgery*. St. Louis, MO, Mosby-Year Book, 1993, pp 159–162.
35. Koutsogiannis E: Treatment of mobile flat foot by displacement osteotomy of the calcaneus. *J Bone Joint Surg* 1971;53B:96–100.
36. Evans D: Calcaneo-valgus deformity. *J Bone Joint Surg* 1975;57B:270–278.
37. Anderson AF, Fowler SB: Anterior calcaneal osteotomy for symptomatic juvenile pes planus. *Foot Ankle* 1984;4:274–283.
38. Phillips GE: A review of elongation of os calcis for flat feet. *J Bone Joint Surg* 1983;65:15–18.
39. Sangeorzan BJ, Mosca V, Hansen ST Jr: Effect of calcaneal lengthening on relationships among the hindfoot, midfoot, and forefoot. *Foot Ankle* 1993;14:136–141.
40. Mann RA: Acquired flatfoot in adults. *Clin Orthop* 1983;181:46–51.
41. Wapner KL, Hecht PJ, Shea JR, et al: Anatomy of second muscular layer of the foot: Considerations for tendon selection in transfer for Achilles and posterior tibial tendon reconstruction. *Foot Ankle Int* 1994;15:420–423.
42. Elbar JE, Thomas WH, Weinfeld MS, et al: Talonavicular arthrodesis for rheumatoid arthritis of the hindfoot. *Orthop Clin North Am* 1976;7:821–826.
43. Fogel GR, Katoh Y, Rand JA, et al: Talonavicular arthrodesis for isolated arthrosis: 9.5-year results and gait analysis. *Foot Ankle* 1982;3:105–113.
44. Thoren K, Ljung P, Pettersson H, et al: Comparison of talonavicular dowel arthrodesis utilizing autogenous bone versus defatted bank bone. *Foot Ankle* 1993;14:125–128.
45. Clain MR, Baxter DE: Simultaneous calcaneocuboid and talonavicular fusion: Long-term follow-up study. *J Bone Joint Surg* 1994;76B:133–136.
46. Johnson WL, Lester EL: Transposition of the posterior tibial tendon. *Clin Orthop* 1989;245:223–227.
47. Graves SC, Mann RA, Graves KO: Triple arthrodesis in older adults: Results after long-term follow-up. *J Bone Joint Surg* 1993;75A:355–362.
48. Sammarco GJ: Technique of triple arthrodesis in treatment of symptomatic pes planus. *Orthopedics* 1988;11:1607–1610.
49. Sangeorzan BJ, Smith D, Veith R, et al: Triple arthrodesis using internal fixation in treatment of adult foot disorders. *Clin Orthop* 1993;294:299–307.
50. Vogler HW: Triple arthrodesis as a salvage for end-stage flatfoot. *Clin Podiatr Med Surg* 1989;6:591–604.
51. Bono JV, Jacobs RL: Triple arthrodesis through a single lateral approach: A cadaveric experiment. *Foot Ankle* 1992;13:408–412.
52. Jahss MH, Godsick PA, Levin H: Quadruple arthrodesis with iliac bone graft, in Bateman JE, Trott AW (eds): *The Foot and Ankle*. New York, NY, Thieme Stratton, 1980, pp 93–102.
53. Horton GA, Olney BW: Triple arthrodesis with lateral column lengthening for treatment of severe planovalgus deformity. *Foot Ankle Int* 1995;16:395–400.

Aging

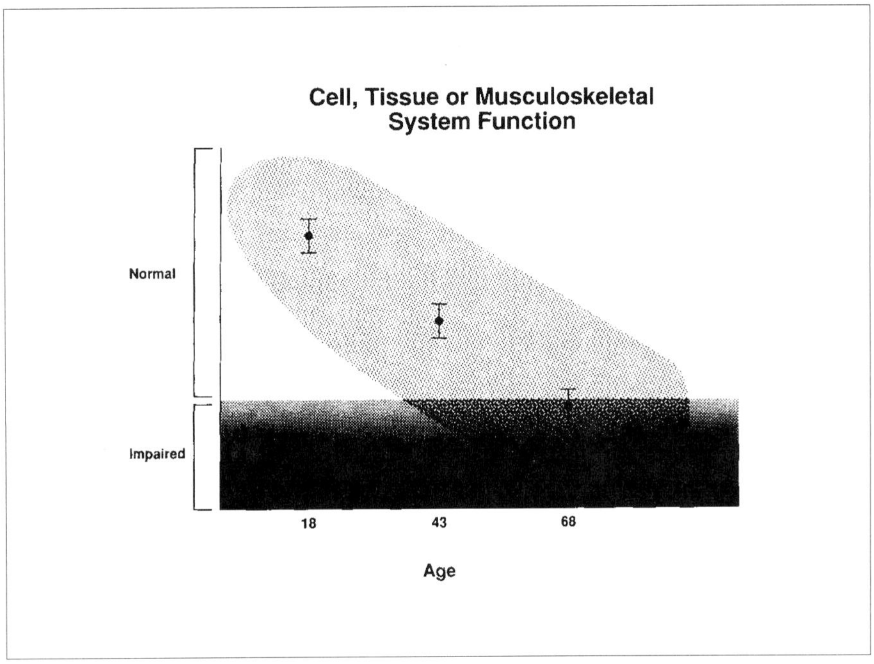
Cell, Tissue or Musculoskeletal System Function
Normal
Impaired
18
43
68
Age

CHAPTER 37

Geriatrics for Orthopaedists

Kenneth Brummel-Smith, MD

The aging of the American population is perhaps the single most important demographic change to affect medical care in the history of the United States. Currently, 13% of the population of the United States is over age 65. By 2040, about 20% will be over 65. The over-85 age group is the fastest growing segment of the population.[1] Traditionally, orthopaedic practice has served two main age-related populations: those between 13 and 18 years old, and those over 65 years old.[2] Geriatric patients will vastly outnumber pediatric patients for the next 30 to 40 years. Except perhaps for those exclusively caring for the pediatric patients or practicing sports medicine, geriatric patients will be the predominant population served for quite some time.

This monograph will address the reasons for this remarkable change in society, provide basic information regarding theories and physiology of aging, and discuss alterations in practice that will be required to serve this burgeoning population. Finally, information regarding the management of common comorbid conditions that the orthopaedist will encounter when dealing with geriatric patients will be presented.

Reasons for the Change in Demographics

Contrary to popular belief, the primary reasons for the marked increase in the number of older persons in our society is not directly related to high quality health care. Most of the change can be attributed to improvements in public health that have led to a decrease in the numbers of infants, children, and mothers dying. Before 1900, almost 25% of the population died before the age of 6 years (Fig. 1).[3] Childbirth was attended by high rates of mortality. Now that childbirth is safer, and almost no infants die of typhoid, cholera, or other contagious diseases, there are many more people alive to live into their later years. Hence, the life expectancy at birth has risen from about 45 years for both males and females in 1900 to almost 80 for females and mid-seventies for males in 1993. However, there has also been a steady rise in life expectancy after age 65.[4] This effect probably owes much to improvements in medical care. It is also the reason that orthopaedists can expect to see more older persons in their practice.

Life expectancy continues to rise as one ages. For instance, at age 65, white males can expect to live 14 more years, and females can anticipate 18 more years. Even at 85, males will have 7 years remaining and females will have 9. Unfortunately, hidden in these numbers is the fact that many will add years that result in increased dependency on others.[5] Chronic disease is extremely common in old age.

Eighty-five percent of the geriatric population has arthritis. Virtually all of the top ten causes of death in those over 65 are chronic diseases, such as heart disease, strokes, and diabetes. This population makes up 13% of the population of the United States, yet uses 33% of all health care dollars and 25% of all prescription drugs.[6] Over 50% of all hospital beds are occupied by elderly patients. The nursing home population is made of almost 95% geriatric residents. The health care system will continue to undergo dramatic shifts—from acute to chronic care, from hospital based to community based, from fee-for-service to managed care, and to dealing with prolonged periods of disability.

What will be the effects on orthopaedic practice as we move into the next millennium? It is clear there will be an increase in the absolute numbers of geriatric patients. The older population is becoming healthier. As baby boomers enter the geriatric population, we can anticipate changes in the expectations of elders, most of whom will want more involvement in health care decisions. Finally, there are likely to be changes in practice patterns. Orthopaedists will extend their practice into nursing homes, subacute units, and possibly even home care.

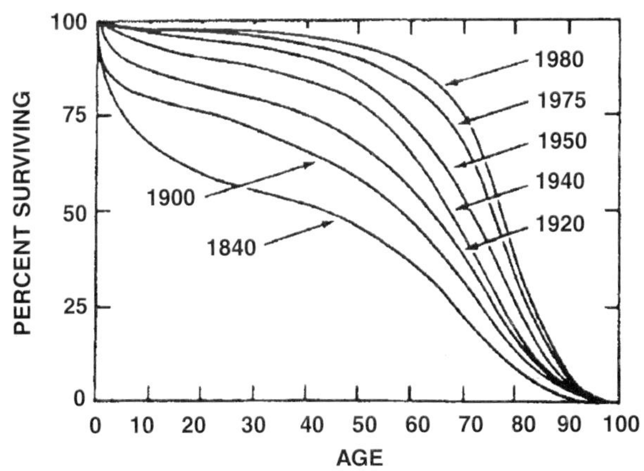

Fig. 1 This figure illustrates how mortality before age 10 was significant before the turn of the century. As a result of fewer children dying in 1980, more people are able to age into the later years. (Reproduced with permission from Cassel CK, Brody JA: Demography, epidemiology, and aging, in Cassel CK, Riesenberg DE, Sorensen LB, et al (eds): *Geriatric Medicine*, ed 2. New York, NY, Springer-Verlag, 1990, pp 16–27.)

Theories of Aging

There are three main theories about why we age.[7] The first deals with cellular aging. Cellular aging takes multiple forms. One of the most prominent is often termed the theory of accumulated accidents. In this model, genetic mistakes accumulate over a lifetime, leading to DNA and RNA transcription errors. Errors in protein synthesis, membrane repair, and a host of other complications ensue. In addition, cells themselves, particularly neural cells, may be damaged, leading to a gradual decline in their numbers. One of the most interesting cellular theories has been promoted by Hayflick.[8] He has demonstrated that human cells grown in vitro have a finite number of divisions. Hence, we may be genetically coded to die. Perhaps this explains the fact that no human has been documented to live longer than approximately 120 years (fixed life span).

Other theories deal with problems that develop in the immune system or neuroendocrine function. Decreases in cell-mediated immunity have been demonstrated. There also may be modulation of the immune system by environmental factors, such as diet or exposure to radiation. Changes in thymic hormone may also affect immune protection systems. Finally, neural and endocrine control of gene activity may lead to multiple end-organ effects. Most experts believe that it is likely that there are numerous interacting causes to aging, expressed to varying degrees within a particular individual.

Changes in the Focus of Medical Care

The aging of America is requiring a shift in the focus of care.[9] Geriatric medicine has advocated an approach that is familiar to many orthopaedists. The focus must shift from simple cure to promoting the patient's functional abilities. Cure is elusive in geriatrics, but function can almost always be enhanced. Furthermore, elders view independence and continued functioning as highly held values, often more important than the prolongation of life itself.

Unfortunately, much of our medical system is focused on diagnosis and cure. Diagnoses have almost no direct relation to function. Functional status may change drastically even when the diagnosis remains the same. For instance, the admission diagnosis of hip fracture does not reveal that one patient fractured her hip crashing her bicycle while participating in the over age 65 group of the Iron Man Triathlon, while another fractured her hip having slipped in the bathroom of a nursing home. Functional status is much more accurate than diagnoses in predicting health care utilization and outcomes following interventions.[10]

The failure to attend to functional status has been shown to lead to many iatrogenic complications, especially when the elder is hospitalized. Elders leave the hospital more functionally disabled than when they are admitted, even when their treatment has been successful.[11] Functional interventions are inadequately funded by reimbursement systems. Yet simple interventions have been shown to be quite rewarding, even in 90-year-old nursing home residents.[12] All geriatric care providers should develop their skills at functional assessment and advocate for interventions to enhance functional abilities. Simple assessments are available that can be incorporated into office and hospital practice, and these can detect the patient at risk and serve to initiate a plan for rehabilitation.

Functional Assessment

Office or preoperative functional assessment should include the major domains of cognition, activities of daily living, and mobility. Simple questions and maneuvers can be used to detect those patients that require more in-depth assessments and possible referral.

Cognition Recall of three words after 2 minutes has been shown to be an effective screen for memory problems.[13] It is far more sensitive than the traditional "alert and oriented times three" method. The patient is given three words (such as garbage, tree, and airplane) and told to remember them. It is important to emphasize that they will be asked what the words were after a few minutes. Failure to remember all three should alert the surgeon that the patient has memory problems and requires further testing. Most patients with dementia serious enough to potentially affect surgical outcomes will miss some of the words. Attention can easily be tested by asking the patient to spell the word "world" backwards. Demented patients usually spell it incorrectly, while patients with delirium often cannot attend well enough to even complete the task. Finally, the patient can be asked to put the numbers of a clock in a circle the examiner has drawn on a piece of paper. Demented patients often complete the task but arrange the numbers in a spatially incorrect manner, and delirious patients cannot complete the task due to poor attention. If the patient is suspected of having either dementia or delirium, the examiner may choose to administer the Mini Mental Status Exam[14] (Fig. 2) or the Confusion Assessment Method,[15] respectively. Consultation with a geriatrician may also be in order.

Activities of Daily Living (ADL) The basic activities of daily living (dressing, feeding, bathing, toileting, transfer, and ambulation) are important factors that can significantly affect surgical outcomes and discharge planning. Deficits in these areas will necessitate further evaluation, often by physical or occupational therapists. Early detection of problems in functional status should alert the surgeon to immediately involve social work in discharge planning.

Mini-Mental State Examination (MMSE)

Add points for each correct response.

		Score	Points
Orientation			
1. What is the:	Year?	____	1
	Season?	____	1
	Date?	____	1
	Day?	____	1
	Month?	____	1
2. Where are we?	State?	____	1
	County?	____	1
	Town or city?	____	1
	Hospital?	____	1
	Floor?	____	1
Registration			
3. Name three objects, taking one second to say each.Then ask the patient to repeat all three after you have said them.		____	3
Attention and calculation			
4. Serial sevens. Give one point for each correct answer. Stop after five answers. Alternate: Spell WORLD backwards.		____	5
Recall			
5. Ask for names of three objects learned in question 3. Give one point for each correct answer.		____	3
Language			
6. Point to a pencil and a watch. Have the patient name them as you point.		____	2
7. Have the patient repeat "No ifs, ands, or buts."		____	1
8. Have the patient follow a three-stage command: "Take a paper in your right hand. Fold the paper in half. Put the paper on the floor."		____	3
9. Have the patient read and obey the following: "CLOSE YOUR EYES." (Write it in large letters.)		____	1
10. Have the patient write a sentence of his or her choice. (The sentence should contain a subject and an object and should make sense. Ignore spelling errors when scoring.)		____	1
11. Have the patient copy the design. (Give one point if all sides and angles are preserved and if the intersecting sides form a quadrangle.)		____	1
		____	1
		____ =	Total 30

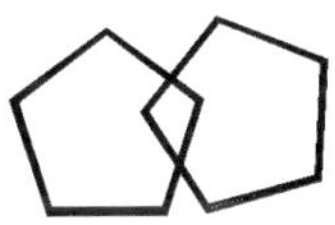

In validation studies using a cut-off score of 23 or below, the MMSE has a sensitivity of 87%, a specificity of 82%, a false-positive ratio of 39.4%, and a false-negative ratio of 4.7%. These ratios refer to the MMSE's capacity to accurately distinguish patients with clinically diagnosed dementia or delirium from patients without these syndromes.

SOURCE: Courtesy of Marshall Folstein, MD. Reprinted with permission.

For additional information on administration and scoring refer to the following references:

1. Anthony JC, LeResche L, Niaz U, et al: Limits of "Mini-Mental State" as a screening test for dementia and delirium among hospital patients. *Psych Med* 1982;12:397–408.
2. Folstein MF, Anthony JC, et al: Meaning of cognitive impairment in the elderly. *J Am Geriatr Soc* 1985;33(4):228–235.
3. Folstein MF, Folstein S, McHugh PR: Mini-Mental State: A practical method for grading the cognitive state of patients for the clinician. *J Psych Res* 1975;12:189–198.
4. Spenser MP, Folstein MF: The Mini-Mental State Examination, *in Keller PA, Ritt LG: Innovations in Clinical Practice: A Source Book.* 1985;4:305–310.

Fig. 2 Mini-Mental State Examination (MMSE). This test can be administered by the physician or trained designee. It is used to establish a baseline cognitive score. Though not a diagnostic test for dementia, low scores should be investigated for dementia, depression or delirium. (Reproduced with permission from Folstein MF, Folstein SE, McHugh PR: "Mini-mental state": A practical method for grading the cognitive state of patients for the clinician. *J Psychiatr Res* 1975;12:189–198.)

Self-report of functional status is a reliable method of assessing ADL capability, as long as the patient has normal cognition. While it is known that elderly patients tend to overrate their abilities, family care givers often underrate their loved one's capacity.[16] Because of possible discrepancies between what is reported and what is actually done by the patient, it may be helpful to have the patient demonstrate simple motor activities that have been shown to be associated with the capacity to perform ADL. The worksheet shown in Figure 3 is a useful way to gather such information.

FUNCTIONAL ASSESSMENT SCREENING TOOL

Functional History: Activities of Daily Living ("B-A-T-T-E-D")

Do you have any trouble with: (if answer is "no," ask "How do you do it?"), score 'yes' if help is needed.

1. Bathing?	Yes ______	No ______
2. Walking (Ambulation)?	Yes ______	No ______
3. Making Transfers?	Yes ______	No ______
4. Using the Toilet?	Yes ______	No ______
5. Eating?	Yes ______	No ______
6. Dressing?	Yes ______	No ______

Instrumental Activities of Daily Living ("S-C-U-M-M")

7. Shopping?	Yes ______	No ______
8. Cooking or cleaning?	Yes ______	No ______
9. Using transportation?	Yes ______	No ______
10. Managing money?	Yes ______	No ______
11. Managing medications?	Yes ______	No ______

Functional Examination

Test	Function tested	Able	Limited	Unable
1. Put both hands together behind head	Hair combing, washing back, etc.	______	______	______
2. Put both hands together behind back	Managing clothing, washing lower back	______	______	______
3. Sitting, touch great toe with opposite hand	Lower extremity dressing and hygiene	______	______	______
4. Squeeze examiner's two fingers with each hand	Approx. 20 lb. grasp needed for functional activities (holding a pan)	______	______	______
5. Hold paper between thumb and lateral side of index finger while examiner tries to pull it out	Approx. 3 lb. grip needed for functional activities (turning a key)	______	______	______
6. Get up from the chair without using your hands, walk down the hall, turn around, stand with eyes closed (nudge), sit down without using hands	Hip strength; gait symmetry and velocity, step height; balance, ability to withstand sudden changes in position; fall risk	______	______	______

Fig. 3 Functional Assessment Screening Tool. By using a standard series of questions, the physician can detect whether the patient has problems with activities of daily living or instrumental activities of daily living. A few standardized physical maneuvers can be used to detect impairments with functional range of motion. (© 1992 Kenneth Brummel-Smith, MD)

Mobility A functional evaluation of gait and balance has been shown to be more sensitive than the standard neurologic exam in detecting problems.[17] The patient, while sitting in a chair, is asked to stand up without using his or her hands, walk 10 to 15 meters down the hall, turn around, and come back to the examiner. Then, while standing with eyes closed, a firm nudge is given on the patient's sternum to test his or her balance (the "nudge" test). Be prepared to catch the patient should he or she fall. Then the patient is directed to sit down without using his or her hands. In a study of nursing home patients, the inability to rise without using hands, a positive "nudge" test, and taking more than four medications was shown to predict with 100% accuracy patients who will fall in the next 6 months.[18] Irregular steps, an unsafe appearing gait, and difficulties with rising and sitting are excellent predictors of gait problems and require further evaluation. A formal scoring system can be applied to the maneuvers but such tests are rarely used in clinical systems.[19]

Psychosocial Status Assessment

Psychological and social problems are among the most powerful predictors of outcomes in elderly surgical patients. A series of simple questions can be used to determine which patients need further evaluation and

Geriatric Depression Scale
(Long Form)

*1.	Are you basically satisfied with your life?	Yes	No
2.	Have you dropped many of your activities and interests?	Yes	No
3.	Do you feel that your life is empty?	Yes	No
4.	Do you often get bored?	Yes	No
*5.	Are you hopeful about the future?	Yes	No
6.	Are you bothered by thoughts you can't get out of your head?	Yes	No
*7.	Are you in good spirits most of the time?	Yes	No
8.	Are you afraid that something bad is going to happen to you?	Yes	No
*9.	Do you feel happy most of the time?	Yes	No
10.	Do you often feel helpless?	Yes	No
11.	Do you often get restless and fidgety?	Yes	No
12.	Do you prefer to stay at home, rather than going out and doing new things?	Yes	No
13.	Do you frequently worry about the future?	Yes	No
14.	Do you feel you have more problems with memory than most?	Yes	No
*15.	Do you think it is wonderful to be alive now?	Yes	No
16.	Do you often feel downhearted and blue?	Yes	No
17.	Do you feel pretty worthless the way you are now?	Yes	No
18.	Do you worry a lot about the past?	Yes	No
*19.	Do you find life very eciting?	Yes	No
20.	Is it hard for you to get started on new projects?	Yes	No
*21.	Do you feel full of energy?	Yes	No
22.	Do you feel that your situation is hopeless?	Yes	No
23.	Do you think that most people are better off than you are?	Yes	No
24.	Do you frequently get upset over little things?	Yes	No
25.	Do you frequently feel like crying?	Yes	No
26.	Do you have trouble concentrating?	Yes	No
*27.	Do you enjoy getting up in the morning?	Yes	No
28.	Do you prefer to avoid social gatherings?	Yes	No
*29.	Is it easy for you to make decisions?	Yes	No
*30.	Is your mind as clear as it used to be?	Yes	No

* Appropriate (non-depressed) answers = yes; all others = no

Score: ______ (Number of "depressed" answers)

*Norms	
Normal	5 + 4
Mildly depressed	15 + 6
Very depressed	23 + 5

Fig. 4 Geriatric Depression Scale (GDS). This test can be taken by the patient or administered by the physician or a trained designee. Though not diagnostic of major depression, scores above 15 are associated with depressive syndromes. (Reproduced with permission from Yesavage J, Brink T: Development and validation of a geriatric screening scale: A preliminary report. *J Psychiatr Res* 1983;17:37-49.)

intervention. When possible (such as before elective procedures) this line of investigation should be conducted before the procedure. Ideally, the primary physician should have assessed these areas before referring the patient.

Depression While not normally considered a part of orthopaedic care, the detection of depression is a task for which all physicians caring for older persons should feel some responsibility. Depression probably has negative effects on surgical outcomes and postoperative recovery. It also can lead to increased pain following surgery, necessitating higher doses of analgesia and the attendant risks. Asking if the patient often feels sad or depressed has been shown to be an effective screening device.[20] If the patient answers positively, a Geriatric Depression Scale questionnaire (Fig.4) can be administered.[21]

Alcoholism It may seem unlikely that a pleasant appearing woman, old enough to be the physician's grandmother, could be an alcoholic. However, the prevalence of alcohol abuse in this population is about the same as it is in younger people. The questions, "Do you have a problem with drinking?" and "When was your last drink?" have been shown to be useful detection methods.[22] The CAGE questionnaire can also be used (Fig. 5).[23]

Social Supports

The absence of social supports is a significant factor in both surgical and rehabilitation outcomes. The question, "Who would help you in your home if you were unable to take care of yourself?" is sensitive at detecting those with limited support systems.[13]

The CAGE Screening Questions

Have you ever felt you ought to **C**ut down?
Have you ever been **A**nnoyed by criticism of your drinking?
Have you ever felt **G**uilty or bad about your drinking?
Have you ever felt the need for an **E**ye-opener?

Fig. 5 The "CAGE" Questionnaire. These four questions can be used to screen for alcoholism. A positive answer to one of the questions has been shown to be indicative of possible alcoholism. The sensitivity rises with the number of positive answers.

Medical Conditions Common in Geriatric Patients

All surgical procedures are stressful. For many geriatric patients, the homeostatic balance between coping with multiple chronic illnesses and developing a "cascade of disasters" after a surgical procedure is a tenuous one. While many of the conditions that raise the risk of surgery are obvious, such as a recent myocardial infarction or chronic obstructive pulmonary disease, many older patients have undetected conditions that can adversely affect outcomes.

Hypothyroidism affects as many as 6% of the disabled elderly population.[24] Screening for this disorder with a serum thyroid-stimulating hormone (TSH) level is advisable for all who are in nursing homes or hospitalized patients. Ejection fractions of less than 30% have been shown to negatively influence rehabilitation, due to poor exercise tolerance.[25]

Many conditions in geriatric patients present with atypical symptoms. Thirty percent of patients with pneumonia present only with confusion, rather than cough, fever, and tachypnea. Forty percent of patients who develop a urinary tract infection will present only with confusion, while another 10% will have only incontinence. In those patients with a myocardial infarction, 20% have silent myocardial infarction, 50% present with secondary symptoms, such as heart block or syncope, and only 30% are classic presentations.[26]

Deconditioning

Deconditioning is an extremely common, unrecognized condition. It is defined as multiple changes in organ system physiology that are caused by inactivity and are reversed by activity.[27] Deconditioning has a rapid onset and long sequelae—it can take 3 to 5 weeks to recover after 1 week of bed rest. This condition affects multiple systems. Cognitive function is decreased, mood is depressed, sleep disturbances are common, and increased anxiety, especially about rehabilitation exercises, is seen. Balance and gait are affected, with increased sway, prolonged reaction time, decreased velocity, and increased fall risk. Cardiovascular function is impaired—increased resting heart rate, decreased blood volume, increased orthostasis, and delayed recovery after exercise are all seen. Decreased strength, increased bone turnover, and increased workload affect the musculoskeletal system. Finally, there are significant metabolic effects with increased calcium loss, dehydration, and increased protein catabolism. Fortunately, minor interventions are preventive. One maximal muscle contraction every 10 minutes will maintain strength, sitting for meals maintains cardiovascular responses, and stretching exercises maintain body awareness and facilitate muscular control.[28]

Delirium

Few things are more distressing to the surgeon than to have an elderly patient become psychotic during the immediate postoperative period. However, delirium more often presents in old age with being withdrawn, lacking initiative, or appearing depressed.[29] The diagnosis depends on a change in consciousness and decreased attentiveness. The classic presentation of hallucinations, delusions, sleep problems, and hyperactivity is less common. The patient appears disoriented and has memory problems, often leading to the mistaken diagnosis of dementia. Unfortunately, a preexisting state of dementia significantly raises the risk of delirium developing postsurgically.

The main causes of delirium are drugs, metabolic conditions, and infections. Benzodiazepines, anticholinergic drugs, certain analgesics (such as pentazocine or meperidine), and cimetadine top the list of offenders. Urinary tract infections and pneumonia are probably the most common causes of infection-related delirium. Hypoxia, electrolyte abnormalities, and occult hypothyroidism are common causes of delirium. Contrary to popular belief, delirium may last for a prolonged period of time, even months.

Falls

Accidents are the sixth leading cause of death in the elderly population, and falls are the most common form of accident. Each year, one third of elders at home and 50% of nursing home patients have a fall.[30] The fall that leads to a fracture is often the last of a series of falls. While most falls are accidental (that is, they are not caused by an arrythmia or syncopal episode), many accidental falls occur in at risk patients.[31] Risk factors include gait and balance disturbances, impaired vision, environmental hazards, and medications.

While the orthopaedic surgeon is likely to meet the "faller" after an untoward complication has occurred, improvements in gait and balance after successful operations may decrease the risk of a future fall. Gait and balance training have been shown to decrease fall rates and injury rates.[32] Muscle strengthening exercises have been shown to increase velocity and decrease fall rates.[33]

Pharmacology and Aging

Because of the high prevalence of disease in old age, virtually all older persons take prescription medications. Adverse drug reactions are the most common cause of iatrogenic complications. As many as 25% of hospitalized elders will suffer an adverse drug reaction.[34] When a person is taking more than six medications, some adverse reaction is almost certain.

There are many reasons for these problems. Drug-drug reactions are common. For instance, warfarin and aspirin enhance the risk of bleeding episodes. Drug-disease interactions also occur. This is seen in demented patients when they are given a drug with anticholinergic properties, such as amitriptyline, and then develop confusion. There are also drug-person interactions. Individuals may have allergic or idiosyncratic reactions to a particular drug, or even a particular brand of a drug. Multiple prescribers may complicate the picture, particularly when the patient does not have a good grasp of his or her own regimen. Finally, because of reductions in renal function and other factors, older persons are more sensitive to the effects of drugs.

Certain drugs are particularly dangerous, especially in their ability to cause falls and increase the fracture rate.[35] Sedative-hypnotics are common offenders. Long-acting benzodiazepines are the most dangerous. Diazepam, chlorazepate, chlordiazepoxide, and prazepam have half lives of 50 to 200 hours in older persons.[34] Flurazepam is similarly dangerous and should be avoided. Tricyclic antidepressants that are highly anticholinergic and highly sedating are the most dangerous. Amitriptyline and doxepin have the highest anticholinergic activity. Because of sedative effects, the low potency antipsychotics, chlorpromazine and thioridazine, are the most dangerous and should be avoided.

Many others can also cause problems. Cimetadine can cause confusion in as many as 30% of elders. Anticholinergic drugs, such as trihexyphenidyl, can cause confusion, urinary retention, and constipation. Antihistamines, such as diphenhydramine, can also cause anticholinergic effects. Centrally acting antihypertensives, such as methyldopa and clonidine, can lead to hypotension and memory loss.

In general, almost any drug can have negative effects and should be suspect. Every effort should be made to limit the number of medications the older patient is given during the perioperative period. When starting a new medication, the maxim, "Start low and go slow" should be followed. If a sedative is needed, low doses (15 to 30 mg) of oxazepam are probably safe.

Iatrogenic Conditions

Thirty-six percent of elderly patients admitted to a hospital suffer an iatrogenic complication.[36] The most common presentations of iatrogenesis are confusion, falls, incontinence, and anorexia.[37] The standard approach to these developments is often iatrogenic. Drugs are given to those who are confused, restraints are used to prevent falls, catheters are inserted in those with incontinence, and tube feedings are started on those who are anorexic. In fact, although it is the most common form of iatrogenesis, medication usage often rises following a medication-induced complication.[38]

These problems can be avoided by carefully reviewing the medication list and discontinuing any that are not absolutely necessary, restricting diagnostic studies to those necessary for the problem for which the patient was admitted, promoting function by encouraging the patient to be up in the chair and ambulate as often as possible, and working with nursing to offer alternatives to Foley catheters and restraints.

Ethical Dilemmas

The question in geriatrics is often not what can be done but what should be done. In ideal situations, the patient will have discussed their advanced directives with their family and primary care physician. Alas, however, this is all too uncommon. Hence, it may be up to the orthopaedic surgeon to explore the patient's wishes. The basis of informed consent is that patients are considered to have the capacity to make a medical decision if they can communicate with you, can understand the risks and benefits of a recommended procedure, and can offer their choice or an expression of their wishes. A disagreement with the opinion of the surgeon is not, by itself, evidence of incapacity.

A case that may be encountered by orthopaedists is the bed-bound demented patient with a fractured hip. There is evidence that such patients may be able to be effectively managed without surgery if they are provided adequate pain relief and comfort care.[39] When there is doubt as to the proper decision, or when the patient's choice may seem unwise, consultation with the hospital ethics committee is a useful option.

Summary

The care of older patients is challenging and fraught with pitfalls, but the orthopaedic surgeon has the opportunity to give the elderly patient a gift that is of the highest value at that time of life, the chance to function better and more independently. By avoiding hospital-induced problems, detecting and managing risk factors, and optimizing physical functioning, orthopaedists make major contributions to elders' lives.

References

1. Fowles DG (ed): *A Profile of Older Americans: 1990.* Washington, DC, American Association of Retired Persons (AARP), 1990.
2. *Orthopaedic Practice in the United States, 1994-1995.* Rosemont, IL, American Academy of Orthopaedic Surgeons, 1995, p 12.
3. Masoro EJ: Biology of aging: Current state of knowledge. *Arch Intern Med* 1987;147:166–169.
4. Cassel CK, Brody JA: Demography, epidemiology, and aging, in Cassel CK, Riesenberg DE, Sorensen LB, et al (eds): *Geriatric Medicine,* ed 2. New York, NY, Springe-Verlag, 1990, pp 16–27.
5. Manton KG, Stallard E: Cross-sectional estimates of active life expectancy for the U.S. elderly and oldest-old populations. *J Gerontol* 1991;46:S170–S182.
6. Vestal RE, Cusack BJ: Pharmacology and aging, in Schneider EL, Rowe JW (eds): *Handbook of the Biology of Aging,* ed 3. San Diego, CA, Academic Press, 1990, pp 349–383.
7. Cristofalo VJ: Biological mechanisms of aging: An overview, in Hazzard WR, Andres R, Bierman EL, et al (eds): *Principles of Geriatric Medicine and Gerontology,* ed 2. New York, NY, McGraw-Hill, 1990, pp 3–14.
8. Hayflick L: Cell biology of aging. *Fed Proc* 1979;38:1847–1850.
9. Brummel-Smith K: Introduction, in Kemp B, Brummel-mith K, Ramsdell JW (eds): *Geriatric Rehabilitation.* Austin, TX, PRO-ED Press, 1990.
10. Stewart AL, Greenfield S, Hays RD, et al: Functional status and well-being of patients with chronic conditions: Results from the Medical Outcomes Study. *JAMA* 1989;262:907–913.
11. Warshaw GA, Moore JT, Friedman SW, et al: Functional disability in the hospitalized elderly. *JAMA* 1982;248:847–850.
12. Fiatarone MA, O'Neill EF, Ryan ND, et al: Exercise training and nutritional supplementation for physical frailty in very elderly people. *N Engl J Med* 1994;330:1769–1775.
13. Lachs MS, Feinstein AR, Cooney LM Jr, et al: A simple procedure for general screening for functional disability in elderly patients. *Ann Intern Med* 1990;112:699–706.
14. Folstein MF, Folstein SE, McHugh PR: "Mini-mental state": A practical method for grading the cognitive state of patients for the clinician. *J Psychiatr Res* 1975;12:189–198.
15. Inouye SK, van Dyck CH, Alessi CA, et al: Clarifying confusion: The confusion assessment method. A new method for detection of delirium. *Ann Intern Med* 1990;113:941–948.
16. Rubenstein LZ, Schairer C, Wieland GD, et al: Systematic biases in functional status assessment of elderly adults: Effects of different data sources. *J Gerontol* 1984;39:686–691.
17. Tinetti ME, Ginter SF: Identifying mobility dysfunctions in elderly patients: Standard neuromuscular examination or direct assessment? *JAMA* 1988;259:1190–1193.
18. Robbins AS, Rubenstein LZ, Josephson KR, et al: Predictors of falls among elderly people: Results of two population-based studies. *Arch Intern Med* 1989;149:1628–1633.
19. Tinetti ME: Performance-oriented assessment of mobility. *Geriatr Rev Syll* 1991;1:480–482.
20. Mahoney J, Drinka TJ, Abler R, et al: Screening for depression: Single question versus GDS. *J Am Geriatr Soc* 1994;42:1006–1008.
21. Sheikh JI, Yesavage JA: Geriatric Depression Scale (GDS): Recent evidence and development of a shorter version. *Clin Gerontol* 1986;5:165–173.
22. Cyr MG, Wartman AS: The effectiveness of routine screening questions in the detection of alcoholism. *JAMA* 1988;259:51–54.
23. Ewing JA: Detecting alcoholism: The CAGE questionnaire. *JAMA* 1984;252:1905–1907.
24. Mokshagundam S, Barzel US: Thyroid disease in the elderly. *J Am Geriatr Soc* 1993;41:1361–1369.
25. Mosqueda LA: Assessment of rehabilitation potential. *Clin Geriatr Med* 1993;9:689–703.
26. Levkoff SE, Cleary PD, Wetle T, et al: Illness behavior in the aged: Implications for clinicians. *J Am Geriatr Soc* 1988;36:622–629.
27. Siebens H: Deconditioning, in Kemp B, Brummel-Smith K, Ramsdell JW (eds): *Geriatric Rehabilitation.* Austin, TX, PRO-ED Press, 1990, pp 177–192.
28. Larson EB, Bruce RA: Health benefits of exercise in an aging society. *Arch Intern Med* 1987;147:353–356.
29. Francis J, Martin D, Kapoor WN: A prospective study of delirium in hospitalized elderly. *JAMA* 1990;263:1097–1101.
30. Tinetti ME, Speechley M, Ginter SF: Risk factors for falls among elderly persons living in the community. *N Engl J Med* 1988;319:1701–1707.
31. Brummel-Smith K: Falls in the aged. *Prim Care* 1989;16:377–393.
32. Tinetti ME, Baker DI, McAvay G, et al: A multifactorial intervention to reduce the risk of falling among elderly people living in the community. *N Engl J Med* 1994;331:821–827.
33. Province MA, Hadley EC, Hornbrook MC, et al: The effects of exercise on falls in elderly patients: A preplanned meta-analysis of the FICSIT Trials. Fraility and injuries: Cooperative studies of intervention techniques. *JAMA* 1995;273:1341–1347.
34. Kane RL, Ouslander JG, Abrass IB (eds): Drug therapy, in *Essentials of Clinical Geriatrics,* ed 2. New York, NY, McGraw-Hill, 1989, pp 341–371.
35. Ray WA, Griffith MR, Schaffner W, et al: Psychotropic drug use and the risk of hip fracture. *N Engl J Med* 1987;316:363–369.
36. Steel K, Gertman PM, Crescenzi C, et al: Iatrogenic illness on a general medical service at a university hospital. *N Engl J Med* 1981;304:638–642.
37. Gillick MR, Serrell NA, Gillick LS: Adverse consequences of hospitalization in the elderly. *Soc Sci Med* 1982;16:1033–1038.
38. Gorbien MJ, Bishop J, Beers MH, et al: Iatrogenic illness in hospitalized elderly people [clinical conference]. *J Am Geriatr Soc* 1992;40:1031–1042.
39. Winter WG: Nonoperative treatment of proximal femoral fractures in the demented, non-ambulatory patient. *Clin Orthop* 1987;218:97–103.

CHAPTER 38

Orthopaedic Challenges in an Aging Population

Victor M. Goldberg, MD
Joseph A. Buckwalter, MD
Wilson C. Hayes, PhD
Kenneth J. Koval, MD

Introduction

Musculoskeletal disorders are prevalent in the elderly population. Musculoskeletal injury and diseases are more likely with increasing age. Limited mobility, stiffness, muscle weakness, soreness and fatigue, and back pain that affects quality of life[1] are major complaints. In 1990 the United States population of people over the age of 65 was 31.7 million, 12.7% of the total population. By the year 2020, the elderly population is predicted to increase to 51.4 million, 17.3% of the total population.[1] Cunningham and Kelsey[2] reported that almost 40% of patients studied had musculoskeletal symptoms while 60% had some musculoskeletal signs. The disparity between the symptoms and signs was related to a number of social factors, including education, income, and marital status. The availability of financial and social resources was also an important factor in determining musculoskeletal impairment and disability.

Specific problems associated with aging of the musculoskeletal system result from changes in both bone and soft tissues. Fractures that are associated with age-related alterations in bone, such as osteoporosis and osteomalacia, cause significant morbidity. Depending on their severity, these fractures can cause death in older people.[3] Loss of muscle strength has been shown to increase the disabilities associated with impairment of joints and ligaments.[4] Although there is good evidence relating increasing age to increasing musculoskeletal impairment, the specific mechanisms of dysfunction of the cells and tissues that make up the musculoskeletal system are less evident.[3]

Experimental work has identified some of the specific age-related changes that affect cell function.[3] Aging differentiated cells are characterized by a decrease in proliferative capacity and ability to perform specialized functions. The diminished proliferative capacity appears to be controlled by the reduction of key transcription factors. Recent investigations have elucidated the changes in gene expression in the senescent cell.[5] Haynesworth and associates[6] have demonstrated that undifferentiated mesenchymal stem cells, which are so critical in the regeneration of the musculoskeletal system, decline with age, although their ability to migrate, proliferate, and differentiate remains intact.

Central to the aspects of musculoskeletal disability is impaired healing, which is related to increasing age.[7] This alternation of function may be a result of a decrease in the proliferative capacity of the cells as well as a diminished ability of the cells to synthesize new matrix. Further, there appears to be a diminished response of the cells and the tissue to specific growth factors such as transforming growth factor-beta.[5] It is clear from both clinical and experimental investigations that the biologic and mechanical characteristics of skeletal muscle, articular cartilage, intervertebral disk, tendon, ligaments, and joint capsules change with age and result in increased vulnerability of these tissues to injury and disease.

The consequences of a specific pathologic process in the elderly, such as osteoarthritis, can have various outcomes. Jette[1] has provided a model called the cycle of disablement, which explains the process of disability in the elderly. For example, osteoarthritis may result in a restricted range of motion and weakness in the knee that is manifested as a slow, unsteady gait and difficulty in rising from a chair. These latter outcomes are functional limitations that in themselves can increase the issues of lower extremity weakness and restriction of the range of motion of other lower extremity joints. Specific physical impairments and functional limitations will result in significant disability and further limitations in activities of daily living, leading to a loss of independence for the individual. In addition, the inactivity that occurs as a result of musculoskeletal impairment can affect the function of other systems, such as the cardiac and/or pulmonary systems.

If disability prevention strategies are to be accomplished, a greater understanding of the underlying mechanism of musculoskeletal disease in the elderly population is critical. Classic attempts at disability prevention have focused on primary prevention of disease. However, diseases such as osteoarthritis may not be preventable, considering the present level of understanding of its etiology. Therefore, secondary and tertiary prevention strategies that affect impairment, functional limitation, and ultimate disability need to be emphasized. For example, secondary prevention efforts designed for early detection of osteoarthritis and the implementation of specific treatment strategies to prevent the pathologic progression of the disease will go a long way toward preventing functional limitations and ultimate loss of independence. Tertiary prevention strategies that attempt to restore functional abilities by employing specific rehabilitation measures may have a wider application to the elderly population. One specific treatment intervention that has had a significant impact on maintenance of musculoskeletal function and prevention of disability is total joint arthroplasty. Although it is difficult to demonstrate a cost-benefit ratio, it is clear that this treatment modality has made significant contributions to maintenance of independence and a reduction in the need for institutionalization in the elderly. The orthopaedic challenges of the aging population require a greater understanding of the function of the aging musculoskeletal system, which will result in an improved basis of treatment of tissue injuries and disease as well as specific strategies to prevent impairment, functional limitation, and disability. There clearly is a need to address the problems of maintaining, improving, and restoring musculoskeletal function in older individuals and to increase our understanding of the prevention and treatment of loss of mobility, tissue trauma, and joint diseases.

Total Joint Arthroplasty in the Elderly

Osteoarthritis (OA) is the most common musculoskeletal disease in the elderly. Its presence has been reported radiographically in more than 80% of individuals older than 55 years, and it may be present in at least 40 million Americans.[4,8] Osteoarthritis of the hip and knee can result in significant impairment, disability, and loss of function. Radiographic evidence of OA of the knee has been reported in 40% of patients 80 years or older.[9] Similarly, radiologic changes of the hip have been reported in almost 12% of patients older than 80 years.[9] However, there is a high degree of variability in regard to specific clinical symptoms as reported by patients with both hip and knee OA. The relationship between the onset of OA and the aging process is poorly understood.[3] There have been reports of structural, biomechanical, and biochemical changes in articular cartilage, which lead to abnormalities of both cell and matrix components of hyaline cartilage.[9] There are a number of factors that increase the disability of the elderly as a result of OA of the hips and knees.[4] These include diminished joint proprioception, increased reaction time, unsteady gait from neurologic impairments, and an altered mental state manifested as significant depression, which can adversely affect the musculoskeletal system.

The advent of total joint replacement has made a significant impact on the treatment of elderly patients with disabling arthritis. Total joint arthroplasty has resulted in significant pain relief, functional improvement, and enhancement of the quality of life for the elderly. Although total joint replacement has significantly altered the treatment of arthritis of the elderly, a number of considerations must be reviewed prior to the recommendation of joint replacement of either the hip or the knee in this population.[10,11]

A number of systemic factors must be considered before total joint replacement can be recommended. Systemic disease, such as diabetes, atherosclerotic heart disease, or pulmonary function abnormalities, can adversely affect musculoskeletal function and may be relative contraindications to joint replacement. Other considerations in deciding whether to proceed with the replacement include hearing and eyesight deficits and the psychological status of the patient. Depression, one of the most frequently missed diagnoses in the elderly, can have a profound effect on musculoskeletal function and on the outcome of total joint replacement. Additional considerations are the patient's living environment and economic status. It is clear that the team approach to the management of musculoskeletal problems of the elderly improves the outcome. Close interaction of the orthopaedic surgeon with a medical-social worker interested in geriatrics, as well as a geriatric physician, is important in preparing the patient for a major surgical intervention. A number of specific factors can adversely affect the outcome of total joint arthroplasty in the elderly. Impaired wound healing, reduction of muscle strength, and incompetent ligaments can compromise the outcome of the arthroplasty and should be carefully considered. Bone stock deficiencies caused by osteoporosis and/or osteomalacia are also important considerations. Aging of the skeleton has a profound affect on the shape of the proximal femur. Noble and associates[12] have demonstrated differences in both the endosteal shape and diaphyseal dimensions of the young and the old female femora. The older female femora had wider canals at the level of the isthmus and a decrease in the canal flair index. Although these factors can adversely affect joint arthroplasty in the elderly, they usually can be managed by attention to technical detail and by having the appropriate component available, and they are not contraindications for the procedure. Although age is an important consideration in patient selection, it is not a contraindication for total joint replacement. A number of studies have reported successful outcome for patients in their 80s or 90s who have undergone total joint arthroplasty.[13-18] The general indications for total joint replacement include significant joint pain and decreased function, mobility, and independence. The patient's lack of response to an optimal medical management program, which includes judicious use of analgesics and rehabilitative considerations, is an important consideration in defining the role of total joint replacement for a specific patient. Because many of the elderly have a significant degree of depression associated with their disability, it is critical to treat the depressive state before undertaking surgical intervention so that the patient has a clear understanding of the goals of the surgery and has the motivation necessary to comply with the postoperative rehabilitative program.

Infection is the most serious contraindication in total joint replacement. Prior to surgery, an exhaustive search should be undertaken to exclude the presence of infection. Infections of the urologic system or of the gums and teeth must be diagnosed and treated prior to surgery. Other contraindications include lack of muscular control, as a result of cerebral vascular accidents, or significant systemic disease, either of which could adversely affect the surgical procedure.

The incidence of medical complications in total joint replacement has been reported to be as high as 70% in patients undergoing total hip replacement. Phillips and associates[15] and, more recently, Newington and associates[19] have indicated that the presence of a significant medical problem, such as chronic venous disease, cardiopulmonary compromise, and/or diminished mental status, may be enhanced by such orthopaedic complications as an intraoperative fracture or a joint dislocation. A preoperative assessment of the general status of the patient who is being considered for total joint replacement is important. Phillips and associates[15] have reported that the preoperative risk rating of the American Society of Anesthesiologists correlated with the postoperative complication rates. Those patients with an American Society of Anesthesiologists Class I had no complications; those of Class III had a 15% complication rate. Before surgery the patient should be comprehensively evaluated for problems in the following areas.[10] Cardiopulmonary status should be assessed and the patient should be evaluated for coronary artery disease, hypertension, and chronic obstructive pulmonary disease. Careful assessment of the urologic system should be performed, with particular emphasis placed on a history of urinary tract infections or benign prostatic hypertrophy. Either condition should be treated prior to surgery. The status of the teeth and gums should be checked for infection, because hematogenous seeding of a joint replacement is not an uncommon occurrence. Patients with a history of venous insufficiency or pulmonary embolism appear to be at a higher risk for recurrence after hip or knee arthroplasty. A patient with a history of recurrent pulmonary embolism may require the use of an inferior vena cava filter prior to surgery. Hematologic evaluation is important, with special emphasis placed on the identification of clotting dysfunctions. Liver abnormalities are not uncommon in the elderly, and specific hepatic functions, including prothrombin time, should be assessed. The comprehensive evaluation of the elderly prior to total joint replacement generally requires a team approach, and to ensure a successful outcome, the patient should be evaluated by both an orthopaedic surgeon and a geriatric physician in order to have optimal perioperative management.

Total Hip Arthroplasty in Patients Over 80 Years of Age

A number of studies have reported the outcome of total hip replacement (THR) in patients over 80 years of age. Levy and associates[20] reported that almost 90% of patients remain community walkers, and 96% of the patients remain independent. Newington and associates[19] reviewed the records of 113 consecutive patients 80 years of age and older who had THR and reported that this patient population had a higher incidence of complications than younger patients. He also reported a mortality of 4% secondary to cardiopulmonary failure during the perioperative period. Those patients who had perioperative complications, such as a dislocation, intraoperative fracture, or perforated shaft, had significantly diminished Harris Hip scores (HHS). Of the patients studied, 76% had a HHS of at least 60 and were considered satisfactory. Interestingly, those patients who were significantly disabled and dependent before surgery had outcomes similar to those of patients who were independent and less disabled. Nevertheless, although THR provided excellent pain relief and continued independence, almost 60% of the patients continued to use ambulatory aids.[19] The use of canes or crutches was required primarily because of unsteady gaits and neurologic disturbances. The incidence of perioperative complications for THR in the elderly appears to be higher than in the younger patients. Acute and chronic dislocations have been reported to have an incidence of between 4% and 15%, while the incidence of intraoperative femoral shaft fractures and perforations was 4.6%.[19] These latter complications resulted in a significantly poorer outcome. Levy and associates[20] reported that 6% of their patients had an early perioperative deterioration in mental status which did cause some difficulty in rehabilitation. However, these patients quickly recovered, and 98% of the patients felt subjectively satisfied with the outcome of the procedure. Perioperative mortality has been reported as high as 28% in patients older than 80 years of age, however, there is a wide discrepancy in the mortality rate for these patients, and, clearly, the incidence of significant complications does correlate directly with the American Society of Anesthesiologists' preoperative risk rating.[15]

Loosening of the components of THR is considered one of the primary causes of failure. In one series, 15% of implants loosened early in the aged population.[16] Levy and associates,[20] however, reported no instances of loosening of the hip in an average follow-up of 5 years with periods of observation as long as 12 years. Other mechanical complications, such as postoperative dislocations and perioperative femoral shaft fracture or perforation, clearly compromised the outcome of THR.[21] Although it has been difficult to evaluate the cost effectiveness of this procedure in the elderly, some assessment may be made. If one assumes an average cost of nursing home care in the United States of about $50,000 per year, preservation of an independent activity level after the joint replacement, rather than institutionalization, makes total joint replacement a very cost-effective treatment. Additionally, the need for secondary care givers is reduced after THR.

We recently evaluated the experience at our institution with THR in patients older than 80 years of age who were operated on between January 1984 and December 1993. During this period of time, we performed 211 THRs in 199 patients. There were 144 females and 55 males with an average age of 84 (range, 80 to 97.7). The diagnoses that necessitated the arthroplasty included 130 patients with osteoarthritis, 46 patients with a hip fracture, 10 patients with previously treated fractures that had failed, and 13 patients with rheumatoid arthritis. The average length of follow-up was 44 months (range, 24 to 132 months). Patients were evaluated pre- and postoperatively using the HHS, which assesses pain, function, and activities of daily living.[22] Early and late mechanical and biologic complications were noted.

During the period of observation, there were ten deaths, and 15 patients were lost to follow-up. Therefore, 186 hip replacements were evaluated in 174 patients. The average preoperative HHS was 26 (range 1 to 50), and the postoperative average was 90 (range 65 to 100). The pain score, which was 18 (range 0 to 35) preoperatively, improved to 40 (range 35 to 44) postoperatively. Results in 85% of the patients were considered excellent or good, and in 15% of the patients they were fair or less (Fig. 1). Those patients who had lower HHS were considered Class C functional patients with multiple joint or other systemic disease.

Complications included a perioperative fracture in two hips; both loosened ultimately and required revisions of the femoral components. Another patient experienced a postoperative neuropraxia of the femoral nerve, from which recovery was incomplete. Of 10 acute dislocations in this series (5%), three ultimately required revision of the acetabular component. During this period of observation, three additional hips required revision because of femoral loosening (Fig. 2).

The results of our review of patients who were 80 years of age or older at the time of primary THR is similar to those reported in the literature. The THR resulted in an outcome that maintained independence of the patient along with reduction in pain. However, when compared to younger patients, there was an increased incidence of perioperative complications, specifically acute dislocations. Reduction in perioperative mortality and complications and improved postoperative outcomes require a careful perioperative assessment of the patient, with particular emphasis on any systemic problems that need to be addressed prior to surgery. However, THR in the elderly can maintain a satisfactory level of independence, with improved pain relief and function.

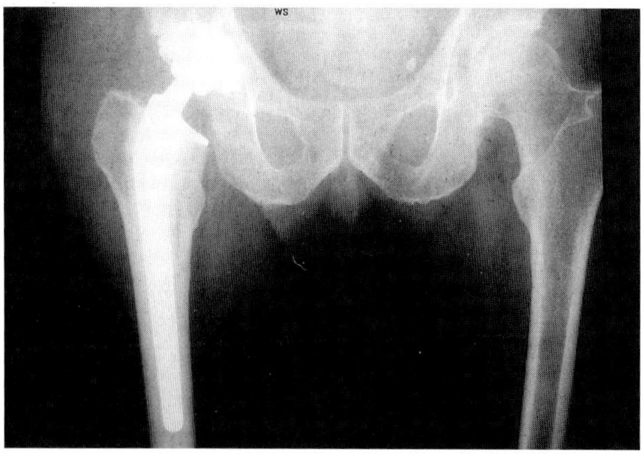

Fig. 1 Anteroposterior radiograph illustrating a well-fixed total hip replacement in an 85-year-old patient with a Harris Hip Score of 95, 8 years postoperative.

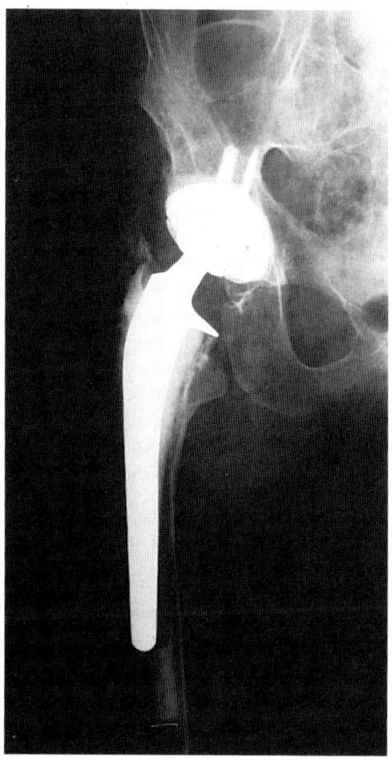

Fig. 2 Anteroposterior radiograph of an 81-year-old patient illustrating femoral loosening 4 years after the procedure. The patient was revised to another cemented femoral stem.

Total Knee Arthroplasty in the Elderly

Total knee arthroplasty has become a highly successful operation with consistent and reproducible outcomes. Recent reports of total knee replacement (TKR) in the very aged have indicated excellent functional and good pain relief with improved quality of life. However, as reported in the total hip population, most patients continue to use ambulatory assistive devices after surgery because of general problems, such as unsteadiness.[13,14] In contrast to the reports delineating increased complications for THR, Zicat and associates[14] and others[13] have reported no increase in complications in the elderly population undergoing TKR, and that pain relief in this group of patients was greater than in younger patients. Overall, good to excellent results have been reported in over 90% of patients who are older than 80 years of age.[13,14,22] TKR in the elderly appears to be a reliable and durable procedure and appears to have a successful outcome when compared to results in younger patients, as well as less risk for mechanical failure of the components. One study compared all-polyethylene tibial components to metal-backed tibial trays and found no difference between the two types of implants.[13] These researchers concluded that perhaps the all-polyethylene tibial component would be a viable alternative for the elderly, less active patient. Zicat and associates[14] compared the preoperative deformities of the patients older than 80 years of age to those of a younger, retiree group. The preoperative deformity of the octogenarian was significant greater, indicating a more advanced disease (Fig. 3). Further, these researchers reported that TKR for osteoarthritis in this elderly group was a reliable and cost-effective procedure. Tankersley and Hungerford[23] recently reported their results, which correlated well with previous reports of TKR in the very aged. Although pain relief was excellent in 18 of the 20 knees, most patients continued to use a cane and three patients required the use of a walker. There was no radiographic or clinical evidence of loosening of the components. They concluded that pain relief was good to excellent in most patients and that the complications were no greater than in a younger patient population. Most importantly, the quality of life for the elderly was significantly improved.

Our clinical experience with total knee arthroplasty in patients over 80 years of age was recently reviewed. All patients older than 80 years of age who underwent total knee replacement from February 1984 through December 1993 were reviewed. There were 257 knees in 203 patients. There were 161 females and 42 males, and the average age was 83.7 (range 80 to 97). Diagnoses were osteoarthritis in 170 patients, posttraumatic arthritis after fractures in 14, rheumatoid arthritis in six patients, and osteonecrosis in 13 patients. The average length of follow-up was 40 months, with a range of 24 to 128 months. The patients were evaluated preoperatively and postoperatively using a modified University Hospitals Knee Score, which assesses pain, function, and activities of daily living.[24] Revisions and complications were noted. During this period of time 12 patients died and five others were lost to follow-up. Therefore, 240 knee arthroplasties in 186 patients were available for the complete study.

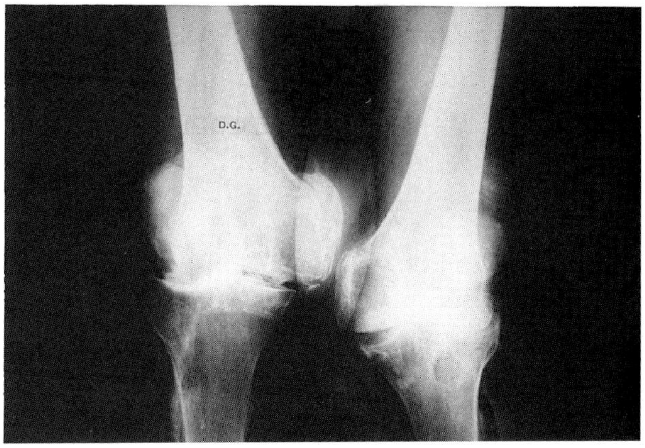

Fig. 3 Weightbearing anteroposterior radiograph of an 84-year-old patient demonstrating significant deformity of both knees.

Results in 80% of the patients were considered excellent or good; in 20% they were fair or less. Once again those patients who had a poorer knee score either had multiple joint involvement or significant systemic disease. Of the patients, 82% continued to use either a cane or walker postoperatively, primarily because of unsteadiness of gait or multiple joint involvement. Complications included symptomatic deep venous thrombosis in eight patients, two of whom had pulmonary emboli. One of these patients died in the immediate postoperative period. One patient with a significant genu valgus deformity had a clinically asymptomatic subluxation of the tibial component posteriorly. This patient has refused revision to the present time.

Revisions were necessary in two patients with two loose tibial components (Fig. 4). Both components were all polyethylene. One of the components loosened after 44 months; the other loosening occurred at 5 years post surgery. Both components were revised to metal-backed components and the patients continue to demonstrate satisfactory results, with knee scores of 76 and 82 respectively.

The results of this review of octogenarians undergoing primary TKR again compares favorably with those reported previously. In general, the patients demonstrated satisfactory functional outcomes with significant pain relief and maintenance of independence. However, a majority of them continued to use assistive

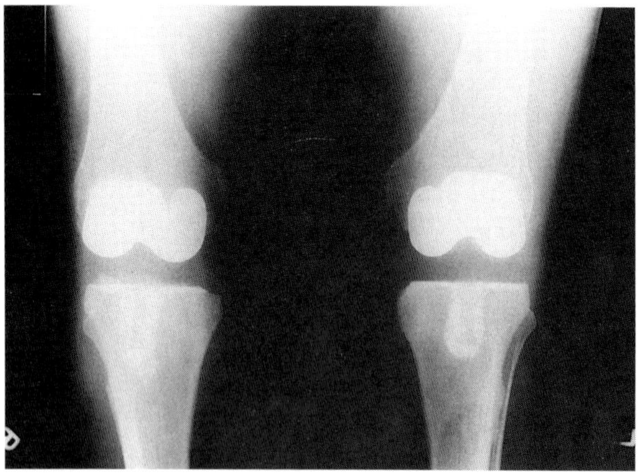

Fig. 4 Anteroposterior weightbearing radiograph of knees of an 86-year-old patient, 6 years after primary procedure, illustrating loosening of the right tibial component, which was revised successfully.

ambulatory devices, such as canes or walkers. By contrast to THR in patients of similar age, these patients demonstrated no increase in perioperative complications, although there was a significant incidence of venous thrombosis and pulmonary emboli.

In conclusion, total knee and hip arthroplasty are cost-effective, reliable, and durable procedures, which are effective in maintaining independence in this elderly patient population. Complications may be minimized by appropriate perioperative medical evaluation, careful planning, and a well-constructed postoperative rehabilitation program. Although pain relief is a consistent outcome, a significant number of these patients continue to use assistive ambulatory devices, primarily because of systemic or multiple joint disease.

References

1. Jette AM: Musculoskeletal impairments and associated physical disability in the elderly: Insights from epidemiological research, in Buckwalter JA, Goldberg VM, Woo SL-Y (eds): *Musculoskeletal Soft-Tissue Aging: Impact on Mobility*. Rosemont, IL, American Academy of Orthopaedic Surgeons, 1993, pp 7–22.
2. Cunningham LS, Kelsey JL: Epidemiology of musculoskeletal impairments and associated disability. *Am J Public Health* 1984;74:574–579.
3. Buckwalter JA, Woo SL, Goldberg VM, et al: Soft-tissue aging and musculoskeletal function. *J Bone Joint Surg* 1993;75A:1533–1548.
4. Schultz AB: Biomechanics of mobility impairment in the elderly, in Buckwalter JA, Goldberg VM, Woo SL-Y (eds): *Musculoskeletal Soft-Tissue Aging: Impact on Mobility*. Rosemont, IL, American Academy of Orthopaedic Surgeons, 1993, pp 23–33.
5. Campisi J: Mechanisms of aging that might contribute to musculoskeletal impairment: Diminished cell proliferative capacity in the elderly, in Buckwalter JA, Goldberg VM, Woo SL-Y (eds): *Musculoskeletal Soft-Tissue Aging: Impact on Mobility*. Rosemont, IL, American Academy of Orthopaedic Surgeons, 1993, pp 73–78.
6. Haynesworth SE, Goldberg VM, Caplan AI: Diminution of the number of mesenchymal stem cells as a cause for skeletal aging in the elderly, in Buckwalter JA, Goldberg VM, Woo SL-Y (eds): *Musculoskeletal Soft-Tissue Aging: Impact on Mobility*. Rosemont, IL, American Academy of Orthopaedic Surgeons, 1993, pp 79–87.
7. Buckwalter JA, Cruess RL: Healing of the musculoskeletal tissues, in Rockwood CA Jr, Green DP, Bucholz RW (eds): *Fractures*. Philadelphia, PA, JB Lippincott, 1991, pp 181–222.
8. Moskowitz RW: Osteoarthritis: Symptoms and signs, in Moskowitz RW, Howell DS, Goldberg VM, et al (eds): *Osteoarthritis: Diagnosis and Medical/Surgical Manage-ment*. Philadelphia, PA, WB Saunders, 1992, pp 255–261.
9. Lohmander S: Osteoarthritis: A major cause of disability in the elderly, in Buckwalter JA, Goldberg VM, Woo SL-Y (eds): *Musculoskeletal Soft-Tissue Aging: Impact on Mobility*. Rosemont, IL, American Academy of Orthopaedic Surgeons, 1993, pp 99–115.
10. Zuckerman JD, Sledge CB: Total joint replacement: Latest developments for the geriatric patient. *Geriatrics* 1985;40:71–85.
11. Goldberg VM: Surgical treatment of osteoarthritis. *J Musculoskelet Med* 1994;11:13–24.
12. Noble PC, Box GG, Kamaric E, et al: The effect of aging on the shape of the proximal femur. *Clin Orthop* 1995;316:31–44.
13. L'Insalata JL, Stern SH, Insall JN: Total knee arthroplasty in elderly patients: Comparison of tibial component designs. *J Arthroplasty* 1992;7:261–266.
14. Zicat B, Rorabeck CH, Bourne RB, et al: Total knee arthroplasty in the octogenarian. *J Arthroplasty* 1993;8:395–400.
15. Phillips TW, Grainger RW, Cameron HS, et al: Risks and benefits of elective hip replacement in the octogenarian. *Can Med Assoc J* 1987;137:497–500.
16. Ekelund A, Rydell N, Nilsson OS: Total hip arthroplasty in patients 80 years of age and older. *Clin Orthop* 1992;281:101–106.
17. Cohn BT, Krackow KA, Hungerford DS, et al: Approaches to senior care: 9. Results of total knee arthroplasty in patients 80 years and older. *Orthop Rev* 1990;19:451–460.
18. Pettine KA, Aamlid BC, Cabanela ME: Elective total hip arthroplasty in patients older than 80 years of age. *Clin Orthop* 1991;266:127–132.
19. Newington DP, Bannister GC, Fordyce M: Primary total hip replacement in patients over 80 years of age. *J Bone Joint Surg* 1990;72B:450–452.
20. Levy RN, Levy CM, Snyder J, et al: Outcome and long-term results following total hip replacement in elderly patients. *Clin Orthop* 1995;316:25–30.
21. Khan MA, O'Driscoll M: Fractures of the femur during total hip replacement and their management. *J Bone Joint Surg* 1977;59B:36–41.
22. Harris WH: Traumatic arthritis of the hip after dislocation and acetabular fractures: Treatment by mold arthroplasty. An end-result study using a new method of result evaluation. *J Bone Joint Surg* 1969;51A:737–755.
23. Tankersley WS, Hungerford DS: Total knee arthroplasty in the very aged. *Clin Orthop* 1995;316:45–49.
24. Goldberg VM, Figgie MP, Figgie HE III, et al: Use of a total condylar knee prosthesis for treatment of osteoarthritis and rheumatoid arthritis: Long-term results. *J Bone Joint Surg* 1988;70A:802–811.

CHAPTER 39

Orthopaedic Challenges in the Aging Population: Trauma Treatment and Related Clinical Issues

Kenneth J. Koval, MD
Joseph D. Zuckerman, MD

Introduction

Fractures in the elderly pose both medical and surgical challenges. More than any other age group, the elderly require individualized fracture management tailored to specific patient needs. Fracture management should be based on patient factors (preinjury medical and functional status) as well as injury factors (fracture level and degree of comminution, soft-tissue status, and multiple organ system involvement). We must avoid placing technology over reason, while trying to fully restore preinjury function.

Patient Factors

Preinjury Status

A detailed history of the patient's preinjury function must be obtained in order to establish a reasonable treatment plan. The management goals for an active community ambulator with a femoral neck fracture differ significantly from goals for an institutionalized nonambulator. In the first instance, surgical treatment is followed by aggressive rehabilitation to return the patient to preinjury ambulatory status. The second patient's situation, limited functional demands and limited rehabilitation potential, calls for a much less aggressive approach, probably nonoperative treatment with early mobilization from bed to wheelchair. In each case, preinjury function may be achieved, but with substantially different approaches.

Systemic Diseases

Elderly fracture patients often have preexisting medical problems that influence fracture management. Cardiopulmonary disease, common in this population segment, affects the patient's ability to tolerate prolonged recumbency, undergo surgery, and participate in rehabilitation. Cardiopulmonary disease is a major determinant of the rating system used by the American Society of Anesthesiologists to assess operative risk.[1] Patients with severe cardiopulmonary disease cannot tolerate prolonged surgery with extensive blood loss; fracture treatment modifications may be required.

Neurologic problems such as Parkinson's disease, Alzheimer's disease, and residual from a previous cerebrovascular accident must be considered during fracture management. In Parkinson's disease, clinical manifestations can range from mild tremors without significant functional limitations to complete incapacitation with severe contractures. Well-controlled disease should not alter choice of fracture treatment. Stroke patients are at increased risk for fracture, primarily because of residual balance and gait problems and osteoporosis of the paretic limb. The fractures usually occur on the affected side.[2,3] Treatment of these patients may be problematic because of the presence of osteoporosis, spasticity, and/or contracture. A worse functional prognosis can be expected if the fracture occurs within 1 week of the stroke. As with Parkinson's disease, the degree of involvement may vary widely, ranging from minimal spasticity without contracture in ambulatory patients to severe spasticity and contracture in nonambulatory patients. The treatment approach must be individualized; a treatment plan that involves a high degree of patient cooperation, for example, would be inappropriate for a patient with Alzheimer's disease.

Endocrinologic problems, particularly diabetes, are common in the elderly. Diabetic patients are generally immunosuppressed and have vascular compromise secondary to small vessel disease.[4] Immunosuppression increases the risk of infection, while vascular compromise increases the risk of wound complications, including skin slough. Diabetic patients have prolonged time to fracture union, especially after open reduction and internal fixation.[4] Nonsurgical treatment of some fractures may be preferable in diabetic patients, particularly if there is a preexisting diabetic ulcer near the planned operative field.

Vascular insufficiency, either venous or arterial, also presents management difficulties in the treatment of the elderly. Arterial insuf-ficiency is manifested by shiny, atrophic skin, absent hair, and diminished or absent pulses. Venous insufficiency is characterized by peripheral edema, skin discoloration, and ulcer formation, particularly around the malleoli. Patients with vascular insufficiency have compromised healing potential of both fractures and surgical incisions. However, they also present the problem of fragile skin, which is susceptible to breakdown even in a well-padded cast.

Bone Quality

Elderly patients are frequently osteopenic. Osteopenia refers to a decrease in bone mass and may be caused by either osteoporosis (decreased bone density with normal bone mineralization) or osteomalacia (decreased bone matrix mineralization with or without a change in bone density). Although senile osteoporosis remains the most common etiology of osteopenia in the elderly, the presence of severe osteopenia necessitates a comprehensive medical evaluation to identify possible treatable causes, such as nutritional deficiencies, hyperparathyroidism, renal disease, Cushing's disease, and tumors.[5]

Osteopenia has a strong influence on fracture management because it decreases the potential for the surgeon to achieve stable fixation and allow early range of joint motion. Plates and screws may provide suboptimal fixation in osteopenic bone secondary to decreased screw pull-out strength. In addition, stress risers, which are created by the screws as well as the end of the plate, may cause subsequent fracture.

Osteopenic patients are at increased risk for the development of delayed union and nonunion. The fracture callus is less dense and less well organized than that formed following fracture in nonosteopenic bone. Immobilization of the injured extremity further exacerbates bone loss. Bone grafts are frequently needed in osteopenic patients at the time of internal fixation. Use of allograft bone is usually necessary because the iliac crest often does not provide enough cancellous bone.

Soft-Tissue Quality

The most characteristic change in muscle tissue related to aging is loss of muscle mass secondary to a decrease in the size and/or number of muscle fibers.[6,7] The functional changes associated with aging of neuromuscular tissue include alterations in strength, reaction time, reflexes and reflex time, speed of contraction, coordination, and endurance.[8,9] Loss of muscle strength affects the lower extremities more than the back and upper extremities. Use of plate and screws in patients with significant muscle atrophy may result in painful prominent hardware.

Soft-tissue status impacts patient care and choice of implant. As a result of aging, the skin becomes more fragile and less tolerant of surgical insult. The presence of decubiti near the fracture site is a relative contraindication to surgery and will dictate the surgical approach. Age-related attrition can compromise soft-tissue repair; aggressive surgical management requiring prolonged rehabilitation may not be warranted in patients with preexisting severe tendinous compromise (ie, rotator cuff disease).

Injury Factors

Polytrauma

Patients older than 65 years of age represent a disproportionate 28% of all fatal injuries in the United States, despite constituting only 12% of the population.[10,11] For a given level of trauma, mortality and morbidity are greater in the geriatric patient than in the younger patient. Traditional trauma rating systems, designed to help triage polytrauma patients and predict mortality, are less reliable and predictive in the elderly.[12,13] The poor reliability and predictability of these scoring systems may be related to the effects of aging and associated medical comorbidities.[12]

Identification of skeletal injuries in the geriatric trauma patient requires vigilance. The presence of fractures should, however, always be considered in major trauma; visceral injuries rarely occur in the absence of orthopaedic injuries in the geriatric polytrauma patient.[14] Long-bone injuries should be immobilized to minimize the risk of fat embolization and reduce the risk of hemorrhage secondary to fragile tissue planes which, in the elderly, may fail to tamponade bleeding. Pelvic fractures represent the greatest acute orthopaedic threat to the patient. Hemorrhage is commonplace in geriatric patients with pelvic fractures; the overall mortality from either the acute or delayed complications of pelvic fractures (hemorrhage or sepsis) is nearly 17%, but approaches 81% in cases of open pelvic fractures in the elderly.[11] Early stabilization of long-bone and pelvic fractures facilitates patient mobilization and optimizes respiratory function.[15]

Open Fractures

Open fractures require emergent treatment. Preexisting vascular insufficiency, diabetes mellitus, immunocompromise, and osteopenia increase the risk of treatment complications in the elderly. To optimize treatment results, the basic principles of open fracture management must be followed.[16,17] The priorities of meticulous soft-tissue and osseous debridement, fracture stabilization, and soft-tissue coverage with early bone grafting, when appropriate, apply to all patients. Open fractures in the elderly, particularly fractures of the lower extremity, should be treated as limb-threatening injuries, with close adherence to established treatment principles.

Special Considerations

Periarticular Fractures

The management of periarticular fractures in the elderly must be individualized. Successful open reduction, with anatomic joint restoration and stable fixation to allow early range of joint motion, is optimal and should be considered in simpler fracture patterns.

Primary prosthetic replacement for comminuted periarticular fractures avoids such early and late fracture complications as delayed nonunion, nonunion, loss of fixation, and osteonecrosis. Prosthetic replacement should be considered for displaced, comminuted fractures of the femoral neck and proximal humerus. The indications for primary prosthetic replacement in the treatment of acute distal femur fractures have not been defined; prosthetic replacement requires use of a modular or custom-designed constrained implant in order to compensate for the loss of bone stock and ligamentous support. However, prosthetic replacement also introduces a new set of potential complications, such as prosthetic dislocation and loosening.

Intra-articular fractures involving an arthritic joint are generally unique to the elderly patient. In this situation, it may be necessary to consider primary total joint arthroplasty. A displaced femoral neck fracture associated with significant hip arthrosis, for example, is an indication for a primary total hip arthroplasty. This is also true of a comminuted proximal humerus fracture with associated glenohumeral arthritis.

Periprosthetic Fractures

Fractures around total joint replacements or other orthopaedic implants are challenging. Fortunately, these fractures are relatively rare, with reported frequency as low as 0.4% to as high as 7.8%.[18,19] They occur more frequently in women than men. Risk factors include osteopenia and previous revision surgery of any type. Treatment of periprosthetic fractures can be simple and straightforward, such as for nondisplaced fractures near total elbow or total shoulder replacements. Treatment of displaced fractures involves a choice between nonsurgical and surgical management and must be individualized (Fig. 1). Treatment goals are early patient mobilization, preservation of the limb mechanical axis, and stability of the bone-implant-cement interface. Nonsurgical treatment may result in mechanical axis malalignment and increased complexity of later revision surgery. In addition, nonsurgical management requiring recumbency increases the likelihood of pulmonary and genitourinary complications, as well as thrombophlebitis. Surgical treatment is complicated by the presence of the prosthesis and cement mantle and may be further complicated by significant osteopenia. Under these circumstances, stable fixation may not be possible and may limit postoperative patient mobilization.

Periprosthetic fractures commonly occur at or near the end of a plate or prosthetic stem, thereby limiting the choice of fixation device or use of fixation entirely. The fracture may also compromise the stability and fixation of the prosthesis within the medullary canal. This is sometimes obvious, such as when the fracture occurs around the prosthesis with subsequent loss of position. When the fracture does not seem to be intimately associated with the prosthesis and its cement mantle, however, traumatic loosening may go undetected until the fracture heals and the patient is weightbearing. In addition, malunion of any degree may exert sufficient abnormal stresses on the prosthesis to cause premature loosening.

A final important factor to consider is the high complication rate following periprosthetic fractures. Compared with fractures not associated with existing

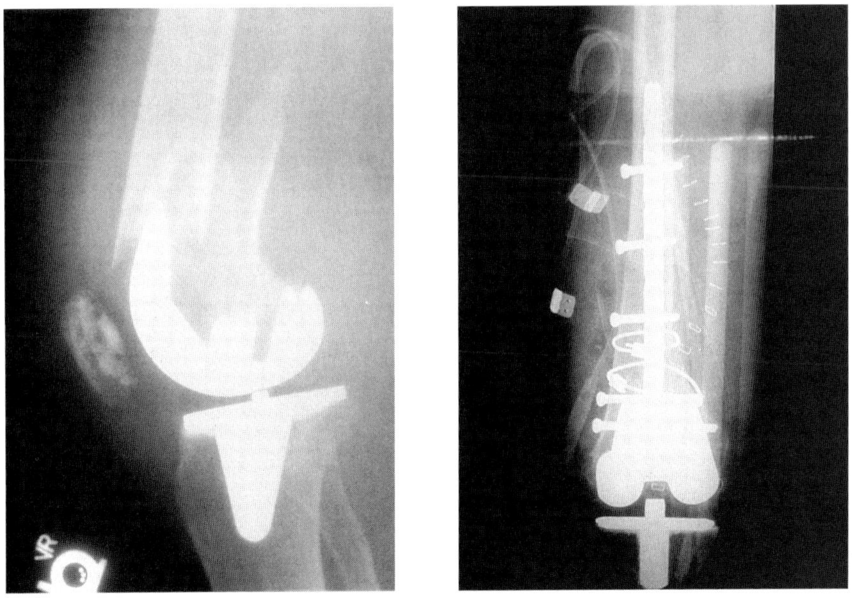

Fig. 1 **Left,** Comminuted supracondylar distal femur fracture proximal to a cemented total knee. **Right,** Stabilized with a locked intramedullary nail and cerclage wire.

implants, there is an increased risk of nonunion, malunion, and infection. The complication rate more closely resembles or exceeds that associated with revision joint replacement.[20] These complications may be secondary to loss of the intramedullary blood supply during the initial joint replacement, compounded by loss of the periosteal blood supply associated with fracture and any subsequent surgery.

Metastatic Disease

The skeleton is the third most common site of distant metastases. The incidence of bone involvement in patients with known malignancy varies in the literature from a low of 12% to as much as 70% in autopsy studies.[21,22] Some metastases predispose to fracture more commonly than others. Breast cancer, for example, results in pathologic fractures in up to 60% of patients with skeletal metastases.[23]

The proximal femur is involved in over 50% of long-bone pathologic fractures, and fractures are more likely to occur here than in other sites because of the significant concentration of mechanical stress in this region.[24] The distribution of metastases to the femoral neck, intertrochanteric, and subtrochanteric regions varies in the literature but appears to be equally divided.

Treatment of pathologic fractures should be directed toward rapid patient mobilization. Surgical management using internal fixation, with or without cement augmentation or prosthetic replacement, is the standard of care in treating pathologic fractures, especially neoplastic fractures of the femur.[25] This treatment approach restores function, alleviates pain, facilitates nursing care, decreases the duration and cost of hospitalization, and improves patient morale. Surgical contraindications are few, and include general condition inadequate to tolerate the anesthesia and surgical procedure; mental obtundation or alteration of consciousness that preclude the need for local measures to alleviate pain; and markedly limited life expectancy, ie, less than 1 to 2 months.

Paget's Disease

Pathologic fractures in Paget's disease are common, occurring most often in the femur, humerus, vertebral column, and pelvis. Controversy exists over union rates in these fractures; some authors report the healing rate to be normal, while most report an increased incidence of delayed union, nonunion, and refracture.[26,27] The treatment goal for patients with Paget's disease is rapid mobilization out of bed; prolonged recumbency can result in hypercalcemia.

Surgical treatment of fractures in patients with Paget's disease is associated with complication rates approaching 50%.[28] This is due in part to the variable quality and characteristics of pagetoid bone encountered at the time of surgery. The bone may be extremely hard, soft, normal, or profusely hemorrhagic, all of which are impossible to predict or anticipate preoperatively. It may be difficult to drill or insert screws into sclerotic bone (which may "explode" on forceful attempts). At the opposite extreme, it may be virtually impossible to achieve secure and stable prosthetic placement in soft bone. Osseous deformity and the tendency for excessive bleeding are often encountered (Fig. 2). Because of the difficulties achieving union and the frequency of surgical complications, management of these fractures must be individualized, with careful preoperative planning and meticulous intraoperative technique.

Surgical Issues

Surgical Indications

Absolute indications for surgical fracture treatment regardless of age are open fracture, compartment syndrome, and neurovascular compromise. Relative surgical indications include displaced intra-articular fractures, diaphyseal fractures in which an acceptable reduction cannot be obtained or maintained nonsurgically, and those fractures that require stabilization in order to mobilize the patient out of bed. Fracture management in the elderly must be individualized and take into consideration all of the injury and patient factors discussed previously. Fracture deformity may not equate with dysfunction, particularly in the upper extremity.

Timing of Surgery

The timing of surgery for isolated fractures in the elderly is controversial. In general, surgery should be performed as soon after injury as possible after stabilization of all comorbid medical conditions, particularly cardiopulmonary and fluid and electrolyte imbalances. In a series of hip fracture patients, Kenzora and associates[29] reported that a surgical delay of less than 1 week that permitted stabilization of medical problems was not associated with an increase in mortality. Interestingly, they found that even healthy patients who underwent surgery within 24 hours had a 34% mortality at 1 year follow-up, compared to only 5.8% for those who underwent surgery between the second and fifth days. On the other hand, Sexson and Lehner[30] found that relatively healthy hip fracture patients (up to two comorbid conditions) who had surgery within 24 hours after admission had a higher survival rate than those relatively healthy patients who had surgery after 24 hours. However, patients with three or more comorbid conditions had a lower survival rate when operated on within 24 hours than did those operated upon after 24 hours. In a prospective series of 367 elderly hip fracture patients, Zuckerman and associates[31] reported that a

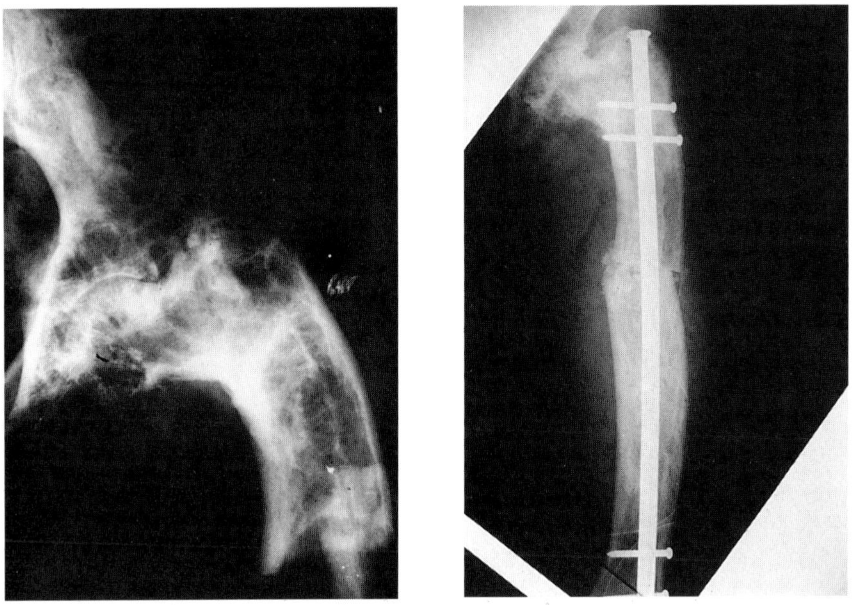

Fig. 2 **Left,** Proximal femur fracture in a patient with Paget's disease and osseous deformity. **Right,** Stabilized with an intramedullary nail after lateral wedge osteotomy.

surgical delay of more than 2 days from hospital admission approximately doubled the risk of the patient dying before the end of the first postoperative year; this relationship was significant when the factors of age, sex, and number of comorbidities were controlled. When the patient's age, sex, and severity of comorbidities were controlled, there was also an increase in mortality associated with surgical delay, but this increase was not statistically significant.

Anesthesia Considerations

Although much has been written on the risks and benefits of the different anesthesia techniques, no significant differences in survival rates have been found in elderly hip fracture patients undergoing surgery under regional or general anesthesia.[32,33] Although many anesthesiologists, internists, and surgeons believe that patients look better following regional anesthesia, studies have documented no difference in postoperative mental status in patients following regional or general anesthesia. Studies have demonstrated the efficacy of regional anesthesia (spinal and epidural) in the prophylaxis of deep vein thrombosis and pulmonary embolus.[34] Because pulmonary embolism is a significant cause of mortality in the elderly, regional anesthesia may be preferable, especially if other medical factors compromise use of thromboprophylaxis.

Implant Choice

The goal of internal fixation is to achieve anatomic joint reduction with stable osseous fixation to allow early range of joint motion. Stability is provided by fracture impaction, not by implant rigidity; fracture impaction restores structural continuity and allows force transmission across the fracture fragments rather than through the implant. This decreases the forces on the implant and protects it from mechanical overload.

The implant of choice for patients with osteopenic bone is an intramedullary device (Fig. 3). Intramedullary nails are positioned closer to the mechanical axis and are thus less likely to fail by fatigue than plates. In addition, they can function as load-sharing devices that align the ends of the bone yet allow force transmission across the fracture. Plates depend on the holding power of the screw in bone to obtain and maintain compression across a fracture surface and provide stable plate-osseous attachment. Bone density is the most important biologic factor affecting holding power. If there is any gap between the fracture ends, the plate will keep the fragments separated, making it a load-bearing device.

Fixation Enhancement

Methylmethacrylate can be used to enhance screw fixation in osteoporotic patients with minimal cortical holding power (Fig. 4).[35] Liquid methylmethacrylate is injected with a syringe into the loose screw hole, and the screw is then inserted. Precooling the cement monomer gives the surgeon increased time for the procedure. If the screw is turned as the methylmethacrylate sets, the holding power is diminished; if the methylmethacrylate hardens and the screw is then tapped, the holding power is also diminished. Therefore, the screw should be fully placed in the cement while it is still soft, and tightened after the cement has

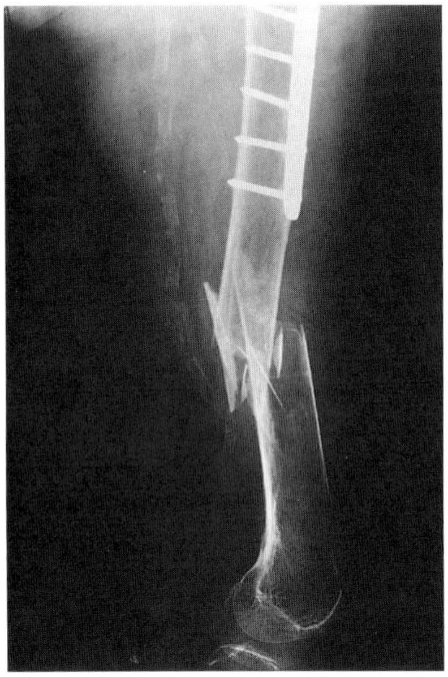

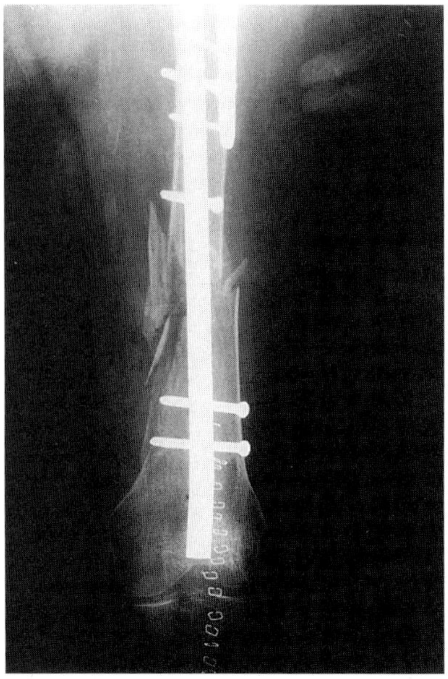

Fig. 3 **Left,** Comminuted distal femur fracture below a fixed angle plate in an 80-year-old female. **Right,** After removing the distal plate screws, the fracture was stabilized with a locked intramedullary nail and the plate screws were then reinserted.

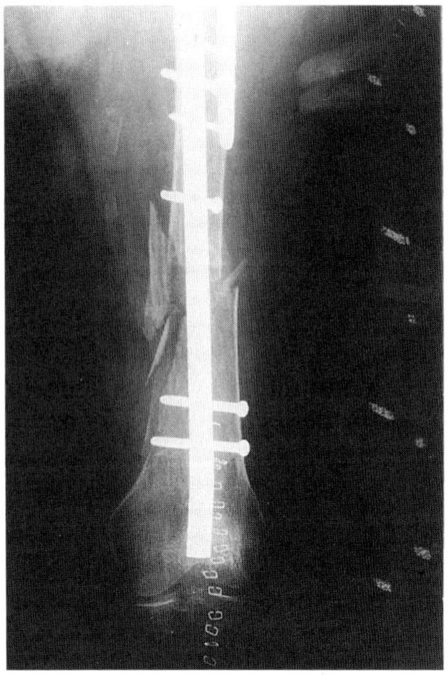

Fig. 4 Cement is used to augment screw fixation in an elderly woman with a distal humeral nonunion.

set.[35] Extravasation of the methylmethacrylate into the fracture site and the surrounding soft tissue is to be avoided.

Placement of a nut on the opposite cortex of a bolted bone screw increases the screw pull-out strength and lessens the risk of screw backout from the plate. Screws can be locked to the plate either with a nut placed under the plate or through use of a tapped hole plate (Fig. 5). Locking the screws to the plate causes the plate-screw construct to act as a fixed-angle device. Toggling of the screws within the plate is prevented, lessening the risk of fracture displacement. Intramedullary devices can be used in conjunction with plates and screws to increase fixation stability. A recent study reported that use of intramedullary Kirschner wires in conjunction with plate and screws provided fixation of comminuted and osteopenic ankle fractures superior to that achieved by plate and screws alone.[36]

Postoperative Management

Postoperative management should focus on early patient mobilization to avoid the complications of recumbency. Thromboembolic prophylaxis should be considered, particularly in patients with lower extremity fractures. The patient's weightbearing status is based on the fracture pattern, implant choice, and fracture stability. Geriatric patients have great difficulty ambulating with restricted weightbearing; this results in significant limitation in their ability to regain their former level of ambulation. Therefore, the goal of fracture management, including implant selection, should be to allow the patient weightbearing ambulation as tolerated.

The contribution of psychosocial factors to an elderly patient's recovery from orthopaedic injury is an important but often neglected aspect of patient care. Most physicians focus on and adequately treat the medical and surgical problems but overlook the psychosocial issues that can adversely affect treatment outcome. Immediately prior to injury, a patient may be

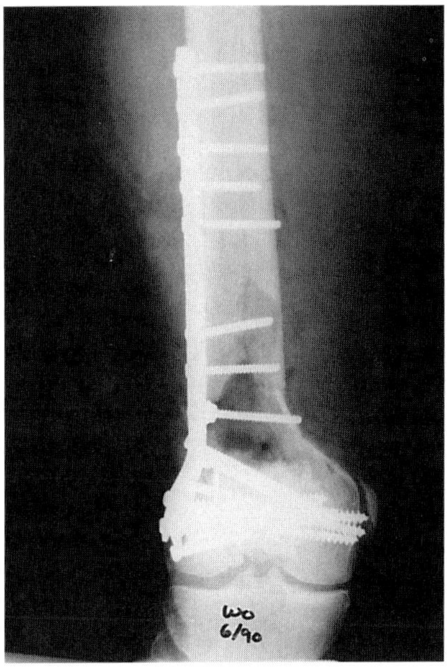

Fig. 5 Use of a nut to lock the screw to the plate.

flourishing within his or her environment with a strong support network, financial security, and a positive outlook. After injury and an extended hospital stay, return home may be possible only if home services can be arranged. The importance of psychosocial factors on treatment outcome in the geriatric population cannot be overestimated and requires close scrutiny by all medical staff involved in the care of these patients.

Maintenance of adequate nutritional status is of primary concern in hospitalized elderly patients, with requirements significantly elevated in the posttraumatic catabolic period marked by increased metabolic demands. Inadequate nutritional status, quantified by hypoalbuminemia, negative nitrogen balance, and anergy, will predispose to immunoincompetence and subsequent wound infection or sepsis. Patterson and associates[37] reported a high incidence (59%) of protein depletion in a series of geriatric hip fracture patients. Protein depletion resulted in an increased incidence of postoperative complications, such as poor wound healing and formation of decubitus ulcers. Parenteral nutrition may thus be warranted at an early stage to assist in musculoskeletal healing and rehabilitation. Once the alimentary tract becomes functional, enteral feeding may be instituted.

Because of the complexities involved in treating hospitalized elderly patients, it has been suggested that their care should be comprehensive and integrated, provided by teams of health-care personnel working in dedicated units. Several studies have documented the efficacy of such collaborative practice in the treatment of the elderly hip fracture patient.[38,39] By improving surgical treatment, beginning weightbearing immediately, and initiating an intensive rehabilitation program in the hospital followed by a home program, Ceder and associates[38] successfully decreased the length of hospital stay and decreased the need for postdischarge institutionalization. Zuckerman and associates[39] compared the results of an interdisciplinary hospital care program treatment of 431 community dwelling geriatric hip fracture patients to a historical set of 60 matched geriatric hip fracture patients treated before the start of the program. The program patients had fewer postoperative complications, significantly fewer intensive care unit transfers, significantly improved ambulatory ability at discharge, and fewer discharges to nursing homes.

Conclusion

Fracture treatment in the elderly must be based on a careful assessment of both the patient and the fracture. Many important patient characteristics impact on fracture management. Conversely, fracture management must be chosen in the context of the patient's preinjury medical and functional status, and should be individualized. Medical stabilization, surgical timing, implant selection, and postoperative management all affect outcome and must be considered as essential elements of patient care.

References

1. Owens WD, Felts JA, Spitznagel EL Jr: ASA physical status classifications: A study of consistency of ratings. *Anesthesiology* 1978;49:239–243.
2. McClure J, Goldsborough S: Fractured neck of femur and contralateral intracerebral lesions. *J Clin Pathol* 1986;39:920–922.
3. Soto-Hall R: Treatment of transcervical fractures complicated by certain common neurological conditions, in Reynolds FC (ed): *Instructional Course Lectures XVII.* St. Louis, MO, CV Mosby, 1960, vol 17, pp 117–120.
4. Loder RT: The influence of diabetes mellitus on the healing of closed fractures. *Clin Orthop* 1988;232:210–216.
5. Lane JM, Vigorita VJ: Osteoporosis. *J Bone Joint Surg* 1983; 65A:274–278.
6. Kalu DN, Masoro EJ: The biology of aging, with particular reference to the musculoskeletal system. *Clin Geriatr Med* 1988; 4:257–267.
7. Tomonaga M: Histochemical and ultrastructural changes in senile human skeletal muscle. *J Am Geriatr Soc* 1977;25:125–131.
8. McCarter R: Effects of age on contraction of mammalian skeletal muscle. *Aging* 1978;6:1–21.
9. Murray MP, Duthie EH Jr, Gambert SR, et al: Age-related differences in knee muscle strength in normal women. *J Gerontol* 1985;40:275–280.
10. Broos PL, Stappaerts KH, Rommens PM, et al: Polytrauma in patients of 65 and older: Injury patterns and outcome. *Int Surg* 1988;73:119–122.
11. Martin RE, Teberian G: Multiple trauma and the elderly patient. *Emerg Med Clin North Am* 1990;8:411–420.
12. DeMaria EJ, Kenney PR, Merriam MA, et al: Survival after trauma in geriatric patients. *Ann Surg* 1987;206:738–743.

13. Horst HM, Obeid FN, Sorensen VJ, et al: Factors influencing survival of elderly trauma patients. *Crit Care Med* 1986; 4:681–684.
14. Oreskovich MR, Howard JD, Copass MK, et al: Geriatric trauma: Injury patterns and outcome. *J Trauma* 1984;4: 565–572.
15. Bone L, Bucholz R: The management of fractures in the patient with multiple trauma. *J Bone Joint Surg* 1986;68A:945–949.
16. Gustilo RB, Anderson JT: Prevention of infection in the treatment of one thousand and twenty-five open fractures of long bones: Retrospective and prospective analyses. *J Bone Joint Surg* 1976;58A:453–458.
17. Gustilo RB, Simpson L, Nixon R, et al: Analysis of 511 open fractures. *Clin Orthop* 1969;66:148–154.
18. Scott RD, Turner RH, Leitzes SM, et al: Femoral fractures in conjunction with total hip replacement. *J Bone Joint Surg* 1975;57A:494–501.
19. Zickel RE, Fietti VG Jr, Lawsing JF, et al: A new intramedullary fixation device for the distal third of the femur. *Clin Orthop* 1977;125:185–191.
20. Johansson JE, McBroom R, Barrington TW, et al: Fracture of the ipsilateral femur in patients with total hip replacement. *J Bone Joint Surg* 1981;63A:1435–1442.
21. Clain A: Secondary malignant disease of bone. *Br J Cancer* 1965;19:15–29.
22. Jaffe HL: *Tumors and Tumerous Conditions of Bones and Joint.* Philadelphia, PA, Lea & Febiger, 1958.
23. Parrish FF, Murray JA: Surgical treatment for secondary neoplastic fractures: A retrospective study of ninety-six patients. *J Bone Joint Surg* 1970;52A:665–686.
24. Harrington KD: Impending pathologic fractures from metastatic malignancy: Evaluation and management, in Anderson LD (ed): American Academy of Orthopaedic Surgeons *Instructional Course Lectures XXXV.* St. Louis, MO, CV Mosby, 1986, pp 357–381.
25. Harrington KD, Sim FH, Enis JE, et al: Methylmethacrylate as an adjunct in internal fixation of pathological fractures: Experience with three hundred and seventy-five cases. *J Bone Joint Surg* 1976;58A:1047–1055.
26. Milgram JW: Orthopedic management of Paget's disease of bone. *Clin Orthop* 1977;127:63–69.
27. Nicholas JA, Killoran P: Fracture of the femur in patients with Paget's disease: Results of treatment in twenty-three cases. *J Bone Joint Surg* 1965;47A:450–461.
28. Dove J: Complete fractures of the femur in Paget's disease of bone. *J Bone Joint Surg* 1980;62B:12–17.
29. Kenzora JE, McCarthy RE, Lowell JD, et al: Hip fracture mortality: Relation to age, treatment, preoperative illness, time of surgery, and complications. *Clin Orthop* 1984;186:45–56.
30. Sexson SB, Lehner JT: Factors affecting hip fracture mortality. *J Orthop Trauma* 1987;1:298–305.
31. Zuckerman JD, Skovron ML, Koval KJ, et al: Postoperative complications and mortality associated with operative delay in older patients who have a fracture of the hip. *J Bone Joint Surg* 1995;77A:1551–1556.
32. Davis FM, Woolner DF, Frampton C, et al: Prospective, multicentre trial of mortality following general or spinal anaesthesia for hip fracture surgery in the elderly. *Br J Anaesth* 1987;59: 1080–1088.
33. Valentin N, Lomholt B, Jensen JS, et al: Spinal or general anaesthesia for surgery of the fractured hip? A prospective study of mortality in 578 patients. *Br J Anaesth* 1986;58:284–291.
34. Modig J, Borg T, Karlstrom G, et al: Thromboembolism after total hip replacement: Role of epidural and general anesthesia. *Anesth Analg* 1983;62:174–180.
35. Cameron HU, Jacob R, Macnab I, et al: Use of polymethylmethacrylate to enhance screw fixation in bone. *J Bone Joint Surg* 1975;57A:655–656.
36. Koval KJ, Petraco D, Kummer F, et al: A new technique for complex ankle fracture fixation: A clinical and biomechanical evaluation. Proceedings of the American Academy of Orthopaedic Surgeons 63rd Annual Meeting, Atlanta, GA. Rosemont, IL, American Academy of Orthopaedic Surgeons, 1996.
37. Patterson BM, Cornell CN, Carbone B, et al: Protein depletion and metabolic stress in elderly patients who have a fracture of the hip. *J Bone Joint Surg* 1992;74A:251–260.
38. Ceder L, Thorngren KG, Wallden B: Prognostic indicators and early home rehabilitation in elderly patients with hip fractures. *Clin Orthop* 1980;152:173–184.
39. Zuckerman JD, Sakales SR, Fabian DR, et al: Hip fractures in geriatric patients: Results of an interdisciplinary hospital care program. *Clin Orthop* 1992;274:213–225.

CHAPTER 40

Biomechanical Considerations of Hip and Spine Fractures in Osteoporotic Bone

Wilson C. Hayes, PhD
Elizabeth R. Myers, PhD

Introduction

Falls and fall-related injuries are among the most serious and common medical problems experienced by the elderly. In the United States each year approximately 30 million falls occur, an average of about one per second.[1-4] Even when no physical injury occurs, a fall can lead to fear of falling,[5] loss of confidence,[6] and functional deterioration.[5,7] Up to 25% of those who have fallen limit their daily activities because they fear falling again.[8,9] As noted by Cummings and Nevitt,[6] a fall can break self-confidence as well as bones.

Hip fracture, one of the most severe consequences of falling in the elderly, occurs in only about 1% of falls.[8,9] In the United States, nearly 300,000 hip fractures occur each year,[10] over 90% of them associated with falls.[11,12] Mortality in patients with a hip fracture is 12% to 20% higher than in persons of similar age, race, and sex who have not fractured a hip. The estimated annual costs of medical and nursing services related to hip fractures in the United States range from 7 to 10 billion dollars.[13,14] Moreover, continued growth in the elderly population can be expected to cause a dramatic increase in the number of hip fractures. If current demographic and incidence trends continue, the number of hip fractures may well double or triple by the middle of the next century.[15,16] Thus, as measured by their frequency, influence on quality of life, and economic cost, hip fractures are a public health problem of crisis proportion.

Identifying those at risk for harmful falls requires an understanding of what kinds of falls result in injury and fracture. Data are just beginning to emerge on what constitutes a fall with a high risk of hip fracture and how factors related to fall severity compare with those related to bone fragility. In a study of falls in elderly nursing home residents, we showed that impact on the hip or side of the leg raised the risk of hip fracture over twentyfold.[17] Nevitt and Cummings[18] reported that among elderly, community-dwelling women, those who sustained hip fractures were more likely to have fallen to the side or straight down and to have landed on or near the hip. By contrast, the risk of hip fracture about doubled for every standard deviation (SD) reduction in bone mineral density (BMD). In a prospective, case-control study in community-dwelling elderly men and women,[19] we showed that simply falling to the side raised the risk of hip fracture sixfold. A decrease of one SD in femoral neck BMD, an increase of one SD in potential energy, and a decrease of one SD in body mass index were all significant and independent risk factors for hip fracture in both sexes. Thus, in elderly persons who fall, in most of whom hip BMD is already more than two standard deviations below peak values, fall severity (as reflected in falling to the side and impacting the hip) and body habitus are important risk factors for hip fracture and touch on a domain of risk entirely missed by knowledge of bone mineral density.

These findings and others[20] clearly suggest that factors related to both loading and bone fragility play important roles in the etiology of hip fracture. In this overview, a strategy based on engineering approaches to fracture risk prediction[21] is provided for determining the relative importance of loading and bone fragility in the etiology of hip and vertebral fracture. From an overview of the complex interplay between the risks associated with the initiation, descent, and impact phases of a fall, we can then suggest an organized approach for evaluating the range of intervention efforts being used to prevent age-related fractures.

The Factor of Risk, Φ

To predict the risk of fracture of any structure, it is necessary to have information on both the imposed loads and the ultimate load-carrying capacity of the structure. This can be formalized by defining a factor of risk Φ as the ratio of the applied loads divided by the loads necessary to cause fracture, which can be written: Φ = Applied Load/Fracture Load,[1] in which Φ is the factor of risk. For a factor of risk much less than 1, fracture is unlikely. For a factor of risk close to or exceeding 1, fracture is considered likely. For either the proximal femur or spine, estimates of the factor of risk require information on the forces to which the skeletal region at risk is subjected and on the forces necessary to cause fracture under the same loading conditions. The forces to which these skeletal regions are subjected have been largely neglected in the literature on age-related fractures and osteoporosis. Instead, the focus has been on densitometric estimates of the denomina-

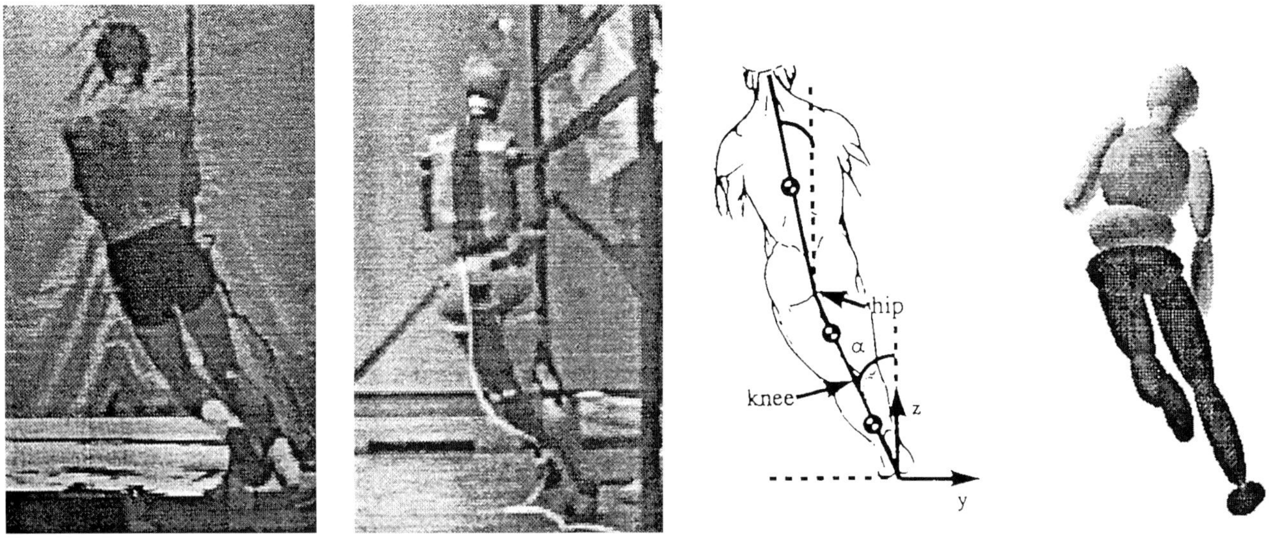

Fig. 1 Experimental and analytical studies of the descent phase of side falls. **Left,** Young adult volunteers; **center left,** 5th percentile Hybrid III crash dummy (Reproduced with permission from Hayes WC, Myers ER, Robinovitch SN, et al: Etiology and prevention of age-related hip fractures. *Bone* 1996;18(suppl):77S-86S.); **center right,** three-link model. (Reproduced with permission from van den Kroonenberg A, Hayes WC, McMahon TA: Dynamic models for sideways falls from standing height. *J Biomech Eng* 1995;117:309-318.); and **Right,** 15-segment Articulated Total Body Model (ATBM). (Reproduced with permission from Hayes WC, Myers ER, Robinovitch SN, et al: Etiology and prevention of age-related hip fractures. *Bone* 1996;18(suppl):77S-86S.)

tor of the factor of risk equation, neglecting the intuitively obvious but largely ignored notion that the applied forces can easily dominate the fracture process.

Side Fall Impact Forces: The Numerator of Φ for Hip Fracture

A fall has four distinct phases: (1) instability that results in a loss of balance; (2) descent; (3) impact; and (4) postimpact (when the subject comes to rest).[17] Previous research on falling in the elderly has focused almost entirely on those factors that result in a loss of balance, ie, the instability phase. By contrast, little is known about the mechanics of the fall itself or about how to define a high-risk fall.[22]

Fall Descent Our group has undertaken a series of experiments and analytical studies (Fig. 1) to determine the configurations and velocities of the body just before the hip strikes the impact surface, and to estimate the force applied to the hip during the impact itself. We have used young adult volunteers (Fig. 1, *left*), a 5th percentile female Hybrid III dummy (Fig. 1, *center left*), analytical models consisting of two- and three-link articulated segments coupled by torsional springs (Fig. 1, *center right*), and a 15-link (3D) model (Articulated Total Body Model, or ATBM) (Fig. 1, *right*) to represent the human body in a fall.[21,23,24]

Fall Impact To estimate the impact forces from a fall, we developed an experimental paradigm that we call the pelvis-release experiment (Fig. 2, *left*).[25] Measures were acquired with subjects in both a state of muscle relaxation and in a state of muscle contraction. The predicted peak forces as a function of fall height demonstrated dramatic increase in peak force for the muscle-active state in men, but not in women (Fig. 2, *right*). At a fall height of 0.7 m (a reasonable average value for a fall from standing height), the peak force in men was 6,100 N in the muscle-relaxed state and 12,100 N in the muscle-active state. Corresponding values for women were 5,050 N in the muscle-relaxed state and 6,370 N in the muscle-active state. Thus, striking the ground in a stiff state increases the impact force. This finding also confirms the widely assumed notion that falling while relaxed reduces the injury potential of a fall. For females, we also found that a threefold increase in soft-tissue thickness reduced predicted peak force by 35%, while no significant relation between peak force and soft-tissue thickness was observed among males. While these data from young subjects must be interpreted with caution when extrapolating to falls among the frail elderly, the findings emphasize the potential for large difference in fall impact forces due to trunk muscle activity and force attenuation in trochanteric soft tissues.[21,26]

Fracture Load of the Proximal Femur: The Denominator of Φ for Hip Fracture

To estimate the factor of risk Φ, the predicted impact force must be divided by the estimated fracture load of the proximal femur. Such estimates of fracture force can be provided by ex vivo studies of cadaveric femora tested in loading configurations that would simulate a fall with impact on the greater trochanter. Courtney and associates[27,28] tested paired specimens of

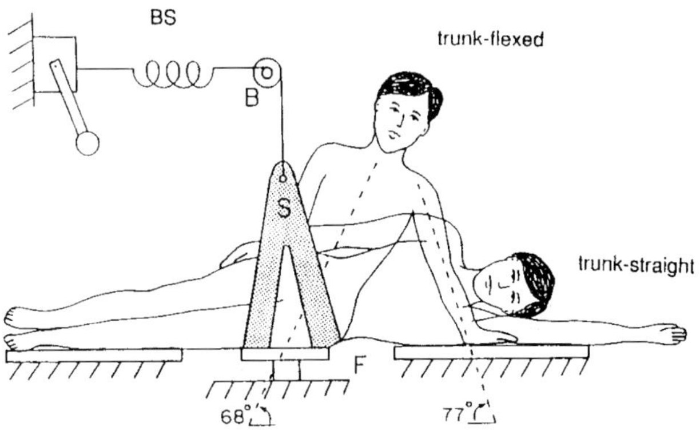

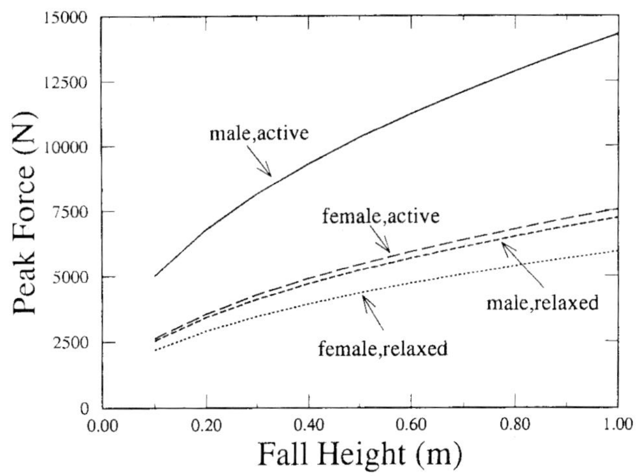

Fig. 2 Pelvis-release experiments for estimating impact forces in falls from standing height. **Left,** Trunk configuration at impact had little influence on impact force predicted using a standard linear solid model (inset) (Reproduced with permission from Hayes WC, Myers ER, Robinovitch SN, et al: Etiology and prevention of age-related hip fractures. *Bone* 1996;18(suppl):77S-86S.); **Right,** Effect of fall height and muscle activity on predicted peak impact force. (Reproduced with permission from Robinovitch SN, Hayes WC, McMahon TA: Prediction of femoral impact forces in falls on the hip. *J Biomech Eng* 1991;113:366-374.)

elderly cadaveric femora in a fall loading configuration under both slow and fast rates, the latter equivalent to those which would occur in a fall. Densitometric variables measured by dual energy x-ray absorptiometry (DXA) were strongly correlated with fracture load (Fig. 3).

Factor of Risk for Hip Fracture in Elderly Fallers

To provide a preliminary estimate of the factor of risk in elderly subjects, we conducted a case-control study to examine the strength of the association between the factor of risk Φ and hip fracture incidence in elderly subjects who fall. Subjects over age 65 who had sustained a fall, either with or without an accompanying hip fracture, were recruited from Boston's Beth Israel Hospital (fracture cases) and from the community or local long-term care facilities (controls without fracture). Bone mineral density of the proximal femur was assessed by DXA using a Hologic QDR-1000. We studied 231 subjects, including 98 hip fracture cases and 133 nonfractured control fallers. The mean age was 84 years, and 80% of the subjects were women. Calculation of the numerator of Φ (applied load) was based on pelvis-release experiments (Fig. 2).[25] Body weight was used to determine effective mass and body height was used to estimate fall height. The denominator (fracture load) was based on the linear association between BMD and femoral failure load in elderly cadaveric hips tested in a configuration simulating a sideways fall. The relationship between the factor of risk and hip fracture incidence was assessed by logistic regression.

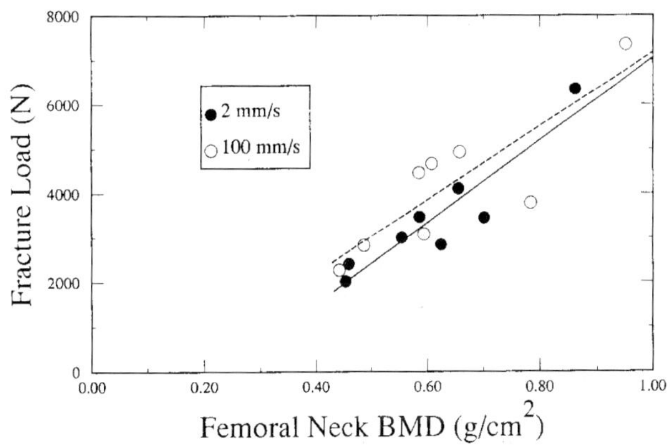

Fig. 3 Bone mineral density (BMD) of the femoral neck assessed with DXA versus fracture load of cadaveric femurs loaded in a fall configuration. Solid circles represent femurs tested at a displacement rate of 2 mm/s, and open circles represent femurs tested at a more realistic rate of 100 mm/s. At each displacement rate, fracture load correlates strongly with BMD (r^2 = 0.85 at 2 mm/s; r^2 = 0.65 at 100 mm/s). (Reproduced with permission from Hayes WC, Myers ER, Robinovitch SN, et al: Etiology and prevention of age-related hip fractures. *Bone* 1996;18(suppl):77S-86S.)

BMD of the femoral neck and estimated failure load of the proximal femur were 10% and 14% lower in fracture cases than in controls, respectively. The estimated load applied to the hip during the fall was slightly higher (4%) in fracture cases than in controls. The average factor of risk was 2.0 in fracture cases and 1.5 in controls, and there was a strong association between factor of risk and hip fracture (χ^2= 40, $p < 0.0001$). The odds of hip fracture increased by 4.8 for every standard deviation increase in the factor of risk (95% CI: 2.7-8.5). The odds ratio for a standard deviation decrease in BMD was 1.9 ($\chi^2 = 20$; 95% CI: 1.4-2.6). However, BMD was not significant in stepwise regression once the factor of risk was entered into the model. These findings indicate that the factor of risk is strongly associated with hip fracture. Furthermore, based on likelihood χ^2 values, the factor of risk is more strongly associated with hip fracture than femoral BMD. It may be that the factor of risk will be a more robust predictor of fracture risk than measures of femoral BMD alone.[29]

Implications for Hip Fracture Prevention

While the factor of risk provides a simple and intuitively satisfying way to examine the relative importance of fall severity and bone fragility in the etiology of hip fracture, it is based on the assumptions that a fall has occurred and that the fall causes the fracture. Thus, the factor of risk does not address the risk factors for falling or for experiencing falls with a high likelihood of injury. Moreover, it does not account for anecdotal reports and some experimental and clinical evidence that suggest spontaneous hip fractures associated with activities of daily living are frequently the precipitating cause of some falls. Although most surveys report a fall event associated with hip fracture in greater than 90% of cases,[30,31] there is some controversy over the role a fall plays in the etiology of hip fracture. Some believe that the proximal femur in the frail elderly can be broken by muscle forces during common activities, and that the fall is then a consequence of the fractured hip.[32,33] In one survey, 24% of hip fracture patients recounted falling as a result of the leg giving way.[32] Furthermore, in a consecutive sample of patients with femoral neck fracture that included 11% with spontaneous fractures, approximately 25% of the spontaneous fractures occurred while getting up or sitting down and an additional 60% occurred during walking.[34] These findings point to the interesting possibility that, in some proportion of cases, hip fractures are the result of loads applied by muscle contractions in common activities. This view of the etiology of hip fracture would suggest that factors related to bone fragility are the most important focus of prevention.

If, on the other hand, we assume that at least the majority of hip fractures are caused by falls, then an assessment of the prospects for hip fracture prevention should encompass those factors that lead to fall initiation as well as to a high factor of risk, Φ (Fig. 4). With respect to fall initiation, falls in the elderly are the consequence of many pathophysiologic processes associated with aging, and of various combinations of intrinsic, activity-related, and environmental factors.[35] In part because falls are such complex, multifactorial events, they have until recently proven remarkably resistant to prevention.[4,7,36] Recently, however, Tinetti and associates[37] reported that an intensive multifactorial risk factor abatement strategy could be used to decrease the percentage of subjects with falls from 47% in the control group to 35% in the intervention group. The cost per injurious fall prevented ($12,392) was high, however. Combined data from a number of intervention studies have also demonstrated that certain exercise programs reduce the fall incidence ratio in elderly patients to 0.83.[3] However, it remains to be determined whether fall prevention can be used successfully to prevent fall-related injuries or hip fracture, in part because falls that cause hip fracture may differ qualitatively from other falls.[17-19] Thus, while exercise for the prevention of falls appears to be a potentially successful intervention strategy, fracture prevention requires an intensive, multifactorial approach and is difficult to target to that

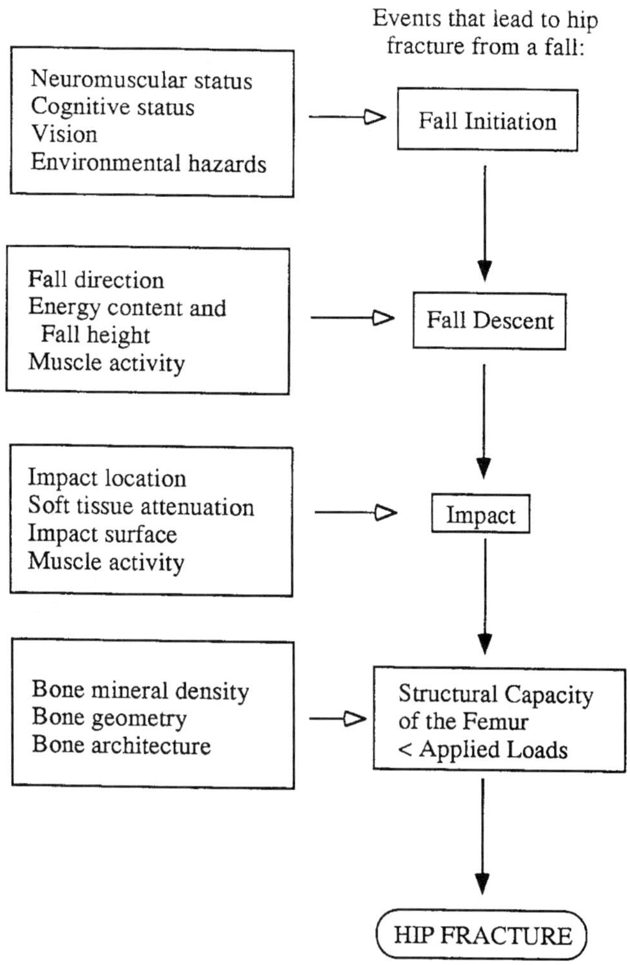

Fig. 4 Schematic view of the events that lead to hip fracture from a fall. Each of the primary determinants of hip fracture is associated with multiple fall, host, and environmental characteristics. (Reproduced with permission from Hayes WC, Myers ER, Robinovitch SN, et al: Etiology and prevention of age-related hip fractures. *Bone* 1996;18(suppl):77S-86S.)

small percentage of fallers who are at risk for fall-associated hip fractures. In light of this, there have also been a few attempts to prevent falls through the use of ceiling-mounted harness systems.[38,39]

With respect to the descent phase of falls (Fig. 4), it appears from available data[17-19] that falling to the side raises the risk of hip fracture roughly sixfold, compared to the threefold increase in relative risk associated with a one standard deviation reduction in hip bone mineral density. Despite this, little is known about the dynamics of falling to the side and, indeed, most research on postural stability, gait, and balance recovery has focused on motion in the plane of progression. During descent, it is also likely that eccentric contraction of the quadriceps and other muscles of the lower extremity is one of the most effective means to reduce velocity at impact and, thereby, the force delivered to the proximal femur. Thus, many of the exercise programs aimed at preventing fall initiation through increased lower extremity strength may also prevent hip fracture by reducing fall severity.[40]

With respect to the impact phase of falls, the primary focus of intervention efforts has been on the use of trochanteric padding systems to attenuate forces delivered to the proximal femur. The results of several recent intervention studies suggest that protective hip padding systems may lower the risk for hip fracture in a fall.[41,42] However, while fractures were prevented when pads were worn, subject compliance in wearing the pads was relatively low (approximately 25% in one study[41]) and user acceptance and compliance are difficult issues.[43] Even so, on an intention to treat basis, Lauritzen and associates[41] reported that their hip protector reduced fracture incidence by 53%.

Finally, as shown in Figure 4, the factor of risk can also be influenced by altering the structural capacity of the femur. While it is clear from our data and those of others that the structural capacity of the femur declines with reduced BMD, the structural consequences of increases in hip BMD that might occur with improved nutrition, pharmacologic agents, or exercise are largely unexplored. Our relationships between femoral neck BMD and fracture load indicate that an increase of more than 20% in BMD would be required to raise the mean fracture load to above the expected impact loads from a worst-case fall on the hip. Controlled trials of pharmacologic interventions have demonstrated increases of only a few percent in femoral neck BMD,[44,45] especially in the older elderly who are at greatest risk of fracture,[46] although recent studies of the bisphosphonate, alendronate, have indicated three-year changes as high as 5.9% in the hip.[47] While these results suggest the possibility of significant reductions in fracture risk through the use of osteodynamic agents, it will be important to understand how these increases in bone density and those associated with improved nutrition and exercise influence the load carrying capacity of the femur.

The Numerator of Φ for Vertebral Fractures

Gaining an understanding of the origin of vertebral fractures can be a more difficult endeavor than the etiology of hip fractures, because vertebral fractures are associated with a multitude of activities[48,49] and a progression of bony injury.[50] As stated by Melton and associates,[51] vertebral fractures have been considered synonymous with osteoporosis, although little is known about fracture epidemiology. The prevalence of vertebral fractures exhibits a rapid rise with age and is associated with low bone density of the spine.[51] Among clinically diagnosed vertebral fractures, 16% are discovered incidentally, indicating a gradual onset with no symptoms.[48] Therefore, it is difficult to attribute a loading activity and to determine a factor of risk for such fractures. Specific activities have been identified, however, for symptomatic vertebral fractures. In a population-based study of 341 fractures, of which 275 were symptomatic, 113 of symptomatic cases (41%) were associated with a fall and 29 (11%) with lifting.[48] In a hospital-based sample of vertebral fracture cases presenting at an emergency ward with back pain, approximately 50% occurred with a fall and 25% with controlled activities such as reaching, bending, lifting, and twisting.[49]

To estimate the forces on the vertebra during controlled activities such as lifting and bending, models of such activities have been adapted from previous studies of the lumbar spine.[52-54] The forces at a vertebral level of interest are found in two steps.[55] First, the forces in a transverse section at a specific spine level are found by static equilibrium. Then, an optimization routine is used to determine muscle forces and vertebral forces that balance the forces from the upper body force balance. Compressive forces on the second lumbar vertebral body for a 50th percentile female are typically 280 N for standing, 900 N for getting up from sitting, and 1660 N for lifting 15 kg. In comparison, compressive forces at the eighth thoracic level are typically lower than in the lumbar spine, with estimates of 200 N for standing, 590 N for getting up from sitting, and 1060 N for lifting 15 kg.[55] By contrast, little is known about the forces generated in the spine during impact from a fall.

Failure Force of the Vertebral Body: The Denominator of Φ for Vertebral Fractures

In parallel with the ex vivo studies of the proximal femur, failure tests of the vertebra have also been conducted. To use the failure force from such tests in the denominator of the factor of risk, the loading conditions in the testing system must mimic the loading conditions of fractures in vivo. In compression, the ultimate load of vertebrae is correlated in a significant and strong manner with densitometric measures from computed tomography and DXA.[56-59] The coefficient of the correlation of the ultimate load of the eleventh thoracic body with lumbar bone mineral density from DXA is 0.94 (Fig. 5).

Factor of Risk for Vertebral Fracture in the Elderly and Implications for Prevention

To provide estimates of the factor of risk for vertebral fracture under controlled activities, the compressive forces on the spine during lifting were compared with the failure load of cadaveric vertebrae in a mechanical test with compression and forward flexion.[55] The numerator of the factor of risk was calculated using the specific body dimensions and weight of the donor. Simple activities, such as lifting a small child, were found to result in forces on the vertebra that come close to the vertebral structural capacity, particularly for those with low bone-mineral density (Fig. 6). These results indicate that fracture prevention efforts should focus on further identification of and education about preventable activities that load the vertebrae beyond safe levels. In addition, treatments that increase bone mineral density of the spine will certainly help increase vertebral failure load and bring the factor of risk below one under lifting activities. As a case in point, alendronate treatment has been found to be associated with a 48% reduction in the proportion of women with new vertebral fractures.[47]

The vertebral fractures that are associated with falls have not been investigated. Models of fall impact and loads to the spine need to be developed to assess the loads on the spine during a fall. In addition, structural

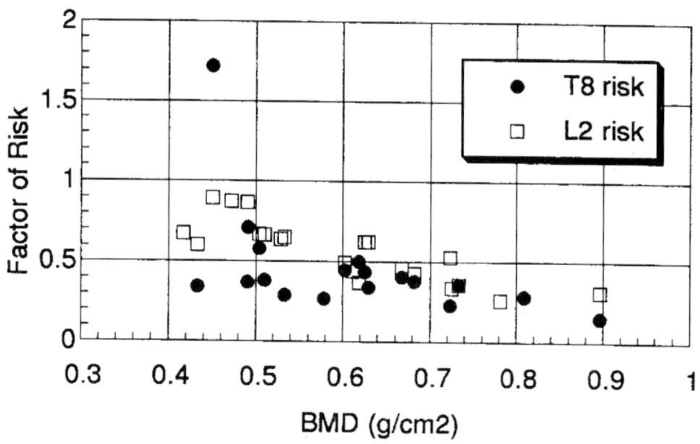

Fig. 6 Estimated factor of risk at two spine levels (T8 and L2) for bending and lifting 15 kg. Factor of risk was calculated for this activity based on body height, weight, and lumbar bone mineral density (BMD) of human cadaveric donors. Solid circles represent the factor of risk at the T8 level. Open squares represent the factor at risk at the L2 level. (Reproduced with permission from Wilson SE, Myers ER: A model to predict the compressive forces associated with age-related vertebral fractures of thoracolumbar vertebrae. *J Bone Joint Surg*, in press.)

capacity of the vertebra during such impact conditions is unknown. Future studies of falls and vertebral fracture may indicate future preventive measures to decrease the incidence of fractures associated with these accidental events.

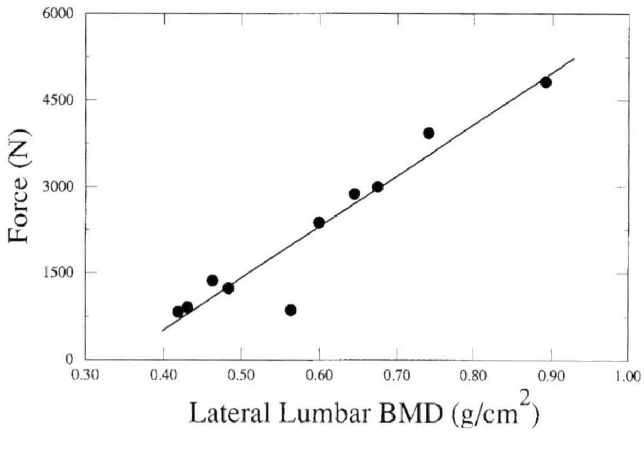

Fig. 5 Bone mineral density of the lumbar spine assessed with DXA versus fracture load of the 11th thoracic vertebra tested in straight compression. Fracture load correlates strongly with bone mineral density ($r^2 = 0.88$).

Summary and Conclusion

Falls and fall-related hip fractures are among the most serious, common, and costly medical problems facing the elderly. Recently, we and others have shown that falls to the side, particularly those that end with impact on the hip, raise the risk of hip fracture from six- to thirtyfold, compared to about threefold increases in risk associated with one SD reduction in BMD at the hip. And yet, despite the apparently crucial importance of sideways falls, little is known about the mechanics of falling to the side. In addition, while previous studies have helped identify those factors that place the elderly at high risk for falling and provided assessment procedures that can be used to identify those at risk for falls, as far as we are aware no previous work has successfully identified subjects at increased risk of falling to the side. Moreover, while rigorous, multifactorial fall prevention efforts have demonstrated moderate reductions in fall incidence, such programs are expensive and potentially inefficient in that they have not consistently demonstrated reductions in the numbers of injurious falls. While trochanteric padding systems show considerable promise for hip fracture prevention by reducing impact force, they involve difficult acceptance and compliance issues and will require large and rigorous clinical trials to demonstrate effectiveness. Finally, while it also appears that osteodynamic agents can be used to increase BMD at the hip and spine, little is known about the local structural consequences of these changes and, in particular, if they are sufficient to prevent hip fracture from a severe fall. The findings reviewed here thus emphasize the continuing need for combined intervention strategies that focus on fall prevention, on reductions in fall severity, and on maintaining or increasing bone mass and strength, either through targeted exercise programs or the use of osteodynamic agents. By developing and refining the factor of risk Φ, a property that captures both the contributions of bone density and the confounding influences of body habitus and fall severity, we believe these intervention strategies can be targeted more appropriately. Based on such approaches and an improved understanding of the complex interplay between fall biomechanics and bone fragility in the etiology of hip fracture, there is hope that the growing worldwide epidemic of hip fractures among the elderly can be substantially abated.

Acknowledgments

This study was supported by grants from the Centers for Disease Control and Prevention (CR102550 and CCR109053), the National Institutes of Health (AR40321, CA41295, AG12349 and AG11985), and by the Maurice E. Mueller Professorship of Biomechanics at Harvard Medical School (WCH). The authors thank Jeanine Dulong for her assistance in manuscript preparation.

References

1. Hinton RY, Lennox DW, Ebert FR, et al: Relative rates of fracture of the hip in the United States: Georgraphic, sex and age variations *J Bone Joint Surg* 1995;77A:695–702.
2. Michelson JD, Myers A, Jinnah R, et al: Epidemiology of hip fractures among the elderly: Risk factors for fracture type. *Clin Orthop* 1995;311:129–135.
3. Province MA, Hadley EC, Hornbrook MC, et al: The effects of exercise on falls in elderly patients: A preplanned meta-analysis of the FICSIT Trials. Frailty and Injuries: Cooperative Studies of Intervention Techniques. *JAMA* 1995;273:1341–1347.
4. Sattin RW: Falls among older persons: A public health perspective. *Annu Rev Public Health* 1992;13:489–508.
5. Tinetti ME, Liu WL, Claus EB: Predictors and prognosis of inability to get up after falls among elderly persons. *JAMA* 1993;269:65–70.
6. Cummings SR, Nevitt MC: Editorial: Falls. *N Engl J Med* 1994; 31:872–873.
7. Wolinsky FD, Johnson RJ, Fitzgerald JF: Falling, health status, and the use of health services by older adults: A prospective study. *Med Care* 1992;30:587–597.
8. Nevitt MC, Cummings SR, Kidd S, et al: Risk factors for recurrent nonsyncopal falls: A prospective study. *JAMA* 1989;261: 2663–2668.
9. Tinetti ME, Speechley M, Ginter SF: Risk factors for falls among elderly persons living in the community. *N Engl J Med* 1988; 319:1701–1707.
10. Apple DF Jr, Hayes WC (eds): *Prevention of Falls and Hip Fractures in the Elderly*. Rosemont, IL, American Academy of Orthopaedic Surgeons, 1994.
11. Grisso JA, Kelsey JL, Strom BL, et al: The Northeast Hip Fracture Study Group: Risk factors for falls as a cause of hip fracture in women. *N Engl J Med* 1991;324:1326–1331.
12. Hedlund R, Lindgren U: Trauma type, age, and gender as determinants of hip fracture. *J Orthop Res* 1987;5:242–246.
13. Holbrook TL, Grazier K, Kelsey JL, et al (eds): *The Frequency of Occurrence, Impact, and Cost of Selected Musculoskeletal Conditions in the United States*. Park Ridge, IL, American Academy of Orthopaedic Surgeons, 1984.
14. Phillips S, Fox N, Jacobs J, et al: The direct medical costs of osteoporosis for American women aged 45 and older, 1986. *Bone* 1988;9:271–279.
15. Kelsey JL, Hoffman S: Editorial: Risk factors for hip fracture. *N Engl J Med* 1987;316:404–406.
16. Parkkari J, Kannus P, Heikkila J, et al: Energy-shunting external hip protector attenuates the peak femoral impact force below the theoretical fracture threshold: An in vitro biomechanical study under falling conditions of the elderly. *J Bone Miner Res* 1995;10:1437–1442.
17. Hayes WC, Myers ER, Morris JN, et al: Impact near the hip dominates fracture risk in elderly nursing home residents who fall. *Calcif Tissue Int* 1993;52:192–198.
18. Nevitt MC, Cummings SR: Letter: Type of fall and risk of hip and wrist fractures: The study of osteoporotic fractures. The study of Osteoporotic Fractures Research Group. *J Am Geriatr Soc* 1993;41:1226–1234.
19. Greenspan SL, Myers ER, Maitland LA, et al: Fall severity and bone mineral density as risk factors for hip fracture in ambulatory elderly. *JAMA* 1994;271:128–133.
20. Cummings SR, Nevitt MC, Browner WS, et al: Risk factors for hip fracture in white women: Study of Osteoporotic Fractures Research Group. *N Engl J Med* 1995;332:767–773.
21. Hayes WC, Myers ER, Robinovitch SN, et al: Etiology and prevention of age-related hip fractures. *Bone* 1996;18(suppl): 77S–86S.
22. Cummings SR, Nevitt MC: A hypothesis: The causes of hip fracture. *J Gerontol* 1989;44:M107–M111.
23. van den Kroonenberg A, Hayes WC, McMahon TA: Dynamic models for sideways falls from standing height. *J Biomech Eng* 1995;117:309–318.
24. van den Kroonenberg A, Hayes WC, McMahon TA: Hip impact velocities and body configurations for experimental falls from standing height. *J Biomech* 1996;29:807–811.
25. Robinovitch SN, Hayes WC, McMahon TA: Prediction of femoral impact forces in falls on the hip. *J Biomech Eng* 1991; 113:366–374.
26. Robinovitch SN, McMahon TA, Hayes WC: Force attenuation in trochanteric soft tissues during impact from a fall. *J Orthop Res* 1995;13:956–962.
27. Courtney AC, Wachtel EF, Myers ER, et al: Effects of loading rate on strength of the proximal femur. *Calcif Tissue Int* 1994;55:53–58.
28. Courtney AC, Wachtel EF, Myers ER, et al: Age-related reductions in the strength of the femur tested in a fall-loading configuration. *J Bone Joint Surg* 1995;77A:387–395.
29. Myers ER, Robinovitch SN, Greenspan SL, et al: Factor of risk is associated with frequency of hip fracture in a case-control study. *Trans Orthop Res Soc* 1994;19:526.
30. Cumming RG, Klineberg RJ: Case-control study of risk factors for hip fractures in the elderly. *Am J Epidemiol* 1994;139: 493–503.

31. Lauritzen JB, Askegaard V: Protection against hip fractures by energy absorption. *Dan Med Bull* 1992;39:91–93.
32. Sloan J, Holloway G: Fractured neck of the femur: The cause of the fall? *Injury* 1981;13:230–232.
33. Yang KH, Shen KL, Demetropoulos CK, et al: The relationship between muscle contraction and fracture of the proximal femur. *Trans Orthop Res Soc* 1995;20:238.
34. Dias JJ: An analysis of the nature of injury in fractures of the neck of the femur. *Age Ageing* 1987;16:373–377.
35. Tinetti ME, Baker DI, Garrett P, et al: Yale FISCIT: Risk factor abatement strategy for fall prevention. *J Am Geriatr Soc* 1993; 41:315–320.
36. Weber T, Yang K, Woo R, et al: Proximal femur strength: Correlation of the rate of loading and bone mineral density. *ASME Adv in Bioeng* 1992;22:111–114.
37. Tinetti ME, Baker DI, McAvay G, et al: A multifactorial intervention to reduce the risk of falling among elderly people living in the community. *N Engl J Med* 1994;331:821–827.
38. Colvin D, Lord C, Bishop G, et al: A fall intervention/mobility aid system for elderly and rehabilitative populations. *Technology for the Aging* 1990;35:1936–1937.
39. Zylke JW: Research focuses not only on where, why, how of falls, but also on preventing them. *JAMA* 1990;263:2022–2023.
40. Nelson ME, Fiatarone MA, Morganti CM, et al: Effects of high-intensity strength training on multiple risk factors for osteoporotic fractures: A randomized controlled trial. *JAMA* 1994;272:1909–1914.
41. Lauritzen JB, Petersen MM, Lund B: Effect of external hip protectors on hip fractures. *Lancet* 1993;341:11–13.
42. Sellberg M, Huston J, Kruger D: The development of a passive protective device for the elderly to prevent hip fractures from accidental falls. *Adv Bioeng BED* 1992;22:505–508.
43. Cameron ID, Quine S: External hip protectors: Likely non-compliance among high risk elderly people living in the community. *Arch Gerontol Geriatr* 1994;19:273–281.
44. Felson DT, Zhang Y, Hannan MT, et al: The effect of post-menopausal estrogen therapy on bone density in elderly women. *N Engl J Med* 1993;329:1141–1146.
45. Riggs BL, Melton LJ III: The prevention and treatment of osteoporosis. *N Engl J Med* 1992;327:620–627.
46. Resnick NM, Greenpan SL: "Senile" osteoporosis reconsidered. *JAMA* 1989;261:1025–1029.
47. Liberman UA, Weiss SR, Broll J, et al: Effect of oral alendronate on bone mineral density and the incidence of fractures in post-menopausal osteoporosis: The Alendronate Phase III Osteoporosis Treatment Study Group. *N Engl J Med* 1995;333: 1437–1443.
48. Cooper C, Atkinson EJ, O'Fallon WM, et al: Incidence of clinically diagnosed vertebral fractures: A population-based study in Rochester, Minnesota, 1985–1989. *J Bone Miner Res* 1992;7: 221–227.
49. Myers ER, Wilson SE, Greenspan SL: Vertebral fractures in the elderly occur with falling and bending. *J Bone Miner Res* 1996; 11:693.
50. Gertzbein SD: Spine update: Classification of thoracic and lumbar fractures. *Spine* 1994;19:626–628.
51. Melton LJ III, Kan SH, Frye MA, et al: Epidemiology of vertebral fractures in women. *Am J Epidemiol* 1989;129:1000–1011.
52. Schultz A, Andersson G, Ortengren R, et al: Loads on the lumbar spine: Validation of a biomechanical analysis by measurements of intradiscal pressures and myoelectric signals. *J Bone Joint Surg* 1982;64A:713–720.
53. Schultz AB, Andersson GB: Analysis of loads on the lumbar spine. *Spine* 1981;6:76–82.
54. Bean JC, Chaffin DB, Schultz AB: Biomechanical model calculation of muscle contraction forces: A double linear programming method. *J Biomech* 1988;21:59–66.
55. Wilson SE, Myers ER: A model to predict the compressive forces associated with age-related vertebral fractures of thoracolumbar vertebrae. *Trans Orthop Res Soc* 1996;21:252.
56. McBroom RJ, Hayes WC, Edwards WT, et al: Prediction of vertebral body compressive fracture using quantitative computed tomography. *J Bone Joint Surg* 1985;67A:1206–1214.
57. Mosekilde L, Bentzen SM, Ortoft G, et al: The predictive value of quantitative computed tomography for vertebral body compressive strength and ash density. *Bone* 1989;10:465–470.
58. Cody DD, Goldstein SA, Flynn MJ, et al: Correlations between vertebral regional bone mineral density (rBMD) and whole bone fracture load. *Spine* 1991;16:146–154.
59. Moro M, Hecker AT, Bouxsein ML, et al: Failure load of thoracic vertebrae correlates with lumbar bone mineral density measured by DXA. *Calcif Tissue Int* 1995;56:206–209.

CHAPTER 41

Outcome Assessment After Fracture in the Elderly

Mary Louise Skovron, DrPH
Kenneth J. Koval, MD
Gina B. Aharonoff, MPH
Joseph D. Zuckerman, MD

Introduction

Because the long-term goal of fracture treatment is to restore the patient to preinjury function, a reliable method must be available to assess functional recovery following treatment. Outcome assessment after orthopaedic interventions has usually focused on physician-defined measures of technical success, such as fracture union, alignment, and range of joint motion, rather than patient function and quality of life. In the literature, however, there are weak and inconsistent correlations among improvements in pain relief, joint motion, functional status, and psychosocial well being.[1-3] A patient's actual quality of life may not reflect the surgeon's clinical evaluation; moreover, clinical and radiographic outcomes often do not parallel functional status, particularly in the elderly.

Recently, the focus of outcome assessment has become patient-oriented functional outcomes.[4,5] With this approach, the patient's broadly defined health status after recovery is the key measure of success. The significance of this approach has only recently been recognized in orthopaedic surgery.[6,7]

In this chapter, we will discuss study designs used in the study of treatment outcomes in elderly fracture patients and then describe selected available outcome assessment instruments that can be used to evaluate fracture treatment in the elderly. We will also review the development of the Functional Recovery Score, a patient-oriented assessment of functional outcome after hip fracture in the elderly.

Observational Study Designs

Observational study designs are applicable in both clinical and etiologic epidemiology. In etiologic epidemiology, one tests whether a hypothesized factor is a determinant or cause of disease development in previously healthy people; in clinical epidemiology, one tests whether particular characteristics, risk factors, or clinical interventions are determinants of the prognosis or outcome in affected patients. Adaptations of three basic etiologic observational study designs can be used for outcome studies—the cohort study, the case-control study, and the cross-sectional study.[8]

Prognostic Cohort Study

The cohort study, when well designed and executed, is the soundest of all the observational study designs. In a prognostic cohort study, a population of elderly people who have had a fracture is identified and characterized with respect to the hypothesized prognostic factor or therapeutic intervention, important covariates, and potential confounders. The population is observed for a period of time adequate for the natural history of recovery from fracture (ie, 6 months to 1 year for hip fracture) and the outcomes are recorded. Prognostic cohort studies are often undertaken by identifying subjects based on existing records and ascertaining outcomes in the more recent past or in the near future. This type of cohort study is called a historical, or retrospective, cohort study because the prognostic events, and possibly the outcome, happened before the study was conducted. When the subjects are enrolled at the time of fracture and followed forward in time, the cohort study may be referred to as a follow-up or prospective cohort study.

Loss to follow-up is a potential problem in cohort studies. If a substantial proportion of subjects are lost to the study for any reason, the number of patients evaluated may be too small to yield stable estimates of the outcome rates and, consequently, the importance of prognostic factors (relative risk). In a cohort study examining the one-year prognostic importance of prior fracture in hip fracture patients, for example, if a large percentage of patients is lost to follow-up, it is not possible to know whether the results in those remaining patients available for follow-up are representative of the entire group. If there have been high proportions lost to follow-up, or higher proportions lost in one exposure category than the other (selective loss to follow-up), biased loss to follow-up may have occurred. The observed prognostic relative risk in that case will underestimate the true relative risk.

Another form of bias—selective attrition or selective survival—can affect what appears to be a cohort study. For example, patients may be enrolled in the study when they come for routine medical care, and those with a history of hip fracture identified to form the prognostic cohort. Information on prognostic factors at the time of fracture is then compiled either from retrieved medical records or by interview. The problem is that the cohort includes only survivors of hip fracture, and nothing is known about the characteristics of those who did not survive. Furthermore, the cohort is limited to survivors of hip fracture who stayed in the area and came for health care, and nothing is known about people who left the area or did not come for health care at the sites being studied.

Outcome studies in which the outcome of interest is rare or develops long after the intervention may require enrollment of a large number of subjects or lengthy follow-up. It can be more efficient, in terms of time and number of subjects studied, to address the hypothesis in a case-control study, as described below.

Case-Control Outcome Study

Case-control prognostic studies differ from the other observational outcome study designs in that individuals are selected for the study based on the presence of the fracture outcome in question (cases) and compared to individuals who do not have the fracture outcome under study (controls). The presence or absence of the hypothesized prognostic factor is then ascertained in both case and control subjects. Although this may appear to be a simple undertaking, the case-control study presents a number of methodologic challenges that must be faced in order for the study results to be valid.

One possible problem in case-control studies occurs when cases and controls are not comparable in "exposure opportunity." That is, cases and controls have been identified in such a way that one group was more or less likely to have the prognostic factor for reasons other than the hypothesis being studied. For example, if in a case-control study of age as a prognostic factor for surgical outcome after fracture, patients who needed revision surgery were identified from Medicare claims while control subjects were identified from workplace medical facility records, the average age of cases and controls would differ because of the way they were selected. It would not be possible to assign causality to an association of age and fracture outcome observed in such a study.

Case-control studies frequently suffer from information biases such as recall bias, in which a case subject is more or less likely to recall an event in the past than is a control subject. Another problem is recall failure, which can occur when subjects are asked to recall events or conditions that took place long ago. It is often difficult to establish that the factor of interest was present long enough before the outcome to be a biologically plausible determinant. This type of problem can be avoided if the case-control study uses prognostic information that was recorded prior to the development of the outcome, for example, in medical or prescription records.

Because of the difficulty in avoiding the problems described above, case-control studies often produce weaker causal evidence than do cohort studies. However, when well designed and well executed to avoid the problems cited above, case-control studies can provide evidence as robust as that of cohort studies at considerably less cost and in less time.

Cross-Sectional Outcome Study

Cross-sectional, or survey, studies simultaneously ascertain the presence of the prognostic factors and outcome in question, in a population sampled without retgard to the presence of either. In contrast to the cohort study, which follows subjects over time and ascertains outcome incidence, the cross-sectional study ascertains conditions present at the moment of study, ie, the prevalence of the outcomes. The estimates of relative risk derived from cross-sectional studies are therefore estimates of prevalence relative risk and are susceptible to distortion by such biases as selective survival or attrition prior to the study, and changes in prognostic factor status prior to the study.

Cross-sectional studies are often undertaken because, unlike case-control studies, they require few a priori decisions with regard to selection of subjects and, unlike cohort studies, it is not necessary to wait for the study outcome. However, cross-sectional studies are vulnerable to some of the problems of both cohort and case-control studies. When uncommon prognostic factors or outcomes are being studied, a large number of people must be included, just as in cohort studies. If information on prognostic determinants of interest is collected at the time of the study rather than from previously existing records, there can be recall biases, recall failures, and problems in establishing the time sequence of events, as with case-control studies. For relatively common outcomes and determinants, cross-sectional studies may be a useful first step. Because of their many limitations, however, cross-sectional studies are rarely sufficient for evaluating the importance of prognostic factors.

Interventional Study Designs: Clinical Trials

In evaluating treatment, observational study designs are susceptible to treatment assignment biases, in which patient treatment is influenced by patient characteristics such as lifestyle or clinical severity that can confound the results. Unrandomized clinical trials, in which the treating physicians or the investigators control the patient treatment, are also susceptible to such biases. Because in randomized control trials only chance influences the treatment that eligible patients receive, these are the standard for evaluating therapeutic interventions.

Validity of randomized control trials depends on all the methodologic features described for the observational study designs. Additionally, analysis of results must be confined to those patients who have agreed to participate. Comparisons of treatment outcomes in patients who agree to participate with those in patients who refuse to participate are not valid. The assignment of patients to different treatments must use accepted methods of randomization, which should be identified in the published report; the resulting comparability of the treatment groups on important covariates should be described, usually in a table summarizing baseline characteristics of the treatment groups. When randomization does not result in comparable groups, potential confounding must be controlled in the statistical analysis.[9]

In randomized trials, the treating physician and the patient should be blinded to treatment assignment. Because this is not possible in trials of surgical techniques, an independent investigator should assess baseline status and outcome, in order to minimize observer (treating surgeon) and participant (patient) biases. This is particularly important when the outcome being assessed is subjective. Information should be collected in a standardized manner at the same time intervals in all treatment groups.[10] Eligibility and exclusion criteria should be detailed, and must be appropriate to the hypothesis addressed. Treatments should be clearly described. Patient compliance, dropouts from the study, and complications should be described and equivalent in both groups. Finally, the outcomes studied should be appropriate to the treatment or condition in question.

On occasion, when surgeons strongly prefer or are more proficient in one surgical technique, it has been suggested that a group of surgeons with proficiency in different techniques be assembled and patients be randomized to different surgeons who perform surgery by their preferred technique. When well designed and executed, this can allow comparability of the patients receiving surgery by the different methods being compared, while avoiding confounding by surgeons' skills and avoiding ethical dilemmas for the participating surgeons.

Disease-Specific Outcome Assessment Instruments

Disease- or condition-specific assessment tools are designed for specific diagnostic groups or patient populations. They are most appropriate for their target patient or disease populations.

Orthopaedic Scales

Many orthopaedic assessment scales are available. Most are intended for use when surgery is undertaken to correct an orthopaedic condition that affected presurgical function. Orthopaedic rating systems are usually weighted for pain, include radiologic results, and assess improvement over preintervention range of motion and strength of the involved limb. Functional abilities are less heavily weighted, and psychosocial well-being is not considered. Orthopaedic rating scales may be less appropriate for postoperative assessment of the elderly fracture patient who had no pain prior to injury and is most concerned about return to prefracture function (ie, activities of daily living).

Medical Assessment Tools

Medical assessment rating scales often measure function and well-being relevant to the disease in question. Two of the instruments available for assessing health status in rheumatoid arthritis are summarized below. These instruments emphasize musculoskeletal function and may be applicable to some orthopaedic patients.

Health Assessment Questionnaire The Health Assessment Questionnaire measures functional status in patients with rheumatoid arthritis.[11] Using a rating scale of 0 to 3, patients rate the amount of difficulty and/or the need for assistive devices to perform activities of daily living in eight areas—eating, dressing and grooming, arising, walking, hygiene, reaching and bending, grip (eg, ability to open jars), and activities (errands and chores). The Health Assessment Questionnaire also includes a Visual Analog Scale to represent the intensity of pain the patient experienced during the previous week. The Health Assessment Questionnaire is self-administered and requires 8 to 10 minutes to complete.

Arthritis Impact Measurement Scale The Arthritis Impact Measurement Scale (AIMS) is another scale that measures the health status of patients with arthritis.[12] Forty-five questions cover nine different categories—mobility, physical activity, social activity, social role, activities of daily living, pain, dexterity, anxiety, and depression. The AIMS is self-administered at home or in a clinical setting and takes 15 to 20 minutes to complete.

General Health Assessment Instruments

General health assessment or generic rating scales are intended for use across the full spectrum of health problems. They are applicable to all types and severity of disease, different medical treatments or health interventions, and varying demographic and cultural subgroups. Advantages of the general health status assessment tools include an ability to detect treatment outcomes and side effects in several aspects of health status, for example, pain and fatigue, and to make comparisons among diseases or condition groups for purposes such as resource allocation. However, they are usually less responsive to changes than disease-specific scales and can be cumbersome, time-consuming, and difficult to conduct as a telephone interview. Three general health assessment instruments have been well-validated and are described below.

SF-36

The SF-36 is a general scale derived from the longer Medical Outcomes Study questionnaire.[13] This scale has eight components—physical functioning, social functioning, role functioning (physical), role functioning (emotional), pain, general health, vitality (energy/fatigue), and mental health (including psychological distress and psychological well-being). The SF-36 can be self-administered in the physician's office and can also be administered by phone, mail, or interview. A shortened form of this assessment, the SF-20, excludes the assessment of vitality and part of reported health.

Sickness Impact Profile

The Sickness Impact Profile consists of 136 questions in 12 major activities of daily living. The activities are organized into three categories: (1) independence (sleep and rest, eating, work, home management, and recreation and pastimes); (2) physical (ambulation, mobility, and body care and movement); and (3) psychosocial (social interaction, alertness behavior, emotional behavior, and communication). The Sickness Impact Profile is self-administered and can be completed in 15 to 30 minutes.[14]

Quality of Well-Being Scale

The Quality of Well-Being (QWB) scale, formerly the Index of Well-Being, emphasizes quality of life and is based on patients' actual performance. This scale has three categories—physical activity, mobility, and social activity—and includes death, therefore indicating a likely prognosis of any medical condition that the patient may have. The QWB scale is a useful tool for assessing the need for health services in both the present and future. The QWB scale is administered by trained interviewers and takes 10 to 15 minutes to complete.[15]

Functional Recovery Score for Elderly Hip Fracture Patients

The Functional Recovery Score (FRS) was developed at the Hospital for Joint Diseases to assess outcome after hip fracture in elderly patients. It is a condition-specific patient-oriented orthopaedic assessment. This instrument reflects the importance that elderly patients place on different functional capacities required in daily life. It was designed for ease of use in clinical practice as well as administration by telephone or mailed questionnaire.

Development

Phase I After review of the orthopaedic, geriatric, and functional status assessment literature, five key functions and health status indicators relevant to quality of life among the elderly and to hip fracture recovery were identified: (1) independence in basic activities of daily living (BADLs),[16] which include the ability to feed oneself, bathe, and use the toilet and dress without help; (2) independence in instrumental activities of daily living (IADLs), which include the ability to shop for food, prepare food, manage personal banking and finances, do light housework and laundry, and use public transportation or get in and out of a vehicle without help;[17] (3) independence in mobility, including the ability to walk indoors or outdoors without help, transfer from bed to chair and chair to bed without help, and climb one or more flights of stairs without help; (4) freedom from pain; and (5) an intact memory.

The relative importance of these components to the elderly was assessed by administering a questionnaire to 260 community-dwelling elderly individuals in three geographically different senior citizen centers (urban, suburban, and rural). There were no significant differences by gender or center in the importance attached to any of the components. Based on the importance assigned by the study subjects, preliminary component weights and a preliminary FRS were developed. The component weights of the preliminary FRS were BADLs (28%), memory (21%), IADLs (18%), mobility (17%), and pain (16%).

Phase II A pilot study of 50 geriatric hip fracture patients was conducted, using the preliminary FRS. Some of the components and items on the preliminary FRS were difficult to measure in the hip fracture population, particularly by telephone interview. As a result of this, the pain and memory components were deleted, as well as the mobility items for transfers and stairs.

Phase III The remaining 11 items were used in a repeat survey of 100 ambulatory, home-dwelling urban elderly, and a revised FRS was developed. The component percentages were BADLs (44%), IADLs (23%), and mobility (33%). The data obtained in the Phase I survey were reanalyzed using only the 11 items of the revised FRS; the component percentages that resulted were essentially identical to those that resulted from the Phase III survey.

Validation

A historical cohort study was performed to assess predictive and discriminant validity and responsiveness of the FRS in 609 geriatric hip fracture patients. The

FRS was found to be responsive to change, as scores following hip fracture plateaued between 6 and 12 months after fracture, consistent with expectation.[18,19] The FRS also has predictive validity; scores before fracture or at early follow-up were predictive of death or nursing home residence 1 to 2 years after fracture. The FRS has discriminant validity; mean scores differed for patients in nursing homes, at home requiring living assistance, and at home not requiring living assistance. In addition, comparison of the FRS with a sex- and age-matched population without hip fracture indicated that hip fracture resulted in a 20% loss of function within the first year.

In a separate study, reliability testing of telephone interviews of patients or proxies as a means of obtaining information indicated very good reliability (correlation coefficient = 0.88).

Conclusion

Outcome assessment is important in the evaluation of orthopaedic treatment of fracture in the elderly. Studies describing outcomes after fracture in the elderly, or evaluating prognostic factors or treatment outcomes, must be conducted according to sound research methods. Outcome assessment instruments should be appropriate to the target population and the type of intervention being evaluated. The instruments should also be reliable, valid, and feasible for the setting in which they are applied (clinical practice or research). The Functional Recovery Score is an example of a disease-specific patient-oriented orthopaedic outcome measure; it was based on an assessment of the functional needs of the elderly and is a reliable and valid method of assessing outcome in elderly hip fracture patients. In addition to its usefulness for research, it may also be useful for monitoring patient care in clinical practice, in order to identify patients needing further intervention.

References

1. MacKenzie EJ, Cushing BM, Jurkovich GJ, et al: Physical impairment and functional outcomes six months after severe lower extremity fractures. *J Trauma* 1993;34:528-539.
2. Gartland JJ: Orthopaedic clinical research: Deficiencies in experimental design and determinations of outcome. *J Bone Joint Surg* 1988;70A:1357-1364.
3. Georgiadis GM, Behrens FF, Joyce MJ, et al: Open tibial fractures with severe soft tissue loss: Limb salvage compared with below the knee amputation. *J Bone Joint Surg* 1993;75A:1431-1441.
4. Gross M: A critique of the methodologies used in clinical studies of hip joint arthroplasty published in the English language orthopaedic literature. *J Bone Joint Surg* 1988;70A:1364-1371.
5. Schroeder AS: Editorial: Outcome assessment 70 years later: Are we ready? *N Engl J Med* 1987;316:160-162.
6. Wright JG, Rudicel S, Feinstein AR: Ask patients what they want: Evaluation of individual complaints before total hip replacement. *J Bone Joint Surg* 1994;76B:229-234.
7. American Academy of Orthopaedic Surgeons, Department of Research: *Fundamentals of Outcome Research.* Rosemont, IL, American Academy of Orthopaedic Surgeons, 1993.
8. Kasser JR (ed): *Orthopaedic Knowledge Update 5*, Rosemont, IL, American Academy of Orthopaedic Surgeons, 1996, pp 71-80.
9. Fleiss JL (ed): *The Design and Analysis of Clinical Experiments.* New York, NY, John Wiley & Sons, 1986.
10. Hulley SB, Cummings SR, Browner WS (eds): *Designing Clinical Research: An Epidemiologic Approach.* Baltimore, MD, Williams & Wilkins, 1988.
11. Fries JF, Spitz P, Kraines RG, et al: Measurement of patient outcome in arthritis. *Arthritis Rheum* 1980;23:137-145.
12. Meenan RF, Gertman PM, Mason JM: Measuring health status in arthritis: The Arthritis Impact Measurement Scales. *Arthritis Rheum* 1980;23:146-152.
13. Ware JE, Snow KK, Kosinski M, et al (eds): *SF-36 Health Survey: Manual and Interpretation Guide.* Boston, MA, New England Medical Center, 1993.
14. Bergner M, Bobbitt RA, Carter WB, et al: The Sickness Impact Profile: Development and final revision of a health status measure. *Med Care* 1981;19:787-805.
15. Guyatt G, Walter S, Norman G: Measuring change over time: Assessing the usefulness of evaluative instruments. *J Chronic Dis* 1987;40:171-178.
16. Katz S, Ford AB, Moskowitz RW, et al: Studies of illness in the aged: The index of ADL. A standardized measure of biological and psychosocial function. *JAMA* 1963;185:914-919.
17. Lawton MP, Brody EM: Assessment of older people: Selfmaintaining and instrumental activities of daily living. *Gerontologist* 1969;9:179-186.
18. Magaziner J, Simonsick EM, Kashner TM, et al: Predictors of functional recovery one year following hospital discharge for hip fracture: A prospective study. *J Gerontol* 1990;45:M101-M107.
19. Mossey JM, Mutran E, Knott K, et al: Determinants of recovery 12 months after hip fracture: The importance of psychosocial factors. *Am J Public Health* 1989;79:279-286.

CHAPTER 42

Osteoporosis: Diagnosis and Treatment

Joseph M. Lane, MD
Edward H. Riley, MD
Philip Z. Wirganowicz, MD

Osteoporosis is characterized by decreased bone mass and increased susceptibility to fracture. Primary osteoporosis occurs in an individual who has no other endocrinopathy or disease state that would account for the changes in bone mass. Osteoporosis affects 20 million individuals in the United States.[1] These individuals sustain more than 1.2 million fractures (including more than 280,000 fractures of the hip) annually; the estimated cost of treatment of such fractures was $10 billion in 1992.[1,2] The absolute number and percentage of persons who have osteoporosis are expected to increase because of the prolonged longevity of the American population. The risk of a fracture of the proximal femur increases with age, especially in women who are more than 50 years old.[3] Fractures of the proximal femur are associated with a high rate of mortality, and most persons who have sustained such a fracture never regain their previous level of function.[4] Emotional morbidity in the form of depression, reclusiveness, and fear of additional fracture may accompany osteoporosis. Advances in our understanding of the etiology and pathophysiology of osteoporosis, as well as progress in the prevention and treatment of this disease, have given the physician the ability to intervene successfully.

Riggs and Melton[5] classified primary osteoporosis on the basis of the patterns of bone loss and fracture. Postmenopausal (type-I), or osteoclast-mediated, osteoporosis is characterized by rapid bone loss and is seen most often in recently postmenopausal women (it affects women six times more frequently than men). This pattern is consistent with high-turnover osteoporosis. There is a rapid phase of bone loss predominantly involving trabecular bone and an association with vertebral and distal radial fractures.

Senile (type-II), or osteoblast-mediated, osteoporosis affects women twice as frequently as men and is related to aging, chronic calcium deficiency, increased parathyroid hormone activity, and decreased bone formation. An individual can display traits of both types of osteoporosis over time.

Osteoporosis is currently the subject of a major interdisciplinary research effort. Consequently, there is a relatively large diversity of opinion regarding the best approach to the management of the osteoporotic patient. The purpose of this chapter is to review the pertinent information regarding the biologic characteristics, physiology, evaluation, treatment, and prevention of osteoporosis. An attempt has been made to present a middle-of-the-road position on the various issues, leaving room for controversy on either side. Some of the information presented undoubtedly will be altered with additional research.

Bone Metabolism

Bone is a living matrix that is in constant flux and under direct cellular control. Bone is formed by osteoblasts, which are cells of marrow stromal origin.[6-9] Newly formed bone contains an organic matrix consisting primarily of type-I collagen that has undergone mineralization. Bone resorption is under the control of osteoclasts. These large, multinucleated cells arise from macrophage precursors. They cause bone resorption by first isolating a segment of bone surface, thereby creating a Howship lacuna. Next, acidification solubilizes the mineral phase by means of a carbonic anhydrase mechanism, and, finally, the production of acid proteases allows for the enzymatic degradation of the organic components, including the collagen.

During the process of continued bone formation, the osteoblasts encase themselves within the bone matrix and become osteocytes. The osteocytes have direct connections to the outer bone surface through microcanaliculi, which play a critical role in calcium flux. Frost[10] first described the bone metabolic unit as a coupled process in which resorption precedes formation.[11] Bone remodeling proceeds throughout life, and an imbalance in this process that either enhances resorption or impairs formation ultimately leads to a net loss of bone mass. The recent Instructional Course Lecture by Buckwalter and associates[12,13] provides a more detailed discussion of bone biology.

Calcium

Calcium is an essential mineral that participates in many important physiological functions. Only the attainment of peak bone mass and the maintenance of the skeleton are considered here. Calcium requirements change throughout life depending on the activity and function of the body as well as on the efficiency of intestinal absorption (Table 1).[14-18] Approximately 25% of the dietary dose of calcium is absorbed, primarily in the upper part of the gut. In young adults, intestinal absorption of calcium is easily accomplished and is the major route by which calcium is provided to

Table 1
Daily Calcium Requirements

Age Group	Calcium (mg/day) Requirements
Youth (1 to 10 yrs. old)	800 to 1,000
Adolescent/young adult (11 to 25 yrs. old)	1,200
Premenopausal (26 to 49 yrs. old)	1,000
Postmenopausal (≥ 50 yrs. old)	1,500
Pregnancy	1,500
Lactation	1,500 to 2,000

the body. In elderly individuals, the intestine is less effective with regard to the absorption of calcium. During periods of negative calcium balance, bone resorption is the principal method of maintaining the serum calcium level. Normal absorption of calcium by the gut requires an appropriate gastric pH, an adequate serum level of 1,25-dihydroxyvitamin D, and an appropriate dietary calcium-phosphate ratio. Inhibitors of calcium absorption in the gut include decreased serum vitamin-D levels; increased dietary phosphates (soft drinks), fat, phytates, and oxalates; sprue and gastrointestinal disorders, such as achlorhydria and blind-loop syndrome; and certain renal disorders. In addition, calcium absorption is compromised by many chronically administered drugs, such as phenytoin, isoniazid, corticosteroids, heparin, tetracycline, and furosemide.

Bone mass increases during childhood, and peak bone mass is obtained by the middle of the third decade.[19-21] Ultimate peak bone mass can be affected adversely by inadequate dietary calcium intake during the years of skeletal growth.[22] Although appealing, the converse has not been demonstrated consistently, and there probably is a threshold level beyond which additional calcium intake during the years of skeletal growth does not affect beneficially the attainment of peak bone mass. A large proportion of girls and women who are more than 13 years old do not have adequate calcium intake and, therefore, have a lower potential peak bone mass.[23-26]

The greater the peak bone mass achieved, the better the chance of avoiding osteoporosis later in life. After peak bone mass is reached, bone loss normally occurs at the rate of 0.3% per year in men and 0.5% per year in women. A rate of bone loss of 2% to 3% per year (an 8% decrease in trabecular bone and a 0.5% decrease in cortical bone) begins at the onset of menopause. This rate continues for a period of 6 to 10 years and then declines to a rate of 0.5% per year. While all adults lose bone with age, osteoporosis develops in only 20% to 30% of women and 10% to 20% of men who are more than 65 years old.[5,27]

Calcitropic Hormones

Vitamin D Many hormones directly affect bone metabolism.[28] A major one is vitamin D, a sterol hormone that plays a critical role in calcium metabolism. Vitamin D is formed from 7-dehydrocholesterol in the skin under the direct stimulation of ultraviolet light (Fig. 1). The vitamin-D precursor is converted to 25-hydroxyvitamin D in the liver before being activated by further hydroxylation to 1,25-dihydroxyvitamin D in the kidneys in response to parathyroid hormone. The 1,25-dihydroxyvitamin D increases absorption of calcium across the gut by maturing the villus lining cells of the intestine and stimulating them to produce calcium-binding protein. Active vitamin D augments parathyroid hormone recruitment of osteoclasts for bone resorption by acting as a maturation hormone for the macrophage stem cell.

Parathyroid Hormone The second prominent hormone in bone metabolism is parathyroid hormone (PTH).[28] PTH responds to low ionic calcium levels by stimulating the retention of calcium and excretion of phosphate by the kidneys. In addition, PTH indirectly increases the absorption of calcium across the gut by stimulating the conversion of 25-hydroxyvitamin D to the active metabolite 1,25-dihydroxyvitamin D in the medullary portion of the kidneys. Indirectly, by means of the osteoblast (the coupling factor that increases osteoclast activation), PTH leads to bone resorption. Hence, PTH indirectly leads to the absorption of calcium across the gut, the resorption of calcium from bone, and increased retention of calcium within the kidneys.[29]

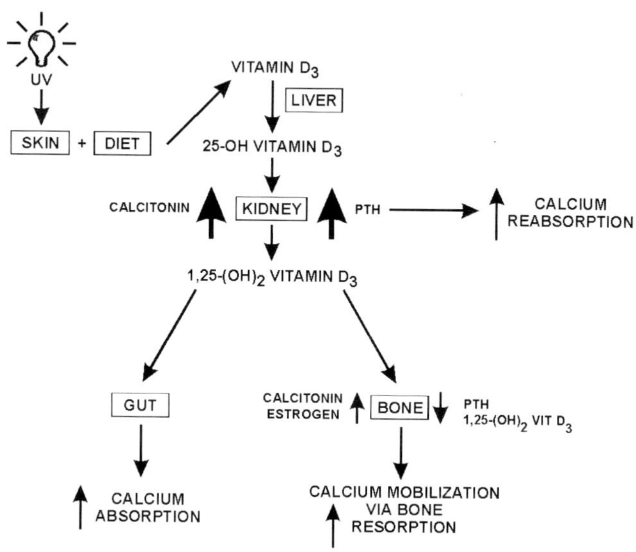

Fig. 1 Illustration of vitamin-D production and the hormonal regulation in the control and coordination of total body calcium. (Reproduced with permission from Mohler DG, Lane JM, Cole BJ, et al: Skeletal failure in osteoporosis, in Lane JM, Healey JH (eds): *Diagnosis and Management of Pathologic Fractures*. New York, NY, Raven Press, 1993, p 24.)

Calcitonin Calcitonin is a calcitropic peptide produced in the parafollicular cells of the thyroid gland. Calcitonin responds to elevated serum ionic calcium levels by decreasing the number and activity of osteoclasts.[30] Calcitonin also functions as a neuropeptide and has analgesic effects, as will be discussed. Its pharmacologic activity primarily decreases bone resorption and secondarily causes a transient increase in bone formation by means of a still unknown mechanism.

Estrogen A normal balance of estrogen and progestin is critical for the maintenance of bone mass. Young women who have episodes of amenorrhea or oligomenorrhea before peak bone mass is attained lose 2% of bone mass per year instead of gaining 2% to 4% per year as they would normally. This loss is estrogen-dependent, and the bone mass that is lost is not regained once normal menstrual cycles are resumed.[31-33] The level of circulating estrogen declines after menopause. Some women have a rapid acceleration of bone loss secondary to increased bone remodeling, with bone resorption exceeding bone formation.[34] Although estrogen has been shown to inhibit bone resorption, the exact mechanism by which this occurs and why it affects only some individuals remain unclear. There is clear evidence that estrogen receptors are present in osteoblast-like cells.[35] The presence of such receptors in osteoclasts and the influence of estrogen on those cells have not been discerned.

Glucocorticoids Glucocorticoids profoundly affect bone metabolism. Exogenously administered corticosteroids impair the function and shorten the lifespan of osteoblasts and contribute to decreased bone formation.[36] Corticosteroids increase the excretion of calcium in the urine and block the resorption of calcium in the gut. These latter two effects create a relative hypocalcemia that induces secondary hyperparathyroidism. The hyperparathyroidism then leads to osteoclastic bone resorption, which proceeds uncoupled from the aforementioned reduced rate of bone formation.[37] The result is a form of osteoporosis that is histologically distinct from postmenopausal osteoporosis in that there is markedly enhanced bone resorption and a profound absence of bone formation. The optimum treatment of this form of osteoporosis is different than that for the postmenopausal form. Minimizing the steroid dose is helpful. Spector and Sambrook[38] as well as Meunier[39] offered additional useful guidelines in the absence of definitive studies.

Thyroid Hormone There have been several reports on the effects of hyperthyroidism and the administration of exogenous thyroid hormone on bone mass.[40-42] Thyroid hormone increases bone-remodeling with osteoclast activity predominating, inducing a net loss of bone.[42] Untreated hyperthyroidism results in high-turnover osteoporosis, which leads to an increased risk of fracture.[40] Questions remain as to the effect of physiologic replacement of thyroid hormone and its potential for inducing osteoporosis. Men and premenopausal women who receive replacement therapy with the lowest possible dose of thyroxine, with the level of thyroid-stimulating hormone kept in the normal range, probably are not at increased risk for fractures.[41,43] In contrast, postmenopausal women who receive such replacement therapy have a dose-dependent decrease in bone mineral density and an increased risk of a fracture of the hip.[44] Estrogen appears to mitigate partially the effects of exogenous thyroid hormone on bone loss.[45]

Bone Biomechanics

Cortical bone has a low ratio of surface area to volume, while trabecular bone proportionately has a much greater surface area. Because bone turnover is a surface event, it affects trabecular bone more profoundly than cortical bone. Consequently, bones and bone regions rich in trabeculae, such as the vertebrae, the calcaneus, and the metaphyseal segments of the long bones, are subject to a loss of structural integrity during the aging process.[46] The body accommodates for bone loss by redistribution. The diameter of the long bones gradually increases with age in both women and men, and a concurrent increase in the medullary diameter leads to a net thinning of the cortical bone. A shift of 10% of the bone mass outward from the epicenter of the bone through this process of enlargement compensates for a 30% decrease in bone mass when bending and torque stresses are applied to the bone. However, this shift of bone mass provides no such protection when an axial load is applied.

The structural strength of bone is related not only to bone mass and its anatomic distribution but also to a concept known as connectivity. Connectivity refers to the degree of trabecular interconnectedness within bone. Mellish and associates[47] and others[48,49] demonstrated that osteoporosis involves a thinning of the cortex as well as a change in the structure of trabecular bone. Within trabecular bone, there are areas in which osteoclasts have created a discontinuity of the trabeculae, shifting the structure of the bone from plates to narrow bars and weakening it in that area. Barth and Lane[50] as well as Grampp and associates[51] reported that as many as three of eight individuals who had an extremely low bone mass in the spine did not sustain vertebral fractures. Thus, the ultimate strength of a specific bone is related to the relative amounts of trabecular and cortical bone, the architectural distribution of the bone mass, and the structural integrity and connectivity of the bone.

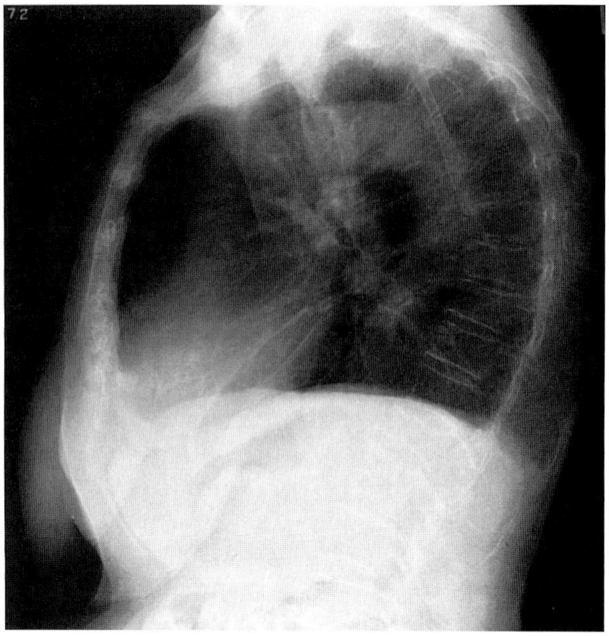

Fig. 2 Lateral radiograph of the chest of a patient who had severe osteoporosis, showing kyphosis due to multiple vertebral wedge fractures.

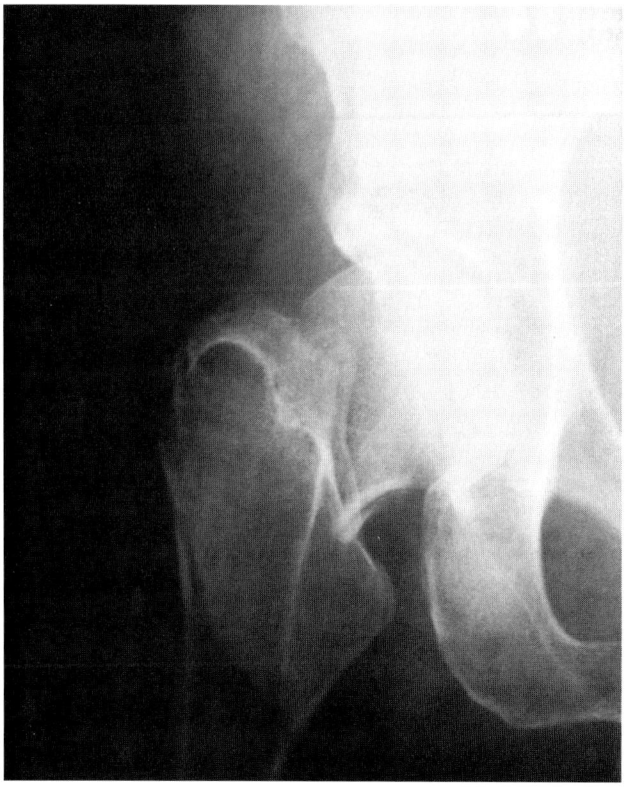

Fig. 3 Anteroposterior radiograph of the proximal femur of a patient who had osteoporosis, showing a fracture of the femoral neck.

Physical Activity

Physical activity is both an important, albeit incompletely understood, factor in bone formation and a common therapeutic intervention. Exercise frequently is prescribed as part of the treatment regimen for patients who have osteoporosis and is recommended for its overall salutary effects in terms of balance, strength, and flexibility. Impact-loading exercises appear to be effective and site-specific in the maintenance of bone mass.[52,53] However, cross-sectional population studies have indicated a more positive relationship between exercise and bone mass than have prospective clinical trials.[54] Selection bias (in that individuals who exercise have greater bone mass than do sedentary individuals) may explain the discrepancies among those studies. The effect of physical activity on peak bone mass is most evident during the years of skeletal growth and is relatively minor in older adults.[55,56] The rate of bone loss among young women who are amenorrheic as the result of chronically high levels of exercise, however, is substantially greater than that among young women who maintain normal menstrual cycles but do not exercise.[57]

As a group, women who exercise and maintain normal menstrual cycles have the greatest bone mass. Eumenorrheic women who do not exercise have less bone mass, and amenorrheic women who exercise have the least. The presumed etiology of the amenorrhea in women who exercise is an inadequate caloric intake.[32] This presumption is supported by the finding that amenorrheic women do not respond to cyclical administration of hormones unless they also gain weight.[31,33] In addition, male marathon runners who have inadequate caloric intake also have low bone mass despite having a normal level of testosterone.[58]

The constellation of disordered eating, amenorrhea, and osteoporosis has been recognized as a serious threat to the health of the female athlete and has been termed the female triad.[59] This triad predisposes the athlete to multiple fractures and other medical problems. Athletes who participate in gymnastics, diving, figure skating, dance, track, and synchronized swimming are affected most frequently.[59] When this triad is identified, the patient should reduce or modify her training regimen, increase caloric and calcium intake, and consider cyclical estrogen and progestin therapy.

Evaluation of Osteoporosis

The evaluation of a patient in whom osteoporosis is suspected should include a thorough medical history, imaging and laboratory studies, and possibly bone histomorphometry. Common fractures due to osteoporosis include wedge fractures of the thoracic spine; central end-plate cupping of the lordotic lumbar vertebral body; and fractures of the proximal and supracondylar regions of the femur as well as of the tibial plateau, the humeral neck, and the distal radius (Figs. 2 and 3). The workup of a patient who has sustained an insufficiency fracture (a fracture that was not the result of noticeable trauma) should proceed in a logical fashion. The possibility of a bone tumor should be evaluated with use of plain radiography, magnetic resonance imaging, computed tomography (CT), or bone scanning. An endocrinopathy or osteomalacia should be ruled out with appropriate laboratory tests (Fig. 4).

History

Risks for Osteoporosis If the patient has a fracture that was not due to noticeable trauma, the clinician first must rule out the presence of a benign, metastatic, or primary malignant bone tumor. Once a tumor has been excluded, the major causes of such a fracture include bone-marrow abnormalities, endocrinopathies, osteomalacia, and osteoporosis.

Risk factors for osteoporosis that the clinician should seek to identify include early natural or operatively induced menopause, prolonged periods of amenorrhea, poor nutrition, a history of limited exercise, genetic factors (a positive family history), and a history of excessive alcohol intake or smoking. Healey and Lane[60] reported that 27 (57%) of 47 women with osteoporosis had scoliosis of at least 10°. Velis and associates[61,62] and Healey and Lane[60] demonstrated that all women who have scoliosis, regardless of whether they are premenopausal or postmenopausal, have lower bone mass than their peers.

Risks for Falls In addition to assessing the risk factors for osteoporosis, the clinician must evaluate the patient's risk of falling. More than 90% of fractures of the hip are associated with falls.[63,64] Hip fractures resulting from falls are due to the interaction of three factors: the strength of the bone, the severity of the fall, and the tendency of the patient to fall. While osteoporosis per se is responsible only for a decrease in bone strength, femoral fractures due to falls account for the preponderance of the morbidity associated with osteoporosis.

Cummings and associates,[65] in a prospective study, found that the risk of a hip fracture increased with every 5 years of aging and that an increased risk was associated with a maternal history of hip fracture, tall height, lack of weight gain with aging, poor health, previously treated hyperthyroidism, the use of anticonvulsants or long-acting benzodiazepines, the lack of walking for exercise, the lack of unsupported standing for 4 hours a day, a pulse rate of more than 80 beats per minute with the patient at rest, a history of any fracture since the age of 50 years, the consumption of caffeine, poor visual depth perception, the inability to rise from a chair without using the arms, and a low bone mass. Those authors reported that if an individual had as many as two of these risk factors, the risk of a hip fracture was one per 1,000 patients per year. If the patient had five risk factors or more in addition to the risk factor of low bone mass, the risk of a hip fracture increased to 27 per 1,000 patients per year. Greenspan and associates[66] also documented that causative factors for these fractures include falls on the side, diminished bone density, a lower bone-mass index, and a higher potential energy of fall.[67]

Courtney and associates[68] showed that the femur of an elderly individual has one half the strength and one third the energy absorption capacity of that of a younger individual. This finding indicates that the hip of an elderly individual is at risk for fracture from a simple fall. Simulated falls from a standing height directly onto the greater trochanter generated an impact force that exceeded femoral strength by 50% in specimens from elderly individuals but was approximately 20%

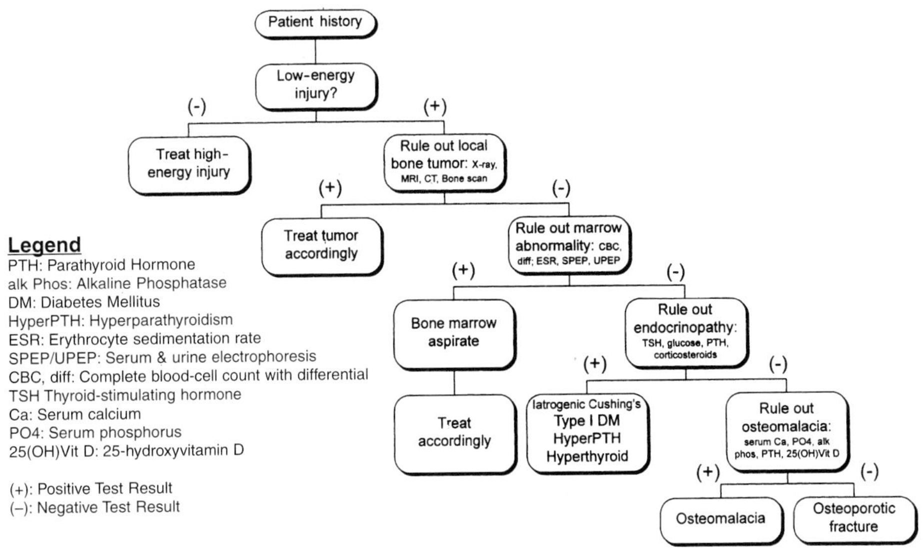

Fig. 4 Workup for an insufficiency fracture.

less than femoral strength in specimens from younger individuals.[68] Factors that increase the risk of a fracture due to a fall include impact on or near the greater trochanter; the lack of protective mechanisms, such as the use of an outstretched arm, to break the fall; and insufficient energy absorption by the local soft tissues.[69] On the basis of a thorough history, the physician can make recommendations to reduce the chances of the patient falling and sustaining a hip fracture. Recommendations may include the removal of environmental hazards such as throw rugs and poor lighting, caution with regard to the use of sedatives, a regular program of exercise, and balance training. Prospective trials are under way to determine if trochanteric padding or energy-absorbent floors can be recommended to reduce the prevalence of hip fractures in susceptible populations.

Imaging Studies and the Measurement of Bone Mineral Density

The primary goal in the treatment of osteoporosis is to prevent bone loss beyond the fracture threshold. Measurements of bone mineral density can be used to assess the risk of a fracture with a high degree of specificity.[70] There is a 1.5 to threefold increase in the fracture rate for each standard deviation of decrease in bone mineral density.[71,72] Thus, if the average remaining lifetime risk of a fracture is 15% in a group of 50-year-old women who have average bone mineral density, then the lifetime risk of a fracture is approximately 30% for a 50-year-old woman in whom the bone mineral density is one standard deviation less than the average and approximately 60% for a 50-year-old woman in whom the bone mineral density is two standard deviations less than the average.[73]

Although the risk of a fracture increases continuously as bone mineral density declines, it is useful, from a practical standpoint, to define cutoff values for the purpose of intervention. Defining osteoporosis as a bone mineral density of 2.5 standard deviations less than the average value for young adults identifies approximately 30% of postmenopausal women who are at the highest risk for a fracture and who need corresponding counseling and treatment.[73] Defining an additional cutoff value as one standard deviation less than the average value for young adults creates another group that includes approximately 15% of postmenopausal women in whom the prevention of bone loss would be most useful as well.

Bone mass can be determined with a number of noninvasive methods.[51,74] The critical elements of any system include precision, accuracy, and sensitivity to changes in bone mass. Radiographs of the spine demonstrate osteopenia (a radiographic term for an apparent decrease in bone mass density) only when 30% of the bone mass has been lost. The preferential loss of horizontal trabeculae in the vertebral body gives the remaining vertical trabeculae a hypertrophic appearance.

Determination of precisely when a vertebral deformation that is due to osteoporosis constitutes a fracture can be difficult with use of standard radiographic techniques. The lack of a universally accepted definition of a fracture has serious implications; as the definition is expanded to include more minor changes, the specific effect of any drug intervention on the disease process becomes more difficult to assess. The technique recommended by Genant requires a 25% change in one dimension or a 40% change in the total cross-sectional area as the minimum criterion for a vertebral fracture.[75,76]

Single-beam densitometry can be used to measure bone mass at the distal third of the forearm.[77] Although the extreme distal end of the radius, termed the ultradistal radius, is more sensitive to changes, reproducibility of results is difficult to achieve at that location.[77] The cortical bone of the distal third of the radius is not very sensitive to changes in bone metabolism, and the findings at that location may not correspond with the changes in the spine or the hip.

Quantitative CT scanning can be used to examine a window within the vertebral body as well as to measure the trabecular bone mass therein. Among radiographic methods, it is the most sensitive to changes in bone mass; however, it is less precise, is more costly, and results in a higher exposure to radiation than dual-energy x-ray absorptiometry.[78,79] Therefore, quantitative CT generally is reserved for research studies. Dual-energy x-ray absorptiometry, commonly called DEXA, has a high rate of precision and subjects the patient to an extremely low dose of radiation; it is currently the most frequently used method of evaluating bone density in clinical practice.[78-80]

Laboratory Studies

Laboratory studies are used to exclude other diseases that can cause osteopenia and to determine the type of osteoporosis.[81] As indicated in the algorithm for the workup of a patient who has an insufficiency fracture (Fig. 4), a complete blood-cell count with differential, determination of the erythrocyte sedimentation rate, and immunoelectrophoresis identify most bone-marrow abnormalities. Such abnormalities are seen in approximately 2% of patients who have osteopenia, and half of these abnormalities are multiple myeloma.[28] If such an abnormality is suspected, a bone-marrow aspiration is performed. If no bone-marrow abnormality is noted, common endocrinopathies are sought. Initially, one should screen for hyperparathyroidism and hyperthyroidism by measuring serum levels of parathyroid hormone and thyroid-stimulating hormone by radioimmunoassay. Corticosteroid-induced osteoporosis, Cushing disease, and diabetes mellitus are sought if they are suspected clinically.

Once endocrinopathies have been excluded, as many as 10% of older individuals who live in northern communities in the United States and who have osteopenia will be found to have varying levels of osteomalacia.[28,46] Osteomalacia can be diagnosed, in more than 50% of these individuals, on the basis of simple blood tests that show low-normal serum calcium levels, low phosphate and 25-hydroxyvitamin-D levels, and high alkaline phosphatase and parathyroid hormone levels. Subtler forms of osteomalacia are more difficult to diagnose and may necessitate bone biopsy.[28]

Advances in the understanding of metabolic bone disease have led to the development of more specific laboratory tests.[82,83] Bone-specific alkaline phosphatase, osteocalcin, and procollagen-I extension propeptides specifically reflect bone formation. Markers of bone degradation are more nonspecific, but urinary pyridinoline and deoxypyridinoline correspond well with histologic indices of bone resorption. These tests can be helpful in complicated cases and in identifying the types of osteoporosis that are difficult to diagnose.

Bone Histomorphometry

Although the more advanced laboratory tests that screen for the presence of markers of bone formation and degradation in blood and urine accurately reflect the metabolic activity of bone in most patients, the determination of bone mass does not characterize the qualitative status of the bone.[81,84] Other methods of assessing the quality of bone are therefore necessary.

A biopsy of tetracycline-labeled, undecalcified, iliac-crest bone is the best method of differentiating among high-turnover and low-turnover osteoporosis, osteomalacia, secondary hyperparathyroidism, and complicated combinations of these conditions. The recent chapter by Mohler and associates[81] provides additional information.

The current candidates for bone biopsy at the University of California at Los Angeles Osteoporosis Center are individuals who are less than 60 years old and in whom bone density is at least 2.5 standard deviations less than that of their peers; individuals who are less than 65 years old, who do not have an apparent metabolic abnormality, and who have sustained a low-energy fracture; and patients who are being managed with chemotherapy, antimetabolites, or corticosteroids because of complex medical problems.

Treatment of Osteoporosis

Pharmacologic Therapy

Calcium Calcium is one of the most widely used agents in the treatment of osteoporosis.[85,86] Because most children have an inadequate calcium intake, the peak bone mass achieved is often less than it might have been. This creates a major risk for osteoporosis later in life.[14-16,85,86] Girls at puberty are probably the optimum population for the early use of calcium to prevent osteoporosis.[87] There is, however, a level of calcium intake beyond which additional supplementation yields no greater ultimate peak bone density. Matkovic and Heaney[88] pointed out that the administration of calcium supplements during growth may only accelerate the attainment of peak bone mass and that there is no evidence that it increases the actual peak bone mass ultimately achieved.

Calcium supplementation does not appear to decrease the 10% loss of bone mass that occurs in the spine during the first several years after menopause, but it is helpful at all ages in enhancing appendicular bone mass.[6,28,46,81] Calcium supplementation in the older population may be most effective when the baseline calcium intake is less than 400 mg/day, for those who have an intestinal malabsorption syndrome, or in combination with an exercise regimen.[89] Calcium supplementation is helpful for patients who have type-II osteoporosis, especially when the therapy is combined with vitamin-D supplementation.[2,90]

A marked decrease in the rate of fractures of the hip was demonstrated in a study[90] of elderly patients from France who had received dietary supplements of calcium and vitamin D. This decrease occurred even though little difference was noted in bone mass, a finding that raises the possibility that the calcium and vitamin-D supplementation had improved the quality of bone or had decreased the prevalence of secondary hyperparathyroidism.

Vitamin D Vitamin-D deficiency is common in elderly individuals who have osteoporosis, in strict vegetarians, and in populations of some northern locations during the winter.[91-93] Individuals who have vitamin-D deficiency typically have poor calcium absorption as well. Vitamin D stimulates bone formation and intestinal calcium absorption; vitamin-D supplementation therefore may improve calcium balance. In addition, by suppressing parathyroid hormone activity, vitamin D may positively influence bone density in healthy individuals who do not have vitamin-D deficiency or osteoporosis.[90,94] This may be especially important during the winter months, during which lower levels of vitamin D and higher levels of parathyroid hormone have been shown to coincide with an increased prevalence of osteoporotic fractures.[81,94] Subjects who had been given a single high dose (100,000 units) of vitamin D in early winter had higher serum vitamin-D concentrations and lower parathyroid hormone levels than did controls after 5 weeks.[94] Several recent studies have shown that the oral administration of calcitriol and some of its synthetic precursors, notably alfacalcidol (1-alpha-hydroxyvitamin D_3), can correct mild secondary hyperparathyroidism, reduce bone loss, and prevent fractures of the hip.[95-97]

Receptors of vitamin D on the osteoblast display phenotypic heterogeneity. This genetic variability was investigated in Australia in an attempt to explain the low levels of vitamin D in individuals who have osteoporosis and the generally positive but inconsistent responses of such individuals to therapy.[98] Additional work in this area may lead to genetic tests for a predisposition to low bone density and allow for the development of more tailored prophylactic interventions.[98] Unfortunately, these results have not been seen consistently in other countries, and the polymorphism of the receptor sites is still under study.

Estrogen Estrogen deficiency plays a prominent role in the pathogenesis of osteoporosis. Estrogen inhibits bone resorption and positively affects calcium balance, either directly, by stimulating the estrogen receptors in bone, or indirectly, by suppressing the production of bone-resorbing cytokines.[99-102] With few exceptions, estrogen therapy protects against postmenopausal osteoporosis regardless of which form of estrogen is administered or which technique is used to measure bone density.[103] The administration of estrogen to postmenopausal women not only prevents bone loss but also protects against vertebral and femoral fractures, with a greater effect on the spine.[28,81,104-106] Discontinuation of the therapy is followed by an immediate resumption of bone loss at a rate similar to that in women who have not received such therapy.[107]

Several different estrogen regimens are available for the treatment of postmenopausal osteoporosis.[108-110] The use of estrogen therapy is increasing worldwide, but even in the countries in which it is used most extensively, no more than one-third of the women accept it over the long term.[109] This situation is the result of side effects, primarily endometrial bleeding, and concern by the public and among physicians about the relative risks of cardiovascular disease as well as endometrial and breast cancer.[111,112] Prolonged use of estrogen appears to increase the risk of breast cancer by 30%,[113-115] an increase roughly from 11 to 14 instances of breast cancer per 100 women. It is important to note that women in whom breast cancer develops during the course of estrogen therapy do not appear to have an increased rate of mortality.[113,115] Therefore, women should have regular gynecologic and breast examinations, including mammography, while receiving estrogen therapy. The concomitant administration of progestin eliminates the risk of uterine cancer, and continuous therapy with a combination of progestin and estrogen can minimize cyclical uterine bleeding in older women.[116] Most of the cardiovascular benefits associated with estrogen are preserved when progestin is given cyclically, but the continuous use of progestin diminishes some of the cardiovascular benefits of estrogen.

Estrogen is an ideal agent for patients who have a high risk of cardiovascular disease, no family history of early breast cancer, a strong family history of osteoporosis or a low bone-mineral density, substantial postmenopausal symptoms, and who are receiving thyroid hormone-replacement therapy. Conversely, patients who do not have osteoporosis or coronary artery disease or substantial risk factors for these diseases, or who have a history of thrombophlebitis or a family history of early breast cancer, are considered poor candidates for estrogen supplementation. The usual daily dose of estrogen required to prevent bone loss is 0.625 mg, but half of this dose may suffice when it is combined with calcium supplementation.[116]

There is an increasing recognition that estrogen therapy may have to be adjusted to the individual patient. About 20% of women who receive conventional doses of estrogen continue to lose bone mass,[117] and such patients might benefit from a higher dose. Women who smoke may need a higher dose because of an increased rate of estrogen degradation.[118] Conversely, obese women who produce substantial amounts of estrogen peripherally may need a lower dose.[119] The use of estrogen during only the early (6- to 10-year) postmenopausal period appears to be inadequate.[120] A study of older women from the Framingham observational group showed that the previous use of estrogen was not protective against fractures of the hip that occurred 10 to 20 years after the termination of treatment.[121] Only use of estrogen for more than 7 years was found to be protective.[35] Some researchers have suggested that estrogen therapy should not be initiated until the patient is 65 years old because prolonged use increases the risk of breast cancer.[114] This approach, however, is unlikely to gain wide acceptance.

Calcitonin Calcitonin can be used to treat osteoporosis, although patients who have osteoporosis do not appear to have a deficiency of this hormone.[122] Calcitonin is used commonly in some countries for the short-term amelioration of pain associated with fractures due to osteoporosis because it has an analgesic property, as a result either of elevating the level of endorphins or of inhibiting the release of neuropeptides.[123] It binds to specific receptors on the osteoclast and exerts an inhibitory effect on its activity. Trabecular bone is affected, but cortical bone is not. Calcitonin has been shown to be a safe alternative for the treatment of osteoporosis in women who cannot take estrogen.[4] Women who have high-turnover osteoporosis or who have pain because of a recent vertebral fracture are likely to benefit most from its use.

Calcitonin, typically administered by means of subcutaneous injection, has also been shown to be effective in intranasal, rectal, and transdermal forms, although there may be erratic patterns of absorption with the nasal route. The analgesic effects of the newly released nasal form are similar to those of the other forms. Reginster and associates[124] conducted a 3-year randomized placebo-controlled study in which women in whom menopause had taken place 6 to 36 months previously were given either calcium alone or the same amount of calcium in addition to calcitonin by means of nasal administration. Lumbar bone-mineral density increased slightly (1.8% ± 5.7% [average and standard deviation]) in the women receiving calcitonin and calcium. In those receiving calcium alone, lumbar bone-mineral density decreased 5.8% ± 4.8%. An evaluation performed at 5 years revealed that the bone mineral density had remained significantly greater ($p < 0.001$) in the patients who had been managed with calcitonin.[125]

Bisphosphonates Bisphosphonates are stable, active analogs of pyrophosphate that both inhibit osteoclastic resorption and depress bone turnover.[126-128] Etidronate has been used for many years for the treatment of Paget disease, but it has not been approved by the Food and Drug Administration for the treatment of osteoporosis. Long-term etidronate therapy creates untoward histologic changes in bone; such abnormalities may be eliminated by intermittent, cyclic use.[129] Etidronate and newer bisphosphonates, including alendronate, pamidronate, residronate, taludrinate, and clonodrate, currently are the most extensively investigated agents in osteoporosis research.[130] Etidronate is most effective during the first 2 years of therapy.[131] Bisphosphonates appear to be effective in the 5-year period of rapid bone turnover that occurs after menopause. Similar to calcitonin, however, bisphosphonates primarily act on trabecular bone and are less effective in preventing the loss of compact bone and hip fractures.[75]

The second-generation agents are more potent and yet cause less inhibition of mineralization than etidronate. These agents appear to have positive effects on vertebral and femoral-neck bone-mineral density.[132] Alendronate, recently approved by the Food and Drug Administration, appears to prevent vertebral bone loss in patients who have osteoporosis and does not alter the mechanical properties of bone.[133] In addition, it appears to continue to work even after it is no longer being administered. Rossini and associates[134] recently reported that lumbar bone-mineral density increased by 3.7% ± 1.7% (average and standard deviation) after 6 months of alendronate therapy and did not change 6 and 12 months after the cessation of treatment.

Fluoride In contrast to the antiresorptive drugs described previously, fluoride causes osteoblast proliferation and stimulates new bone formation. Researchers have found substantial increases in trabecular bone in patients who had received fluoride.[135,136] Enthusiasm for fluoride has been tempered by studies that have shown impaired bone mineralization and increased rates of fractures of the hip and vertebrae despite increased bone density in the lumbar spine.[137,138]

Early clinical trials involved the administration of high doses of fluoride (more than 75 mg/day).[137] Analysis of patients who sustained hip fractures during the course of fluoride treatment revealed that the patients had been receiving excessive doses of fluoride; patients who had high-turnover osteoporosis were not excluded from that study.[28] Patients in whom osteoporosis is treated with fluoride often have a calcium deficiency because of the increased mineralization of trabecular bone. This situation renders the patients vulnerable to secondary hyperparathyroidism. Vitamin-D supplementation can correct the calcium deficiency while potentiating the effect of fluoride on the osteoblast; this allows the dose of fluoride to be decreased and thereby minimizes its side effects.[139]

Proponents of fluoride use suggest that better results are possible with lower doses (approximately 50 mg/day) in a delayed-release form.[138,140] Riggs and associates[138] reviewed their original study,[113] in which high doses of fluoride had been used. A subset of patients from that study were managed with a lower dose of fluoride to avoid side effects. Analysis of the rate of vertebral fractures revealed a complex relationship between bone mineral density and the serum fluoride level. The rate of vertebral fractures decreased as the bone mineral density increased, except when the higher bone mineral density was associated with a rapid rate of increase of bone mineral density in the spine or a large increase in the level of serum fluoride from baseline. These findings imply that bone formation due to fluoride therapy decreases the rate of vertebral fractures as long as bone production proceeds slowly enough to allow for proper mineralization and as long as the fluoride level does not exceed a toxic threshold.

Pak and associates[141] recently reported that patients in whom postmenopausal osteoporosis had been treated with a preparation of slow-release sodium fluoride had a lower rate of vertebral fractures and a higher fracture-free rate (defined as the absence of fractures during the trial) compared with a group of controls who had received calcium. A substantial increase in the bone mass of the lumbar vertebrae of 4% to 5% per year for 4 years, an average increase in the bone density of the femoral neck of 2.4% per year, and no change in the bone density of the radial shaft were observed in the patients who had received fluoride. The frequency with which minor side effects and appendicular fractures occurred was similar in the two groups. Pak and associates[141] concluded that slow-release sodium fluoride and calcium citrate administered for 4 years inhibits new vertebral fractures, augments spinal and femoral-neck bone mass, and is safe to use.

The ideal role of fluoride in the future may be to augment bone density at the initiation of therapy before switching to antiresorptive agents for the long-term maintenance of bone density. At present, however, the use of fluoride is considered experimental.

Our current treatment protocol for osteoporosis in women at the University of California at Los Angeles Osteoporosis Center involves the separation of premenopausal and postmenopausal patients into two groups (Outline 1). Premenopausal women who are eumenorrheic should have a physiologic calcium intake (700 to 1,300 mg/day), vitamin-D supplementation (400 IU/day), and appropriate exercise. Premenopausal women who are amenorrheic should be managed as just described and should also consider cyclical estrogen and progestin therapy and have an appropriate caloric intake.

All postmenopausal women should have a calcium intake of 1,500 mg/day and vitamin-D supplementation of 400 IU/day. Post-menopausal women are subdivided according to their bone mineral density. For women who have a bone mineral density that is within one standard deviation less than that of their peers, cyclical estrogen and progestin supplementation should be considered. Women who have a bone mineral density that is one to 2.5 standard deviations less than that of their peers, who do not have a fracture, and who are less than 70 years old should receive estrogen (0.625 mg/day) and progestin (2.5 to 10.0 mg/day). Women who have a fracture or a bone mineral density that is more than 2.5 standard deviations less than that of their peers should receive calcitonin (50 to 100 units subcutaneously, 3 to 7 days per week) acutely, for as long as 18 months, in addition to calcium and vitamin-D supplements. Once the administration of calcitonin is discontinued, either estrogen and progestin (if the patient is less than 70 years old) or alendronate (10.0 mg/day if the bone mineral density is more than 2.5 standard deviations less than that of the patient's peers) should be given.

Outline 1
Osteoporosis treatment protocol

I. Premenopause
   A. Eumenorrheic
      1. Physiologic calcium (700 to 1,300 mg/day)
      2. Vitamin D (400 IU/day)
      3. Exercise
   B. Amenorrheic
      1. Physiologic calcium (700 to 1,300 mg/day)
      2. Consider cyclical estrogen and progestin*
      3. Vitamin D (400 IU/day)
      4. Appropriate caloric intake
      5. Exercise
II. Postmenopause
   A. Bone mineral density within 1 standard deviation less than that of peers
      1. Calcium (1,500 mg/day)
      2. Vitamin D (400 IU/day)
      3. Consider cyclical estrogen and progestin* if patient < 70 yrs. old
   B. Bone mineral density 1 to 2.5 standard deviations less than that of peers and no fracture
      1. Calcium (1,500 mg/day)
      2. Vitamin D (400 IU/day)
      3. Cyclical estrogen and progestin* if patient < 70 yrs. old
   C. Bone mineral density > 2.5 standard deviations less than that of peers, or fracture
      1. Calcium (1,500 mg/day)
      2. Vitamin D (400 IU/day)
      3. Calcitonin (50 to 100 units subcutaneously, 3 to 7 days/wk) acutely, for as long as 18 months
      4. Then, cyclical estrogen and progestin* if patient < 70 yrs. old, or alendronate (10.0 mg/day) if bone mineral density > 2.5 standard deviations less than that of peers, as per Food and Drug Administration recommendations

*A typical regimen consists of 0.625 milligram of estrogen per day and 2.5 to 10.0 milligrams of progestin per day

Conclusion

A review of the treatment of osteoporosis indicates that, at the present time, prevention is clearly the best solution. Maximization of peak bone mass and reduction of postmenopausal and age-associated bone loss are both crucial. Adequate calcium intake during growth as well as calcium and vitamin-D supplementation postmenopausally constitute the fundamental strategy applicable to essentially all patients. A lifetime habit of physical exercise and the elimination of falls as well as attenuation of the severity of falls are important for the elderly. Estrogen is the drug of choice for the prevention of postmenopausal bone loss. Calcitonin is the agent of choice for patients who cannot take estrogen or who have pain due to a fracture. The newly approved bisphosphonate, alendronate, appears to have substantial antiresorptive properties with minimum side effects. Fluoride has been shown to affect bone formation positively and may have a role in treatment in the future.

References

1. American Academy of Orthopaedic Surgeons: Position statement: Prevention of hip fractures. Rosemont, IL, American Academy of Orthopaedic Surgeons, 1993.
2. Riggs BL, Melton LJ III: The prevention and treatment of osteoporosis. *N Engl J Med* 1992;327:620–627.
3. Meunier PJ: Prevention of hip fractures. *Am J Med* 1993; 95:75S–78S.
4. Kleerekoper M, Avioli LV: Evaluation and treatment of postmenopausal osteoporosis, in Favus MJ (ed): *Primer on the Metabolic Bone Diseases and Disorders of Mineral Metabolism*, ed 2. New York, NY, Raven Press, 1993, pp 223–229.
5. Riggs BL, Melton LJ III: Evidence for two distinct syndromes of involutional osteoporosis. *Am J Med* 1983;75:899–901.
6. Lane JM, Cornell CN, Healey JH: Orthopaedic consequences of osteoporosis, in Riggs BL, Melton LJ III (eds): *Osteoporosis: Etiology, Diagnosis and Management.* New York, NY, Raven Press, 1988, pp 433–455.
7. Peck WA, Woods WL: The cells of bone, in Riggs BL, Melton LJ III (eds): *Osteoporosis: Etiology, Diagnosis and Management.* New York, NY, Raven Press, 1988, pp 1–44.
8. Rodan GA, Rodan SB: Expression of the osteoblast phenotype, in Peck WA (ed): *Bone and Mineral Research*, ed 2. Amsterdam, The Netherlands, Elsevier Science, 1983, pp 244–285.
9. Stein GS, Lian JB: Molecular mechanisms mediating proliferation/differentiation interrelationships during progressive development of the osteoblast phenotype. *Endocr Rev* 1993; 14:424–442.
10. Frost HM (ed): *Bone Remodelling Dynamics.* Springfield, IL, Charles C Thomas, 1963.
11. Gallagher JC, Melton LJ, Riggs BL, et al: Epidemiology of fractures of the proximal femur in Rochester, Minnesota. *Clin Orthop* 1980;150:163–171.
12. Buckwalter JA, Glimcher MJ, Cooper RR, et al: Bone biology: Part I. Structure, blood supply, cells, matrix, and mineralization. *J Bone Joint Surg* 1995;77A:1256–1275.
13. Buckwalter JA, Glimcher MJ, Cooper RR, et al: Bone biology: Part II. Formation, form, modeling, remodeling, and regulation of cell function. *J Bone Joint Surg* 1995;77A:1276–1289.
14. Heaney RP: Calcium intake and bone health, in Coissac P (ed): *Postmenopausal Osteoporosis: Prevention and Treatment.* Davos, Switzerland, Sandoz, 1985.
15. Heaney RP: Calcium, bone health, and osteoporosis, in Peck WA (ed): *Bone and Mineral Research.* Amsterdam, The Netherlands, Elsevier Science, 1986, vol 4, pp 255–301.
16. Heaney RP, Recker RR, Saville PD: Calcium balance and calcium requirements in middle-aged women. *Am J Clin Nutr* 1977; 30:1603–1611.
17. Heaney RP, Recker RR, Saville PD: Menopausal changes in calcium balance performance. *J Lab Clin Med* 1978;92:953–963.
18. National Institutes of Health: Optimal calcium intake. *NIH Consensus Statement* 1994;12:1–31.
19. Matkovic V, Fontana D, Tominac C, et al: Factors that influence peak bone mass formation: A study of calcium balance and the inheritance of bone mass in adolescent females. *Am J Clin Nutr* 1990;52:878–888.
20. Slemenda C, Hui SL, Johnston CC: Patterns of bone loss and physiologic growing: Prospects for prevention of osteoporosis by attainment of greater peak bone mass, in Christiansen C, Overgaard K (eds): *Osteoporosis 1990: International Symposium on Osteoporosis.* Copenhagen, Denmark, Osteopress, 1990, vol 2, pp 948–953.
21. Teegarden D, Proulx WR, Martin BR, et al: Peak bone mass in young women. *J Bone Miner Res* 1995;10:711–715.
22. Johnston CC Jr, Miller JZ, Slemenda CW, et al: Calcium supplementation and increases in bone mineral density in children. *N Engl J Med* 1992;327:82–87.
23. Johnston CC Jr, Slemenda CW: Peak bone mass, bone loss and risk of fracture. *Osteoporos Int* 1994;4(suppl 1):43–45.
24. Matkovic V, Jelic T, Wardlaw GM, et al: Timing of peak bone mass in Caucasian females and its implication for the prevention of osteoporosis: Inference from a cross-sectional model. *J Clin Invest* 1994;93:799–808.
25. Recker RR: Bone biopsy and histomorphometry in clinical practice, in Favus MJ (ed): *Primer on the Metabolic Bone Diseases and Disorders of Mineral Metabolism*, ed 2. New York, NY, Raven Press, 1993, pp 146–150.
26. Recker RR, Davies KM, Hinders SM, et al: Bone gain in young adult women. *JAMA* 1992;268:2403–2405.
27. Cummings SR, Kelsey JL, Nevitt MC, et al: Epidemiology of osteoporosis and osteoporotic fractures. *Epidemiol Rev* 1985; 7:178–208.
28. Lane JM, Healey JH (eds): *Diagnosis and Management of Pathological Fractures.* New York, NY, Raven Press, 1993.
29. Wong GL: Skeletal effects of parathyroid hormone, in Peck WA (ed): *Bone and Mineral Research.* Amsterdam, The Netherlands, Elsevier Science, 1986, vol 4, pp 103–129.
30. Austin LA, Heath H III: Calcitonin: Physiology and pathophysiology. *N Engl J Med* 1981;304:269–278.
31. Cann CE, Cavanaugh DJ, Schnurfield K, et al: Menstrual history is the primary determinant of trabecular bone density in women runners. *Med Sci Sports Exerc* 1988;20(suppl):559.
32. Loucks AB: Effects of exercise training on the menstrual cycle: Existence and mechanisms. *Med Sci Sports Exerc* 1990;22: 275–280.
33. Warren MP, Fox RP, DeRogatis AJ, et al: Osteopenia in hypothalamic amenorrhea: A 3-year longitudinal study. *Endocrine Soc Ann Meet* 1994;76:461.
34. Heaney RP, Recker RR, Saville PD: Menopausal changes in bone remodeling. *J Lab Clin Med* 1978;92:964–970.
35. Eriksen EF, Colvard DS, Berg NJ, et al: Evidence of estrogen receptors in normal human osteoblast-like cells. *Science* 1988; 241:84–86.
36. Hahn TJ: Steroid and drug-induced osteopenia, in Favus MJ, Christakos S, Kleerekoper M, et al (eds): *Primer on the Metabolic Bone Diseases and Disorders of Mineral Metabolism*, ed 2. New York, NY, Raven Press, 1993, pp 250–255.
37. Healey LH: Glucocorticoid-induced osteoporosis. *Curr Opin Orthop* 1994;5:33–38.
38. Spector TD, Sambrook PN: Editorial: Steroid osteoporosis. *Br Med J* 1993;307:519–520.
39. Meunier PJ: Editorial: Is steroid-induced osteoporosis preventable? *N Engl J Med* 1993;328:1781–1782.
40. Diamond T, Vine J, Smart R, et al: Thyrotoxic bone disease in women: A potentially reversible disorder. *Ann Intern Med* 1994; 120:8–11.
41. Franklyn JA, Betteridge J, Daykin J, et al: Long-term thyroxine treatment and bone mineral density. *Lancet* 1992;340:9–13.
42. Mosekilde L, Eriksen EF, Charles P: Effects of thyroid hormones on bone and mineral metabolism. *Endocrinol Metab Clin North Am* 1990;19:35–63.
43. Marcocci C, Golia F, Bruno-Bossio G, et al: Carefully monitored levothyroxine suppressive therapy is not associated with bone loss in premenopausal women. *J Clin Endocrinol Metab* 1994; 78:818–823.
44. Bauer DC, Browner WS, Cauley JA, et al: Factors associated with appendicular bone mass in older women: The study of Osteoporotic Fractures Research Group. *Ann Intern Med* 1993;118:657–665.
45. Schneider DL, Barrett-Connor EL, Morton DJ: Thyroid hormone use and bone mineral density in elderly women: Effects of estrogen. *JAMA* 1994;271:1245–1249.
46. Lane JM, Cornell CN, Healey JH: Osteoporosis: The structural and reparative consequences for the skeleton, in Griffin PP

(ed): *Instructional Course Lectures XXXVI.* Park Ridge, IL, American Academy of Orthopaedic Surgeons, 1987, pp 71–83.
47. Mellish RW, Ferguson-Pell MW, Cochran GV, et al: A new manual method for assessing two-dimensional cancellous bone structure: Comparison between iliac crest and lumbar vertebra. *J Bone Miner Res* 1991;6:689–696.
48. Compston JE: Editorial: Connectivity of cancellous bone: Assessment and mechanical implications. *Bone* 1994;15: 463–466.
49. Shen V, Dempster DW, Birchman R, et al: Loss of cancellous bone mass and connectivity in ovariectomized rats can be restored by combined treatment with parathyroid hormone and estradiol. *J Clin Invest* 1993;91:2479–2487.
50. Barth RW, Lane JM: Osteoporosis. *Orthop Clin North Am* 1988; 19:845–858.
51. Grampp S, Jergas M, Gluer CC, et al: Radiologic diagnosis of osteoporosis: Current methods and perspectives. *Radiol Clin North Am* 1993;31:1133–1145.
52. Madsen OR, Schaadt O, Bliddal H, et al: Relationship between quadriceps strength and bone mineral density of the proximal tibia and distal forearm in women. *J Bone Miner Res* 1993; 8:1439–1444.
53. Revel M, Mayoux-Benhamou MA, Rabourdin JP, et al: One-year psoas training can prevent lumbar bone loss in postmenopausal women: A randomized controlled trial. *Calcif Tissue Int* 1993;53:307–311.
54. Drinkwater BL, Grimston SK, Raab-Cullen DM, et al: ACSM position stand on osteoporosis and exercise. American College of Sports Medicine. *Med Sci Sports Exerc* 1995;27:745–750.
55. Cooper C, Cawley M, Bhalla A, et al: Childhood growth, physical activity, and peak bone mass in women. *J Bone Miner Res* 1995;10:940–947.
56. Lohman T, Going S, Pamenter R, et al: Effects of resistance training on regional and total bone mineral density in premenopausal women: A randomized prospective study. *J Bone Miner Res* 1995;10:1015–1024.
57. Jacobson PC, Beaver W, Grubb SA, et al: Bone density in women: College athletes and older athletic women. *J Orthop Res* 1984;2:328–332.
58. Hetland ML, Haarbo J, Christiansen C: Low bone mass and high bone turnover in male long distance runners. *J Clin Endocrinol Metab* 1993;77:770–775.
59. Flawn LB: Amenorrhea, anorexia, and osteoporosis: The female triad. *Curr Opin Orthop* 1994;5:16–20.
60. Healey JH, Lane JM: Structural scoliosis in osteoporotic women. *Clin Orthop* 1985;195:216–223.
61. Velis KP, Healey JH, Schneider R: Osteoporosis in unstable adult scoliosis. *Clin Orthop* 1988;237:132–141.
62. Velis KP, Healey JH, Schneider R: Peak skeletal mass assessment in young adults with idiopathic scoliosis. *Spine* 1989;14:706–711.
63. Cummings SR, Black DM, Nevitt MC, et al: Appendicular bone density and age predict hip fracture in women: The Study of Osteoporotic Fractures Research Group. *JAMA* 1990;263: 665–668.
64. Grisso JA, Kelsey JL, Strom BL, et al: Risk factors for falls as a cause of hip fracture in women: The Northeast Hip Fracture Study Group. *N Engl J Med* 1991;324:1326–1331.
65. Cummings SR, Nevitt MC, Browner WS, et al: Risk factors for hip fracture in white women: Study of Osteoporotic Fractures Research Group. *N Engl J Med* 1995;332:767–773.
66. Greenspan SL, Myers ER, Maitland LA, et al: Fall severity and bone mineral density as risk factors for hip fracture in ambulatory elderly. *JAMA* 1994;271:128–133.
67. Hayes WC, Myers ER, Morris JN, et al: Impact near the hip dominates fracture risk in elderly nursing home residents who fall. *Calcif Tissue Int* 1993;52:192–198.
68. Courtney AC, Wachtel EF, Myers ER, et al: Age-related reductions in the strength of the femur tested in a fall-loading configuration. *J Bone Joint Surg* 1995;77A:387–395.
69. Cummings SR, Nevitt MC: A hypothesis: The causes of hip fractures. *J Gerontol* 1989;44:M107–M111.
70. WHO Study Group on Assessment of Fracture Risk and its Application to Screening for Postmenopausal Osteoporosis: Assessment of fracture risk and its application to screening for postmenopausal osteoporosis. Geneva, Switzerland, World Health Organization, 1994.
71. Cummings SR, Black DM, Nevitt MC, et al: Bone density at various sites for prediction of hip fractures: The Study of Osteoporotic Fractures Research Group. *Lancet* 1993;341:72–85.
72. Hui SL, Slemenda CW, Johnston CC Jr: Baseline measurement of bone mass predicts fracture in white women. *Ann Intern Med* 1989;111:355–361.
73. Kanis JA, Melton LJ III, Christiansen C, et al: The diagnosis of osteoporosis. *J Bone Miner Res* 1994;9:1137–1141.
74. Jergas M, Genant HK: Current methods and recent advances in the diagnosis of osteoporosis. *Arthritis Rheum* 1993;36: 1649–1662.
75. Storm T, Thamsborg G, Steiniche T, et al: Effect of intermittent cyclical etidronate therapy on bone mass and fracture rate in women with postmenopausal osteoporosis. *N Engl J Med* 1990;322:1265–1271.
76. Watts NB, Harris ST, Genant HK, et al: Intermittent cyclical etidronate treatment of postmenopausal osteoporosis. *N Engl J Med* 1990;323:73–79.
77. Kelly TL, Crane G, Baran DT: Single x-ray absorptiometry of the forearm: Precision, correlation, and reference data. *Calcif Tissue Int* 1994;54:212–218.
78. American College of Physicians: Radiologic methods to evaluate bone mineral content. *Ann Intern Med* 1984;100:908–911.
79. Schneider R, Math K: Bone density analysis, an update. *Curr Opin Orthop* 1994;5:66–72.
80. Mazess RB: Bone densitometry of the axial skeleton. *Orthop Clin North Am* 1990;21:51–63.
81. Mohler DG, Lane JM, Cole BJ, et al: Skeletal failure in osteoporosis, in Lane JM, Healey JH (eds): *Diagnosis and Management of Pathologic Fractures.* New York, NY, Raven Press, 1993, pp 13–36.
82. Price CP, Thompson PW: The role of biochemical tests in the screening and monitoring of osteoporosis. *Ann Clin Biochem* 1995;32:244–260.
83. Sanchez CP, Salusky IB: Biochemical markers in metabolic bone disease. *Curr Opin Orthop* 1994;5:43–49.
84. Uebelhart D, Schlemmer A, Johansen JS, et al: Effect of menopause and hormone replacement therapy on the urinary excretion of pyridinium cross-links. *J Clin Endocrinol Metab* 1991;72:367–373.
85. Heaney RP: Calcium in the prevention and treatment of osteoporosis. *J Intern Med* 1992;231:169–180.
86. Heaney RP: Bone mass, nutrition, and other lifestyle factors. *Am J Med* 1993;95:29S–33S.
87. Matkovic V: Calcium and peak bone mass. *J Intern Med* 1992; 231:151–160.
88. Matkovic V, Heaney RP: Calcium balance during human growth: Evidence for threshold behavior. *Am J Clin Nutr* 1992;55:992–996.
89. Dawson-Hughes B, Dallal GE, Krall EA, et al: A controlled trial of the effect of calcium supplementation on bone density in postmenopausal women. *N Engl J Med* 1990;323:878–883.
90. Chapuy MC, Arlot ME, Duboeuf F, et al: Vitamin D3 and calcium to prevent hip fractures in elderly women. *N Engl J Med* 1992;327:1637–1642.
91. Komar L, Nieves J, Cosman F, et al: Calcium homeostasis of an elderly population upon admission to a nursing home. *J Am Geriatr Soc* 1993;41:1057–1064.

92. Lamberg-Allardt C, Karkkainen M, Seppanen R, et al: Low serum 25-hydroxyvitamin D concentrations and secondary hyperparathyroidism in middle-aged white strict vegetarians. *Am J Clin Nutr* 1993;58:684–689.
93. Need AG, Morris HA, Horowitz M, et al: Effects of skin thickness, age, body fat, and sunlight on serum 25 hydroxyvitamin D. *Am J Clin Nutr* 1993;58:882–885.
94. Khaw KT, Scragg R, Murphy S: Single dose cholecalciferol suppresses the winter increase in parathyroid hormone concentrations in healthy older men and women: A randomized trial. *Am J Clin Nutr* 1994;59:1040–1044.
95. Menczel J, Foldes J, Steinberg R, et al: Alfacalcidol (alpha D3) and calcium in osteoporosis. *Clin Orthop* 1994;300:241–247.
96. Orimo H, Shiraki M, Hayashi T, et al: Reduced occurrence of vertebral crush fractures in senile osteoporosis treated with 1 alpha (OH)-vitamin D3. *Bone Miner* 1987;3:47–52.
97. Tilyard MW, Spears GF, Thomson J, et al: Treatment of postmenopausal osteoporosis with calcitriol or calcium. *N Engl J Med* 1992;326:357–362.
98. Morrison NA, Qi JC, Tokita A, et al: Prediction of bone density from vitamin D receptor alleles. *Nature* 1994;367:284–287.
99. Girasole G, Jilka RL, Passeri G, et al: 17 beta-estradiol inhibits interleukin-6 production by bone marrow-derived stromal cells and osteoblasts in vitro: A potential mechanism for the antiosteoporotic effect of estrogens. *J Clin Invest* 1992;89:883–891.
100. Jilka RL, Hangoc G, Girasole G, et al: Increased osteoclast development after estrogen loss: Mediation by interleukin-6. *Science* 1992;257:88–91.
101. Oursler MJ, Osdoby P, Pyfferoen J, et al: Avian osteoclasts as estrogen target cells. *Proc Natl Acad Sci USA* 1991;88:6613–6617.
102. Pacifici R, Rifas L, McCracken R, et al: Ovarian steroid treatment blocks a postmenopausal increase in blood monocyte interleukin 1 release. *Proc Natl Acad Sci USA* 1989;86:2398–2402.
103. Weiss NS, Ure CL, Ballard JH, et al: Decreased risk of fractures of the hip and lower forearm with postmenopausal use of estrogen. *N Engl J Med* 1980;303:1195–1198.
104. Ettinger B, Genant HK, Cann CE: Long-term estrogen replacement therapy prevents bone loss and fractures. *Ann Intern Med* 1985;102:319–324.
105. Kiel DP, Felson DT, Anderson JJ, et al: Hip fracture and the use of estrogens in postmenopausal women: The Framingham study. *N Engl J Med* 1987;317:1169–1174.
106. Lindsay R, Hart DM, Forrest C, et al: Prevention of spinal osteoporosis in oophorectomised women. *Lancet* 1980;2:1151–1154.
107. Christiansen C, Christensen MS, Transbol I: Bone mass in postmenopausal women after withdrawal of oestrogen/gestagen replacement therapy. *Lancet* 1981;1:459–461.
108. Barrett-Connor E: Estrogen and estrogen-progestogen replacement: Therapy and cardiovascular diseases. *Am J Med* 1993; 95:40S–43S.
109. Consensus Development Conference: Diagnosis, prophylaxis, and treatment of osteoporosis. *Am J Med* 1993;94:646–650.
110. Lindsay R: Hormone replacement therapy for prevention and treatment of osteoporosis. *Am J Med* 1993;95:37S–39S.
111. American College of Physicians: Guidelines for counseling postmenopausal women about preventive hormone therapy. *Ann Intern Med* 1992;117:1038–1041.
112. Hemminki E, Topo P, Malin M, et al: Physicians' views on hormone therapy around and after menopause. *Maturitas* 1993;16:163–173.
113. Belchetz PE: Hormonal treatment of postmenopausal women. *N Engl J Med* 1994;330:1062–1071.
114. Colditz GA, Egan KM, Stampfer MJ: Hormone replacement therapy and risk of breast cancer: Results of epidemiologic studies. *Am J Obstet Gynecol* 1993;168:1473–1480.
115. Colditz GA, Hankinson SE, Hunter DJ, et al: The use of estrogens and progestins and the risk of breast cancer in postmenopausal women. *N Engl J Med* 1995;332:1589–1593.
116. Session DR, Kelly AC, Jewelewicz R: Current concepts in estrogen replacement therapy in the menopause. *Fertil Steril* 1993;59:277–284.
117. Rozenburg S, Gevers R, Peretz A, et al: Decrease of bone mineral density during estrogen substitution therapy. *Maturitas* 1993;17:205–210.
118. Hollenbach KA, Barrett-Connor E, Edelstein SL, et al: Cigarette smoking and bone mineral density in older men and women. *Am J Public Health* 1993;83:1265–1270.
119. Tremollieres FA, Pouilles JM, Ribot C: Vertebral postmenopausal bone loss is reduced in overweight women: A longitudinal study in 155 early postmenopausal women. *J Clin Endocrinol Metab* 1993;77:683–686.
120. Ettinger B, Grady D: Editorial: The waning effect of postmenopausal estrogen therapy on osteoporosis. *N Engl J Med* 1993;329:1192–1193.
121. Felson DT, Zhang Y, Hannan MT, et al: The effect of postmenopausal estrogen therapy on bone density in elderly women. *N Engl J Med* 1993;329:1141–1146.
122. Body JJ: Calcitonin: From the determination of circulating levels in various physiological and pathological conditions to the demonstration of lymphocyte receptors. *Horm Res* 1993; 39:166–170.
123. Gennari C, Agnusdei D, Camporeale A: Use of calcitonin in the treatment of bone pain associated with osteoporosis. *Calcif Tissue Int* 1991;49(suppl 2):S9–S13.
124. Reginster JY, Denis D, Deroisy R, et al: Long-term (3 years) prevention of trabecular postmenopausal bone loss with low-dose intermittent nasal salmon calcitonin. *J Bone Miner Res* 1994; 9:69–72.
125. Reginster JY, Meurmans L, Deroisy R, et al: A 5-year controlled randomized study of prevention of postmenopausal trabecular bone loss with nasal salmon calcitonin and calcium. *Eur J Clin Invest* 1994;24:565–569.
126. Endo Y, Nakamura M, Kikuchi T, et al: Aminoalkyl-bisphosphonates, potent inhibitors of bone resorption, induce a prolonged stimulation of histamine synthesis and increase macrophages, granulocytes, and osteoclasts in vivo. *Calcif Tissue Int* 1993;52:248–254.
127. Sahni M, Guenther HL, Fleisch H, et al: Bisphosphonates act on rat bone resorption through the mediation of osteoblasts. *J Clin Invest* 1993;91:2004–2011.
128. Shinoda H, Adamek G, Felix R, et al: Structure-activity relationships of various bisphosphonates. *Calcif Tissue Int* 1983;35: 87–99.
129. Storm T, Steiniche T, Thamsborg G, et al: Changes in bone histomorphometry after long-term treatment with intermittent, cyclic etidronate for postmenopausal osteoporosis. *J Bone Miner Res* 1993;8:199–208.
130. Ott SM: Clinical effect of bisphosphonates in involutional osteoporosis. *J Bone Miner Res* 1993;8(suppl 2):S597–S606.
131. Harris ST, Watts NB, Jackson RD, et al: Four-year study of intermittent cyclic etidronate treatment of postmenopausal osteoporosis: Three years of blinded therapy followed by one year of open therapy. *Am J Med* 1993;95:557–567.
132. Toolan BC, Shea M, Myers ER, et al: Abstract: The effect of long-term alendronate treatment on vertebral strength in ovariectomized baboons and rats. *J Bone Miner Res* 1991;(suppl 1):S248.
133. Balena R, Markatos A, Gentile M, et al: Abstract: Bone turnover in the cortical bone of primates. Effects of the aminobisphosphonate alendronate. *Calcif Tissue Int* 1993;52(suppl 1):S73.
134. Rossini M, Gatti D, Zamberlan N, et al: Long-term effects of a treatment course with oral alendronate of postmenopausal osteoporosis. *J Bone Miner Res* 1994;9:1833–1837.
135. Boivin G, Dupuis J, Meunier PJ: Fluoride and osteoporosis, in

Simopoulos AP, Galli C (eds): *Osteoporosis: Nutritional Aspects.* Basel, Switzerland, Karger, 1993, pp 80–103.
136. Farley SM, Wergedal JB, Farley JR, et al: Spinal fractures during fluoride therapy for osteoporosis: Relationship to spinal bone density. *Osteoporos Int* 1992;2:213–218.
137. Riggs BL, Hodgson SF, O'Fallon WM, et al: Effect of fluoride treatment on the fracture rate in postmenopausal women with osteoporosis. *N Engl J Med* 1990;322:802–809.
138. Riggs BL, O'Fallon WM, Lane A, et al: Clinical trial of fluoride therapy in postmenopausal osteoporotic women: Extended observations and additional analysis. *J Bone Miner Res* 1994; 9:265–275.
139. Kassem M, Mosekilde L, Eriksen EF: 1,25-dihydroxyvitamin D3 potentiates fluoride-stimulated collagen type I production in cultures of human bone marrow stromal osteoblast-like cells. *J Bone Miner Res* 1993;8:1453–1458.
140. Pak CY, Sakhaee K, Piziak V, et al: Slow-release sodium fluoride in the management of postmenopausal osteoporosis: A randomized controlled trail. *Ann Intern Med* 1994;120:625–632.
141. Pak CY, Sakhaee K, Adams-Huet B, et al: Treatment of post-menopausal osteoporosis with slow-release sodium fluoride: Final report of a randomized controlled trial. *Ann Intern Med* 1995;123:401–408.

CHAPTER 43

Maintaining and Restoring Mobility in Middle and Old Age: The Importance of the Soft Tissues

Joseph A. Buckwalter, MD

Increasing age serves to make us more aware of the importance of free, painless movement in making full use of our abilities in pursuit of leisure activities or work. Most individuals want to, and should, remain physically active throughout life. Yet weakness, stiffness, and musculoskeletal pain that limit mobility are among the most frequent complaints of middle-aged and older people. Decreasing strength and flexibility, often combined with pain that occurs with movement, prevent many of these people from participating in the regular physical activity necessary to maintain optimal general health. For some individuals, declining mobility leads to loss of independence and the ability to participate in social and recreational activities.

Age-related decline in musculoskeletal function leading to loss of mobility may result from bone fractures or changes in the soft tissues that form the muscles, articular cartilages, intervertebral disks, tendons, ligaments, and joint capsules. Fractures associated with age-related alterations in bone cause significant morbidity, including exacerbating age-related loss of function in the musculoskeletal soft tissues. Although fractures can initiate a sequence of events leading to death, they do not cause impairment for as many older people as do weakness, pain with movement, and restriction of motion due to changes in the soft tissues.[1] In addition to the decrease in musculoskeletal function due to age-related changes in the soft tissues, loss of tissue strength with age[2] may increase the probability and severity of soft-tissue damage from a given injury. Healing following soft-tissue injuries or surgical repair or reconstruction of bones, joints, tendons, and ligaments often requires more time with increasing age.[3] These changes can accelerate the age-related loss of mobility, further compromising the quality of life.

If changes in musculoskeletal soft tissues and in musculoskeletal function progressed relentlessly with age in everyone, there would be little reason to invest effort in trying to understand the aging processes and develop strategies to maintain or restore musculoskeletal function in older individuals. However, recent research[1] has demonstrated that age-related changes in musculoskeletal tissues and function do not progress uniformly and that certain interventions may temporarily reverse or slow the progression of these changes. For these reasons, there is a clear need to disseminate and advance knowledge of the basic processes of aging and methods of maintaining or improving musculoskeletal function for older individuals. This chapter summarizes current understanding of age-related changes in musculoskeletal function; the specific age-related changes in skeletal muscle, articular cartilage, intervertebral disk, and tendon, ligament, and joint capsule; mechanisms that alter tissue composition, structure, and function with age; and interventions that may alter the age-related loss of mobility.

Age-Related Changes in Musculoskeletal System Function

Despite the evidence showing a direct correlation between increasing age and increasing musculoskeletal impairment,[4] the relationships between age and function are proving to be extremely complex. Figure 1, *left*, illustrates how age-related deterioration of cell, tissue, and musculoskeletal system function following skeletal maturity may result in impairment. As a cell, tissue, or organ system ages, function gradually declines, susceptibility to disease and injury increases, and the ability to recover from disease or injury decreases. The affected functions extend from the cellular level (for example, chondrocyte synthetic function) to the organ system level (for example, lower extremity strength and flexibility). At some point, the progressive decline in function reaches a level recognized as impairment, although the boundary between adequate function and impairment usually is not sharp. Further decline in function increases the severity of the impairment. Even though mean values at different ages may be strikingly different, there is considerable individual variability of cell, tissue, and musculoskeletal system function at every age. This variability in function at any age is so great that some individuals could have a higher level of function at age 68 than some individuals at age 18.

Most studies of age-related changes in function are cross-sectional—they examine organ systems, tissues, or cells at different ages but do not follow an individual or sample longitudinally. Thus, the function of a person, organ system, tissue, or cell may not progressively decline with age even though the population sampled at different ages shows a steady decline in function. Age-related changes in cell, tissue, or musculoskeletal function for all individuals do not necessarily progress uniformly, nor do they necessarily lead to impairment. Although the mean values for a function may decline

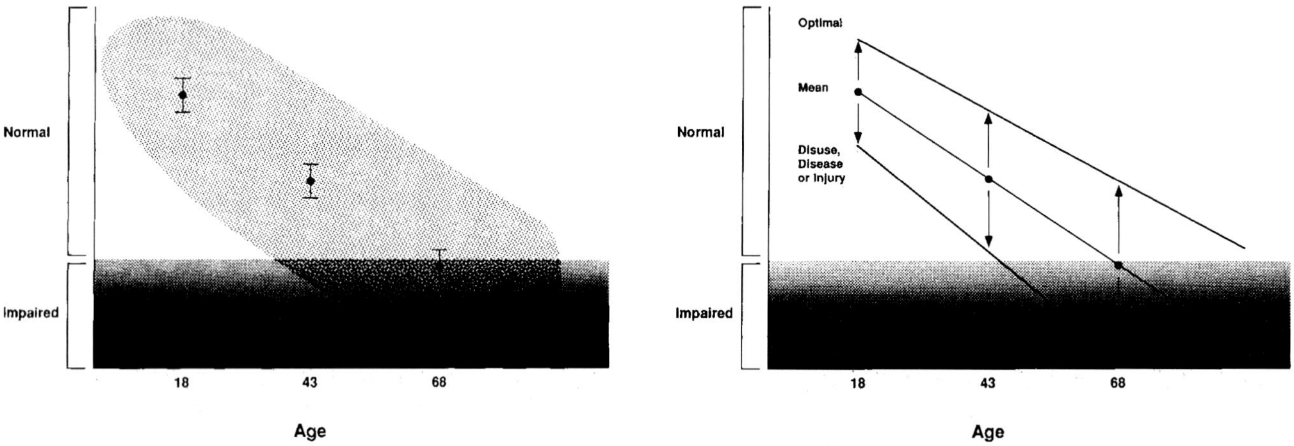

Fig. 1 Schematic representations of the change in cell, tissue, or musculoskeletal function with age. **Left,** The dots and error bars plotted at 18, 43, and 68 years of age represent the mean values and standard errors for function at each age. The shaded elongated oval area represents the range of values. With increasing age the average level of function declines, but at any age a broad range of functional levels exists. **Right,** The level of function at the ages represented can decrease because of disuse, disease of injury. A number of studies indicated that function can also be improved at any age by interventions that include restoring tissue structure, physical activity, and use of trophic hormones. (Reproduced with permission from Buckwalter JA, Woo SL, Goldberg VM, et al: Soft tissue aging and musculoskeletal function. *J Bone Joint Surg* 1993;75A: 1533–1548.)

progressively, the rate of decline varies among individuals, and function at any age can increase or decrease relative to the mean value (Fig. 1, *left*). Disuse, disease, or injury may decrease function, and interventions such as exercise or hormonal replacement may maintain or improve function (Fig. 1, *right*). For these reasons, stating that a given function uniformly declines with age is usually an oversimplification.

The concepts presented above are based on current understanding of age-related changes in some cells, tissues, and organ systems, and the evidence that changes in muscle and joint function cause significant impairment; however, impairments due to other causes also contribute to declining mobility. Age-related changes in reaction time, proprioception, vision, hearing, postural balance, pulmonary function, central nervous system function, and cardiovascular performance can affect mobility. Other variables that can influence mobility over time include living conditions, systemic diseases, nutrition, and social, psychologic, and economic factors.

Age-Related Changes in Soft Tissues

The biologic and mechanical behaviors of all the musculoskeletal soft tissues—skeletal muscle, articular cartilage, intervertebral disk, tendon, ligament, and joint capsule—change with age. Although these changes follow similar patterns in each tissue, they must be considered individually because the tissues differ in composition, structure, and function.

Skeletal Muscle

Beginning in middle age, or earlier, most individuals notice a progressive decline in strength; measurements of the force that major muscle groups can generate show that between 30 and 80 years of age, the strength of muscle groups in the arms, back, and legs decreases by as much as 60%.[5] Decreased strength not only limits mobility, it increases the probability of injuries, including falls.[6]

Loss of muscle mass resulting from decreases in the number and size of muscle cells appears to be the major cause of the age-related decline in strength.[7] Starting at 25 years of age, skeletal muscle mass declines at an average rate of 4% per decade until 50 years of age.[5,8] Thereafter, the rate of loss increases to 10% of the remaining skeletal muscle per decade. In elderly individuals with low plasma growth hormone and insulin-like growth factor I (IGF-I) levels, skeletal muscle mass may be lost at a rate of 35% per decade.[8-10] In addition to decreasing strength and increasing the risk of injury, marked loss of muscle mass may lower body temperature and increase the risk of hypothermia during cold stress.[11] Factors that contribute to the loss of muscle mass with age include decreased exercise, especially fewer contractions against high loads; decreases in hormonal levels, including growth hormone, testosterone, and thyroxin; and neuromuscular changes, including structural and functional changes in spinal motor neurons and neuromuscular junctions.

In addition to the decrease in strength, the ability of some muscles to provide sustained power during repeated contractions may decline with age. Brooks and Faulkner[12] found that the muscles of older animals had a 50% decrease in sustained power, primarily due to the inability of the older muscles to maintain their energy balance with frequent contractions. This may result from a decline in the muscle enzyme systems associated with oxidative capacity.[5,12-15]

Age-related changes in skeletal muscle may also increase the probability of muscle injury and decrease the ability of muscle to heal. Skeletal muscles are frequently injured by their own contractions, especially when they are lengthened during contraction. Zerba and associates[16] showed that immediately following contraction-induced injury, maximum muscle force decreases due to direct mechanical damage to the sarcomeres, and then partially recovers. Three days following injury, muscle force drops to the lowest level, probably due to damage caused by oxygen free radicals.[16] Older muscles appear to have an increased susceptibility to contraction-induced mechanical and free radical injury and decreased ability to regenerate damaged tissue.[5,13,14,16] Muscles from younger animals recover from severe contraction injury completely in less than a month, but muscles from older animals continue to have deficits in mass and force generation for months after injury and possibly indefinitely.[14] The combination of increased vulnerability to injury and slower healing may contribute to the increased weakness and fatigability of older muscles.

Although loss of skeletal muscle mass and declining strength and endurance with age appear to be inevitable, a number of interventions can slow these changes. Some studies show beneficial effects of hormone supplementation or replacement therapy, including growth hormone and testosterone,[10,17,18] but these therapies also have a variety of potential complications.[18] Multiple investigations provide convincing evidence that exercise increases the strength of older individuals by increasing muscle mass, cross-sectional areas, contractile proteins, motor unit recruitment, and oxidative capacity.[1] However, minor musculoskeletal injuries and pain with exercise, primarily joint and back pain, occur more commonly in older people, especially with aerobic training.[19] These problems occur less frequently with lower intensity strength and flexibility training programs, and usually respond quickly to conservative treatment. Obesity, previous joint injuries, osteoarthritis, foot deformity, weakness, and limited hip and ankle motion are associated with increased frequency of exercise-related musculoskeletal pain and minor injuries.[19] For these reasons, older people should have a medical evaluation before starting an exercise program.

Articular Cartilage

Articular cartilage undergoes significant age-related changes in cell function and matrix tensile properties, composition, and molecular organization that precede and may lead to degeneration of the tissue (fraying or fibrillation of the articular surface). In addition, like other collagenous tissues, articular cartilage develops a yellow-brown tinge with increasing age. This color change may result from posttranslational modification of the matrix proteins,[20,21] but its significance remains unknown.

Basic investigations have identified significant alterations in cartilage that occur during skeletal maturation, and cross-sectional studies of human joints show that focal articular cartilage degenerative changes first appear near skeletal maturity.[1,22] The degenerative changes increase progressively in prevalence, extent, and severity with increasing age. The increasing prevalence of cartilage degeneration with age parallels the striking age-related increase in the prevalence of the clinical syndrome of osteoarthritis, ie, joint pain and stiffness associated with cartilage degeneration, increased subchondral bone density, and osteophytes. These observations suggest that in some individuals, age-related superficial cartilage fibrillation progresses into deep clefts, fissures, fragmentation of the cartilage, and eventually large erosions that leave exposed subchondral bone and cause symptoms of osteoarthritis.

Despite the strong correlations among age, increased prevalence of cartilage degenerative changes, and increased prevalence of osteoarthritis, the relationships between the age-related tissue changes and the clinical syndrome of osteoarthritis remain poorly understood. The prevalence and severity of cartilage fibrillation varies among joints and among different regions of the same joint. Not all degenerative changes in articular cartilage are associated with joint pain and loss of motion, and not all people with symptoms of osteoarthritis have radiographic evidence of osteoarthritis, nor do all degenerative changes progress with age, even in people with the clinical and radiographic diagnosis of osteoarthritis. Furthermore, age-related alterations in other tissue components of synovial joints—the synovium, subchondral bone, menisci, ligaments, and joint capsules—may contribute to joint symptoms and musculoskeletal impairment.

The relationships between age changes in chondrocytes and degeneration of articular cartilage also remain unclear. Cell density declines sharply with skeletal maturity, but most studies suggest that it remains relatively constant in adult life.[23] However, with increasing age, cell morphology and synthetic function change. The cells accumulate intracytoplasmic filaments and may lose some of their endoplasmic reticulum. They change their synthetic patterns to produce different, more variable matrix proteoglycans.[1,24] These changes may make the cells less effective in replacing degraded matrix macromolecules and in repairing the matrix following injury.[1,3,25]

Studies of the mechanical properties of cartilage have not found age-related changes in compressive properties, but they have shown significant age-related decreases in tensile stiffness, fatigue resistance, and strength.[26-28] Although the underlying matrix alterations responsible for the age-related changes in matrix tensile properties have not been identified, the water content generally decreases with age[29,30] and both the proteoglycans and collagens that form the primary components of the articular cartilage matrix macromolecular framework undergo age-related changes.[1]

The large aggregating matrix proteoglycans, aggrecan molecules responsible for giving the tissue its stiffness in compression and resiliency, undergo significant changes with skeletal maturation. They become much smaller and more variable in size (Fig. 2), their keratan sulfate content increases, their chondroitin sulfate content decreases, and the proportion of these molecules that form large aggregates declines.[1,24] As these changes in aggrecan molecules occur, the size of proteoglycan aggregates decreases because of the decrease in aggrecan size and in the number of aggrecan molecules per aggregate.

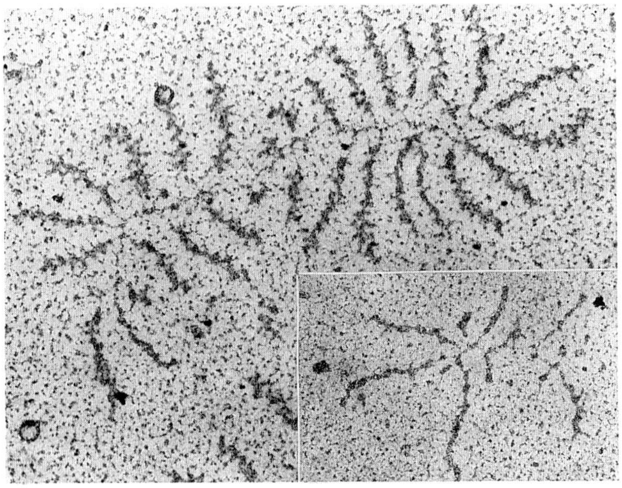

Fig. 2 Electron micrographs of human articular cartilage proteoglycan aggregates consisting of central hyaluronan filaments and multiple attached aggrecan molecules. The large micrograph shows proteoglycan aggregate from a human newborn containing 30 aggrecan molecules. The insert shows proteoglycan aggregate from a 22-year-old human containing 12 aggrecan molecules. Note that the aggrecan molecules vary more in length than those from the younger person. (Reproduced with permission from Buckwalter JA, Woo SL, Goldberg VM, et al: Soft tissue aging and musculoskeletal function. *J Bone Joint Surg* 1993;75A:1533-1548.)

The decline in aggregation and aggregate size probably results from several changes in the molecules and in the matrix. Proteolytic degradation leaves molecular fragments in the matrix that occupy space and that may bind to hyaluronan where they can inhibit aggregation of fully functional molecules.[31] Link proteins, the protein molecules responsible for stabilizing and organizing large proteoglycan aggregates, also undergo increasing proteolytic modification with age, and the altered molecules accumulate in the matrix.[32-34] Although the altered link proteins bind to hyaluronan and aggrecan, they may be less effective in stabilizing aggregates. Hyaluronan, the glycosaminoglycan that forms the central core molecules of proteoglycan aggregates, decreases in size and increases in concentration with increasing age.[35,36] It is not certain if the increased concentration of hyaluronan results from increased synthesis or accumulation of degraded molecules. Since aggregation helps organize and stabilize proteoglycans within the matrix, the decline in aggregation and in aggregate size may alter the stability and mechanical properties of the matrix.

The cartilage matrix also contains nonaggregating proteoglycans, including decorin, biglycan, and fibromodulin. Decorin and fibromodulin interact with collagen fibrils, and biglycan accumulates in the pericellular regions.[37,38] Age-related changes in fibromodulin have not been established. The biglycan concentration remains relatively constant, while the concentration of decorin increases from about half the concentration of biglycan in newborns to twice the concentration of biglycan in adults.[39,40] Although the functions of these proteoglycans have not been well defined, they affect the formation, organization, and stability of the matrix and can inhibit cell adhesion and migration.[41] Thus, an increasing concentration of decorin may affect matrix turnover and inhibit repair.[40]

The cartilage collagens also undergo age-related changes that may alter the tissue properties. During aging, cross-linking of collagen molecules may increase through nonenzymic glycation reactions. The matrix collagen fibrils tend to increase in diameter with age, a change thought to be related at least in part to the decreased content of type XI collagen relative to type II collagen.[42] Larger diameter collagen fibrils with a greater degree of cross-linking may be less flexible and make the cartilage matrix more rigid. The increased rigidity combined with decreased water content[29,30] could limit the ability of the macromolecular framework to deform repetitively when loaded without damaging its structure.[42] Increasing rigidity of the collagen framework and decreased water content might also interfere with the matrix turnover necessary to replace degraded molecules.

Maintaining articular cartilage function and synovial joint range of movement, even for elderly people, requires regular joint loading and motion.[43-45] Marked decreased joint use decreases chondrocyte synthetic activity and adversely alters matrix composition and cartilage mechanical properties. It also decreases joint range of motion and may contribute to the age-related loss of muscle mass. However, repetitive high-intensity impact and torsional loading of joints may cause or accelerate joint degeneration. For these reasons, middle-aged and older people, including people with mild joint degeneration, should participate in regular physical activity that requires joint loading and motion and maintains joint range of motion. In general, they should avoid activities that result in high-intensity impact and torsional loading of joints.

Intervertebral Disk

Back and neck stiffness and pain are among the most common complaints of middle-aged and older people.[46] The relationship of these clinical problems to age-related changes in the soft tissues of the spine remains unknown, but no musculoskeletal tissue undergoes more dramatic age-related changes than the intervertebral disk.[25] The most extensive changes occur in the central regions of the disk, the inner anulus fibrosus, and nucleus pulposus. During skeletal growth and maturation, the clear gelatinous nucleus pulposus of childhood becomes a firm fibrous plate. In early adult life, fissures and cracks appear in the disk and then extend from the periphery to the central regions. A decrease in proteoglycan and water concentration and an increase in noncollagenous protein concentration accompany these morphologic changes.[1,25] Disk volume and shape also change, although these alterations have not been as well defined as the alterations in disk structure and composition. The age-related alterations in disk tissue appear to increase the probability of disk herniation,[47] and the age-related changes in the disk shape and volume can affect spine mobility and alter the alignment and loads applied to the facet joints, spinal ligaments, and paraspinous muscles. These alterations may contribute to age-related loss of spine mobility and strength, spinal stenosis, and degeneration of the facet joints.[1,25]

Morphologic studies show that cell types and the number of viable cells change dramatically with age in the central regions of the disk.[1,25] In infants, syncytial cords and clusters of notochordal cells occupy the central region of the nucleus pulposus, but by adolescence few of these cells remain. As the notochordal cells disappear, chondrocyte-like cells take their place. Following skeletal maturity, the number of viable cells in all regions of the disk declines sharply, but especially in the central regions (Fig. 3).

Electron microscopic studies of disk matrix show a progressive increase in mean collagen fibril diameter and in the variability of collagen fibril diameter with age.[48-50] At the same time, dense granular filamentous osmophilic material accumulates throughout the matrix (Fig. 3).[48-50] This material concentrates in the regions immediately surrounding the cells of the central disk regions. Its composition has not been defined, but it may consist of degraded matrix molecules and noncollagenous proteins.

As the ultrastructure of the disk matrix changes and the proteoglycan concentration in the central regions of the disk declines, the proportion of proteoglycans that form aggregates and proteoglycan aggrecan size decrease. Proteoglycan aggregates from human infant intervertebral disk anulus fibrosus and vertebral cartilage end plate consist of a long central hyaluronan filament and multiple attached aggrecan molecules, a structure identical to the aggregates of hyaline cartilages.[51-53] However, in human infants only about one third of nucleus pulposus proteoglycan aggregates resemble these large aggregates; the other two thirds consist of monomer clusters that frequently lack a visible central hyaluronan filament. By adolescence, the proteoglycan population of the nucleus pulposus consists almost entirely of clusters of short aggrecan molecules and nonaggregated proteoglycans. A decline in the concentration of functional link protein may cause at least some of these change in proteoglycan aggregates.[54,55]

The most critical variable responsible for the changes in central disk cells and their matrices appears to be declining nutrition.[1,25,56] The disk cells rely on diffusion of nutrients through the disk matrix from blood vessels on the periphery of the anulus fibrosus and within the vertebral bodies. The progressive age-related decline in the number of arteries supplying the region of the intervertebral disk presumably contributes to declining cell viability and biosynthetic function. At the same time, accumulation of degraded matrix macromolecules and decreasing matrix water content may interfere with diffusion through the matrix, further compromising cell nutrition.

Factors that may accelerate the rate and increase the severity of age-related changes in intervertebral disk by altering the tissue or tissue nutrition include increased disk loading due to demanding physical activities, vibration, or spinal deformity, and factors that directly compromise the vascular supply, such as smoking, vascular disease, and diabetes.[1,24,25]

Despite the apparent inevitability of age-related changes in the human intervertebral disk, regeneration of disk tissue may be possible. Experimental studies of the effects of enzymatic degradation of the normal central disk region extracellular matrix suggest that the cells can regenerate a matrix even in older animals.[57-59] Re-expansion of narrowed human disks after injection of enzymes has not occurred consistently.[60] Factors that may limit restoration of degenerated

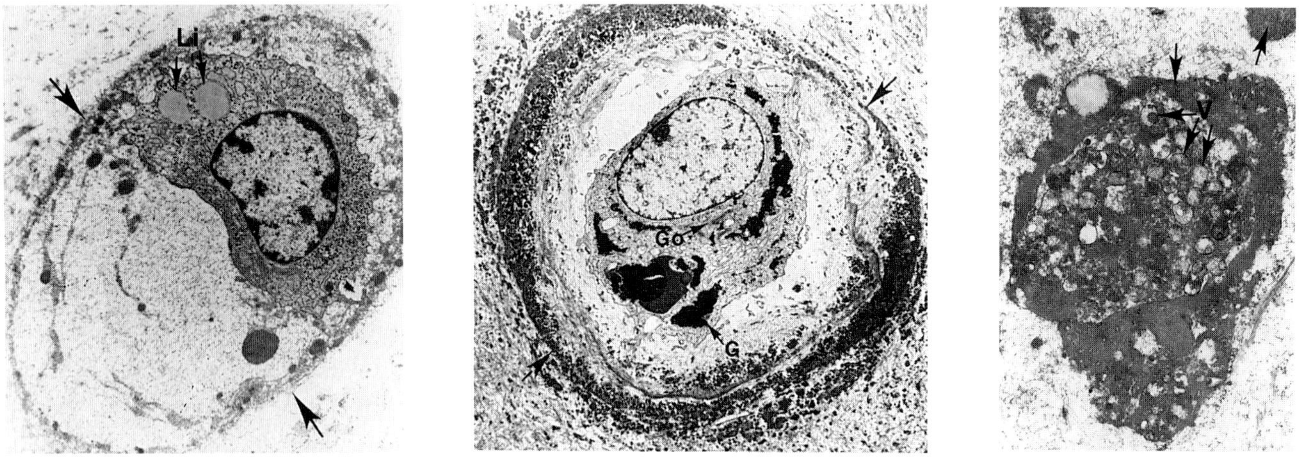

Fig. 3 Electron micrographs of human nucleus pulposus cells. **Left,** Electron micrograph of a cell from the central region of a child's nucleus pulposus. Li indicates lipid and the arrows mark the edge of the accumulation of electron dense matrix material. **Center,** Electron micrograph of a cell from the central region of an elderly adult's nucleus pulposus. Go indicates Golgi membranes, G indicates glycogen, and the arrows mark the edge of the accumulation of dense matrix material. Note the increased thickness of the rim of accumulated granular material surrounding this cell compared with the cell from the younger individual. **Right,** Electron micrograph showing the remains of a necrotic nucleus pulposus cell from an adult. V indicates vacuoles and the unlabeled arrows indicate electron dense material.

human disks include severity of disk degeneration including near complete loss of disk tissue, limited diffusion of enzymes in degenerated narrowed disks, inadequate number of remaining viable cells or cells that are capable of responding by producing new disk tissue, and mechanical constraints, including soft tissue contractures due to disk narrowing that prevent re-expansion.

Tendon, Ligament, and Joint Capsule

Age-related changes in the dense fibrous tissues have received less attention than the changes in skeletal muscle, articular cartilage, and intervertebral disk, but middle-aged and older persons can develop significant impairment as a result of alterations in tendons, ligaments, and joint capsules. Degenerative changes in dense fibrous tissues may result in spontaneous or low-energy level ruptures of the shoulder rotator cuff, the long head of the biceps, tibialis posterior, patellar and Achilles tendons, and sprains and ruptures of joint capsules and ligaments, including those of the spine and wrist. It is likely that at least some of the soreness following physical activity in middle-aged and older people or chronic activity-related musculoskeletal pain results from injuries to the fibrous components of muscle tendon junctions or tendon, ligament, and joint capsule insertions into bone.

The tensile mechanical properties of at least some ligament-bone complexes deteriorate significantly with age.[61-66] Investigation of the mechanical properties of the human anterior longitudinal ligament showed that the strength of the ligament-bone complex decreased approximately twofold from age 21 years to 79 years.[66] A study of the mechanical properties of human femur-anterior cruciate ligament-tibia complexes from three age groups showed a progressive decline in tensile stiffness and ultimate load to failure with increasing age.[67] The decrease in ultimate load to failure occurred most rapidly between the third decade of life (22 to 35 years) and middle age (40 to 50 years). Following middle age, ultimate load to failure continued to decrease; ligament-bone complexes from older individuals (60 to 97 years) failed at less than one third the ultimate load to failure of the younger ligament complexes. In another study of anterior cruciate ligament complexes, the elastic modulus, ultimate tensile stress, and strain energy to failure were two to three times greater for complexes from young adults (age range 16 to 25 years) than for older people (age range 48 to 86 years).[65] In older ligament-bone complexes, tensile failure occurred more frequently by rupture of the ligament substance than by avulsion from the bone, suggesting that the ligament substance may deteriorate more rapidly than the bone; however, this possibility needs further study. Study of dog and rabbit medial collateral ligaments shows that their mechanical properties also deteriorate with increasing age following skeletal maturity, but the decline is more gradual than in the anterior cruciate ligament bone complexes.[61,68,69] Therefore, the rate and extent of change in mechanical properties may vary among ligaments.

Detailed mechanical studies of the age-related changes in tendons and joint capsules have not been reported, but the similarities in structure, composition, and mechanical function between these tissues and ligaments, and the available evidence,[2] suggest that their mechanical properties also deteriorate with age. Furthermore, histologic degenerative changes in tendons appear more frequently with increasing age.[70]

The tissue changes responsible for the age-related decline in the strength of dense fibrous tissues have not been clearly identified. In at least some locations, including the rotator cuff, the nutrition of dense fibrous tissue cells may decrease with age due to decreased vascular perfusion. The resulting decline in cell function may lead to tissue degeneration. Changes in the cell function, matrix composition, and organization of the matrix macromolecules that occur independently of alterations in nutrition may also contribute to the decline in mechanical properties.

Aging fibroblasts flatten and elongate, losing most of their rough endoplasmic reticulum and Golgi membranes. A study of tendon also showed that tissue from young animals had a high level of aerobic glycolysis, but the level of aerobic glycolysis declined with age to the point that it could not be detected in tissues from older animals.[71] These changes may be associated with decreasing biosynthetic activity[72] and, possibly, a decreased ability to participate in tissue turnover or respond to injury. Recent work also indicates that ligament cells are less able to respond to exercise in older animals.[69]

Highly oriented fibrillar collagens form the bulk of the matrix in the dense fibrous tissues. Therefore, it seems reasonable to expect that the age-related decrease in tissue mechanical properties results from an alteration in the collagens. Although biochemical analyses have not shown dramatic age-related changes in tendon or ligament matrix composition, the collagen and water concentration of these tissues may decline slightly with age as the labile reducible collagen cross links decrease and the more stable nonreducible cross links increase.[72] The properties of the tissues could also be affected by alterations in the organization and molecular structure of the collagens, and animal studies have suggested that the collagen fibril alignment and fiber bundle organization decrease with increasing age.[62,72,73] Posttranslational modifications of the collagens may also contribute to the age-related decline in mechanical properties.[20,21]

Given the magnitude of the age-related changes in the mechanical properties of knee ligaments, and probably in other dense fibrous tissues, and the known changes in the cells and matrices of these tissues, it is surprising that older individuals do not have more frequent ligament, joint capsule, and tendon injuries. To some extent, decreasing levels of vigorous physical activity with increasing age may prevent injuries to these tissues.

Causes of Age-Related Changes in Soft Tissues

Taken together, cell, extracellular matrix, tissue, organ system, and systemic changes with age can contribute to declining musculoskeletal function, increase the vulnerability of the musculoskeletal soft tissues to injury, and lead to slower, less effective healing. Although experimental work has identified a variety of specific mechanisms of age-related changes, the importance of each of these mechanisms in producing changes in tissues and musculoskeletal function has not been established.[1] Senescence of differentiated cells, characterized by declining proliferative capacity and ability to perform specialized functions, and decreasing numbers of mesenchymal stem cells alter the behavior of the cell populations. In particular these changes may decrease the ability of the cells to maintain the tissues and repair tissue damage. An age-related decrease in blood supply may contribute to a decline in the function of cells in skeletal muscle, dense fibrous tissue structures, and the intervertebral disk. Posttranslational modification of matrix proteins and accumulation of degraded matrix macromolecules change the organization and properties of extracellular matrices. Systemic changes, including declining levels of trophic hormones, alter the tissue environment and the response of the tissue to use and injury. Decreased physical activity appears to accelerate the age-related loss of skeletal muscle mass and contributes to loss of flexibility. Although each of these mechanisms of age-related change is usually studied as an isolated event, understanding the interactions among them will be essential in explaining their impact on the tissues and musculoskeletal function.[1]

Methods of Restoring and Maintaining Mobility

A variety of surgical procedures can restore mobility for middle-aged and elderly people with musculoskeletal injuries or diseases. Few, if any, treatments restore mobility as rapidly and effectively as secure internal stabilization of fractures and joint replacement. Other surgical treatments, including joint and spinal fusions and tendon and ligament reconstructions, can also restore or help maintain mobility. In many instances, gaining the optimal results of these procedures depends on maintenance or recovery of soft-tissue function, in particular muscle strength and full movement of muscle tendon units, ligaments, and joint capsules. Furthermore, the results of surgical reconstruction or replacement of bones, joints, and soft tissues could be improved by methods that accelerated or improved recovery of musculoskeletal soft-tissue function, and these procedures do not slow the age-related changes in other tissues.

Despite many recent advances in understanding of the aging process, specific methods of preventing or slowing age-related changes remain poorly understood. However, it is clear that the appropriate type and level of regular physical activity can help maintain or restore musculoskeletal system function. Physicians can help middle-aged and older people maintain mobility by assessing their level of musculoskeletal function and risks of injury, and then recommending specific physical activities. To decrease the risk of injury, even healthy older individuals should have a careful evaluation before initiating an exercise program. For most people, regular low-impact physical activity, including resistance exercises that help maintain or increase muscle mass, have the potential to slow age-related loss of muscle mass and flexibility. Maintaining or increasing muscle mass in elderly patients may also decrease their risk of injury, including falls, and help maintain body temperature and the ability to respond to cold stress. Older individuals are more vulnerable to soft-tissue injuries during exercise, but the risk can be decreased by modifying activity, use of orthoses or supports, and activity programs that emphasize stretching, range of motion, and muscle strengthening. Because controlled activity can promote healing of soft tissues and bone in people of any age,[43,74] older patients who have been treated for musculoskeletal injuries should be advised of the need for regular physical activity to restore function. Most patients with joint replacements can also benefit from regular exercise, and even some sports, without significantly increasing the risk of joint failure.

Experimental methods of slowing age-related tissue changes in older individuals include use of trophic hormones. In a group of men aged 61 to 81 years with low levels of IGF-I, 1 month of human growth hormone treatment increased IGF-I levels to the normal range for young men, and 6 months of treatment increased average lean body mass to 105% of the baseline value and decreased adipose body mass to 87% of the baseline value.[10] These changes in body composition persisted during another 6 months of treatment and then returned to the initial baseline values 3 months after cessation of treatment. Although this study did not measure changes in muscle function, investigations of growth hormone-deficient adults and elderly adults with chronic lung disease and markedly reduced muscle mass show that growth hormone replacement can increase exercise capacity and muscle strength.[9,75,76] Studies of growth hormone supplementation in normal adults indicate that it can have a favorable effect on body composition.[18] Unfortunately, growth hormone replacement and supplementation can adversely affect glucose metabolism and blood pressure and have been associated with carpal tunnel syndrome and gynecomastia.[18] In an effort to avoid the adverse effects of growth hormone administration, investigators have begun assessing the use of growth hormone-releasing hormone to increase growth hormone levels. Testosterone supplementation in older males has produced improvements in lean body mass and strength in some studies but not in others; in one study, prostatic specific antigen levels increased in older men receiving testosterone supplementation.[18] At the present time, use of trophic hormones to maintain or restore muscle mass and strength should be considered experimental.

Improved soft-tissue healing in older patients would accelerate recovery following injuries and surgery. Despite the theoretical potential of androgenic hormones to improve soft-tissue healing, this effect has not been demonstrated.[77] Experimental work, however, indicates that local or possibly even systemic administration of growth factors has the potential to promote bone and soft-tissue healing.[3] In one set of experiments, administration of transforming growth factor beta (TGF-ß) systemically 24 hours before making a skin incision reversed the age-related decline in wound healing in rats (E. Amento, MD, personal communication, 1993). TGF-ß has generally been considered a paracrine or autocrine factor, but the reported beneficial effect of systemic TGF-ß indicates that it might work as an endocrine factor through a circulating inactive form. These observations suggest that other autocrine and paracrine factors might also facilitate healing in older individuals.

Other possible future methods of maintaining or restoring musculoskeletal function include tissue regeneration, inhibition of modification of matrix macromolecules, and alteration of transcription factors to restore cell function. One possible cause of age-related impaired healing is a decline in the concentration of undifferentiated mesenchymal cells that can migrate into regions of tissue injury or degeneration, proliferate, and form new tissue.[1,3]

Mesenchymal stem cells can be identified from a number of locations, even in older individuals.[78] Isolating these cells from bone marrow or other sites, expanding them in culture, and then transplanting them into sites of age-related tissue degeneration or damage could provide a method of facilitating tissue repair or regeneration in older individuals. Recent work indicates that inhibition of glycation reactions can prevent at least some of the adverse age-related changes in collagenous tissues, including blood vessel and nerve.[21] This approach might also be effective in musculoskeletal soft tissues. There is increasing evidence that the age-related change in cell proliferative capacity is controlled by key transcription factors, proteins that bind to DNA and control gene expression.[79] In particular, recent work suggests that the changes in gene expression that cause cellular senescence result from alterations in the action of selected transcription factors.[79,80] This observation raises the possibility of identifying one or a few genes responsible for cell senescence and then targeting specific transcription factors to arrest or reverse age-related changes in cell function.

Summary and Conclusions

For many older individuals, impairment of musculoskeletal function, especially weakness, stiffness, and pain, cause progressive disability, thereby limiting mobility and decreasing the quality of life. With advancing age, musculoskeletal soft tissue function declines, susceptibility to degenerative diseases and injuries increases, and the ability to recover from disease or injury declines; these changes increase the probability of impairment (Fig. 1). However, the function of individual cells, tissues, or organ systems may remain stable or even improve temporarily with age, and a number of interventions have the potential to maintain or improve musculoskeletal function. Age-related changes in cells, tissues, and musculoskeletal function are not necessarily unidirectional or uniform among individuals, organ systems, tissues, or cells, nor are they necessarily irreversible. Surgical procedures can restore mobility for many patients with age-related musculoskeletal injuries or degenerative diseases. Regular resistance and range-of-motion exercises can decrease the age-related loss of strength and help maintain or restore flexibility. However, exercise programs can also cause injury. Older individuals should have a careful medical evaluation before starting an exercise program, and the program should be selected based on this evaluation. This is especially important for individuals with systemic illness and for individuals at greater risk of musculoskeletal injury, including people with previous joint injuries, obesity, osteoarthritis, joint deformity, weakness, or restricted joint motion. Trophic hormone replacement or supplementation may also modify age-related changes in the soft tissues, including loss of strength, but these hormones have adverse effects. Systemic or local use of growth factors and cell transplantation after expanding the population of mesenchymal stem cells in culture could improve healing in older people. Other potential methods of slowing or reversing age-related deterioration of the soft tissues include inhibition of posttranslational modification of matrix proteins and alteration of the activity of selected transcription factors. In particular, better understanding of the role of transcription factors in cell senescence may make it possible to devise methods of delaying or reversing age-related loss of cell proliferative and synthetic capacity.

Acknowledgment

Many of the concepts presented in this chapter were developed during a symposium entitled "Age-Related Changes in the Musculoskeletal Soft Tissues" held November 14–17, 1992, and sponsored by the American Academy of Orthopaedic Surgeons, the National Institute of Arthritis and Musculoskeletal and Skin Diseases, and the National Institute on Aging. The results of the symposium have been previously published.[1,24]

References

1. Buckwalter JA, Woo SL, Goldberg VM, et al: Soft-tissue aging and musculoskeletal function. *J Bone Joint Surg* 1993;74A: 1533–1548.
2. Yamada H: *Strength of Biological Materials*. Baltimore, MD, Williams & Wilkins, 1970.
3. Buckwalter JA, Einhorn TA, Bolander ME, et al: Healing of the musculoskeletal tissues, in Rockwood CA Jr, Green DP, Bucholz RW, et al (eds): *Fractures*, ed 4. Philadelphia, PA, Lippincott-Raven, 1996, vol 1, pp 261–304.
4. Jette AM: Musculoskeletal impairments and associated physical disability in the elderly: Insights from epidemiological research, in Buckwalter JA, Goldberg VM, Woo SL-Y (eds): *Musculoskeletal Soft-Tissue Aging: Impact on Mobility*. Rosemont, IL, American Academy of Orthopaedic Surgeons, 1993, pp 7–22.
5. Faulkner JA, Brooks SV: Age-related immobility: The roles of weakness, fatigue, injury and repair, in Buckwalter JA, Goldberg VM, Woo SL-Y (eds): *Musculoskeletal Soft-Tissue Aging: Impact on Mobility*. Rosemont, IL, American Academy of Orthopaedic Surgeons, 1993, pp 187–194.
6. Wolfson L, Judge J, Whipple R, et al: Strength is a major factor in balance, gait, and the occurrence of falls. *J Gerontol A* 1995; 50:64–67.
7. Brown M, Hasser EM: Complexity of age-related change in skeletal muscle. *J Gerontol A* 1996;51:B117–B123.
8. Booth FW, Weeden SH: Structural aspects of aging human skeletal muscle, in Buckwalter JA, Goldberg VM, Woo SL-Y (eds): *Musculoskeletal Soft-Tissue Aging: Impact on Mobility*. Rosemont, IL, American Academy of Orthopaedic Surgeons, 1993, pp 195–200.
9. Clemmons DR, Underwood LE: Role of growth hormone and IGF-I in mediating the anabolic response, in Buckwalter JA, Goldberg VM, Woo SL-Y (eds): *Musculoskeletal Soft-Tissue Aging: Impact on Mobility*. Rosemont, IL, American Academy of Orthopaedic Surgeons, 1993, pp 229–237.
10. Shetty KR, Gupta KL, Rudman D: New clinical applications for recombinant human growth hormone, in Buckwalter JA, Goldberg VM, Woo SL-Y (eds): *Musculoskeletal Soft-Tissue Aging: Impact on Mobility*, Rosemont, IL, American Academy of Orthopaedic Surgeons, 1993, pp 61–72.
11. Kenney WL, Buskirk ER: Functional consequences of sarcopenia: Effects on thermoregulation. *J Gerontol A* 1995;50:78–85.
12. Brooks SV, Faulkner JA: Maximum and sustained power of extensor digitorum longus muscles from young, adult, and old mice. *J Gerontol* 1991;46:B28–B33.
13. Faulkner JA, Brooks SV, Zerba E: Skeletal muscle weakness and fatigue in old age: Underlying mechanisms. *Ann Rev Gerontol Geriatr* 1990;10:147–166.
14. Brooks SV, Faulkner JA: Contraction-induced injury: Recovery of skeletal muscles in young and old mice. *Am J Physiol* 1990; 258:C436–C442.
15. Brooks SV, Faulkner JA: Contractile properties of skeletal muscles from young, adult, and aged mice. *J Physiol* 1988;404:71–82.
16. Zerba E, Komorowski TE, Faulkner JA: Free radical injury to

skeletal muscles of young, adult, and old mice. *Am J Physiol* 1990; 258:C429–C435.
17. Rudman D, Feller AG, Nagraj HS, et al: Effects of human growth hormone in men over 60 years old. *N Engl J Med* 1990;323:1–6.
18. Schwartz RS: Trophic factor supplementation: Effect on the age-associated changes in body composition. *J Gerontol* 1995; 50:151–156.
19. Brown M: Physical and orthopaedic limitations to exercise in the elderly, in Buckwalter JA, Goldberg VM, Woo SL-Y (eds): *Musculoskeletal Soft-Tissue Aging: Impact on Mobility*. Rosemont, IL, American Academy of Orthopaedic Surgeons, 1993, pp 209–216.
20. Monnier VM, Kohn RR, Cerami A: Accelerated age-related browning of human collagen in diabetes mellitus. *Proc Natl Acad Sci USA* 1984;81:583–587.
21. Monnier VM, Sell DR, Pokharna HK, et al: Posttranslational protein modification by the Maillard reaction: Relevance to aging of extracellular matrix molecules, in Buckwalter JA, Goldberg V, Woo SL-Y (eds): *Musculoskeletal Soft-Tissue Aging: Impact on Mobility*. Rosemont, IL, American Academy of Orthopaedic Surgeons, 1993, pp 49–59.
22. Bullough PG, Brauer FU: Age-related changes in articular cartilage, in Buckwalter JA, Goldberg VM, Woo SL-Y (eds): *Musculoskeletal Soft-Tissue Aging: Impact on Mobility*. Rosemont, IL, American Academy of Orthopaedic Surgeons, 1993, pp 117–135.
23. Stockwell RA (ed): *Biology of Cartilage Cells*. Cambridge, England, Cambridge University Press, 1979.
24. Buckwalter JA, Goldberg VM, Woo SL-Y (eds): *Musculoskeletal Soft-Tissue Aging: Impact on Mobility*. Rosemont, IL, American Academy of Orthopaedic Surgeons, 1993.
25. Buckwalter JA: Aging and degeneration of the human intervertebral disc. *Spine* 1995;20:1307–1314.
26. Kempson GE: Relationship between the tensile properties of articular cartilage from the human knee and age. *Ann Rheum Dis* 1982;41:508–511.
27. Kempson GE: The mechanical properties of articular cartilage, in Sokoloff L (ed): *The Mechanical Properties of Articular Cartilage*, New York, NY, Academic Press, 1980, pp 177–238.
28. Kempson GE: Age-related changes in the tensile properties of human articular cartilage: A comparative study between the femoral head of the hip joint and the talus of the ankle joint. *Biochim Biophys Acta* 1991;1075:223–230.
29. Venn MF: Variation of chemical composition with age in human femoral head cartilage. *Ann Rheum Dis* 1978;37:168–174.
30. Maroudas A: Physicochemical properties of articular cartilage, in Freeman MAR (ed): *Adult Articular Cartilage*, ed 2. Kent, England, Pitman Medical, 1979, pp 215–290.
31. Roughley PJ, White RJ, Poole AR: Identification of a hyaluronic acid-binding protein that interferes with the preparation of high-bouyant-density proteoglycan aggregates from adult human articular cartilage. *Biochem J* 1985;231:129–138.
32. Nguyen Q, Liu J, Roughley PJ, et al: Link protein as a monitor in situ of endogenous proteolysis in adult human articular cartilage. *Biochem J* 1991;278:143–147.
33. Mort JS, Poole AR, Roughley PJ: Age-related changes in the structure of proteoglycan link proteins present in normal human articular cartilage. *Biochem J* 1983;214:269–272.
34. Mort JS, Caterson B, Poole AR, et al: The origin of human cartilage proteoglycan link-protein heterogeneity and fragmentation during aging. *Biochem J* 1985;232:805–812.
35. Thonar EJ, Sweet MB, Immelman AR, et al: Hyaluronate in articular cartilage: Age-related changes. *Calcif Tissue Res* 1978; 26:19–21.
36. Holmes MW, Bayliss MT, Muir H: Hyaluronic acid in human articular cartilage: Age-related changes in content and size. *Biochem J* 1988;250:435–441.
37. Bianco P, Fisher LW, Young MF, et al: Expression and localization of the two small proteoglycans biglycan and decorin in developing human skeletal and non-skeletal tissues. *J Histochem Cytochem* 1990;38:1549–1563.
38. Hedbom E, Heinegard D: Interaction of a 59-kDa connective tissue matrix protein with collagen I and collagen II. *J Biol Chem* 1989;264:6898–6905.
39. Poole AR, Reiner A, Inonescu M, et al: Immunochemical analyses of the small proteoglycans decorin and biglycan in normal and osteoarthritic human cartilages. *Trans Combined Ortho Res Soc USA, Japan, Canada* 1993;1:80.
40. Rosenberg LC, Choi H, Johnson T, et al: Structural changes in proteoglycans in aging articular cartilages. in Peyron JG (ed): *Osteoarthritis: Current Clinical and Fundamental Problems*. Paris, France, Ciba-Geigy, 1985, pp 179–191.
41. Rosenberg L, Choi HU, Neame PJ, et al: Proteoglycans of soft connective tissues, in Leadbetter WB, Buckwalter JA, Gordon SL (eds): *Sports-Induced Inflammation: Clinical and Basic Science Concepts*. Park Ridge, IL, American Academy of Orthopaedic Surgeons, 1990, pp 171–188.
42. Roughley PJ: Articular cartilage: Matrix changes with aging, in Buckwalter JA, Goldberg VM, Woo SL-Y (eds): *Musculoskeletal Soft-Tissue Aging: Impact on Mobility*. Rosemont, IL, American Academy of Orthopaedic Surgeons, 1993, pp 151–164.
43. Buckwalter JA: Activity vs. rest in the treatment of bone, soft tissue and joint injuries. *Iowa Orthop J* 1995;15:29–42.
44. Buckwalter JA, Woo SL–Y: Effects of repetitive loading and motion on the musculoskeletal tissues, in DeLee JC, Drez D Jr (eds): *Orthopaedic Sports Medicine: Principles and Practice*. Philadelphia, PA, WB Saunders, 1994, vol 1, pp 60–72.
45. Buckwalter JA, Lane NE, Gordon SL: Exercise as a cause of osteoarthritis, in Kuettner KE, Goldberg VM (eds): *Osteoarthritic Disorders*. Rosemont, IL, American Academy of Orthopaedic Surgeons, 1995, pp 405–417.
46. Praemer A, Furner S, Rice DP (eds): *Musculoskeletal Conditions in the United States*. Park Ridge, IL, American Academy of Orthopaedic Surgeons, 1992.
47. Andersson GBJ: Intervertebral disk: Clinical aspects, in Buckwalter JA, Goldberg VM, Woo SL-Y (eds): *Musculoskeletal Soft-Tissue Aging: Impact on Mobility*. Rosemont, IL, American Academy of Orthopaedic Surgeons, 1993, pp 331–347.
48. Trout JJ, Buckwalter JA, Moore KC: Ultrastructure of the human intervertebral disc: II. Cells of the nucleus pulposus. *Anat Rec* 1982;204:307–314.
49. Trout JJ, Buckwalter JA, Moore KC, et al: Ultrastructure of the human intervertebral disc: I. Changes in notochordal cells with age. *Tissue Cell* 1982;14:359–369.
50. Buckwalter JA: The fine structure of human intervertebral disc, in White AA III, Gordon SL (eds): American Academy of Orthopaedic Surgeons *Symposium on Idiopathic Low Back Pain*. St Louis, MO, CV Mosby, 1982, pp 108–143.
51. Buckwalter JA, Pedrini-Mille A, Pedrini V, et al: Proteoglycans of human infant intervertebral disc: Electron microscopic and biochemical studies. *J Bone Joint Surg* 1985;67A:284–294.
52. Buckwalter JA, Rosenberg LC: Electron microscopic studies of cartilage proteoglycans. *Electron Micro Rev* 1988;1:87–112.
53. Buckwalter JA, Smith KC, Kazarien LE, et al: Articular cartilage and intervertebral disc proteoglycans differ in structure: An electron microscopic study. *J Orthop Res* 1989;7:146–151.
54. Pearce RH, Mathieson JM, Mort JS, et al: Effect of age on the abundance and fragmentation of link protein of the human intervertebral disc. *J Orthop Res* 1989;7:861–867.
55. Donohue PJ, Jahnke MR, Blaha JD, et al: Characterization of link protein(s) from human intervertebral-disc tissues. *Biochem J* 1988;251:739–747.
56. Urban JPG: The effect of physical factors on disk cell metabolism, in Buckwalter JA, Goldberg VM, Woo SL-Y (eds): *Musculoskeletal Soft-Tissue Aging: Impact on Mobility*. Rosemont, IL, American Academy of Orthopaedic Surgeons, 1993, pp 391–412.
57. Bradford DS, Oegema TR Jr, Cooper KM, et al: Chymopapain, chemonucleolysis, and nucleus pulposus regeneration: A biochemical and biomechanical study. *Spine* 1984;9:135–147.
58. Bradford DS, Cooper KM, Oegema TR Jr: Chymopapain, chemonucleolysis, and nucleus pulposus regeneration. *J Bone Joint Surg* 1983;65A:1220–1231.

59. Nitobe T, Harata S, Okamato Y, et al: Degradation and biosynthesis of proteoglycans in the nucleus pulposus of canine intervertebral disc after chymopapain treatment. *Spine* 1988; 13:1332–1339.
60. Deutman R: The case for chemonucleolysis in discogenic sciatica: A review. *Acta Orthop Scand* 1992;63:571–575.
61. Woo SL, Orlando CA, Gomez MA, et al: Tensile properties of the medial collateral ligament as a function of age. *J Orthop Res* 1986;4:133–141.
62. Vasseur PB, Pool RR, Arnoczky SP, et al: Correlative biomechanical and histologic study of the cranial cruciate ligament in dogs. *Am J Vet Res* 1985;46:1842–1854.
63. Tkaczuk H: Tensile properties of human lumbar longitudinal ligaments. *Acta Orthop Scand* 1968;115(suppl):8–69.
64. Nachemson AL, Evans JH: Some mechanical properties of the third human lumbar interlaminar ligament (ligamentum flavum). *J Biomech* 1968;1:211–220.
65. Noyes FR, Grood ES: The strength of the anterior cruciate ligament in humans and rhesus monkeys: Age-related and species-related changes. *J Bone Joint Surg* 1976;58A:1074–1082.
66. Neumann P, Ekstrom LA, Keller TS, et al: Aging, vertebral density, and disc degeneration alter the tensile stress-strain characteristics of the human anterior longitudinal ligament. *J Orthop Res* 1994;12:103–112.
67. Woo SL, Hollis JM, Adams DJ, et al: Tensile properties of the human femur-anterior cruciate ligament-tibia complex: The effects of specimen age and orientation. *Am J Sports Med* 1991; 19:217–225.
68. Woo SL, Ohland KJ, Weiss JA: Aging and sex-related changes in the biomechanical properties of the rabbit medial collateral ligament. *Mech Ageing Dev* 1990;56:129–142.
69. Wang CW, Weiss JA, Albright JP, et al: Life-long exercise and aging effects on the canine medial collateral ligament (MCL). *Orthop Trans* 1990;14:488–489.
70. Kannus P, Jozsa L: Histopathological changes preceding spontaneous rupture of a tendon: A controlled study of 891 patients. *J Bone Joint Surg* 1991;73A:1507–1525.
71. Floridi A, Ippolito E, Postacchini F: Age-related changes in the metabolism of tendon cells. *Connect Tissue Res* 1981;9:95–97.
72. Amiel D, Kuiper SD, Wallace CD, et al: Age-related properties of medial collateral ligament and anterior cruciate ligament: A morphologic and collagen maturation study in the rabbit. *J Gerontol* 1991;46:B159–165.
73. Strocchi R, De Pasquale V, Guizzardi S, et al: Human Achilles tendon: Morphological and morphometric variations as a function of age. *Foot Ankle* 1991;12:100–104.
74. Buckwalter JA: Editorial: Should bone, soft-tissue, and joint injuries be treated with rest or activity? *J Orthop Res* 1995; 13:155–156.
75. Pape GS, Friedman M, Underwood LE, et al: The effect of growth hormone on weight gain and pulmonary function in patients with chronic obstructive lung disease. *Chest* 1991; 99:1495–1500.
76. Salomon F, Cuneo RC, Hesp R, Sonksen PH, et al: The effects of treatment with recombinant human growth hormone on body composition and metabolism in adults with growth hormone deficiency. *N Engl J Med* 1989;321:1797–1803.
77. Buckwalter JA: Pharmacological treatment of soft-tissue injuries. *J Bone Joint Surg* 1995;77A:1902–1914.
78. Haynesworth SE, Goldberg VM, Caplan AI: Diminution of the number of mesenchymal stem cells as a cause for skeletal aging, in Buckwalter JA, Goldberg VM, Woo SL-Y (eds): *Musculoskeletal Soft-Tissue Aging: Impact on Mobility.* Rosemont, IL, American Academy of Orthopaedic Surgeons, 1993, pp 79–87.
79. Campisi J: Mechanisms of aging that might contribute to musculoskeletal impairment: Diminished cell proliferative capacity, in Buckwalter JA, Goldberg VM, Woo SL-Y (eds): *Musculoskeletal Soft-Tissue Aging: Impact on Mobility.* Rosemont, IL, American Academy of Orthopaedic Surgeons, 1993, pp 73–78.
80. Seshadri T, Campisi J: Repression of c-fos transcription and an altered genetic program in senescent human fibroblasts. *Science* 1990;247:205–209.

Growth Factors

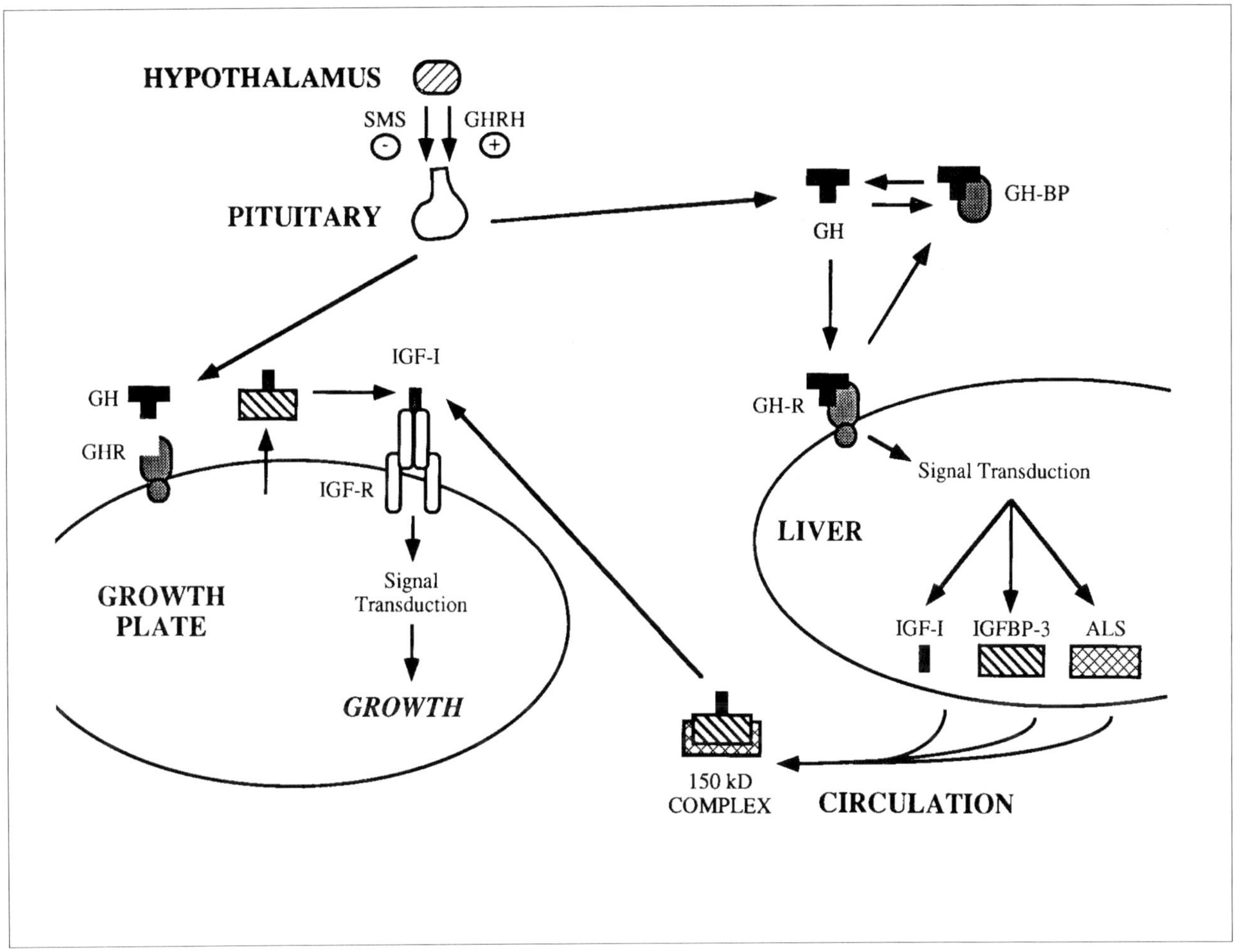

CHAPTER 44

Growth Factors as Therapeutic Agents

Stephen B. Trippel, MD

Many, if not most, of the diseases treated by orthopaedic surgeons reflect a failure of function of specific populations of cells, particularly those that comprise the musculoskeletal system. From this perspective, osteoporosis occurs when the cells that form bone fail to maintain normal bone mass and architecture. Arthritis represents a diminished ability of the cells of diarthrodial joints to balance the repair and degradation of articular cartilage. Many of the skeletal deformities of childhood (and hence of adulthood) stem directly or indirectly from the abnormal function of the cells of the growth plate and preosseous cartilage. Similarly, impaired healing after trauma represents a failure of resident and immigrant cells to restore the tissue at the trauma site. Thus, an understanding of the regulation of cell behavior may provide important insight into the cause of orthopaedic diseases, and the ability to control cell behavior would be a powerful tool in treating these diseases. Recent advances in cell biology and molecular biology have brought us to the point that manipulating cell behavior is both plausible and feasible.

One of the principal candidates for therapeutically altering cell behavior is the class of molecules known as growth factors. Growth factors are small proteins that serve as signaling agents for cells. The discovery of these substances revolutionized the field of cell biology by revealing the mechanism of regulation of a broad range of cell activities. Despite the fact that growth factors are present in plasma or tissue at concentrations that are generally measured in billionths of a gram, they are the principal effectors of such critical cellular functions as cell division, matrix synthesis, and tissue differentiation in virtually every organ system yet investigated, including musculoskeletal tissues.

Growth Factors

To date, no comprehensive taxonomy has been developed for the factors that regulate cells. As a result, general terms, such as hormone, cytokine, and growth factor, are principally of historical interest. Specific terms, such as insulin-like growth factor, fibroblast growth factor, and platelet-derived growth factor, are carried over from early descriptions of a factor's action or source. Thus, to avoid confusion, the names given to these substances are best viewed not as meaningful descriptors of function, but rather as identifiers that are accepted by tradition. Some of the principal contributors to the regulation of the skeleton are the insulin-like growth factors (IGFs), fibroblast growth factors (FGFs), transforming growth factor-beta (TGF-ß), platelet-derived growth factor (PDGF), and bone morphogenetic proteins (BMPs) (Table 1).

Two classes of insulin-like growth factor, IGF-I and IGF-II, have been identified to date. IGF-I mediates many of the stimulatory effects of growth hormone on the skeleton, while IGF-II helps regulate fetal growth.[1] IGF-I stimulates cell division and matrix synthesis by many of the cells of the musculoskeletal system, including those of cartilage,[1] bone,[2,3] tendon,[4] and muscle.[5]

Although identified as a product of platelets that is released at sites of injury, PDGF has emerged as a potent regulator of bone cells both on its own[6,7] and in concert with other factors.[7,8] Its role in cartilage, if any, remains unclear.

The FGFs are a group of heparin-binding polypeptides that were originally discovered on the basis of their mitogenic effect on fibroblasts.[9] Members of the FGF family regulate cell functions as diverse as mitogenesis, differentiation, protease production, receptor modulation, and cell maintenance.[10] Acidic FGF and basic FGF (also termed FGF-1 and FGF-2 respectively), the first FGFs to be identified, have both been implicated in cartilage and bone cell regulation.[11]

The TGF-ß family of polypeptides is composed of at least five molecules ($TGF\text{-}ß_1$ to $TGF\text{-}ß_5$) and is itself a member of a superfamily that includes the BMPs, activins, inhibins, Mullerian inhibiting substance, Drosophila decapentaplegic gene complex, growth and differentiation factors, and several other molecules that regulate morphogenesis in early development. Although originally discovered because of their ability to promote cellular transformation from a normal to a neoplastic growth pattern, the TGF-ß family members are now recognized as multifunctional signaling molecules that can act both as inhibitors and stimulators of cell replication.[12]

Close cousins of the TGF-ßs, the BMPs comprise a family of at least 15 growth factors originally identified for their ability to stimulate de novo bone formation.[13,14] Specifically, when implanted into soft tissues, most BMPs are capable of stimulating a cascade of cellular events that closely mimics the process of endochondral ossification seen in the growth plate and in normal fracture healing. Precursor cells are recruited and differentiate into chondrocytes that manufacture cartilage matrix. The cartilage is then gradually replaced by bone as osteoblasts populate the site. Eventually, marrow elements fill the newly formed

Table 1
Selected growth factors that regulate skeletal tissue

Growth Factor	Principle Actions
IGFs (somatomedins)	
IGF-I,* somatomedin-C (Sm-C)	Mitogenic, anabolic, mediates some growth hormone actions
IGF-II,* multiplication stimulating activity (MSA), skeletal growth factor (SGF)	Mitogenic, anabolic, generally less potent than IGF-I
FGFs	
FGF-1† (acidic fibroblast growth factor)	Mitogenic, angiogenic, regulates cell differentiation
FGF-2† (basic fibroblast growth factor)	Mitogenic, angiogenic, regulates cell differentiation
TGF-ß‡	Context-dependent, multifunctional
BMPs‡	Prototypes induce bone formation
PDGF§	Mitogenic

*IGF-I and IGF-II are structurally and biologically related to insulin
† FGF-1 and FGF-2 are the prototypes of the fibroblast growth factor family, of which there are at least nine members
‡ The TGF-ßs and BMP families are representatives of a large superfamily that includes at least five TGF-ßs and fifteen BMPs, the activins, the inhibins, and other factors involved in morphogenesis
§ PDGF occurs as a dimer of subunits, termed A and B, and may therefore take three forms: AA, AB, or BB

intertrabecular spaces. In the absence of further stimuli, as when BMP is placed in subcutaneous tissue, the new bone is resorbed and ultimately disappears. In bony defects, such as in calvarial drill holes[15] or femoral segmental resection defects,[16] the newly formed bone is incorporated into the structure of the host bone and subsequently remodels. Members of the BMP family have been reported to also regulate other cell types, including chondrocytes,[13] limb bud cells,[17] and bone-marrow stromal cells.[17]

Receptors

Growth factors elicit their cellular actions by binding to specific, large, transmembrane molecules on their target cells. These receptors serve as information transducers. They convert information carried by a growth factor into a form usable by the cell. The receptor's presence or absence defines whether or not a cell can respond to the information in its external environment. In addition, receptors may add to the information content carried by the signal molecule by integrating the message with information from the intracellular environment.

Phylogenetically, receptors probably had their origin in unicellular organisms. As they evolved, these cells needed a means of sorting materials around them, admitting some and excluding others. Receptor precursors may have also been used for intracellular communication. With the development of multicellular organisms, cells had to develop a system for communicating with each other. Even in early multicellular organisms, some method of conveying organizational signals would be required to coordinate cell activities. Transmission of these signals has fallen to growth factors and other signaling molecules, and the role of interpreting these signals for the cells has been assumed by receptors.

Growth factor receptors are linked by cascades of chemical reactions in the cytoplasm to various genes in the nucleus (Fig. 1).[18] Often these cascades activate several genes at a time. As a result, when considering the use of a growth factor for treatment of a specific cell defect, it is well to be aware that the factor may generate multiple effects even within a single cell type. While this may be advantageous, as when both cell division and matrix synthesis are desired for a repair response, it is a theoretical disadvantage if "mismatched" effects (for example, cell division and matrix degradation) are stimulated simultaneously.

Each family of growth factors has its own corresponding family of receptors. Despite marked differences in structure among receptor families, many of the key links in the gene-activating chain of reactions are shared by these families. It is therefore not surprising that binding of different growth factors to their respective receptors may lead to the same cellular response (eg, cell division). Much more impressive than the similarities among post-receptor pathways, and much less well understood, are their differences. Many growth factors display pleiotropic activity, eliciting a variety of effects in different cell types, or even in the same cell type at different stages of development. Although it is not yet clear how this remarkable versatility is achieved, the mechanisms responsible will probably be important in designing growth factor therapies that are capable of activating only certain genes and not others.

Knowledge about receptors is crucial to the successful application of factors as therapeutic agents. Clearly, treatment with a growth factor will not help a problem caused by an abnormality in that growth factor's receptor. For example, knowledge that the receptor for one factor is nonfunctional may form the basis for therapy with another factor that regulates some of the same cellular activities.

Challenges to Clinical Application

Growth Factor Interactions

The enormously complex task of operating the machinery of a cell, and of maintaining its activities in precise homeostatic balance, requires multiple levels of control and multiple controlling factors. It is unlikely that cell-signaling molecules act independently of each other or are present in isolation from each other at their sites of action. Therefore, understanding the regulation of cell behavior requires an understanding of the interactions between regulatory molecules. In some cases, these interactions may produce additive or even synergistic cell responses.[19,20] Thus, although therapeutic measures that employ single agents may be expected to be efficacious in some circumstances, it seems likely that maximizing the clinical benefit of cell-regulatory molecules will require the development of combination or serial treatment regimens.

Interactions between cell-signaling molecules may also help determine those specific disorders for which the signaling molecules may be therapeutically used. Consider, for example, the therapeutic potential of FGF-2 in disorders of articular cartilage. As a potent mitogen for articular chondrocytes,[21] FGF-2 would be expected to promote articular cartilage repair. However, FGF-2 also upregulates the receptor for interleukin-1,[22] a potent inhibitor of cartilage matrix synthesis and a central mediator of cartilage degradation.[23] Thus, in the presence of joint inflammation or other stimulus of IL-1 production, the net action of FGF-2 might be to exacerbate degradation,[24] just the opposite of the effect desired. Because the specific actions of many, if not most, growth factors are context-dependent, care will be required in distinguishing appropriate from inappropriate indications in the clinical setting.

Target Cells

The therapeutic application of growth factors must also accommodate the fact that most factors have a widespread and varied distribution of target cells. A growth factor that is administered to elicit a desired response from one cell type will also influence other cell types, possibly in unintended or undesirable ways. Therapies designed, for example, to influence articular cartilage must accommodate the reaction to the growth factor(s) both of the articular chondrocytes and of the synovial cells that line the joint. This problem of specificity is, of course, true of any pharmaceutical agent. Nonspecific actions in the form of toxicity or side effects have historically been a common reason to abandon otherwise attractive drug candidates and may be expected to do the same for some potentially attractive growth factors. The discovery of methods to target growth factors to specific tissues or specific cell types will likely be an important aspect of growth factor therapy development.

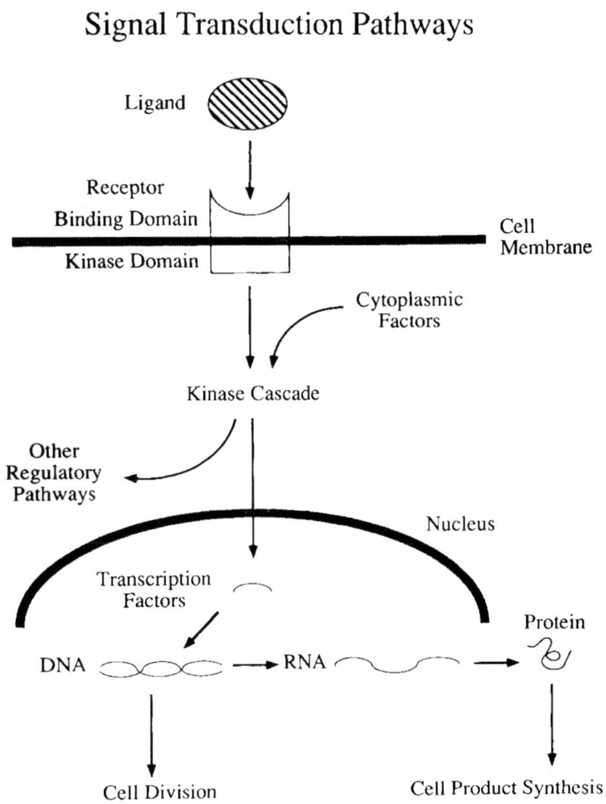

Fig. 1 Schematic illustration of the mechanism by which growth factors regulate cell behavior. A cell-signaling molecule in the extracellular environment binds to the extracellular domain of its receptor. This ligand-receptor interaction activates the intracellular domain of the receptor. For many growth factor receptors, this kinase domain possesses the enzymatic ability to transfer phosphate groups to proteins (kinase activity), an important signaling step in intracellular communication. The activated receptor in turn activates a series of additional phosphorylation steps (the kinase cascade) in association with other regulatory factors in the cytoplasm. This cascade culminates in the nucleus with the binding of transcription factors (proteins that bind to specific regulatory sequences of DNA) to activate gene transcription into messenger RNA (mRNA). The mRNA is then transcribed into protein to be used within the cell or exported for matrix production or other tissue functions.

Pharmaceutical Development

Bringing a molecule from the test tube to the bedside is a remarkably involved and protracted process. IGF-I is a case in point. This growth factor was first identified as a stimulatory activity (termed sulfation factor) in serum in 1957.[20] The molecule, later named IGF-I, that was responsible for this stimulatory activity was gradually purified and finally sequenced in 1978.[25] The IGF-I gene was cloned in 1983,[26] which made possible the production by recombinant DNA methodology of sufficient quantities of IGF-I to test the factor in vivo. The first human studies with IGF-I were reported in 1987,[27] exactly three decades after its discovery.

Advances in molecular biology have accelerated the basic science components of this discovery process, but the subsequent development of growth factors as pharmaceutical products remains a major undertaking. Safety and efficacy must be firmly established, as for any new drug, to obtain approval for clinical use. The requisite preclinical animal investigations and clinical human studies take several years and scores to hundreds of millions of dollars to complete. Currently several growth factors, including IGF-I, TGF-ß, BMP-2, and BMP-7 are in this investigative stage, and some may soon become a part of our orthopaedic armamentarium.

Acknowledgments

Supported by NIH grant AR31068. The author wishes to thank Ms. Allie McGuinness for assistance in manuscript preparation.

References

1. Trippel SB: Role of insulin-like growth factors in the regulation of chondrocytes, in Adolphe M (ed): *Biological Regulation of the Chondrocytes.* Boca Raton, FL, CRC Press, 1992, pp 161–190.
2. Canalis EM, Hintz RL, Dietrich JW, et al: Effect of somatomedin and growth hormone on bone collagen synthesis in vitro. *Metabolism* 1977;26:1079–1087.
3. Scheven BA, Hamilton NJ, Fakkeldij TM, et al: Effects of recombinant human insulin-like growth factor I and II (IGF-I/-II) and growth hormone (GH) on the growth of normal adult human osteoblast-like cells and human osteogenic sarcoma cells. *Growth Regul* 1991;1:160–167.
4. Florini JR, Roberts SB: A serum-free medium for the growth of muscle cells in culture. *In Vitro* 1979;15:983–992.
5. Bowen-Pope DF, Ross R: Platelet-derived growth factor. *Clin Endocrinol Metab* 1984;13:191–205.
6. Hock JM, Canalis E: Platelet-derived growth factor enhances bone cell replication, but not differentiated function of osteoblasts. *Endocrinology* 1994;134:1423–1428.
7. Pfeilschifter J, Oechsner M, Naumann A, et al: Stimulation of bone matrix apposition in vitro by local growth factors: A comparison between insulin-like growth factor I, platelet-derived growth factor, and transforming growth factor beta. *Endocrinology* 1990;127:69–75.
8. Lynch SE, Trippel SB, Finkelman RD, et al: The combination of platelet-derived growth factor-BB and insulin-like growth factor-I stimulates bone repair in adult Yucatan miniature pigs. *Wound Rep Reg* 1994;2:182–190.
9. Gospodarowicz D: Localisation of fibroblast growth factor and its effect alone and with hydrocortisone on 3T3 cell growth. *Nature* 1974;249:123–127.
10. Trippel SB: Biologic regulation of bone growth, in Brighton CT, Friedlaender GE, Lane JM (eds): *Bone Formation and Repair.* Rosemont, IL, American Academy of Orthopaedic Surgeons, 1994, pp 39–60.
11. Froger-Gaillard B, Charrier AM, Thenet S, et al: Growth-promoting effects of acidic and basic fibroblast growth factor on rabbit articular chondrocytes aging in culture. *Exp Cell Res* 1989;183:388–398.
12. Sporn MB, Roberts AB: Transforming growth factor-beta: Recent progress and new challenges. *J Cell Biol* 1992; 119:1017–1021.
13. Reddi AH: Regulation of cartilage and bone differentiation by bone morphogenetic proteins. *Curr Opin Cell Biol* 1992; 4:850–855.
14. Urist MR: Bone: Formation by autoinduction. *Science* 1965; 150:893–899.
15. Hollinger J, Mark DE, Bach DE, et al: Calvarial bone regeneration using osteogenin. *J Oral Maxillofac Surg* 1989;47:1182–1187.
16. Gerhart TN, Kirker-Head CA, Kriz MJ, et al: Healing segmental femoral defects in sheep using recombinant human bone morphogenetic protein. *Clin Orthop* 1993;293:317–326.
17. Wozney JM : The bone morphogenetic protein family and osteogenesis. *Mol Reprod Dev* 1992;32:160–167.
18. Johnson GL, Vaillancourt RR: Sequential protein kinase reactions controlling cell growth and differentiation. *Curr Opin Cell Biol* 1994;6:230–238.
19. Osborn KD, Trippel SB, Mankin HJ: Growth factor stimulation of adult articular cartilage. *J Orthop Res* 1989;7:35–42.
20. Trippel SB, Wroblewski J, Makower A-M, et al: Regulation of growth-plate chondrocytes by insulin-like growth-factor I and basic fibroblast growth-factor. *J Bone Joint Surg* 1993;75A: 177–189.
21. Sah RL, Chen AC, Grodzinsky AJ, et al: Differential effects of bFGF and IGF-I on matrix metabolism in calf and adult bovine cartilage explants. *Arch Biochem Biophys* 1994;308:137–147.
22. Chandrasekhar S, Harvey AK: Induction of interleukin-1 receptors on chondrocytes by fibroblast growth factor: A possible mechanism for modulation of interleukin-1 activity. *J Cell Physiol* 1989;138:236–246.
23. Howell DS, Treadwell BV, Trippel SB: Etiopathogenesis of osteoarthritis, in Moskowitz RW, Howell DS, Goldberg VM, et al (eds): *Osteoarthritis: Diagnosis and Medical/Surgical Management,* ed 2. Philadelphia, PA, WB Saunders, 1992, pp 233–252.
24. Chin JE, Hatfield CA, Krzesicki RF, et al: Interactions between interleukin-1 and basic fibroblast growth factor on articular chondrocytes: Effects on cell growth, prostanoid production, and receptor modulation. *Arthritis Rheum* 1991;34:314–324.
25. Rinderknecht E, Humbel RE: The amino acid sequence of human insulin-like growth factor I and its structural homology with proinsulin. *J Biol Chem* 1978;253:2769–2776.
26. Jansen M, van Schaik FM, Ricker AT, et al: Sequence of cDNA encoding human insulin-like growth factor I precursor. *Nature* 1983;306:609–611.
27. Guler HP, Zapf J, Froesch ER: Short-term metabolic effects of recombinant human insulin-like growth factor I in healthy adults. *N Engl J Med* 1987;317:137–140.

Growth Factor Treatment of Disorders of Skeletal Growth

Stephen B. Trippel, MD
Ron G. Rosenfeld, MD

Disorders of skeletal growth have long been a focus of orthopaedics. To date the options available to orthopaedists for the treatment of these abnormalities have been limited by a lack of knowledge about their underlying causes. Recent advances in cellular and molecular biology are beginning to provide this missing information. From the cellular standpoint, disorders of skeletal growth are disorders in the function of cells in the developing skeleton. Many cell functions are regulated by cell-signaling molecules, and it has become clear that substances such as growth factors play an important role in both normal and abnormal skeletal growth and development. Indeed, some of the most dramatic successes in the treatment of pediatric skeletal growth disorders have resulted from the identification of deficiencies in cell-signaling molecules that are crucial to skeletal development. These substances include vitamin D in the treatment and prevention of the skeletal deformities of rickets, thyroid hormone for the skeletal developmental failure of cretinism, and growth hormone for the skeletal growth deficiency of hypopituitarism. The importance of growth factors in skeletal development is emphasized by the recent discoveries that the skeletal deformities of achondroplasia,[1,2] Apert syndrome,[3] Cruzon syndrome,[4] Pfeiffer syndrome,[5] and Jackson-Weiss syndrome[6] are all caused by mutations in receptors for the fibroblast growth factor (FGF) family of signaling molecules.

The Growth Hormone–IGF-I Axis

Of the hormonal and growth factor systems that regulate skeletal growth, perhaps the best understood is the growth hormone-IGF-I (insulin-like growth factor I) axis (Fig. 1). The hypothalamus, at the top of the regulatory hierarchy, elaborates growth hormone-releasing hormone, which stimulates growth hormone secretion by the cells of the anterior pituitary.[7] Growth hormone released into the systemic circulation is then carried to such target tissues as the liver and the growth plate. Binding of growth hormone to specific cell-surface receptors stimulates these cells to produce IGF-I, which may then enter the circulation to be carried to its target cells (endocrine action), or may act locally by binding to cell surface receptors on the same cells that produced it (autocrine action) or on neighboring cells (paracrine action)[8,9] (Fig. 2). IGF-I helps regulate its own synthesis by negative feedback on both the pituitary and hypothalamus.[10]

In the circulation and other tissue fluids, most IGF-I is bound to carrier proteins, termed insulin-like growth factor binding proteins (IGFBPs). The IGFBP family consists of at least six structurally related proteins that transport IGF-I and modulate its actions on target tissues. Normally, IGFBP-3 is the major binding protein in plasma. IGFBP-3 production, like that of IGF-I, is growth-hormone dependent.[11,12]

Alteration of any step in this growth regulating system can be expected to disrupt normal skeletal development. If a specific abnormal site in the sequence can be identified, corrective treatment becomes a possibility. For example, classic hypopituitary dwarfism, which is caused by deficient production of growth hormone by the cells of the anterior pituitary, is readily treated by growth hormone replacement.

Growth Hormone Resistance

Discovery

The cause of growth failure in individuals without growth hormone deficiency has not been clear until recently. In 1966, Laron and associates[13] identified a family with many features of growth hormone insufficiency but who, paradoxically, were found to have elevated circulating levels of growth hormone. In its classic form, this syndrome, known as Laron dwarfism, is characterized by severe growth failure, normal or elevated secretion of growth hormone, and markedly reduced serum concentrations of both IGF-I and IGFBP-3.[14] Several possible etiologies were ruled out, including an abnormality in the growth hormone molecule, circulating anti-growth hormone antibodies, and anti-growth hormone receptor antibodies. The defect was eventually traced to the growth hormone receptor itself by demonstrating that cells from these patients were unable to bind growth hormone.[15]

Etiology

With the advent of molecular biologic methods and the sequencing of the human growth hormone receptor gene, several growth hormone receptor gene abnormalities that cause Laron dwarfism have been identified. The specific genetic defect responsible for the growth hormone resistance varies considerably

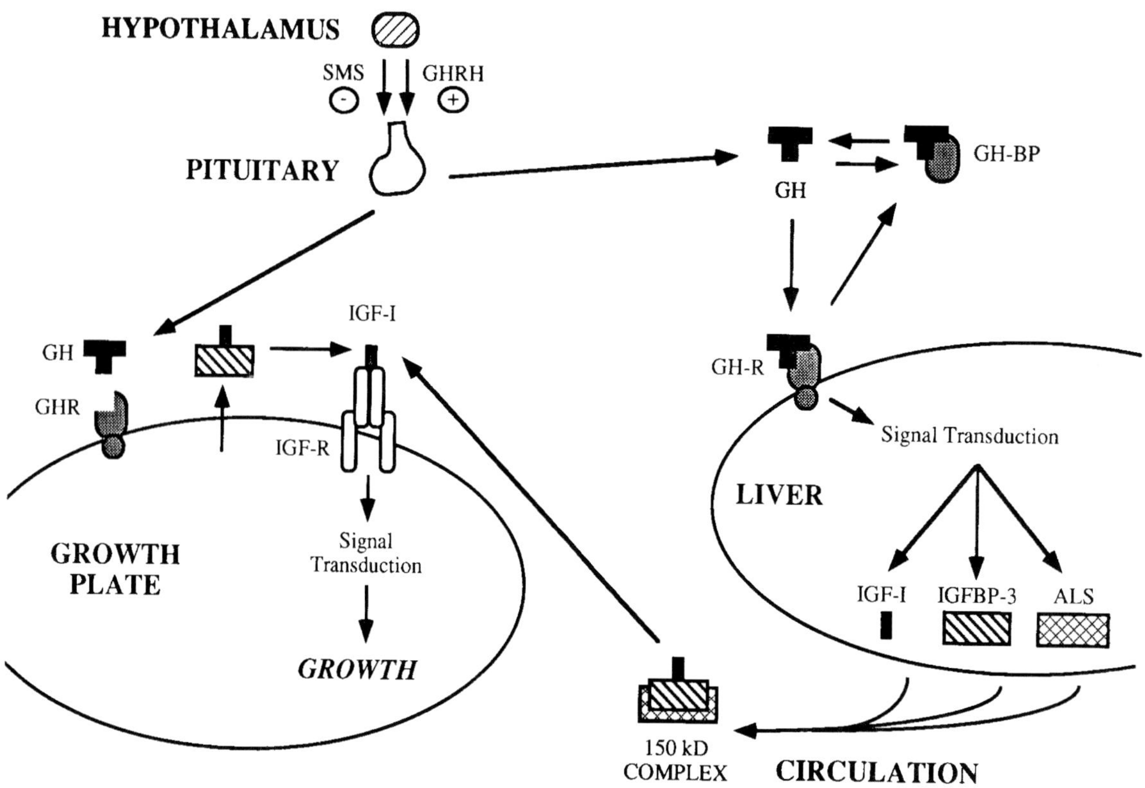

Fig. 1 Schematic illustration of the regulation of bone growth by the growth hormone–IGF-I axis. The hypothalamus produces growth hormone-releasing hormone (GHRH) or somatostatin (SMS). GHRH stimulates and SMS inhibits growth hormone (GH) release by the anterior pituitary. GH enters the systemic circulation in equilibrium with a binding protein (GH-BP) derived from the GH receptor. GH binds to GH receptors on liver cells, activating the synthesis of IGF-I and its predominant carrier protein, insulin-like growth factor binding protein-3 (IGFBP-3). A second carrier protein, the acid labile subunit (ALS) combines with IGF-I and IGFBP-3 to form a tripartite circulating complex (150 kd complex) that conveys IGF-I to its target tissues, including the growth plate. There IGF-I is transferred to IGF receptors (IGF-R) on the chondrocyte membrane, initiating a cascade of intracellular reactions that regulate cell division and maturation. Growth hormone may also bind to GH receptors on growth plate chondrocytes, stimulating IGF-I production by these cells for local regulation.

among affected individuals. Some patients have large deletions of the extracellular hormone-binding domain of the growth hormone receptor. Most have only a point mutation, in which one of the many (approximately 87,000) nucleotide bases spanned by the receptor gene is replaced by an alternative nucleotide. More than 20 such point mutations have been identified to date, almost all of them affecting the extracellular domain of the receptor.[7] Each of these mutations alters the amino acid sequence of the receptor, presumably interfering with the ability of the receptor to recognize or bind to growth hormone and thereby preventing growth hormone from initiating the signal-transducing function of the receptor. In some cases, the mutation appears to disrupt the dimerization, or pairing, of growth hormone receptors that is required for signal transduction.[16]

Not all children with mutations of the growth hormone receptor gene manifest the features of complete growth hormone insensitivity. Recent studies have revealed that heterozygous mutations in the growth hormone receptor, in which only one of the patient's two gene copies is abnormal, may produce skeletal growth deficiency. These patients appear to have a partial growth hormone insensitivity. Indeed, it is plausible that there is a continuum of growth hormone responsiveness ranging from complete insensitivity, as in Laron dwarfism, to short stature with partial insensitivity.[17] Currently, it is not clear what percentage of children diagnosed with idiopathic growth failure actually are suffering from heterozygosity for a mutation in the growth hormone receptor.[7]

Patients with growth hormone insensitivity are unresponsive or only marginally responsive to growth hormone therapy.[17] However, because the stimulatory effects of growth hormone on skeletal growth are thought to be mediated by IGF-I and because individuals with growth hormone receptor abnormalities have low serum concentrations of IGF-I, these patients are candidates for treatment with IGF-I. Several clinical tri-

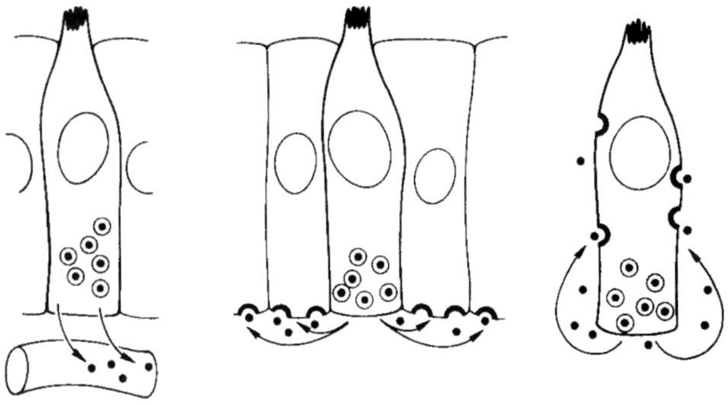

Fig. 2 Diagrammatic representation of endocrine, paracrine, and autocrine cell regulation. In the endocrine pathway, the cell-signaling molecules are released into the circulation by the secreting cell to act on distant target cells. In the paracrine pathway, the cell-signaling molecules are secreted locally to act on neighboring cells. The autocrine pathway is characerized by cellular self-activation. Cell-signaling molecules are represented by dots and their receptors by thickened semicircles in the cell membrane. (Reproduced with permission from Sporn MB, Todaro GJ: Autocrine secretion and malignant transformation of cells. *N Eng J Med* 1980;303:878-880.)

als have been undertaken to test this possibility. To our knowledge, these trials represent the first reported use of a growth factor to correct an abnormality in skeletal development.

IGF-I Treatment

Initial studies of IGF-I effects in humans were conducted in normal volunteers.[18] Rapid intravenous administration of recombinant human IGF-I produced pronounced hypoglycemia, with a nadir of 50% of baseline glucose at 30 minutes and a return to normal glucose levels by 120 minutes. In order to avoid this complication, the rate of infusion was reduced to 100 µg/kg/hr. A 6-day subcutaneous infusion at 20 µg/kg/hr increased systemic protein synthesis and produced feedback inhibition of growth hormone secretion.[19] The half-life of the administered IGF-I was short. Even after subcutaneous injection, free IGF-I was estimated to have a half-life of 10 to 12 minutes, and IGF-I disappeared from serum within 18 hours after administration.

Unfortunately, in initial studies of patients with growth hormone receptor deficiency, the intravenous administration of IGF-I caused even more severe hypoglycemia, and the IGF-I was eliminated more rapidly than in normal subjects.[20] An intravenous bolus of 75 µg/kg produced hypoglycemia to an average of 45% of baseline, comparable to that observed in normal subjects. In these patients, however, hypoglycemia persisted at 120 minutes, until a meal was given to restore glucose levels. This effect was presumed to result from the deficiency of growth hormone-dependent IGFBP-3 in these individuals. Normally, approximately 95% of the IGF-I in plasma is bound to IGFBP-3, which serves both to prolong its half-life and to modulate its access to extravascular target cells.

A subcutaneous preparation of 40 µg/kg IGF-I was administered to adult patients with growth hormone receptor deficiency twice daily for 1 week.[21] This regimen normalized serum IGF-I levels and appropriately decreased serum growth hormone levels. With regular meal consumption, no hypoglycemia was observed.

To determine whether IGF-I treatment could bypass the effect of the growth hormone receptor defect and directly stimulate growth in affected skeletally immature individuals, several investigators have attempted long-term treatment of pediatric patients who have growth hormone receptor deficiency.[22-27] In two patients treated with 120 µg/kg IGF-I twice daily, height velocity increased from an average of 2.9 cm/yr to 7.0 cm/yr during 1 year of treatment. Interestingly, this beneficial response occurred despite a failure of the treatment to increase circulating IGFBP-3 levels or to improve the half-life of IGF-I.[26]

Similarly, treatment for 3 to 10 months with a single daily injection of 150 µg/kg IGF-I produced a growth velocity of 8.8 to 13.6 cm/yr, a rate comparable to that seen with growth hormone treatment of patients with growth hormone deficiency.[24] In another study, children with growth hormone receptor deficiency were treated with 80 to 120 µg/kg IGF-I subcutaneously twice a day for periods of 3 to 18 months.[22] This regimen generated catch-up growth, a phenomenon characterized by skeletal growth that is faster than normal. This is a particularly encouraging observation because catch-up growth tends to restore normal height, rather than simply producing a transiently normal growth rate.

The largest study of IGF-I therapy reported to date involved 30 patients, age 3 to 23 years, who were treated for 6 to 12 months.[27] All patients except the two oldest (20 and 23 years old) responded with growth rates that were an average of 2 cm/yr greater than the rates before treatment. Although a few of these patients responded to the relatively low dose of 40 µg/kg of IGF-I twice daily, most required up to 120 µg/kg IGF-I twice daily to achieve this degree of growth acceleration.

One randomized, prospective, double-blind placebo-controlled study has to our knowledge been reported.[23] Children with growth hormone receptor deficiency were treated with twice-daily subcutaneous injections of IGF-I (120 µg/kg) for 12 months, or with 6 months of placebo followed by 6 months of IGF-I. IGF-I treatment produced a significant ($p < 0.05$) increase in growth rate from an average of 2.9 cm/yr before treatment to an average of 8.6 cm/yr after treatment. This response was sustained over the 1-year course of therapy. IGF-I therapy also resulted in noticeable increases in foot size and lower segment length compared to measurements in the placebo group. No significant changes were seen in head circumference, brachial circumference, arm span, or weight. Interestingly, in subjects receiving IGF-I therapy for the full 12 months, the mean cumulative increase in bone age was only 9 months. This finding suggests that this regimen of IGF-I treatment does not cause an accelerated skeletal maturation that would result in premature termination of growth and hence a shortening of ultimate stature. Currently, however, the effect of IGF-I on ultimate stature remains unknown.

In addition to its effect on linear growth, growth hormone insensitivity is associated with abnormal craniofacial development. Patients with growth hormone insensitivity have a characteristic facial phenotype that is recognizable at birth.[28] Such features include a prominent forehead, depressed nasal bridge, and hypoplasia of the midface. IGF-I therapy was associated with striking changes in the craniofacial bones, with lengthening of the face and partial correction of head length, skull height, and head width. In addition, IGF-I therapy produced a loss of subcutaneous fat, and an increase in hair growth and changes in its texture.[29]

Clinical trials of IGF-I in growth hormone receptor deficiency and other syndromes of growth hormone insensitivity are still in their early stages. While IGF-I therapy has been shown to stimulate growth acceleration (in the short term at least), information about the optimum dose and frequency of administration must await further studies.

Complications of IGF-I Therapy

With any novel therapy, side effects and toxicity can limit the usefulness of the therapeutic agent. With IGF-I, a variety of side effects and complications have been noted. Most, but not all, have been minor. In uncontrolled studies, side effects and complications included electrolyte shifts, changes in serum concentrations of insulin and growth hormone, hypoglycemia (sometimes severe enough to cause convulsions), hypercalciuria, pseudotumor cerebri, convulsions, papilledema, facial nerve palsy, parotid swelling, and tachycardia.[30] In the only available placebo-controlled trial that we know of, the IGF-I treatment group experienced a higher incidence of upper respiratory infections, transient elevation of liver function tests, anti-IGF-I antibodies, and transient papilledema.[23] Curiously, the most common (occurring in six of seven patients) complication of IGF-I therapy was hair loss, which was followed by regrowth of thick, curly hair that was coarser in texture than the original hair.

In other reports, complications have been more prevalent. In the long-term study of Wilton and associates,[27] more than half the patients experienced hypoglycemia; in two out of 17, it was severe enough to cause convulsions. Twelve out of 30 patients reported mild to moderate headache, which in one case was severe and accompanied by vomiting and bilateral papilledema that resolved after cessation of treatment. One patient had hypotension, a decrease in serum potassium, and fatigue following each injection, and treatment was stopped. Partial peripheral paresis of the right facial nerve in one child appeared after 10 days of therapy and resolved within 2 weeks. In some patients, an asymptomatic increase in heart rate has been observed. Mean heart rate of patients in one study rose from 101 ± 1.9 beats per minute before treatment to 116 ± 2.3 beats per minute during treatment.[31] Heart rate increased with dose escalation and was not associated with changes in glucose or electrolytes. The etiology of this effect remains unknown. The administration of any mitogen (IGF-I is mitogenic for multiple cell types) raises the concern of tumorigenicity, but this does not currently appear to be a side effect of IGF-I therapy.

Insulin-Like Growth Factor Binding Protein-3 (IGFBP-3)

The relatively low dosages of IGF-I employed in the early clinical trials were based, in part, on safety issues (eg, possibility of a hypoglycemic reaction), and concerns about a short IGF-I half-life resulting from the deficiency in IGFBP-3, which failed to be corrected by IGF-I treatment. Indeed, it is remarkable that growth acceleration occurred in the absence of a normalization of IGFBP-3 levels or an increase in the half-life of IGF-I to more than a few minutes.

One approach to resolving the failure of IGFBP-3 to respond to IGF-I therapy is to administer both agents together. In preliminary studies in cynomolgus monkeys, administration of an intravenous bolus of the relatively high dose of 2 mg/kg (2000 μg/kg) of IGF-I bound to IGFBP-3 did not result in hypoglycemia (Sommer A, Bagi CM, DeLeon E, unpublished data, 1995). Thus, this approach appears to suppress the acute insulin-like effects associated with the administration of IGF-I alone.

Direct Action of IGF-I

The growth response to exogenous IGF-I incidentally clarifies the mechanism of IGF-I action on the cells responsible for skeletal growth. The clinical data discredit the previously popular dual effector theory of growth regulation.[32] This theory postulated that precursor cells in the epiphyseal growth plate could respond to the mitogenic action of IGF-I only after they had been induced to differentiate by a prior exposure to growth hormone. The current data suggest that IGF-I, by itself, is fully capable of stimulating skeletal growth.

On the other hand, a role for growth hormone has not been excluded. At the very least, growth hormone stimulates production of IGFBP-3 and a protein termed the acid labile subunit, the two of which combine with IGF-I to form the 150 kd ternary complex in which most IGF is transported. It is also of note that in most studies of IGF-I treatment of growth hormone insensitivity, the growth response does not quite equal that observed with growth hormone treatment of naive growth hormone deficient children. This may be caused by the failure of IGF-I therapy to increase serum concentrations of IGFBP-3 and acid labile subunit, resulting in a continued short half-life for serum IGF polypeptides.

Although preliminary results from studies involving the use of IGF-I in regulating skeletal growth and development have been encouraging, it remains to be established whether this growth response will be sustained over the full course of normal skeletal development or lead to significantly increased adult stature.

Role of Fibroblast Growth Factors

Progress in the application of other growth factors to skeletal disorders is much less advanced than for those involving the growth hormone-IGF-I axis, partly because of the relatively recent recognition of the role of growth factors in the etiology of specific disorders. For example, the fibroblast growth factor (FGF) family of polypeptides was named for its ability to stimulate fibroblasts but subsequently was found to influence multiple cell types, including cartilage. The cells responsible for skeletal growth, the chondrocytes of the epiphyseal growth plate, have been known for some time to be under the mitogenic influence of FGF.[33,34] However, it has only been in the last few years that FGF receptors on these cells have been identified[35] and characterized[36] or that cloning of the mammalian FGF receptor family[37] has permitted gene analysis. Thus, it was not until 1994 that mutations in the receptors for the FGF family were discovered to be the cause of an expanding group of chondrodysplasias, including achondroplasia, the most common genetic form of dwarfism.

Unlike those of the growth hormone-IGF-I axis, the actions of the FGF family do not appear to involve a cascade of events involving multiple tissues and multiple mediators. There is no currently available means of "bypassing" the FGF receptor defect in achondroplastic dwarfism in a fashion analogous to the use of IGF-I to circumvent the growth hormone receptor defect in Laron dwarfism. Similarly, even the elegant gene therapy methodologies that have been developed for delivering cell-signaling molecules cannot resolve problems caused by abnormalities in the receptors for these signaling molecules. Methods will be required that can activate postreceptor pathways through means other than the cognate receptor. For this, we must await the elucidation of these pathways and their mechanisms of regulation.

Ethics of Intervention

The availability of therapeutic agents that enhance skeletal growth raises several ethical questions. At what height is a person to be considered "too short"? In an era of increasing focus on the cost effectiveness of all therapies, what is the value of a centimeter of stature? If growth factor treatment proves to be capable of increasing normal growth to supranormal levels, should this therapy be used to augment height that is not abnormal but would become "desirably abnormal" with treatment? Clearly, progress in the application of growth factors to disorders of skeletal development will require advances in ethics and socioeconomics as well as in the necessary science and technology.

Acknowledgments

Supported by NIH Grant AR31068 (SBT) and Pharamacia, Inc. (RGR). The authors thank Ms. Allie McGuinness for assistance in manuscript preparation.

References

1. Rousseau F, Bonaventure J, Legeai-Mallet L, et al: Mutations in the gene encoding fibroblast growth factor receptor-3 in achondroplasia. *Nature* 1994;371:252–254.
2. Shiang R, Thompson LM, Zhu Y-Z, et al: Mutations in the transmembrane domain of FGFR3 cause the most common genetic form of dwarfism, achondroplasia. *Cell* 1994;78: 335–342.
3. Wilkie AO, Slaney SF, Oldridge M, et al: Apert syndrome results from localized mutations of FGFR2 and is allelic with Crouzon syndrome. *Nat Genet* 1995;9:165–172.
4. Reardon W, Winter RM, Rutland P, et al: Mutations in the fibroblast growth factor receptor 2 gene cause Crouzon syndrome. *Nat Genet* 1994;8:98–103.
5. Muenke M, Schell U, Hehr A, et al: A common mutation in the fibroblast growth factor receptor 1 gene in Pfeiffer syndrome. *Nat Genet* 1994;8:269–274.
6. Jabs EW, Li X, Scott AF, et al: Jackson-Weiss and Crouzon syndromes are allelic with mutations in fibroblast growth factor receptor 2. *Nat Genet* 1994;8:275–279.
7. Rosenfeld RG, Rosenbloom AL, Guevara-Aguirre J: Growth hormone (GH) insensitivity due to primary GH receptor deficiency. *Endocr Rev* 1994;15:369–390.
8. Sporn MB, Todaro GJ: Autocrine secretion and malignant transformation of cells. *N Engl J Med* 1980;303:878–880.
9. Trippel SB: Role of insulin-like growth factors in the regulation of chondrocytes, in Adolphe M (ed): *Biological Regulation of the Chondrocytes.* Boca Raton, FL, CRC Press, 1992, pp 161–190.
10. Berelowitz M, Szabo M, Frohman LA, et al: Somatomedin-C mediates growth hormone negative feedback by effects on both the hypothalamus and the pituitary. *Science* 1981;212: 1279–1281.
11. Cohen P, Fielder PJ, Hasegawa Y, et al: Clinical aspects of insulin-like growth factor binding proteins. *Acta Endocrinol* 1991;124(suppl 2):74–85.

12. Lamson G, Giudice LC, Rosenfeld RG: Insulin-like growth factor binding proteins: Structural and molecular relationships. *Growth Factors* 1991;5:19–28.
13. Laron Z, Pertzelan A, Mannheimer S: Genetic pituitary dwarfism with high serum concentration of growth hormone: A new inborn error of metabolism? *Isr J Med Sci* 1966;2:152–155.
14. Rosenfeld RG: Editorial: Broadening the growth hormone insensitivity syndrome. *N Engl J Med* 1995;333:1145–1146.
15. Eshet R, Laron Z, Brown M, et al: Immunoreactive properties of the plasma hGH from patients with the syndrome of familial dwarfism and high plasma IR-hGH. *J Clin Endocrinol Metab* 1973;37:819–821.
16. Kelly PA, Postel-Vinay MC, Finidori J, et al: Growth hormone receptor structure, dimerization and function. *Acta Paediatr Suppl* 1994;399:107–111.
17. Goddard AD, Covello R, Luoh S-M, et al: The Growth Hormone Insensitivity Study Group: Mutations of the growth hormone receptor in children with idiopathic short stature. *N Engl J Med* 1995;333:1093–1098.
18. Guler HP, Zapf J, Froesch ER: Short-term metabolic effects of recombinant human insulin-like growth factor I in healthy adults. *N Engl J Med* 1987;317:137–140.
19. Guler HP, Schmid C, Zapf J, et al: Effects of recombinant insulin-like growth factor-I on insulin secretion and renal function in normal human subjects. *Proc Natl Acad Sci USA* 1989;86:2868–2872.
20. Laron Z, Klinger B, Erster B, et al: Effect of acute administration of insulin-like growth factor I in patients with Laron-type dwarfism. *Lancet* 1988;2:1170–1172.
21. Vaccarello MA, Diamond FB Jr, Guevara-Aguirre J, et al: Hormonal and metabolic effects and pharmacokinetics of recombinant insulin-like growth factor-I in growth hormone receptor deficiency/Laron syndrome. *J Clin Endocrinol Metab* 1993;77:273–280.
22. Backeljauw PF, Underwood LE: Abstract: Effects of prolonged IGF-I treatment in children with growth hormone insensitivity syndrome (GHIS). *Pediatr Res* 1993;33(suppl):S56.
23. Guevara-Aguirre J, Vasconez O, Martinez V, et al: A randomized, double blind, placebo-controlled trial on safety and efficacy of recombinant human insulin-like growth factor-I in children with growth hormone receptor deficiency. *J Clin Endocrinol Metab* 1995;80:1393–1398.
24. Laron Z, Anin S, Klipper-Aurbach Y, et al: Effects of insulin-like growth factor on linear growth, head circumference, and body fat in patients with Laron-type dwarfism. *Lancet* 1992;339:1258–1261.
25. Walker JL, Van Wyk JJ, Underwood LE: Stimulation of statural growth by recombinant insulin-like growth factor-I in a child with growth hormone insensitivity syndrome (Laron type). *J Pediatr* 1992;121:641–646.
26. Wilson KF, Fielder PJ, Guevara-Aguirre J, et al: Long-term effects of insulin-like growth factor (IGF)-I treatment on serum IGFs and IGF binding proteins in adolescent patients with growth hormone receptor deficiency. *Clin Endocrinol* 1995;42:399–407.
27. Wilton P: Kabi Pharmacia Study Group on Insulin-like Growth Factor I Treatment in Growth Hormone Insensitivity Syndromes: Treatment with recombinant human insulin-like growth factor I of children with growth hormone receptor deficiency (Laron syndrome). *Acta Paediatr Suppl* 1992;383:137–142.
28. Guevara-Aguirre J, Rosenbloom AL, Fielder PJ, et al: Growth hormone receptor deficiency in Ecuador: Clinical and biochemical phenotype in two populations. *J Clin Endocrinol Metab* 1993;76:417–423.
29. Leonard J, Samuels M, Cotterill AM, et al: Effects of recombinant insulin-like growth factor I on craniofacial morphology in growth hormone insensitivity. *Acta Paediatr Suppl* 1994;399:140–141.
30. Otten BJ, Rotteveel JJ, Cruysberg JRM: Abstract: Pseudotumour cerebri following treatment with growth hormone. *Horm Res* 1992;37(suppl 4):16.
31. Vasconez O, Martinez V, Martinez AL, et al: Heart rate increases in patients with growth hormone receptor deficiency treated with insulin-like growth factor I. *Acta Paediatr Suppl* 1994;399:137–139.
32. Green H, Morikawa M, Nixon T: A dual effector theory of growth-hormone action. *Differentiation* 1985;29:195–198.
33. Kato Y: Roles of fibroblast growth factor and transforming growth factor beta families in cartilage formation, in Adolphe M (ed): *Biological Regulation of the Chondrocytes.* Boca Raton, FL, CRC Press, 1992, pp 141–160.
34. Trippel SB, Wroblewski J, Makower A-M, et al: Regulation of growth-plate chondrocytes by insulin-like growth-factor I and basic fibroblast growth factor. *J Bone Joint Surg* 1993;75A:177–189.
35. Iwamoto M, Shimazu A, Nakashima K, et al: Reduction of basic fibroblasts growth factor receptor is coupled with terminal differentiation of chondrocytes. *J Biol Chem* 1991;266:461–467.
36. Trippel SB, Whelan MC, Klagsbrun M, et al: Interaction of basic fibroblast growth factor with bovine growth plate chondrocytes. *J Orthop Res* 1992;10:638–646.
37. Johnson DE, Williams LT: Structural and functional diversity in the FGF receptor multigene family. *Adv Cancer Res* 1993;60:1–41.

CHAPTER 46

Growth Factor Treatment of Fractures

Thomas A. Einhorn, MD
Stephen B. Trippel, MD

The response of bone to structural damage is nearly unique in biology. The vast majority of tissues, when traumatized, heal with a fibrous scar, the cells and structure of which are not normal for the tissue and are unable to assume that tissue's function. In contrast, bone and a few other tissues (eg, cornea and to a limited extent, liver) are capable of true cellular, morphologic, and functional restoration. The initial phase of fracture healing is characterized by an inflammatory response and the consolidation of hematoma within the fracture site. This is followed by proliferation of periosteal, endosteal, and marrow stromal cells adjacent to the fracture, and the recruitment of undifferentiated mesenchymal cells from nearby soft tissues. These cells and their progeny differentiate to become chondroblasts, chondrocytes, osteoblasts, and osteocytes. The cartilage thus formed is eventually replaced by bone and the early woven bone is remodeled to a more mature lamellar bone.[1]

Although 90% to 95% of the estimated 5.6 million fractures that occur annually in the United States heal satisfactorily, the remaining 5% to 10% progress to delayed union or nonunion.[2] The specific cause of impaired healing is often unknown. However, a host of conditions have been identified as risk factors. These include site of fracture, instability, soft-tissue trauma, infection, and distraction. Under adverse circumstances, agents with the ability to ensure or accelerate the repair process would be of great benefit. Growth factors are, by virtue of their ability to regulate cell behavior, excellent candidates to serve as such agents.

Several growth-promoting substances have been identified at the site of healing fractures and hence are believed to play a role in the healing process. Among these are the transforming growth factor betas (TGF-ßs), bone morphogenetic proteins (BMPs), fibroblast growth factors (FGFs), insulin-like growth factors (IGFs), and platelet-derived growth factors (PDGFs).[3,4]

Transforming Growth Factor-Beta

The TGF-ßs are a family of polypeptide growth factors encoded by closely related genes. This family includes at least five molecules known as TGF-ß (TGF-$ß_1$, TGF-$ß_2$, TGF-$ß_3$, TGF-$ß_4$, and TGF-$ß_5$) as well as several other molecules including the BMPs (discussed below).

The broad range of cellular activities regulated by the TGF-ßs themselves include the proliferation and expression of the differentiated phenotype of many of the cell populations that comprise the skeleton. Among these are the mesenchymal precursor cells for chondrocytes, osteoblasts, and osteoclasts.[5] In vivo studies have shown that, during endochondral ossification, chondrocytes and osteoblasts synthesize TGF-ß, which accumulates in the extracellular matrix.[6] Indeed, the largest source of TGF-ß in the body is the extracellular matrix of bone.[7]

In vitro studies using fracture callus organ cultures have demonstrated TGF-ß mRNA in the soft callus (which is mostly cartilage) approximately 14 days after fracture and in the hard callus (which is mostly bone) on days 5 and 15.[8] Recent in situ hybridization studies of normal human fracture healing in vivo have localized TGF-ß mRNA to areas of proliferating mesenchymal tissue, cartilage, and bone. Messenger RNA levels were lower in cells in the fracture hematoma and in hypertrophic chondrocytes.[9] Because mRNA levels generally reflect gene activity and because mRNA is the template from which protein is synthesized, these data suggest that fracture activates the genes for TGF-ß, increasing TGF-ß mRNA levels and hence the synthesis and release of TGF-ß protein.

The presence of TGF-ß in normal fracture healing suggests that this factor plays a role in the repair process. Several studies have tested the hypothesis that exogenous administration of TGF-ß can stimulate repair of bone defects.[10-12] Exogenously applied recombinant human TGF-ß stimulated the recruitment and proliferation of osteoblasts in defects in the skulls of rabbits. In the presence of TGF-ß, rapid deposition of bone matrix and normal remodeling occurred. In the absence of growth factor, the defects failed to heal.[10] In another study, native human TGF-ß (obtained from platelets) augmented the healing of tibial fractures in rats. Four or 40 ng of TGF-ß were administered every other day for 40 days. TGF-ß induced a dose-dependent increase in the cross-sectional area of the callus and bone at the site of the fracture. Mechanical testing showed an accompanying increase in maximal load-bearing capacity without affecting ultimate stress, stiffness or energy-storage capacity. In a plated mid-diaphyseal tibial osteotomy model in adult rabbits, the continuous administration of TGF-ß in doses of 1 mg to 10 mg per day for 6 weeks increased maximal bending strength and callus formation in the groups receiving TGF-ß compared to the group receiving the control delivery vehicle substance. In this study, TGF-ß had no effect on bending, stiffness, bone mineral content, cortical thickness, or Haversian canal diameter.[11]

Bone Morphogenetic Proteins

Bone graft has long been known to stimulate bone repair. In 1965, Urist[13] demonstrated that the demineralized matrix of bone graft was capable of inducing de novo bone formation. Purification of the active component of the demineralized bone graft led to the discovery of a family of regulatory molecules termed bone morphogenetic proteins (BMPs). Although the BMPs were originally studied in their crude form (as demineralized bone matrix),[14,15]the availability of recombinant human BMPs has permitted the use of pure agents in more recent in vivo bone repair studies. The clinical utility of the BMPs has been explored by several investigators in animal models and is presently under investigation in human trials.

Recombinant human BMP-2 (rhBMP-2), in combination with an inactive demineralized bone matrix carrier, induced dose-dependent formation of endochondral bone in 5-mm segmental defects in the femora of rats.[16] Radiographic union was achieved in eight of ten defects treated with 11 mg of rhBMP-2 and in none of the defects treated by either carrier alone or by 1.4 mg of rhBMP-2. Similar results have been obtained in a sheep model employing a 2.5-cm nonhealing osteoperiosteal segmental defect stabilized with a plate and screws. Defects were treated with rhBMP-2 plus carrier, carrier alone, autogenous bone graft, or no treatment. Radiographic evaluation showed union of all six defects that had been treated with rhBMP-2 and of both defects that had been treated with autogenous bone graft. In the groups that had been treated with carrier alone (three defects) or the group that had been left untreated (three defects) no unions occurred. On biomechanical testing, the femora that had been treated with rhBMP-2 or autogenous bone graft manifested bending strengths that were comparable to those of the unoperated contralateral femora.[17] The closely related protein, osteogenic protein-1 (OP-1 or BMP-7) has been analyzed in a 1.5-cm ulnar defect model in rabbits. Recombinant human OP-1 or naturally occurring bovine osteogenic protein induced complete radiographic union and histologic evidence of new bone formation. In addition, the torsional strength and energy-absorptive capacities of these treated bones were comparable to those of the unoperated contralateral ulnae. Untreated defects and defects that had been treated with collagen carrier alone showed no evidence of healing.[18]

Recently, BMP-1, another polypeptide isolated from the osteogenetic fractions of bone, has been identified not as a growth factor, but rather as the procollagen C-proteinase that cleaves the carboxy termini of procollagens I, II, and III to yield the major fibrous components of bone and cartilage matrix. Thus the BMPs are involved not only in the support of cellular activities that result in cartilage and bone formation, but also in the chemical modification of the extracellular matrix as well.[19]

Curiously, there appear to be no published reports describing the effects of BMPs on the healing of fresh fractures (as opposed to segmental defects) or on nonunions, despite the fact that it is in these two human situations that these molecules would be expected to find their greatest clinical utility. Conversely, the clinical circumstance that is analogous to the segmental defect model, in which the BMPs have proved so efficacious, is generally associated with ablative surgery for musculoskeletal neoplasms. This indication for the BMPs (and for other repair molecules) is, to our knowledge, not currently considered a clinical option due to concern over tumor recurrence.

Fibroblast Growth Factors

Members of the fibroblast growth factor (FGF) family, like those of the TGF-ß and BMP families, are both present in and act upon bone. The local injection of FGF-1 (acidic FGF) in a rat fracture model produced an enlargement of the fracture callus in the cartilage-formation stage of repair. The enlargement was produced with 1 mg of FGF-1 delivered either daily or every other day for 9 days and persisted until 4 weeks after the fracture. This apparent stimulation occurred despite an inhi-bition of cartilage matrix gene expression (type II procollagen and proteoglycan core protein mRNA).[20]

bFGF-2 (basic FGF) has been evaluated using a rat fibular fracture model both in normal rats and in streptozotocin-induced diabetic rats, a model in which fracture healing is impaired. Immunohistochemical staining for FGF-2 showed that endogenous FGF-2 was widely distributed around the fracture site in normal rats 1 and 3 weeks after fracture but was reduced in diabetic rats. A single application of FGF-2 in fibrin gel immediately after fracture was noted to facilitate the repair process in normal rats and also to restore the impaired healing process in diabetic rats. The callus volume and mineral content increased in a dose-dependent manner in response to the FGF-2 treatment.[21] The action of FGF-2 on bone, as on cartilage,[22] appears to be complex, as illustrated by the observation that a low dose of FGF-2 (15 ng) stimulated bone induction while a high dose (1,900 ng) had a profoundly inhibitory effect when injected into the marrow cavity of rat bone implants.[23]

Insulin-Like Growth Factors

The pivotal role of insulin-like growth factor-I (IGF-I) in regulating the endochondral ossification of skeletal growth[24] suggests that this growth factor may also participate in the endochondral ossification of fracture repair. In vitro studies have demonstrated that, in bone cells, IGF-I regulates both bone matrix formation and cell replication.[25] In vivo, systemic IGF-I has been shown to stimulate healing of 5-mm defects in the zygomatic arches of rats. Half of the animals were treated with IGF-I, administered subcutaneously by osmotic infusion pump, and half with physiologic saline. Although IGF-I potentiated the repair process based on radiographic and histologic criteria, the control defects were also found to heal.[26] It is therefore not known from these studies whether IGF-I is capable of inducing repair under circumstances in which healing would otherwise not occur. This question has been partly answered by the evaluation of IGF-I in the treatment of critical-size calvarial defects in rats. Eight-millimeter, full-thickness calvarial defects (which do not heal spontaneously) were treated systemically with either IGF-I or saline via a subcutaneous osmotic infusion pump. The defects in animals receiving 2 mg of IGF-I over 14 days healed by proliferation of cortical bone from the margins of the surgical defect.[27] These data suggest that IGF-I may accelerate the repair of intramembranous bone defects, but its therapeutic potential in endochondral fracture repair remains unknown.

The putative stimulatory effect of IGF-I on bone repair may also be invoked indirectly. Because IGF-I is growth-hormone dependent, IGF-I levels may be increased in vivo by growth hormone administration. Several studies have investigated the question whether growth hormone augments fracture repair. Some have found that growth hormone stimulates healing,[28] while others have shown no growth hormone effect.[29] A recent investigation of the biomechanics of fracture healing in a rabbit tibial model revealed that growth hormone treatment produced no statistically significant effect on serial in vivo measurements of fracture stiffness or on ex vivo measurements of load to failure. In addition, there was no significant correlation between the biomechanical properties of the healing fracture and the serum levels of IGF-I. In this rabbit model, as in some human fractures, there was a persistent nutritional deficit, which may account, at least in part, for the observed failure of growth hormone to significantly increase circulating IGF-I levels.[30] Taken together, these data indicate that further studies will be required to establish a therapeutic role for either growth hormone-elicited or direct IGF-I treatment of fracture repair.

IGF-II, a close relative of IGF-I, is among the most abundant growth factors in bone.[31] The biologic actions of IGF-II are similar or identical to those of IGF-I, probably because they are transduced largely or exclusively by the same cell surface receptor. Although IGF-II binds with lower affinity than IGF-I to the type I IGF-receptor and is generally less potent than IGF-I in stimulating cells, it circulates at higher concentrations than IGF-I. It is thus possible that IGF-II plays a role in fracture healing. Of considerable interest in this regard is the recent observation that externally applied magnetic fields stimulate IGF-II production in both human osteoblast-like cell cultures and explanted rat fracture callus cultures.[32]

Platelet-Derived Growth Factor

Platelet-derived growth factor (PDGF) is another polypeptide-signaling molecule with the ability to regulate bone cells. In a rabbit tibial osteotomy model, a single injection of PDGF increased callus density and volume compared to growth-factor-free collagen controls. In addition, nonquantitative histologic analysis suggested that there may have been a more advanced stage of osteogenesis in the PDGF-treated osteotomies. However, mechanical testing by three-point bending to failure showed no improvement of strength in response to PDGF treatment.

The therapeutic potential of PDGF (and indeed of all growth factors) will likely be best realized in the presence of other growth factors. As a case in point, PDGF, IGF-I, and TGF-ß have each been shown to generate a dose-dependent increase in bone matrix apposition in an in vitro fetal rat calvarial model of bone formation. In combination, however, the stimulatory effect of these factors was greater than that of any of the individual factors alone.[33] Similar results have been observed in vivo. The combination of PDGF and IGF-I, delivered locally in a methocellulose gel to cortical defects in adult Yucatan miniature pigs, significantly increased the area ($p < 0.05$), perimeter ($p < 0.01$), and percentage ($p < 0.05$) of mineralized tissue within the callus. No significant differences in the measured parameters of callus formation were found in defects treated with either PDGF or IGF-I alone.[34]

Treatment of Fractures

The therapeutic application of growth factors to fracture healing faces a variety of challenges. Not only must the growth factors lack immunogenicity, side effects, and toxicity, they must also be available in a delivery system that is user-friendly both to the cells at the fracture site and to the orthopaedic surgeon managing the fracture. A second challenge is the convincing demonstration of efficacy. To establish, for example, that the incidence of nonunions is reduced by growth factor treatment requires large numbers of patients and carefully designed experimental protocols that standardize the many variables associated with the development of nonunions. Similarly, to demonstrate that growth factor treatment accelerates the rate of healing of fresh fractures requires both large numbers of patients and meticulous objective and reproducible follow-up to document the progress of healing. In any fracture study, quantitating fracture healing or even showing that a fracture is healed by noninvasive means can be a challenging task. Additionally, in this era of cost-consciousness in health care, the cost-effectiveness of any new treatment must be demonstrated along with efficacy. As these challenges are met, it is plausible, if not probable, that better ways of treating patients with difficult fractures will be available in the foreseeable future.

References

1. Ham AW (ed): *Histology*, ed 6. Philadelphia, PA, JB Lippincott, 1969.
2. Praemer A, Furner S, Rice DP (eds): *Musculoskeletal Conditions in the United States*. Park Ridge, IL, The American Academy of Orthopaedic Surgeons, 1992, pp 83–124.
3. Bolander ME: Regulation of fracture repair by growth factors. *Proc Soc Exp Biol Med* 1992;200:165–170.
4. Cotran RS, Kumar V, Robbins SL: Inflammation and repair, in Cotran RS, Kumar V, Robbins SL (eds): *Robbins' Pathologic Basis of Disease*, ed 4. Philadelphia, PA, WB Saunders, 1989, pp 39–86.
5. Sporn MB, Roberts AB: Peptide growth factors are multifunctional. *Nature* 1988;332:217–219.
6. Joyce ME, Roberts AB, Sporn MB, et al: Transforming growth factor-beta and the initiation of chondrogenesis and osteogenesis in the rat femur. *J Cell Biol* 1990;110:2195–2207.
7. Centrella M, McCarthy TL, Canalis E: Transforming growth factor-beta and remodeling of bone. *J Bone Joint Surg* 1991; 73A:1418–1428.
8. Joyce ME, Jingushi S, Bolander ME: Transforming growth factor-beta in the regulation of fracture repair. *Orthop Clin North Am* 1990;21:199–209.
9. Andrew JG, Hoyland J, Andrew SM, et al: Demonstration of TGF-beta 1 mRNA by in situ hybridization in normal human fracture healing. *Calcif Tissue Int* 1993;52:74–78.
10. Beck LS, Amento EP, Xu Y, et al: TGF-beta 1 induces bone closure of skull defects: Temporal dynamics of bone formation in defects exposed to rhTGF-beta. *J Bone Min Res* 1993;8:753–761.
11. Lind M, Schumacker B, Soballe K, et al: Transforming growth factor-beta enhances fracture healing in rabbit tibiae. *Acta Orthop Scand* 1993;64:553–556.
12. Nielsen HM, Andreassen TT, Ledet T, et al: Local injection of TGF-beta increases the strength of tibial fractures in the rat. *Acta Orthop Scand* 1994;65:37–41.
13. Urist MR: Bone: Formation by autoinduction. *Science* 1965;150:893–899.
14. Bolander ME, Balian G: The use of demineralized bone matrix in the repair of segmental defects: Augmentation with extracted matrix proteins and a comparison with autologous grafts. *J Bone Joint Surg* 1986;68A:1264–1274.
15. Einhorn TA, Majeska RJ, Rush EB, et al: The expression of cytokine activity by fracture callus. *J Bone Miner Res* 1995; 10:1272–1281.
16. Yasko AW, Lane JM, Fellinger EJ, et al: The healing of segmental bone defects, induced by recombinant human bone morphogenetic protein (rhBMP-2): A radiographic, histological, and biomechanical study in rats. *J Bone Joint Surg* 1992; 74A:659–670.
17. Gerhart TN, Kirker-Head CA, Kriz MJ, et al: Healing segmental femoral defects in sheep using recombinant human bone morphogenetic protein. *Clin Orthop* 1993;293:317–326.
18. Cook SD, Baffes GC, Wolfe MW, et al: The effect of recombinant human osteogenic protein-1 on healing of large segmental bone defects. *J Bone Joint Surg* 1994;76A:827–838.
19. Kessler E, Takahara K, Biniaminov L, et al: Bone morphogenetic protein-1: The type I procollagen C-proteinase. *Science* 1996;271:360–362.
20. Jingushi S, Heydemann A, Kana SK, et al: Acidic fibroblast growth factor (aFGF) injection stimulates cartilage enlargement and inhibits cartilage gene expression in rat fracture healing. *J Orthop Res* 1990;8:364–371.
21. Kawaguchi H, Kurokawa T, Hanada K, et al: Stimulation of fracture repair by recombinant human basic fibroblast growth factor in normal and streptozotocin-diabetic rats. *Endocrinology* 1994;135:774–781.
22. Sah RL, Chen AC, Grodzinsky AJ, et al: Differential effects of bFGF and IGF-I on matrix metabolism in calf and adult bovine cartilage explants. *Arch Biochem Biophys* 1994;308:137–147.
23. Wang JS, Aspenberg P: Basic fibroblast growth factor and bone induction in rats. *Acta Orthop Scand* 1993;64:557–561.
24. Trippel SB, Rosenfeld RG: Growth factor treatment of disorders of skeletal growth, in Springfield DS (ed): *Instructional Course Lectures 46*. Rosemont, IL, American Academy of Orthopaedic Surgeons, 1997.
25. Hock JM, Centrella M, Canalis E: Insulin-like growth factor I has independent effects on bone matrix formation and cell replication. *Endocrinology* 1988;122:254–260.
26. Thaller SR, Hoyt J, Tesluk H, et al: Effect of insulin-like growth factor-1 on zygomatic arch bone regeneration: A preliminary histological and histometric study. *Ann Plast Surg* 1993;31: 421–428.
27. Thaller SR, Dart A, Tesluk H: The effects of insulin-like growth factor-1 on critical-size calvarial defects in Sprague-Dawley rats. *Ann Plast Surg* 1993;31:429–433.
28. Koskinen EVS, Lindholm RV, Nieminen RA, et al: Human growth hormone in delayed union and non-union of fractures. *Int Orthop* 1978;1:317–322.
29. Northmore-Ball MD, Wood MR, Meggitt BF: A biomechanical study of the effects of growth hormone in experimental fracture healing. *J Bone Joint Surg* 1980;62B:391–396.
30. Carpenter JE, Hipp JA, Gerhart TN, et al: Failure of growth hormone to alter the biomechanics of fracture-healing in a rabbit model. *J Bone Joint Surg* 1992;74A:359–367.
31. Frolik CA, Ellis LF, Williams DC: Isolation and characterization of insulin-like growth factor-II from human bone. *Biochem Biophys Res Commun* 1988;151:1011–1018.
32. Ryaby JT, Fitzsimmons RJ, Khin NA, et al: A growth factor dependent model for magnetic field regulation of bone formation. *Trans Orthop Res Soc* 1994;19:518.
33. Pfeilschifter J, Oechsner M, Naumann A, et al: Stimulation of bone matrix apposition, in vitro by local growth factors: A comparison between insulin-like growth factor I, platelet-derived growth factor, and transforming growth factor beta. *Endocrinology* 1990;127:69–75.
34. Lynch SE, Trippel SB, Finkelman RD, et al: The combination of platelet-derived growth factor-B and insulin-like growth factor-I stimulates bone repair in adult Yucatan micro pigs. *Wound Repair Regen* 1994;2:182–190.

CHAPTER 47

Effect of Growth Factors on Cartilage Repair

Richard D. Coutts, MD
Robert L. Sah, MD, ScD
David Amiel, PhD

Introduction

Hyaline cartilage is a hypocellular, avascular, alymphatic, and insensate tissue with an abundant collegen/proteoglycan matrix that provides a low-friction, wear-resistant bearing surface on the ends of bones where they meet to form a joint. Because the cells in cartilage are imprisoned in their matrix, and cells capable of supporting repair cannot be delivered other than from a vascular source, the capacity of cartilage to heal after sustaining damage from injury or disease is severely limited. Cartilage damage and repair have been studied by a number of investigators.[1-17] These investigators are in general agreement on the classification of articular cartilage damage and the relationship between the damage pattern and the repair response. A brief review of this work will set the stage for a discussion of the effect of growth factors on cartilage repair.

Acute Mechanical Damage

Superficial Penetrating Injury

In this type of injury, the surface skin of the cartilage (the lamina splendens) is disrupted and the lesion extends a variable distance into the matrix, but no further than the subchondral bone. In other words, the lesion is contained completely within the cartilage matrix. The lesion could be small, such as might occur by penetration by an ice pick, or it could be extensive, as occurs with traumatic avulsion of a segment of cartilage with high velocity impact or patellar dislocation. As with any injury, severity and extent can vary.

The repair response to a superficial lesion is minimal, because vascular elements have no access to the defect. The chondrocytes in the matrix adjacent to the defect will divide, as evidenced by the presence of grouping of cells (clones) in this area. However, the cells have no capability to move through the matrix, and they remain entrapped. Cellular production of matrix constituents occurs in the cartilage adjacent to the defect and, if there is minimal gapping, presumably these matrix products could heal the defect. In addition to the role that the size of the lesion has on this process, it can be presumed that the local mechanical environment will influence the repair process also. If the loading patterns constantly disrupt the matrix at the injury site, there is less likelihood that a fusion of the matrix walls will occur. Whether the deterring factor is the size of the lesion or mechanical factors, these lesions confined to the cartilage matrix usually do not heal, and remain an "open sore" on the cartilage topography. Again, if the mechanical environment is hostile, the lesion can progress to involve a larger area of the cartilage and/or the opposing articular surface. Alternatively, if the stresses on the surrounding cartilage are below injury level, the lesion will remain unchanged for several years.[1,2,4,5,7,9-11,18-21]

The superficial lesion just described is in some ways analogous to the lesions of osteoarthritis. In osteoarthritis, it is believed that the initial lesion is fissuring of the articular surface, with the fissures extending to the subchondral bone over time. The major difference is that osteoarthritis is a progressive disorder, wherein the fibrillated matrix wears down, with eventual exposure of the subchondral bone on both sides of the joint. The same type of cellular response described for lacerations occurs at the edges of the fissures in osteoarthritis, with cell mitosis and increased production of proteoglycans representing the inadequate attempts by the cartilage to repair the damage. There is no bridging of the fissures by new matrix or granulation tissue. Instead, the matrix loses its proteoglycans and the collagenous structure wears away. With the added consideration of age and the known decrease in cell number and density that accompanies aging in cartilage, there is progressive likelihood that cartilage degeneration will occur with advancing years.[22,23]

Deep Penetrating Injury

In circumstances in which the damage to the joint surface penetrates through the supporting subchondral bone, an entirely different repair response occurs. Lesions that access the marrow provide a route for cellular migration and vascular invasion. A granulation tissue is laid down, just as occurs in most wound healing circumstances. Mesenchymal stem cells can move from the marrow to the repair site, and in turn differentiate along the lineage of a chondroblast. Under the influence of the joint environment, a fibrocartilaginous repair tissue is formed, as well as a new supporting subchondral bone plate. Unfortunately, the repair matrix produced by the cells effecting the repair usually fails to restore all the damaged cartilage, and the repair tissue lacks the organizational structure of native

Outline 1
Variables that can influence the results of growth factor studies

Culture conditions
- Primary
- Passaged
- Explant
- In vivo

Growth factor issues
- Concentration
- Form
- Source

Species
- Murine
- Rabbit
- Pig
- Cow
- Avian
- Human

Cell Types
- Growth plate
- Hyaline articular

Age of cell donors
- Fetal
- Immature
- Adult

Cell differentiation

Cell culture media

cartilage. Despite the ability of these cells to produce type II collagen, the matrix is always a mixture of types I and II collagen, hence the name of fibrocartilage. Proteoglycan is also elaborated by these repair cells, but the percentage of proteoglycan in the repair matrix is lower than normal. This repair tissue characteristically degrades over time, ultimately breaking down and leaving an arthrotic lesion in its place.[4-6,8,10,14,15,19,20,24,25]

It is not clear why lesions that penetrate bone heal in the fashion just described. The cells effecting that repair clearly express a chondroblastic phenotype by producing type II collagen. And the wound site presumably contains the cytokines required to signal the cells to proliferate, differentiate, and produce the appropriate matrix. One can speculate that the random macropattern in which the repair tissue is formed may doom it to failure. Or perhaps the microarchitecture of the repair tissue is somehow flawed, making it susceptible to breakdown. To date, little has been done to characterize the microstructure of this repair tissue to clearly define its differences from normal cartilage.

Blunt Trauma

Cartilage can be traumatized by a direct blow, such as a dashboard injury, which injures the tissue without breaking the surface of the cartilage. The trauma can lead to cell death and disruption of the matrix. The severity of the changes in the cartilage will reflect the intensity of the force applied and the strain experienced by the matrix. It can be severe enough to cause swelling and cyst formation within the cartilage. Healing can occur in this circumstance, because there is no void that cells and matrix must fill.[17,26-29]

Inflammatory Disease

Infection and the inflammatory arthritides lead to destruction of the cartilage matrix through enzymatic pathways. The disruption of the matrix integrity and the enzymatic action of cytokines release the proteoglycans from the cartilage, and a degradation of the entire structure ensues. Only if the cause of inflammation is removed before the cartilage surface is violated is there a chance that the cartilage will survive. As a rule, this survival is possible only when an infection is treated early with the appropriate antibiotic and surgical intervention. Lacking a treatment that will cure the common inflammatory arthritides means that there will be a relentless assault upon the cartilage, until it is ultimately destroyed. The capacity to repair in this circumstance is feeble and inadequate against the forces of destruction directed at the cartilage.[30-34]

Summary of Cartilage Repair Capacity

Chondrocytes are capable of elaborating the matrix elements that are lost by virtue of injury or disease of cartilage. However, lacking mobility and adequate numbers, the chondrocytes are unable to mount an effective repair at sites of destruction. Cells brought to a repair site by virtue of vascular exposure can produce a repair matrix, but unfortunately one that only partially recreates the missing hyaline cartilage as measured by morphologic, chemical, and mechanical methods.

What is missing, one might ask? If the cells responding to an injury are uncommitted stem cells, why are they not influenced by the local environment to become chondroblasts? And why do they not then produce a healthy, architecturally accurate hyaline articular cartilage, assuming there are factors in the local milieu that will direct the cells to produce such a normal tissue? Could it be that the appropriate molecular signals are not present or operative in these cells? And would the addition of these factors somehow magically turn the tide in favor of a satisfactory repair? The remainder of this chapter will be spent on reviewing what is known about these molecular agents of growth and repair, and speculating on their promise to provide the missing link in the evolving cartilage repair story.

By way of definition, a growth factor is a polypeptide that will direct a cell to migrate, divide, differentiate, or produce matrix. A growth factor can produce all, one, or some combination of these effects on a cell.

Before attempting a description of growth factor effects on cartilage, it is important to recognize the limitations on assembling the knowledge that exists currently on the subject. The variables that are present between studies of growth factors in cartilage are numerous and are listed in Outline 1.

The following discussion will survey the variables that apply, with the purpose of giving the reader a sense of the difficulty that exists in sorting out the results of experiments. Most of the studies performed on cartilage are on cultured cells, and it is a long-established fact that cultured cells in the cartilage line very quickly lose the cartilage phenotype under standard passaged monolayer conditions and convert to a fibroblastic form. This can be prevented by a variety of culturing techniques, including use of a three-dimensional or suspension culture medium, high cell density, primary culture, short culture duration, or a combination of these, but this methodology is used only in the minority of studies. With cells in monolayer, which is the most common method of study of chondroid cells, there is always the question of whether any measured response truly represents the in vivo behavior of chondrocytes. Tissue or explant culture, wherein pieces of cartilage are maintained in a nurturing medium, is a more life-like model of chondrocyte behavior, because the matrix interactions with the cells are preserved and the cartilage phenotype is not lost. Best, of course, is an in vivo study, in which the cartilage cells are functioning in a normal environment. Progressing from the culture of individuals cells to the in vivo models carries with it the increasingly difficult problem of controlling variables, hence the attractiveness of using cell cultures where a single perturbation is apt to be the factor that changes the cell behavior. In this circumstance, cells that are grown in primary culture are the most likely to represent the cartilage phenotype behavior. With each subsequent passage (subculture), the chondrocytic cells become more fibroblastic.[35]

When studying growth factors, the investigator must choose a dose and decide when and how long to maintain the presence of the growth factor. This can vary from study to study. The investigator must also choose which animals from which to obtain cells, with the favorites being mice, rats, fowl, rabbits, pigs, dogs, cows, horses, or humans. Obviously, human tissue has the most significant relevance to human cell behavior and, if there were not a barrier to the harvest of this tissue, it might be the only relevant and appropriate tissue to study.

In addition to studying different species, investigators harvest cartilage cells from a variety of sites, such as a joint, growth plate, or the cartilaginous portion of the rib. They use embryonal limb buds, fetal cartilage, or cartilage from immature or mature animals. And they choose from a variety of culture media to nurture the cells and may or may not add serum to the culture, which itself contains a variety of growth factors. All of these variables can result in a different cellular response to the same growth factor. Add to the above the fact that some growth factors produce different results when used alone or in combination with other cytokines, or that the effect of a growth factor will vary according to the maturational stage of the cell in culture, and one can appreciate the difficulty that investigators have in sorting out the mystery of growth factor/cell interaction.

Under normal circumstances, cartilage, like bone, exists in a steady state of matrix degradation and rejuvenation. The collagen in cartilage turns over slowly, but the proteoglycans have a fairly rapid half-life, ranging from 8 days to several months.[36] The processes of matrix breakdown and replacement are mediated by catabolic and anabolic cytokines. The identification of the anabolic cytokines or growth factors and the determination of their genetic code has led to the production of purified growth factors that can be tested in a variety of experimental setups. The following growth factors have been tested against cartilage.

Insulin-Like Growth Factor (IGF-I)

IGF-I is a circulating cytokine that reaches articular cartilage via the synovial fluid.[37] Its major effect is the stimulation of matrix production in a dose-dependent manner as evidenced by increases in sulfate incorporation in bovine explant cultures.[38-41] IGF-I does not appear to have a comparable effect on collagen production,[41,42] although another study did show a dose-dependent stimulation of tritiated hydroxyproline (a constituent of collagen) incorporation in cow cartilage.[43]

It has been shown in humans that there is a decrease in serum IGF-I levels, as well as a decrease in chondrocyte responsiveness to IGF-I, with age.[44,45] The obvious conclusion from these findings would suggest that aging chondrocytes slowly lose their ability to produce the matrix constituents necessary to maintain cartilage function due to a decrease in the effect of IGF-I. This in turn may be an etiologic factor in the development of osteoarthritis. In osteoarthritis, IGF-I binding to the chondrocyte is made less effective by the presence of alternative IGF-I binding sites on the surfaces of the cells. These binding sites are not specific for the growth factor, effectively rendering the growth factor inactive.[46] In the final analysis, IGF-I seems to be an important factor for the maintenance of matrix proteoglycan, and its deficiency may contribute to the development of osteoarthritis.

Basic Fibroblastic Growth Factor (bFGF)

Basic fibroblastic growth factor is produced by cartilage cells, as well as by the pituitary. In connective tissues, bFGF is a powerful mitogen, and it has this effect on cartilage cells in culture.[38,47] It can also stimulate proteoglycan and collagen synthesis by chondrocytes. There are, however, some interesting variations in the response of cartilage to bFGF, depending on the age of the tissue. In young bovine explants, low doses of bFGF stimulated anabolic processes, and higher doses stimulated catabolic processes. In adult cartilage, low concentrations of bFGF accelerated release of proteoglycan, but with increasing concentrations, stimulation of proteoglycan, protein, and collagen synthesis was observed. In adult cartilage, chondrocyte mitotic activity was not observed, but in cell culture, bFGF is very effective in stimulating cell proliferation.[43]

In addition, bFGF has an interesting contradiction, in that it will stimulate catabolic behavior in cartilage. It has been shown that bFGF will stimulate interleukin 1 (IL-1), which in turn induces a host of catabolic reactions in cartilage.[48] It seems almost paradoxical that a growth factor would also stimulate degradative functions, and the phenomenon remains unexplained.

Clearly, bFGF is a potent stimulator of cell mitosis in a culture environment, and it can be a useful tool to accelerate cell replication in culture. In vivo, it may express the mitotic potential if circumstances would allow it (ie, a large population of cells needed for repair) but, more likely, its major effect is expressed as a stimulation of cartilage matrix production.

Transforming Growth Factor Beta (TGF-ß)

TGF-ß, a ubiquitous protein cell regulator, has been identified in bone matrix, cartilage, platelets, activated lymphocytes, and other tissues. It is multifunctional, and in most cells it acts to stabilize or enhance the differentiated phenotype. It is produced by articular chondrocytes and exists in the matrix of cartilage, albeit in a latent form. It can be activated by decreased local pH or degradation by proteases.[49-55]

TGF-ß in cartilage is enigmatic, with different cellular responses reported by different investigators. Many of these differences depend on the cell type and the assay system used. TGF-ß has been found to increase the production of collagen,[56,57] proteoglycan,[42,51,58] and inhibitors of matrix breakdown,[59] while at the same time inhibiting cell proliferation.[54] Injected subperiosteally, TGF-ß results in cartilage formation.[60] It has also been demonstrated to have the opposite effects in other studies. For example, TGF-ß has been shown to inhibit, rather than promote, chondrocyte differentiation as reflected by decreased collagen[61-63] and proteoglycan[64] production, albeit in different culture models using different sources of cells. TGF-ß has also been shown to stimulate, instead of inhibit, cell proliferation,[65,66] and it has been demonstrated that TGF-ß has different and possibly opposite effects depending on the stage of differentiation of the target cell.[63,67,68] Thus, investigators may have been studying the same cells but in different phases of growth, producing varying results.

In studies using human cultured chondrocytes, Gueıne and associates[35] showed that TGF-ß is the most potent stimulator of chondrocyte proliferation when tested against a panel of growth factors, including platelet-derived growth factor (PDGF), bFGF, and IGF-I. This same group of investigators also showed that in humans there is an age-related decrease in the mitotic response of chondrocytes from more aged donors (up to age 83).[69] This has also been noted for IGF. This decreased responsiveness of adult human chondrocytes to TGF-ß could play a role in cartilage degeneration.

In bovine tissue culture, TGF-ß stimulates proteoglycan production, while decreasing proteoglycan catabolism.[42] It appears to have little effect on collagen production. Human osteoarthritis cartilage explants are much more sensitive to TGF-ß, producing more proteoglycan than normal human cartilage. However, in keeping with the contradictory nature of this growth factor, a recent report on the effect of TGF-ß on human osteoarthritic cartilage explants failed to find any evidence for stimulation.[70]

TGF-ß, more than any other growth factor in cartilage, has a strong interdependency with other growth factors. In human chondrocyte cell culture, bFGF and PDGF both stimulate TGF-ß production or release from chondrocytes. In fact, TGF-ß will stimulate additional TGF-ß production.[71] In ear cartilage, both bFGF and TGF-ß are required to stimulate a full chondrogenic response.[72] Frazer and associates[73] found that the proliferative effect of TGF-ß required an interaction with other factors in serum. TGF-ß also will suppress the cytokines that mediate catabolic responses.[74]

In summary, TGF-ß in cartilage has multiple effects, depending on the culture conditions under which it is tested. It promotes the cartilaginous differentiation of cells and can be a potent stimulator of mitosis. It will also promote matrix synthesis, most notably when evaluated in explant culture. It will inhibit catabolism, but it can also suppress chondrocytic matrix production, especially type II collagen, under certain circumstances. It exists in cartilage matrix in latent form, presumably to be activated when repair is needed. In circumstances calling for repair, the chondrocytes are more responsive to TGF-ß.

Growth Factors as Agents of Cartilage Healing

Studies using growth factors as agents of repair have been performed. Basic fibroblastic growth factor has been shown to facilitate the healing of superficial cartilage lacerations in vivo in a rabbit model.[75,76] IGF-I has been administered intra-articularly in association with the intramuscular injection of sodium pentosan polysulfate (an inhibitor of matrix catabolism) in a dog anterior cruciate ligament insufficiency model. These agents were able to reduce the severity of the cartilage breakdown. The levels of neutral metalloproteinase, tissue inhibitor of metalloproteinase (TIMP), collagenase, uronate, and hydroxyproline were maintained at near normal levels compared to controls.[77] To date, TGF-ß has not been tested in an in vivo healing model, even though it would appear to be one of the more likely candidates as an agent for repair.

A recent report on the use of cultured cells to produce repairs of articular cartilage offers another opportunity for the use of growth factors for cartilage healing.[78] In this system, autologous chondrocytes are harvested and multiplied in culture, then reimplanted in a cartilage defect under a periosteal flap. The known ability of growth factors to promote mitosis and preserve phenotype could be used during the culture process. O'Driscoll has used TGF-ß successfully to promote cartilage phenotypic expression in explant cultures of periosteum, and it is conceivable that these cultured explants could be used as a graft material to heal chondral defects.[79,80]

Growth Factor Carriers

If growth factors have the potential to assist in cartilage repair, then a significant requirement for their use is the development of a suitable carrier. Growth factors are soluble proteins that are absorbed rapidly. In the study by Cuevas and associates,[75] an Alzet osmotic pump was implanted to provide a continuous supply of bFGF to the rabbit knee. Rogachefsky and associates[77] injected IGF-1 repeatedly into the dog knee repair model that they tested. Unfortunately, it is not known how long a growth factor needs to be administered to achieve a desirable healing response, but the presumption is that this time period would be measured in days as opposed to hours.

Table 1 lists a variety of substances that could be used or have been tried as carriers of growth factors. The choice of carrier will depend on the mechanical characteristics demanded by the implantation site and the rate of degradation required. If the carrier must perform as a load-bearing construct, then it must be stronger than a carrier that might be placed free in the joint to release the growth factor. In addition, the carrier must be able to assist in the evolution of the

Table 1
Substances as carriers of growth factors

Substance	Pros	Cons*	Time In Vivo*
Zyderm II (bovine dermal collagen)	Clinically used in plastic surgery for scars, skin defects	Immune reactions reported[81-84]	Reinjections required after 8 to 12 mos. May persist up to 4 yrs[89]
Fibrin	Resides naturally in body. Present in blood clot	Never reported as a carrier of exogenous growth factors	Two half-lives, cleared from serum rapidly first, $t_{0.5}$ = 5.5 ± SD 3.5 hrs then gradually $t_{0.5}$ = 10 ± SD 3.5 hrs[90]
Fibrinogen	Resides naturally in body. Present in blood clot	Never reported as a carrier of exogenous growth factors	$t_{0.5}$ = 24 to 72 hrs[91] and 62 ± SD 19 hrs[90] in serum
Hyaluronic acid	Resides naturally in body. Has been used as a carrier for growth factors.[85-87] Present in fibrin clot[92]	Was similar to phosphate-buffered saline in holding ^{125}I-EGF at dermal wound site, 23% after 1 d and 16% after 2 d[85]	$t_{0.5}$ = 12 hrs[93] after injection into rabbit knee
Liposomes (single lamellar)	Lipids used, phosphatidylglycerol, phosphatidylcholine, cholesterol [1:4:5][88]	Up to 65% of aqueous material encapsulated only[94]	^{125}I-EGF formulated into single lamellar liposomes. 37% of the EGFf was retained in the incision in the backs of adult male Sprague-Dawley rats (n=12). 30% was retained after 2 d, & 4% after 3 d[85]
Liposomes (multilamellar)			^{125}I-EGF formulated in multilamellar liposomes. 62% of the growth factor was retained in the incision in the backs of adult male Sprague-Dawley rats (n=12) 1 d after surg. 48% was retained after 2 d, & 11% after 3 d[5]
Polylactic/polyglycolic acid	Currently used as suture material. Degrades into natural waste products by hydrolysis	Reported to induce an inflammatory reaction. Nature of growth factor binding not known	Variable, depending on formulation of material

* EGF, epidermal growth factor

repair tissue, or at least not impede the repair process. The ability to manufacture the carrier in a variety of architectures may prove to be essential in this regard.

One of the intriguing strategies being explored to effect cartilage healing is to transfect progenitor cells with the genetic code for one of the growth factors described above. These cells will presumably overexpress the growth factor gene and produce extra growth factor. If such cells were to be placed in a repair site, they presumably could more effectively induce a repair. This is a novel and unique way to provide a carrier for the growth factor, although the cells themselves may require a carrier to ensure their placement at a repair site. Chu and associates[95] reported on the use of a polylactic acid carrier for chondroblasts to heal articular cartilage defects. This carrier, used so far only for cells, could presumably serve double duty as a carrier for growth factors as well. However, an advantage of having the cell act as the carrier for the growth factor is that the cell can exert control over the expression of the growth factor gene, presumably enhancing the timing of the growth factor production, as well as being subject to the autocrine and paracrine controls of cell function. Interactions with other growth factors might be idealized as well.

The era of biologic manipulation of basic cellular processes is dawning, and in the circumstance of cartilage, the potential to effect repair, which until now has been a near impossibility, appears promising. The expectation is that the lesions of cartilage produced by trauma will be the most responsive to this treatment modality and that the processes of degeneration and inflammatory destruction will be less responsive, or at least more difficult to influence. Stay tuned, for the moment is pregnant with promise and the expectation is that the actions and interactions of growth factors will be deciphered and harnessed to manage disease more effectively.

References

1. Bennett GA, Bauer W: The study of the repair of articular cartilage and the reaction of normal joints of adult dogs to surgically created defects of articular cartilage, "joint mice" and patellar displacement. *Am J Pathol* 1932;8:499–524.
2. Bennett GA, Bauer W: Further studies concerning the repair of articular cartilage in dog joints. *J Bone Joint Surg* 1935; 17:141–150.
3. Buckwalter JA: Articular cartilage, in Evarts CM (ed): American Academy of Orthopaedic Surgeons *Instructional Course Lectures XXXII.* St Louis, MO, CV Mosby, 1983, pp 349–370.
4. Calandruccio RA, Gilmer WS Jr: Proliferation, regeneration, and repair of articular cartilage of immature animals. *J Bone Joint Surg* 1962;44A:431–455.
5. Campbell CJ: The healing of cartilage defects. *Clin Orthop* 1969;64:45–63.
6. Convery FR, Akeson WH, Keown GH: The repair of large osteochondral defects: An experimental study in horses. *Clin Orthop* 1972;82:253–262.
7. DePalma AF, McKeever CD, Subin DK: Process of repair of articular cartilage demonstrated by histology and autoradiography with tritiated thymidine. *Clin Orthop* 1966; 8:229–242.
8. Furukawa T, Eyre DR, Koide S, et al: Biochemical studies on repair cartilage resurfacing experimental defects in the rabbit knee. *J Bone Joint Surg* 1980;62A:79–89.
9. Ghadially FN, Thomas I, Oryschak AF, et al: Long-term results of superficial defects in articular cartilage: A scanning electron-microscope study. *J Pathol* 1977;121:213–217.
10. Mankin HJ: Localization of tritiated thymidine in articular cartilage of rabbits: II. Repair in immature cartilage. *J Bone Joint Surg* 1962;44A:688–698.
11. Mankin HJ: The reaction of articular cartilage to injury and osteoarthritis: Parts I and II. *N Engl J Med* 1974;291:1285–1292 and 1335–1340.
12. Mankin HJ: The response of articular cartilage to mechanical injury. *J Bone Joint Surg* 1982;64A:460–466.
13. Meachim G: The effect of scarification on articular cartilage in the rabbit. *J Bone Joint Surg* 1963;45B:150–161.
14. Meachim G, Roberts C: Repair of the joint surface from sub-articular tissue in the rabbit knee. *J Anat* 1971;109: 317–327.
15. Mitchell N, Shepard N: The resurfacing of adult rabbit articular cartilage by multiple perforations through the subchondral bone. *J Bone Joint Surg* 1976;58A:230–233.
16. Rubak JM: Reconstruction of articular cartilage defects with free periosteal grafts: An experimental study. *Acta Orthop Scand* 1982; 53:175–180.
17. Thompson RC Jr: An experimental study of surface injury to articular cartilage and enzyme responses within the joint. *Clin Orthop* 1975;107:239–248.
18. Bailey RW, Habel DW: The fate of surgically created osteochondral fractures in adult and young dogs. *Surg Forum* 1960; 11:438–440.
19. Frost GE: Cartilage healing and regeneration. *J S Afr Vet Assoc* 1979;50:181–187.
20. Fuller JA, Ghadially FN: Ultrastructural observations on surgically produced partial-thickness defects in articular cartilage. *Clin Orthop* 1972;86:193–205.
21. Mankin HJ, Boyle CJ: The acute effects of lacerative injury on DNA and protein synthesis in articular cartilage, in Bassett CAL (ed): *Cartilage Degradation and Repair.* Washington DC, National Research Council, 1967, pp 185–199.
22. Stockwell RA: The cell density of human articular and costal cartilage. *J Anat* 1967;101:753–763.
23. Stockwell RA, Meachim G: The chondrocytes, in Freeman MAR (ed): *Adult Articular Cartilage,* ed 2. Tunbridge Wells, England, Pitman Medical, 1979, pp 69–144.
24. Cheung HS, Cottrell WH, Stephenson K, et al: In vitro collagen biosynthesis in healing and normal rabbit articular cartilage. *J Bone Joint Surg* 1978;60A:1076–1081.
25. Mitchell N, Shepard N: Healing of articular cartilage in intra-articular fractures in rabbits. *J Bone Joint Surg* 1980;62A: 628–634.
26. Dekel S, Weissman SL: Joint changes after overuse and peak overloading of rabbit knees in vivo. *Acta Orthop Scand* 1978; 49:519–528.
27. Radin EL, Paul IL, Lowy M: A comparison of the dynamic force transmitting properties of subchondral bone and articular cartilage. *J Bone Joint Surg* 1970;52A:444–456.
28. Radin EL, Ehrlich MG, Chernack R, et al: Effect of repetitive impulsive loading on the knee joints of rabbits. *Clin Orthop* 1978;131:288–293.
29. Repo RU, Finlay JB: Survival of articular cartilage after controlled impact. *J Bone Joint Surg* 1977;59A:1068–1076.
30. Curtiss PH Jr: Cartilage damage in septic arthritis. *Clin Orthop* 1969;64:87–90.
31. Donohue JM, Buss D, Oegema TR Jr, et al: The effects of indirect blunt trauma on adult canine articular cartilage. *J Bone Joint Surg* 1983;65A:948–957.
32. Parsons JR, McManus E, Johnson E: Time dependent histologic and mechanical alteration of articular cartilage with joint sepsis. *Trans Orthop Res Soc* 1982;7:217.

33. Reagan BF, McInerny VK, Treadwell BV, et al: Irrigating solutions for arthroscopy: A metabolic study. *J Bone Joint Surg* 1983;65A:629–631.
34. Reimann I, Christensen SB, Diemer NH: Observations of reversibility of glycosaminoglycan depletion in articular cartilage. *Clin Orthop* 1982;168:258–264.
35. Guerne PA, Sublet A, Lotz M: Growth factor responsiveness of human articular chondrocytes: Distinct profiles in primary chondrocytes, subcultured chondrocytes, and fibroblasts. *J Cell Physiol* 1994;158:476–484.
36. Mankin HJ, Lippiello L: The turnover of adult rabbit articular cartilage. *J Bone Joint Surg* 1969;51A:1591–1600.
37. Schalkwijk J, Joosten LA, van den Berg WB, et al: Insulin-like growth factor stimulation of chondrocyte proteoglycan synthesis by human synovial fluid. *Arthritis Rheum* 1989;32:66–71.
38. Osborn KD, Trippel SB, Mankin HJ: Growth factor stimulation of adult articular cartilage. *J Orthop Res* 1989;7:35–42.
39. Luyten FP, Hascall VC, Nissley SP, et al: Insulin-like growth factors maintain steady-state metabolism of proteoglycans in bovine articular cartilage explants. *Arch Biochem Biophys* 1988;267:416–425.
40. Tyler JA: Insulin-like growth factor 1 can decrease degradation and promote synthesis of proteoglycan in cartilage exposed to cytokines. *Biochem J* 1989;260:543–548.
41. Barone-Varelas J, Schnitzer TJ, Meng Q, et al: Age-related differences in the metabolism of proteoglycans in bovine articular cartilage explants maintained in the presence of insulin-like growth factor 1. *Connect Tissue Res* 1991;26:101–120.
42. Morales TI, Roberts AB: Transforming growth factor-beta regulates the metabolism of proteoglycans in bovine cartilage organ cultures. *J Biol Chem* 1988;263:12828–12831.
43. Sah RL, Chen AC, Grodzinsky AJ, et al: Differential effects of bFGF and IGF-I on matrix metabolism in calf and adult bovine cartilage explants. *Arch Biochem Biophys* 1994;308:137–147.
44. Florini JR, Roberts SB: Effect of rat age on blood levels of somatomedin-like growth factors. *J Gerontol* 1980;35:23–30.
45. Kumar N: Unresponsiveness of cartilage to serum somatomedins: Further observations. *Indian J Exp Biol* 1979;17: 571–573.
46. Dore S, Pelletier JP, DiBattista JA, et al: Human osteoarthritic chondrocytes possess an increased number of insulin-like growth factor I binding sites but are unresponsive to its stimulation: Possible role of IGF-1-binding proteins. *Arthritis Rheum* 1994;37:253–263.
47. Sachs BL, Goldberg VM, Moskowitz RW, et al: Response of articular chondrocytes to pituitary fibroblast growth factor (FGF). *J Cell Physiol* 1982;112:51–59.
48. Chin JE, Hatfield CA, Krzesicki RF, et al: Interactions between interleukin-1 and basic fibroblast growth factor on articular chondrocytes: Effects on cell growth, prostanoid production and receptor modulation. *Arthritis Rheum* 1991;34:314–324.
49. Assoian RK, Komoriya A, Meyers CA, et al: Transforming growth factor-beta in human platelets: Identification of a major storage site, purification, and characterization. *J Biol Chem* 1983;258: 7155–7160.
50. Bonewald LF, Mundy GR: Role of transforming growth factor-beta in bone remodeling. *Clin Orthop* 1990;250:261–276.
51. Morales TI, Joyce ME, Sobel ME, et al: Transforming growth factor-beta in calf articular cartilage organ cultures: Synthesis and distribution. *Arch Biochem Biophys* 1991;288:397–405.
52. Roberts AB, Anzano MA, Lamb LC, et al: New class of transforming growth factors potentiated by epidermal growth factor: Isolation from non-neoplastic tissues. *Proc Natl Acad Sci USA* 1981;78:5339–5343.
53. Roberts AB, Anzano MA, Meyers CA, et al: Purification and properties of a type beta transforming growth factor from bovine kidney. *Biochemistry* 1983;22:5692–5698.
54. Sporn MB, Roberts AB, Wakefield LM, et al: Transforming growth factor-beta: Biological function and chemical structure. *Science* 1986;233:532–534.
55. Sporn MB, Roberts AB, Wakefield LM, et al: Some recent advances in the chemistry and biology of transforming growth factor-beta. *J Cell Biol* 1987;105:1039–1045.
56. Hill DJ, Han VK: Paracrinology of growth regulation. *J Dev Physiol* 1991;15:91–104.
57. Ignotz RA, Massague J: Transforming growth factor-beta stimulates the expression of fibronectin and collagen and their incorporation into the extracellular matrix. *J Biol Chem* 1986; 261:4337–4345.
58. Schonfeld H-J, Poschl B, Wessner B, et al: Altered differentiation of limb bud cells by transforming growth factors-beta isolated from bone matrix and from platelets. *Bone Miner* 1991;13:171–189.
59. Laiho M, Saksela O, Andreasen PA, et al: Enhanced production and extracellular deposition of the endothelial-type plasminogen activator inhibitor in cultured human lung fibroblasts by transforming growth factor-beta. *J Cell Biol* 1986;103:2403–2410.
60. Joyce ME, Roberts AB, Sporn MB, et al: Transforming growth factor-beta and the initiation of chondrogenesis and osteogenesis in the rat femur. *J Cell Biol* 1990;110:2195–2207.
61. Horton WE Jr, Higginbotham JD, Chandrasekhar S: Transforming growth factor-beta and fibroblast growth factor act synergistically to inhibit collagen II synthesis through a mechanism involving regulatory DNA sequences. *J Cell Physiol* 1989;141:8–15.
62. Rosen DM, Stempien SA, Thompson AY, et al: Transforming growth factor-beta modulates the expression of osteoblast and chondroblast phenotypes in vitro. *J Cell Physiol* 1988;134: 337–346.
63. Rosier RN, O'Keefe RJ, Crabb ID, et al: Transforming growth factor beta: An autocrine regulator of chondrocytes. *Connect Tissue Res* 1989;20:295–301.
64. Chen P, Carrington JL, Hammonds RG, et al: Stimulation of chondrogenesis in limb bud mesoderm cells by recominant human bone morphogenetic protein 2B (BMP-2B) and modulation by transforming growth factor-beta 1 and beta 2. *Exp Cell Res* 1991;195:509–515.
65. Rosen DM, Stempien SA, Thompson AY, et al: Differentiation of rat mesenchymal cells by cartilage-inducing factor: Enhanced phenotypic expression by dihydrocytochalasin B. *Exp Cell Res* 1986;165:127–138.
66. Gelb DE, Rosier RN, Puzas JE: The production of transforming growth factor-beta by chick growth plate chondrocytes in short term monolayer culture. *Endocrinology* 1990;127:1941–1947.
67. Carrington JL, Reddi AH: Temporal changes in the response of chick limb bud mesodermal cells to transforming growth factor beta (-) type 1. *Exp Cell Res* 1990;186:368–373.
68. van der Kraan PM, Vitters EL, van den Berg WB: Inhibition of proteoglycan synthesis by transforming growth factor beta in anatomically intact articular cartilage of murine patellae. *Ann Rheum Dis* 1992;51:643–647.
69. Guerne P-A, Blanco F, Kaelin A, et al: Growth factor responsiveness of human articular chondrocytes in aging and development. *Arthritis Rheum* 1995;38:960–968.
70. Posever J, Phillips FM, Pottenger LA: Effects of basic fibroblast growth factor, transforming growth factor-beta 1, insulin-like growth factor-1, and insulin on human osteoarthritic articular cartilage explants. *J Orthop Res* 1995;13:832–837.
71. Villiger PM, Lotz M: Differential expression of TGF beta isoforms by human articular chondrocytes in response to growth factors. *J Cell Physiol* 1992;151:318–325.
72. Frenz DA, Liu W, Williams JD, et al: Induction of chondrogenesis: Requirement for synergistic interaction of basic fibroblast growth factor and transforming growth factor-beta. *Development* 1994;120:415–424.
73. Frazer A, Bunning RA, Russell RG: Effects of transforming growth factor beta and interleukin-1 beta on [3H] thymidine incorporation by human articular chondrocytes in vitro. *Biochim Biophys Acta* 1994;1226:193–200.
74. Campbell IK, Wojta J, Novak U, et al: Cytokine modulation of plasminogen activator inhibitor-1 (PAI-1) production by human articular cartilage and chondrocytes: Down-regulation by tumor necrosis factor alpha and up-regulation by transforming growth factor-B basic fibroblast growth factor. *Biochim Biophys Acta* 1994;1226:277–285.
75. Cuevas P, Burgos J, Baird A: Basic fibroblast growth factor (FGF) promotes cartilage repair in vivo. *Biochem Biophys Res Commun* 1988;156:611–618.
76. Wellmitz G, Petzold E, Jentzsch KD, et al: The effect of brain fraction with fibroblast growth factor activity on regeneration

and differentiation of articular cartilage. *Exp Pathol* 1980;18:282–287.
77. Rogachefsky RA, Dean DD, Howell DS, et al: Treatment of canine osteoarthritis with sodium pentosan polysulfate and insulin-like growth factor-1. *Ann NY Acad Sci* 1994;732:392–394.
78. Brittberg M, Lindahl A, Nilsson A, et al: Treatment of deep cartilage defects in the knee with autologous chondrocyte transplantation. *N Engl J Med* 1994;331:889–895.
79. Dounchis JS, Monosov A, Harwood F, et al: Abstract: Effect of TGFß1 on the Proliferation and Chondrogenic Phenotype of Perichondrocytes in Primary Culture. *Med Sci Sports Exerc* 1996;28:S184.
80. Miura Y, Fitzsimmons JS, Commisso CN, et al: Enhancement of periosteal chondrogenesis in vitro: Dose-response for transforming growth factor-beta 1 (TGF-beta 1). *Clin Orthop* 1994; 301:271–280.
81. Moscona RR, Bergman R, Friedman-Birnbaum R: An unusual late reaction to Zyderm I injections: A challenge for treatment. *Plast Reconstr Surg* 1993;92:331–334.
82. Overholt MA, Tschen JA, Font RL: Granulomatous reaction to collagen implant: Light and electron microscopic observations. *Cutis* 1993;51:95–98.
83. Hanke CW, Higley HR, Jolivette DM, et al: Abscess formation and local necrosis after treatment with Zyderm or Zyplast collagen implant. *J Am Acad Dermatol* 1991;25:319–326.
84. Frank DH, Vakassian L, Fisher JC, et al: Human antibody response following multiple injections of bovine collagen. *Plast Reconstr Surg* 1991;87:1080–1088.
85. Brown GL, Curtsinger LJ, White M, et al: Acceleration of tensile strength of incisions treated with EGF and TGF-beta. *Ann Surg* 1988;208:788–794.
86. Rich LF, Hatfield JM, Louiselle T: The influence of epidermal growth factor on cat corneal endothelial wound healing. *Curr Eye Res* 1991;10:823–830.
87. Raphael B, Kerr NC, Shimizlu RW, et al: Enhanced healing of cat corneal endothelial wounds by epidermal growth factor. *Invest Opthalmol Vis Sci* 1993;34:2305–2312.
88. Szoka F Jr, Papahadjopoulos D: Procedure for preparation of liposomes with large internal aqueous space and high capture by reverse-phase evaporation. *Proc Natl Acad Sci USA* 1978; 75:4194–4198.
89. Tolleth H: Long-term efficacy of collagen. *Aesthetic Plast Surg* 1985;9:155–158.
90. Nilsen DW, Brosstad F, Holm B, et al: Thrombus-related uptake and vascular clearance of ^{131}I-fibrin des-AABB as compared to ^{125}I-fibrinogen in patients with established venous thrombosis. *Thromb Haemost* 1984;51:165–168.
91. Mosher DF: Physiology of fibronectin. *Ann Rev Med* 1984; 35:561–575.
92. Weigel PH, Fuller GM, LeBoeuf RD: A model for the role of hyaluronic acid and fibrin in the early events during inflammatory response and wound healing. *J Theor Biol* 1986; 119:219–234.
93. Laurent UB, Fraser JR, Engstrom-Laurent A, et al: Catabolism of hyaluronan in the knee joint of the rabbit. *Matrix* 1992;12: 130–136.
94. Athanasiou KA, Singhal AR, Agrawal CM, et al: In vitro degradation and release characteristics of biodegradable implants containing trypsin inhibitor. *Clin Orthop* 1995;315:272–281.
95. Chu CR, Monosov AZ, Amiel D: In situ assessment of cell viability within biodegradable polylactic acid polymer matrices. *Biomaterials* 1995;16:1381–1384.

CHAPTER 48

Growth Factors as Potential Therapeutic Agents in Osteoporosis

Gregory R. Mundy, MD

Introduction

Osteoporosis is characterized by progressive loss of bone mass and increased fragility of bone that predisposes to fracture. Osteoporotic fractures are a major source of morbidity and mortality among the elderly, and agents that can prevent such fractures are increasingly needed as the population ages.

Although patients with established osteoporosis require treatment with agents that will substantially increase bone formation, no widely acceptable agent is currently available. The development of such agents will likely come from an increased understanding of the physiologic factors that control normal bone formation. The complex and highly integrated process of bone formation in human adults generally occurs at sites of previous osteoclastic bone resorption. However, endochondral bone formation occurs in growing long bones, and appositional bone formation may appear without prior local resorption (particularly on periosteal surfaces) during growth and adolescence. Among the cellular events involved in bone formation are chemotaxis of osteoblast precursors; proliferation of committed osteoblast precursors; differentiation, including expression of growth regulatory factors and the structural proteins of bone such as osteocalcin, osteopontin, and type-I collagen; and, lastly, mineralization of the proteinaceous extracellular matrix formed by osteoblasts. Tight regulatory control is essential in these cellular events, which can be modulated by systemic hormones. Such modulators include the calciotropic hormones, parathyroid hormone and 1,25 dihydroxyvitamin D, and other systemic hormones (such as the pituitary and thyroid hormones and sex steroids), but the predominant regulators are likely to be local factors or cytokines generated in the bone-cell microenvironment.

Regulatory Control of Bone Formation

Identifying the factors that control normal bone formation is one of the most important goals of bone cell biologists, because, among other things, these may represent potential therapies for all diseases of bone insufficiency, including osteoporosis. In this chapter, what is currently known of the relative importance of the bone-active growth regulatory factors will be discussed. Recent research demonstrates that the bone matrix serves as a storehouse for growth regulatory factors for bone.[1,2] Some of these growth factors may be released in active form during the process of bone resorption, as has been shown in organ culture experiments. In conditioned media from resorbing bone organ cultures, transforming growth factor beta (TGF-ß) is present, having been released from the binding protein complex that masks its biologic activity.[3] The bone matrix, moreover, houses all of the major families of growth regulatory factors, and the possibility of unidentified family members still exists. Among these families are the TGF-ß superfamily (including activin and the bone morphogenetic proteins), platelet-derived growth factor, the insulin-like growth factors, and the acidic and basic heparin-binding fibroblast growth factor.[1] All of these growth regulatory factors stimulate bone formation in vivo, although they act at different sites in the osteoblast lineage.

In addition to being stored in the bone matrix, all of these growth regulatory factors are also present at other sites in the bone microenvironment. Some are stored in the alpha granules of the platelet; some are expressed by the osteoclast; and some are expressed by other types of bone cells or mesenchymal stromal cells.

Transforming Growth Factor-Beta

TGF-ß is one of the most abundant of these factors. During bone resorption, TGF-ß is released from matrix-binding proteins in active form, making it capable of targeting cells for specific biologic effects.[3] The effects on osteoblasts are complex. TGF-ß's major effect is apparently to stimulate osteoblast proliferation, presumably increasing the pool of committed osteoblast precursors.[4-6] TGF-ß has also been shown to cause osteoblast chemotaxis.[7] Histomorphometry studies demonstrate that when TGF-ß is injected into the subcutaneous tissue over the calvarium of rodents or is infused into the marrow cavity of rats, it causes a prominent increase in bone formation in vivo.[5,6,8] Effects on osteoclasts are even more complex. TGF-ß appears to stimulate some osteoclasts while inhibiting others. We have shown that TGF-ß inhibits osteoclast formation.[9,10] Moreover, TGF-ß promotes osteoclast apoptosis.[11] However, TGF-ß may actually increase osteoclastic bone resorption under special circumstances. For example, when injected locally over the calvarium, TGF-ß may stimulate osteoclastic bone resorption within the adjacent marrow cavity.[5] Presumably, this effect is the result of TGF-ß stimulation of local prostaglandin synthesis.[9,10] Moreover, TGF-ß inhibits osteoblast differentiation in vitro, although it stimulates osteoblast proliferation.[4,12] TGF-ß's stimulatory effects on bone formation in vivo are evidently due to its powerful mitogenic effects on osteoblast precursors.

Binding proteins apparently regulate TGF-ß by inhibiting its activity. Latent transforming growth factor binding protein (LTBP) exists in the extracellular bone matrix along with TGF-ß in the form of fibrils.[13] This latent TGF-ß binding protein is produced by bone cells in parallel with TGF-ß and has a molecular weight of 130 kD. LTBP possesses many domains in the molecule characteristic of other extracellular matrix molecules, particularly fibrillin. A recent study shows LTBP antibodies to inhibit osteoblast differentiation and bone nodule formation in primary bone cell cultures.[13] LTBP may target TGF-ß for storage in bone or even influence bone cell migration in the bone microenvironment.

Bone Morphogenetic Proteins

Although they are members of the extended TGF-ß family, bone morphogenetic proteins (BMPs) have markedly different effects on bone cells from those of TGF-ß. In vitro studies show BMPs actually enhance bone cell differentiation.[4,12] Additionally, BMPs may play a role in directing cells along the osteoblast lineage. In vivo studies show that BMPs also possess the unique property of stimulating ectopic bone formation.[2,14,15] Once injected into the subcutaneous tissue of rats, BMPs produce local accumulation of ectopic bone, forming an ossicle with a marrow cavity and marrow cell constituents. Such findings have spurred the current interest in developing BMPs as therapeutic agents in diseases in which there is a need for enhanced bone formation.

As bone cells differentiate, the expression of BMP-2 and BMP-4 occurs inversely.[4,12] BMP-4 has two promoters, one of which is expressed preferentially in osteoblasts.[16] Several unique response elements characterize this promoter. These apparently functional elements bind to the nuclear extracts of fetal rat calvarial cells.[16]

Fibroblast Growth Factors

Like TGF-ß, the fibroblast growth factors (FGFs) enhance cell proliferation. The likelihood is that they increase the pool of osteoblast precursors, which then differentiate down the osteoblast lineage.[17] They do not share TGF-ß's effects on bone resorption. Once again, these agents effectively restore bone mass and stimulate new bone formation. A recent study indicates that in certain skeletal defects, members of the FGF receptor family may be abnormal.[18,19] For instance, achondroplasia, a growth cartilage disorder that produces short-limbed dwarfism, has recently been shown in most cases to be the result of a single point mutation in the transmembrane domain of the type-3 receptor for the FGF family.[19] Moreover, Crouzon's syndrome, an autosomal-dominant condition associated with premature fusion of the cranial sutures, is connected with mutations in the FGF receptor-2 gene.[18] Lastly, we have also discovered that an N-terminal extended form of basic FGF stimulates bone growth factor activity produced by a human tumor associated with bone formation in vivo.[17]

Platelet-Derived Growth Factor

Another powerful bone cell mitogen is platelet-derived growth factor (PDGF). Although PDGF's receptors are frequently expressed in bone cells, the reported actions of PDGF in vivo are variable.[20-22] When delivered systemically in an osteoporotic rat model, PDGF increased the compressive strength of the vertebral bodies and the torsional stiffness of the femoral shaft.[23] However, when injected locally over mouse calvarium, PDGF stimulates both new bone formation and an increase in bone resorption. This dual effect may well limit PDGF's therapeutic potential.

Insulin-Like Growth Factors

For many years, studies of insulin-like growth factors (IGFs) have focused on their potential effects on bone formation. In vivo studies have demonstrated powerful bone formation results with both IGF-I and IGF-II.[24] IGF-II is the most abundant growth factor yet discovered in the bone matrix. Systemic hormones such as parathyroid hormone (PTH) apparently regulate IGF-I,[25] although there is no evidence they have similar effects on IGF-II. Currently, both agents are being used in patients in clinical trials in an attempt to increase bone mass.

In vitro studies[24] have demonstrated powerful bone formation in response to IGF-I. In vivo studies[26] have provided additional support to the idea that IGF-I has an anabolic effect on bone. In an ovariectomized rat model of osteoporosis, the systemic administration of recombinant human IGF-I for 8 weeks promoted periosteal and endosteal bone formation, reduced the endosteal resorption induced by oophorectomy, and increased trabecular thickness.[26] IGF-I did not increase the number of trabeculae. Interestingly, the delivery of IGF-I complexed to its carrier protein, IGF-binding protein-3, may augment these actions.

The actions of IGF-I on human bone are beginning to be elucidated. When delivered by subcutaneous injection to 18 postmenopausal women for 6 days, IGF-I produced dose-dependent increases in serum concentrations of type-I procollagen carboxyl-terminal propeptide, an index of collagen synthesis, as well as in urinary excretion of deoxypyridinolone, an index of bone collagen breakdown.[27] These results demonstrate that short-term systemic administration of IGF-I increases bone turnover in normal women. These actions of IGF-I appear to be similar in osteoporotic men.[28] Although long-term studies are not available, 6 months of treatment with IGF-I in a patient who had osteoporosis associated with Werner syndrome produced an increase in the bone mineral density of the vertebral bodies, suggesting that IGF-I generated a net increase in bone formation.[29]

IGF-II, like IGF-I, stimulates bone cells in vitro[30] and is abundant in bone matrix. Systemic hormones, such as PTH, apparently regulate production of IGF-I by bone cells and may have similar effects[31] on the production of IGF-II. Currently, both agents are being used in patients in clinical trials in an attempt to increase bone mass. It is hoped that it will be demonstrated that factors such as IGF and the BMPs, as well as other growth factors, can produce beneficial effects without the limitations of toxicity and be a useful therapy for osteoporosis in the near future.

Cascade Theory of Bone Formation

Bone formation is a complex but highly ordered process. The process is most likely triggered as osteoclasts discontinue resorbing bone. However, the signal that triggers bone formation is apparently brief and leads to sequential changes within the cells themselves, changes that produce subsequent cellular and molecular effects. As bone is resorbed, active growth factors are released, presumably including active TGF-ß. These factors may have chemotactic and proliferative effects on osteoblast precursors. Such a process is a likely description of bone formation in its incipient stage. However, once bone cells begin to differentiate, they express other growth factors, which may produce later osteoblast differentiation. Primary cultures of fetal rat calvarial osteoblasts, for instance, express the BMPs as they differentiate to form mineralized bone nodules.[4,12] Enhanced new bone formation is the result of exogenous addition of the bone morphogenetic proteins to these osteoblast cultures. The orderly formation of bone that occurs under normal physiologic conditions may be the result of endogenous expression of BMPs by differentiating bone cells.

Therapeutic Potential

The outstanding therapeutic need in most common bone diseases, including osteoporosis, segmental bone defects, and periodontal disease, is agents that will stimulate the growth of new bone. Agents of this sort that are acceptable for use are sadly lacking at the present time. However, the naturally occurring endogenous signals for bone formation are all potential therapeutic agents for such diseases. If it could be demonstrated that the BMPs or the FGFs cause beneficial effects without associated toxicity, the systemic administration of such bone growth factors could be a useful therapy for osteoporosis. Additionally, these agents may be useful when administered locally, to help in the repair of nonunited fractures or segmental bone defects, with or without allografts. It remains to be seen whether these agents will become accepted for therapeutic use, but since the advent of their availability as recombinant molecules in sufficient amounts, their clinical utility should soon be known. Ultimately, even if these agents do not produce the desired clinical effects, understanding the sequence of molecular events and the process of regulation involved in bone formation should lead to novel targets in bone for the development of therapeutic agents.

Acknowledgments

I am grateful to Nancy Garrett and Gavin Mundy for their help with the preparation of this review. This work is supported by grants P01-CA40035, P01-AR39529, R37-AR28149, RO1-DK45239, and RO1-AR42372.

References

1. Hauschka PV, Mavrakos AE, Iafrati MD, et al: Growth factors in bone matrix: Isolation of multiple types by affinity chromatography on heparin-sepharose. *J Biol Chem* 1986;261:12665–12674.
2. Urist MR: Bone: Formation by autoinduction. *Science* 1965;150: 893–899.
3. Pfeilschifter J, Mundy GR: Modulation of type beta transforming growth factor beta activity in bone cultures by osteotropic hormones. *Proc Natl Acad Sci USA* 1987;84:2024–2028.
4. Harris SE, Bonewald LF, Harris MA, et al: Effects of transforming growth factor beta on bone nodule formation and expression of bone morphogenetic protein 2, osteocalcin, osteopontin, alkaline phosphatase, and type I collagen mRNA in long-term cultures of fetal rat calvarial osteoblasts. *J Bone Miner Res* 1994;9:855–863.
5. Marcelli C, Yates AJ, Mundy GR: In vivo effects of human recombinant transforming growth factor beta on bone turnover in normal mice. *J Bone Miner Res* 1990;5:1087–1096.
6. Noda M, Camilliere JJ: In vivo stimulation of bone formation by transforming growth factor-beta. *Endocrinology* 1989;124: 2991–2994.
7. Pfeilschifter J, Chenu C, Bird A, et al: Interleukin-1 and tumor necrosis factor stimulate the formation of human osteoclast-like cells in vitro. *J Bone Miner Res* 1989;4:113–118.
8. Mackie EJ, Trechsel U: Stimulation of bone formation in vivo by transforming growth factor-beta: Remodeling of woven bone and lack of inhibition by indomethacin. *Bone* 1990;11: 295–300.
9. Pfeilschifter J, Seyedin SM, Mundy GR: Transforming growth factor beta inhibits bone resorption in fetal rat long bone cultures. *J Clin Invest* 1988;82:680–685.
10. Tashjian AH Jr, Voelkel EF, Lazzaro M, et al: Alpha and beta human transforming growth factors stimulate prostaglandin production and bone resorption in cultured mouse calvaria. *Proc Natl Acad Sci USA* 1985;82:4535–4538.
11. Hughes DE, Wright KR, Mundy GR, et al: Abstract: TGFß1

induces osteoclast apoptosis in vitro. *J Bone Miner Res* 1994; 9(suppl 1):S138.
12. Harris SE, Sabatini M, Harris MA, et al: Expression of bone morphogenetic protein messenger RNA in prolonged cultures of fetal rat calvarial cells. *J Bone Miner Res* 1994; 9:389–394.
13. Dallas SL, Mundy GR, Skerry TM, et al: Abstract: The latent TGFb binding protein (LTBP) appears to be a fibrillar extracellular matrix protein which plays a role in bone formation. *J Bone Miner Res* 1994;9(suppl 1):S312.
14. Wozney JM, Rosen V, Celeste AJ, et al: Novel regulators of bone formation: Molecular clones and activities. *Science* 1988;242: 1528–1534.
15. Wozney JM: The bone morphogenetic protein family and osteogenesis. *Mol Reprod Dev* 1992;32:160–167.
16. Feng JQ, Harris MA, Cooney AJ, et al: Abstract: Transcriptional regulation of bone morphogenetic protein 4 (BMP–4) by COUP-TFI. *J Bone Miner Res* 1994;9 (suppl 1):S123.
17. Izbicka E, Dunstan C, Esparza J, et al: Abstract: A human amniotic tumor which induces new bone formation in vivo produces a growth regulatory activity in vitro for osteoblasts identified as basic fibroblast growth factor (FGF). *J Bone Miner Res* 1993; 8(suppl 1):S140.
18. Reardon W, Winter RM, Rutland P, et al: Mutations in the fibroblast growth factor receptor 2 gene cause Crouzon syndrome. *Nat Genet* 1994;8:98–103.
19. Rousseau F, Bonaventure J, Legeai-Mallet L, et al: Mutations in the gene encoding fibroblast growth factor receptor-3 in achondroplasia. *Nature* 1994;371:252–254.
20. Graves DT, Antoniades HN, Williams SR, et al: Evidence for functional platelet-derived growth factor receptors on MG-63 human osteosarcoma cells. *Cancer Res* 1984;44:2966–2970.
21. Graves DT, Owen AJ, Barth RK, et al: Detection of c-sis transcripts and synthesis of PDGF-like proteins by human osteosarcoma cells. *Science* 1984;226:972–974.
22. Graves DT, Valentin-Opran A, Delgado R, et al: The potential role of platelet-derived growth factor as an autocrine or paracrine factor for human bone cells. *Connect Tissue Res* 1989;23:209–218.
23. Mitlak FH, Finkelman RD, Hill EL, et al: The effect of systemically administered PDGF-BB on the rodent skeleton. *J Bone Miner Res* 1996;11:238–247.
24. Hock JM, Centrella M, Canalis E: Insulin-like growth factor I has independent effects on bone matrix formation and cell replication. *Endocrinology* 1988;122:254–260.
25. Canalis E, Centrella M, Burch W, et al: Insulin-like growth factor I mediates selective anabolic effects of parathyroid hormone in bone cultures. *J Clin Invest* 1989;83:60–65.
26. Bagi CM, DeLeon E, Bromage R, et al: Treatment of ovariectomized rats with the complex of rhIGF-I/IGFBP-3 increases cortical and cancellous bone mass and improves structure in the femoral neck. *Calcif Tissue Internat* 1995;57:40–46.
27. Ebeling PR, Jones JD, O'Fallon WM, et al: Short-term effects of recombinant human insulin-like growth factor I on bone turnover in normal women. *J Clin Endocrinol Metab* 1993;77: 1384–1387.
28. Johansson AG, Lindh E, Ljunghall S: Letter: Insulin-like growth factor I stimulates bone turnover in osteoporosis. *Lancet* 1992;339:1619.
29. Rubin CD, Reed B, Sakhaee K, et al: Treating a patient with the Werner syndrome and osteoporosis using recombinant human insulin-like growth factor. *Ann Intern Med* 1994;121:665–668.
30. Schmid D, Steiner T, Froesch ER: Insulin-like growth factors stimulate synthesis of nucleic acids and glycogen in cultured calvaria cells. *Calcif Tissue Internat* 1983;35:578–585.
31. Linkhart TA, Mohan S: Parathyroid hormone stimulates release of insulin-like growth factor-I (IGF-I) and IGF-II from neonatal mouse calvaria in organ culture. *Endocrinology* 1989;125: 1484–1491.

Amputation

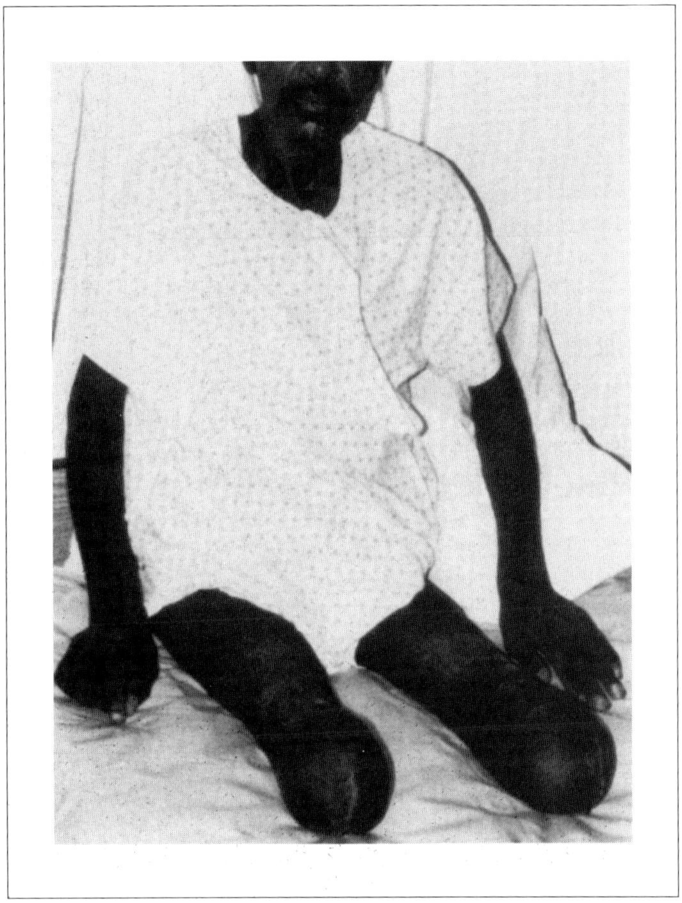

CHAPTER 49

Current Concepts: Amputation Surgery in Peripheral Vascular Disease

Michael S. Pinzur, MD

Introduction

Burgess and Zettl[1] have long stressed amputation surgery as reconstructive surgery, the first step in the rehabilitation of a patient where functional restoration of a limb cannot be achieved. In the present environment, outcome has become the watchword and needs to be measured based on level of functional independence, as opposed to the amount of salvaged tissue and limb length. A multidisciplinary team approach assures restoration of the patient's maximum level of independence. A successful outcome-oriented program should be led by a function-based, outcome-oriented orthopaedic or peripheral vascular surgeon, and supported by the disciplines of physical medicine and rehabilitation, prosthetics, physical therapy, psychology, social work, and nursing, in order for rehabilitation to be successful.

Most of the recent technical advances in prosthetics have been accomplished in the use of componentry geared to enhance the performance of young, active traumatic and tumor amputees. While restoration of function in this group of patients is highly challenging and rewarding, the more pressing challenge to our health care system is the geriatric patient with peripheral vascular disease. When undertaking transtibial amputation in these patients, the financial cost to the third-party payor for hospitalization and surgery, physicians' fees, rehabilitation unit treatment, prosthetics, and physical therapy, exceeds $50,000 per patient. The American Diabetes Association estimates that in patients with diabetes, from 40 to 50 thousand lower extremity amputations are performed annually. These figures represent approximately 50% of amputations performed yearly. The cost to the health care system becomes staggering when the cost of institutionalization in a nursing home is compared to that of a successful return to independent living.

The medical care of these patients is further complicated by multiple organ system involvement in the disease process. In order to develop a systematic approach to this complex group of patients, a basic understanding of their unique biologic environment is necessary before creating critical pathways that will optimize their eventual functional independence.

Joints are Energy Couples

Self-selected walking speed is decreased and the oxygen consumption per meter walked is increased with proximal level amputations, being inversely proportional to the length of the residual limb and the number of joints preserved. The metabolic cost of walking becomes so severe in transfemoral amputees with peripheral vascular disease that maximum energy is expended during normal walking[2-4] (Fig. 1). Considering that this data was generated in a laboratory on a walkway or treadmill, the metabolic demands

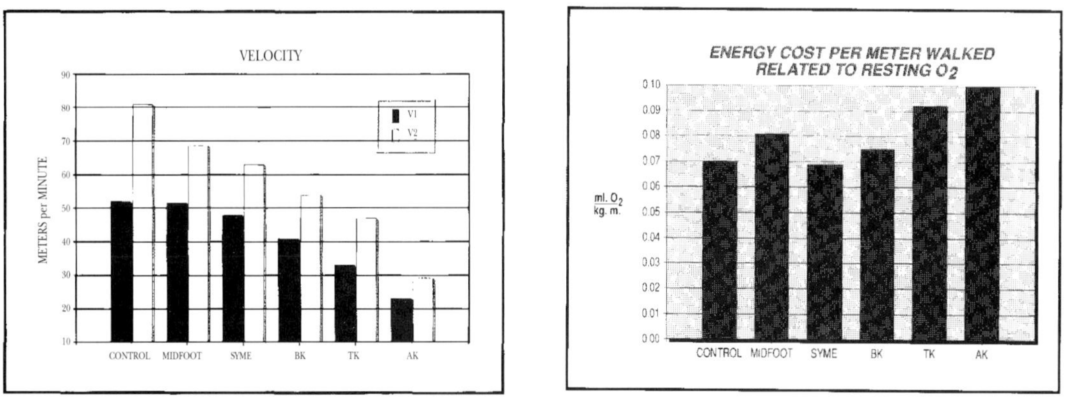

Fig. 1 Walking velocity (**left**) and oxygen consumption per meter walked in peripheral vascular amputees at the midfoot, ankle disarticulation, transtibial (bk), knee disarticulation (tk), and transfemoral (ak) amputation levels. (Reproduced with permission from Pinzur M, Gold J, Schwartz D, et al: Energy demands for walking in dysvascular amputees as related to the level of amputation. *Orthopaedics* 1992;15:1033–1037.)

for walking distances or duration are likely greater still. It is not surprising that functional independence is inversely proportional to the length of the amputee's residual limb and number of joints preserved. In geriatric transfemoral amputees with peripheral vascular disease, the metabolic cost of walking is so great that high levels of walking independence are rarely achieved.[5,6]

Cognitive and Psychological Requirements for Walking in Amputees

In order for patients to learn to walk with a prosthesis and care for their residual limb and prosthesis, they must possess the cognitive capacities of memory, attention, concentration, and organization. Patients with cognitive deficits or psychiatric disease have a low likelihood of success in using a prosthesis. The prospective amputee with peripheral vascular disease should be evaluated for cognitive capacity and motivation before deciding on the appropriate amputation level because of the preponderance of cerebrovascular disease as a comorbidity.[7]

Load Transfer

The soft-tissue envelope of the amputee's residual limb acts as an interface between the bone of the residual limb and the prosthetic socket. The soft-tissue envelope should be composed of a mobile, nonadherent muscle mass and full thickness skin that will tolerate the direct pressures of weightbearing and the shearing forces resulting from pistoning within the prosthetic socket, which often causes ulceration of the residual limb (Fig. 2).

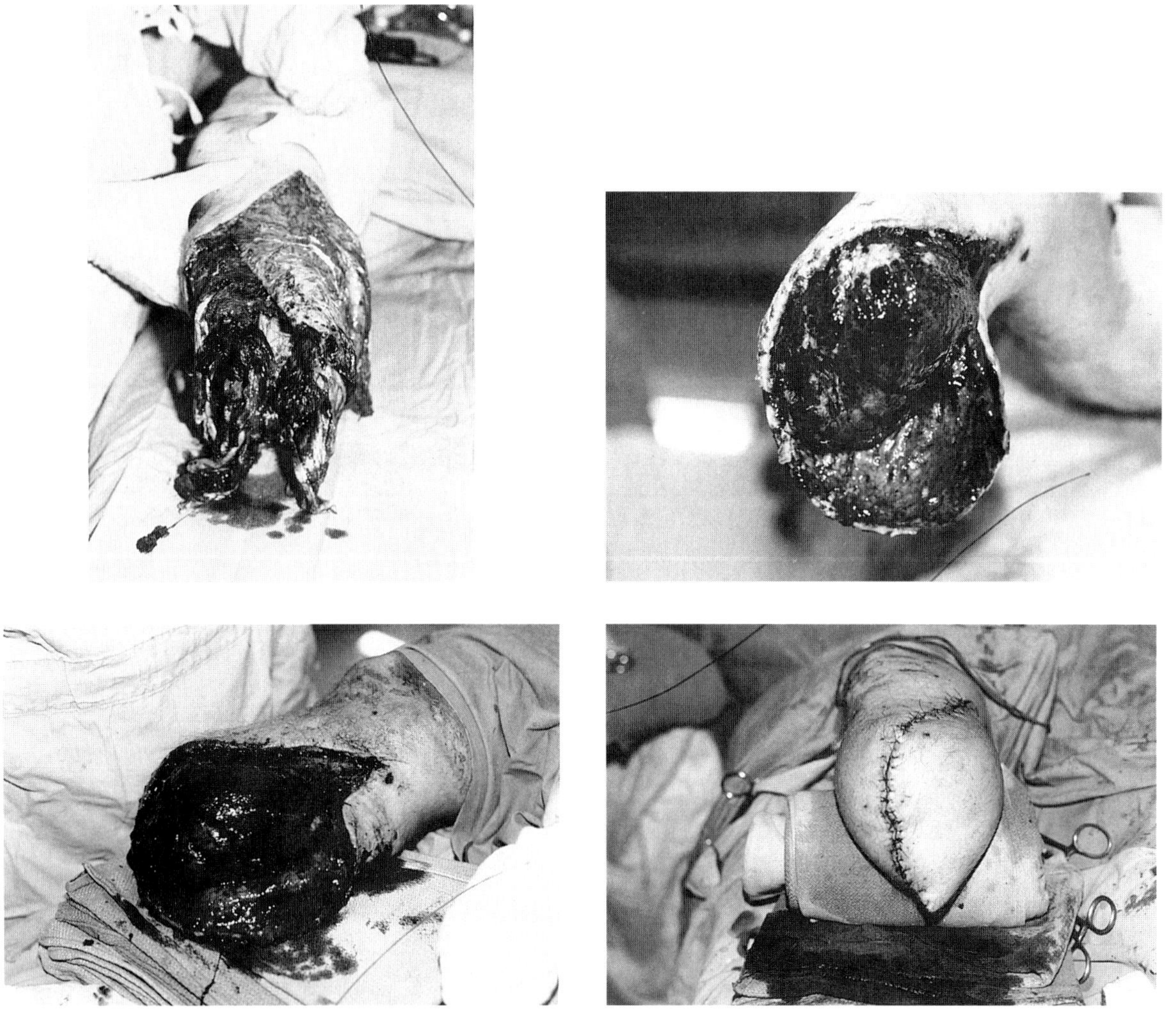

Fig. 2 Creation of a soft tissue envelope. **Top left,** Traumatic amputation from railroad injury. The first step is debridement of nonviable tissue, followed by open wound care. **Top right,** The medial gastrocnemius was wrapped about the tibia to create a soft-tissue envelope comprised of a mobile muscle mass, and full thickness skin. **Bottom left,** Prior to skin closure. **Bottom right,** Final wound closure. Note that while the wound overlies the distal anterior tibia, the soft tissue envelope is composed of a mobile muscle mass and full thickness skin. This durable residual limb has functioned without tissue breakdown in a laborer for over 10 years.

Load transfer (weightbearing) is accomplished by either direct or indirect load transfer. Direct load transfer (end weightbearing) is accomplished with knee or ankle (Syme) disarticulation. The weightbearing surfaces of these bones are expanded to allow dissipation of weightbearing stresses over a larger surface area, and the elastic modulus of the metaphyseal bone allows stress dissipation at initial loading, ie, heel strike. Intimacy, or the snugness of prosthetic socket fit, is not crucial for weightbearing, but only for suspension. When the amputation is performed through the diaphysis of a long bone, as in transfemoral or transtibial levels, the end of the bone and residual limb must be unloaded, transferring the load indirectly by the total contact method. This requires an intimate prosthetic socket fit and 7° to 10° of flexion of the tibia below, or adduction of the femur above the knee joint[8] (Fig. 3).

Amputation Wound Healing

More than oxygenated blood is necessary to create an environment favorable to support amputation wound healing. Patients are malnourished when their serum albumin is below 3.5 g/dl, and immune deficiency occurs when the total (absolute) lymphocyte count is below 1500/mm^3. Both conditions are frequently overlooked in trauma and peripheral vascular disease patient populations. Malnourished or immune-deficient patients have a 40% to 50% risk for wound failure or infection, as compared with patients with corrected wound healing environments, where a wound healing rate of 90% can be expected.[9,10] Surgery in such patients can be delayed until these values are improved, usually by oral hyperalimentation, to support wound healing. When infection or gangrene dictates urgent surgery, open drainage of infection or open amputation at the most distal viable level, followed by open wound care, culture-specific antibiotic therapy, and metabolic support, can be accomplished until wound healing potential can be optimized (Fig. 4).

Oxygenated blood is a prerequisite to wound healing in both ischemic and traumatized limbs. Consultation with the vascular surgeon is essential, if only to determine if the limb can be salvaged. There are presently many options available to the vascular surgeon. Interventional therapy can range from angioplasty with balloon, laser, or coring device, to in situ bypass using locally available veins, to standard bypass surgery using autologous vein or synthetic graft material. If improvement of vascular inflow is an option, a

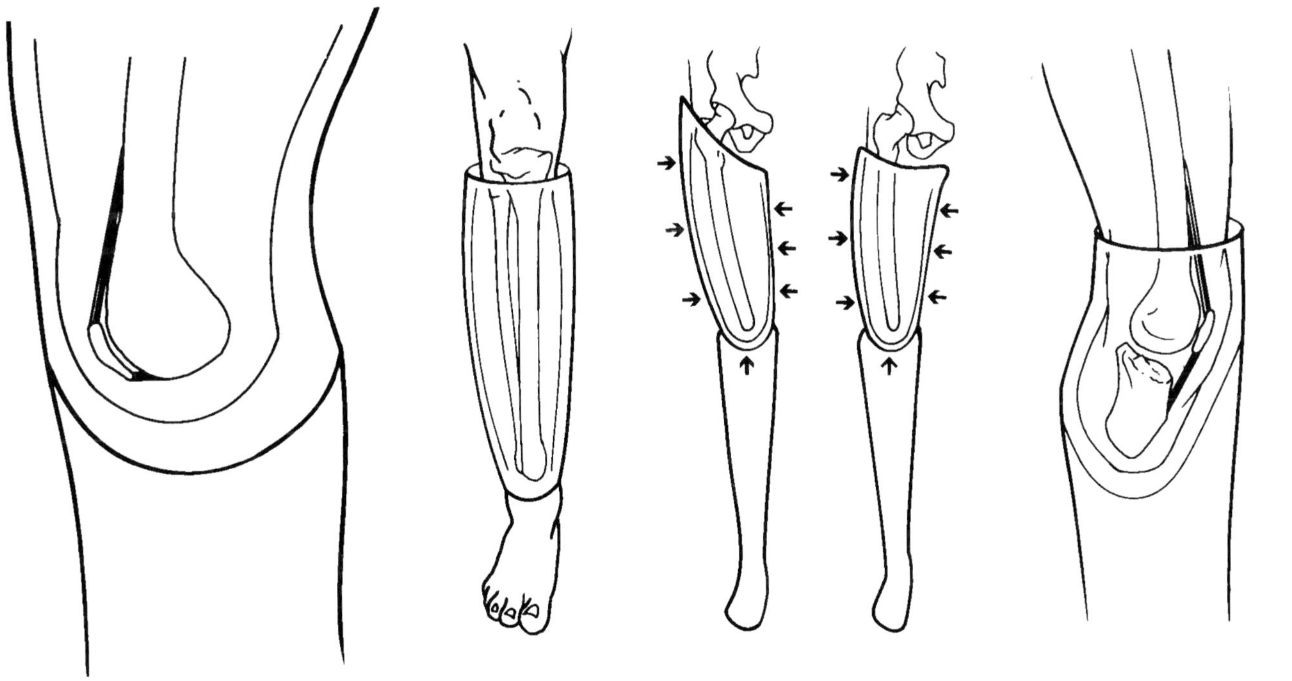

Fig. 3 Direct load transfer, ie, endbearing, is accomplished in knee **(left)**, and ankle **(center left)** disarticulations. Since load is transferred directly to the weightbearing surface of the limb, intimate prosthetic fit is not crucial. This is not the case in indirect, ie, total contact, load transfer where load is transmitted to the entire residual limb surface area while unloading the bony ends, as in transfemoral **(center right)** and transtibial **(right)** amputations. (Reproduced with permission from Pinzur M: New concepts in lower-limb amputation and prosthetic management, in Greene WB (ed): *Instructional Course Lectures XXXIX*. Park Ridge, IL, American Academy of Orthopaedic Surgeons, 1990, pp 361–365.)

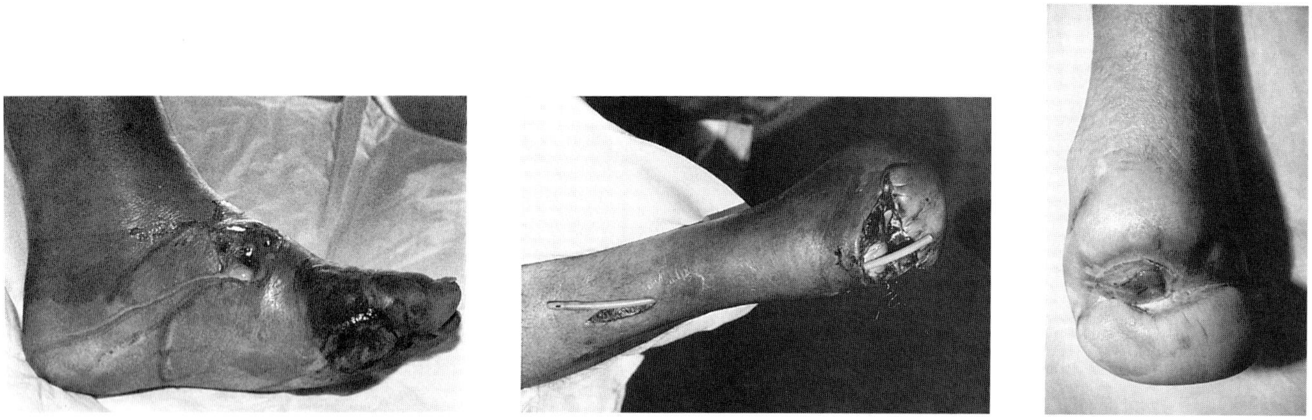

Fig. 4 **Left,** This patient presented with sepsis that tracked proximally into the anterior compartment of the leg. An open forefoot amputation was performed. Compression of the calf "milked" pus from the compartment. It was not necessary to amputate through the leg. The anterior compartment was debrided and treated with open wound management. **Right,** The patient's medical condition precluded a timely return to the operating room for wound closure. The wound was allowed to heal by secondary intention. The patient now walks with a modified high top shoe.

risk-benefit ratio can be established to determine if the potential benefits of therapeutic intervention justify the risks involved with treatment.

Amputation wounds generally heal by collateral blood flow in the peripheral vascular disease population, so arteriography is rarely a useful tool in assessing the vascular inflow available to support wound healing. The ultrasound Doppler has historically been used as the measure of vascular inflow to the ischemic limb. The Doppler measures arterial pressure, and only indirectly measures vascular inflow. The ischemic index is the ratio of the Doppler pressure at the level being tested, to the brachial systolic pressure. The most commonly reported value is the ischemic index recorded at the ankle level, the ankle-brachial index (ABI). An absolute Doppler pressure of 70 mm Hg, or an ischemic index of 0.5, has been accepted as the minimum necessary measure of inflow to support amputation wound healing.[11] In the normal limb, the area under the Doppler waveform is a measure of the inflow. These values can be falsely elevated, and nonpredictive, in at least 15% of patients with peripheral vascular disease, because of noncompressible, noncompliant, calcified atherosclerotic peripheral arteries.[12]

Determination of the transcutaneous partial pressure of oxygen ($TcpO^2$) at the level in question is the present "gold standard" measurement of vascular inflow in ischemic limbs. Transcutaneous oximetry actually measures the oxygen-delivering capacity of the vascular system to the level of surgery. Values of 20 to 30 mm Hg are correlated with acceptable wound healing rates, apparently without false positive values[13,14] (Fig. 5).

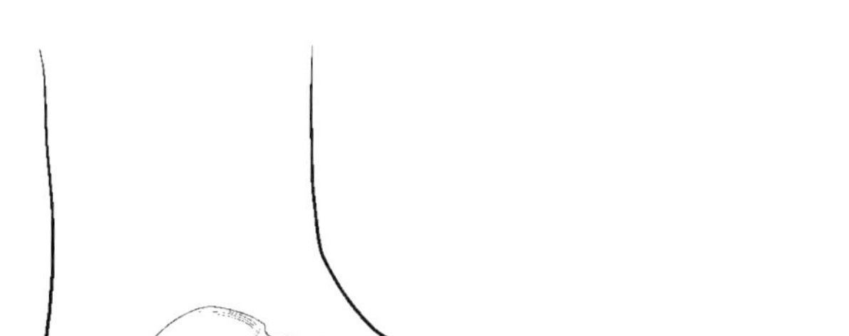

Fig. 5 The long plantar flap for midfoot amputation. Metatarsal transection at the level of the proximal metaphysis.

Selection of Amputation Level

The first step in selection of the appropriate amputation level is the evaluation of rehabilitation potential of the patient. The young trauma patient with a nonreconstructible extremity injured by trauma should have residual limb salvage at the most distal amputation level compatible with providing a serviceable soft-tissue envelope and residual limb capable of accomplishing load transfer. Retaining limb length may allow acceptance of a less than optimal residual limb, with the thought of late reconstruction, if necessary, which might require bony lengthening, plastic surgery free flaps, or use of a tissue expander.

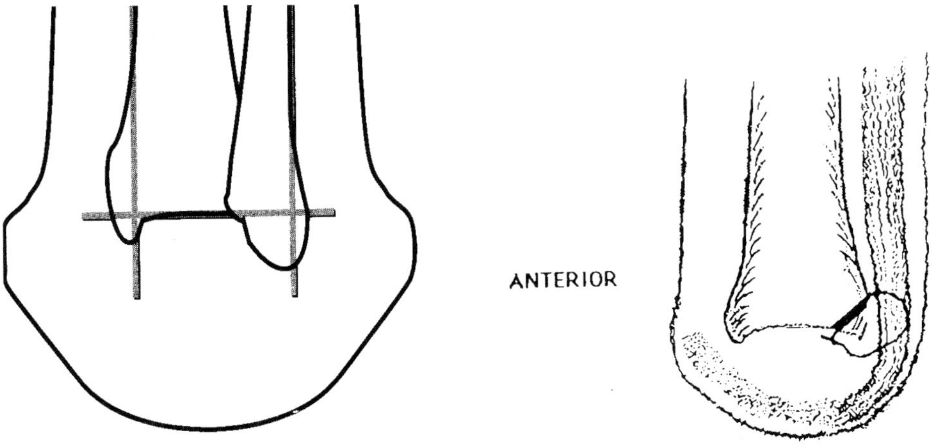

Fig. 6 **Left,** One stage ankle disarticulation is performed with an incision similar to two stage procedure. The malleoli are transected at the joint line and the metaphyseal flares are narrowed in line with the shafts of the tibia and fibula. (Reproduced with permission from Pinzur MS, Smith D, Osterman H: Syme ankle disarticulation in peripheral vascular disease and diabetic foot infection: The one-stage versus two-stage procedure. *Foot Ankle Int* 1995;16:124-127.) **Right,** Tenodesis of the Achilles tendon prevents posterior migration of the heel pad while retaining the articular surface of the distal tibia. (Reproduced with permission from Smith DG, Sangeorzan BJ, Hansen ST, et al: Achilles tendon tenodesis to prevent heel pad migration in the Syme's amputation. *Foot Ankle Int* 1994;15:14–17.)

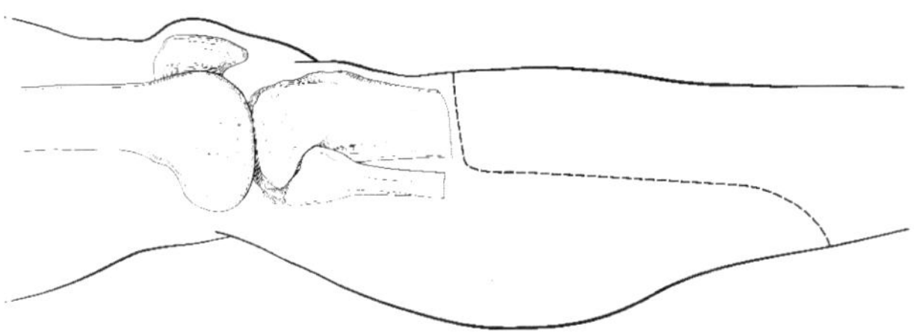

Fig. 7 Long posterior myocutaneous flap in transtibial amputation. Bone level is 12 to 15 cm distal to the knee joint.

The rehabilitation potential of the patient with peripheral vascular disease is very different. If patients have vascular disease sufficient to necessitate amputation, they are likely to have concomitant cardiovascular and cerebrovascular disease. In addition, their life expectancy is limited, so less time is available for late reconstructive procedures.[15] A reasonable assessment of their premorbid ambulatory status and projection of their functional independence following amputation is crucial. The physical therapist, psychologist, social worker, and physiatrist provide key input into the decision-making algorithm whether patients should undergo vascular reconstruction, amputation, or a combination to preserve limb length.

The biologic amputation level is the most distal functional amputation level with a high probability of supporting wound healing. Once the decision is made to proceed, the biologic amputation level is determined by clinical examination, adequate vascular inflow measured by Doppler or transcutaneous oximetry, serum albumin of 3.0 to 3.5 g/dl as a measure of total body nutrition, and total lymphocyte count of 1500/mm^3 as a measure of immunocompetence.

The rehabilitation amputation level is then determined by combining the biologic amputation level with the rehabilitation potential to determine the amputation level that will maximize the functional independence of the patient, without subjecting that patient to undue surgical/anesthetic risk.

Functional Amputation Levels

Great Toe

The great toe acts as a stabilizer during the stance phase of normal walking. Patients with ischemic peripheral vascular disease generally have an apropulsive gait pattern and notice little functional deficit following amputation of the great toe. A long plantar flap is optimal, but can be modified based on the available tissue. If possible, the base of the proximal phalanx with the insertion of the flexor hallucis brevis should be retained for stability.

Lesser Toes

The lesser toes serve little function in patients with ischemic peripheral vascular disease, so extended effort should not be expended for salvage, nor should salvage of a single protruding toe be attempted. Retaining the base of the second toe proximal phalanx will prevent lateral drift of the great toe.

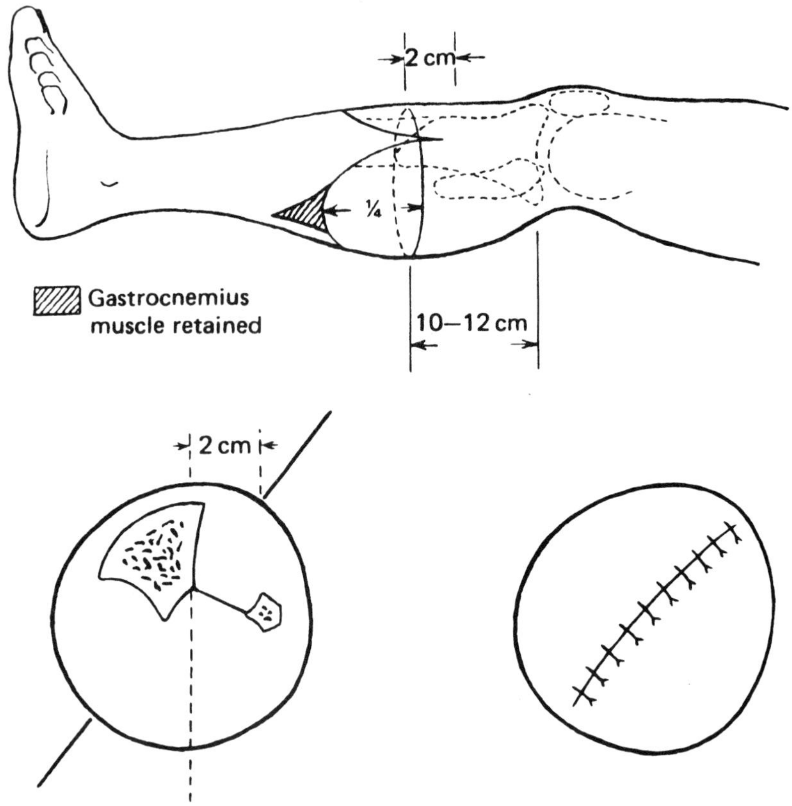

Fig. 8 **Top,** Drawing of anteromedial and posterolateral skew flaps as seen from the lateral side. **Bottom,** Drawings of the distal portion of the left leg show the orientation of skew flaps in relation to the tibia and fibula and the axis of the sutured wound. (Reproduced with permission from Robinson KP: Skew flap myoplastic below-knee amputation: A preliminary report. *Br J Surg* 1982;69:554.)

Ray Resection

Ray resection should be limited to a single outer ray for bony infection, not for gangrene. Single central ray resection should only be performed if wound closure can be achieved, as the open wound created takes appreciable time and effort to affect healing. Resection of more than one ray produces a narrow residual forefoot frequently complicated by equinus that will not outperform midfoot amputation.[16]

Midfoot Amputation

Amputation at this level allows walking with a standard oxford shoe with an orthotic toe filler. The long plantar flap is preferable to equal dorsal-plantar flaps, but is dictated by the available viable tissue. When the bone cuts are performed at the level of the proximal metaphyses, a low potential exists for recurrent plantar ulceration under longer residual metatarsal shafts, which will retain a longer lever arm for push-off. Lisfranc tarsal-metatarsal amputation functions well, but percutaneous Achilles tendon lengthening should be performed to prevent the late development of ankle equinus[10] (Fig. 5).

Hindfoot Amputation (Boyd, Chopart)

Procedures at this level should generally be avoided in adults because they often lead to severe residual limb equinus and varus, require custom high top shoe gear, and provide a very short lever arm for propulsion and stability during terminal stance phase.

Ankle Disarticulation (Syme)

This level provides a durable residual limb that allows direct load transfer, is rarely complicated by the development of late residual limb ulcers, and requires minimal prosthetic training. The procedure can be performed in one stage, trimming the malleoli at the joint surface, and narrowing the metaphyseal flares to allow comfortable prosthetic use[17,18] (Fig. 6).

Transtibial

Transtibial amputation is best performed at 12 to 15 cm distal to the knee joint, allowing adequate residual limb length for load transfer, and creating a durable soft-tissue envelope by using a long posterior myocutaneous flap. In longer length residual limbs, the poserior flap will be performed through the Achilles tendon and not allow production of a durable soft-tissue envelope, and the knee will need to be extended to contain the residual limb within the shank of the prosthesis producing end residual limb weightbearing (Fig. 7). The skew flap has recently become popular in limbs with severe peripheral vascular disease.[19] While touting improved biologic vascular supply, it performs much like a standard long posterior myocutaneous flap (Fig. 8).

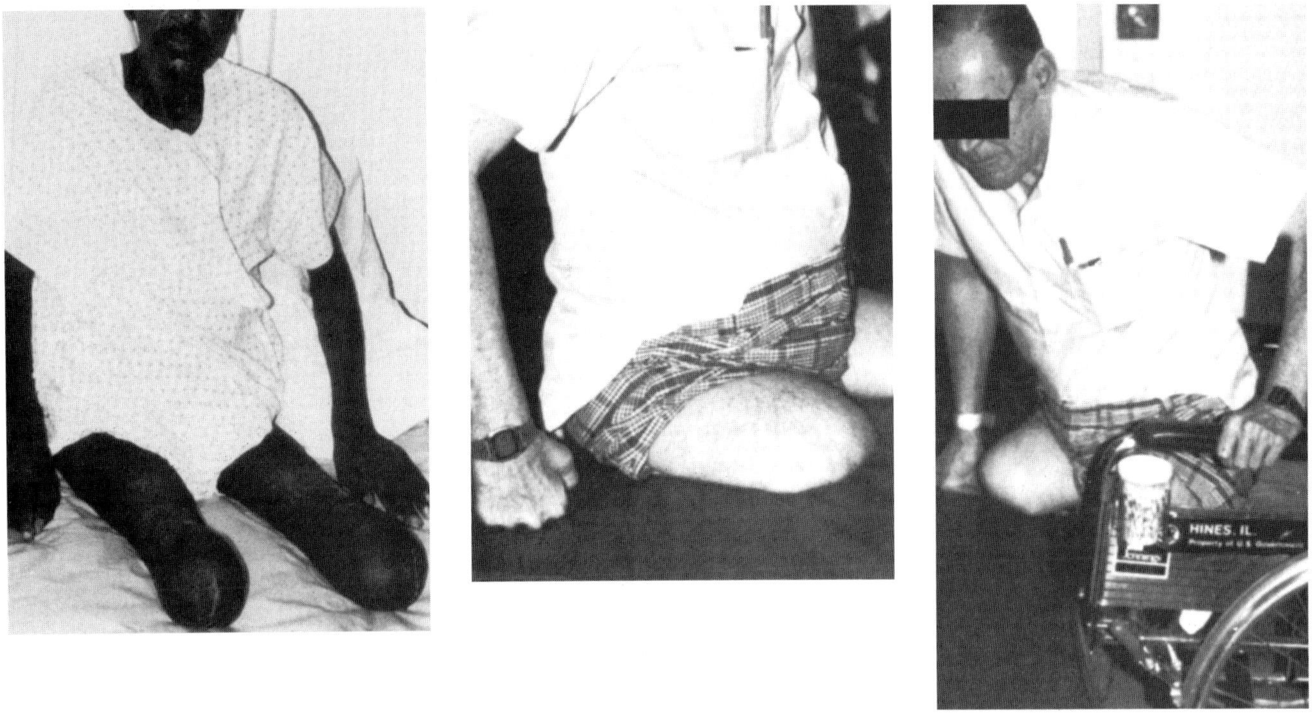

Fig. 9 **Left,** Bilateral knee disarticulation patient exhibiting excellent platform for sitting and lever arm for transfer as opposed to **(center)** small weightbearing platform and **(right)** short lever arm available with transfemoral amputation. (Reproduced with permission from Pinzur MS: Knee disarticulation: Surgical procedures, in Bowker JH, Michael JW (eds): American Academy of Orthopaedic Surgeons *Atlas of Limb Prosthetics*. St Louis, MO, Mosby-Year Book, 1992, pp 479-486.)

Knee Disarticulation

Amputation at this level is generally performed on the patient with the ability to achieve wound healing at the transtibial level, but who will not become a prosthetic walker. The procedure is muscle balanced, so the patient will not develop late joint contractures, and provides an excellent platform for sitting and lever arm for transfers (Fig. 9). When used in walking patients, it allows use of the intrinsically stable four-bar linkage prosthetic knee joint.[20] Wagner popularized use of a soft-tissue envelope comprised of the gastrocnemius muscle and sagittal skin flaps. Recent experience has shown a decreased risk of wound morbidity with use of a long posterior myocutaneous flap similar to the flap used in transtibial amputation. The flaps are created at the level of the midpatellar tendon. The length of the flap is equal to a diameter of the limb at the knee joint plus 1 cm. The thickness of the flap should be approximately one third the distance from posterior to anterior. The patellar tendon is incised at its insertion and sutured into the stumps of the cruciate ligaments, which have been incised at their insertion. The posterior fascia of the gastrocnemius muscle is sutured to the knee joint retinaculum, creating a durable soft-tissue envelope[21] (Fig. 10).

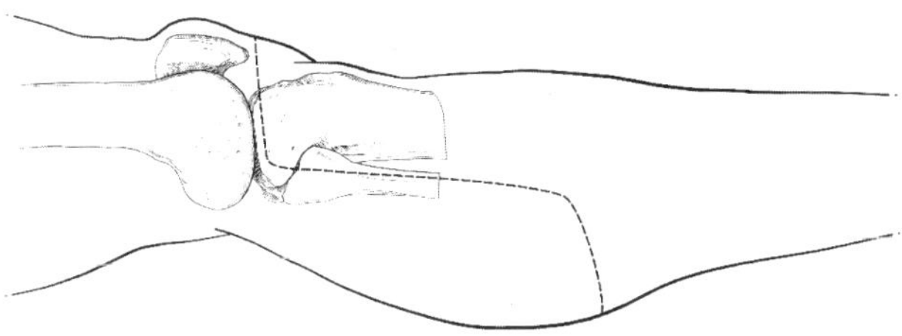

Fig. 10 Long posterior myocutaneous flap used in knee disarticulation.

Transfemoral

Because geriatric patients with peripheral vascular disease will have limited walking potential, there is little room for error in the transfemoral type of amputation. Gottschalk and associates[22] have shown that the prosthetic socket is not capable of maintaining the normal biomechanical axis with the femur aligned in adduction. In order to create a normal biomechanical axis in walking with a prosthesis, they developed the adductor-based myofasciocutaneous flap. A long, medial-based sagittal flap is created, dissecting the adductor muscle from the femur, which is transected approximately 12 cm above the knee joint. The adductor magnus muscle is secured to the lateral cortex

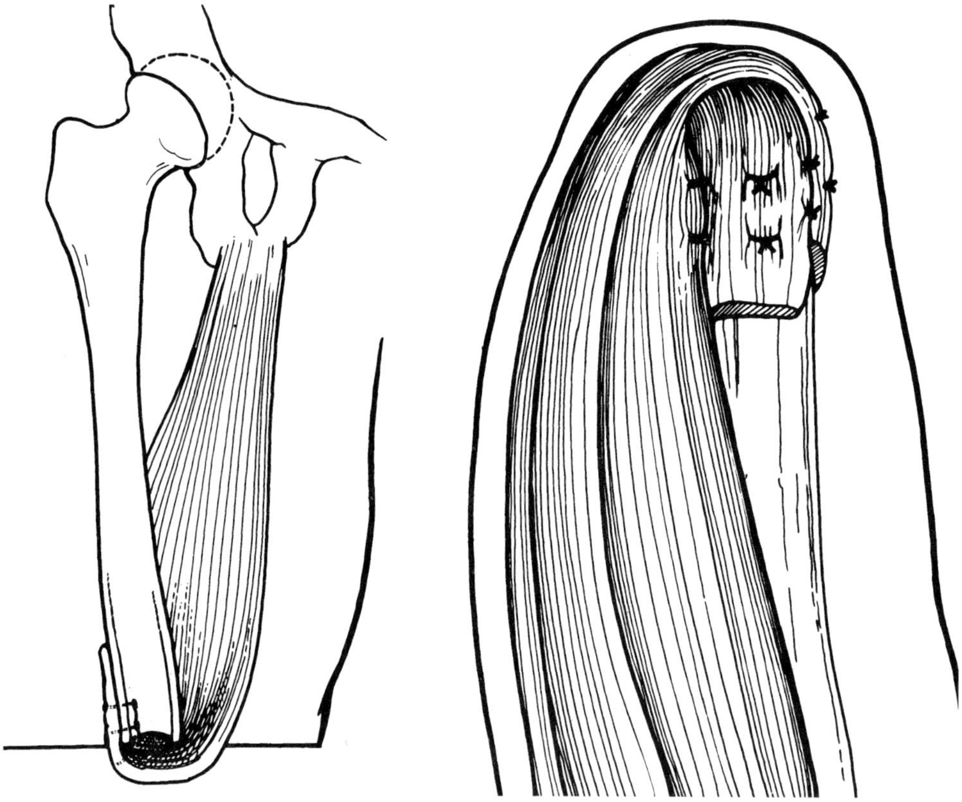

Fig. 11 **Left,** Diagram depicting the proposed skin flaps and level of bone section. **Right,** Diagram to show attachment of the adductor magnus to the lateral part of the femur. (Reproduced with permission from Gottschalk F: Transfemoral amputation, in Bowker JH, Michael J: American Academy of Orthopaedic Surgeons *Atlas of Limb Prosthetics*, ed 2. St. Louis, MO, CV Mosby, 1992, pp 501–507.)

of the femur through drill holes. The quadriceps is transected just proximal to its tendinous attachment to the patella, and sutured to drill holes in the posterior cortex of the residual femur, with the femur maintained in normal extension, to prevent the creation of an iatrogenic hip flexion contracture. The posterior muscles are anchored to the posterior border of the adductor magnus[23] (Fig. 11).

Upper Limb

Gangrene of the upper limb in a patient with diabetes occurs in those with end stage disease. Limited distal amputation surgery will generally fail. These patients will likely die before the wound heals, or within 2 years of diagnosis.[24]

Rehabilitation

Rehabilitation should not be delayed until the stump matures. Prolonged sitting leads to aerobic deconditioning, joint contractures, and decubitus ulcers. Ambulation and weightbearing should be initiated early in the rehabilitation period. Foot and ankle amputations should be immobilized in plaster casts, with weightbearing initiated at 10 to 14 days following surgery, unless the condition of the residual limb dictates otherwise. Transtibial and knee disarticulation residual limbs can also be initially managed with rigid plaster dressings, with weightbearing being started at 5 to 21 days following surgery, based on the condition of the residual limb and the experience of the rehabilitation team. Because of difficulty in suspension of the rigid dressing, transfemoral amputees are managed with soft compressive bandages.

The goal of treatment in peripheral vascular disease is to return the patient to a maximum level of independent function, whether by vascular bypass surgery or judicious amputation. Because outcomes are based on function, early rehabilitation is critical to achieving results that are concerned with functional outcome measures.

References

1. Burgess EM, Zettl JH: *The Management of Lower Extremity Amputations.* Washington, DC, US Government Printing Office, 1969.
2. Fisher SV, Gullickson G Jr: Energy cost of ambulation in health and disability: A literature review. *Arch Phys Med Rehabil* 1978;59:124–133.
3. Pinzur MS, Gold J, Schwartz D, et al: Energy demands for walking in dysvascular amputees as related to the level of amputation. *Orthopedics* 1992;15:1033–1037.
4. Waters RL, Perry J, Antonelli D, et al: Energy cost of walking of amputees: The influence of level of amputation. *J Bone Joint Surg* 1976;58A:42–46.

5. Pinzur MS, Littooy F, Daniels J, et al: Multidisciplinary preoperative assessment and late function in dysvascular amputees. *Clin Orthop* 1992;281:239–243.
6. Volpicelli LJ, Chambers RB, Wagner FW Jr: Ambulation levels of bilateral lower-extremity amputees: Analysis of one hundred and three cases. *J Bone Joint Surg* 1983;65A:599–605.
7. Pinzur MS, Graham G, Osterman H: Psychologic testing in amputation rehabilitation. *Clin Orthop* 1988;229:236–240.
8. Pinzur MS: New concepts in lower-limb amputation and prosthetic management, in Greene WB: *Instructional Course Lectures XXXIX.* Park Ridge, IL, American Academy of Orthopaedic Surgeons, 1990, pp 361–366.
9. Dickhaut SC, DeLee JC, Page CP: Nutritional status: Importance in predicting wound-healing after amputation. *J Bone Joint Surg* 1984;66A:71–75.
10. Pinzur M, Kaminsky M, Sage R, et al: Amputations at the middle level of the foot: A retrospective and prospective review. *J Bone Joint Surg* 1986;68A:1061–1064.
11. Wagner FW Jr: Management of the diabetic-neurotrophic foot: Part II. A classification and treatment program for diabetic, neuropathic, and dysvascular foot problems, in Cooper RR (ed): American Academy of Orthopaedic Surgeons *Instructional Course Lectures XXVIII.* St. Louis, MO, CV Mosby, 1979, pp 143–165.
12. Emanuele MA, Buchanan BJ, Abraira C: Elevated leg systolic pressures and arterial calcification in diabetic occlusive vascular disease. *Diabetes Care* 1981;4:289–292.
13. Pinzur MS, Sage R, Stuck R, et al: Transcutaneous oxygen as a predictor of wound healing in amputations of the foot and ankle. *Foot Ankle Int* 1992;13:271–272.
14. Wyss CR, Harrington RM, Burgess EM, et al: Transcutaneous oxygen tension as a predictor of success after an amputation. *J Bone Joint Surg* 1988;70A:203–207.
15. Pinzur MS, Gottschalk F, Smith D, et al: Functional outcome of below-knee amputation in peripheral vascular insufficiency: A multicenter review. *Clin Orthop* 1993;286:247–249.
16. Pinzur MS, Sage R, Schwaegler P: Ray resection in the dysvascular foot: A retrospective review. *Clin Orthop* 1984;191:232–234.
17. Pinzur MS, Morrison C, Sage R, et al: Syme's two-stage amputation in insulin-requiring diabetics with gangrene of the forefoot. *Foot Ankle Int* 1991;11:394–396.
18. Pinzur MS, Smith D, Osterman H: Syme ankle disarticulation in peripheral vascular disease and diabetic foot infection: The one-stage versus two-stage procedure. *Foot Ankle Int* 1995; 16:124–127.
19. Robinson KP, Hoile R, Coddington T: Skew flap myoplastic below-knee amputation: A preliminary report. *Br J Surg* 1982; 69:554–557.
20. Radcliffe CW.: Four-bar linkage prosthetic knee mechanisms: Kinematics, alignment and prescription criteria. *Prosthet Orthot Int* 1994;18:159–173.
21. Pinzur MS, Smith DG, Daluga DJ, et al: Selection of patients for through-the-knee amputation. *J Bone Joint Surg* 1988;70A: 746–750.
22. Gottschalk FA, Kourosh S, Stills M, et al: Does socket configuration influence the position of the femur in above-knee amputation? *J Prosthet Orthot* 1989;2:94–102.
23. Gottschalk F: Transfemoral amputation: Surgical procedures, in Bowker JH, Michael JW (eds): *Atlas of Limb Prosthetics: Surgical Prosthetic and Rehabilitatiaon Principles,* ed 2. St. Louis, MO, Mosby-Year Book, 1992, pp 501–507.
24. Lagaard SW, McElfresh F: Gangrene of the upper extremity in diabetic patients. *J Bone Joint Surg* 1989;71A:257–264.

CHAPTER 50

Amputation Versus Limb Salvage

Paul Tornetta III, MD
Steven A. Olson, MD

Introduction

The decision to attempt limb salvage versus amputation of a severely injured limb is often one of the most difficult faced by the orthopaedic traumatologist. Because these injuries are relatively uncommon, it is difficult for the practicing orthopaedic surgeon to gain extensive clinical experience in this area. With few exceptions, these decisions are not clear-cut. Factors relating to the extremity injury, the overall injury, and the individual patient's lifestyle and support system must all influence the decision to salvage or amputate the limb.

The goal after limb-threatening injury is to provide the best outcome for the patient. We have all seen patients who have undergone multiple surgeries over a period of several years to "heroically" save a leg only to render the patient depressed, divorced, unemployed, and significantly disabled. These patients would obviously be better off if amputation was performed at the time of injury. The question is, can these patients be identified in the immediate postinjury period?

This chapter will attempt to provide an objective and subjective framework upon which to make these decisions in the case of acute injuries. Inherent in this discussion is the patient's psychological status and family situation. The same treatment may not be appropriate for the same injury in two different patients.

Which Injuries?

For which injuries should amputation be considered? All high grade open fractures with severe soft-tissue injury may be considered, including type IIIB injuries (requiring soft-tissue reconstruction) and blunt type IIIC injuries (requiring vascular repair).[1] The distinction between these two levels of injury is not always clear. Fractures with severe soft-tissue injury that have one or two vessels injured but still have adequate perfusion to maintain foot viability fall in between these categories. A vascular repair is not mandated, but the nonrepaired vascular injury may have a profound effect on outcome.[2] Open fractures that do not require vascular or significant soft-tissue reconstruction should not be considered for early amputation.

Factors Affecting Salvage

Ideally, the best indication for early amputation is an injury that precludes successful salvage and will ultimately result in a late amputation. Thus, multiple authors have tried to identify the factors that will predict the failure of salvage attempts.

One of these factors is vascular injury. The natural history of blunt type IIIC open fractures is amputation in the majority of cases (Table 1). Ischemia has such a profound effect on outcome that warm ischemia time of more than 6 hours has been suggested as an absolute indication for amputation.[7] However, successful salvage has been reported after more than 6 hours of ischemia.[9] The level and mechanism of the vascular injury is also of particular importance. Padberg and associates[4] reported an 83% amputation rate for patients with blunt infrapopliteal vascular injuries; this included 100% of those patients who had three vessels injured. They concluded that at least one tibial artery is necessary for salvage. In addition, Lazarides and associates[9] reported a 100% amputation rate for blunt trifurcation injuries.

A blunt vascular injury associated with a significant muscular crush component is very different from a vascular injury without significant soft-tissue damage.[4] In these cases, long bypass procedures may be capable of maintaining viability of the foot, but blood supply to the leg musculature is completely compromised. This condition frequently leads to difficulty obtaining union, a high incidence of infection, and a dysfunctional leg.[2,7] Even patients who present with a viable foot in the face of vascular injury are at risk to develop infection and nonunion, and amputation is likely.[2,10]

The degree of soft-tissue damage is the next important aspect of the injury. Successful coverage is needed to avoid infection. Inability to provide coverage with a good vascular supply will lead to infected nonunions

Table 1
Amputation rates for type IIIC injuries

Author	Percent Amputations
Georgiadis et al[3]	88%
Padberg et al[4]	88%
Caudle and Stern[5]	78%
Katzman and Dickson[6]	73%
Lange et al[7]	61%
Gustilo et al[1]	42%
Helfet et al[8]	40%

(Reproduced with permission from Turen CH, Di Stasio AJ: Treatment of grade III B and III C open tibial fractures. *Orthop Clin N Am* 1994;25:561-571.)

and eventual amputation in many cases. Even delays in obtaining coverage are associated with much higher rates of infection.[11,12]

Associated injuries and patient factors also have a bearing on the ability to salvage a mangled extremity. Patient age, overall injury score, the presence of shock or compartment syndrome, fluid balance, comorbidities, and preoperative status of the leg all have important prognostic implications.[3,13-18]

Scoring Systems

Several investigators have attempted to create scoring systems by quantifying the factors that predict failure of salvage attempts. These scores were devised based on the factors known to be important in predicting failure as reviewed in the preceding paragraphs. In general, the scores were then retrospectively applied to a series of patients in whom salvage was attempted to determine the critical score that predicts amputation.

Gregory and associates[13] defined the term "mangled extremity" as an extremity with injury to three or more of its organ systems: integument, nerves, vessels, and bone. They developed the mangled extremity severity index (MESI), as described in Table 2. This index considers ten different factors: injury severity score, injury to integument, nerve, and bone, both arterial and venous injury, delay of more than 6 hours in treatment, patient age, preexisting disease, and shock. A score of less than 20 was believed to be indicative of limb salvage. Of the 17 cases reviewed in this series, 12 were lower extremity injuries, and five were upper extremity injuries. Vascular injury was present in 16 of 17 cases. The MESI is cumbersome to use, because multiple injuries, eg, segmental arterial injuries, are scored more than once.

Howe and associates[14] studied 21 lower extremity injuries associated with vascular disruptions. These included 12 tibia fractures, five femur fractures, two knee dislocations, and two symphysis pubis diastasis. They found four criteria useful in predicting limb salvage versus amputation: level of arterial injury (suprapopliteal to infrapopliteal), degree of bone injury, degree of muscle injury, and interval from injury until arrival in the operating room. Each of these four factors was scored in a predictive salvage index (PSI) (Table 3). A score of 8 or more was 78% sensitive and 100% specific for eventual amputation. The authors found that infrapopliteal arterial injuries and associated venous injuries had a poor prognosis for salvage.

Russell and associates[18] reviewed 70 lower extremity injuries with major arterial trauma. An associated musculoskeletal injury was found in 57 cases; 22 were considered type IIIC open fractures. These authors developed the limb salvage index (LSI) (Table 4). This index considers seven factors: arterial injury, injury to nerve, bone, skin, and muscle, deep vein injury, and warm ischemia time. The authors consider absolute indications for amputation to be (1) limb salvage index of 6 or greater; and (2) a type IIIC open fracture with an associated nerve injury. The patient with a severely traumatized extremity with an associated sciatic or tibial nerve injury is a candidate for amputation.

Johansen and associates[19] reviewed the experience of 26 type IIIC open fractures and developed the mangled extremity severity score (MESS), presented in Table 5. The score is based on four factors: skeletal/soft-tissue injury, shock, patient age, and ischemia. The MESS was applied in a prospective manner to an additional 26 lower extremity type IIIC open fractures. In both the retrospective and prospective evaluations a MESS greater than 7 was 100% predictive of amputation. The authors stress that the MESS should be used to aid in decision-making along with, and not in place of, clinical judgment.

Table 2
Mangled extremity syndrome index (MESI) grading system

Injury Severity Score:	
0-25	1
25-50	2
> 50	3
Integument	
Guillotine	1
Crush/burn	2
Avulsion/degloving	3
Nerve	
Contusion	1
Transection	2
Avulsion	3
Vascular	
Artery	
Transected	1
Thrombosed	2
Avulsed	3
Vein	1
Bone	
Simple Fx*	1
Segmental Fx	2
Segmental-comminuted Fx	3
Segmental-comminuted Fx with bone loss < 6 cm	4
Segmental Fx intra- or extra-articular	5
Segmental Fx intra- or extra-articular with bone loss > 6 cm	6
(If bone loss is greater than 6 cm, add 1)	
Lag time (1 point for every hr > 6)	
Age	
40 to 50 years	1
50 to 60 years	2
60 to 70 years	3
Preexisting disease	1
Shock	2
Total score (Mangled Extremity Severity Index)	

*Fx, fracture

(Reproduced with permission from Gregory RT, Gould RJ, Peclet M, et al: The mangled extremity syndrome (MES): A severity grading system for multisystem injury of the extremity. *J Trauma* 1985;25:1147–1150.)

An attempt to modify the MESS has separated the skeletal/soft-tissue score into separate categories of nerve injury, skeletal injury, and soft-tissue (muscle) injury,[20] resulting in the NISSSA score (Table 6), an acronym for Nerve injury, Ischemia, Soft-tissue contamination, Skeletal, Shock, and Age.

Effectiveness of Scoring

Attempts by other investigators to apply these scoring systems have not met with the same success that the original authors described. Bonanni and associates[21] reported a review of 58 patients with severe lower extremity injuries who had undergone attempted limb salvage, and compared the actual outcome with that predicted by the MESI, PSI, LSI, and MESS. The authors modified the definition of a mangled extremity from that of Gregory and associates[13] to include injuries with more than 5 cm of segmental bone loss and those requiring muscle flap coverage. Forty-five of the 58 patients required a vascular repair. The sensitivity and specificity, respectively, of each score were MESI, 0.06 and 0.90; PSI, 0.33 and 0.70; LSI, 0.61 and 0.43; and MESS, 0.22 and 0.53 (Table 7). The authors found that none of the scoring systems performed satisfactorily in their patient population.

Poole and associates[22] reported on 48 mangled lower extremities with associated arterial injuries. Amputation was best predicted by injury to the sciatic or tibial nerves and failed vascular repair. The overall accuracy of limb salvage scoring systems was PSI, 71%; MESS, 77%; and LSI, 85%. Robertson[15] reported on 164 severely injured lower extremities. Of the 121 limbs eventually amputated, early amputation was performed on 30. Vascular repair was required in 18 patients. Robertson evaluated only the MESS and found that 100% of limbs with a score greater than 7 were amputated. However, 43 limbs with a MESS less than 7 were amputated.

Table 3
Point system for Predictive Salvage Index

Variable	Points
Level of arterial injury	
Suprapopliteal	1
Popliteal	2
Infrapopliteal	3
Degree of bone injury	
Mild	1
Moderate	2
Severe	3
Degree of muscle injury	
Mild	1
Moderate	2
Severe	3
Interval from injury until arrival in the operating room	
< 6 hours	0
6 to 12 hours	2
> 12 hours	4

Total points = Predictive Salvage Index

(Reproduced with permission from Howe HR Jr, Poole GV Jr, Hansen KJ, et al: Salvage of lower extremities following combined orthopedic and vascular trauma: A predictive salvage index. *Am Surg* 1987;53:205–208.)

Roessler and associates[16] reported on 14 patients with isolated lower extremity fractures and arterial injury who underwent attempted limb salvage. Three deaths were related to the attempted limb salvage. A positive fluid balance of greater than 3 liters at 24 hours after revascularization was found to be associated with mortality following limb salvage. The authors also compared the actual outcomes with those predicted by the various scoring systems. The PSI predicted salvage for five limbs that were amputated, and amputation in two limbs that were salvaged. The MESI predicted salvage in four limbs that were amputated, and amputation in five limbs that were salvaged. The MESS predicted salvage in five limbs that were amputated, and amputation in two limbs that were salvaged.

These evaluations of scoring systems indicate that none of the systems are accurate in all cases, at least partly because any scoring system is affected by the subjective nature of the determination of the degree of soft-tissue injury, as well as extent of ischemia, and true venous injury. Large variations have been documented in interobserver agreement of classification of open fractures, emphasizing the subjective nature of soft-tissue injury assessment.[23] The more specific the assessment of soft tissue becomes, and the more objective data that scoring systems incorporate, the harder these scoring systems will become to apply. These systems are a good beginning in the decision-making process, but should not be applied rigidly.

Finally, it must also be understood that scoring systems are an attempt to assess our technical ability to salvage an extremity. As such, institutional and technical considerations as well as resource availability and individual surgeon experience play a large role. A surgeon who treats only a small number of trauma patients without backup from a multidisciplinary team cannot expect to have the same results as those obtained in a level 1 trauma center where significant resources are devoted to treating these injuries. Even in major centers, availability of special personnel can affect outcome on a patient to patient basis.

Factors Affecting Outcome

Until recently, attempts at limb salvage were considered to be desirable if at all possible. Planned protocols of multiple operations including serial debridements, bony stabilization, soft-tissue reconstruction, and one or more bone grafts leading to limb salvage were viewed as heroic. From a surgical viewpoint, the suc-

Table 4
Limb Salvage Index

Location	Points	Extent of Injury
Artery	0	Contusion, intimal tear, partial laceration or avulsion (pseudoaneurysm) with no distal thrombosis and palpable pedal pulses; complete occlusion of one of three shank vessels or profunda.
	1	Occlusion of two or more shank vessels, complete laceration, avulsion or thrombosis of femoral or popliteal vessels without palpable pedal pulses.
	2	Complete occlusion of femoral, popliteal, or three of three shank vessels with no distal runoff available.
Nerve	0	Contusion or stretch injury; minimal clean laceration of femoral, popliteal, or tibial nerve.
	1	Partial transection or avulsion of sciatic nerve; complete or partial transection of femoral, peroneal, or tibial nerve.
	2	Complete transection or avulsion of sciatic nerve; complete transection or avulsion of both peroneal and tibial nerves.
Bone	0	Closed fracture one or two sites; open fracture without comminution or with minimal displacement; closed dislocation without fracture; open joint without foreign body; fibula fracture.
	1	Closed fracture at three or more sites on same extremity; open fracture with comminution or moderate to large displacement; segmental fracture; fracture dislocation; open joint with foreign body; bone loss < 3 cm
	2	Bone loss > 3 cm; type IIIB or IIIC fracture (open fracture with periosteal stripping, gross contamination, extensive soft-tissue injury-loss).
Skin	0	Clean laceration, single or multiple, or small avulsion injuries, all with primary repair; first degree burn.
	1	Delayed closure due to contamination; large avulsion requiring split thickness skin graft or flap closure. Second and third degree burns.
Muscle	0	Laceration or avulsion involving a single compartment or single tendon.
	1	Laceration or avulsion involving two or more compartments; complete laceration or avulsion of two or more tendons.
	2	Crush injury.
Deep vein	0	Contusion, partial laceration, or avulsion; complete laceration or avulsion if alternate route of venous return is intact; superficial vein injury.
	1	Complete laceration, avulsion, or thrombosis with no alternate route of venous return.
Warm ischemia time	0	< 6 hours
	1	6 to 9 hours
	2	9 to 12 hours
	3	12 to 15 hours
	4	> 15 hours

(Reproduced with permission from Russell WL, Sailors DM, Whittle TB, et al: Limb salvage versus traumatic amputation: A decision based on a seven-part predictive index. *Ann Surg* 1991;213:473–481.)

cesses of these protocols represent a true technical achievement.[24,25] However, the functional results obtained in some cases may prove to demonstrate a triumph of technology over reason. The desired outcome is for the patient to resume preinjury activity; in some instances, this end may be better met with an amputation rather than prolonged salvage. An example of this is in the case of neurologic impairment, particularly of the posterior tibial nerve. Because the posterior tibial nerve provides plantar sensation, salvage may not be advisable if this nerve is damaged. Lange and associates[7] recommended amputation for these patients.

Multiple reports describing the functional results after prolonged salvage reveal less than perfect results. Francel and associates[26] reported a 93% salvage rate after soft-tissue reconstruction in 72 patients with type IIIB injuries. The functional assessment of these limbs demonstrated decreased ankle motion in 66%, the use of ambulation aids in 50%, problems with edema in 44%, and return to work in only 28%. The same group of authors was able to increase the rate of return to work to 65% using a more aggressive protocol of earlier soft-tissue reconstruction.[27] Variables relating to the patient, rather than the injury, were found to correlate with return to work. Age younger than 40, higher education, and a white collar job were predictors of return to work. In a smaller series, Laughlin and associates[28] reported seven of nine patients to return to work after

Table 5
Mangled Extremity Severity Score

Type	Characteristics	Injuries*	Points
Skeletal/soft-tissue			
Group			
1	Low energy	Stab wounds, simple closed fractures, small-caliber gunshot wounds	1
2	Medium energy	Open or multiple-level fractures, dislocations, moderate crush injuries	2
3	High energy	Shotgun blast (close range), high-velocity gunshot wounds	3
4	Massive crush	Logging, railroad, oil rig accidents	4
Shock			
Group			
1	Normotensive hemodynamics	BP stable in field and in OR	0
2	Transiently hypotensive	BP unstable in field but responsive to intravenous fluids	1
3	Prolonged hypotension	Systolic BP less than 90 mmHg in field and responsive to intravenous fluid only in OR	2
Ischemia			
Group			
1	None	A pulsatile limb without signs of ischemia	0†
2	Mild	Diminished pulses without signs of ischemia	1†
3	Moderate	No pulse by Doppler, sluggish capillary refill paresthesia, diminished motor activity	2†
4	Advanced	Pulseless, cool, paralyzed and numb without capillary refill	3†
Age			
Group			
1	< 30 years		0
2	> 30 < 50 years		1
3	> 50 years		2

*OR, operating room; BP, blood pressure
†Points × 2 if ischemic time exceeds 6 hours
(Reproduced with permission from Johansen K, Paines M, Howey T, et al: Objective criteria accurately predict amputation following lower extremity trauma. *J Trauma* 1990;30:568-573.)

free-flap coverage. However, infection was present in six of the nine.

Georgiadis and associates[3] compared 27 patients in whom salvage was attempted with 18 patients who had an early amputation for the treatment of tibia fractures with severe soft-tissue injuries. Five of the salvage attempts resulted in amputation. The patients with successfully salvaged legs were found to have had more surgeries, longer hospital stays, and a longer time to weightbearing. They were less willing to work, more likely to consider themselves severely disabled, and had greater problems with recreational activities.

The outcome of patients who had an early amputation as definitive treatment was reviewed by Purry and Hannon.[29] Twenty-five patients younger than age 45 when injured were evaluated 2 to 12 years after injury. Ninety-six percent returned to work and 84% did not consider themselves significantly disabled. These patients routinely wore their prosthesis for more than 13 hours a day. However, it took approximately 1 year to reach this functional level and 72% of these patients complained of phantom limb or stump pain at follow-up.

Another retrospective series of amputation versus salvage was reported by Dahl and associates.[30] They used a matched cohort of 30 patients found in an amputation database to compare with 49 patients in whom salvage was done using free-flap soft-tissue reconstruction. Many of these patients were treated with a flap for osteomyelitis (36%) or exposed bone (30%). The patients treated with free flaps had higher rates of pain and edema. However, there were no significant differences in long-term functional or social outcomes. The authors also concluded that early rather than reconstructive soft-tissue reconstruction should lead to even better results. Pedersen and Damholt[31] evaluated 22 patients who underwent amputation at an average of 2 months after lower extremity injury. Sixty-seven percent returned to work. Eleven of the 22 (50%) were completely independent, six could manage their own personal care, and five required help with personal care. Older patients did not fare as well as younger patients in terms of return to work or the need for help with activities of daily living.

Associated Injuries

In addition to determining the possibility of salvage and the resultant long-term outcome, the immediate effects of salvage attempts require evaluation. Patients with other severe injuries may be better served with

Table 6
NISSSA rating criteria

Type of injury	Degree of injury	Points	Description†
Nerve injury N	Sensate	0	No major nerve injury
	Dorsal	1	Deep or superficial peroneal nerve, femoral nerve injury§
	Plantar partial	2	Tibial nerve injury§
	Plantar complete	3	Sciatic nerve injury§
Ischemia I	None	0	Good to fair pulses, no ischemia
	Mild	1*	Reduced pulses, perfusion normal
	Moderate	2*	No pulse(s), prolonged capillary refill, Doppler pulses present
	Severe	3*	Pulseless, cool, ischemic, no Doppler pulses
Soft-tissue/ contamination S	Low	0	Minimal to no ST contusion, no contamination [Gustilo type I]
	Medium	1	Moderate ST injury, low-velocity GSW, moderate contamination, minimal crush [Gustilo type II]
	High	2	Moderate crush, deglove, high velocity GSW, moderate ST injury may require soft-tissue flap, considerable contamination [Gustilo type IIIA]
	Severe	3	Massive crush, farm injury, severe deglove, severe contamination, requires soft-tissue flap [Gustilo type IIIB]
Skeletal S	Low energy	0	Spiral fracture, oblique fracture, no or minimal displacement [Winquist and Hansen type I, Johner and Wruhs A_1, A_2]
	Medium energy	1	Transverse fracture, minimal comminution, small caliber GSW [Winquist and Hansen type II, Johner and Wruhs A_3, B_1]
	High energy	2	Moderate displacement, moderate comminution, high velocity GSW, butterfly fragment(s) [Winquist and Hansen type III-IV, Johner and Wruhs B_1, B_2, B_3]
	Severe energy	3	Segmental, severe comminution, bony loss [Winquist and Hansen type IV, Johner and Wruhs C_1, C_2, C_3]
Shock S	Normotensive	0	Blood pressure normal, always > 90 mm Hg systolic
	Transient hypotension	1	Transient hypotension in field or emergency center
	Persistent hypotension	2	Persistent hypotension despite fluids
Age A	Young	0	< 30 yrs
	Middle	1	30 to 50 yrs
	Old	2	> 50 yrs
Total score (N + I + S + S +S + A)			

*Score doubles with ischemia > 6 h
† GSW, gunshot wound; ST, soft tissue
§ Nerve injury as assessed primarily in emergency room
(Reproduced with permission from McNamara MG, Heckman JD, Corley FG: Severe open fractures of the lower extremity: A retrospective evaluation of the Mangled Extremity Severity Score (MESS). *J Orthop Trauma* 1994;8:8–87.)

an immediate amputation rather than prolonged surgery to reestablish perfusion of a limb that will contribute to the patient's overall catabolic state.[32] Indeed, Tscherne and associates in Hanover have recommended that patients with a severely injured extremity, ie, a type III open fracture as well as a closed fracture with Tscherne type IV soft-tissue injury, undergo a primary amputation when the polytrauma score is greater than 3 (roughly equivalent to an Injury Severity Score of greater than 40).[17] The concept of damage control via amputation to help save a patient's life cannot be overemphasized. These considerations are even more important in the face of chronic comorbidities such as diabetes, cardiac history, or pulmonary compromise.

Ipsilateral ankle and foot injuries may also make amputation more likely.[33] The prognosis for isolated high grade open foot injuries is poor, and this type of injury in combination with a high grade open tibia fracture makes salvage more difficult. Preinjury status of the leg has similar implications. Many preinjury variables, including vascular insufficiency, age, smoking, and sensation, also affect the ability to salvage the limb.

Social Considerations

The final area that impacts on the decision to amputate is related to the patient's social situation. This includes the patient's wishes, desires, occupation, social support system, reliability, and financial status. These factors are difficult to quantitate during the initial

Table 7
Predictive value of scoring systems[21]

Score	Sensitivity	Specificity
MESI	6%	90%
MESS	22%	53%
PSI	33%	70%
LSI	61%	43%

surgery, but family members may be of some help. A patient who cannot afford to be out of work for a prolonged period, has little or no social support system, and is not reliable is a poor candidate for prolonged salvage attempts.

Cost

As managed care becomes more of a force in determining the treatment of patients, the cost/benefit ratio will also become more important. More of the responsibility for the cost of treatments will be assumed by the patient. The estimated cost of an acute amputation was $29,000 and a late amputation $54,000 in 1988.[34] Identification of patients who will require or benefit from amputation as opposed to limb salvage may help to enable physicians to maintain some control over these decisions.

Summary

The decision to attempt salvage or to amputate a severely injured leg is among the most difficult that the orthopaedist must face. Even surgeons with tremendous trauma experience cannot agree on a standard course of action. In the face of such injuries, physician consultation regarding the treatment decision, including all of those members of the team that are needed for a successful salvage, is necessary. In the best circumstances, the trauma surgeon, vascular surgeon, orthopaedist, and a soft-tissue specialist are all involved.

From a psychological perspective, the timing of an amputation is important. Although each patient's case is unique, immediate amputation is often viewed by the patient and family as a result of the injury. Conversely, a delayed amputation may be viewed as a failure of treatment. It is imperative that the surgeon have a detailed discussion with the patient and the family whenever possible before making these decisions.

Scoring systems are of some help in estimating the chances of a successful salvage. However, the ultimate decision to amputate or attempt salvage is based on such patient factors as preinjury function and social situation, and on associated injuries, surgeon experience, available resources, projected physical abilities, and the patient's projected physical requirements. These decisions are difficult and tax the judgment and emotions of the patient, family, and physician.

References

1. Gustilo RB, Mendoza RM, Williams DN: Problems in the management of type III (severe) open fractures: A new classification of type III open fractures. *J Trauma* 1984;24:742–746.
2. Shah DM, Corson JD, Karmody AM, et al: Optimal management of tibial arterial trauma. *J Trauma* 1988;28:228–234.
3. Georgiadis GM, Behrens FF, Joyce MJ, et al: Open tibial fractures with severe soft-tissue loss: Limb salvage compared with below-the-knee amputation. *J Bone Joint Surg* 1993;75A:1431–1441.
4. Padberg FT Jr, Rubelowsky JJ, Hernandez-Maldonado JJ, et al: Infrapopliteal arterial injury: Prompt revascularization affords optimal limb salvage. *J Vasc Surg* 1992;16:877–886.
5. Caudle RJ, Stern PJ: Severe open fractures of the tibia. *J Bone Joint Surg* 1987;69A:801–807.
6. Katzman SS, Dickson K: Determining the prognosis for limb salvage in major vascular injuries with associated open tibial fractures. *Orthop Rev* 1992;21:195–199.
7. Lange RH, Bach AW, Hansen ST Jr, et al: Open tibial fractures with associated vascular injuries: Prognosis for limb salvage. *J Trauma* 1985;25:203–208.
8. Helfet DL, Howey T, Sanders R, et al: Limb salvage versus amputation: Preliminary results of the Mangled Extremity Severity Score. *Clin Orthop* 1990;256:80–86.
9. Lazarides MK, Arvanitis DP, Kopadis GC, et al: Popliteal artery and trifurcation injuries: Is it possible to predict the outcome? *Eur J Vasc Surg* 1994;8:226–230.
10. Dickson K, Katzman S, Delgado E, et al: Delayed unions and nonunions of open tibial fractures: Correlation with arteriography results. *Clin Orthop* 1994;302:189–193.
11. Fischer MD, Gustilo RB, Varecka TF: The timing of flap coverage, bone grafting, and intermedullary nailing in patients who have a fracture of the tibial shaft with extensive soft-tissue injury. *J Bone Joint Surg* 1991;73A:1316–1322.
12. Ostermann PA, Henry SL, Seligson D: Timing of wound closure in severe compound fractures. *Orthopedics* 1994;17:397–399.
13. Gregory RT, Gould RJ, Peclet M, et al: The mangled extremity syndrome (MES): A severity grading system for multisystem injury of the extremity. *J Trauma* 1985;25:1147–1150.
14. Howe HR Jr, Poole GV Jr, Hansen KJ, et al: Salvage of lower extremities following combined orthopedic and vascular trauma: A predictive salvage index. *Am Surg* 1987;53:205–208.
15. Robertson PA: Prediction of amputation after severe lower limb trauma. *J Bone Joint Surg* 1991;73B:816–818.
16. Roessler MS, Wisner DH, Holcroft JW: The mangled extremity: When to amputate? *Arch Surg* 1991;126:1243–1249.
17. Sudkamp N, Haas N, Flory PJ, et al: Criteria for amputation, reconstruction and replantation of extremities in multiple trauma patients. *Chirurg* 1989;60:774–781.
18. Russell WL, Sailors DM, Whittle TB, et al: Limb salvage versus traumatic amputation: A decision based on a seven-part predictive index. *Ann Surg* 1991;213:473–481.

19. Johansen K, Daines M, Howey T, et al: Objective criteria accurately predict amputation following lower extremity trauma. *J Trauma* 1990;30:568–573.
20. McNamara MG, Heckman JD, Corley FG: Severe open fractures of the lower extremity: A retrospective evaluation of the Mangled Extremity Severity Score (MESS). *J Orthop Trauma* 1994;8:81–87.
21. Bonanni F, Rhodes M, Lucke JF: The futility of predictive scoring of mangled lower extremities. *J Trauma* 1993;34:99–104.
22. Poole GV, Agnew SG, Griswold JA, et al: The mangled lower extremity: Can salvage be predicted? *Am Surg* 1994;60:50–55.
23. Brumback RJ, Jones AL: Interobserver agreement in the classification of open fractures of the tibia: The results of a survey of two hundred and forty-five orthopaedic surgeons. *J Bone Joint Surg* 1994;76A:1162–1166.
24. Edwards CC: Staged reconstruction of complex open tibial fractures using Hoffmann external fixation: Clinical decision and dilemmas. *Clin Orthop* 1983;178:130–161.
25. Tornetta P III, Bergman M, Watnik N, et al: Treatment of grade IIIB open tibial fractures: A prospective randomised comparison of external fixation and non-reamed locked nailing. *J Bone Joint Surg* 1994;76B:13–19.
26. Francel TJ, Vander Kolk CA, Hoopes JE, et al: Microvascular soft-tissue transplantation for reconstruction of acute open tibial fractures: Timing of coverage and long-term functional results. *Plast Reconstr Surg* 1992;89:478–489.
27. Francel TJ: Improving reemployment rates after limb salvage of acute severe tibial fractures by microvascular soft-tissue reconstruction. *Plast Reconstr Surg* 1994;93:1028–1034.
28. Laughlin RT, Smith KL, Russell RC, et al: Late functional outcome in patients with tibia fractures covered with free muscle flaps. *J Orthop Trauma* 1993;7:123–129.
29. Purry NA, Hannon MA: How successful is below-knee amputation for injury? *Injury* 1989;20:32–36.
30. Dahl B, Andersson AP, Andersen M, et al: Functional and social long-term results after free tissue transfer to the lower extremity. *Ann Plast Surg* 1995;34:372–375.
31. Pedersen P, Damholt V: Rehabilitation after amputation following lower limb fracture. *J Trauma* 1994;36:195–197.
32. Hervé C, Gaillard M, Andrivet P, et al: Treatment in serious lower limb injuries: Amputation versus preservation. *Injury* 1987;18:21–23.
33. Sanders R, Pappas J, Mast J, et al: The salvage of open grade IIIB ankle and talus fractures. *J Orthop Trauma* 1992;6:201–208.
34. Bondurant FJ, Cotler HB, Buckle R, et al: The medical and economic impact of severely injured lower extremities. *J Trauma* 1988;28:1270–1273.

Additional Areas of Interest

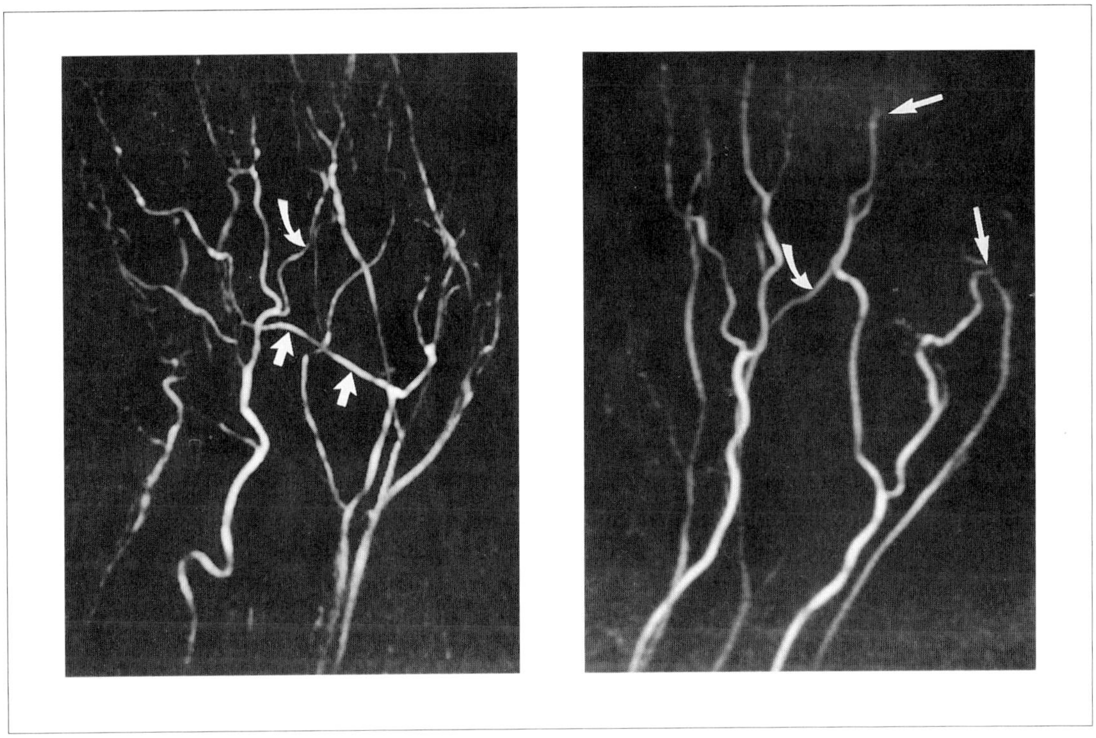

CHAPTER 51

Advanced Imaging in Orthopaedics: Current Pitfalls and New Applications

Hollis G. Potter, MD
Mark E. Schweitzer, MD
David W. Altchek, MD

Current opinion suggests that magnetic resonance imaging (MRI) is limited by poor specificity[1,2] and does not aid in patient management. Careful scrutiny of many studies, however, shows little attempt to standardize MR pulse sequences, while a review of studies performed with more vigilant attention to sequence standardization demonstrates significantly higher sensitivity and specificity[3,4] in detecting meniscal tears, rotator cuff tears, and labral pathology. While this improved accuracy in the detection of joint pathology is encouraging, it is important to correlate the MRI with the clinical examination, because abnormal MRI findings are moderately prevalent in asymptomatic individuals, particularly in those of advancing age.[5] In an increasingly cost conscious medical environment, the clinical value of advanced imaging tests is placed into question. On an individual joint-by-joint basis, MRI techniques will be presented that facilitate accurate diagnosis, describe recent MRI advancements, and aid in clinical management. High-resolution, high-contrast techniques will be demonstrated that obviate the need for intra-articular contrast injection, particularly in the upper extremity, thus maintaining the noninvasive advantage of MRI.

Shoulder Imaging

Rotator Cuff

Previous authors have reported high sensitivity and specificity of noncontrast MRI of the shoulder in assessing tears of the rotator cuff tendons.[3,4] In the setting of a partial tear, however, the accuracy of noncontrast MRI has been placed into question.[6] Using high field strength MR units, fat-suppression techniques, and higher resolution fast spin echo sequences, noncontrast MRI may provide an accurate depiction of both the articular and bursal side of the rotator cuff (Fig. 1). Given the tomographic nature of the technique, MRI can assess the size of the tear and the quality of the underlying tissue, and thus help to identify those patients who are suitable candidates for arthroscopic or open tendon repair. Oblique sagittal T1-weighted images may be used as a "survey view," to assess for disproportionate atrophy of muscle, distinguishing chronic tear from primary denervation.

A pitfall of MRI evaluation of the rotator cuff is the overlooked subscapularis tendon,[7-9] which is best visualized in the axial plane. On axial images, localization of the long head of the biceps tendon posterior to the subscapularis indicates a tear of the subscapularis tendon (Fig. 2).

Glenohumeral Ligaments/Labrum

Increasing attention has been directed toward preoperative evaluation of the glenoid labrum and capsular mechanism. Previous anatomic studies[10] have outlined the importance of the glenohumeral ligaments in providing both translational and rotational stability, particularly at the extremes of motion. The concavity of the relatively shallow glenoid fossa is increased by the fibrocartilaginous labrum. Because clinically apparent glenohumeral instability may be due to primary capsular stretch and/or a true Bankart lesion involving the labrum, appropriate clinical management of the instability depends both on clinical findings and on imaging techniques that provide accurate visualization of the

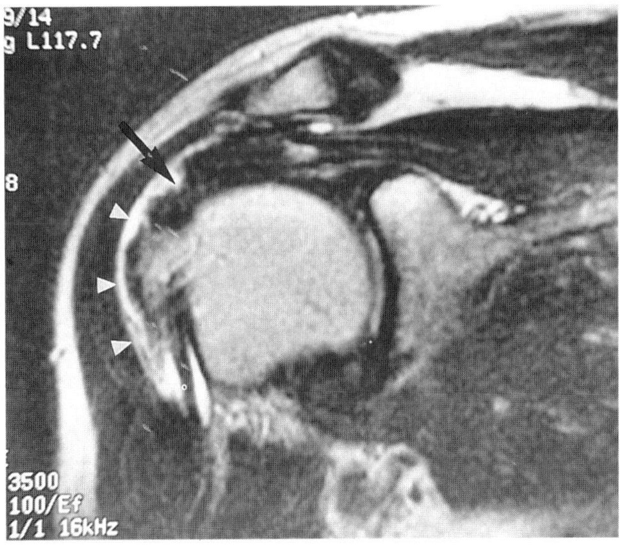

Fig. 1 Oblique coronal T2-weighted MRI of the right shoulder in a 65-year-old patient demonstrates an arthroscopically confirmed bursal side partial thickness tear of the supraspinatus tendon (black arrow). Associated fluid is seen in the subacromial/subdeltoid bursa (arrowheads).

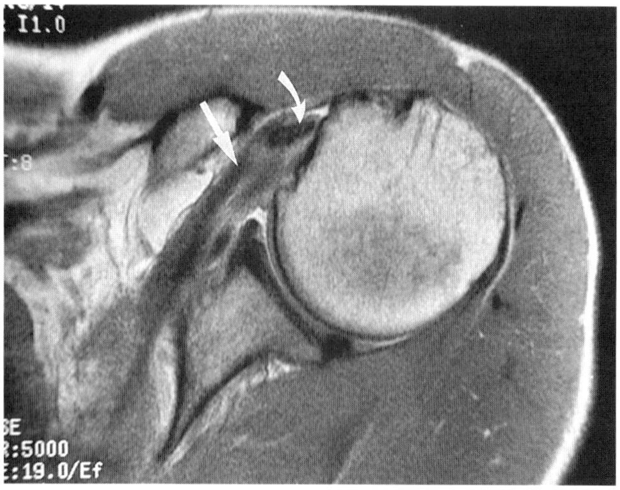

Fig. 2 Axial high resolution fast spin echo image through the left shoulder demonstrating medial subluxation of the long head of the biceps tendon (curved arrow), which lies posterior to the subscapularis tendon (straight arrow). This finding indicates a complete tear of the subscapularis tendon, which was confirmed at surgery.

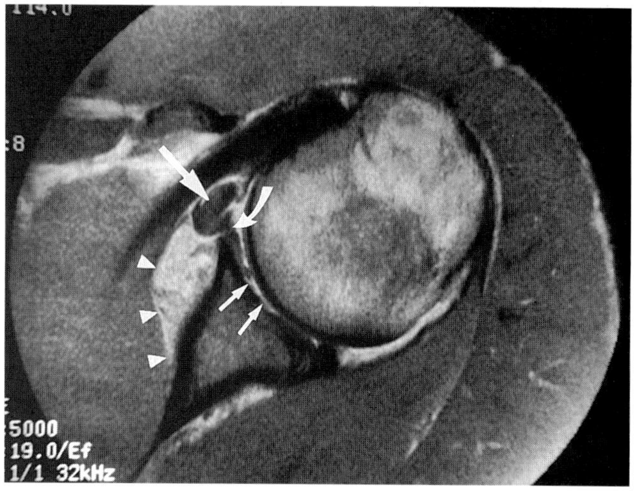

Fig. 3 Axial high resolution fast spin echo image demonstrates detached anterior labral tear (curved arrow), as well as complete stripping of the anterior capsule off the scapula (arrowheads). Additional injury is seen to the middle glenohumeral ligament (straight arrow) which appears thickened and hyperintense. Also of note is severe chondral shear injury off the glenoid, with marked thinning of the articular cartilage (small straight arrows). At surgery, a Bankart lesion was confirmed, as well as the associated articular cartilage injury.

supporting structures of the shoulder. The differentiation between capsular laxity and a Bankart lesion may not be readily apparent on clinical examination, and the distinction may have prognostic significance in patient outcome and predisposition to recurrent dislocation.[11]

Recent MRI research has been dedicated to the development of sequences that differentiate clearly between hyaline and fibrocartilage, and the adjacent capsule and glenohumeral ligaments. MRI arthrography has been promoted in the detection of labral injuries, using both saline and gadolinium as contrast agents.[12-14] While MRI arthrography does provide contrast between the high signal intensity joint fluid and low signal labral-capsular complex, it converts MRI into an invasive procedure and increases the cost of the study. Recent advances in MRI technology allow for faster imaging times, improved spatial resolution, and soft-tissue contrast, which may be achieved without the use of intra-articular contrast agents (Fig. 3). In a prospective evaluation of 103 patients, all of whom had arthroscopic evaluation, overall accuracy of MRI was 95% in the detection and localization of labral tears, differentiating between anterior, superior, and posterior labral tears.[15] The ability to detect superior labral tears is of particular interest, because these injuries may be clinically occult, with no consistently reliable clinical test to detect the presence of the SLAP lesion. The controversy of noncontrast MRI versus MRI arthrography in the detection of primary capsular injuries still exists, with no broad-based acceptance for the use of MRI arthrography.

Elbow Imaging

The use of three-dimensional volumetric gradient echo and fast spin echo techniques have been added to the software advances in MRI, enabling thin (less than 3 mm) section imaging of structures of the elbow, including the collateral ligaments and the extensor and flexor tendons. Such sequences impart improved visualization of partial tears of ligaments and musculotendinous units (Fig. 4). On the medial side of the elbow, the medial collateral ligament has been found to be the primary stabilizer of the elbow.[16] Biomechanical studies have determined that, in particular, the anterior bundle of the medial collateral ligament is the prime stabilizer to valgus stress.[17,18] Although well described in the competitive throwing athlete,[19] injury to the medial collateral ligament in recreational athletes may also impart significant disability in normal elbow function. Rupture is typically the result of chronic overuse,[20] with repetitive stresses leading to collagen degeneration and microscopic attritional tears.

Despite the significance of such injury, physical examination is often limited in the detection of medial collateral ligament injury. Furthermore, distinction between medial collateral ligament injury and common flexor/pronator pathology (medial epicondylitis) may not be possible in all patients. Whereas complete disruptions of the medial collateral ligament often result in clinically apparent valgus instability, partial disruptions are typically clinically occult injuries. As

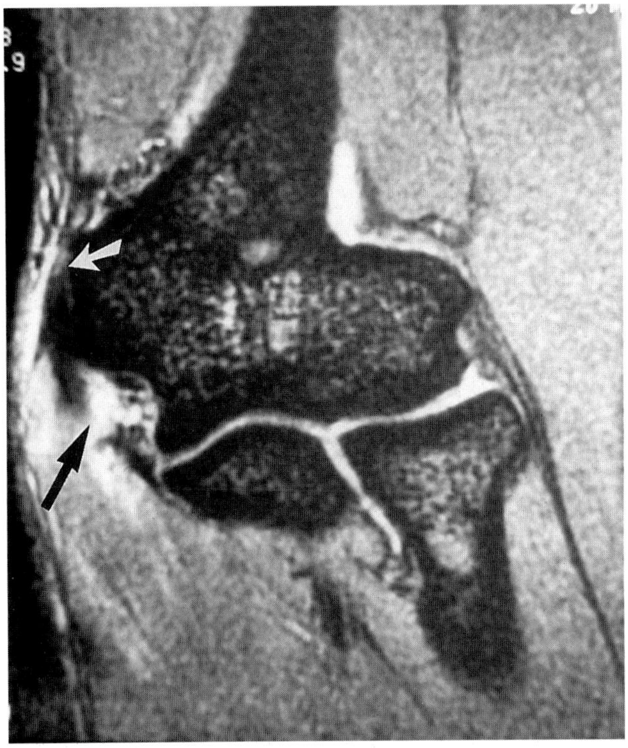

Fig. 4 Coronal gradient recalled MRI, using a 1.5-mm section through the right elbow in a competitive throwing athlete. MRI demonstrates a complete tear of the medial collateral ligament (black arrow). The patient had pain and tenderness at the medial epicondyle, at the origin of the common flexor/pronator mass. MRI examination confirmed that the flexor/pronator origin was preserved (white arrow).

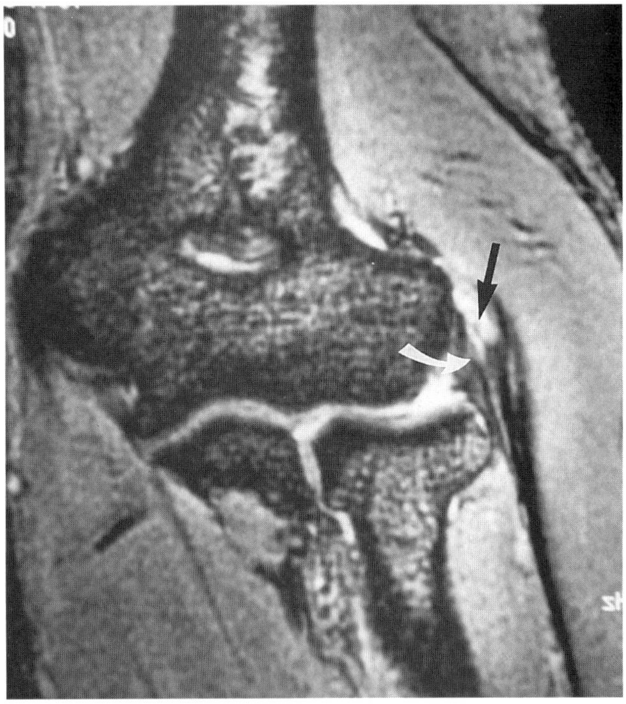

Fig. 5 Coronal gradient recalled MRI section (1.5 mm) through the left elbow in a patient with clinically diagnosed recalcitrant lateral epicondylitis. MRI demonstrates frank detachment of the degenerated extensor carpi radialis brevis origin (black arrow). Note the intact radial collateral ligament (curved white arrow).

increasing emphasis has been placed on ligament preservation rather than primary reconstruction, preoperative localization of the site of ligament tear aids in surgical planning. Arthroscopic evaluation of the medial collateral ligament has been shown to be limited in the visualization of the anterior bundle and humeral or ulnar insertions,[21,22] emphasizing the need to provide accurate imaging techniques.

Previous authors have advocated the use of saline or gadolinium contrast to assess the undersurface of the collateral ligament, particularly in the detection of small undersurface tears contained within the capsule of the joint.[23,24] While MRI arthrography provides greater contrast between the low signal intensity ligament and surrounding joint, it converts the noninvasive MRI to an invasive procedure, limiting its wide acceptance.

Evaluation of the lateral aspect of the elbow similarly requires high contrast thin section techniques, in order to distinguish the extensor carpi radialis longus and brevis tendons from the adjacent radial collateral ligament. On such pulse sequences, the classic appearance of lateral epicondylitis is a focus of increased signal at the origin of the extensor carpi radialis brevis (Fig. 5), indicating intrasubstance degeneration. Studies providing histologic correlation have demonstrated that the increased signal intensity on MRI correlates to neovascularization, disruption of collagen, and mucoid degeneration, without an inflammatory component.[25] The value of the MRI is in assessing the severity of clinically established disease, and, in particular, the degree of partial or complete thickness tendon tear. Those patients with frank tendon rupture may be refractory to conservative management, and require open tendon debridement and subsequent repair. In addition, high resolution techniques allow for depiction of subtle articular cartilage injuries, which may prompt preliminary elbow arthroscopy, prior to open tendon debridement.

Wrist and Hand Imaging

The thin section high contrast volumetric techniques used in the elbow have also proven efficacious in evaluating the ligamentous complexes of the wrist[26-28] as well as the articular disk[29] (Fig. 6). Using such imaging techniques, both the size and localization of the triangular fibrocartilage (TFC) tear may be preoperatively determined, thus directing management towards either primary debridement and/or open pri-

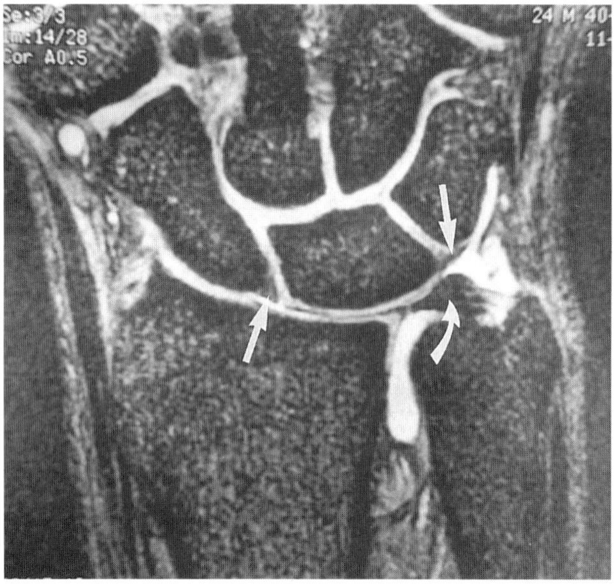

Fig. 6 Coronal volumetric MRI technique through the wrist, using a 1-mm slice thickness, demonstrates the normal appearance of the articular disk (curved white arrow). Note the intact scapholunate and lunotriquetral ligaments (straight arrows).

mary repair (Fig. 7). Degenerative change, traumatic detachments, and associated ligamentous and chondral injuries can be detected.

Additional areas of research in MRI of the hand and wrist include noninvasive vascular imaging. Conventional contrast angiography of the hand is a costly procedure, with a potential risk of contrast reaction and osmotic overload in older patients, and it also subjects the patient to a moderate dose of ionizing radiation. Noninvasive MRI angiography obviates these risks, and is helpful in directing patient management. While experience is limited, continuing research in this area is being performed, yielding satisfactory MRI angiograms which simulate conventional arteriography (Fig. 8). It is important to note that MRI angiography requires no catheterization or intravenous contrast agent. Effective contrast in blood vessels is afforded by the natural contrast between the high signal intensity of inflowing, unsaturated, but fully magnetized protons in blood, and the low signal intensity of saturated stationary tissue. Either selective venography or arteriography may be performed.

Foot and Ankle: Recent Advances

Subluxation/Dislocation/Splits

Common disorders of the peroneal tendons include tendon subluxations and dislocations, which are a partial or complete incongruity, respectively, between peroneal tendons and their groove in the posterior aspect of the distal fibula. Dislocations may be induced by tears or by avulsion of the superior retinaculum, congenital hypoplasia of the superior reticulum, abnormally shaped fibular grooves, and calcaneal fractures.

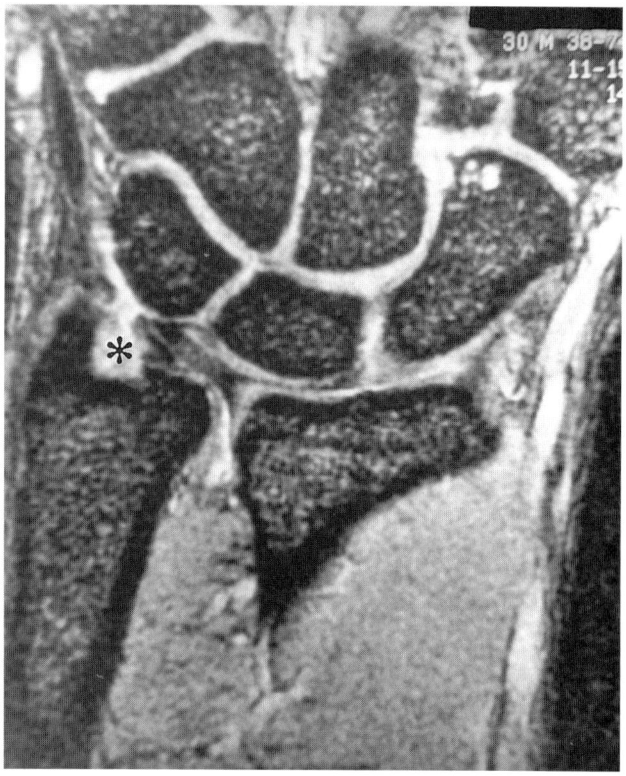

Fig. 7 Coronal volumetric gradient recalled MRI of the right wrist in a patient with ulnar sided wrist pain. There is complete detachment of the ulnar aspect of the articular disk (asterisk). The patient underwent primary arthroscopic repair with good results.

Repetitive subluxation associated with ankle instability can result in peroneal splits syndrome, manifested as a bisection of the peroneus brevis tendon, with occasional hypertrophy of the longus tendon that appears as "Mickey Mouse ears" (Fig. 9) on MRI. MRI may also demonstrate atresia or hyperplasia of the tendon: an axial image with a ratio of longus to brevus other than one-to-one may indicate a tendon disorder, typically of the brevis.

Because the peroneus brevis tendon may normally flatten at the fibula, true peroneal splits should be viewed at least to this point. Of note, the peroneal quartus tendon may simulate a split peroneal brevis, but it is smaller than the brevis and continuous with its own muscle belly. In contrast, splits syndrome demonstrates two halves of the brevis that are similar in size.[30]

Stenosing Tenosynovitis

Analogous to adhesive capsulitis in the shoulder or de Quervain's stenosing tenosynovitis in the wrist, stenosing tenosynovitis appears in any tendon having a fibro-osseous tunnel. On MRI, stenosing tenosynovitis

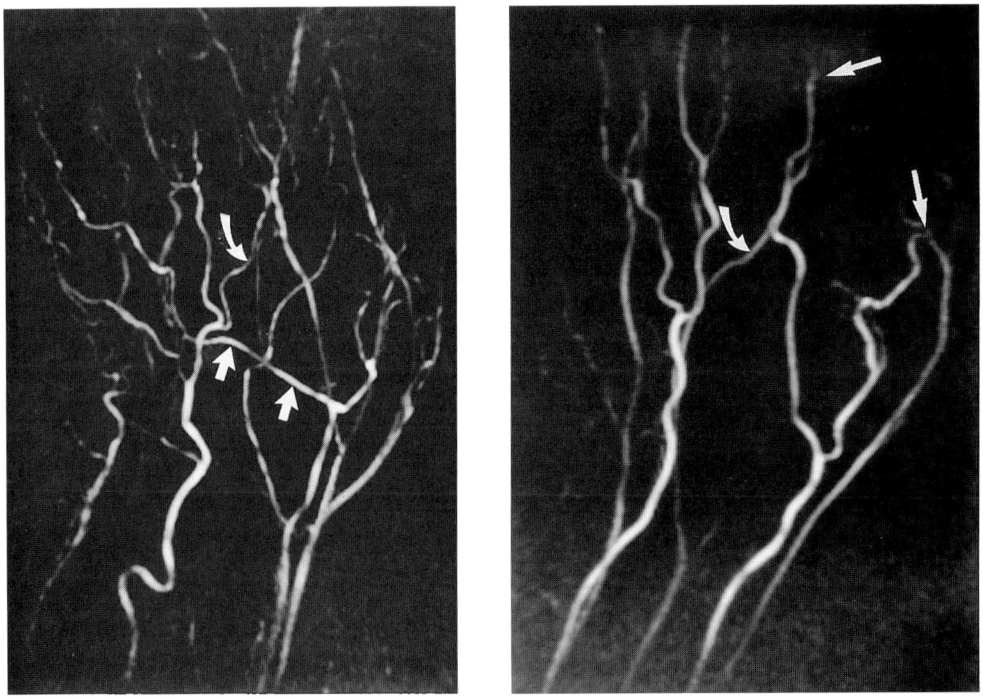

Fig. 8 MR arteriography. **Left,** Two-dimensional-phase contrast MRI arteriogram in a normal patient demonstrates a patency of both the deep (straight arrows), and superficial (curved arrow) palmar arches. **Right,** Two-dimensional phase contact MRI arteriogram in a patient with clinically suspected scleroderma and cold fingers, some of which had clinically apparent tip ulcerations. In contrast to the patient in the figure to the left, diminutive flow is seen distal to the metacarpal branches, particularly those to the index finger and thumb (straight arrows). The patient has an intact superficial arch (curved arrow), but no patent deep palmar arch is seen.

demonstrates adhesions manifested as low signal septae forming loculations of joint sheath fluid.[31] More specific findings appear on sagittal images when proximal tendon sheath fluid is truncated distally (Fig. 10).

Peroneal Tendinitis/Tears

Peroneal tendinitis is uncommon and typically appears at the level of the calcaneal cuboid joint in the axial plane. While peroneal tendon tears typically demonstrate retraction on MRI, tendinitis does not. Peroneal tendinitis extends longitudinally, involves approximately 80% to 90% of an axial cross section in diameter, and appears only faintly or as a bull's-eye on long T2-weighted images. Unlike peroneal tendon tears, peroneal tendinitis does not induce morphologic alterations, so that the peroneus brevis and longus tendons remain similar in size.[31]

Peroneal tendon tears appear more often in the peroneus brevis than in the peroneus longus, and typically occur at the level of the calcaneal cuboid joint (Fig. 11). Plain radiography routinely demonstrates posterior displacement of the os peroneum proximal to the calcaneal cuboid joint.[31]

Osteomyelitis

Scintigraphy is usually sensitive in the diagnosis of osteomyelitis, with the exception of acute osteomyelitis and septic arthritis which, due to increased intramedullary or intra-articular pressure, may reduce upake on scintigraphy. Bone scintigraphy demonstrates only modest specificity. Results may be improved by using additional gallium scans or indium-labeled white blood cell scans, but costs and delays in diagnosis are increased concomitantly.[32] A more cost-effective approach, MRI is the preferred method for evaluating osteomyelitis.[33]

Studies show that 92% accuracy may be achieved with the use of intravenous contrast agents in MR imaging, in part due to the superior anatomic resolution of MRI. In addition to a nonspecific bone marrow edema pattern (low signal on T1-weighted, high signal on T2-weighted or STIR), secondary changes, including soft-tissue sinus tracts, soft-tissue and osseous abscesses, periosteal reaction, and adjacent skin or soft-tissue ulcerations, may be seen, and increase diagnostic specificity.

While gadolinium enhancement usually denotes infection,[34] marrow edema is nonspecific, as a variable amount of sympathetic edema often accompanies osteomyelitis and/or septic arthritis. Marrow changes must be present with adjacent soft-tissue changes to indicate infection. A knowledge of compartmental foot anatomy is essential, because infections can occur in the medial, central, or lateral compartments, and they spread along, rather than between, compartments.

Signs of patient predisposition to infection include bright signal in the deep muscles of the foot on STIR (fat suppressed) images, indicative of diabetic myopathy. To differentiate reactive edema and neuropathic changes from infection, it is important to recog-

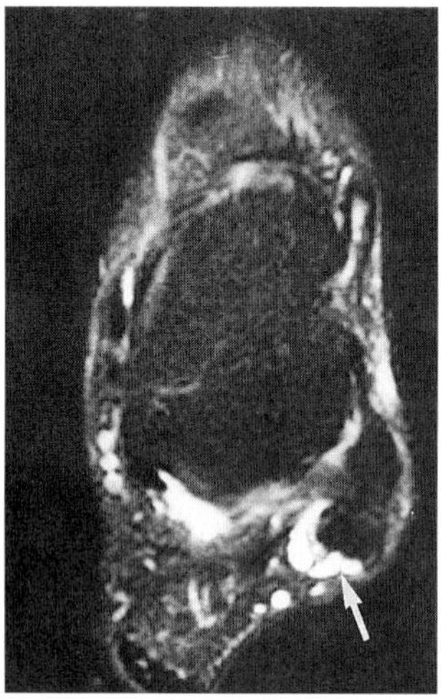

Fig. 9 T2-weighted MRI demonstrates bisection of the peroneus brevis tendon. An excessive amount of fluid is seen in the common peroneal tendon sheath (arrow) consistent with splits syndrome.

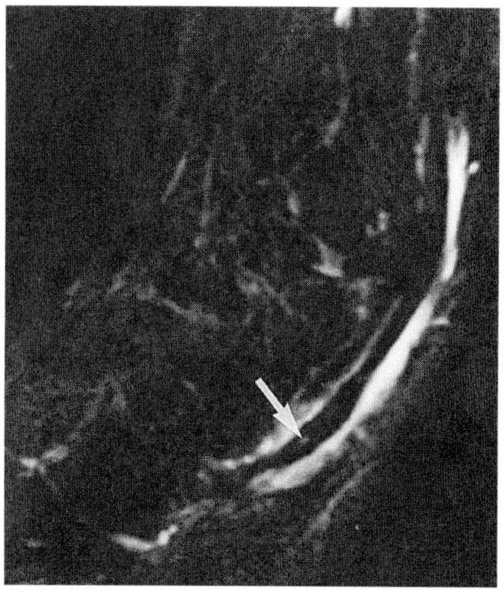

Fig. 11 Sagittal fast-STIR image demonstrates an interstitial tear of the peroneus brevis (arrow).

nize that most neuropathic joints are not frequently affected by osteomyelitis. Rather, osteomyelitis occurs most often in regions of ulceration. The "ghost sign," present with extensive disruption in the shape of tarsal bones on T1- or T2-weighted images, is useful in distinguishing osteomyelitis from neuroarthropathy. When using gadolinium or STIR images, the appearance of a normal shadow indicates infection. Neuropathic joints, however, demonstrate joint disorganization on all imaging sequences and never appear as a normal "ghost" bone. The reactive changes in adjacent soft tissue may impart greater diagnostic specificity, because soft tissue tumor-like masses occur frequently with infection and infrequently with neuropathic joints. Periosteal reaction, contiguous articular extension, and adjacent joint effusions, however, are nonspecific findings.

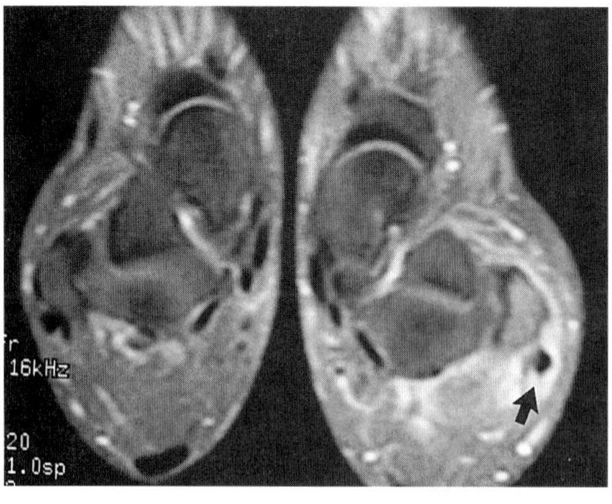

Fig. 10 Fat-suppressed image following intravenous gadolinium administration shows enhancement of peroneal tendon sheath (arrow), consistent with peroneal stenosing tenosynovitis.

Occult Fractures

Marrow edema is a nonspecific finding, seen in infection, tumoral infiltration, and posttraumatic change. Manifestations of acute trauma differ from the more repetitive, stress-type injury. The mature periosteal reaction of radiographically occult fractures appears low signal on MRI, and is less frequently seen than the more aggressive acute periosteal reaction, which is bright on T2-weighted or STIR sequences, and enhances thickly and prominently following intravenous gadolinium administration.

Stress fractures may have an appearance similar to occult fractures on MRI. A characteristic finding in the tibia and fibula is multiple horizontally oriented low signal lines. The bone bruise, or stress response, of a stress fracture is similar in appearance to an occult fracture, but is more poorly defined. Because normal physiologic adaptation to stress is part of this continuum, it is important to note that the biomechanics from altered weightbearing can cause the appearance of a stress fracture.

Knee Imaging

Biomechanical Disorders of the Patellofemoral Joint

Anterior knee pain is frequently associated with patellofemoral biomechanical disorders and chondromalacia patella. Evaluating for the presence of biomechanical disorders of the patella is problematic, because the optimal position (between 10° and 30° of flexion) is difficult to obtain with radiographs. While computed tomography (CT) scanning is less costly than MRI, CT without concomitant arthrography is not capable of evaluating articular cartilage.

Kinematic MRI, a sequential or stepped imaging technique, and dynamic imaging, which is performed during motion, are frequently employed in MRI and may be used with the patient in either prone or supine position, with or without quadriceps contraction.[35] While either technique will correctly diagnose patellofemoral biomechanical disorders, the preferred method is dynamic MRI, using a range of motion of 0° to 40° in the supine position. Use of thick slices improves signal-to-noise and facilitates measurement. Both knees are typically imaged due to the frequency of bilateral pathology and the necessity of a large field-of-view. Axial images are obtained from the top of the patella to 1.5 cm below the patella to allow for the normal migration of the patella with flexion. Images can then be displayed on the cine loop, simulating dynamic tracking.

Several measurements are used to evaluate for the presence of either patella tilt (Excessive Lateral Pressure Syndrome (ELPS)), or patellar subluxation, and include patella tilt angle, bisect offset, and congruence angle. An abnormally angulated or tilted patella (ELPS) is oriented past midline, as described by the above measurements (Fig. 12). ELPS is sometimes accompanied by subluxation; isolated subluxation is less common. As patella tilt and subluxation may be normal on hyperextended images or images obtained in 0° of flexion, pathologic alteration should only be described on images obtained between 10° and 30° of flexion. Malposition of the patella frequently resolves following 30° of flexion, obviating the need for imaging past 30°.

Evaluation for patella alta should be performed on sagittal images, measuring the relative height of the patellar tendon to the patella (Insall-Salvati ratio), with a normal range of 1.02 (SD = 0.13).

Chondromalacia

Detection of chondromalacia has been an area of recent research in MRI. Articular cartilage is a highly organized structure, separated into four discrete layers. These are the tangential zone, a superficial layer consisting of densely packed collagen fibers that lie parallel to the joint surface and provide the gliding suface of the joint; the intermediate zone with randomly distributed fibers; the deeper noncalcified radial zone, made of the largest fibers, which are oriented perpendicular to the joint surface; and the deepest layer, which consists of calcified cartilage.[36] On most imaging sequences, hyaline cartilage is usually intermediate in signal intensity. Fat suppression techniques improve visibility of cartilage because they enhance the dynamic range and give superior tissue contrast.[37]

Gradient echo or fast spin echo images with T2-weighting and/or fat suppression use synovial fluid to obtain an arthrographic effect. In early chondromalacia, the cartilage may thicken to more than 4 mm and has low signal secondary to desiccation. Subtle defects with surface fibrillation may be seen, as well as larger defects, including focal surface flaps. It is important to note that changes in subchondral marrow signal may exist in the absence of full-thickness cartilage defects, due to a sympathetic response.

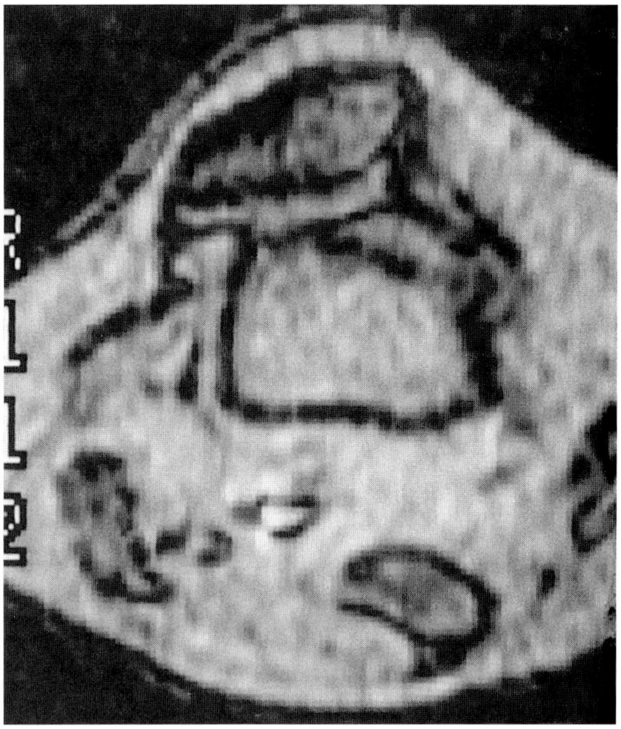

Fig. 12 Dynamic gradient echo axial image through the knee demonstrates subluxation of the patella with excessive lateral pressure syndrome.

Infected Arthroplasty

Because laboratory cultures can be false negative in the presence of an infected arthroplasty, it is necessary to ascertain the extent of infection.[38] Traditionally, MRI following total joint arthroplasty is limited by the presence of susceptibility artifacts. Newer fast spin echo techniques demonstrate fewer artifacts, particularly with a short echo train, diminished interecho spacing, and relatively short repetition times. Fat suppression should be avoided due to the increased magnetic field inhomogeneity in the presence of the arthroplasty. With appropriate pulse sequences, MRI can be accurate in determining the extent of infection.

Hip Imaging

Advances in hip imaging include higher resolution techniques using small surface coils, which impart

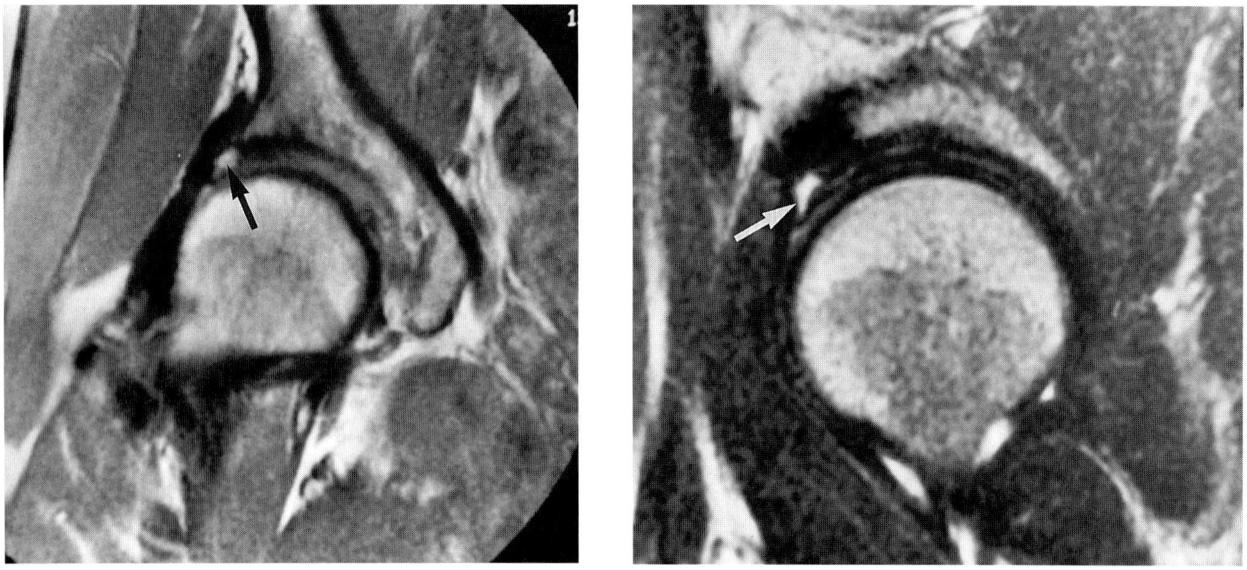

Fig. 13 **Left,** High resolution surface coil imaging of the hip in a 36-year-old woman with right hip clicking and pain. **Right,** Coronal fast spin echo surface coil image demonstrates a globular focus of signal hyperintensity within the substance of the labrum (arrow), indicating a labral tear. The abnormal signal is seen to better advantage in this figure, which represents a sagittal T2 image. At arthroscopy, a labral tear was successfully debrided.

smaller fields of view and improved spatial resolution. With appropriate pulse sequences, adequate contrast is achieved between bone, articular cartilage, fibrocartilaginous labrum, capsule, and joint fluid. Using such sequences, subtle osteochondral injuries, isolated chondral injuries, and labral tears may be detected (Fig. 13).

Conclusion

In summary, with vigilant attention to proper imaging technique, and due to recent technologic developments in MRI software, a high degree of accuracy can be obtained in detecting tendon ligament and cartilage injuries. High contrast thin section techniques permit improved visualization of small or closely opposed structures, including flexor and extensor tendons in the elbow, collateral ligaments, the ligaments and triangular fibrocartilage of the wrist, and articular cartilage of all joints. Kinematic MRI provides insight into normal patellofemoral tracking disorders of the knee, and new fast spin echo techniques allow visualization of adjacent soft-tissue structures surrounding total joint arthroplasty, which was not previously possible. With improved software and hardware imaging technology on the horizon, faster scanning times will be achieved with improved spatial resolution and an anticipated cost reduction.

References

1. Falconiero RP, Balduini FC, Marcelli EA, et al: The accuracy of MRI for the knee in a community setting. *Orthop Trans* 1994; 18:1013.
2. Gelb HJ, Glasgow SG, Sapega AA, et al: The clinical value and cost-effectiveness of magnetic resonance imaging (MRI) in the management of knee disorders in a sports medicine practice. *Orthop Trans* 1994;18:1012–1013.
3. Iannotti JP, Zlatkin MB, Esterhai JL, et al: Magnetic resonance imaging of the shoulder: Sensitivity, specificity, and predictive value. *J Bone Joint Surg* 1991;73A:17–29.
4. Zlatkin MB, Iannotti JP, Roberts MC, et al: Rotator cuff tears: Diagnostic performance of MR imaging. *Radiology* 1989;172: 223–229.
5. Sher JS, Uribe JW, Posada A, et al: Abnormal findings on magnetic resonance images of asymptomatic shoulders. *J Bone Joint Surg* 1995;77A:10–15.
6. Hodler J, Kursunoglu-Brahme S, Snyder SJ, et al: Rotator cuff disease: Assessment with MR arthrography versus standard MR imaging in 36 patients with arthroscopic confirmation. *Radiology* 1992;182:431–436.
7. McAuliffe TB, Dowd GS: Avulsion of the subscapularis tendon: A case report. *J Bone Joint Surg* 1987;69A:1454–1455.
8. Gerber C, Krushell RJ: Isolated rupture of the tendon of the subscapularis muscle: Clinical features in 16 cases. *J Bone Joint Surg* 1991;73B:389–394.
9. Patten RM: Tears of the anterior portion of the rotator cuff (the subscapularis tendon): MR imaging findings. *Am J Roentgenol* 1994;162:351–354.
10. O'Brien SJ, Neves MC, Arnoczky SP, et al: The anatomy and histology of the inferior glenohumeral ligament complex of the shoulder. *Am J Sports Med* 1990;18:449–456.
11. Baker CL, Uribe JW, Whitman C: Arthroscopic evaluation of acute initial anterior shoulder dislocations. *Am J Sports Med* 1990; 18:25–28.

12. Tirman PF, Stauffer AE, Crues JV III, et al: Saline magnetic resonance arthrography in the evaluation of glenohumeral instability. *Arthroscopy* 1993;9:550–559.
13. Chandnani VP, Yeager TD, DeBerardino T, et al: Glenoid labral tears: Prospective evaluation with MR imaging, MR arthrography, and CT arthrography. *Am J Roentgenol* 1993;161:1229–1235.
14. Palmer WE, Caslowitz PL: Anterior shoulder instability: Diagnostic criteria determined from prospective analysis of 121 MR arthrograms. *Radiology* 1995;197:819–825.
15. Gusmer PB, Potter HG, Schatz JA, et al: Labral injuries: Accuracy of detection with unenhanced MR imaging of the shoulder. *Radiology* 1996;200:519–524.
16. Morrey BF, An KN: Functional anatomy of the ligaments of the elbow. *Clin Orthop* 1985;201:84–90.
17. Hotchkiss RN, Weiland AJ: Valgus stability of the elbow. *J Orthop Res* 1987;5:372–377.
18. Schwab GH, Bennett JB, Woods GW, et al: Biomechanics of elbow instability: The role of the medial collateral ligament. *Clin Orthop* 1980;146:42–52.
19. Jobe FW, Ciccotti MG: Lateral and medial epicondylitis of the elbow. *J Am Acad Orthop Surg* 1994;2:1–8.
20. Jobe FW, Stark H, Lombardo SJ: Reconstruction of the ulnar collateral ligament in athletes. *J Bone Joint Surg* 1986;68A:1158–1163.
21. Field LD, Callaway GH, O'Brien SJ, et al: Arthroscopic assessment of the medial collateral ligament complex of the elbow. *Am J Sports Med* 1995;23:396–400.
22. Timmerman LA, Schwartz ML, Andrews JR: Preoperative evaluation of the ulnar collateral ligament by magnetic resonance imaging and computed tomography arthrography: Evaluation in 25 baseball players with surgical confirmation. *Am J Sports Med* 1994;22:26–32.
23. Timmerman LA, Andrews JR: Undersurface tear of the ulnar collateral ligament in baseball players: A newly recognized lesion. *Am J Sports Med* 1994;22:33–36.
24. Schwartz ML, al-Zahrani S, Morwessel RM, et al: Ulnar collateral ligament injury in the throwing athlete: Evaluation with saline-enhanced MR arthrography. *Radiology* 1995;197:297–299.
25. Potter HG, Hannafin JA, Morwessel RM, et al: Lateral epicondylitis: Correlation of MR imaging, surgical, and histopathologic findings. *Radiology* 1995;196:43–46.
26. Totterman SM, Miller R, Wasserman B, et al: Intrinsic and extrinsic carpal ligaments: Evaluation by three-dimensional Fourier transform MR imaging. *Am J Roentgenol* 1993;160:117–123.
27. Smith DK: Scapholunate interosseous ligament of the wrist: MR appearances in asymptomatic volunteers and arthrographically normal wrists. *Radiology* 1994;192:217–221.
28. Smith DK: Dorsal carpal ligaments of the wrist: Normal appearance on multiplanar reconstructions of three-dimensional Fourier transform MR imaging. *Am J Roentgenol* 1993;161:119–125.
29. Totterman SM, Miller RJ: Triangular fibrocartilage complex: Normal appearance on coronal three-dimensional gradient-recalled-echo MR images. *Radiology* 1995;195:521–527.
30. Schweitzer ME, Eid ME, Deely DM: MR imaging of the peroneal splits syndrome. *Am J Roentgenol*, in press.
31. Schweitzer ME, Karasick D: MRI of the ankle and hindfoot. *Semin Ultrasound CT MR* 1994;15:410–422.
32. Eckman MH, Greenfield S, Mackey WC, et al: Foot infections in diabetic patients: Decision and cost-effectiveness analyses. *JAMA* 1995;273:712–720.
33. Morrison WB, Schweitzer ME, Wapner KL, et al: Osteomyelitis in feet of diabetics: Clinical accuracy, surgical utility, and cost-effectiveness of MR imaging. *Radiology* 1995;196:557–564.
34. Morrison WB, Schweitzer ME, Bock GW, et al: Diagnosis of osteomyelitis: Utility of fat-suppressed contrast-enhanced MR imaging. *Radiology* 1993;189:251–257.
35. Shellock FG, Mink JH, Deutsch AL, et al: Patellar tracking abnormalities: Clinical experience with kinematic MR imaging in 130 patients. *Radiology* 1989;172:799–804.
36. Recht MP, Resnick D: MR imaging of articular cartilage: Current status and future directions. *Am J Roentgenol* 1994;163:283–290.
37. Recht MP, Resnick D: Magnetic resonance imaging of articular cartilage: The state of the art. *J Rheumatol Suppl* 1995;43:52–55.
38. Manaster BJ: Total knee arthroplasty: Postoperative radiologic findings. *Am J Roentgenol* 1995;165:899–904.

CHAPTER 52

Bioresorbable Implants: Applications in Orthopaedic Surgery

R. Dale Blasier, MD, FRCS(C)
Robert Bucholz, MD
William Cole, PhD, FRACS, FRCSC
Lanny L. Johnson, MD
E. Antero Mäkelä, MD

Historic Overview

The existence of absorbable implants depends on the fact that naturally occurring substances can be formed into structural plastics. Specifically, organic molecules can be polymerized to form strong fibers and solid components. Once implanted in the body, these structures will break down and be absorbed, metabolized, and excreted, safely.

The use of resorbable implants has always been attractive to surgeons. The need to remove implants after they have served their function has always been a nuisance to the surgeon and patient, so the idea of a device that can be implanted and will later dissolve is appealing. The use of resorbable material for surgery is not a new idea. Galen, the Greek physician, initiated the use of resorbable gut suture in 175 A.D.

It was not until 1,800 years later that the first synthetic resorbable material was introduced into the United States for surgical use. This was Dexon®, a polymer of glycolic acid produced by Davis & Geck Division of American Cyanamid. Other resorbable materials soon followed, including Vicryl® and PDS® (polydioxanone).

It was found that these materials could be sintered together, using heat and pressure, or melt-molded to form solids, in much the same way products can be fabricated from nonresorbable plastics. Meshes, vascular clips, staples, and bowel anastomotic rings have been formulated from polymers for use by general surgeons.

The use of resorbable materials for bone fixation has a short history, only a quarter century. Maxillofacial surgeons were the first to experiment with resorbable devices,[1,2] using sutures, rods, and sheets of polymers. While these devices were relatively well-tolerated by their animal hosts, with minimal inflammatory response, they clearly were not as strong as metallic implants. The first use of resorbable material to repair fracture in humans was described in 1974[3] for use in the mandible.

The use of resorbable materials for repair of extremity fractures lagged by several years. PLA (polylactic acid), PGA (polyglycolic acid), and PHBA (poly-beta-hydroxybutyric acid) implants were used to fix tibial osteotomies in rabbits with success (Fig. 1).[4] Cancellous bone fractures were successfully fixed with PGA rods in dogs and cats.[5]

The first internal fixation of an extremity fracture in a human was performed in 1985 in Finland, where malleolar fractures[6] were repaired using rods of Polygalactin 910®, a copolymer of PGA and PLA. In 1987, PDS pins were introduced into the United States market by Johnson & Johnson Orthopaedics. Initial problems with strength and biocompatibility were addressed by improvements in the materials.

Small diameter pins were found to be safe when placed across the physis in the treatment of children's fractures.[7] In 1990, resorbable pins and rods of PGA were released in the United States by Bioscience,

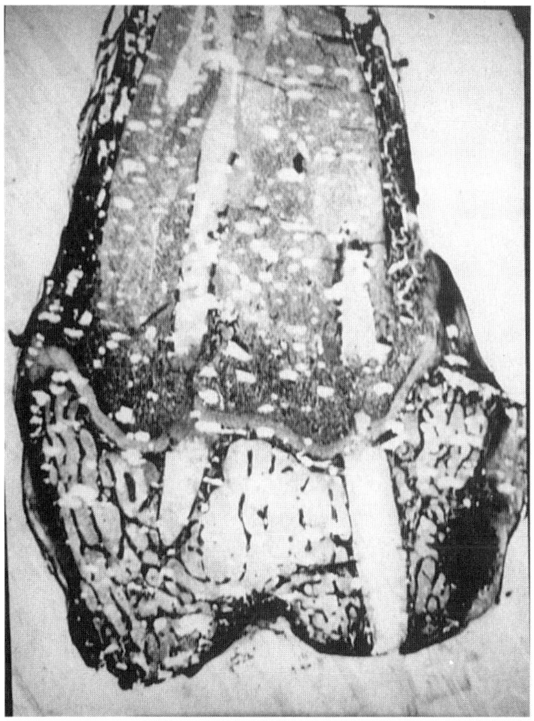

Fig. 1 New bone is seen to form around PGA implants in distal rabbit femur at 12 weeks after implantation.

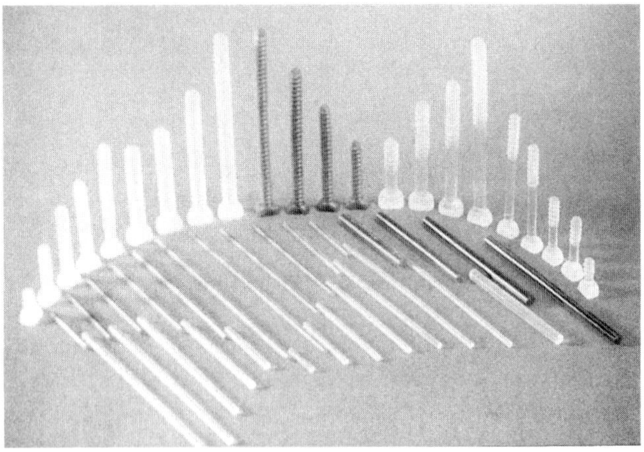

Fig. 2 Assortment of PLA and PGA pins, rods, and screws available today.

Ltd. In 1991, the Suretac® staple was released for use in shoulder capsulorrhaphy.

Polyglycolide pins were described to be comparable to Kirschner wires (K-wires) in the treatment of hand fractures.[8] In 1992, the Instrument Makar ACL staple was released for use. In 1993, Danek released a porous PLA cement plug for use in total hip arthroplasty, and Bioscience released PGA bone screws.

In 1994, a randomized, prospective, multicenter study of fixation of the medial malleolus in ankle fractures compared polylactide screws with metallic screws and showed that the degradable screws were a reasonably safe and effective alternative.[9] In the same year, Bioscience released PLA pins and rods, and Linvatec introduced a PLA interference screw for ACL fixation. New devices are gradually gaining approval from the FDA as clinical trials prove their safety and efficacy.

The plastics from which these devices are manufactured are of considerable interest. Organic molecules such as glycolic acid, lactic acid, or paradioxanone can be polymerized under proper conditions in the presence of a catalyst to form solid structures. They can be cast into sheets or films, spun into fibers, extruded into pins, or melt-molded into complex structures (Fig. 2).

These implants can be completely absorbed after implantation into bone. New bone is formed on and within the implant as it degrades.[10-15] The materials degrade by hydrolysis in the presence of water. Degradation is accelerated in vivo by heat, movement, and nonenzyme action.[15] In the case of PGA or PDS, the monomer is then degraded to glycine or oxalic acid. PLA degrades to pyruvic acid, which is consumed in the tricarboxalic acid cycle. Eventually, the breakdown products are excreted in urine, feces, or respiration. The rate of degradation is influenced by the molecular weight, crystallinity, thermal history, geometry, and surface coating.[16] Useful mechanical strength is maintained for weeks to months after implantation.

Outline 1
Some important bioresorbable implant materials described in the scientific literature

Polyglycolide (PGA)

Copolymers of glycolide
- Glycolide/L-lactide copolymers (PGA/PLLA)
- Glycolide/trimethylene carbonate copolymers (PGA/TMC)

Polylactides (PLA)

Stereocopolymers of PLA
- Poly-L-lactide (PLLA)
- Poly-DL-lactide (PDLLA)
- L-lactide/DL-lactide copolymers

Copolymers of PLA
- Lactide/tetramethylglycolide copolymers
- Lactide/trimethylene carbonate copolymers
- Lactide/δ-valerolactone copolymer
- Lactide/ε-caprolactone copolymer
- Polydepsipeptides
- PLA/polyethylene oxide copolymers
- Unsymmetrically 3,6-substituted poly-1,4-dioxane-2,5-diones

Poly-β-hydroxybutyrate (PHBA)
- PHBA/β-hydroxyvalerate copolymers (PHBA/HVA)

Others
- Poly-p-dioxanone
- Poly-δ-valerolactone
- Poly-ε-caprolactone
- Methylmethacrylate-N-vinyl pyrrolidine copolymers
- Polyesteramides
- Polyorthoesters
- Polydihydropyrans
- Polyalkyl-2-cyanoacrylates
- Polyurethanes (PU)
- Polyvinylalcohol (PVA)
- Poly-β-malic acid (PMLA)
- Poly-β-alkanoic acids
- Polyphosphazenes
- Polypeptide

Initial attempts to use resorbable implants were complicated by relatively low implant strength, inflammatory tissue reactions, and sinus formation. However, materials improvements, including the introduction of fiber-reinforced composite polymer structures by a Finnish group,[16] advanced material purification, and the development of new copolymers have allowed the development of implants that are better tolerated. Even now, these implants are far from perfect and are not likely to obviate the need for metallic implants in bone fixation. More information will be given later regarding the specific advantages and disadvantages of resorbable implants.

Properties and Characteristics

Introduction

The various words used to designate these polymer implants are only general terms: bioresorbable, bioabsorbable, biodegradable, resorbable, and absorbable. Although more than 30 polymers are claimed to be bioresorbable (Outline 1), the polymers with the greatest potential for use in orthopaedic surgery are polyglycolic acid, poly-L-lactic acid, poly-DL-lactic acid (PDLLA), poly-p-dioxanone, glycolide/trimethylenecarbonate copolymers (PGA/TMC), and poly-beta-hydroxybutyric acid (Fig. 3). These terms do not describe the exact composition or varying physical properties, the absorption rate, or potential for inflammation of the different materials. Therefore, a more extensive description is necessary to reveal the properties of any given bioresorbable implant. The biochemical composition may be based on either glycolic acid or lactic acid. These chemicals vary in several ways. For instance, lactic acid may be the L or DL racemic form. The polymer chain may be of one substance (monomer) or of two chemicals (copolymer). The percentages of each chemical may vary in the copolymers. For example, the implant may be designated with the prefix 50/50, which means that each monomer makes up one half of the copolymer chain. If the designation is 85/15, the first monomer is 85% of the chain, and the second contributes 15%. In addition, there are many potential variables in bioresorbable devices; the molecules, the chemical form, the percentage of each, and the physical properties. The absorption rates of a bioresorbable implant are affected by the geometry, mass, and surface area. The absorption rate may also vary with host tissue type. The chemical and physical nature of the implant influence the amount of induced inflammation.

Bioresorbable Polymers

Polyglycolic Acid (PGA) Polyglycolic acid is synthesized by a ring-opening method from glycolide, often referred to as hydroxyacetic acid. PGA with a high molecular weight (MW 10,000 d or more) is a hard, tough, crystalline polymer with a melting point of 224° to 266°C and a glass-transition temperature (T_g) of 36°C. For fiber extrusion, a molecular weight between 20,000 and 145,000 d is suitable.[17] Unlike other closely related poly-alpha-hydroxyacids (PLA, PHBA), PGA is insoluble in most common polymer solvents.

Polylactic Acid (PLA) Polylactic acid is produced by anionic ring-opening polymerization of the cyclic diester, the lactide under the influence of a catalyst. PLA is a pale polymer with four different compound forms, depending on the L- and D- configuration of the lactic moieties forming the polymer molecules. The melting point and the glass transition temperature (T_g) of poly-L-lactic acid (PLLA) are 173°C and 58°C, respectively.[18] Polymers with a molecular weight between 180,000 and 260,000 are used to produce melt-spun fibers. Polymers with a molecular weight from 350,000 to 530,000 are suitable for the production of solution-spun fibers. High-molecular-weight copolymers of L-lactide and glycolide are produced by heating a mixture of the monomers at 200°C in the presence of a stannous octoate catalyst.

Poly-p-dioxanone (PDS) Poly-p-dioxanone is a colorless, crystalline polymer with a high molecular weight. It is characterized by a melting temperature (T_m) of 110°C and a glass-transition temperature (T_g) of -16°C. Para-p-dioxanone monomer is prepared by reacting ethylene glycol, metallic sodium, and chloroacetic acid. The resulting lactone monomer is purified to 99% by multiple distillations and recrystallizations to obtain a high-molecular-weight polymer. The purified monomer is then polymerized at a temperature of 20°C to 130°C in the presence of an organometallic catalyst to yield high-molecular-weight poly-p-dioxanone (Fig. 3).[19]

Poly-beta-hydroxybutyric Acid (PHBA) Poly-beta-hydroxybutyric acid is an optically active polymer formed by certain bacteria (*Alcaligenes eurtophus, Bacillus megaterium, Rhodopirillium rubrum*) in a D-stereoisomeric form.[20] The characteristics of PHBA are as follows: crystalline melting temperature (T_m) 175°C, glass-transition temperature (T_g) 15°C, and molecular weight 500,000 d.

Manufacturing Methods

Production of Bioresorbable Polymers

By definition, bioresorbable materials are synthetic or modified materials used in medical devices and intended to interact with biologic systems. These materials are designed to degrade in vivo to nonharmful by-products and to be finally excreted or assimilated depending on the chemical and physical structure of the material. Therefore, bioresorbable polymers require a hydrolytically labile bond in the polymer chain and they cannot be synthesized by chain-growth mechanism, which is used to make vinyl polymers. Instead, bioresorbable polymers have to be prepared by a poly-condensation (step-growth) mechanism (with the exception of the ring-opening polymerization). Orthopaedic applications of bioresorbable implants impose formidable strength requirements on polymers, that is, the implants should be sufficiently strong when implanted, and they must lose their mechanical strength at an appropriate rate. The high demands of initial strength that are required can only be met with high-molecular-weight polymers. Unfortunately, it is a rather challenging task to obtain high-molecular-weight polymers with the step-growth mechanism. A technique that can yield molecular weights comparable to those obtained by chain-growth polymerization is ring-opening polymerization, the mechanism most often used to produce high-molecular-weight bioresorbable polymers.

Processing of Bioresorbable Polymers

Maintenance of their molecular weight appears to be a major problem in the processing of bioresorbable

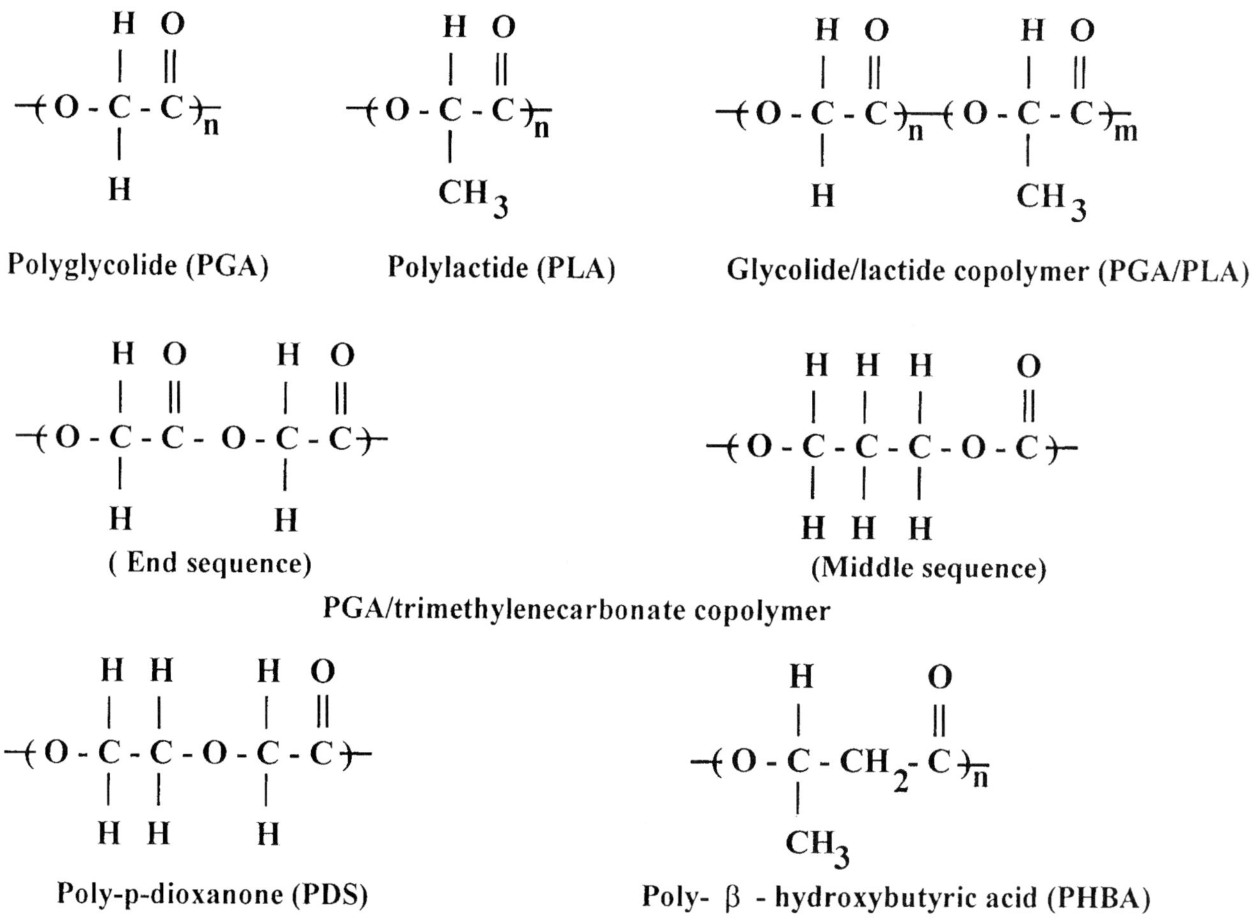

Fig. 3 Structural formulas of the bioresorbable polymers with the greatest potential for use in orthopaedic surgery at the moment.

polymers. In particular, processing them at temperatures above the melting temperature of the polymer material will significantly change the properties of the material. The molecular weight itself correlates directly with the final properties of the implants. When the molecular weight diminishes, so do the mechanical properties and vice versa. Standard methods used to process these polymers can be classified into nonreinforcing techniques and reinforcing techniques.

Nonreinforcing Techniques The nonreinforcing techniques involve as-polymerization and melt-molding processes, like injection molding, compression molding, extruded or compression-molded polymeric implants. When bioresorbable polymers are processed by the conventional melt-molding processes to implants, the end products generally have mechanical strength values between 30 and 80 MPa. These implants usually are brittle and too flexible to allow safe fixation in demanding orthopaedic applications. In conclusion, partially crystalline, linear-chain absorbable polymers, such as PGA and PLLA, show only modest mechanical strength values when manufactured using nonreinforcing techniques.[21]

Reinforcing Techniques The reinforcing techniques involve solid-state transformation methods, like hot drawing and die drawing, and sintering of polymer fibers followed by the consolidation of the form of the sample under elevated pressure.[16] Both solid-state reinforcing and sintering give so-called self-reinforced structures. Self-reinforced (SR-) bioresorbable composites are polymeric materials in which the reinforcing elements and the matrix material have the same chemical element composition. (A composite is a material made up of different types of material components, such as reinforcing fibers, which are held together by the binding matrix.)

Bioresorbable composites can also be made by combining different bioresorbable materials with each other. For example, a bioresorbable polymer matrix can be reinforced with ceramic fibers, such as bioresorbable glass fibers. However, there is poor adhesion between the reinforcing fibers and the matrix material. These adhesion problems between the matrix and the reinforcing elements can probably be avoided by using self-reinforced structures.[22] In any case, the presence of reinforcing structures in polymers makes a significant improvement in their initial mechanical properties. The high demands of strength that are imposed by orthopaedic applications of bioresorbable fixation materials may best be fulfilled by the use of reinforcing techniques in the manufacture of bioresorbable composites.

Sterilization of Bioresorbable Implants

The only two techniques used to sterilize bioresorbable implants are high-energy gamma irradiation (with doses in the range of 1.5 to 2.5 MRad) and ethylene oxide gas sterilization. Because most bioresorbable polymers are highly hygroscopic, implants made of these polyesters cannot be sterilized using heated steam under pressure (autoclaving). Even the residual moisture that remains after processing and packing definitely results in degradation. Although irradiation sterilization is effective, it cannot be used with all polymers because of the risk of polymer decomposition and a significant loss of mechanical strength. However, irrespective of the decrease of the molecular weight of the SR-PLLA implants, sterilization by gamma irradiation with a minimum dose of 2.5 MRads (25 kGy) does not significantly affect their initial strength.

Bioresorbable implants can be sterilized with ethylene oxide gas, but they must always be thoroughly degassed to remove any ethylene oxide, which is toxic, that may remain in the implant. Due to the nature of these bioresorbable materials, the most reliable methods of sterilization currently are ethylene oxide gas sterilization for PGA implants and gamma irradiation for PLA implants.

Mechanical Properties of Bioresorbable Materials

When discussing mechanical properties, the data most often reported are bending strength, bending modulus, tensile strength, and tensile modulus (Young's modulus). They are usually measured in $N/mm^2 = 1$ MPa [1 MPa = 156 psi (pounds per square inch); 1 psi = 0.0064 MPa; 1 GPa = 1,000 MPa]. The specific properties of the implant can be calculated from the stress-strain curve and the size of the implant.

The mechanical properties of bioresorbable polymers show a considerable variation, not only between polymers, but also within the same polymer of a different origin. These properties are strongly dependent on the chemical structure and the molecular weight of the polymer, the orientation of the polymer chains, the crystallinity, the amount of free monomers, and the stereotatic configuration. In addition, the material purity and the presence or absence of defects, voids, and/or reinforcing elements in the implant material are all factors that affect the mechanical properties of the bioresorbable implants. In short, the increase in polymer crystallinity and polymer chain orientation accompanied by fibrillation enhances the mechanical properties of the material in the direction of the orientation.

Nonreinforced PGA, PLLA, PDS, PHBA, and PGA/TMC implants have an initial tensile strength of between 30 and 70 MPa. The corresponding value of bending strength is approximately 60 to 120 MPa. Composites made of polymeric fibers and a matrix of the same (self-reinforced) or another bioresorbable material possess significantly higher tensile and bending strength values because of the orientation of the molecules in the fiber. In comparison, self-reinforced (SR-) implants made of high-molecular-weight polyglycolide and poly-L-lactide have initial bending strength values of 410 MPa and 300 MPa, respectively (Table 1).[11,23]

Biodegradation of the Bioresorbable Implants

The Mechanism of the Biodegradation

Bioresorbable biomaterials decompose and/or disintegrate in living tissues within a period that can range from 1 month to as long as 6 years by means of the metabolic activity of the living cells. In vivo and in aqueous media, bioresorbable polyesters undergo hydrolytic degradation to endogenous substances or to compounds with well-known metabolic pathways. The majority of bioresorbable polyesters are highly

Table 1
Mechanical properties of implant materials and bone

Material*	Tensile Strength (MPa)	Bending Strength (MPa)	Young's Modulus (MPa)
Polyglycolide	57		6,500
Poly-L-lactide	70	120	4,000
Poly-DL-lactide	50	200	3,000
Glycolide/lactide copolymer	†	265	
Poly-p-dioxanone	76[11]	60	1
Polymethylmethacrylate	80	140	3,000
Steel	200-1,000	310-690	200,000
Cortical bone	80-150	120-210	20,000
Cancellous bone		120-210	100-1,700
Glycolide/trimethylene carbonate copolymer	65	120	4
SR-polyglycolide	-	410	18,000
SR-poly-L-lactide	450	300	10,000

*SR= self-reinforced
† Tensile strength of the 90/10 polyglycolide/lactide copolymer suture 450 MPa

Table 2
Bioresorption rates of selected bioresorbable polymers

Polymer	Time of Complete Strength Loss (Months)	Time of Complete Resorption (Months)
Poly-p-dioxanone	2	6
SR-polyglycolide	1	3
SR-poly-L-lactide	12	up to 5-6 years
Poly-D, L-lactide	6	up to 3 years
Glycolide/trimethylene-carbonate copolymer	2-5	6

hygroscopic, and it is well established that the degradation proceeds via a random, bulk hydrolysis of the ester bonds in the polymer chains. Tissue enzymes may be involved in the degradation of the monomeric byproducts formed. At the early stage of the bioresorption, the depolymerization results in the decrease of the molecular weight of the polymer but no change is seen in the appearance of the implant nor is there any cellular response. For example, the SR-PLLA implants with initial molecular weight of 260,000 show an average molecular weight of 10,000 d after 36 weeks of implantation in the subcutis of the rabbit. Parallel with the reduction of the molecular weight, the mechanical strength of the implant also decreases.

When the molecular weight of the polymer goes below about 5,000 d, the implant disintegrates into small particles (debris), which trigger the nonspecific foreign body reaction. These small particles (less than 50 mm) are surrounded by inflammatory cells, including macrophages, giant cells (multinuclear cells that digest the polymer debris), and leukocytes. When the polymer bioresorption is complete, the inflammatory cells disappear, leaving only scar tissue. This bioresorption process takes place with PGA in approximately 6 to 24 months. A bioresorption time of several years is needed for implants made of PLA, depending on the chemical structure and size of the implant. The bioresorption rate of PHBA is controversial. Recent studies suggest a very low degradation rate in vivo, exceeding 6 months.[24] Bioresorption times of bioresorbable polymers with potential use as implant materials in orthopaedic surgery are given in Table 2. In general, large size implants degrade more slowly than implants with small crosssections, and copolymers degrade faster than homopolymers. With regard to the site of implantation, bioresorption takes place more rapidly in soft tissues than in bone, depending on the vascularity. Bioresorption is also accelerated when a load is applied to the implant material.

The Metabolic Routes of the Biodegradation of Polyhydroxides

Polyglycolic Acid PGA is degraded by hydrolysis to glycolic acid. The glycolic acid molecules are then acted upon by glycolate oxidase and are transformed into glyoxylate, which reacts with glycine transaminase to form glycine. The glycine can be used for protein synthesis or for the synthesis of serine, which may be incorporated into the tricarboxylic acid cycle after transformation into pyruvate. The breakdown products of the PGA are mainly excreted from the body in exhaled carbon dioxide and in urine.[25]

Polylactic Acid In hydrolysis, PLA is depolymerized to lactic acid, which in turn is transformed to pyruvate by lactate dehydrogenase. Decarboxylation of pyruvate yields acetyl-CoA, which enters the tricarboxylic acid cycle.[25]

Poly-p-dioxanone Poly-p-dioxanone degrades by hydrolysis. The degradation products are mainly excreted in urine (94%) but also in exhaled carbon dioxide (3%) and in feces (2%).[26]

Poly-beta-hydroxybutyric Acid Poly-beta-hydoxybutyric acid polymers implanted in living tissues within the body are attacked by esterase enzymes and degrade slowly. The esterase enzymes break the polymer down to beta-hydroxy carboxylic acids, which are oxidized to acetoacetate and transformed to acetoacetyl-CoA. This in turn is cleaved by thiolase to yield acetyl-CoA, which is incorporated into the tricarboxylic acid cycle.[27]

Advantages and Disadvantages of Resorbable Implants for Orthopaedic Surgery

Introduction

There are several advantages and disadvantages in using bioresorbable implants in orthopaedic surgery. The surgeon needs to be familiar with each in order to determine if such implants should be incorporated into his practice.

Advantages of Resorbable Devices

No Second Surgery for Hardware Removal Obviously, the main attraction for resorbable implants is elimination of the need to return the patient to the operating room for the removal of deep implants. This is cost beneficial and results in the reduction of patient discomfort and periods of temporary disability. For superficial implants that could be removed in the office setting, not having to remove the implant eliminates the pain of extraction for the patient.

Additionally, the presence of metal in the body may disqualify an otherwise acceptable candidate for the military service. This may also be the reason for an unplanned second operation.

Decreased Load Sharing Prolonged retention of metallic implants can lead to weakening and partial resorption of the underlying bone.[28,29] It is felt that resorbable implants, which are less rigid initially and soften with time, would lessen stress shielding in healing bone.

Drill-Through Potential When conventional metallic implants are used in bone, revision of fixation generally requires removal of the implant. Removal can be challenging, especially if the implant is overgrown with bone, is interosseous, or is broken. Revision of a resorbable fixation implant can be accomplished by simply drilling through the old implant and placing a new one. This would be beneficial in revision of both fracture fixation and ligament reconstruction surgery.

Multi-Tasking The advantages of multi-tasking are largely theoretical, although the potential clearly exists for melt-mixing antibiotics with the polymer.[30] It is conceivable that resorbable devices for internal fixation could be created that would elute antibiotics for the prevention or treatment of infection. Experimental studies have been performed with some success that attempt to use resorbable polymer as a carrier for bone morphogenetic protein.[31] It is possible that an implant that contains growth factors could enhance or accelerate healing.

Cost-Effective One of the benefits of not removing hardware is the elimination of the cost for return to the operating room and the associated costs for anesthesia, medications, and supplies. As long as there would otherwise be a requirement for hardware removal, the additional cost of a resorbable implant may be more than offset by eliminating the need for second surgery.[32]

No Metal Toxicity Orthopaedic implants of metals or alloys are known to have drawbacks such as corrosion and carcinogenesis.[33] Tissue staining and encapsulation around metallic implants have been seen at surgical removal. The risks of long-term implantation are not fully known. The use of resorbable devices may negate these risks.

Disadvantages of Resorbable Devices

Cost One of the current drawbacks of resorbable implants is price. The high cost of raw materials, manufacture, and handling can make the price of a resorbable implant as much as 15 times the price of a comparable metallic implant.[34] As manufacturing techniques improve and production increases, these prices may decrease in the future.

Strength The strength and stiffness of resorbable implants are less than those of metallic implants but more closely resemble those of bone. Self-reinforced rods of PGA or PLA have a bending strength of 180 to 290 MPa, a bending modulus of 7 to 10 GPa, and a shear strength of 110 to 190 MPa.[35] Intact cortical bone has a bending strength of 180 to 195 MPa, a bending modulus of 9.5 to 11.5 GPa[36] and a shear strength of 68 MPa.[37] The shear strength of cancellous bone has been estimated at 6.6 MPa.[38] Nonreinforced resorbable implants are not as strong as the reinforced implants. These implants are suitable for fixation of fracture types in bones such as cancellous bone and epiphyses in which shear loads comprise the major strains.[39] The use of resorbable implants in long bones, which are subject to high loads, is not advised.

Even when the polyester is machined in the shape of a screw, it provides less interfragmental compression than comparably designed metallic screws. Some of this loss of compression may be attributable to the surgical technique, which requires tapping of the full length of the bioresorbable screw canal to decrease the torque during screw insertion.

Foreign Body Reactions A minority of patients will have a clinically manifested foreign body reaction at an average of 3 months after implantation of resorbable implants. Bostman and associates[40] reported such a reaction in 7.9% of 516 patients treated with rods of polyglycolide or lactide-glycolide copolymer for the internal fixation of fractures or osteotomies. The reaction seemed to be related to the presence of particulate polymeric debris. Evacuation of the debris by aspiration or incision relieved the problem. Bony healing was not affected. Elimination of an aromatic quinone dye from the implants was associated with a decrease in the incidence of this reaction. No deleterious long-term effect was seen after this complication.[41]

Delayed Tissue Reaction It has been estimated that it may take 3 years, or even longer, for PLLA implants to fully resorb from the body.[42] Symptomatic intermittent swelling has occurred 3 years after implantation of poly(L-lactide) bone plates and screws for zygomatic fractures. At debridement and removal, a nonspecific foreign body reaction with crystalline-like PLLA material in the cytoplasm of various cells was seen.[43] The reaction did not interfere with fracture healing.

Extrusion Eitenmüller and associates (Eitenmüller J, David A, Muhr G, personal communication, 1990) described extrusion of fragments of poly(L-lactide) in four out of 25 cases in which poly(L-lactide) plates and screws were implanted about the ankle for the surgical treatment of fractures. It is felt that the risk of adverse tissue reactions may be decreased by using small amounts of implant material, by keeping them away from the skin, by using them interosseously if possible, and by avoiding regions subject to considerable soft-tissue motion. (Rokkanen P, personal communication, 1995).

Osteolysis Osteolysis may be seen around resorbable implants on postoperative radiographs starting about 3 months after implantation in about half of adult patients. Osteolysis was seen in 82% of patients with foreign body reactions and 40% of patients without. The bone structure returns to normal after about a year.[44] Osteolysis has also been seen in children, though less frequently than in adults. Growth plate function is unaffected.[45]

Sinus Formation Sinus formation may occur in association with an inflammatory reaction after implantation. Nine of 516 patients treated for a variety of fractures

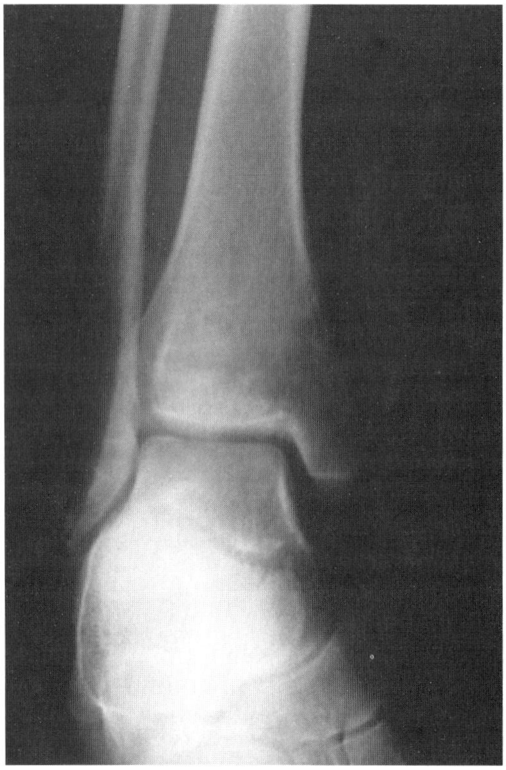

Fig. 4 Sclerosis is seen around radiolucent pin tracts traversing the distal tibia.

and osteotomies presented with a sinus after surgery. Others had persistent drainage after aspiration or incision of a local fluctuance. On average, the drainage had subsided by the fifth week, but in some cases it continued for up to 2 months. Debris from the wound includes giant cells, macrophages, and polymeric debris. Cultures were uniformly negative.[40] Sinus formation, seen after absorbable screw fixation in 10 of 152 operated patients, did not influence healing or functional recovery.[46] Patients must be warned of this possibility prior to surgery with these implants.

Radiolucency Resorbable implants are not visible on plain radiographs, although frequently the implant tract in bone can be seen (Fig. 4). In North America, many surgeons, for medical or legal reasons, prefer to visualize the location of the implant on radiographs. For these surgeons, the radiolucency of the implants is a drawback.

Shelf Life Unlike those of metallic implants, the mechanical properties of resorbable implants degrade with time. For this reason, many implants have a limited shelf life and, in fact, are given an expiration date, by which time the implant should be used or discarded. Because this can add to the cost of maintaining an inventory of components, the overall cost of using these implants is increased.

Material Deterioration with Manipulation Unlike metallic implants, which have relatively constant material properties, resorbable implants are made up of high-molecular-weight polymers, which determine the mechanical properties. Any manipulation of the individual implant, such as heating, sterilization, or machining, decreases its molecular weight and causes its mechanical properties to deteriorate.

Synovitis with Intra-Articular Use Recent reports from Scandinavian surgeons have documented protracted synovitis after using resorbable pins of PLA or PGA to fixate intra-articular fragments in the knee.[47-49] The exact cause of this synovitis, predisposing factors, and the frequency are not known.

Summary Obviously, there are many pros and cons involved in the use of resorbable implants in orthopaedics. The surgeon must be aware of these factors when determining whether to use them in a particular application.

Applications of Bioresorbable Implants in Orthopaedic Surgery in Adults

The major focus of clinical trials to date has been fracture fixation. Because of the mechanical limitations of the implants, only low load metaphyseal or periarticular fractures have been treated. Ankle fractures represent by far the most common clinical application. Böstman and associates[50] reported on the use of polyglycolide rods for the treatment of unstable bimalleolar fractures. Despite a high union rate in the 64 fractures treated, he noted that nine (15%) redisplaced following fixation, and five (8%) developed an inflammatory sinus. Screws made of polyglycolide were subsequently found to have a lower prevalence of loss of reduction. Partio and associates,[46] however, reported that 10 of 152 ankles treated with PGA screws still developed spontaneous drainage of liquefied polyester and sterile sinuses 2 to 6 months following surgery. Copolymers of polyglycolide and polylactide were first used in ankle fractures by Böstman in the mid-1980s. He compared PGA/PLA rods to stainless steel screws and plates in the treatment of unstable ankle fractures.[51] Despite the inability to achieve interfragmental compression, he noted at 1 year no major differences in the study and control patients.

Pure polylactide in the form of rods and screws has also been studied as implants in ankle fractures. In a randomized, prospective study of 155 patients with unstable medial malleolar, bimalleolar, or trimalleolar fractures, 4.0 mm orientruded PLA screws were compared to comparable sized stainless steel screws for fixation of the medial malleolar fractures.[8] (Orientrusion is a manufacturing process that, by aligning the polymeric chains in parallel, enhances the material's strength.) At follow-ups of greater than 8 years, no sig-

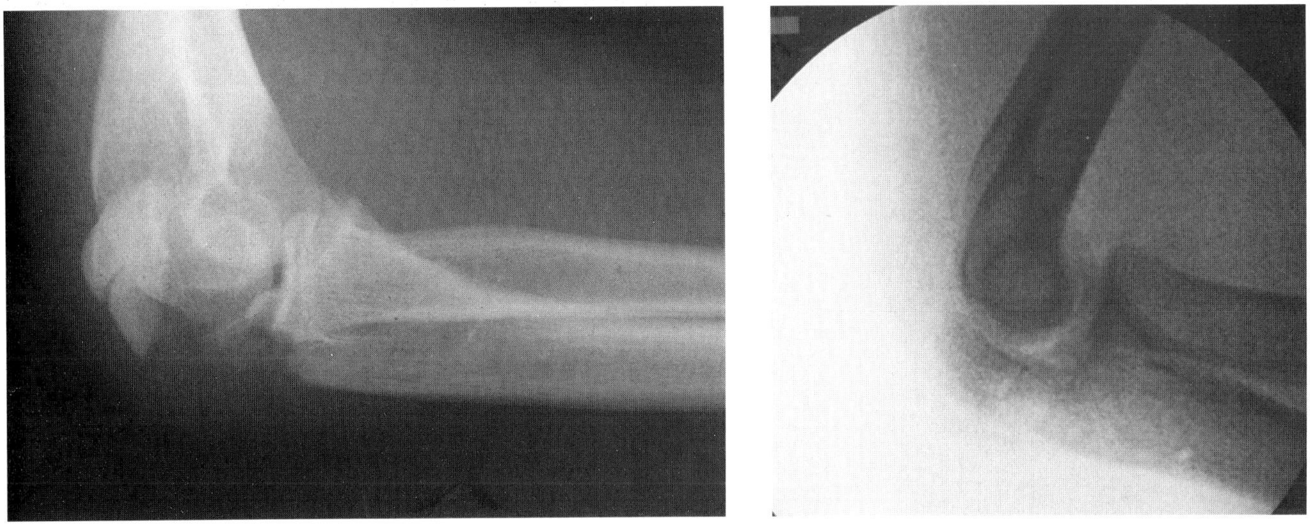

Fig. 5 Olecranon fracture after internal fixation with PGA pins and circlage of Vicryl® suture.

nificant differences in the radiographic or functional results or in the rates of operative and postoperative complications were noted in the two groups. Of 83 patients treated with PLA screws, only one patient had an inflammatory reaction, and in no case was sinus formation present. The lack of inflammatory reaction was attributed to the slow rate of degradation of the PLA implant compared to that of polyglycolide.

Other low load fractures have also been treated using the bioresorbable implants. Fractures about the elbow, including simple fractures of the radial head, olecranon (Fig. 5), and capitellum, have been fixed with bioresorbable rods and screws. In olecranon fractures, the surgical constructs are designed to obtain bicortical purchase with screws, because the thread purchase on the medullary canal is inadequate compared to that achieved with cancellous stainless steel screws. Distal radius fractures, especially those involving the radial styloid, have also been stabilized with these implants. In cases where polyglycolide screws or pins have been used, there appears to be a high prevalence of sinus formation, probably attributable to the subcutaneous location of the implants in this particular application.[15] Fixation of patellar fractures has also been a popular application for these implants because of problems associated with prominent metallic hardware in these fractures. Small bioresorbable pins or rods also can be used in selected metatarsal and phalangeal fractures, and bioresorbable screws have also been used for fixation of corticocancellous bone grafts to recipient sites. Other possible fracture applications not yet reported include fractures of the greater tuberosity of the humerus, the glenoid fossa, the greater trochanter of the femur, the acetabulum, the tibial plateau, the calcaneus, and the talus.

The use of bioresorbable implants for fixation of osteotomies has been largely limited to the foot. They have been found useful in fixation of Chevron and comparable osteotomies for hallux valgus. Their use for major long-bone osteotomies is limited by the poor mechanical properties of the screws and rods. Partio and associates[52] reported the use of bioresorbable screws for stabilization of ankle arthrodeses. Both PGA and PLA interfragmental screws were inserted obliquely from the tibia to the talus for fixation of the arthrodesis site. A short leg cast is worn for 8 weeks, but early weightbearing is allowed. In an initial series of 12 patients, fusion was achieved in all but one.[52]

The first decade of clinical use of bioresorbable rods and screws has ended with their application essentially limited to low load, cancellous fractures, osteotomies, and arthrodeses. Major improvements in the mechanical properties of these implants are needed prior to their wider application to the adult population.

Applications of Bioresorbable Implants in Children's Orthopaedics

In children, many osteotomies and fractures are fixed with K-wires. In many instances, the K-wires are smooth and are left protruding from the skin for removal in the Outpatient Clinic or office. The latter treatment is frequently used for supracondylar fractures of the humerus. In contrast, K-wires, when used to treat fractures of the lateral condyle of the humerus, often are buried beneath the skin to avoid the risk of infection. Under these circumstances, the child, who is usually young, has to be readmitted for removal of the wires under general anesthesia. Threaded K-wires are frequently used to fix osteotomies, such as innominate

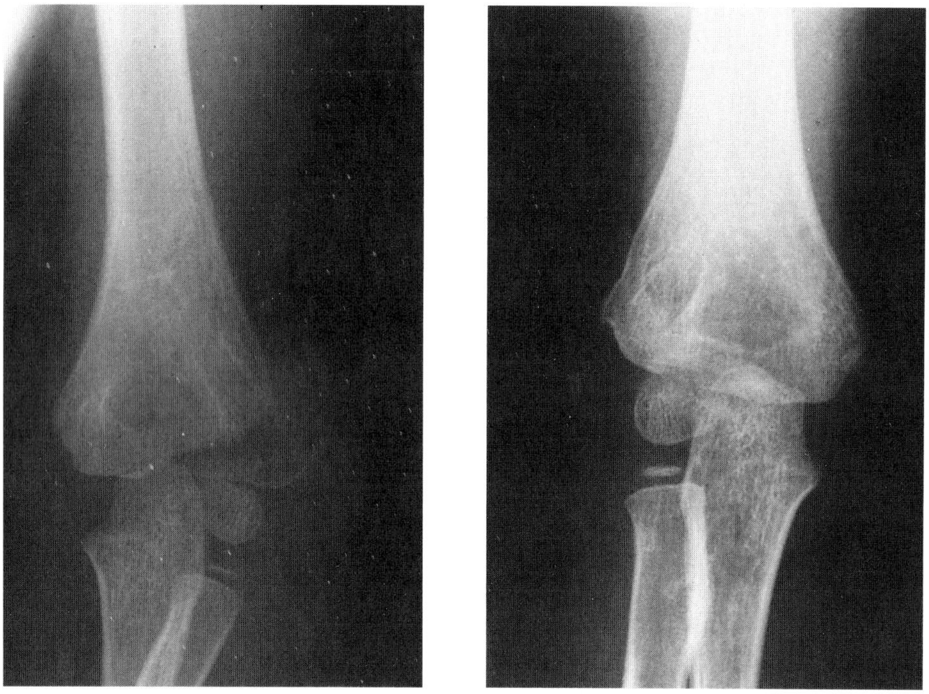

Fig. 6 **Left,** Displaced lateral condyle fracture in a child. **Right,** After internal fixation with PGA pins.

osteotomies. In this case, the pins are also buried and require subsequent removal under a general anesthetic. Use of bioresorbable implants as an alternative to buried K-wires in the fixation of fractures and osteotomies avoids the necessity for readmission and general anesthesia.

Pediatric Fractures

Indications Most elbow fractures that require open reduction and K-wire fixation are suitable for fixation with bioresorbable rods. They include fractures of the lateral and medial condyles of the humerus (Fig. 6), the medial epicondyle, and the olecranon. Shear fractures of the capitellum and fractures of the phalanges and metacarpals can also be stabilized with bioresorbable rods.

Materials The implant only needs to provide stability for about 3 weeks, as the fracture callus provides stability beyond that time. The bioresorbable rods used are fine, with diameters of 1.5 and 2 mm, because the fracture fragments are often small.[53] Polyglycolic acid rods meet these specifications. When fixing fractures of the olecranon, a supplemental tension band of polyglycolic acid suture may also be used.

Outcome Fracture union is radiographically normal. After 3 to 6 weeks, the rod tracts can often be seen due to osteolysis.[45] The lytic areas heal over the following few months. Seromas and granulomas are infrequent, probably because of the small amount of bioresorbable material in the short thin rods used to fix most fractures.

Pediatric Osteotomies

Indications Metaphyseal osteotomies of small bones, such as the base of the first metatarsal in the treatment of hallux valgus, are suitable for fixation with bioresorbable implants. Osteotomies of cancellous bone of the pelvis in the treatment of developmental dysplasia of the hip, Perthes disease, and epiphyseal dysplasias can also be stabilized with bioresorbable fixation.

Materials In weightbearing bones, such as the metatarsals and ilium, the osteotomies must be stabilized with an implant that will last at least 6 weeks. For this reason, the rapidly degrading polyglycolic acid rods are unsuitable, and the slowly degrading polylactide rods are used instead. For the Salter osteotomy, we recommend the use of 2-mm PLA rods in smaller children and 3.2-mm PLA rods in older children.

Outcome Osteotomies of metatarsals and other small bones are protected with casts. Innominate (Salter) osteotomies undertaken alone need not be supported with a hip spica. The children can use crutches with non-weightbearing for 6 weeks. The bioresorbable implants appear to provide adequate fixation of small bone and iliac osteotomies and do not appear to alter the rate of bone healing. Seromas are rare with the PLA rods.

Bioresorbable Implants in Anterior Cruciate Ligament Reconstruction

The first bioresorbable implant to gain FDA marketing approval was a staple made of 85/15 DL glycolide/lactide (Fig. 7). This approval was based on clinical studies, which established that the bioresorbable device is safe and effective and was substantially equivalent to an existing metal device. This bioresorbable staple was compared to a metal staple made by the same company (Instrument Makar) for autogenous hamstring tendon graft reconstruction.[54] During laboratory testing, the resistance to pull-out from bone was the same for both staples. A prospective, randomized, single center study was performed in 1989. Follow-up was maintained long enough for complete absorption of the device (about 6 months). Symptomatic complaints were minimal and were similar for both groups. The Lachman test was trace positive in four out of 12 of the bioresorbable group and five out of 12 for the metal group. The average knee joint stability at 30° flexion and 40 pounds pull was zero (range +6 to -4 mm) for the bioresorbable group and same (range +4 to -4 mm) for the metal group.

The second bioresorbable device reported for anterior cruciate ligament (ACL) graft fixation was an interference screw made of a monomer of poly L-lactide.[55] The study supporting equivalence was a randomized, prospective multicenter comparison of the bioresorbable screw with a metal screw produced by the same company (Linvatec). The study included 110 patients, with an average follow-up of 19 months. In 42 of the patients, a bioresorbable implant was used in the operation. The operative times were similar. The Tegner and Lysholm scores were the same. The pivot shift was absent in 83% of the knees with the bioresorbable device and 90% of knees with the metal screw. The measured knee joint stability averaged 1.6 mm for each group with maximum manual force. Seven percent of the 7-mm absorbable screws were broken on initial insertion. No lytic bone changes were reported on plain film radiographs. It should be noted that the complete absorption time for this implant (minimum 2 years) is such that little breakdown had occurred by the time of the average follow-up. Therefore, if inflammation was to occur, it would have been beyond the average follow-up of this study.

In 1995, another bioresorbable implant was introduced for ACL bone-patellar tendon-bone graft fixation. This implant was an interference screw made of copolymer 85/15 DL lactide/glycolide. The screw was compared to a metal screw of similar geometry manufactured by the same company (Instrument Makar) (Fig. 7). This unique screw design included a blunt nose to avoid self carrying of the screw past the graft. The flutes were blunted to avoid cutting or fracturing the graft. There was no cannulation in the screw. The design geometry was such that the combination of a blunted nose, short thick lines, and absence of cannulation hole resulted in less surface area to mass than a conventional cannulated screw. This design change accommodated the use of this specific bioabsorbable material. It was believed that if the material was changed, the design should also be changed to accommodate the different physical properties of the new material. The shorter and blunted tines of the new design would not produce the same fixation as a conventional screw. Therefore, a new surgical method was introduced to enhance the density of the bone tunnel for the screw. This method, which compacts the cancellous bone with a series of dilators of successively larger diameter,[55] also removes the necessity for cannulation and use of a guide wire. Laboratory testing showed the resistance to pull-out of a screw of this configuration, inserted by this method, was the same for both metal or biodegradable material.[56] A similar observation has been reported by others concerning the effect of material on fixation.[57] Three studies on the clinical use of this screw have been completed.

Stahelin and associates[58] reported on 36 patients with 36 such bioabsorbable screws with mean follow-up of 1 year. The study included computed tomographic scans, magnetic resonance imaging (MRI), and selected biopsy. There were no fixation failures, and no distortion was seen on MRI. There was good knee joint stability. Selected biopsy showed only minimal bone tissue reaction to this implant.

Toljan and Orthner[59] reported on a prospective, randomized clinical trial with 60 patients. Bioabsorbable screws were inserted in 30 patients, using the bone compaction method of insertion. There was excellent fixation and no clinical problems. There were no abnormalities on plain radiographs. MRI studies were

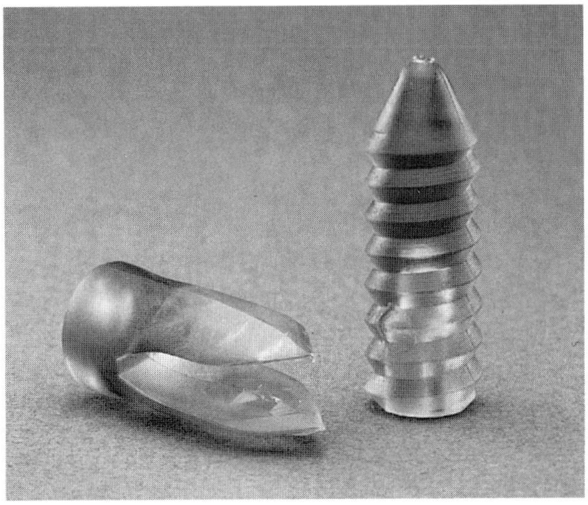

Fig. 7 Bioresorbable staple and screw for ACL reconstruction.

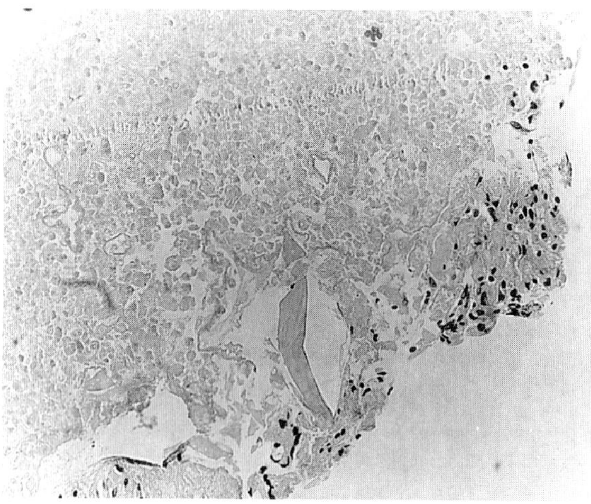

Fig. 8 Inflammatory cells as observed in fibrous tissue.

performed at 6 weeks, and at 3, 6, and 12 months. The MRIs showed increased fluid around the absorbing screws. Forty-one percent showed edema or cysts on MRI in early stages of absorption. There was decreasing tissue reaction by 12 months. There were no adverse clinical observations. Because of the changes seen on MRI, final recommendations will not be made until completion of long-term follow-up.

Kousa and associates[57] reported on their 100-case prospective, multiple center trial. This study also compared the bioresorbable interference screw with the traditional metal screw. Occasional intraoperative bioresorbable screw breakage was experienced during the initial cases by all surgeons. The cause of such breakage was angulation forces applied with a stirring motion of the screw driver. The broken screws were removed and replaced without compromise of the procedure. After a short learning curve on the part of the surgeons, this intraoperative complication was eliminated. Follow-up clinical evaluations and plain radiographs were made monthly through the sixth month, at 1 year, and at 2 years in both groups. The clinical assessment was statistically the same for both groups. Graft fixation was not lost in any case. All patients had restoration of ACL functional stability. The average postoperative injured-to-uninjured measurement of knee ligament laxity was the same for both groups with a Stryker® knee ligament laxity tester; there was 1.3-mm displacement difference at 20 pounds pull and, interestingly, a 1.2-mm difference at 40 pounds. The plain radiographs showed no evidence of bone cyst formation in the bioabsorbable screw group. An MRI was taken in three patients for clinical management reasons in the bioabsorbable group. The imaging was performed at a time when implant absorption was near completion (5 and 8 months) or, in one case, complete (19 months). There was no evidence of edema or bone cyst formation on these incidental MRIs. Four reoperations were necessary in the bioresorbable group to restore full knee extension. The second look arthroscopies, at an average of 6 months, revealed no intra-articular reaction related to the bioresorbable implant. Exploration of the previous screw site showed no gross evidence of the implant. The implant sites were filled with fibrous tissue. Biopsies were made of the previous screw site in each case. Histologic sections showed fibrous tissue filling the space where the implant had been placed. There was a small amount of bioabsorbable material in the fibrous tissue. A few areas of chronic inflammatory cells were observed in the fibrous tissue (Fig. 8). There were no reoperations in the metal group.

Summary

The early experience with bioresorbable fixation devices in ACL reconstructive surgery has provided graft fixation and clinical results comparable to those seen with metal screws. The potential for device breakage during insertion is readily eliminated with surgical experience. Plain radiographs have not shown any bone cyst formation. MRI evaluation may show edema, due to the hydrophilic nature of the material during the absorption phase, and radiolucency in areas previously occupied by the implant, but without any associated adverse clinical affects.[59] The bioresorbable fixation device appears to be a reasonable alternative for use in ACL reconstructive surgery.

The Future of Bioresorbable Implants for Orthopaedics

New Implants

Several resorbable implants for various uses will be expected to reach the American market in the near future. Included among these will be implants awaiting FDA approval, implants already in use in other countries, implants still under development, and conceptually new implants that have not yet been tested.

In the near future, several types of resorbable suture anchors will be available for attaching soft tissue to bone. These devices will have the advantages of not interfering with MR imaging of joints and of disappearing after their function is complete. Resorbable devices that resemble expansion bolts, which have an inner core that expands against a serrated outer sleeve, should provide marked improvements in pull-out strength when attaching soft tissues to bone. Furthermore, it is likely that these devices can be placed percutaneously or arthroscopically. Absorbable clips and small barbed tacks are being developed for meniscus repair, and these should obviate the need for intra-articular knot-tying or the risks to neurovascular structures associated with tying sutures outside the capsule at the back of the knee (Fig. 9). Small tacks have been developed for attaching ligaments to bone without the need to place complex stitches, tie over buttons, or use pull-out wire in such procedures as the repair of the gamekeeper's thumb. There is considerable interest in the use of resorbable membranes for osseous reconstruction in oral surgery, and experimentation is underway to determine if resorbable membranes can be used to provoke or contain osteogenesis in long-bone defects.

Solid resorbable polymeric implants can be created by melt-molding or by machining of molded or extruded pieces. Material properties are improved by solid state transformation such as hot drawing or die drawing, processes that introduce fibers into the material and tend to reinforce it. In the process of material manufacture, it may be possible to introduce additives, which may alter the mechanical properties of the implant or impart multiple functions. Conceivably, antibiotic could be added to the material, which could then be used to release the antibiotic locally to fight infection or to create a fixation device with anti-infective properties. Adding barium to an implant could make it radiopaque in portions or in its entirety. The addition of gas to the polymer may create structural foams that could be used as fillers and would disintegrate with time. There is considerable interest in adding growth factors or hormones to resorbable polymeric implants for the local delivery of these factors to tissues. Hydroxyapatite could be incorporated to create an osteoinductive effect.

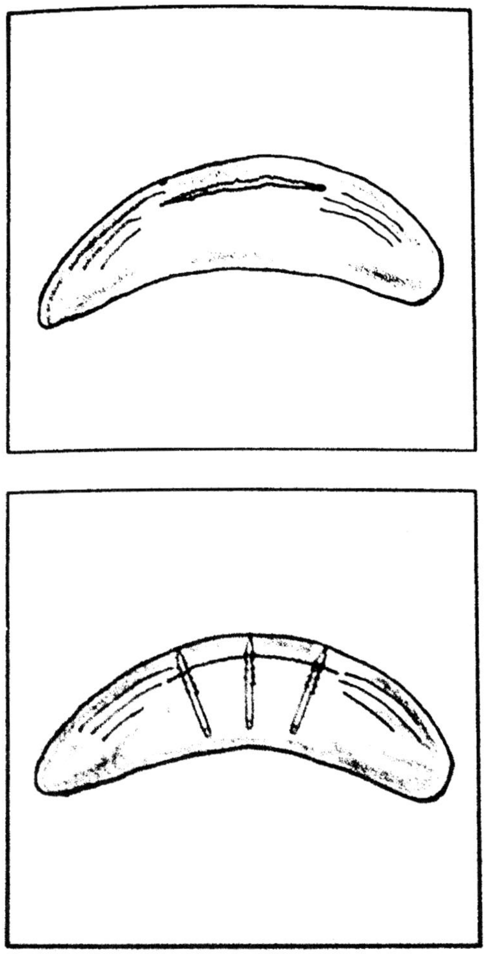

Fig. 9 Bioresorbable barbed tack for meniscus repair.

Possiblities for the Future

There are several innovative potential uses for resorbable implants.

Acetabular Cup Fixation Particulate debris is known to be a contributor to failure in hip replacement arthroplasty. Particles are generated at the junctions of dissimilar materials that are subject to motion. Screws used to fix the acetabular cup to the pelvis may generate wear debris at their interface with the metallic cup. If these screws were constructed of a resorbable material, they could serve their short-term function of cup fixation until bony stabilization had occurred and then resorb without generating particulate debris. Such cup fixation screws are currently under development.

Bone Graft Substitute Generally, in order to achieve successful spinal arthrodesis, large quantities of autogenous bone graft are required. Considerable morbidity is associated with the harvest of autogenous graft, including pain, operative time, blood loss, and potential for infection. Furthermore, in cases of repeat surgery, there may not be a good source of donor graft. The use of allograft carries a risk of infectious disease and less surety of successful fusion. It would be attractive to be able to achieve fusion without having to harvest autogenous graft. Interest has been expressed in the use of resorbable polymers as replacements for bone graft. Such implants would have osteoinductive potential and would also allow addition of decalcified bone matrix or hydroxyapatite.[60] Experimental studies, which attempted to achieve fusion without bone graft by implanting bone morphogenetic protein (BMP) carried in a polymer matrix, have proven successful in a dog model.[61]

Anti-Adhesion Membrane Free motion of muscle and tendon is necessary for normal joint function. After tendon injury and repair, there is a risk of scar and adhesion formation, which can impede range of motion. This is commonly associated with Zone 2 flexor tendon injury and repair in the hand. It is conceivable that an area of injury and repair could be protected by a thin resorbable membrane that would be permeable to nourishing fluids but would keep the repair from adhering to surrounding tissue during healing. This

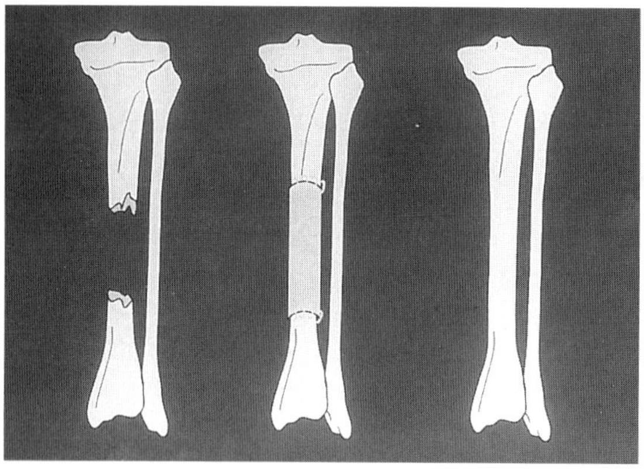

Fig. 10 Tubular polymeric membrane for enhanced bone healing in diaphyseal defects.

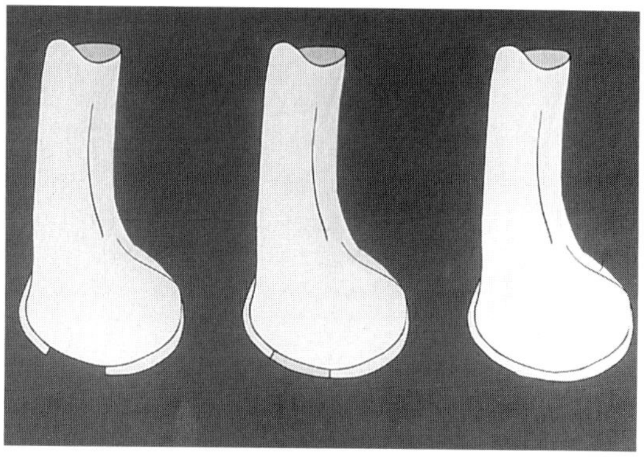

Fig. 12 Delivery of chondrocytes with absorbable scaffolding to cartilage deficient distal femur. Scaffolding disappears leaving living cells enmeshed in natural matrix.

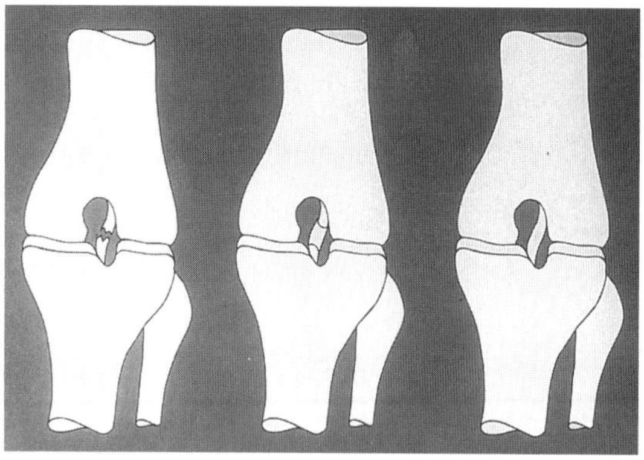

Fig. 11 Splinting of repaired ligament during healing. Absorbable ligament prosthesis gradually disappears.

membrane would then gradually resorb and disappear from the tendon sheath once its function had been completed. Anti-adhesion membranes may be useful in other locations as well.

Osteosynthesis There is considerable interest in the use of resorbable implants to fill in discontinuities in bone, especially in craniofacial applications,[62] in which implants have shown a limited osteoinductive potential. Experiments in small animals have shown that tubular polymeric membranes may enhance bone healing in diaphyseal defects by maintaining a suitable environment for osteogenic cells (Fig. 10).[63] Studies continue to focus on the use of resorbable implants to contain or enhance osteogenic reaction.

Ligament Augmentation Surgical efforts to repair acutely torn ACLs have not met with success due to the intra-articular location and relative hypovascularity. Attempts have been made to augment repairs with autogenous tissues and ligament prostheses. The use of autogenous tissue generally is associated with some donor site morbidity. Prosthetic ligaments have failed to withstand the mechanical demands of the knee. The use of absorbable ligament prosthesis is attractive in that it could be used to splint a repaired ligament during healing and then would gradually disappear as the natural ligament became able to withstand more stress with time (Fig. 11). Initial studies in augmenting repair of canine ACL have shown some promise.[64]

Tissue Engineering Considerable interest is currently being directed toward tissue engineering. Hopefully, deficient tissues such as bone, ligament, and cartilage can be replaced using derivatives of autogenous tissue. For instance, if there is a localized deficiency of cartilage in a joint, it may be possible to harvest chondrocytes from a safe location, culture the chondrocytes to increase their number and volume, and then deliver them to the area of deficiency, where they will heal to the surrounding tissue and resume normal function (Fig. 12). One area of difficulty in developing such a technique is how to deliver the cells to the intended site of implantation, and it may be possible to use an absorbable scaffolding to hold the cells in place. With time the scaffolding would disappear, leaving the living cells enmeshed in their naturally elaborated matrix. The goal would be the return of normal tissue at the original site of defect.

Multi-Tasking Multi-tasking is a theoretical possibility for resorbable implant materials. Because these materials can be formed into structural devices, such as pins, rods, screws, tacks, and staples, and can also be fabricated to contain antibiotics, growth factors, and hormones, there would appear to be possibilities for multi-tasking. For instance, a screw for internal fixation could elute antibiotic which would prevent or fight infection locally at the site of implantation. Similarly, a device containing BMP may be expected to promote bone healing at high-risk sites or in the treatment of established nonunion. The prospects for multi-tasking are many and exciting.

Summary There are several new and potential uses for absorbable implants. Some will provide exciting options in the future. Ongoing animal and clinical studies will help focus future areas of development.

References

1. Cutright DE, Hunsuck EE, Beasley JD: Fracture reduction using a biodegradable material, polylactic acid. *J Oral Surg* 1971;29: 393–397.
2. Kulkarni RK, Moore EG, Hegyeli AF, et al: Biodegradable poly(lactic acid) polymers. *J Biomed Mater Res* 1971;5:169–181.
3. Roed-Petersen B: Absorbable synthetic suture material for internal fixation of fractures of the mandible. *Int J Oral Surg* 1974;3:133–136.
4. Vainionpää S, Vihtonen K, Mero M, et al: Biodegradable fixation of rabbit osteotomies. *Acta Orthop Scand* 1986;57:237–239.
5. Axelson P, Raiha J, Sittnikow K, et al: The use of biodegradable implants in the fixation of small animal cancellous bone fractures. *Acta Vet Scand* 1988;29:469–476.
6. Böstman O, Mäkelä EA, Törmälä P, et al: Transphyseal fracture fixation using biodegradable pins. *J Bone Joint Surg* 1989;71B: 706–707.
7. Kumta SM, Spinner R, Leung PC: Absorbable intramedullary implants for hand fractures: Animal experiments and clinical trial. *J Bone Joint Surg* 1992;74B:563–566.
8. Bucholz RW, Henry S, Henley MB: Fixation with bioabsorbable screws for the treatment of fractures of the ankle. *J Bone Joint Surg* 1994;76A:319–324.
9. Christel P, Chabot F, Leray JL, et al: Biodegradable composites for internal fixation, in Winter GD, Gibbons DF, Plenk H Jr (eds): *Biomaterials 1980*. Chichester, England, John Wiley & Sons, 1982, pp 271–280.
10. Cutright DE, Hunsuck EE: The repair of fractures of the orbital floor using biodegradable polylactic acid. *Oral Surg Oral Med Oral Pathol* 1972;33:28–34.
11. Greve H, Holste J: Refixation of osteochondral fragments using absorbable plastic pins. *Aktuelle Traumatol* 1985;15: 145–149.
12. Miller RA, Brady JM, Cutright DE: Degradation rates of oral resorbable implants (polyactates and polyglycolates): Rate modification with changes in PLA/PGA copolymer ratios. *J Biomed Mater Res* 1977;11:711–719.
13. Sedel L, Chabot F, Christel P, et al: Biodegradable implants in orthopedic surgery. *Rev Chir Orthop Reparatrice Appar Mot* 1978;64(suppl 2):92–96.
14. Vainionpää S, Vihtonen K, Mero M, et al: Fixation of experimental osteotomies of the distal femur of rabbits with biodegradable material. *Arch Orthop Trauma Surg* 1986;106:1–4.
15. Böstman OM: Absorbable implants for the fixation of fractures. *J Bone Joint Surg* 1991;73A:148–153.
16. Törmälä P, Vainionpää S, Kilpikari J, et al: The effects of fibre reinforcement and gold plating on the flexural and tensile strength of PGA/PLA copolymer materials *in vitro*. *Biomaterials* 1987;8:42–45.
17. Frazza EJ, Schmitt EE: A new absorbable suture. *J Biomed Mater Res* 1971;5:43–58.
18. Vert M, Chabot F, Leray J, et al: Bioresorbable polymers for bone surgery. *Makromol Chem* 1981;5:30–41.
19. Doddi N, Versfelt CC, Wasserman D: Synthetic absorbable surgical devices of polydioxanone. US Patent, 4 052 988, 1977.
20. Grace WR: Absorbable prosthetic devices and surgical sutures. British Patent 1034123, 1966.
21. Vainionpää S, Rokannen P, Törmälä P: Surgical applications of biodegradable polymers in human tissues. *Progr Polym Sci* 1989;14:679–716.
22. Zimmerman M, Parsons JR, Alexander H: The design and analysis of a laminated partially degradable composite bone plate for fracture fixation. *J Biomed Mater Res* 1987;21(suppl A3):345–361.
23. Claes LE: Mechanical characterization of biodegradable implants. *Clin Mater* 1992;10:41–46.
24. Miller ND, Williams DF: On the biodegradation of poly-beta-hydroxybutyrate (PHB) homopolymer and poly-beta-hydroxybutyrate-hydroxyvalerate copolymers. *Biomaterials* 1987;8: 129–137.
25. Hollinger JO, Battistone GC: Biodegradable bone repair materials: Synthetic polymers and ceramics. *Clin Orthop* 1986; 207:290–305.
26. Ray JA, Doddi N, Regula D, et al: Polydioxanone (PDS), a novel monofilament synthetic absorbable suture. *Surg Gynecol Obstet* 1981;153:497–507.
27. Lehninger AL (ed): *Principles of Biochemistry*. New York, NY, Worth Publishers, 1982.
28. Woo SL, Simon BR, Akeson WH, et al: An interdisciplinary approach to evaluate the effect of internal fixation plate on long bone remodeling. *J Biomech* 1977;10:87–95.
29. Uhthoff HK, Finnegan M: The effects of metal plates on post-traumatic remodelling and bone mass. *J Bone Joint Surg* 1983; 65B:66–71.
30. Wei G, Kotoura Y, Oka M, et al: A bioabsorbable delivery system for antibiotic treatment of osteomyelitis: The use of lactic acid oligomer as a carrier. *J Bone Joint Surg* 1991;73B:246–252.
31. Miyamoto S, Takaoka K, Okada T, et al: Evaluation of polylactic acid homopolymers as carriers for bone morphogenetic protein. *Clin Orthop* 1992;278:274–285.
32. Böstman O, Hirvensalo E, Partio E, et al: Impact of the use of absorbable fracture fixation implants on consumption of hospital resources and economic costs. *J Trauma* 1991;31:1400–1403.
33. Ward JJ, Thornbury DD, Lemons JE, et al: Metal-induced sarcoma: A case report and literature review. *Clin Orthop* 1990;252: 299–306.
34. Böstman OM: Absorbable implants for the fixation of fractures. *J Bone Joint Surg* 1991;73A:148–153.
35. Pohjonen T, Manninen MJ, Törmälä P, et al: The in vitro and in vivo strength retention of fibrillated self-reinforced poly-L-lactide rods, in *Transactions of the Fourth World Biomaterials Congress*. Berlin, Germany, European Society for Biomaterials, 1992, p 269.
36. Tonino AJ, Davidson CL, Klopper PJ, et al: Protection from stress in bone and its effects: Experiments with stainless steel and plastic plates in dogs. *J Bone Joint Surg* 1976;58B: 107–113.
37. Reilly DT, Burstein AH: The elastic and ultimate properties of compact bone tissue. *J Biomech* 1975;8:393–405.
38. Stone JL, Beaupre GS, Hayes WC: Multiaxial strength characteristics of trabecular bone. *J Biomech* 1983;16:743–752.
39. Törmälä P, Vasenius J, Vainionpää S, et al: Ultra-high-strength absorbable self-reinforced polyglycolide (SR-PGA) composite rods for internal fixation of bone fractures: In vitro and in vivo study. *J Biomed Mater Res* 1991;25:1–22.
40. Böstman O, Hirvensalo E, Mäkinen J, et al: Foreign-body reactions to fracture fixation implants of biodegradable synthetic polymers. *J Bone Joint Surg* 1990;72B:592–596.
41. Böstman O, Partio E, Hirvensalo E, et al: Foreign-body reactions to polyglycolide screws: Observations in 24/216 malleolar fracture cases. *Acta Orthop Scand* 1992;63:173–176.
42. Bos RR, Rozema FR, Boering G, et al: Degradation of and tissue reaction to biodegradable poly(L-lactide) for use as internal fixation of fractures: A study in rats. *Biomaterials* 1991;12:32–36.
43. Bergsma EJ, Rozema FR, Bos RR, et al: Foreign body reactions to resorbable poly(L-lactide) bone plates and screws used for the fixation of unstable zygomatic fractures. *J Oral Maxillofac Surg* 1993;51:666–670.
44. Böstman OM: Osteolytic changes accompanying degradation of absorbable fracture fixation implants. *J Bone Joint Surg* 1991; 73B:679–682.
45. Fraser RK, Cole WG: Osteolysis following biodegradable pin fixation of fractures in children. *J Bone Joint Surg* 1992;74B: 929–930.
46. Partio EK, Bšstman O, Hirvensalo E, et al: Self-reinforced absorbable screws in the fixation of displaced ankle fractures: A prospective clinical study of 152 patients. *J Orthop Trauma* 1992; 6:209–215.
47. Barfod G, Svendsen RN: Synovitis of the knee after intra-articular fracture fixation with Biofix®: Report of two cases. *Acta Orthop Scand* 1992;63:680–681.

48. Friden T, Rydholm U: Severe aseptic synovitis of the knee after biodegradable internal fixation: A case report. *Acta Orthop Scand* 1992;63:94–97.
49. Tegnander A, Engebretsen L, Bergh K, et al: Activation of the complement system and adverse effects of biodegradable pins of polylactic acid (Biofix®) in osteochondritis dissecans. *Acta Orthop Scand* 1994;65:472–475.
50. Böstman O, Hirvensalo E, Vainionpää S, et al: Degradable polyglycolide rods for the internal fixation of displaced bimalleolar fractures. *Int Orthop* 1990;14:1–8.
51. Böstman O, Vainionpää S, Hirvensalo E, et al: Biodegradable internal fixation for malleolar fractures: A prospective randomised trial. *J Bone Joint Surg* 1987;69B:615–619.
52. Partio EK, Hirvensalo E, Partio E, et al: Talocrural arthrodesis with absorbable screws: 12 cases followred for 1 year. *Acta Orthop Scand* 1992;63:170–172.
53. Hope PG, Williamson D, Coates CJ, et al: Biodegradable pin fixation of elbow fractures in children: A randomised trial. *J Bone Joint Surg* 1991;73B:965–968.
54. Johnson LL (ed): *Arthroscopic Surgery: Principles and Practice*, ed 3. St. Louis, MO, CV Mosby, 1986, vol 2, pp 1101–1238.
55. Barber FA, Elrod BF, McGuire DA, et al: Preliminary results of an absorbable interference screw. *Arthroscopy* 1995;11: 537–548.
56. Johnson LL, van Dyk GE: Arthroscopically monitored ACL reconstruction: Compaction drilling and compression screw fixation, in Feagin JA Jr, Applewhite LB (eds): *The Crucial Ligaments: Diagnosis and Treatment of Ligamentous Injuries About the Knee*, ed 2. New York, NY, Churchill Livingstone, 1994, pp 555–593.
57. Kousa P, Jarvinen TL, Pohjonen T, et al: Fixation strength of a biodegradable screw in anterior cruciate ligament reconstruction. *J Bone Joint Surg* 1995;77B:901–905.
58. Stahelin AC, Feinstein R, Friederich NF: Clinical experience using a bioabsorbable interference screw for ACL reconstruction. *Orthop Trans* 1995;19:287–288.
59. Toljan MA, Orthner E: Abstract: Bioresorbable interference screws in ACL surgery. *Arthroscopy* 1995;11:381–382.
60. Coombes AGA, Meikle MC: Resorbable synthetic polymers as replacements for bone graft. *Clin Mater* 1994;17:35–67.
61. Sandhu HS, Kanim LEA, Zeegen EN, et al: Evaluation of rhBMP-2 with an OPLA carrier in a canine posterolateral spinal fusion model. Proceedings of the American Academy of Orthopaedic Surgeons 62nd Annual Meeting, Orlando, FL. Rosemont, IL, American Academy of Orthopaedic Surgeons, 1995, p 189.
62. Hollinger JO, Schmitz JP: Restoration of bone discontinuities in dogs using a biodegradable implant. *J Oral Maxillofac Surg* 1987;45:594–600.
63. Gogolewski S, Mainil-Varlet P, Pineda L, et al: Bone regeneration with resorbable polymeric membranes: Effect of membrane chemistry on the bone healing process. *Trans Orthop Res Soc* 1995;20:257.
64. Cabaud HE, Feagin JA, Rodkey WG: Acute anterior cruciate ligament injury and repair reinforced with a biodegradable intraarticular ligament: Experimental studies. *Am J Sports Med* 1982;10:259–265.

CHAPTER 53

Patient Management During Limb Lengthening

Stuart A. Green, MD

Introduction

The technique of limb lengthening with external fixation has permitted surgeons to offer hope to patients with limbs that have been stunted during development or growth or as a result of trauma or disease. While limb elongation has been a part of orthopaedic surgery for many decades, Gavriil A. Ilizarov's method of distraction osteogenesis[1] has eliminated the need to use bone grafting to fill the skeletal defect that would ordinarily result when stretching an extremity. What have not been eliminated by Ilizarov's techniques, however, are the many complications of external skeletal fixation in general,[2] and the problems associated with the forcible separation of bone fragments.[3] Indeed, surgeons, no longer bound by the need for autogenous bone graft material, now attempt to elongate limbs by 100% or more of the original length—a likely source of severe soft-tissue complications.

Unlike most other surgical operations, in which the work is done when the patient leaves the operating room, an external fixation procedure takes months to complete. For this reason, success or failure depends on postoperative management—the subject of this chapter.

Principles of Management

The principles of postoperative management described below apply to any treatment protocol in which an external skeletal fixator is used to distract bone fragments, whether for lengthening, deformity correction, or bone transport for a skeletal defect. Each of these therapies involves the distraction of bone and soft tissues and the subsequent filling in of the resulting defect with regenerate new bone tissue. My suggestions for patient management thus apply to any type of fixator—unilateral, biplanar, or circular. Prior to surgery, a considerable amount of time is spent with the patient, advising him or her of the commitment needed for a successful application of the fixator.

This description of the postoperative care of a patient undergoing limb lengthening starts, naturally enough, on the day after an external fixator has been applied to a patient, and it assumes that the frame has been aligned properly and is sufficiently stable to properly secure the osteotomized bone fragments. With suboptimal fixation, the patient will frequently complain of feeling motion at the osteotomy site—often accompanied by clicking—as the fragments move against each other. Although the clicking will disappear as the bone ends are pulled apart, and increasing tension on stretched soft tissues will impart some stability to the bone-fixator configuration, early instability inhibits a patient's initial functional capacity, and slows down rehabilitation substantially.

Physical therapy is started on the first postoperative day.[4] The patient must work to prevent contractures before lengthening begins. The important elements of every postoperative physical therapy treatment plan designed to prevent deformities and contractures include elastic splinting, passive stretching, active use of the limb, and appropriate nighttime positioning.

Splinting

Both static and dynamic splinting have a role in the management of patients undergoing elongation of soft tissues. Static splints include fixed position orthoses and straps, ropes, and other nonelastic devices that hold a limb in position. I frequently use a canvas strap to connect a patient's footwear to the front of the fixator frame (Fig. 1). Such devices are especially helpful at night, when the constant pressure of a dynamic splint can become uncomfortable for the patient.

Dynamic splinting can be as simple as elastic or rubber bands from the foot to the fixator (Fig. 2, *left*) or as

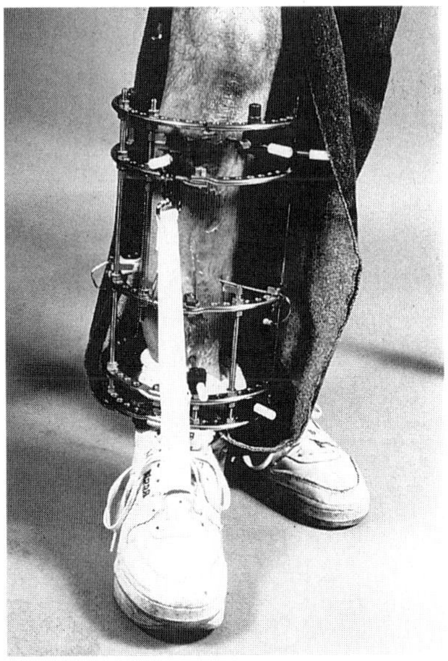

Fig. 1 Static strap to prevent plantarflexion of ankle.

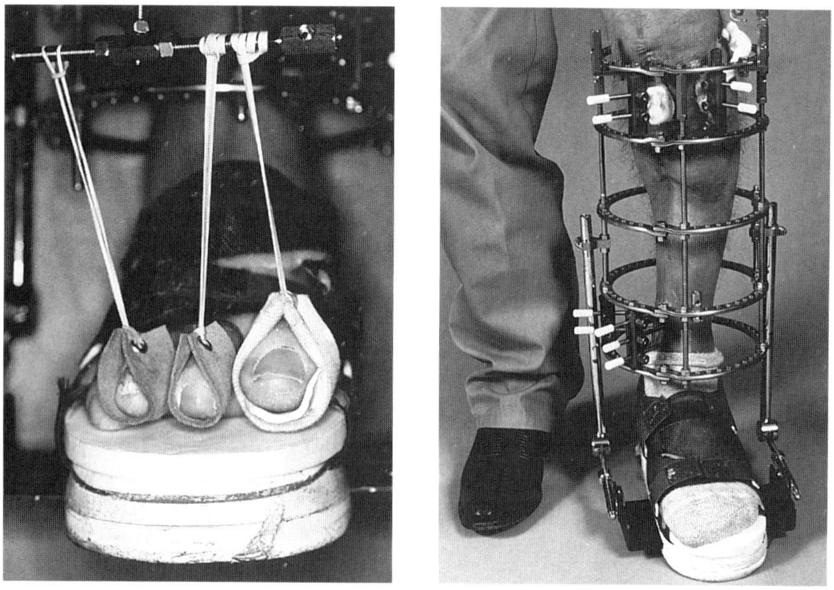

Fig. 2 **Left,** Elastic slings for toes. **Right,** Dynasplint attached to external fixator.

elaborate (and expensive) as a spring-loaded clamp-on dynamic extension splint (Fig. 2, *right*). In either case, dynamic splinting should always be a part of any application that involves muscle stretching.

Night Positioning

The 7 or 8 hours a patient spends in bed may be the most important hours of the day for a patient wearing an external fixator. Joints that are allowed to fall into suboptimal positions during that time will resist correction during daylight. For most lower extremity applications, the foot must be supported and prevented from dropping into plantarflexion. Likewise, the knee joint should be gently forced into full extension, usually by the proper placement of pillows. If left alone, a ring fixator surrounding the lower leg will flex the knee and permit the foot to drop into plantarflexion when a patient is supine (Fig. 3, *top*). Propping up the fixator under its most distal ring will extend the knee; a shoe on the foot can be tied to the frame to support the ankle (Fig. 3, *bottom*).

With thigh lengthenings, the tendency for hip flexion at night can be overcome by placing the patient prone. (A special mattress may be needed if the fixator is located anteriorly.) A pillow can be placed under the knee to extend that joint.

Stretching

Passive muscle stretching is another essential measure designed to prevent contractures. The physical therapist must teach patients and family members how to stretch the calf, the hamstrings, and other muscle groups. At least 2 or 3 hours a day should be devoted to this activity, especially in cases involving substantial

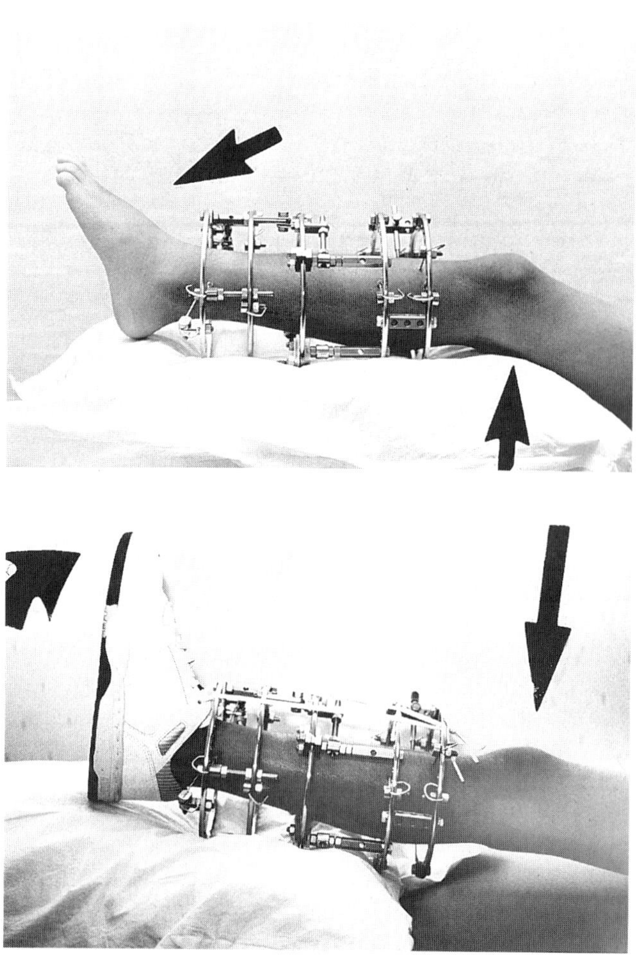

Fig. 3 **Top,** Pillow under calf encourages knee flexion and ankle equinus deformities during limb lengthening. **Bottom,** Correct position with pillow under foot to dorsiflex foot and extend knee.

lengthenings. In fact, the greater the anticipated elongation, the more time per day that must be devoted to passive muscle stretching.

Active muscle exercises do not help much in preventing contractures, because contractures appear to arise from the fascial, rather than the contractile, limb tissues. For example, active dorsiflexion of the ankle is not nearly as effective as passive stretching of the calf musculature in limiting equinus contractures.

Joint Mobility

Intensive physiotherapy is also necessary to prevent the joint contractures and subluxations often associated with limb elongation and the correction of deformities. Even if the fixator is applied to deal with a fracture or a nonunion—conditions not ordinarily associated with stretching of tissues—irritation of muscles impaled by pins or wires can lead to restriction of joint mobility. Thus, joint mobilization has an important place in the management of all patients in external fixation.

Whenever bone fragments are moved with respect to one another, soft tissues are placed under tension: the greater the movement, the greater the tension. For this reason, it is important for the surgeon to consider every external fixator application that involves movement of bone fragments as a form of limb lengthening, even if the extremity does not end up longer as a result of the procedure.

Functional Use

Ambulation and upper extremity use promote ossification of the regenerate bone tissue and, at the same time, help prevent contractures, subluxations, and dislocations. Weightbearing, for example, serves as a means of passive calf muscle stretching while maintaining tone and stimulating circulation in the limb. Eating, hair combing, gymnastics, dance therapy, and other similar activities are also useful adjuncts to therapy. The rhythmic movements involved with swimming, cycling, and walking are among the best therapeutic exercises available.

Ambulation

For a successful lengthening, a limb stabilized in an external fixator must be used in a physiologic manner throughout the time the frame is in place. Mechanical stimulation is essential for the proper ossification of the newly formed regenerate bone in a distraction gap and for the optimum maturation of healing fractures and pseudarthroses.

To achieve this goal, a patient must bear weight on a lower limb in an external fixator and use upper extremities in fixator frames as normally as possible (Fig. 4). Implicit in this requirement is the need to preserve joint mobility through the strategic placement of fixator wires and pins at the time that the fixator is applied. Moreover, the configuration should be stable enough to eliminate movement of the bone with respect to the fixator, because such movement can cause patient discomfort, pin loosening, and decreased neo-osteogenesis. Constant encouragement by the physical therapist and surgeon will do much to insure rapid ossification of healing bone.

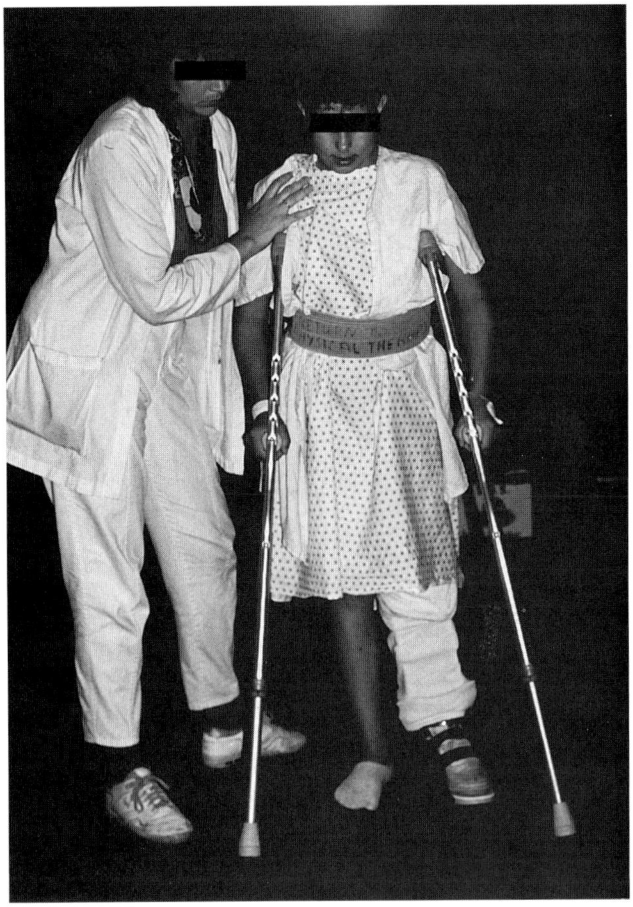

Fig. 4 Ambulation with weightbearing should start as soon as possible after the external fixator is applied.

If, during the course of postoperative fixator management, a patient's walking ability decreases, the surgeon must immediately determine the cause. Usually, there is a clear-cut reason why the patient is having difficulty with ambulation. The most common source of pain with weightbearing is wire or pin site sepsis. At times, the infection may not drain to the surface, but the patient will indicate which implant is causing the pain. The surgeon must not ignore such a development. If antibiotics cannot control the infection, the offending pin or wire should be changed.

Whenever a patient wearing an external fixator stops walking, bone density decreases. The osteoporosis reduces anchorage of wires or pins in the bone, leading

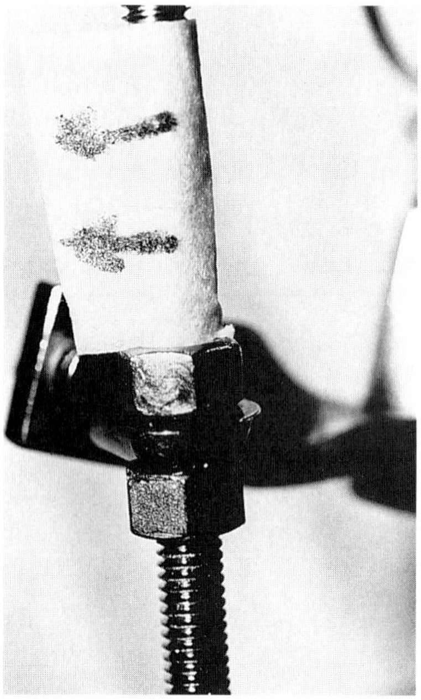

Fig. 5 Marked tape indicates the direction of rotation of the lengthening elements of the fixator and also blocks the patient from turning the lengthening assembly in the wrong direction.

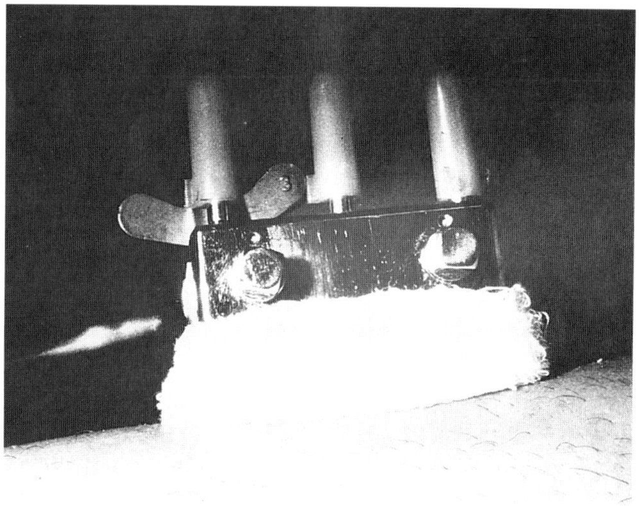

Fig. 6 A bulky wrap prevents the soft tissues from sliding back and forth along the pins.

to loss of fixation. The resultant pin-bone motion encourages microbial invasion, resulting in more sepsis, pain, and a further decline in ambulatory capacity. This vicious cycle should not be allowed to occur. Treat every pin or wire site infection aggressively. A loose fixator must be reapplied.

Management in External Fixation

Postoperative Day 1

Evaluate the pin and wire sites at the first postoperative visit. This can be done without necessarily unwrapping any pins or wires. A patient will complain of excessive wire or pin site pain if there is undue pressure or tension on the skin. If intense pain at an implant site occurs, it may be necessary either to remove the wire or pin and reinsert one elsewhere in a more neutral position, or to release the skin (with a scalpel) adjacent to the wire.

Bleeding from a pin or wire site that persists beyond 1 or 2 days suggests that the implant has penetrated a vascular structure. If this happens, replace the pin or wire with one in a more satisfactory position.

The patient's bed must be flat, not elevated behind the knee, because knee elevation can lead to a knee flexion deformity (Fig. 3, *top*). Place a pillow, instead, under the most distal ring (for a circulator fixator) or under the ankle (for a unilateral fixator) to force the knee into extension (Fig. 3, *bottom*).

Postoperative Days 2, 3, and 4

The patient's physical therapy program continues with progressive weightbearing and range of motion of the joints. Passive stretching is an important part of the physiotherapy program.

Often, patients are discharged from the hospital on postoperative day 2, 3, or 4. At the time of discharge, the patient must be off parenteral pain medication, taking only oral pain killers. The patient is routinely given a prescription for oral antibiotics—usually cephalexin. The patient is instructed to begin taking the antibiotics as soon as any symptoms of pin or wire site sepsis develop. Patients are encouraged to be as active as possible once they leave the hospital.

Latency Interval

The latency interval, which is the delay after application of the fixator and before beginning distraction, allows the first stage of fracture healing to commence. The latency interval commonly used is 5 days, but this can vary considerably, depending on a number of circumstances. For young children, the latency interval may be only 4 days. For bone distraction in adults, the delay often is 7 days before commencing limb lengthening. With very dense cortical bone at the site of distraction (due, perhaps, to old fracture callus), the delay before distraction may be 10 or even 20 days. Because the method of Ilizarov involves callus distraction, it is essential to wait until callus starts to form before beginning the lengthening process. The day that distraction begins, whether it is postoperative day 5, 6, 7, or later, is one of the most important days for the patient wearing a lengthening fixator.

Distraction

Following the latency interval, the patient is taught to distract the corticotomy gap 0.25 mm every 6 hours. This rate and frequency may be altered, depending on the clinical circumstances. For an adult with dense bone and suboptimal surrounding tissues, a more appropriate initial rate and frequency would be 0.25 mm every 8 or 12 hours.

Separating a fixator's pin or wire gripping clamps 0.25 mm does not immediately stretch the tissues the same length; instead, the fixator's wires or pins initially bend toward the middle of the frame as fascia and other dense soft tissues resist elongation.

When distraction starts, it is important to take up the slack in the wires or pins. At the initial lengthening session, the implants will deflect somewhat without causing the bone fragments to separate. It is usually necessary to distract the bone 1 or 2 mm before the bone fragments begin to move apart. The patient will usually feel pain when the bone fragments start to separate. I back the frame up (compressing the fragments) 0.25 mm at a time until the distraction pain subsides. I always mark the frame with adhesive tape to remind the patient in which direction to turn the lengthening component of the apparatus. I place the tape against the element of the frame that will prevent the patient from turning the lengthening unit in the wrong direction (Fig. 5).

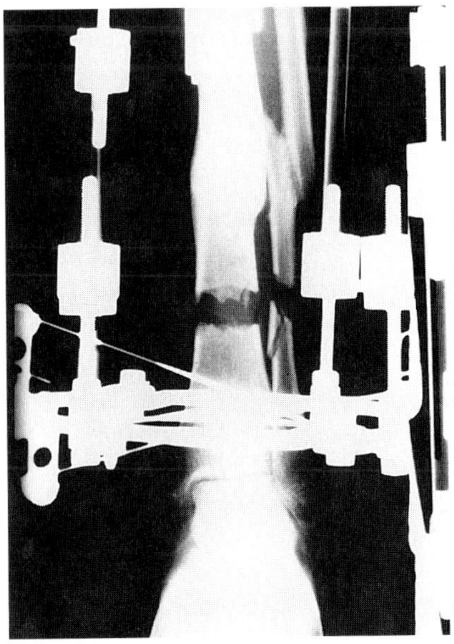

Fig. 7 At 1 month of distraction, hazy ossification must be observed within the widening distraction gap; if not, the distraction should be reversed, and the fragments brought together again, but for twice the latency interval before beginning the distraction again. The rate of distraction should be halved thereafter.

Pin Sites

I do not unwrap the pin or wire site dressings until the day that the sutures are removed—usually on the seventh to tenth day after surgery. Thereafter, the patient is instructed to rewrap certain implant sites after a shower. Specifically, implant wrapping is important in regions where pins or wires penetrate a bulky soft-tissue location, such as the upper thigh (Fig. 6).[5] I recommend avoiding antiseptics, hydrogen peroxide, or any other types of disinfectants for the implant sites, because these substances can actually inhibit the host tissue in its battle with invading microbes at the pin hole.[6] Simply cleansing with a mild soap and water in the shower seems adequate. I have my patients apply Bactroban® ointment each day after they shower, after having cleansed about the pin or wire sites with a detergent soap, such as Dial.

After 1 Week of Distraction

The first set of radiographs should show a gap between the bone fragments that corresponds in width to the rate and frequency of distraction. If the bone fragments are not separating, the corticotomy or osteotomy is probably incomplete. At times, a residual bridge of bone holding the fragments together can be pulled apart by continuing distraction, thereby disrupting the bridge. The patient must be warned that he or she may experience acute severe pain in the limb if the bone suddenly yields to the forces generated by the fixator. When this occurs, the fixator should be backed up to the point close to where distraction began, to start limb lengthening anew. In any case, the frame must not be distracted for more than 10 mm if the bone is not separating to ensure that the sudden elongation will not damage nerves or vessels.

After 2 Weeks of Distraction

After 2 weeks of distraction, the gap should be 14 mm wide (or less if the limb is being elongated at a rate slower than 1 mm per day). Regenerate new bone may not be visible at this stage of distraction.

After 3 Weeks of Distraction

By the third week of distraction, some regenerate new bone should be visible in the distraction gap—usually as a cloudy haze in adults or a fully formed regenerate (with striations and an early interzone) in children. At this stage, the absence of any evidence of regenerate new bone means that the rate of distraction should be slowed down—perhaps to 0.25 mm every 8 or 12 hours.

After 4 Weeks of Distraction

At the end of the fourth week of distraction, the gap will be up to 28 mm wide (with a rate of 1 mm per day). By this time, regenerate new bone must be clearly

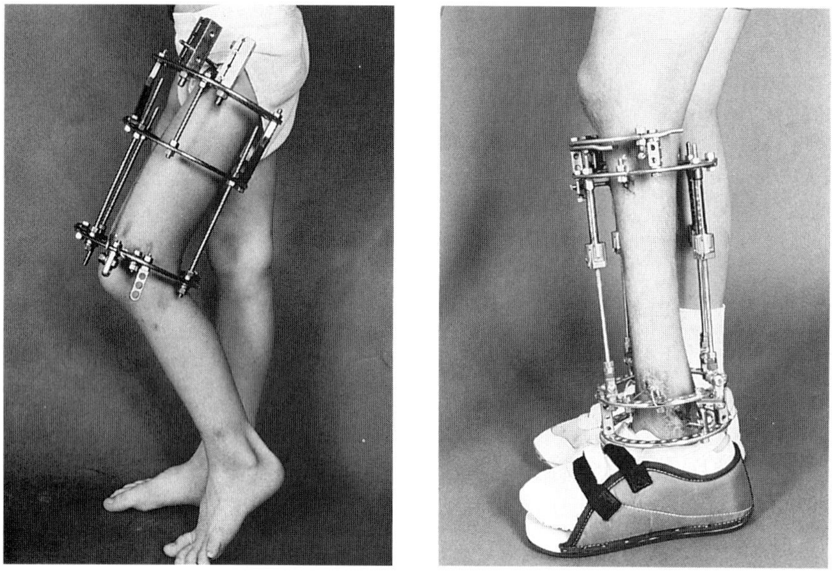

Fig. 8 **Left,** A dangerous situation during limb lengthening: progressive flexion and posteriorward subluxation of the knee joint, often combined with either a progressive hip flexion deformity, or increasing ankle equinus. Lengthening should not proceed lest the knee (and possibly the hip as well) dislocate. **Right,** A knee flexion deformity with only one quarter-inch needed to achieve limb length equality. We stopped distraction at this point, and allowed consolidation, leaving the last quarter-inch to another fixator application—after full knee motion has been restored.

evident in the distraction gap (Fig. 7). If not, reverse the distraction, closing the gap at a rate that is tolerable to the patient—generally about 1 or 2 mm per day in divided doses of 0.25 to 0.5 mm every 6 hours. Usually, regenerate new bone will form and be visible before the gap is completely closed, especially if the patient has been bearing weight on the limb. If no bone forms by the time the gap is fully closed, wait a longer latency interval than initially used (doubling the initial latency interval), and begin distracting again at a slower rate. Follow the postdistraction tactics as before.

Weekly Visits During Distraction

With good regenerate formation, the patient is evaluated on a weekly basis. Assess the quality of the regenerate radiographically, slowing down, speeding up, or even stopping distraction, depending on the quality of bone forming in the distraction gap. Professor Ilizarov recommends resting the limb (stopping distraction) 1 or even 2 days for every 10 days of distraction.

During the weekly visits, check the range of joint motion of the limb. It is critically important to check the joints for any evidence of subluxation—a problem that could lead to complete dislocation if not noticed (Fig. 8, *left*). It is both safer and wiser to stop lengthening a limb that develops a contracture, and plan a second stage procedure at a later time to complete limb elongation (Fig. 8, *right*).

During lengthening, the bone may deform. When this occurs, correct the deviation or it will get worse. Often, these angular deformities are combined with translation of one fragment with respect to another. To correct such a deviation, determine the true apex of the deformity in the usual way for a deformity correction, and correct the evolving deformity as the limb elongation proceeds.

When Length is Achieved

When the patient's limb has reached the goal of lengthening, the frame must be neutralized, thereby transferring weightbearing stresses to the newly formed regenerate osseous tissue. At this point, Ilizarov recommends training the regenerate by overlengthening the limb 7 to 10 mm, and then compressing this overlong regenerate back down to proper length at a rate of 0.25 to 0.5 mm every 12 hours. In this manner, extra bulk of regenerate new bone will be available to participate in consolidation.

Neutralization

Neutralization of the frame is achieved by reversing distraction 2 or 3 mm until the tension on the pins or wires no longer bends them under tension away from the center of the configuration.[7] At this point, the frame is in neutral fixation. Throughout the course of neutral fixation, the patient must be encouraged to bear weight on the limb, lest the regenerate (distraction tissue) not ossify.

Visits During Neutral Fixation

The patient's weightbearing and functional capacity should increase steadily during this period. Investigate any decline in the patient's ability to use the elongated or corrected limb. Often, pin or wire site sepsis will be the problem. If the infection cannot be suppressed, the implant site may have to be changed.

Fixator instability is a frequent and important cause of diminished limb function. The protracted period of

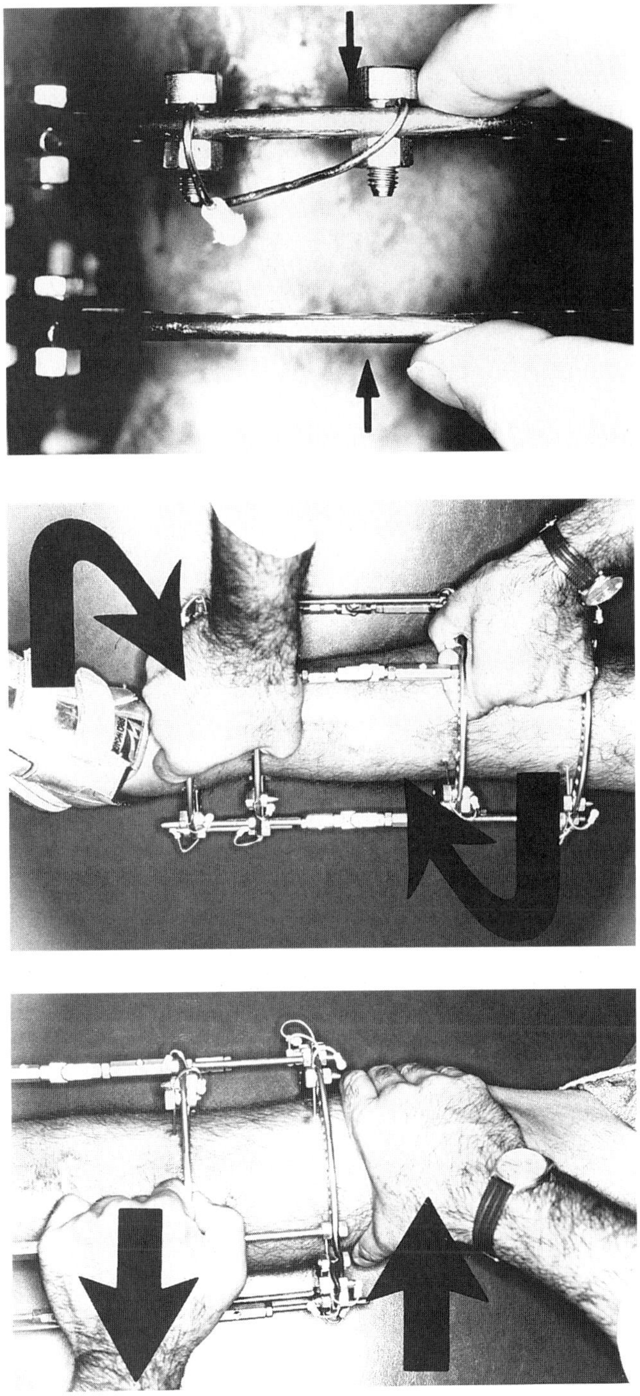

Fig. 9 Frame instabilities that cause pain for the patient and poor quality of regenerate during elongation. **Top,** Ring-to-ring instability. **Center,** Proximal group-to-distal group torsional instability. **Bottom,** Fixator-to-limb instability, causing shifting of the fixator on the limb.

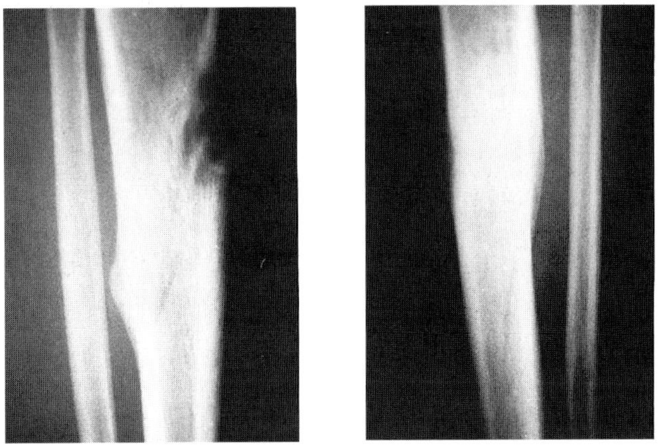

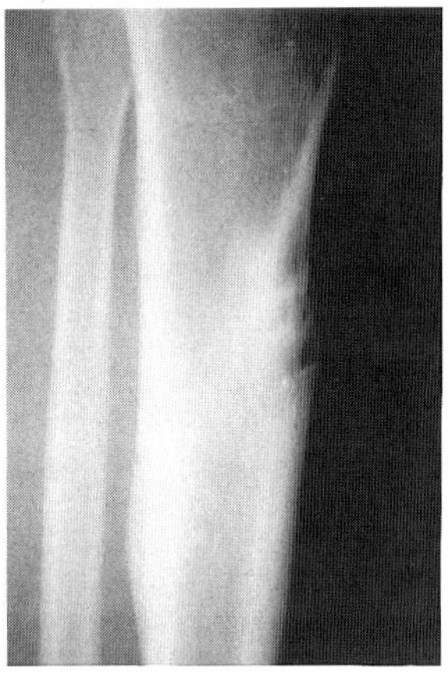

Fig. 10 Assessing the quality of the regenerate. **Top left,** Lateral view shows a large defect in osteogenesis along the anterior cortex, but the posterior cortex is mature. **Top right,** Anteroposterior view shows maturation of the medial and lateral cortices. The regenerate was deemed solid enough to begin dynamization by sequential rod removal. **Bottom,** Four months later (3 months after frame removal), the anterior cortex has filled in with new bone.

time that accompanies slow regenerate ossification may lead to gradual absorption of bone from around the implants. This is most likely to occur with transfixion wires, but can also happen with threaded pins. In my experience, titanium pins resist osteolysis better than any other implant. Indeed, titanium pins often bond to the bone, necessitating general anesthesia for pin removal.

With fixator instability, the patient may describe clicking or wobbling of the frame. Confirm the instability by grasping the limb with one hand and the fixator with the other and trying to displace the frame on the limb (Fig. 9). If such a movement occurs, the frame must be secured to the limb with additional wires or pins. It is unlikely that retensioning a wire (or advancing a tapered pin) will stabilize a loose fixator, because osteolysis at the bone-implant interface will preclude secure fixation.

Dynamization

The final phases of ossification prior to removal can be stimulated by gradually dynamizing the fixator. The process of dynamization cannot begin until the regenerate new bone is fully corticalized on three sides (Fig. 10). With circular fixation frames, the nuts on the connecting rods are released in a sequence at 1- or 2-week intervals. Other strategies are available to dynamize tubular fixators. I start to dynamize a circular fixator with a rod loosening pattern that will leave the final rod

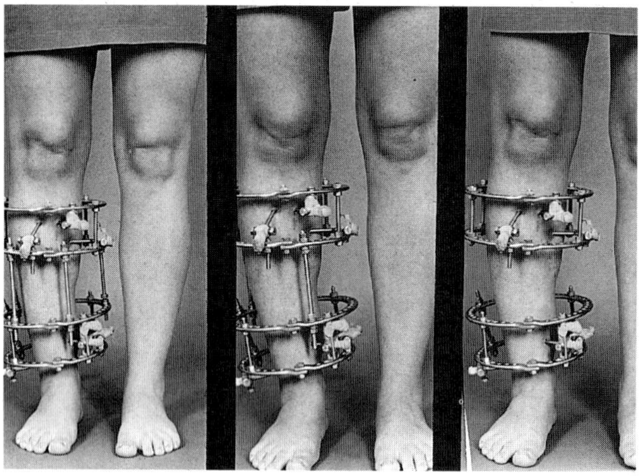

Fig. 11 Sequential rod removal over a period of 1 month. **Left**, Four rods. **Center**, Two rods. **Right**, No rods.

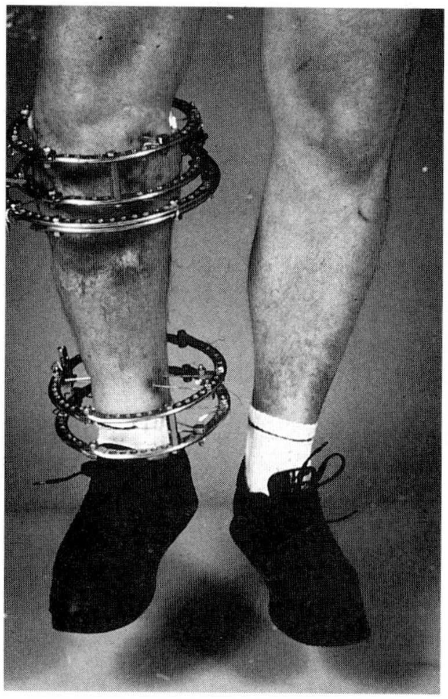

Fig. 12 Patient jumping up and down in a ring fixator prior to frame removal. Note that there are no longitudinal connecting rods left in the frame.

in place adjacent to the weakest portion of the regenerate new bone (Fig. 11). In the lower leg, for example, the regenerate will ossify last along the anteromedial cortex, where the soft tissue overlying the bone is thinnest and where the osteotome was inserted for the corticotomy. Thus, I will first loosen the longitudinal rod in the posteromedial corner of the frame, followed in a week or two by the anterolateral corner, leaving the two oblique rods at the anteromedial and posterolateral corners in place. Next, I remove the posterolateral rod, leaving the patient with a "unilateral fixator."

At the time that the final rod is removed, test the limb manually. The bone should feel quite solid, resisting deflection in any plane. Ilizarov claims that, following a successful physiotherapy program, the patient should be able to "jump up and down" while the fixator is still in place (Fig. 12). I usually have the patient test the stability of the limb by standing on it. He or she should report no difference in the sense of stability, compared to having the longitudinal elements in place. I require the patient to walk around for a week with the pins or wires and fixator still connected to the limb, but with no longitudinal connecting elements in place. Most often, the patients prefer crutches for assisted ambulation during this period of time, although it should not be necessary, since the regenerate new bone is solid at this point in the treatment protocol.

Post Fixator Management

After the frame is removed, it should not be necessary to apply a splint, orthosis, or cast to the patient's limb. In my experience, only one patient in 50 has needed a cast or orthosis after fixator removal. Professor Ilizarov has told me that "physiotherapy should be finished on the day that the frame comes off," although this is often not the case. Instead, intensive physiotherapy must frequently be started to insure restoration of the normal range of motion of the joints surrounding the elongated bone.

Although following the principles outlined in this chapter does not ensure a successful outcome, the measures recommended above will do much to reduce many of the problems, obstacles, and complications ordinarily associated with limb lengthening in both children and adults.

References

1. Ilizarov GA, Green SA (eds): *Transosseous Osteosynthesis: Theoretical and Clinical Aspects of the Regeneration and Growth of Tissue.* Berlin, Germany, Springer-Verlag, 1992.
2. Green SA (ed): *Complications of External Skeletal Fixation: Causes, Prevention and Treatment.* Springfield, IL, Charles C Thomas, 1981.
3. Paley D: Problems, obstacles, and complications of limb lengthening by the Ilizarov technique. *Clin Orthop* 1990;250:81–104.
4. Green SA: Physiotherapy during Ilizarov fixation. *Tech Orthop* 1990;5:61–65.
5. Green SA: The use of wires and pins. *Tech Orthop* 1990;5:19–25.
6. Branemark PI, Ekholm R: Tissue injury caused by wound disinfectants. *J Bone Joint Surg* 1967;49A:48–62.
7. Aronson J, Harp JH Jr: Mechanical considerations in using tensioned wires in a transosseous external fixation system. *Clin Orthop* 1992;280:23–29.

CHAPTER 54

Prevention of Deep Periprosthetic Joint Infection

Arlen D. Hanssen, MD
Douglas R. Osmon, MD
Carl L. Nelson, MD

Although the prevalence of postoperative deep wound infection after total joint arthroplasty has decreased over the past few decades, it remains a feared consequence for both surgeons and patients.[1] Moynihan stated that "every operation in surgery is an experiment in bacteriology."[2] This statement provides remarkable insight into the seemingly variable and unpredictable nature of infection. Often, the specific mechanism and timing of bacterial delivery in a given wound is unknown, and it is usually extremely difficult to prove the exact cause of the infection in an individual situation. Despite improved outcomes of treatment for established deep periprosthetic infection, prevention remains a meaningful objective. The estimated cost of treatment[3] of an infection at the site of a total hip or total knee arthroplasty exceeds $50,000.

A thorough appreciation of and respect for the innumerable factors that may contribute to an infection is essential in the development of an overall approach to prevention. The concept of an interdependent relationship among the triad of bacteria, host, and wound is helpful when considering prevention (Fig. 1). Infection depends on the number and virulence of the bacteria introduced into a wound, the host's ability to eliminate these bacteria, and the status or viability of the wound environment. Within this triad, multiple variables can contribute to the deposition of bacteria into the wound, many conditions may impair the patient's ability to eliminate bacteria, and numerous vagaries of the wound milieu can facilitate the infectious process (Table 1). Every variable may be influenced by the other variables within the triad. For example, the effect of a foreign body on the absolute number of bacteria required to facilitate the infectious process is well known.[4]

When developing an approach toward the prevention of deep periprosthetic infection, the entire health-care team must integrate its disciplined prevention efforts into the preoperative, operative, and postoperative time-periods and direct them toward all three areas of the triad by optimizing the wound environment, augmenting the host's ability to fight infection, and minimizing the number of bacteria in the wound. Preventive measures include both methodologies that have been proved in a scientific manner and techniques that are considered to be reasonable despite the fact that their effectiveness in the clinical setting probably cannot be proved. It is important to emphasize the need to educate all members of the health-care team and to make them aware of the importance of their participation in the preventive efforts.

Preoperative Period

Efforts during this time-period should concentrate on assessment of patients who have impaired host defenses, evaluation of operative sites that may provide a poor wound environment, and identification of remote sources of infection (Table 1). In general, conditions such as impairment of the immune system or malnutrition may not be entirely reversible but need to be decreased as much as possible before the arthroplasty. Some studies have suggested that patients who are managed with immunosuppressive medications;[5] who have diabetes mellitus,[6-9] rheumatoid arthritis,[7,10-12] or an advanced age;[13-15] or who are obese,[16-18] at high risk for anesthesia-related complications,[19] or malnourished[5,14,20,21] should be considered high-risk hosts. Open reduction and internal fixation of fractures in patients who have acquired immunodeficiency syndrome is

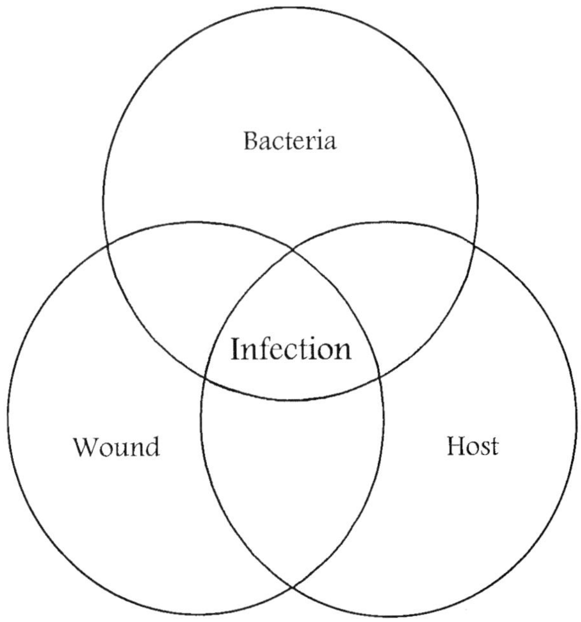

Fig. 1 Venn diagram demonstrating the dependent nature of bacteria, host factors, and wound environment on the development of infection.

Table 1
Variables influencing deep periprosthetic infection

	Preoperative Period	Operative Period	Postoperative Period
Bacteria	Urinary tract infection, skin ulcers, other remote infections, poor dental hygiene, shaving of operative site, prolonged hospitalization, prophylactic antibiotics	Instrument sterilization; operating-room traffic; personnel; dispersers; face masks or hoods; body-exhaust suits; ultraviolet light; laminar airflow; skin preparation; surgical scrub, gloves, drapes, or gowns; plastic surgical drape; wound irrigation; suction tips; splash basins	Urinary tract management, remote sites of infection, intravenous catheters, invasive procedures, possibly prophylactic antibiotics
Host	Altered immune system, immunosuppressive medications, diabetes mellitus, rheumatoid arthritis, advanced age, malnutrition, anesthetic risk		Rheumatoid arthritis, altered immune system
Wound environment	Extensive scarring, previous operation, previous infection, obesity, vascular disease, anatomical site, local skin conditions, thin atrophic skin	Duration of procedure, operative technique, suture selection, implant selection, antibiotic bone cement, structural bone graft, hemostasis, surgical drains, wound closure	Wound hematoma, wound drainage, skin necrosis, reoperation, loose prostheses, particulate debris

associated with an increased risk of infection, but the effect of the syndrome on elective joint replacement has not been established.[22] Prolonged hospitalization just before the surgical procedure has been associated with an increased prevalence of infection.[23] In a study of 23,649 surgical wounds by Cruse and Foord,[23] the prevalence of deep infection was 1.1% for patients who were admitted on the day of the operation or who were hospitalized for only 1 day preoperatively, 1.6% for patients who were hospitalized for 2 to 6 days preoperatively, 2% for patients who were hospitalized for 7 to 13 days preoperatively, and 4.3% for patients who were hospitalized for at least 14 days preoperatively. Whether this represents a selection bias for high-risk patients with other serious medical illness or is due to skin colonization with nosocomial organisms resistant to antibiotics commonly used for prophylaxis is unknown.

Preoperative laboratory assessment of nutritional status should be individualized and may include appraisal on the basis of anthropometric indicators (circumference of the arm to indicate the muscle mass, thickness of the triceps skin fold, and weight-height ratio), immunologic indicators (total lymphocyte count), or biochemical indicators (levels of serum albumin and transferrin, total iron-binding capacity, and nitrogen balance).[5,20,21,24] A preoperative total lymphocyte count of less than 1,500 cells/mm^3 (1.5×10^9/l) and an albumin level of less than 35 g/l have been associated with an increased prevalence of wound complications.[5] Serum transferrin levels have been shown to be an even more sensitive indicator of wound complications after hip arthroplasty than lymphocyte counts and serum albumin levels.[14] Currently, there is no accepted standard of or definition for nutritional depletion in patients who are scheduled to have an elective total joint arthroplasty; however, the nutritional index of Rainey-MacDonald and associates and the total lymphocyte count have been helpful for predicting which patients will not have a postoperative infection and serve as baselines for future studies.[25]

The local wound environment is often suboptimum in patients who have advanced vascular disease, a history of multiple surgical procedures, extensive scarring, or a history of wound infection (Table 1). Although conditions such as extensive scarring cannot be altered, careful preoperative assessment may allow modification of the surgical approach and technique to minimize the risk of infection.

Preoperative shaving of the operative site results in rapid colonization of the small nicks left by the razor and is associated with an increased risk of deep infection.[26,27] Shaving should be avoided until immediately before the surgical procedure or depilatory agents should be used.[27] Psoriatic plaques in the region of the operative site may increase the risk of infection, although reports on the effect of this condition have been conflicting.[28-30] Preoperative assessment of psoriatic lesions, when classified on the basis of severity and treated accordingly by a dermatologist, will probably minimize the risk of postoperative infection.[28] Certain anatomic sites, such as the elbow and knee, are associated with a higher prevalence of deep infection, and although the exact reasons are unknown it has been suggested that this vulnerability may be due to the relatively subcutaneous position of these joints.[11,31-33]

Cognizance of this anatomic susceptibility suggests the need for meticulous wound closure and attentive wound care in the postoperative period for patients who have a knee or elbow arthroplasty. Likewise, thin atrophic skin at any site should be particularly noted for special wound care both in the operating room and postoperatively.

Remote sites of infection, such as the oral cavity, the genitourinary tract, the pulmonary system, and skin ulcers, increase the risk of postoperative infection.[3,12,15] A disciplined and consistent physical examination preoperatively is advised for every patient who is scheduled to have an arthroplasty. Abrasions or follicular infection at the intended operative site, venous stasis ulcers, skin breaks in the web spaces of the toes, infections under toenails, poor dentition, and infections of the pulmonary system or urinary tract should be identified and eliminated before the operation whenever possible.

Prophylactic Antibiotics

Prophylactic administration of antibiotics is probably the single most effective method for reducing the prevalence of postoperative wound infection.[34-37] Despite limitations in the designs of most published studies, most consensus panels support the routine use of systemic antimicrobial prophylaxis because the consequences of infection about a prosthetic joint are so severe. Most clinicians routinely use systemic antibiotic prophylaxis at the time of total joint arthroplasty.[38,39] The current controversies with regard to such prophylaxis include identification of the optimum antibiotic, the appropriate timing and duration of antimicrobial prophylaxis, and whether or not antimicrobial prophylaxis and ultraclean operating rooms used concurrently are additive in their ability to reduce the prevalence of infection.

The ideal prophylactic antimicrobial agent would have excellent in vitro activity against staphylococci and streptococci, penetrate tissue well, have a relatively long serum half-life to provide coverage for the duration of the entire surgical procedure, be relatively nontoxic, and be inexpensive.[38,40] The penicillinase-resistant penicillins and cephalosporins have been studied most extensively; however, no single agent has been shown to be superior.[16,17,41-44] It should be recognized that there is no universal agreement on the optimum antimicrobial agent, and some have advocated the prophylactic use of broad-spectrum antimicrobials such as cefamandole and cefuroxime because of concern regarding organisms resistant to the spectrum of coverage provided by first-generation cephalosporins.[16,17,42] To our knowledge, no data have shown the efficacy or cost-effectiveness of this approach. Cefazolin, a first-generation cephalosporin that has been studied extensively, has a long serum half-life, is relatively nontoxic, and is inexpensive compared with other agents; it is thus a prudent choice for antimicrobial prophylaxis.[38,40] For patients who have a type-I hypersensitivity reaction to penicillin (an IgE-mediated hypersensitivity reaction manifested by immediate urticaria; laryngeal edema; and bronchospasm, with or without cardio-vascular shock), vancomycin is an excellent alternative for antimicrobial prophylaxis.

It is important to note that some deep periprosthetic infections, such as late hematogenous infections, are due to causes that occur after the effective time-period of perioperative antibiotic prophylaxis.[1,3,11,45-52] These infections should not be included in the intended spectrum of antibiotic coverage for the initial surgical procedure. Furthermore, the entire spectrum of nosocomial infections within a given institution should not be considered collectively when the type of antibiotic prophylaxis for a total joint arthroplasty is determined. Rather, the susceptibility patterns of surgical wound infections, with special emphasis on the infections that have occurred after implantation of a prosthesis, should be reviewed with the local infection control officer. Decisions should then be individualized and based on the susceptibility patterns demonstrated in that particular institution.

The appropriate time to administer antimicrobials prophylactically is just before the skin is incised.[53] A large prospective clinical trial of 2,847 patients who had a variety of clean and clean-contaminated surgical procedures revealed the lowest rate of surgical wound infection when prophylactic antimicrobials had been administered within 2 hours before the skin incision was made as compared with administration after or more than 2 hours before the incision.[54] Currently, we recommend that systemic antimicrobial prophylaxis be given within 30 to 60 minutes before the skin incision is made and at least 5 to 10 minutes before inflation of a tourniquet, to allow proper penetration of the tissues by the antibiotic.[55] For prolonged procedures exceeding one to two times the half-life of the antibiotic or for procedures associated with extensive blood loss, an additional intraoperative dose of antibiotic is advised.[38]

The optimum duration of systemic antimicrobial prophylaxis has been addressed in several clinical trials but has not been definitively established.[17,43,56] In these studies, a short duration of administration of the prophylactic agent was as efficacious as longer time-periods. In a randomized clinical trial involving 2,651 total hip arthroplasties, deep infection developed in 11 (0.8%) of 1,327 patients who had received one postoperative dose of cefuroxime, compared with six (0.5%) of 1,324 patients who had received three postoperative doses.[57] Although this difference was not significant, the power to detect meaningful statistical differences between the patient groups was low and therefore it was difficult to provide any definitive conclusions. Because of the extremely low rate of infection after total joint arthroplasty, the calculation of the statistical power of a study and the limitations that it imposes on any conclusions must always be remembered. In fact, this concern applies to many available reports that discuss possible risk factors for deep periprosthetic infection.[58,59]

Most authorities recommend a single preoperative dose of antibiotics followed by two or three postoperative doses to reduce the possibility of antimicrobial toxicity, prevent selection of resistant organisms, and minimize the expense associated with antimicrobial prophylaxis.[35,37,38] For example, the estimated reduction in annual health-care costs for 100,000 patients would be $7,700,000 if prophylactic antibiotics were administered in only one intraoperative dose rather than for 48 hours postoperatively.[15] Furthermore, these costs escalate substantially when a more expensive antibiotic is selected or if the duration of prophylaxis is extended.

The use of antibiotic-impregnated bone cement for prophylaxis in primary total joint arthroplasty has been shown to be effective in experimental models,[60] and it has been used extensively for antibiotic prophylaxis outside of the United States. However, its use for primary total joint arthroplasty in North America remains controversial.[61-65] Potential disadvantages of the routine use of antibiotics in bone cement include a possible allergic reaction that may lead to a second operation to remove the implant and all bone cement, emergence of resistant organisms, and weakening of the bone cement. Although it seems reasonable to add antibiotics to cement for high-risk patients, such as those who have a history of infection at the operative site, the proper role of antibiotic-impregnated cement for use as prophylaxis during primary total joint arthroplasty has not been clearly defined and requires additional study.

Operating-Room Environment

Clean-Air Technology

The use of ultraviolet light to sterilize air particles carrying bacteria was initiated in 1936, but the absolute effectiveness of this technology in the clinical setting has not been definitively determined, as studies to date have been retrospective, with comparison of clinical experiences and historical controls.[66-68] The lack of conclusive clinical studies combined with concern regarding exposure of operating-room personnel to ultraviolet light has led to only tentative acceptance of this methodology. However, recent cost-effectiveness comparisons have created a resurgent interest in ultraviolet-light technology because it is considerably less expensive than laminar airflow systems.[68,69]

In 1969, Charnley and Eftekhar[10] reported a dramatic reduction in the prevalence of postoperative infection after total hip arthroplasty, from 9% (17 of 190) to 1% (nine of 708), with the implementation of a clean-air operating theater. Careful analysis of their data suggested that multiple factors over the course of the study, such as the method of subcutaneous wound closure and the use of antibiotics, may also have contributed to the reduced rate of infection. In a subsequent report that attempted to clarify these other variables, Charnley[70] concluded that clean air was the most important factor but was not the sole reason for this reduction in the prevalence of infection. It should be noted that he suggested that clean air is optimally provided by a combination of laminar airflow, with a room-air-exchange turnover rate of more than 300 times an hour; the use of a vertical airflow system; and the use of personnel isolator suits. He also stressed that horizontal laminar airflow systems should be used with body-exhaust systems and impermeable gowns.[70] Finally, he stated: "I most certainly do not wish to be reported as advocating clean air as a panacea for all surgeon's problems of sepsis in total hip replacement."[70]

Subsequently, substantial interest developed in the use of clean-air technology as a method of preventing infection in association with total joint arthroplasty. Many initial studies retrospectively evaluated the efficacy of laminar airflow systems by comparing historical rates of infection, and a thorough review by Nelson and associates[71] detailed many of these studies. A large multicenter prospective randomized clinical trial[32] evaluating the effect of laminar airflow during 6,781 hip arthroplasties and 1,274 knee arthroplasties performed between 1974 and 1979 was published in 1982. Infection occurred in 63 (1.5%) of 4,129 patients in the control group and in only 23 (0.6%) of 3,923 patients in the ultraclean-air group ($p < 0.001$).[32] Although these results seemed to provide irrefutable evidence as to the efficacy of laminar airflow systems, the study design had flaws that included randomization irregularities and lack of patient stratification, and, furthermore, the use of prophylactic antibiotics was not controlled.[72] This study did demonstrate clearly that body exhaust suits reduced the bacterial counts in the room air and, in general, that vertical airflow systems performed better than horizontal airflow systems. The inconsistency in the use of prophylactic antibiotics in this study[32] was a major problem because, in the presence of prophylactic antibiotics, the independent effect of laminar airflow was reduction of the prevalence of infection further from 24 (0.8%) of 2,968 in the control group to ten (0.3%) of 2,863 in the ultraclean-air group, which was not significant ($p < 0.1$) (Table 2). However, in the absence of prophylactic antibiotics, the rate of infection was reduced from 39 (3.4%) of 1,161 to 13 (1.2%) of 1,060, which was significant ($p < 0.01$) (Table 2). These data suggest that both factors have an independent effect on the reduction of infection but leave open the question of whether laminar airflow is necessary when prophylactic antibiotics are used.

A large retrospective study of 2,384 total hip arthroplasties resulted in additional doubt about the absolute efficacy of laminar airflow technology when prophylactic antibiotics are used.[73] Between 1975 and 1978, when none of the patients received prophylactic antibiotics, infection developed after nine (3.1%) of 289 arthroplasties performed in a conventional operating room, compared with nine (2.5%) of 363 arthroplasties performed in a laminar airflow room ($p = 0.5$). After the use of prophylactic antibiotics was initiated in 1979, infection developed following six (0.9%) of 669 arthroplasties performed in the conventional operating room, compared with three (0.3%) of 1,063 arthroplasties performed in a laminar airflow room. Again, these differences were not significant ($p = 0.1$). The difference in the rates of infection between the two study periods (2.8% without antibiotic prophylaxis, compared with 0.5% with antibiotic prophylaxis) was highly significant ($p < 0.00001$).[73] Although retrospective, the study was limited to patients who had had the arthroplasty performed by the same surgeons in one hospital and who had received the same prosthesis, and it was based on excellent documentation of the use of prophylactic antibiotics and consistent use of vertical laminar airflow and body-exhaust suits.[73]

A large retrospective study by Salvati and associates[74] of 3,175 total hip and knee replacements, performed with or without a horizontal unidirectional filtered airflow system, demonstrated a detrimental effect of laminar airflow. It is extremely important to note that personnel isolator suits were not used in this study. The paradoxical increase in the rate of infection after total knee arthroplasty performed in the laminar airflow rooms was attributed to positioning of the operating team between the patient and the airflow unit, with subsequent entrainment of air containing particulate matter and bacteria from the operating-room personnel into the surgical wound.

Table 2
Effects of clean air and use of prophylactic antibiotics on the rate of infection after total hip and total knee arthroplasty[32]

Prophylactic Antibiotics	Laminar Airflow No	Laminar Airflow Yes	
No	39 of 1161 (3.4%)	13 of 1060 (1.2%)	($p < 0.01$)
Yes	24 of 2968 (0.8%)	10 of 2863 (0.3%)	($p < 0.1$)
	($p < 0.001$)	($p < 0.01$)	

Preliminary results were recently reported for a randomized blinded prospective study of 7,305 patients who had a total hip or knee arthroplasty with use of horizontal unidirectional airflow and no personnel isolator suits.[75] All of the patients received antibiotic prophylaxis. Although there was no significant difference in the rate of deep periprosthetic infection between the patients who had the procedure in a room with activated laminar airflow and those who had it in the presence of conventional airflow, it should be noted that these preliminary results essentially parallel the results of Salvati and associates,[74] in that there was a trend toward a higher rate of infection in some groups with laminar airflow but not in others.

These recent studies emphasize the need for appropriate application of clean-air technology and the paradoxical effects that can occur with the misunderstanding of clean-air concepts. Although there is still considerable controversy regarding the necessity of laminar airflow for the performance of total joint arthroplasty if prophylactic antibiotics are used, the following points can be reasonably drawn from the available literature: (1) Vertical laminar airflow units generally reduce airborne contamination better than horizontal airflow units. This is especially true when personnel isolator suits are not used. (2) Strict attention to laminar airflow protocol is essential, and there can be paradoxical increases in the rates of infection if these concepts are disregarded. (3) During the past few decades, the appropriate use of clean-air technology to reduce airborne contamination has reduced the prevalence of infection after total hip and knee arthroplasty. (4) The current literature has not established that clean-air technology can greatly reduce the prevalence of infection when prophylactic antibiotics are also used. However, if the rate of early postoperative infection following the procedures performed by an individual surgeon or at a specific institution exceeds four or five per 1,000 total hip arthroplasties and six, seven, or eight per 1,000 total knee arthroplasties, the use of some method of clean-air technology should be considered to reduce further the prevalence of infection.[10,32,70,75-78] It is important to remember that, with this low prevalence of infection of less than 1%, analysis of more than 6,000 patients is required to achieve the statistical power necessary to determine the effect of any one independent variable, such as airflow, on the rate of infection after total joint replacements.

Other Methods of Reducing Bacterial Contamination

Reduction of bacterial contamination should be a primary focus of the entire operating-room team. Proper sterilization of instruments, careful preparation of the operative site, avoidance of contact with objects outside the sterile field, and maintenance of fundamental aseptic protocols are all essential. When the patient is transported into the operating room, ward bedding should be excluded. Traffic in and out of the operating room should be restricted, and the number of personnel in the operating room should be minimized.[15] In one study, microbiologic counts in an unoccupied operating room increased significantly ($p < 0.05$) when the door was left open to the hallway, and the addition of five operating-room personnel further increased the microbiologic counts by more than sixfold.[79] Although many bacteria are normally shed every minute by all individuals, some individuals, known as dispersers, shed substantially more bacteria, and their presence in the operating room has been associated with an increased prevalence of wound infection.[80,81]

There is conflicting evidence regarding the efficacy of face masks, because some studies have demonstrated that their use does not make any difference in the number of colony-forming units deposited on culture plates in an operating room or in the prevalence of postoperative wound infection.[79,82,83] Conversely, one study demonstrated that the method with which a mask was used when combined with a surgical hood was an important factor in the reduction of airborne contamination.[84] In this study, airborne contamination was most effectively reduced when the surgical mask was donned beneath an overlapping hood rather than over the hood, which allows dispersal of bacteria along the sides of the mask. Minimizing conversation also decreased airborne contamination.[84]

The operative site should be prepared with an antiseptic agent or isopropyl alcohol; however, superiority of an actual agent or the optimum duration of the surgical preparation has not been established.[85,86] A one-step water-insoluble iodophor-in-alcohol solution effectively reduces bacterial counts on the skin as does the traditional two-step scrub-and-paint skin preparation.[85] Iodophor sprays have also demonstrated excellent bactericidal action and are less time-consuming than the traditional scrub.[86] Although antiseptic agents effectively eliminate the immediate bacterial count at the operative site, hair follicles prevent complete sterilization of the skin and, within 30 minutes, the bacteria on the skin begin to recolonize.[87]

Compared with a cloth drape, a plastic surgical adhesive drape reduces wound contamination (as measured on culture of deep wound specimens taken just before closure), probably by preventing lateral migration of the skin bacteria.[88] However, a simple plastic skin drape allows normal recolonization of the skin beneath it within 30 minutes, and microbial counts reach normal levels within 3 hours.[87] In contrast, a plastic drape impregnated with slow-release iodophor effectively eliminates any skin colonization for as long as 3 hours; therefore, this drape seems preferable.[87] At the end of long operative procedures, when the edges of the plastic drape are peeled away from the incision, it seems reasonable to swab the exposed skin with a povidone-iodine solution to reduce the bacterial colony count again before wound closure. Finally, plastic adhesive drapes can avulse or harm thin, friable skin, and the use of a one-step water-insoluble iodophor-in-alcohol solution without the use of a drape offers a satisfactory alternative for sterilization of the skin.[85]

The optimum antiseptic agent and proper duration for the surgical hand scrub has not been established; however, application of a hexachlorophene foam compound provides excellent bactericidal action and is also less time-consuming than traditional scrubbing methods.[89]

The use of double gloves is advisable because of the large number of perforations that routinely occur during an orthopaedic procedure. In one study, use of double latex gloves resulted in a significantly higher rate ($p < 0.0001$) of puncture of the inner glove during orthopaedic procedures, compared with that incurred when a cloth outer glove was used over an inner latex glove.[90] With the use of double latex gloves, the number of punctures correlated directly with the duration of the operation, and all gloves had punctures after procedures that lasted more than 180 minutes.[90] It has been reported that the rates of wound contamination are similar with single or double-gloving routines and that contamination is due to sources other than puncture of the glove.[91] Despite this observation, routine changing of the outer gloves during procedures that last more than several hours is probably still advisable to protect both the surgeon and the patient.

Surgical gowns and drapes should prevent the spread of bacteria by airborne dispersion or direct contamination through the gown by capillary action.[10,92,93] Some materials are more effective than others; for example, Gore-Tex (W.L. Gore and Associates, Flagstaff, AZ) prevents the dispersion of bacteria 1,000 times more effectively than ordinary cotton.[93] Because bacteria invariably do progress to the surface of the gown, the members of the operating team should avoid repetitive touching of the surgical gown with their gloves.

The suction tip is a recognized source of operative contamination, because large volumes of air pass through it and the airborne bacteria that collect on the suction tip can be transferred to the wound.[94-96] In one study, after an average of 100 minutes of operative time, 12 (55%) of 22 suction tips were contaminated.[96] In another study, 11 (37%) of 30 were contaminated at the end of a hip arthroplasty, compared with only one (3%) of 31 when the tip had been exchanged before preparation of the femoral canal.[94] Placement of the suction tip into the medullary canal for prolonged periods of time effectively draws airborne contaminants into the surgical wound, and this common practice should be avoided. Changing the suction tip at 30-minute intervals, using a clean femoral tip, and turning the suction system on only before its actual use help to minimize this source of bacterial contamination.

Another demonstrated source of bacterial contamination is the splash basin. In one study, 58 (74%) of 78 splash basins were culture-positive at the end of the orthopaedic procedure.[97] Thirty-four (59%) of the 58 positive cultures yielded multiple organisms, and the most common organism was coagulase-negative staphylococcus—the organism most frequently associated with deep periprosthetic infection. Contrary to usual practice, instruments that have been placed into the splash basin should not be returned to the surgical wound.

Operative sites are invariably contaminated with bacteria to some degree, despite fastidious attempts to minimize the bacteria during the surgical procedure. Copious irrigation with a syringe, pulsatile lavage, application of antiseptic agents, and use of antibiotic irrigating solutions are all reasonable methods of wound decontamination. Pulsatile lavage has the potential to remove as many as 99% of wound contaminants, but high-pressure lavage may damage tissue.[98] When applied to the wound, concentrated antiseptic agents may also damage tissue. Furthermore, many of these agents are deactivated by plasma products present in the wound.[99,100] Chlorhexidine is not deactivated in the wound, and a 0.05% solution applied with syringe lavage has been shown to remove as many as 99.8% of wound contaminants.[101] Antibiotic irrigating solutions have been shown to be effective in the reduction of bacterial contamination of experimental wounds.[60,102-104] The potential for systemic aminoglycoside toxicity must be remembered, particularly when intraoperative blood transfusion retrieval systems and antibiotic irrigation fluid containing an aminoglycoside are used concomitantly. Repetitive irrigation to prevent tissue desiccation, reduce bacterial colonization, and remove clot or tissue debris should be a part of the overall prevention approach.

Optimization of the Wound Environment

The extensive dissection and long operative time necessary for total joint arthroplasty, combined with the implantation of a large foreign body, create a fertile environment for infection. Quantification of the many variables related to surgical technique is difficult and emotionally laden; however, the importance of adept and proficient surgical technique cannot be overstated. Prolonged operating time influences the rate of deep periprosthetic infection.[7,14] Utilization of existing scars to avoid postoperative skin necrosis is especially essential about the knee joint. If possible, pre-existing scars should be excised, unless doing so compromises wound closure. Appropriately placed incisions avoid the need for excessive tissue retraction. Gentle handling of tissue and avoidance of devitalization of tissue are essential. Dissection of subcutaneous tissue from the underlying fascia devitalizes the subcutaneous tissue layer, and awareness of this tissue fragility suggests that retractors should be placed carefully along fascial planes rather than in the subcutaneous tissue plane. Prolonged use of self-retaining retractors may also produce large areas of devitalized tissue.

Inappropriate placement of sutures strangles tissue and facilitates infection. Careful suturing of tissue layers to eliminate dead space, attentive hemostasis (while avoiding tissue destruction by excessive diathermy), and the use of surgical drains are generally considered to be effective in minimizing the postoperative wound hematoma. A tense hematoma can compromise the surrounding soft tissues and prevent antibiotic access.[105] It should be emphasized that, although recent reports have suggested that the routine use of surgical drains is not indicated for total hip and total knee arthroplasty,[58,59] the numbers of patients evaluated in these studies were far too small for an assessment of the effect of this practice on the prevalence of infection. Careful epidermal apposition is essential for early wound-sealing, and a hasty wound closure with overlapped skin often leads to prolonged postoperative wound drainage and a potential portal for the retrograde introduction of bacteria into the surgical wound.

The increased susceptibility of the wound to infection in the presence of a foreign body is well known.[4] Initial studies, with the use of silk suture as the foreign body, revealed that 2×10^2 staphylococci were required to create an abscess in the presence of a silk suture; however, 2 to 8×10^6 staphylococci were required to create a subcutaneous abscess in its absence.[4] Subsequently, it was demonstrated that the chemical composition of the suture is an important determinant of infection in the contaminated wound.[106] Monofilament absorbable synthetic suture is associated with a lower rate of infection than braided absorbable synthetic suture, which is, in turn, better than nonabsorbable braided suture or nonsynthetic natural suture, such as catgut or silk.[107-109] Therefore, careful choice of suture, particularly for a high-risk wound, seems advisable.

As the surgeon selects from a large array of implant alternatives for total joint arthroplasty, the effect of the specific physical and chemical properties of many of these foreign materials on the development of infection has been investigated extensively.[108,110-117] Although the exact role of most of these variables in the genesis of deep periprosthetic infection in the clinical setting is unknown, it is helpful to review some of these investigative efforts. For example, the physical and chemical characteristics of a specific biomaterial affect the efficiency of bacterial adhesion to the surface, so that coagulase-negative staphylococci exhibit preferential adhesion to polymers whereas coagulase-positive staphylococci adhere more readily to metals.[111] The metabolic characteristics of bacteria can also be altered when they adhere to a biomaterial, changing the susceptibility of the bacteria to antibiotics.[113] This metabolic effect appears to be independent of the presence of a glycocalyx, or slime covering; instead, it is dependent on the properties of the biomaterial, as bacteria that are adherent to methylmethacrylate demonstrate a remarkably higher resistance to antibiotics than do bacteria that are adherent to metals.[113]

In experimental models, it has been demonstrated that the prevalence of infection is increased in the presence of various foreign implants commonly used in total joint arthroplasty.[117,118] Polymethylmethacrylate promoted infection with coagulase-negative staphylococcus at a rate that was four times higher than the rate associated with high-density polyethylene and 15 times higher than that associated with stainless steel or aluminum.[118] Furthermore, the rate of infection associated with polymethylmethacrylate cured in vivo was higher than that associated with polymethylmethacrylate that had been first cured and then placed into the experimental model.[117] Polymethylmethacrylate has been shown to impair the chemotactic and phagocytic functions of human leukocytes.[116]

On the basis of these observations, it has been postulated that infection might occur less often with implants that rely on tissue integration for fixation than with those that are fixed with bone cement. A large clinical series revealed a significant difference ($p < 0.01$) between the rates of infection associated with total hip and knee arthroplasties, with deep periprosthetic infection developing after 21 of 2,575 knee arthroplasties and after only six of 2,392 hip arthroplasties.[76] However, comparison of the rate for implants inserted with cement with that for porous-coated implants revealed no significant differences in either the hip or knee groups: deep infection developed after two of 958 hip arthroplasties with a porous implant and after four of 1,434 hip arthroplasties with cement ($p = 0.19$), while deep infection developed after three of 201 knee arthroplasties with a porous implant and after 18 of 2,374 knee arthroplasties with cement ($p = 0.71$).[76] One possible explanation for this finding was provided by a recent experimental rabbit model.[110] The bacterial concentrations of *Staphylococcus aureus* required to cause infection were similar for hips with a polished titanium implant and those with a cobalt-chromium implant, but the concentration was reduced by a factor of 2.5 for hips with a porous-coated titanium implant and by a factor of 40 for those with a porous-coated cobalt-chromium implant.[110] This increased susceptibility to infection is probably due to the marked increase in the surface area of porous-coated implants, as described by Gristina.[111]

In another in vitro study, adherence of coagulase-negative staphylococci to stainless-steel, titanium alloy, hydroxyapatite-coated titanium, and sintered hydroxyapatite implants was evaluated.[115] Assays revealed that the sintered hydroxyapatite had a higher level of bacterial adherence than the other three materials. This increased adherence may reduce the susceptibility of bacteria to antibiotics or to the host's bacterial clearance mechanisms. Another study revealed that the ability of bacteria to adhere to polymethylmethacrylate is inhibited by the presence of antibiotics within the bone cement.[114] As previously mentioned, the clinical importance of these experimental findings is not yet known; however, discoveries like these may be used to support the use of certain methods under the surgeon's control or they may affect the decision about the type of implants used in high-risk individuals.

Postoperative Period

In the postoperative period, one must be vigilant for the development of infection and address the many factors that may contribute to it. Careful positioning of the patient and padding of osseous prominences should be undertaken to prevent the development of skin ulcerations. Hematomas are commonly identified as important factors in the development of postoperative infection.[7,15,31] A rapidly expanding hematoma necessitates formal evacuation and debridement in the operating room, because the pressure from it can devitalize adjacent tissues and prevent the influx of antibiotic into the operative site.[105] Benign neglect of superficial skin necrosis all too commonly allows it to progress to a deep periprosthetic wound infection. Therefore, superficial skin necrosis should also be treated intensively with formal excision and debridement in the operating room. Serous wound drainage may be treated initially with compressive dressings and antimicrobial coverage to prevent retrograde introduction of bacteria into the wound; however, continued drainage mandates a return of the patient to the operating room for formal debridement.[7,119] Persistent wound drainage portends a 3.2 times higher risk of eventual deep infection.[120] Surgical intervention itself for a complication in the immediate postoperative period, such as evacuation of a hematoma or open reduction of a dislocated hip, increases the risk of infection by a factor of more than four.[120]

Although the true prevalence of early or late hematogenous seeding of the sites of total joint prostheses is unknown, there is no question that this phenomenon occurs.[1,3,11,45-52] In the early postoperative period, the operative hematoma at the site of a total joint arthroplasty is susceptible to hematogenous seeding; therefore, when possible, conditions that may create an episode of bacteremia should be avoided during this period.[121] For instance, as it has been suggested that peripheral intravenous catheters made of Teflon (polytetrafluoroethylene) may be a distant source of bacterial contamination of the operative site, these catheters should be removed as soon as feasible.[122]

Urinary tract management is a frequent problem in the postoperative period, and there is no universal agreement on the proper postoperative protocol. If possible, patients who have difficulties related to the urinary tract should be identified and managed before the total joint arthroplasty.[123] The short-term use of an indwelling urinary catheter, placed while the patient is in the operating room, reduces the prevalence of urinary retention and prevents overdistention of the bladder.[124] There does not appear to be an increased risk of urinary tract infection if the indwelling catheter is used for only a short time in the immediate postoperative period.[124,125] Although no data are available, it seems reasonable to maintain antimicrobial coverage for manipulation of the genitourinary tract in the early postoperative period.

In most of the reported cases of periprosthetic joint infection attributed to hematogenous seeding, it has been difficult to document the bacteremia preceding the infection.[1,3,11,45-52] It seems prudent to diagnose and to treat intensively remote infections of the urinary tract, respiratory tract, and skin, as well as overt dental infection in order to prevent hematogenous seeding. Effective selection of the antimicrobial agent in these situations depends on the site of infection, the in vitro susceptibility of the microorganism causing the infection, and the patient's history of intolerance to antibiotics.

Many reports of hematogenous infection have detailed the importance of the host's ability to resist infection. Patients who have rheumatoid arthritis are frequently cited as being susceptible to hematogenous infections.[3,31,45-47,50,70] There are many other predisposing factors as well. The presence of structural bone graft, the use of metal-metal prostheses, and the use of constrained prostheses have all been cited as additional risk factors.[11,12,47,78] These additional risk factors are actually variables related to the wound environment that impair the host's ability to clear bacteria seeded in the wound. It has been demonstrated that total joint implants are surrounded by an immunoincompetent, fibroinflammatory zone.[112] Within this zone, there is an increased susceptibility to infection because of repeated macrophage stimulation by particulate debris, which leads to the formation of superoxide radicals and cytokine-mediated tissue damage. A self-perpetuating cytokine cascade is initiated, leading to progressive enlargement of the immunoincompetent fibroinflammatory zone surrounding the implant. In advanced stages, this zone is recognized on radiographs as osteolysis. The production of reactive oxygen intermediates, macrophage exhaustion, and continual tissue damage around these implants may result in aseptic loosening, but hematogenous seeding of the immunoincompetent zone may lead to periprosthetic infection. Progressive osteolysis caused by polyethylene, polymethylmethacrylate, or metallic particulate debris, or a combination of these, is therefore an additional factor that may predispose the patient to hematogenous infection. We have observed this phenomenon in patients who had asymptomatic loosening of a prosthesis and who were being followed closely to monitor the progress of periprosthetic osteolysis. There is an acute onset of pain and the patients are diagnosed with a deep periprosthetic infection, presumably from a hematogenous source. To our knowledge, there are currently no data available to quantify the risk for these patients, and substantial investigative efforts are necessary to identify the various risk factors associated with the host and wound environment for late hematogenous infection as well as the appropriate antibiotic prophylaxis.

Antimicrobial prophylaxis for patients with a prosthetic joint who have a dental procedure or an invasive procedure, such as endoscopy of the gastrointestinal tract or cystoscopy of the genitourinary tract, is extremely controversial.[3,18,37,46,48,49,126-128] The rate of bacteremia after dental and certain diagnostic or therapeutic procedures has been well documented,[129] and the frequency and intensity of bacteremia is generally high in association with oral procedures, lower in association with genitourinary manipulation, and lowest in association with diagnostic procedures of the gastrointestinal tract.[129] Because it is possible that bacteremia can lead to hematogenous deposition of bacteria around the total joint prosthesis, the questions that remain unanswered are (1) what types of procedures or conditions result in bacteremia that can lead to hematogenous infection around a prosthetic joint, (2) which prostheses put the hip at risk for infection when there is bacteremia, and (3) what type of interventions can prevent infection?

Reports of periprosthetic infection caused by flora indigenous to the body and temporally related to these invasive procedures have documented that late hematogenous infection can occur.[48,51,52] The difficult issue is whether the prevalence of hematogenous infection caused by these procedures is sufficiently high to outweigh the risks and cost of antimicrobial prophylaxis. Currently, the answer to this question is unknown.[37,126] Furthermore, the efficacy of antibiotic prophylaxis for these procedures in patients with a prosthetic joint has not been studied.

The controversial issues of antibiotic prophylaxis for patients who have a prosthetic joint parallel the controversy surrounding the use of antibiotic prophylaxis to prevent infective endocarditis.[129-131] The compliance with recommended guidelines for the prevention of infective endocarditis has continued to improve with time, primarily because of the continued education of health-care providers and ongoing investigations of this disease.[129] It must be noted that the information obtained from investigations into the prevention of infective endocarditis has been much more extensive than that for patients who have a prosthetic joint.[129-131] Although it is helpful to review the current treatment guidelines for antibiotic prophylaxis to prevent infective endocarditis, direct extrapolation of study results and recommendations to a patient who has a prosthetic joint is probably not appropriate. Despite the large amount of knowledge that has been assimilated regarding infective endocarditis, the following issues have not been resolved: (1) No prospective studies have definitively proved the efficacy of antibiotic prophylaxis for the prevention of infective endocarditis; (2) many cases of apparent failure of antibiotic prophylaxis have been reported; and (3) based on cost-effectiveness studies, routine antibiotic prophylaxis is probably not justified and should be reserved only for patients with high-risk cardiac disorders.[129]

With these considerations in mind, Osmon and associates (unpublished data, 1993) as well as Steckelberg and Osmon[132] identified the rates of periprosthetic infection of the hip and knee that could be epidemiologically linked to an oral source. They demonstrated that the presence of teeth was a risk factor for infections caused by *Streptococcus viridans* after total hip and knee arthroplasty (odds ratio = 6.4; 95% confidence interval, 2.2 to 18.0; $p \leq 0.001$) but not for infection caused by *S aureus* or peptostreptococci.[90] It must be emphasized that the infections with *S viridans* were due to all oral sources and not just clean dental procedures. The rate of deep periprosthetic infection was highest in the first 2 years after an arthroplasty, occurring at a frequency of 0.14 cases per 1,000 joint-years (confidence interval; 0.07 to 0.25), whereas the annual rate after the first 2 years was only 0.03 cases per 1,000 joint-years (confidence interval, 0.01 to 0.07). The rate after the first 2 years is similar to that for infective endocarditis caused by *S viridans* among patients in the general population who do not have a heart murmur or endocarditis, patient groups for which the American Heart Association currently recommends no antimicrobial prophylaxis because the toxicity outweighs the potential benefit.[130,131]

On the basis of these data, a blanket recommendation for antimicrobial prophylaxis for routine, clean dental procedures in all patients who have had an arthroplasty of a large joint does not appear warranted for the rest of the patient's life. These preliminary data suggest that in the first postoperative year, during which soft-tissue healing occurs and inflammation subsides, prophylactic antibiotics may be appropriate in an effort to prevent deep periprosthetic infection with *S viridans*. It is important to note, however, that *S viridans* causes only a small proportion of deep periprosthetic infections. Furthermore, data are currently inadequate to formulate recommendations regarding prophylaxis for genitourinary or gastrointestinal procedures in the absence of infection.

Medicolegal considerations cloud this issue further. The decision to provide antibiotic prophylaxis for invasive procedures in patients who have a prosthetic joint is more complex than that associated with infective endocarditis because of the paucity of information available for patients who have a prosthetic joint compared with for those who have infective endocarditis. Because the patients who are at risk for a deep periprosthetic infection after an invasive procedure have not yet been clearly identified, it is difficult to make any definitive recommendations. The following statement, as applied to infective endocarditis, is worthy of review. "A reasonable standard of care requires that a physician or dentist know the connection between procedure-induced bacteremia and endocarditis; ask whether the patient has a predisposing heart disorder; inform patients of the small risk; and decide whether to advise prophylaxis according to the perceived risks and benefits. If these steps are taken and documented, claims based on the later development of endocarditis should not succeed."[129]

As is the current practice with regard to infective endocarditis, rational recommendations regarding antimicrobial prophylaxis for clean dental procedures, genitourinary procedures, or gastrointestinal procedures in patients who have a large orthopaedic implant depend on the identification of groups of patients who are at substantially increased risk for infection after these procedures. If a physician elects to recommend antimicrobial prophylaxis for the prevention of hematogenous infection, the antibiotic should be chosen on the basis of the flora expected at the site of the procedure, and potentially rare but life-threatening adverse reactions as well as the more common drug toxicities should be considered by both physician and patient.

Overview

In conclusion, few areas in orthopaedic surgery are the subject of as much controversy, myth, and dismay as deep periprosthetic infection. Prevention of such an infection is complex, with many unresolved issues that require considerable investigation. The attentive application of reasonable principles of infection control with the goals of optimization of the wound environment, augmentation of the host response, and minimization of bacterial contamination in the preoperative, operative, and postoperative time-periods is essential to the overall reduction of the prevalence of infection.

References

1. Schmalzried TP, Amstutz HC, Au MK, et al: Etiology of deep sepsis in total hip arthroplasty: The significance of hematogenous and recurrent infections. *Clin Orthop* 1992;280:200–207.
2. Moynihan BG: Infection acquired in hospitals. *Lancet* 1880; 2:885.
3. Maderazo EG, Judson S, Pasternak H: Late infections of total joint prostheses: A review and recommendations for prevention. *Clin Orthop* 1988;229:131–142.
4. Elek SD, Conen PE: The virulence of staphylococcus pyogenes for man: A study of the problems of wound infection. *Br J Exper Pathol* 1957;38:573–586.
5. Greene KA, Wilde AH, Stulberg BN: Preoperative nutritional status of total joint patients: Relationship to postoperative wound complications. *J Arthroplasty* 1991;6:321–325.
6. England SP, Stern SH, Insall JN, et al: Total knee arthroplasty in diabetes mellitus. *Clin Orthop* 1990;260:130–134.
7. Fitzgerald RH Jr, Nolan DR, Ilstrup DM, et al: Deep wound sepsis following total hip arthroplasty. *J Bone Joint Surg* 1977;59A: 847–855.
8. Menon TJ, Thjellesen D, Wroblewski BM: Charnley low-friction arthroplasty in diabetic patients. *J Bone Joint Surg* 1983;65B: 580–581.
9. Moeckel B, Huo MH, Salvati EA, et al: Total hip arthroplasty in patients with diabetes mellitus. *J Arthroplasty* 1993;8:279–284.
10. Charnley J, Eftekhar N: Postoperative infection in total prosthetic replacement arthroplasty of the hip-joint: With special reference to the bacterial content of the air of the operating room. *Br J Surg* 1969;56:641–649.
11. Poss R, Thornhill TS, Ewald FC, et al: Factors influencing the incidence and outcome of infection following total joint arthroplasty. *Clin Orthop* 1984;182:117–126.
12. Wilson MG, Kelley K, Thornhill TS: Infection as a complication of total knee-replacement arthroplasty: Risk factors and treatment in sixty-seven cases. *J Bone Joint Surg* 1990;72A:878–883.
13. Fernandez MC, Gottlieb M, Menitove JE: Blood transfusion and postoperative infection in orthopedic patients. *Transfusion* 1992;34:318–322.
14. Gherini S, Vaughn BK, Lombardi AV Jr, et al: Delayed wound healing and nutritional deficiencies after total hip arthroplasty. *Clin Orthop* 1993;293:188–195.
15. Nelson CL: Prevention of sepsis. *Clin Orthop* 1987;222:66–72.
16. Bryan CS, Morgan SL, Caton RJ, et al: Cefazolin versus cefamandole for prophylaxis during total joint arthroplasty. *Clin Orthop* 1988;228:117–122.
17. Mauerhan DR, Nelson CL, Smith DL, et al: Prophylaxis against infection in total joint arthroplasty: One day of cefuroxime compared with three days of cefazolin. *J Bone Joint Surg* 1994;76A: 39–45.
18. Stern SH, Insall JN: Total knee arthroplasty in obese patients. *J Bone Joint Surg* 1990;72A:1400–1404.
19. Gordon SM, Culver DH, Simmons BP, et al: Risk factors for wound infections after total knee arthroplasty. *Am J Epidemiol* 1990;131:905–916.
20. Jensen JE, Jensen TG, Smith TK, et al: Nutrition in orthopaedic surgery. *J Bone Joint Surg* 1982;64A:1263–1272.
21. Smith TK: Nutrition: Its relationship to orthopedic infections. *Orthop Clin North Am* 1991;22:373–377.
22. Hoekman P, van de Perre P, Nelissen J, et al: Increased frequency of infection after open reduction of fractures in patients who are seropositive for human immunodeficiency virus. *J Bone Joint Surg* 1991;73A:675–679.
23. Cruse PJ, Foord R: A five-year prospective study of 23,649 surgical wounds. *Arch Surg* 1973;107:206–210.
24. Dreblow DM, Anderson CF, Moxness K: Nutritional assessment of orthopedic patients. *Mayo Clin Proc* 1981;56:51–54.
25. Puskarich CL, Nelson CL, Nusbickel FR, et al: The use of two nutritional indicators in identifying long bone fracture patients who do and do not develop infection. *J Orthop Res* 1990;8: 799–803.
26. Mishriki SF, Law DJ, Jeffery PJ: Factors affecting the incidence of postoperative wound infection. *J Hosp Infect* 1990;16:223–230.
27. Seropian R, Reynolds BM: Wound infections after preoperative depilatory versus razor preparation. *Am J Surg* 1971;121: 251–254.
28. Beyer CA, Hanssen AD, Lewallen DG, et al: Primary total knee arthroplasty in patients with psoriasis. *J Bone Joint Surg* 1991; 73B:258–259.
29. Menon TJ, Wroblewski BM: Charnley low-friction arthroplasty in patients with psoriasis. *Clin Orthop* 1983;176:127–128.
30. Stern SH, Insall JN, Windsor RE, et al: Total knee arthroplasty in patients with psoriasis. *Clin Orthop* 1989;248:108–111.
31. Glynn MK, Sheehan JM: An analysis of the causes of deep infection after hip and knee arthroplasties. *Clin Orthop* 1983; 178:202–206.
32. Lidwell OM, Lowbury EJ, Whyte W, et al: Effect of ultraclean air in operating rooms on deep sepsis in the joint after total hip or knee replacement: A randomized study. *Br Med J* 1982;285: 10–14.
33. Morrey BF, Bryan RS: Infection after total elbow arthroplasty. *J Bone Joint Surg* 1983;65A:330–338.
34. Doyon F, Evrard J, Mazas F: An assessment of published trials on antibiotic prophylaxis in orthopaedic surgery. *Fr J Orthop Surg* 1989;3:49–53.
35. Heath AF: Antimicrobial prophylaxis for arthroplasty and total joint replacement: Discussion and review of published clinical trials. *Pharmacotherapy* 1991;11:157–163.
36. Hill C, Flamant R, Mazas F, et al: Prophylactic cefazolin versus placebo in total hip replacement: Report of a multicentre double-blind randomised trial. *Lancet* 1981;1:795–796.
37. Norden CW: Antibiotic prophylaxis in orthopedic surgery. *Rev Infect Dis* 1991;13(suppl 10):S842–S846.
38. Dellinger EP, Gross PA, Barrett TL, et al: Quality standard for antimicrobial prophylaxis in surgical procedures. *Clin Infect Dis* 1994;18:422–427.
39. Wilson NI: A survey, in Scotland, of measures to prevent infection following orthopaedic surgery. *J Hosp Infect* 1987;9:235–242.
40. Fitzgerald RH Jr, Thompson RL: Cephalosporin antibiotics in the prevention and treatment of musculoskeletal sepsis. *J Bone Joint Surg* 1983;65A:1201–1205.
41. DeBenedictis KJ, Rowan NM, Boyer BL: A double-blind study comparing cefonicid with cefazolin as prophylaxis in patients undergoing total hip or knee replacement. *Rev Infect Dis* 1984;6(suppl 4):S901–S904.
42. Evrard J, Doyon F, Acar JF, et al: Two-day cefamandole versus five-day cephazolin prophylaxis in 965 total hip replacements: Report of a multicentre double blind randomised trial. *Int Orthop* 1988;12:69–73.
43. Pollard JP, Hughes SP, Scott JE, et al: Antibiotic prophylaxis in total hip replacement. *Br Med J* 1979;1:707–709.
44. Soave R, Hirsch JC, Salvati EA, et al: Comparison of ceforanide and cephalothin prophylaxis in patients undergoing total joint arthroplasty. *Orthopedics* 1986;9:1657–1660.
45. Ahlberg A, Carlsson AS, Lindberg L: Hematogenous infection in total joint replacement. *Clin Orthop* 1978;137:69–75.
46. Ainscow DA, Denham RA: The risk of haematogenous infection in total joint replacements. *J Bone Joint Surg* 1984;66B:580–582.
47. Bengtson S, Blomgren G, Knutson K, et al: Hematogenous infection after knee arthroplasty. *Acta Orthop Scand* 1987;58: 529–534.
48. Lindqvist C, Slatis P: Dental bacteremia: A neglected cause of arthroplasty infections? Three hip cases. *Acta Orthop Scand* 1985;56:506–508.
49. Maniloff G, Greenwald R, Laskin R, et al: Delayed postbacteremic prosthetic joint infection. *Clin Orthop* 1987;223: 194–197.
50. Stinchfield FE, Bigliani LU, Neu HC, et al: Late hematogenous infection of total joint replacement. *J Bone Joint Surg* 1980; 62A:1345–1350.
51. Strazzeri JC, Anzel S: Infected total hip arthroplasty due to Actinomyces Israelii after dental extraction: A case report. *Clin Orthop* 1986;210:128–131.

52. Sullivan PM, Johnston RC, Kelley SS: Late infection after total hip replacement, caused by an oral organism after dental manipulation: A case report. *J Bone Joint Surg* 1990;72A:121–123.
53. Burke JF: The effective period of preventive antibiotic action in experimental incisions and dermal lesions. *Surgery* 1961;50: 161–168.
54. Classen DC, Evans RS, Pestotnik SL, et al: The timing of prophylactic administration of antibiotics and the risk of surgical-wound infection. *N Engl J Med* 1992;326:281–286.
55. Bannister GC, Auchincloss JM, Johnson DP, et al: The timing of tourniquet application in relation to prophylactic antibiotic administration. *J Bone Joint Surg* 1988;70B:322–324.
56. Heydemann JS, Nelson CL: Short-term preventive antibiotics. *Clin Orthop* 1986;205:184–187.
57. Wymenga A, van-Horn J, Theeuwes A, et al: Cefuroxime for prevention of postoperative coxitis: One versus three doses tested in a randomized multicenter study of 2,651 arthroplasties. *Acta Orthop Scand* 1992;63:19–24.
58. Beer KJ, Lombardi AV Jr, Mallory TH, et al: The efficacy of suction drains after routine total joint arthroplasty. *J Bone Joint Surg* 1991;73A:584–587.
59. Ritter MA, Keating EM, Faris PM: Closed wound drainage in total hip or total knee replacement: A prospective, randomized study. *J Bone Joint Surg* 1994;76A:35–38.
60. Petty W, Spanier S, Schuster JJ: Prevention of infection after total joint replacement: Experiments with a canine model. *J Bone Joint Surg* 1988;70A:536–539.
61. Carlsson AK, Lidgren L, Lindberg L: Prophylactic antibiotics against early and late deep infections after total hip replacements. *Acta Orthop Scand* 1977;48:405–410.
62. Josefsson G, Gudmundsson G, Kolmert L, et al: Prophylaxis with systemic antibiotics versus gentamicin bone cement in total hip arthroplasty: A five-year survey of 1,688 hips. *Clin Orthop* 1990; 253:173–178.
63. Lynch M, Esser MP, Shelley P, et al: Deep infection in Charnley low-friction arthroplasty: Comparison of plain and gentamicin-loaded cement. *J Bone Joint Surg* 1987;69B:355–360.
64. McQueen M, Littlejohn A, Hughes SP: A comparison of systemic cefuroxime and cefuroxime loaded bone cement in the prevention of early infection after total joint replacement. *Int Orthop* 1987;11:241–243.
65. Trippel SB: Antibiotic-impregnated cement in total joint arthroplasty. *J Bone Joint Surg* 1986;68A:1297–1302.
66. Goldner JL, Allen BL Jr: Ultraviolet light in orthopedic operating rooms at Duke University: Thirty-five years' experience, 1937–1973. *Clin Orthop* 1973;96:195–205.
67. Hart D: Sterilization of the air in the operating room by bactericidal radiant energy: Results in over eight hundred operations. *Arch Surg* 1938;37:956–972.
68. Berg M, Bergman BR, Hoborn J: Ultraviolet radiation compared to an ultra-clean air enclosure: Comparison of air bacteria counts in operating rooms. *J Bone Joint Surg* 1991;73B: 811–815.
69. Lowell JD, Kundsin RB, Schwartz CM, et al: Ultraviolet radiation and reduction of deep wound infection following hip and knee arthroplasty. *Ann N Y Acad Sci* 1980;353:285–293.
70. Charnley J: Postoperative infection after total hip replacement with special reference to air contamination in the operating room. *Clin Orthop* 1972;87:167–187.
71. Nelson JP, Glassburn AR Jr, Talbott RD, et al: Clean room operating rooms. *Clin Orthop* 1973;96:179–187.
72. Laurence M: Ultra-clean air. *J Bone Joint Surg* 1983;65B:375–377.
73. Marotte JH, Lord GA, Blanchard JP, et al: Infection rate in total hip arthroplasty as a function of air cleanliness and antibiotic prophylaxis: 10-year experience with 2,384 cementless Lord Madreporic prostheses. *J Arthroplasty* 1987;2:77–82.
74. Salvati EA, Robinson RP, Zeno SM, et al: Infection rates after 3,175 total hip and total knee replacements performed with and without a horizontal unidirectional filtered air-flow system. *J Bone Joint Surg* 1982;64A:525–535.
75. Fitzgerald RH Jr: Total hip arthroplasty sepsis: Prevention and diagnosis. *Orthop Clin North Am* 1992;23:259–264.
76. Hanssen AD, Fitzgerald RH Jr: Infection rates following cemented and uncemented primary total hip and total knee arthroplasty. Proceedings of the American Academy of Orthopaedic Surgeons 58th Annual Meeting, Anaheim, CA. Park Ridge, IL, American Academy of Orthopaedic Surgeons, 1991, p 153.
77. Lidwell OM: Clean air at operation and subsequent sepsis in the joint. *Clin Orthop* 1986;211:91–102.
78. Schutzer SF, Harris WH: Deep-wound infection after total hip replacement under contemporary aseptic conditions. *J Bone Joint Surg* 1988;70A:724–727.
79. Ritter MA, Eitzen H, French ML, et al: The operating room environment as affected by people and the surgical face mask. *Clin Orthop* 1975;111:147–150.
80. Davies RR, Noble WC: Dispersal of bacteria on desquamated skin. *Lancet* 1962;2:1295–1297.
81. Walter CW, Kundsin RB: The airborne component of wound contamination and infection. *Arch Surg* 1973;107:588–595.
82. Mitchell NJ, Hunt S: Surgical face masks in modern operating rooms: A costly and unnecessary ritual? *J Hosp Infect* 1991;18: 239–242.
83. Tunevall TG: Postoperative wound infections and surgical face masks: A controlled study. *World J Surg* 1991;15:383–388.
84. Letts RM, Doermer E: Conversation in the operating theater as a cause of airborne bacterial contamination. *J Bone Joint Surg* 1983;65A:357–362.
85. Gilliam DL, Nelson CL: Comparison of a one-step iodophor skin preparation versus traditional preparation in total joint surgery. *Clin Orthop* 1990;250:258–260.
86. Ritter MA, French ML, Eitzen HE, et al: The antimicrobial effectiveness of operative-site preparative agents: A microbiological and clinical study. *J Bone Joint Surg* 1980;62A:826–828.
87. Johnston DH, Fairclough JA, Brown EM, et al: Rate of bacterial recolonization of the skin after preparation: Four methods compared. *Br J Surg* 1987;74:64.
88. French ML, Eitzen HE, Ritter MA: The plastic surgical adhesive drape: An evaluation of its efficacy as a microbial barrier. *Ann Surg* 1976;184:46–50.
89. Eitzen HE, Ritter MA, French ML, et al: A microbiological in-use comparison of surgical hand-washing agents. *J Bone Joint Surg* 1979;61A:403–406.
90. Sanders R, Fortin P, Ross E, et al: Outer gloves in orthopaedic procedures: Cloth compared with latex. *J Bone Joint Surg* 1990; 72A:914–917.
91. Ritter MA, French ML, Eitzen H: Evaluation of microbial contamination of surgical gloves during actual use. *Clin Orthop* 1976; 117:303–306.
92. Moylan JA, Fitzpatrick KT, Davenport KE: Reducing wound infections: Improved gown and drape barrier performance. *Arch Surg* 1987;122:152–157.
93. Whyte W, Bailey PV, Hamblen DL, et al: A bacteriologically occlusive clothing system for use in the operating room. *J Bone Joint Surg* 1983;65B:502–506.
94. Greenough CG: An investigation into contamination of operative suction. *J Bone Joint Surg* 1986;68B:151–153.
95. Meals RA, Knoke L: The surgical suction tip: A contaminated instrument. *J Bone Joint Surg* 1978;60A:409–410.
96. Strange-Vognsen HH, Klareskov B: Bacteriologic contamination of suction tips during hip arthroplasty. *Acta Orthop Scand* 1988; 59:410–411.
97. Baird RA, Nickel FR, Thrupp LD, et al: Splash basin contamination in orthopaedic surgery. *Clin Orthop* 1984;187: 129–133.
98. Hamer ML, Robson MC, Krizek TJ, et al: Quantitative bacterial analysis of comparative wound irrigations. *Ann Surg* 1975; 181:819–822.
99. Branemark PI, Ekholm R: Tissue injury caused by wound disinfectants. *J Bone Joint Surg* 1967;49A:48–62.
100. Zamora JL, Price MF, Chuang P, et al: Inhibition of povidone-iodine's bactericidal activity by common organic substances: An experimental study. *Surgery* 1985;98:25–29.
101. Taylor GJ, Leeming JP, Bannister GC: Effect of antiseptics, ultraviolet light and lavage on airborne bacteria in a model wound. *J Bone Joint Surg* 1993;75B:724–730.
102. Benjamin JB, Volz RG: Efficacy of a topical antibiotic irrigant in decreasing or eliminating bacterial contamination in surgical wounds. *Clin Orthop* 1984;184:114–117.
103. Rosenstein BD, Wilson FC, Funderburk CH: The use of bacitracin irrigation to prevent infection in postoperative skeletal

wounds: An experimental study. *J Bone Joint Surg* 1989;71A: 427–430.
104. Scherr DD, Dodd TA: In vitro bacteriological evaluation of the effectiveness of antimicrobial irrigating solutions. *J Bone Joint Surg* 1976;58A:119–122.
105. Nelson CL, Bergfeld JA, Schwartz J, et al: Antibiotics in human hematoma and wound fluid. *Clin Orthop* 1975;108:138–144.
106. Edlich RF, Panek PH, Rodeheaver GT, et al: Physical and chemical configuration of sutures in the development of surgical infection. *Ann Surg* 1973;177:679–688.
107. Chu C-C, Williams DF: Effects of physical configuration and chemical structure of suture materials on bacterial adhesion: A possible link to wound infection. *Am J Surg* 1984;147: 197–204.
108. Katz S, Izhar M, Mirelman D: Bacterial adherence to surgical sutures: A possible factor in suture induced infection. *Ann Surg* 1981;194:35–41.
109. Sharp WV, Belden TA, King PH, et al: Suture resistance to infection. *Surgery* 1982;91:61–63.
110. Cordero J, Munuera L, Folgueira MD: Influence of metal implants on infection: An experimental study in rabbits. *J Bone Joint Surg* 1994;76B:717–720.
111. Gristina AG: Biomaterial-centered infection: Microbial adhesion versus tissue integration. *Science* 1987;237:1588–1595.
112. Gristina AG: Implant failure and the immuno-incompetent fibro-inflammatory zone. *Clin Orthop* 1994;298:106–118.
113. Naylor PT, Myrvik QN, Gristina A: Antibiotic resistance of biomaterial-adherent coagulase-negative and coagulase-positive staphylococci. *Clin Orthop* 1990;261:126–133.
114. Oga M, Arizono T, Sugioka Y: Inhibition of bacterial adhesion by tobramycin-impregnated PMMA bone cement. *Acta Orthop Scand* 1992;63:301–304.
115. Oga M, Arizono T, Sugioka Y: Bacterial adherence to bioinert and bioactive materials studied in vitro. *Acta Orthop Scand* 1993;64:273–276.
116. Petty W: The effect of methylmethacrylate on bacterial phagocytosis and killing by human polymorphonuclear leukocytes. *J Bone Joint Surg* 1978;60A:752–757.
117. Petty W, Spanier S, Schuster JJ, et al: The influence of skeletal implants on incidence of infection: Experiments in a canine model. *J Bone Joint Surg* 1985;67A:1236–1244.
118. Oga M, Sugioka Y, Hobgood CD, et al: Surgical biomaterials and differential colonization by Staphylococcus epidermidis. *Biomaterials* 1988;9:285–289.
119. Weiss AP, Krackow KA: Persistent wound drainage after primary total knee arthroplasty. *J Arthroplasty* 1993;8:285–289.
120. Surin VV, Sundholm K, Bäckman L: Infection after total hip replacement with special reference to a discharge from the wound. *J Bone Joint Surg* 1983;65B:412–418.
121. Blomgren G, Lindgren U: The susceptibility of total joint replacement to hematogenous infection in the early postoperative period: An experimental study in the rabbit. *Clin Orthop* 1980;151:308–312.
122. Wilkins J, Patzakis MJ: Peripheral teflon catheters: Potential source for bacterial contamination of orthopedic implants? *Clin Orthop* 1990;254:251–254.
123. Wroblewski BM, del Sel HJ: Urethral instrumentation and deep sepsis in total hip replacement. *Clin Orthop* 1980;146:209–212.
124. Michelson JD, Lotke PA, Steinberg ME: Urinary-bladder management after total joint-replacement surgery. *N Engl J Med* 1988;319:321–326.
125. Ritter MA, Faris PM, Keating EM: Urinary tract catheterization protocols following total joint arthroplasty. *Orthopedics* 1989; 12:1085–1087.
126. Gillespie WJ: Infection in total joint replacement. *Infect Dis Clin North Am* 1990;4:465–484.
127. Nelson JP, Fitzgerald RH Jr, Jaspers MT, et al: Editorial: Prophylactic antimicrobial coverage in arthroplasty patients. *J Bone Joint Surg* 1990;72A:1.
128. Wahl MJ: Myths of dental-induced prosthetic joint infections. *Clin Infect Dis* 1995;20:1420–1425.
129. Durack DT: Prevention of infective endocarditis. *N Engl J Med* 1995;332:38–44.
130. Dajani AS, Bisno AL, Chung KJ, et al: Prevention of bacterial endocarditis: Recommendations by the American Heart Association. *JAMA* 1990;264:2919–2922.
131. Steckelberg JM, Wilson WR: Risk factors for infective endocarditis. *Infect Dis Clin North Am* 1993;7:9–19.
132. Steckelberg JM, Osmon DR: Prosthetic joint infections, in Bisno AL, Waldvogel FA (eds): *Infections Associated with Indwelling Medical Devices*, ed 2. Washington, DC, American Society for Microbiology, 1994, pp 259–290.

CHAPTER 55

Tendon Problems in Athletic Individuals

Carol C. Teitz, MD
William E. Garrett, Jr, MD, PhD
Anthony Miniaci, MD, FRCSC
Moo-Hyung Lee, MD
Roger A. Mann, MD

Tendons attach muscle to bone and transmit the forces generated by muscles across joints to bone in order to achieve movement or stability of the body in space. Even when the muscle-tendon unit is not shortening, it can be performing a useful function when activated under conditions of constant length (isometric) or lengthening (eccentric) contractions. The compliance of tendons varies. Tendons of the digital flexors and extensors are very stiff, and their length changes very little when muscle forces are applied through them. In contrast, the tendons of some muscles, particularly those involved in locomotion and ballistic performance, are more elastic. The Achilles tendon, for example, is stretched in late stance phase as the triceps surae contracts and the ankle dorsiflexes. Near the beginning of plantarflexion, the muscle activation ceases and energy stored in the stretched tendon helps to initiate plantarflexion. Tendons that transmit large loads under eccentric and elastic conditions are more subject to injury.[1]

A muscle has a much larger cross-sectional area than does its tendon near its attachment to bone. The tendon fans out into a much broader and thinner structure as it joins the muscle. This junctional area is the location of most injuries caused by tensile forces in a normal muscle-tendon unit, and it is the site of most common muscle strains in the active population.[2]

Histologically, the tendon is seen to be a densely packed connective-tissue structure, consisting of a matrix of many type-I collagen-fiber bundles that are oriented along the axis of the tendon.[3] The tightly packed and highly oriented collagen-fiber matrix makes the tendon ideal for sustaining tensile load.[1] Between the bundles are spindle-shaped fibroblasts that are responsible for creating and maintaining the matrix.

A loose connective-tissue matrix surrounds the bundles of collagen fibrils and is organized within the primary collagen bundles as well as between the bundles and surrounding them. A peritendinous connective-tissue sheath (paratenon) surrounds the entire tendon. This sheath consists of two layers: an inner (visceral) layer and an outer (parietal) layer with occasional connecting bridges (mesotenon). If there is synovial fluid between these two layers, the paratenon is called tenosynovium; if not, it is termed tenovagium.

Pathophysiology

Histologic Findings

Painful areas of tendon are traditionally diagnosed by clinicians as tendinitis. This term implies an inflammatory nature of the lesion. However, histologic studies of surgical specimens do not show the characteristic signs of an inflammatory response as there are few inflammatory cells such as macrophages or polymorphonuclear leukocytes. There is little formation of granulation tissue. Rather, the histologic pattern is more characteristic of a degenerative condition. The matrix is very disorganized and lacks the usual axial, tightly woven collagen bundles. Fibroblasts are more numerous, and vascularity is generally increased. The degenerative pattern can assume fatty, mucoid, or hyaline features histologically. The better and more commonly used term for this degenerative condition is tendinosis.[3,4]

Necropsy studies have shown that these degenerative changes may also be present in asymptomatic tendons.[5] The degree of degeneration increases with age and may represent part of the normal aging process. The degeneration appears to be activity-related as well. Surgical specimens obtained from younger or middle-aged patients who put high demands on the involved muscle-tendon units through recreational or occupational activities, such as using a strong grip to hold a tennis racquet or a hammer, often show degenerative changes in the affected tendon.[6]

Tendon Failure

High forces created by eccentric muscle activation usually are responsible for tendon failure.[4,6,7] Biomechanical studies of the effect of loading on normal bone-tendon-muscle-tendon-bone preparations have shown that failure rarely occurs in the tendon.[8] Biopsy specimens obtained soon after the spontaneous failure of tendons showed degenerative changes in the ruptured tendon ends.[5] Specimens of Achilles tendon obtained on exploration for surgical repair almost always demonstrate that degenerative changes were present within the tendon before it failed. These changes presumably weakened the tendon to such a degree that it became the weakest link in the chain.

Research aimed at understanding the pathophysiology and treatment of tendinosis has been limited by the lack of a good and affordable animal model.[9] Injection of collagenase into the center of an equine tendon produces a histologic picture similar to that seen in biopsy specimens of human tendinosis.[10] However, this lesion tends to heal and, therefore, may be more of a model for tendon sprain than for chronic tendinosis. Perhaps the model most closely resembling tendinosis occurs in the superficial digital flexor tendon of the horse. Lesions in this tendon are responsible for poor performance or lameness, especially in racehorses. The condition is characterized by fusiform swelling of the tendon with a degenerative core lesion and more normal tissue in the tendon peripherally. The tendon undergoes rapid loading and high strains in the galloping horse. Tendons store energy on stretching and return most of it when released. However, the energy that is not returned is dissipated as heat within the tendon, and the temperature in the central area of the tendon can reach nearly 45°C. Fibroblast viability is at risk at this temperature, and death of the central fibroblasts may create the central core degeneration that is seen histologically.

In summary, the pathophysiology of tendinosis has not been well studied and is not well understood. Susceptible tendons are those that undergo large loads in an eccentric or stretching mode in which the tendons are storing and releasing energy. Susceptibility appears to be related both to activity and to age. The basic lesion can be identified within the tendon core and is characterized as degenerative rather than inflammatory. The term tendinitis is, therefore, less applicable than tendinosis. Possible factors in the etiology include age-related changes in tendon structure and exercise-related hyperthermia within the tendon.

Tendinosis of the Rotator Cuff

Disorders of the rotator cuff occur commonly. Overuse or repetitive stress of the upper extremity in the overhead position may be an important cause of rotator cuff tendinosis.[11-14] Poor vascularity and primary degenerative changes also may contribute to the development of the lesion. Codman[11] described a so-called critical zone, located approximately 1 cm medial to the supraspinatus tendon insertion, where tears usually occur. Rathbun and Macnab[15] showed that there was relative avascularity in this critical zone, and they hypothesized that this was the reason for the degenerative changes. Lohr and Uhthoff[16] also found this to be an area of hypovascularity, but they noted that the articular side of the tendon was poorly vascularized whereas the bursal side was well vascularized. Ogata and Uhthoff[17] suggested that primary tendinosis was also an important etiologic factor, especially for the deep-surface or intratendinous tears that are seen more often than tears on the bursal side.

Shoulder pain and rotator cuff tendinosis are frequently seen in athletes who are involved in sports, such as baseball, tennis, and swimming, that require overhead actions. Jobe and associates[18] suggested that subtle glenohumeral instability was one of the causes of rotator cuff tendinosis in this group. The overhead throwing motion of baseball pitchers and the service motion of tennis players require eccentric muscle contractions as the rotator cuff and shoulder-girdle muscles attempt to maintain stability of the glenohumeral joint.[18-20] These eccentric contractions can injure structures such as the biceps-labrum complex.[21]

Because the static stabilizers in patients who have shoulder laxity or multidirectional instability are reltively incompetent, the rotator cuff and other shouder-girdle muscles must work harder to limit glenohumeral translation. This may lead to overuse tendinosis. Fowler and Webster[22] as well as Richardson and associates[23] observed a close relationship between rotator cuff tendinosis and shoulder laxity in competitive swimmers. Neuromuscular imbalance, especially between the internal and external rotators, also may result in rotator cuff tendinosis.[19] For athletes who use the arms overhead, an imbalance between the internal and external rotators may compromise the stabilizing function of the rotator cuff, causing secondary impingement as the humeral head migrates superiorly. The internal rotators usually are stronger than the external rotators, causing further migration of the humeral head anteriorly and superiorly.

Shoulder pain is a common presenting symptom for many conditions about the shoulder. Although most patients who have rotator cuff tendinosis report pain, others may describe clicking, catching, weakness, stiffness, crepitation, or symptoms of instability. In addition, problems of the neck and the shoulder often have overlapping symptoms, and they may exist concomitantly, complicating diagnosis and management. The age and occupation of the patient; the duration and location of the symptoms; and the radiation, timing, quality, and severity of the pain can be important differentiating factors. The patient should be asked about any alleviating or aggravating factors as well as about any specific traumatic event that precipitated the problem. Athletes should be questioned about the level and intensity of their participation in sports activities, particularly those that require overhead use of the upper extremity, such as baseball, tennis, volleyball, and swimming. They should be questioned about the time that the pain occurs during each activity and asked to note specific movements or other factors, such as the position of the upper limb, that induce the symptoms.

The shoulder examination should be approached systematically for every patient by following the consecutive steps of inspection, palpation, assessment of the range of motion, strength-testing, neurologic assessment, and the performance of special tests. In addition, the physical examination should include a thorough assessment of the cervical spine and the rest of the upper extremity.

During inspection, scapular winging may be noted, which suggests an underlying scapulothoracic dysfunction that may be associated with shoulder instability, muscle imbalance, or muscle fatigue. Scapular winging may become more evident with range-of-motion and strength testing. Osseous and soft-tissue structures are palpated in order to identify specifically any areas of tenderness. The range of motion, both active and passive, should then be assessed and documented in all planes. When there is pain, its severity and the arc of motion at which it occurs should be noted. An attempt should be made to determine if any loss of motion is secondary to pain or to capsular contracture. Loss of internal rotation may be due to posterior capsular contracture, a condition that is often associated with glenohumeral instability.[24]

Muscles should be isolated and tested specifically for strength. Special tests may be helpful for differentiating the etiology of the shoulder pain. Impingement tests such as the Neer[25] test and the test of Hawkins and Kennedy[26] may be positive regardless of the cause of the rotator cuff tendinosis. Pain during crossed-arm adduction at 90° suggests a lesion in the acromioclavicular joint. The tests of Yergason[27] and of Speed[28] are used to check for a lesion in the biceps. Tests for instability include the apprehension sign and the relocation test.[29] The load and shift test, as described by Hawkins and associates,[30] assesses the degree of translation in all planes. A sulcus sign may indicate multidirectional instability.[30] Field and Savoie[31] described a test to check for labral tears involving the anchoring point of the long head of the biceps.

Radiographic evaluation should consist of an anteroposterior, a transscapular lateral, and an axillary radiograph. The supraspinatus outlet radiograph, a lateral radiograph of the erect scapula with a downward tilt of 10°, can help in the assessment of acromial morphology.[32] The examiner should note any osseous abnormalities, such as a variation in the shape and slope of the acromion, osteoarthrosis of the acromioclavicular joint, spurring of the distal aspect of the clavicle, and calcification of the rotator cuff tendons. The examiner should also look for evidence of an osseous Bankart lesion or a Hill-Sachs lesion. Cystic changes or sclerosis in the region of the greater tuberosity, proximal migration of the humeral head, decreased acromiohumeral distance, or glenohumeral osteoarthrosis may be indicative of a rotator cuff tear. Arthrography, ultrasonography, and magnetic resonance imaging (MRI) can be helpful in the diagnosis of full-thickness tears of the rotator cuff, but their clinical value in the assessment of rotator cuff tendinosis remains questionable.[33-36] In our experience, shoulder arthroscopy has been extremely useful in demonstrating the exact location and extent of partial-thickness tears of the rotator cuff and in identifying other pathologic conditions in the shoulder, such as labral tears or ligamentous laxity.

Regardless of the etiology of the condition, patients who have rotator cuff tendinosis have similar symptoms and most can be managed conservatively with an appropriate rehabilitation program. Physiotherapists often play an important role in this program, using a variety of modalities such as heat, cold, ultrasound, laser, friction, and transcutaneous electrical nerve stimulation. Good communication between the physician, the patient, and the physiotherapist is essential for a successful outcome. The role of the patient in the treatment program should be clearly defined at the onset, and realistic goals and expectations of therapy also should be established at the start.

The first phase of the rehabilitation process is pain control, which is achieved by having the patient rest the shoulder and modify or avoid activities that aggravate the pain. Anti-inflammatory medications may be helpful. Subacromial injections of corticosteroids may be considered, but they usually are used only in the later stages of the conservative treatment protocol. We limit treatment to a maximum of three injections.

The second phase of the rehabilitation protocol is restoration of the range of motion. Patients are instructed in circumduction exercises and in the use of pulleys to improve motion. Specific stretching exercises also are taught as a standard part of this program.

The third phase is muscle-strengthening. Emphasis is placed on the strength of the rotator cuff, the deltoid, and the scapular stabilizing muscles. Overhead activities should be avoided, especially during the early phases of treatment. A progressive resistive program is initiated with use of Therabands (DePuy, Warsaw, IN), elastic tubing, free weights, or a combination of these. Therabands and elastic tubing are easily adapted for use at home. They create a closed kinetic system, which may be preferable to the high torque stresses generated at the shoulder by free weights. Restoration of the power, endurance, and smooth coordination of the shoulder muscles is emphasized and should be sport-specific. Any muscle imbalance, especially one between the internal and external rotators, must be identified and addressed. Glenohumeral instability should be identified early, and a proper strengthening program should be directed at improving the dynamic stabilizers of the shoulder. If symptomatic glenohumeral instability continues despite a comprehensive rehabilitation program, surgical intervention should be considered to restore stability.

Surgical intervention for rotator cuff tendinosis should be considered only after all attempts at conservative treatment have failed. For patients who demonstrate primary mechanical impingement, the surgical procedures available are resection of the coracoacromial ligament,[26,37-39] anterior acromioplasty, resection of the distal part of the clavicle, and resection of inferior osteophytes from the acromioclavicular joint, depending on the specific underlying disorder. Glenohumeral instability that is unresponsive to a program of muscle-strengthening and balancing should be treated with surgical stabilization.

The use of shoulder arthroscopy has enhanced the ability to diagnose and evaluate various pathologic conditions in the shoulder, including rotator cuff tendinosis and, in particular, partial-thickness tears. Although we agree with those investigators[40,41] who have advocated repair of sizable or delaminated partial-thickness tears of the rotator cuff, there is little in the literature describing the treatment of partial-thickness tears of the rotator cuff and controversy still exists regarding the effectiveness of treatment. Snyder[41] described an arthroscopic suture-repair technique for partial-thickness tears as well as for small full-thickness tears of the rotator cuff.

Tendinosis of the Elbow

The term tennis elbow is widely used to describe a series of overuse injuries that are characterized by pain and tenderness in the region of the humeral epicondyles and that involve the extensors or flexors of the wrist. The peak prevalence of tennis elbow is in the fourth decade of life, when it is four times higher than the prevalence in any other decade.[42] The lateral epicondyle is involved seven times more often than is the medial epicondyle. Although it is termed tennis elbow, the condition occurs very commonly in nonathletes.

Lateral Tendinosis of the Elbow

Although lateral epicondylitis was first described in 1873,[43] some controversy still exists regarding the etiology and the pathogenesis of this condition. The basic underlying lesion seems to be a macroscopic or microscopic tear in the origin of the extensor carpi radialis brevis tendon that heals with immature reparative tissue.[44] Gross examination of this region characteristically shows grayish, gelatinous, friable immature scar tissue that appears shiny and edematous. Light microscopy reveals a characteristic invasion of fibroblasts and vascular granulation, which has been described as so-called angiofibroblastic hyperplasia.[45] Although lateral tendinosis of the elbow most commonly involves the origin of the extensor carpi radialis brevis, the origins of the extensor digitorum communis, the extensor carpi radialis longus, and the supinator can also be involved in the process. Inflammation of the lateral collateral and orbicular ligaments also can be observed.

The patient usually is first seen because of the gradual onset of aching pain in the region of the lateral epicondyle and in the proximal muscles of the forearm. The pain often is related to flexion and extension of the wrist and to pronation and supination activities. Other conditions that should be considered in the differential diagnosis include nerve entrapment (radial tunnel syndrome) and intra-articular disorders such as radiocapitellar osteoarthrosis, osteochondritis disscans, and an osseous tumor.

Physical examination usually reveals localized tenderness directly over the lateral epicondyle in the region of the origin of the extensor carpi radialis brevis; however, the area of tenderness often is quite diffuse. Pain may increase with resisted wrist or finger extension, particularly with the forearm in pronation. Patients may have a positive coffee-cup test, described by Coonrad,[42] in which grasping or pinching with the wrist in extension reproduces the pain at the point of maximum tenderness. They also may have a positive chair test, described by Gardner,[46] in which the patient has pain in the region of the lateral epicondyle while lifting a chair with one hand with the forearm pronated. Isokinetic strength deficits also may be observed.

Anteroposterior and lateral radiographs of the elbow should be made routinely, as they are helpful for ruling out other conditions such as radiocapitellar osteoarthrosis or the presence of a loose body or an osseous tumor. Oblique radiographs occasionally demonstrate calcifications in the region of the lateral epicondyle. The findings of electromyographic studies are usually normal, even for patients who have radial tunnel syndrome. MRI may demonstrate abnormal changes in signal intensity at the extensor origin on the lateral aspect of the elbow, but a change in signal intensity does not necessarily correlate with the histologic findings or with the symptoms.[47]

The pain needs to be brought under control before the patient can start any extensive rehabilitation. Pain control can be achieved with the use of nonsteroidal anti-inflammatory medications, rest, and modification of activity. Physical modalities such as ice or heat, ultrasound, and electrical stimulation may help to control the pain; phonophoresis with 10% hydrocortisone cream has been found to be useful.[48] Injections of corticosteroids can be tried in resistant cases, with a maximum of three injections during a period of 1 year. Care should be taken to inject the medications directly into the area of maximum tenderness. Counterforce braces have been shown to be effective in the treatment of elbow tendinosis as well.[49] These braces are straps, approximately 5 to 6 cm wide, that are applied just distal to the elbow over the origin of the common extensor tendon. Biomechanical and electromyographic analysis has shown inhibition of maximum contraction of the wrist and finger extensors by use of a counterforce brace.[49] For the tennis player, stroke mechanics should be evaluated and modified as necessary to help control symptoms. When the pain has been controlled, an exercise program that focuses on eccentric strengthening (as described by Stanish and associates[50]) and the restoration of flexibility and endurance can be initiated.

Of 1,213 elbows in one series,[45] 7% (88) had resistant lateral tendinosis that needed surgical intervention. Surgical treatment should be considered only after nonsurgical treatment has failed for at least 1 year. The principles of surgical treatment were previously described by Nirschl and Pettrone.[45] The origin of the extensor carpi radialis brevis is exposed, and tears as well as any granulation tissue that is seen on the underside of the extensor carpi radialis brevis tendon are excised. A small area of the lateral condyle can be decorticated or drilled to improve the blood supply for healing of the detached tendon. Intra-articular examination usually is not necessary unless an associated abnormality was anticipated presurgically. Usually, the elbow is splinted in 90° of flexion for three weeks postsurgically. Then, range-of-motion and gradual strengthening exercises of the hand and wrist are performed daily for 3 additional weeks. From 6 to 12 weeks postsurgically, resisted and eccentric exercises of the wrist are performed. Weights are gradually increased to a maximum of 5 pounds (2.3 kg). After 12 weeks, patients should return gradually to full activities. They may return to sports activities at 4 to 6 months after surgery or when strength and endurance are approximately 80% of normal.

Medial Tendinosis of the Elbow

Medial tendinosis of the elbow occurs much less commonly than lateral tendinosis of the elbow and results from overuse of the forearm flexor muscles or from repetitive valgus stress in throwing athletes. The condition is seen also in patients who play racquet sports, such as tennis, squash, and racquetball, in which the forehand stroke creates excessive stress on the medial elbow structures. In medial tendinosis of the elbow, the tendons of the pronator teres, the flexor carpi radialis, and occasionally the flexor carpi ulnaris are principally affected.

Patients who have medial tendinosis of the elbow usually report aching pain that originates from the region of the medial epicondyle and radiates into the muscles of the forearm. They may also report decreased grip strength, but this problem is usually related to pain rather than to an injury of nerve or muscle. Some of these patients are seen with an acute disruption of the common flexor origin or the ulnar collateral ligament, or both. These conditions, chronic tendinosis and acute disruption, must be differentiated clinically because acute rupture of the ulnar collateral ligament is best treated surgically, especially in an athlete who uses overhead motion. In medial tendinosis of the elbow, the pain increases with resisted wrist flexion when the forearm is held in pronation. With a disruption of the ulnar collateral ligament, a valgus stress test of the elbow produces pain. Ulnar-nerve entrapment can also cause medial pain in the elbow, and it should be included in the differential diagnosis. Nirschl[51] reported ulnar-nerve dysfunction in 60% of patients who had surgical treatment for medial epicondylitis. Entrapment of the ulnar nerve usually is found in zone 3, distal to the medial epicondyle.

Nonsurgical treatment of medial tendinosis of the elbow should follow the same steps as those described for lateral tendinosis of the elbow. Surgical treatment involves a medial longitudinal incision with the surgeon carefully avoiding the medial antebrachial cutaneous nerve. The tendons of the pronator teres and flexor carpi radialis are split longitudinally, distal from their origin on the medial epicondyle. Care should be taken not to detach the common flexor origin, as this can lead to posteromedial instability of the elbow. All abnormal, torn, or degenerative tissue should be sharply excised. If there is evidence of ulnar neuropathy presurgically, a formal ulnar-nerve transposition should be performed because the results of cubital tunnel decompression alone have not been satisfactory.[52]

Tendinosis About the Hip (Snapping Hip)

Two distinct conditions, which have been characterized as internal and external, can cause symptomatic snapping with motion of the hip. The internal type is due to the iliopsoas tendon snapping over the femoral head, over the iliopectineal eminence, or, less commonly, over a ridge on the lesser trochanter. Internal snapping hip often is found in athletes who frequently flex and extend this joint, especially in association with abduction and external rotation, as occurs commonly in dance and in the martial arts. The patient is first seen because of the gradual onset of a reproducible, audible, and palpable low-pitched clunk in the groin. Typically, the problem is unilateral. On physical examination, there is no tenderness and no pain when the rectus femoris works against resistance. Occasionally, the examiner can elicit pain with resisted use of the iliopsoas muscle.

Although arthrography or MRI can be considered in order to rule out a loose body or a labral tear within the hip joint, no workup is necessary when the clinical findings are typical. The diagnosis can be made definitively by iliopsoas bursography, which will demonstrate the snapping tendon.[53]

The internal snapping hip is treated first by encouraging the patient to stop intentional snapping. Nonsteroidal anti-inflammatory medications may be helpful in relieving any inflammation that may have resulted from repeated snapping. Stretching and strengthening exercises of the iliopsoas are helpful as is repatterning muscle use during the affected motions. Surgical lengthening of the iliopsoas tendon is rarely necessary.[54]

The external snapping hip is caused by the iliotibial band snapping over the greater trochanter. This condition is most common in cyclists and runners, particularly those who run up and down hills. Anatomic factors that maintain the iliotibial band in a stretched position and make it more likely to rub as it passes over the greater trochanter include genu varum, a true limb-length discrepancy or a functional short limb (the downhill limb while an individual is running on a canted surface), and a crossover running style. Occasionally, a causative factor for external snapping hip in cyclists is the position of the cleat or other shoe-fixation device on the bicycle.

When these patients are first seen, they report the gradual onset of pain and a high-pitched snapping over the greater trochanter. Typically, the problem is unilateral and is sometimes difficult to distinguish from greater trochanteric bursitis. The patient has tenderness to palpation over the greater trochanter when tendinosis is present and behind it when bursitis is present. In either case, the patient has pain when the lower extremity is adducted across the midline. The hip usually is painful to lie on when the patient has bursitis, but not when the patient has iliotibial tendinosis. Resisted abduction is painful when tendinosis is present, but not when the patient has bursitis alone. An Ober test reveals tightness of the iliotibial band (Fig. 1).

The initial treatment of both bursitis and tendinosis includes the use of nonsteroidal anti-inflammatory drugs and ice-friction massage. Stretching the iliotibial band is helpful, but it may aggravate bursitis initially. The physician should look for and correct any training, biomechanical, or anatomic factors that may have contributed to the problem. Differentiation of bursitis from tendinosis is more important when initial treatment is unsuccessful. When a patient has chronic bursitis of the greater trochanter, an injection of steroids into the bursa often relieves symptoms. When the problem is chronic iliotibial tendinosis, however, injections of steroids are less likely to provide relief, and lengthening of the iliotibial band should be considered in order to achieve long-lasting relief.[55]

Lateral Runner's Knee (Iliotibial Band Tendinosis)

The condition that is termed lateral runner's knee is caused by the iliotibial band rubbing over the lateral femoral epicondyle. This is most commonly an overuse condition with the same predisposing biomechanical and anatomic factors as those noted previously for the iliotibial band snapping over the greater trochanter. In addition, a mild varus position of the heel can predispose a runner to iliotibial band tendinosis at the knee because of the varus moment imposed by this deformity on the knee during heel-strike and midstance.[56]

The patient is first seen with unilateral pain in the lateral aspect of the knee, proximal to the joint line, at the level of the lateral femoral epicondyle. Occasionally, a patient reports snapping as well. The pain is insidious in onset, but it is made worse by going up or down stairs, riding a bicycle, or running. Tenderness to palpation at the epicondyle and, sometimes, crepitation are noted. The Ober test is positive for tightness of the iliotibial band (Fig. 1). The examiner should also check the shoes of the runner for abnormal wear along the lateral part of the midsole and forefoot.

The treatment for this condition is identical to that for external snapping hip, as described previously. One way to correct the common biomechanical problems is to encourage the patient to run in alternate directions on the track or on alternate sides of the road to avoid always having the same lower extremity in the downhill position. In addition, a lateral wedge in the shoe of a patient who has varus heels or knees can help to decrease the varus moment during running. If all else fails, an injection of steroids into the area of maximum tenderness may produce relief, as an inflamed bursa may have developed deep to the tendon. Lengthening of the iliotibial band may be performed, but it is rarely necessary.[57]

Jumper's Knee

Jumper's knee, or so-called patellar tendinosis, results from microtears of the patellar ligament followed by a chronic inflammatory response. It is an overuse injury that is most commonly seen in athletes who participate in sports that require a great deal of jumping or kicking, such as basketball, volleyball, and soccer. Symptoms may occur during an adolescent growth spurt, perhaps because the ligament does not lengthen as fast or as much as the adjacent bones are growing.

The patient is first seen with tenderness over the patellar ligament. The area may be red, swollen, or crepitant. Resisted use of the quadriceps and full passive flexion of the knee produce pain. Quadriceps tightness is frequently present.

Treatment includes decreasing or stopping the inciting activity, use of nonsteroidal anti-inflammatory drugs, and ice-friction massage. A program of quadriceps stretching is critical, particularly for the adolescent. Isometric exercises to strengthen the quadriceps can be started immediately, but isotonic or isokinetic exercises for strengthening the quadriceps should begin only when the tenderness has subsided. It is very

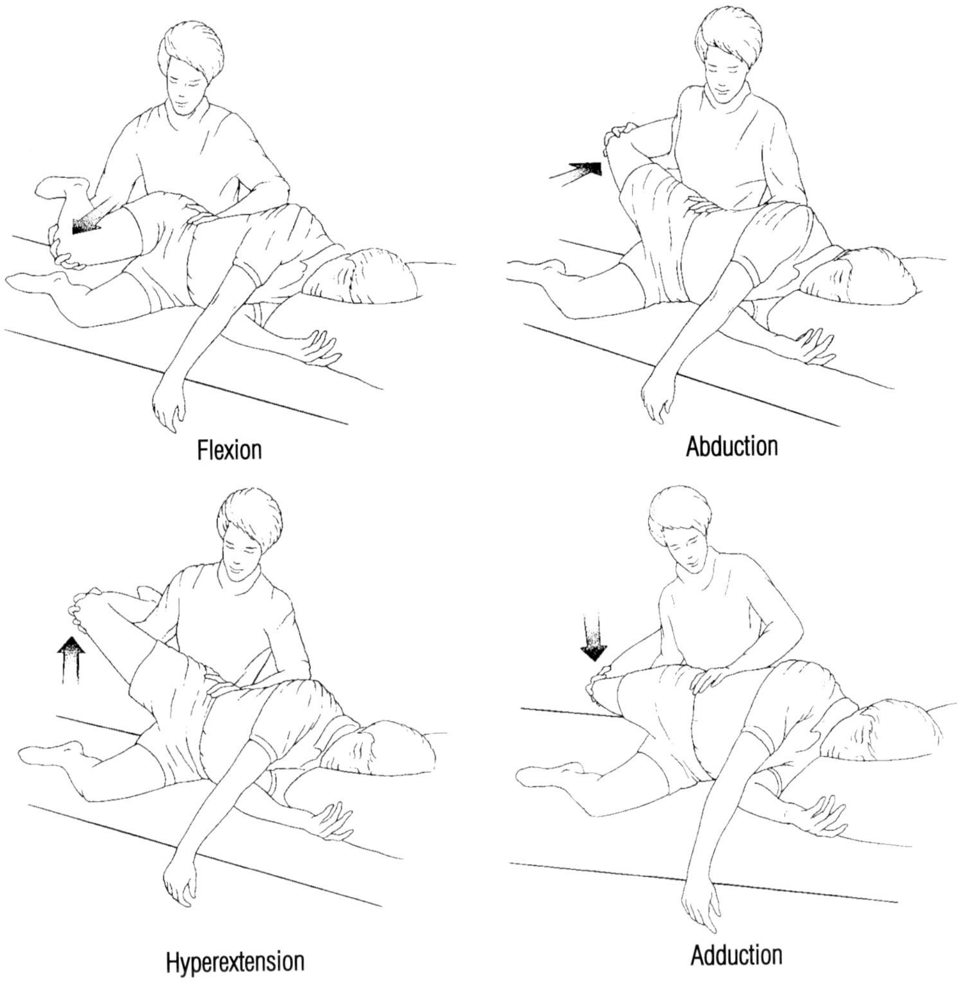

Fig. 1 The Ober test is used to assess contracture of the iliotibial band. The patient lies on the unaffected side with the unaffected hip and knee flexed enough to eliminate lumbar lordosis. The examiner holds the extremity to be tested with the knee flexed. The examiner's other hand stabilizes the pelvis. The hip is then flexed, abducted, and hyperextended to catch the iliotibial band on the greater trochanter. The limb is then adducted. If the iliotibial band is tight, the limb cannot be adducted back down to the examining table or to the contralateral limb but remains passively abducted.

important that the athlete eventually advance to eccentric quadriceps strengthening in order to train for his or her sport. Although the precise reason for its clinical effectiveness is not known, application of a brace that contains a pad over the patellar ligament is useful when the pain has resolved and the athlete wishes to return to participation in sports (Fig. 2).

When patellar tendinosis does not respond to nonsurgical intervention, diagnostic ultrasonography may reveal an area of angiofibroblastic hyperplasia and fibrinoid necrosis deep within the ligament (Fig. 3, *top*). With use of a local anesthetic, excision of this area can be carried out by splitting the ligament longitudinally (Fig. 3, *bottom*), and the surgeon should look for gelatinous material between normal fibers. This material should be excised, and the remainder of the ligament should be closed with absorbable sutures. Roels and associates[58] reported that surgical treatment allowed all ten patients in their series to return to participation in sports.

Dysfunction of the Posterior Tibial Tendon

The posterior tibial muscle is the main invertor of the subtalar joint. The short fiber length of this muscle produces a great deal of force on its five insertions into the plantar aspect of the foot. The posterior tibial tendon has an excursion of 2 cm.[59] If the hindfoot is in an abnormal amount of valgus or the forefoot is in too much varus, excessive tension is placed on the posterior tibial tendon, a situation that may lead to tenosynovitis.

Dysfunction of the posterior tibial tendon can be acute or chronic. Most commonly, the condition consists of an acute tenosynovitis secondary to overuse, without any structural change in the hindfoot. In one series, this condition was reported in 58 (6%) of 974 runners.[60] Chronic tenosynovitis, which usually is found in the nonathletic population, is associated with tendinosis and structural changes in the hindfoot. An acute rupture of the posterior tibial tendon before the age of 30 years has been reported in only four

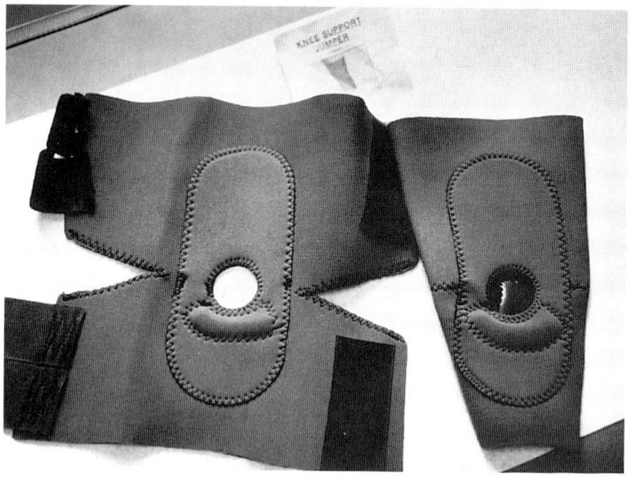

Fig. 2 A brace for jumper's knee. The pad must be positioned directly over the patellar ligament.

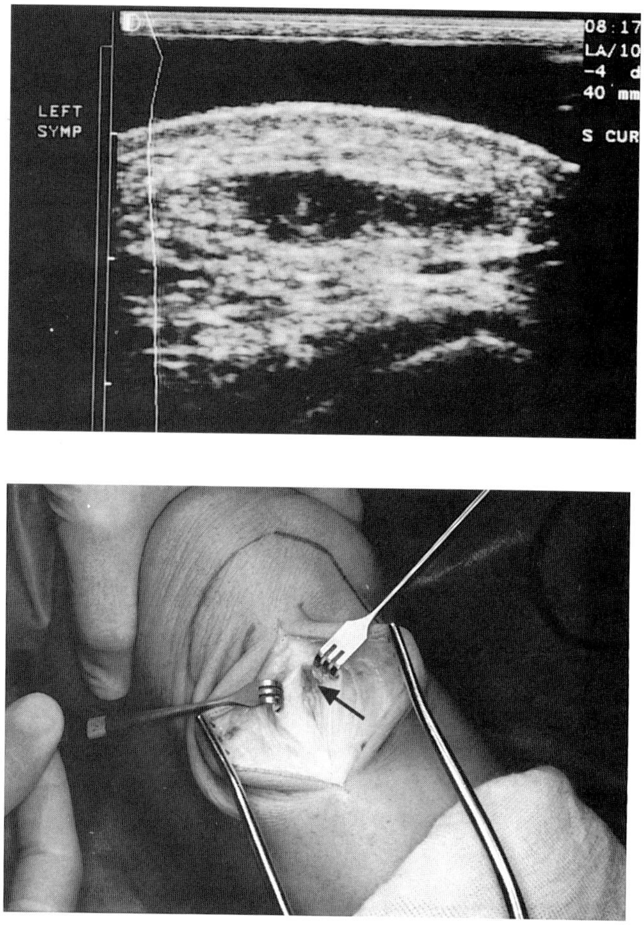

Fig. 3 A patient who had jumper's knee. **Top,** This ultrasonogram shows the hypoechoic area (arrow) within the fibers of the patellar ligament. This area corresponds to the area of angiofibroblastic hyperplasia and fibrinoid necrosis in the ligament. **Bottom,** The gross appearance of the patellar ligament. Note the discoloration and the loss of fibrous integrity in the damaged area deep in the ligament (arrow).

patients.[61] Woods and Leach[62] reported one other series of six patients who had had an acute rupture (complete or partial) of the posterior tibial tendon and emphasized the necessity for early recognition and treatment.

Patients who have tenosynovitis of the posterior tibial tendon report pain along the posteromedial aspect of the foot and ankle. The pain is minor at first, but swelling and progressive disability develop as the condition progresses. The evaluation should begin with careful questioning regarding history, with particular attention paid to the onset of the condition, changes in training habits, the nature and frequency of training, the type of footwear, and the use of orthotic devices. The single most important aspect in the assessment of a patient who has suspected dysfunction of the posterior tibial tendon is the physical examination. The hindfoot should be observed with the patient standing. A patient who has posterior tibial tendon dysfunction may have an increased valgus posture of the calcaneus and a fullness that is seen just distal to the medial malleolus. The patient should be asked to stand on tiptoe so that the examiner can assess the degree of active inversion of the calcaneus that occurs at the subtalar joint. Lack of heel inversion usually indicates dysfunction or weakness of the posterior tibial tendon. Next, the patient should be asked to repeat a toe-rise on one foot approximately eight to ten times. The examiner should carefully observe how high the patient is able to rise on the toes as well as the degree of heel inversion that occurs. Frequently, during an acute episode of tenosynovitis, the patient is unable to stand on tiptoe at all because of pain.

The examiner should carefully note the degree of dorsiflexion and plantarflexion of the ankle (specifically looking for any lack of dorsiflexion), the range of subtalar joint motion (looking particularly for diminished inversion), and the motion of the transverse tarsal joint. The tendon sheath should be palpated carefully, with the examiner looking for thickening, increased warmth, and crepitation. The strength of the tendon should be evaluated by having the patient both bring the foot actively from a fully everted position into inversion and attempt to hold the foot in an inverted position against resistance.

Weightbearing anteroposterior, lateral, and oblique radiographs of the foot should be made. The anteroposterior radiograph can demonstrate subluxation of the talonavicular joint and the relationship of the talus to the calcaneus. The lateral radiograph should be studied for any sagging of the talonavicular, naviculocuneiform, or first metatarsal-cuneiform joint. No single specific pattern of radiographic changes is observed in these patients.

Treatment

Acute Tenosynovitis When acute tenosynovitis is mild, it can be treated with a decrease in the level of activities. However, when the symptoms are moderate, the extremity should be rested and stressful activities should be stopped. An anti-inflammatory medication or ice, or both, should be used at this stage. If the symptoms do not respond within 4 to 6 weeks, immobilization in a weightbearing below-the-knee cast for 4 to 6 weeks is recommended. If the symptoms still fail to respond, surgical treatment should be recommended. The surgical procedure consists of exploration of the tendon between the medial malleolus and the tendon insertion. Most frequently, varying degrees of synovial proliferation are found. The tendon and sheath should be carefully debrided of the exuberant synovial tissue. If necessary, the debridement may be continued proximal to the medial malleolus, but a 1-cm section of sheath should be left in place to act as a pulley behind the medial malleolus. Occasionally, when the posterior tibial tendon is explored, the tendon itself appears to be intact, but the abnormality lies at the insertion of the tendon into the navicular. Although excision of the affected portion and advancement of the posterior tibial tendon into the navicular is preferable in this situation, often there is not enough excursion of the musculotendinous unit to allow the advancement of the tendon into the navicular. Therefore, we have found that it is better to carry out a reconstruction with use of the flexor digitorum longus tendon as a transfer into the navicular and then to suture the end of the posterior tibial tendon into the flexor digitorum longus.

Acute Rupture A patient who sustains an acute rupture of the posterior tibial tendon, a rare injury, demonstrates no active inversion of the subtalar joint. A defect in the tendon may be palpable because the rupture usually occurs between the medial malleolus and the navicular. However, blood in the tendon sheath may mask this finding. When an acute rupture is present, a reconstruction with use of the flexor digitorum longus should be performed as soon as possible in order to avoid the development of a flatfoot deformity.[63]

Chronic Tenosynovitis A patient who has had tenosynovitis of the posterior tibial tendon for more than a year probably has a mild to moderate degree of tendinosis. The foot probably has structural changes (such as flattening of the longitudinal arch secondary to sagging of the talonavicular joint), although the deformities may be mild and usually are not fixed. These patients retain fair-to-good strength of the posterior tibial muscle and can be managed with an orthosis. The orthosis should include a varus heel-wedge and a medial forefoot post. When the symptoms persist and interfere with activities of daily living or athletic activities, exploration, decompression, and reconstruction of the tendon with use of the flexor digitorum longus is indicated.

Chronic Rupture Patients who have chronic rupture of the posterior tibial tendon note a flatfoot deformity that has progressed over a period of several years. The physical examination often demonstrates loss of subtalar joint motion, especially inversion, and a fixed varus deformity of the forefoot that usually exceeds 15°. When this is the case, tendon decompression and transfer is not effective and a double or triple arthrodesis is indicated. It should be realized that fusion of this type can be a substantial impediment to running activities; however, walking, golf, and doubles tennis are still feasible.

Dysfunction of the Achilles Tendon

The gastrocnemius-soleus complex spans two joints and is the largest and strongest muscle in the calf. It is a stance-phase muscle that undergoes both eccentric (lengthening) and concentric (shortening) contractions during walking and running. Normally, the Achilles tendon twists as it passes to its insertion, particularly in the area approximately 2 to 6 cm proximal to the insertion. This anatomic configuration results in increased internal stress on the tendon.[64] In addition, the blood supply to this area has been demonstrated to be tenuous.[65,66] Problems that commonly occur in the area that is proximal to the insertion of the tendon and to the level of the retrocalcaneal bursa are termed noninsertional problems. These include Achilles tendinitis, which is an inflammation of the tendon sheath without intrinsic tendinous changes; Achilles tendinosis, which is the occurrence of intrinsic tendinous changes with or without associated tendinitis; and Achilles tendon rupture.[67,68] Another set of problems occurs in the area posterior to the retrocalcaneal bursa and at the insertion of the tendon. Termed insertional problems, these include calcification within the Achilles tendon at its insertion into the calcaneus without tendinosis; Achilles tendinosis at its insertion with or without associated calcification; and Achilles dysfunction associated with a Haglund deformity, which is a prominence of the posterosuperior aspect of the calcaneus. Such categorization of the various pathologic entities that occur about the Achilles tendon is important for accurate diagnosis, prognosis, and treatment.

The prevalence of Achilles tendinitis has been estimated to be 11% in runners,[69] 9% in dancers,[70] 5% in gymnasts,[71] 2% in tennis players,[72] and less than 1% in football players.[73] Tendinitis is brought about most frequently by training-related errors, although mechanical factors, such as hyperpronation of the foot, contracture of the gastrocnemius-soleus complex, or faulty footwear, may be involved as well. Conversely, Achilles tendinosis represents a degenerative process of the tendon and probably has nothing to do with training errors or other mechanical problems. Achilles tendon ruptures, which are not described in the present report, are thought to be due to underlying tendinosis,[74,75] although usually the tendinosis is subclinical.

Evaluation of a patient who has a painful Achilles tendon begins with careful questioning regarding the history, including the onset of the condition, the level of activities, the training techniques, the type of footwear, and the previous treatment. The patient is asked to place a finger on the area of maximum pain. The patient should then stand while the examiner notes the posture of the foot. Next, a toe-rise should be done three, four, or five times on each foot individually. A patient who has tendinosis often is unable to do a single toe-rise, whereas a patient who has tendinitis can perform a toe-rise without as much difficulty. The tendon should be palpated for thickening, increased warmth along the tendon sheath, and crepitation. The range of motion of the ankle and the subtalar joint should be determined carefully.

The physical findings in tendinitis consist of inflammation that is limited to the peritenon, as demonstrated by increased warmth and tenderness and, possibly, by crepitation. Nodularity is not present with acute Achilles tendinitis. During dorsiflexion and plantarflexion, the fingertips of the examiner feel no nodules in the Achilles tendon.

When tendinosis is present, the tendon is thickened over a length of 2 to 5 cm. This area may or may not demonstrate increased warmth, depending on the extent and duration of the tendinosis. Squeezing the area of tendinosis often causes substantial pain. Tendinosis may limit the ability of a patient to stand on tiptoe.

On occasion, an inflamed retrocalcaneal bursa may be the cause of pain. In this case, most of the pain is located between the calcaneus and the Achilles tendon but proximal to the insertion of the tendon. There may be focal tenderness over the bursal area anterior to the Achilles tendon, but usually there is no substantial thickening of the tendon per se. Palpation of the tendon does not cause pain. Sometimes, the swollen bursa can be palpated.

Insertional tendinosis includes two basic types. The first type is characterized by generalized thickening of the tendon at its insertion, where there is an area of increased warmth, frequently an osseous prominence, and marked tenderness to palpation. Performing a single toe-rise is often difficult for patients who have this type of tendinosis, and only rarely can these patients repeat a toe-rise more than two or three times. The second type of insertional tendinosis involves a well-localized area that a patient can pinpoint at the insertion of the Achilles tendon. Frequently, the tendon itself is not particularly thickened except in the localized area where the pain is located. Patients who have this type of tendinosis usually can perform a single toe-rise without difficulty. Radiographs often demonstrate calcification about the insertion of the tendon (Fig. 4, *left*). The radiographs of a patient who has a focal area of pain usually show a localized area of calcification, as op-posed to a large area, which is frequently seen in a patient who has generalized tendinosis. Computed tomography (CT) scans of a patient who has localized calcification frequently demonstrate an area of calcification that corresponds to the area of the pain (Fig. 4, *right*). For patients who have generalized tendinosis, an MRI may demonstrate cystic areas within the substance of the tendon, either proximal to or at the level of the insertion (Fig. 5). The extent of the involvement varies greatly among patients.

Treatment of all of these conditions depends on the severity of the problem. The initial treatment consists of rest, ice massages, nonsteroidal anti-inflammatory medication, and stretching of the Achilles tendon. Athletes may need to change their training program or footwear. Effective modifications of footwear may include a softer heel-counter, an orthotic device to correct severe pronation if it is present, or a softer heel-cushion. If the symptoms fail to respond to these measures, we have found that immobilization in a weightbearing cast, particularly for a patient who has insertional tendinosis, is extremely useful. If the symptoms respond to the use of a below-the-knee cast and subsequently recur but the patient is not a good candidate for surgery, a polypropylene ankle-foot orthosis with no motion of the ankle joint often provides effective long-term relief.

Surgical management should be undertaken only after conservative treatment has been exhausted. In a patient who has Achilles tendinitis, chronic inflammation may create a thickening of the tendon sheath. Release of the tendon sheath has been reported to be successful,[76] but we have not found the procedure to be necessary for these patients because tendinitis virtually always responds to nonsurgical treatment. In patients who have recalcitrant Achilles tendinosis, we explore the area of tendinosis but rarely find any substantial lesion or cyst formation other than an occasional area of cholesterol deposition. We do not attempt to excise small lesions of 2 cm or less but rather we weave the plantaris tendon back and forth through the area to stimulate an inflammatory healing response. Postsurgically, the leg is kept in a nonweightbearing below-the-knee cast for 1 month and in a weightbearing below-the-knee cast for another month. During the second month, a removable cast is used to allow the patient to work on range-of-motion exercises and to use an elastic band to keep some tone in the muscles during the later healing phase. The enlarged area of tendinosis usually does not disappear, but it often becomes much less painful. We do not permit a patient to resume unrestricted activities until the enlarged area

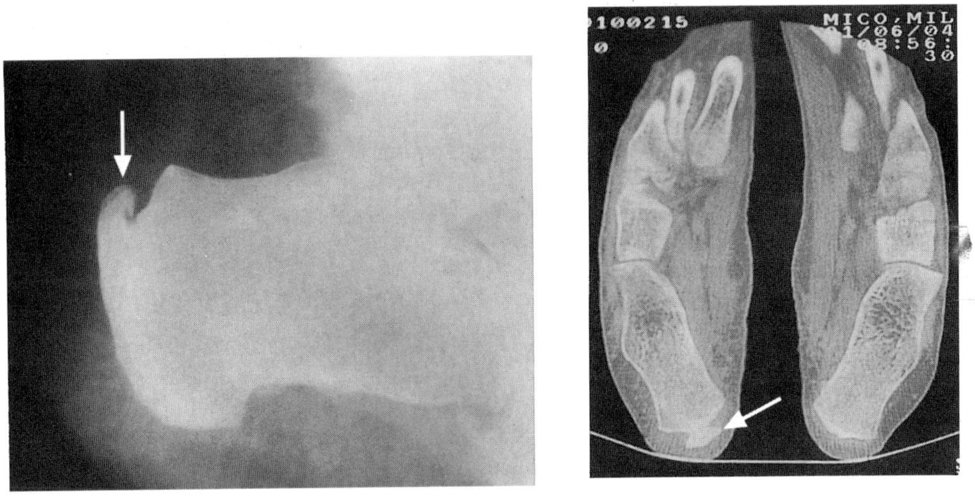

Fig. 4 Insertional tendinosis. **Left,** The radiograph demonstrates calcification at the insertion of the Achilles tendon (arrow). **Right,** The computed tomography scan localizes the area of calcification (arrow).

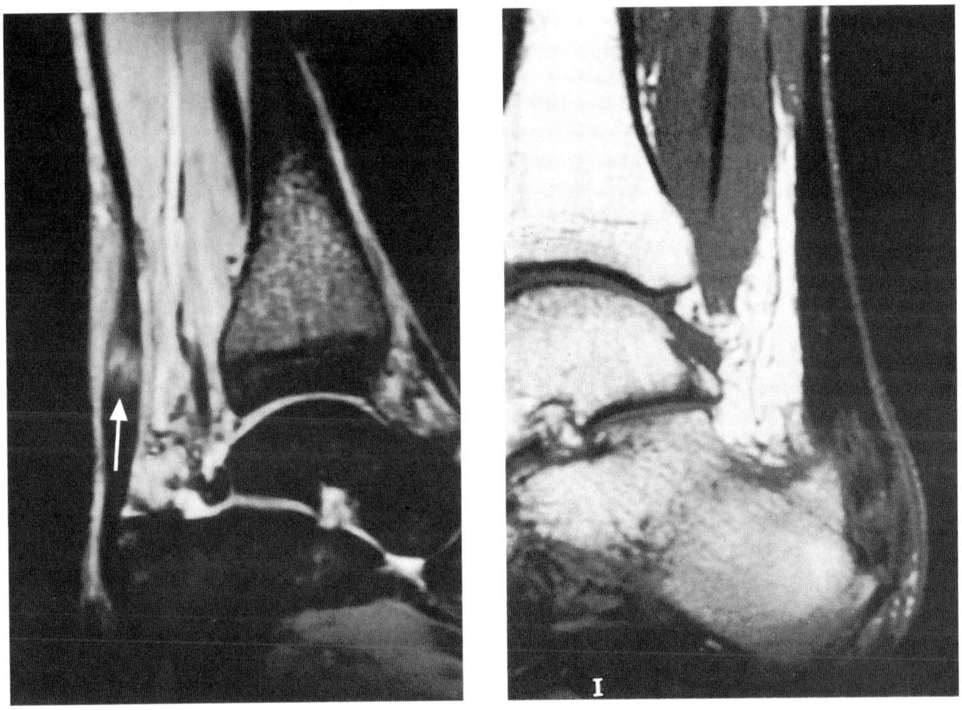

Fig. 5 Abnormalities within the Achilles tendon. **Left,** A defect in the mid-substance of the Achilles tendon, representing the area of tendinosis (arrow). **Right,** Insertional tendinosis with probable obliteration of the retrocalcaneal bursa because of adhesion of the tendon to the calcaneus.

is no longer warm or tender to palpation. For some patients, this may take 3 to 6 months. Eight of our ten patients who were managed with this technique had a successful result.

When the tendinosis involves the entire segment of tendon and has failed to respond to conservative treatment, a procedure is used to bypass the involved area, whether it is in the midsubstance or at the level of the insertion of the tendon into the calcaneus.[63] In this procedure, either the flexor hallucis longus or the flexor digitorum longus is transplanted from the plantar aspect of the foot and is used to bypass the segment of tendinosis (Fig. 6, *left*). Depending on the severity and the length of the segment involved, a portion of the Achilles tendon may need to be excised. The tendon of the flexor hallucis longus or flexor digitorum longus is freed from the midfoot and tunneled through the calcaneus to reinforce the reconstructed tendon and to create one stable musculotendinous unit. The transferred tendon acts as a splint for the area of the Achilles tendon where the segment has been advanced and, in this way, a sort of scaffolding is created to support the Achilles tendon until it heals. Next, the central portion of the Achilles tendon is advanced across the excised area, either into the calcaneus if the distal portion of the Achilles tendon was resected or into the substance of the tendon if a more proximal area was excised (Fig. 6, *right*).[67,68] This procedure is technically demanding. Caution must be used in handling the skin, as it has a marginal blood supply and a skin slough may occur. Postsurgically, the patient is not allowed to bear weight on the limb for 3 months. Afterward, progressive weightbearing is begun, but full mobilization without a cast is not permitted until the involved area is no longer warm or painful to palpation.

When there is a well-localized area of calcification within the tendon, a transverse incision is made in the skin. Then, a longitudinal incision is made over the area of calcification, and the calcified area is shelled out. Postsurgically, a below-the-knee nonweightbearing cast is worn for 3 weeks and then a weightbearing cast is worn for an additional 3 weeks. The result is usually successful for these patients as the problem is well localized and extensive tendinosis usually is not present. This surgical approach cannot be used for a large area of calcification within the substance of the tendon, as that type of lesion usually is located in the anterior aspect of the tendon and cannot be reached from a posterior approach.

A patient who has chronic retrocalcaneal bursitis, with or without an associated Haglund deformity but with no tendinosis, often is managed successfully with simple excision of the posterosuperior aspect of the calcaneus in order to decompress the bursa.[76] Not infrequently, it has been observed that the Achilles tendon actually has become adherent to the posterior aspect of the calcaneus. Relieving this irritation of the Achilles tendon usually benefits the patient.

Overview

Tendinitis, although not life-threatening, is an extremely common problem that interferes with an active lifestyle. Although it is used often, the term tendinitis is probably a misnomer. Tendinosis should be used to describe problems that are predominantly degenerative, such as those that occur in the rotator cuff and in the extensor tendons of the wrist. In tendons with a tenosynovial layer, such as the posterior tibial tendon, the visceral layer of paratenon can become inflamed in response to microtrauma or to degenerative changes in the tendon proper. The semantic difficulties arise from a paradox between the histologic and the clinical findings. The results of histologic examination of chronically painful tendons are more consistent with tendinosis, revealing angiofibroblastic hyperplasia and fibrinoid necrosis with few or no inflammatory

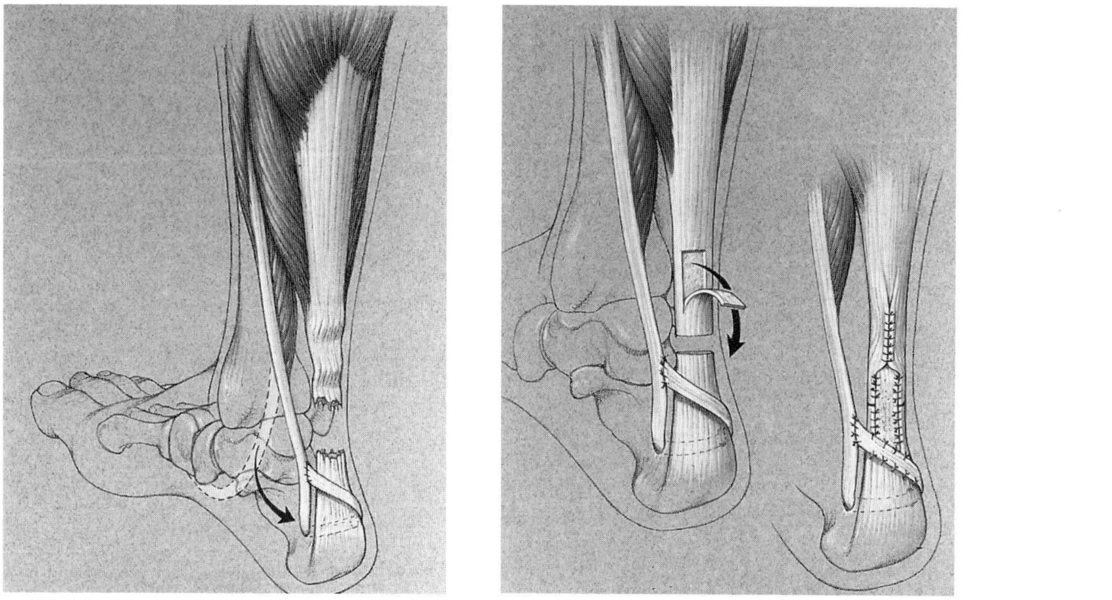

Fig. 6 Reconstruction of the Achilles tendon with use of a flexor digitorum transfer. **Left,** The flexor digitorum longus or the flexor hallucis longus is freed from the plantar aspect of the foot and brought posteriorly through a drill-hole in the calcaneus, after which it is sutured back onto itself. It is important to tension the transplant to approximate the tension felt with manual dorsiflexion of the contralateral extremity. Usually, this procedure will hold the foot in approximately 10° of plantarflexion. **Right,** A flap of the Achilles tendon is developed either by the turndown method, as demonstrated, or by some type of advancement somewhat more proximally, depending on the nature of the abnormality. The flap is brought down under tension in order to reconstruct the Achilles tendon. Sutures are then placed between the transferred tendon and the Achilles tendon.

cells. These findings are seen, perhaps, because surgical treatment is rarely undertaken early in the process. Yet, early in the clinical setting, the symptoms in many patients respond favorably to anti-inflammatory drugs and modalities. One can speculate that these drugs are acting solely as pain relievers, much as they do in osteoarthrosis. Alternatively, perhaps in some patients, a microscopic tear in the tendon initiates an inflammatory response that, if not treated, is replaced by tissue that resembles a failed repair or degenerative process: it is poorly organized, has numerous blood vessels, and contains fibro-blasts and areas of hyaline or mucoid degeneration. Questions remain about the exact pathophysiology and appropriate terminology for what are predominantly overuse problems in the tendon.

In the evaluation of a patient who has a tendon problem, it is important to obtain a detailed history of the onset of pain and the examiner must look carefully for contributing anatomic or biomechanical factors. As we have pointed out, most of these tendon problems are due to overuse caused by errors in training by either a younger enthusiastic athlete or an older, unconditioned recreational athlete. Most tendon problems can be treated nonsurgically by changing the training routine and by adjusting or modifying predisposing anatomic and biomechanical factors. Additional treatment elements include the use of rest, circulatory stimulants, and anti-inflammatory modalities, such as contrast therapy, ice-friction massage, and nonsteroidal anti-inflammatory drugs. When the initial pain has subsided and while new collagen fibers at the site of injury are remodeling, the involved musculotendinous unit should be stretched and strengthened to avoid recurrence. For a recalcitrant problem, surgical treatment can be considered.

References

1. Woo SL-Y, An K-N, Arnoczky SP, et al: Anatomy, biology, and biomechanics of tendon, ligament, and meniscus, in Simon SR (ed): *Orthopaedic Basic Science.* Rosemont, IL, American Academy of Orthopaedic Surgeons, 1994, pp 45–87.
2. Garrett WE Jr: Muscle strain injuries: Clinical and basic aspects. *Med Sci Sports Exerc* 1990;22:436–443.
3. Clancy WG Jr: Tendon trauma and overuse injuries, in Leadbetter WB, Buckwalter JA, Gordon SL (eds): *Sports-Induced Inflammation: Clinical and Basic Science Concepts.* Park Ridge, IL, American Academy of Orthopaedic Surgeons, 1990, pp 609–618.
4. Puddu G, Ippolito E, Postacchini F: A classification of Achilles tendon disease. *Am J Sports Med* 1976;4:145–150.
5. Kannus P, Jozsa L: Histopathological changes preceding spontaneous rupture of a tendon: A controlled study of 891 patients. *J Bone Joint Surg* 1991;73A:1507–1525.
6. Jozsa L, Kvist M, Balint BJ, et al: The role of recreational sport activity in Achilles tendon rupture: A clinical, pathoanatomical, and sociological study of 292 cases. *Am J Sports Med* 1989;17:338–343.
7. Lehto MU, Jarvinen M, Suominen P: Chronic Achilles peritendinitis and retrocalcanear bursitis: Long-term follow-up of surgically treated cases. *Knee Surg Sports Traumatol Arthrosc* 1994;2:182–185.
8. Garrett WE Jr, Nikolaov PK, Ribbeck BM, et al: The effect of muscle architecture on the biomechanical failure properties of skeletal muscle under passive extension. *Am J Sports Med* 1988;16:7–12.
9. Okuda Y, Gorski JP, An KN, et al: Biochemical, histological, and biomechanical analyses of canine tendon. *J Orthop Res* 1987;5:60–68.
10. Williams IF, McCullagh KG, Goodship AE, et al: Studies on the pathogenesis of equine tendonitis following collagenase injury. *Res Vet Sci* 1984;36:326–328.
11. Codman EA (ed): *The Shoulder.* Boston, MA, Thomas Todd, 1934.
12. Keyes EL: Anatomical observations on senile changes in the shoulder. *J Bone Joint Surg* 1935;17:953–960.
13. Meyer AW: Chronic functional lesions of the shoulder. *Arch Surg* 1937;35:646–674.
14. Morrison DS, Bigliani LU: The clinical significance of variations in acromial morphology. *Orthop Trans* 1987;11:234.
15. Rathbun JB, Macnab I: The microvascular pattern of the rotator cuff. *J Bone Joint Surg* 1970;52B:540–553.
16. Lohr JF, Uhthoff HK: The microvascular pattern of the supraspinatus tendon. *Clin Orthop* 1990;254:35–38.
17. Ogata S, Uhthoff HK: Acromial enthesopathy and rotator cuff tears: A radiologic and histologic postmortem investigation of the coracoacromial arch. *Clin Orthop* 1990;254:39–48.
18. Jobe FW, Moynes DR, Tibone JE, et al: An EMG analysis of the shoulder in pitching: A second report. *Am J Sports Med* 1984;12:218–220.
19. Glousman R, Jobe F, Tibone J, et al: Dynamic electromyographic analysis of the throwing shoulder with glenohumeral instability. *J Bone Joint Surg* 1988;70A:220–226.
20. Ryu RK, McCormick J, Jobe FW, et al: An electromyographic analysis of shoulder function in tennis players. *Am J Sports Med* 1988;16:481–485.
21. Andrews JR, Carson WG Jr, McLeod WD: Glenoid labrum tears related to the long head of the biceps. *Am J Sports Med* 1985;13:337–341.
22. Fowler PJ, Webster MS: Shoulder pain in highly competitive swimmers. *Orthop Trans* 1983;7:170.
23. Richardson AB, Jobe FW, Collins HR: The shoulder in competitive swimming. *Am J Sports Med* 1980;8:159–163.
24. Lombardo SJ, Jobe FW, Kerlan RK, et al: Posterior shoulder lesions in throwing athletes. *Am J Sports Med* 1977;5:106–110.
25. Neer CS II: Anterior acromioplasty for the chronic impingement syndrome in the shoulder: A preliminary report. *J Bone Joint Surg* 1972;54A:41–50.
26. Hawkins RJ, Kennedy JC: Impingement syndrome in athletes. *Am J Sports Med* 1980;8:151–158.
27. Yergason RM: Supination sign: Case report. *J Bone Joint Surg* 1931;13:160.
28. Crenshaw AH, Kilgore WE: Surgical treatment of bicipital tenosynovitis. *J Bone Joint Surg* 1966;48A:1496–1502.
29. Hunter-Griffin LY (ed): The shoulder, in *Athletic Training and Sports Medicine,* ed 2. Park Ridge, IL, The American Academy of Orthopaedic Surgeons, 1991, pp 231–266.
30. Hawkins RJ, Abrams JS, Schutte J: Multidirectional instability of the shoulder: An approach to diagnosis. *Orthop Trans* 1987;11:246.
31. Field LD, Savoie FH III: Arthroscopic suture repair of superior labral detachment lesions of the shoulder. *Am J Sports Med* 1993;21:783–790.
32. Neer CS II, Poppen NK: Supraspinatus outlet. *Orthop Trans* 1987;11:234.
33. Farley TE, Neumann CH, Steinbach LS, et al: Full-thickness

tears of the rotator cuff of the shoulder: Diagnosis with MR imaging. *Am J Roentgenol* 1992;158:347–351.
34. Iannotti JP, Zlatkin MB, Esterhai JL, et al: Magnetic resonance imaging of the shoulder: Sensitivity, specificity, and predictive value. *J Bone Joint Surg* 1991;73A:17–29.
35. Miniaci A, Dowdy PA, Willits KR, et al: Magnetic resonance imaging evaluation of the rotator cuff tendons in the asymptomatic shoulder. *Am J Sports Med* 1995;23:142–145.
36. Neumann CH, Holt RG, Steinbach LS, et al: MR imaging of the shoulder: Appearance of the supraspinatus tendon in asymptomatic volunteers. *Am J Roentgenol* 1992;158:1281–1287.
37. Jackson DW: Chronic rotator cuff impingement in the throwing athlete. *Am J Sports Med* 1976;4:231–240.
38. Kessel L, Watson M: The painful arc syndrome: Clinical classification as a guide to management. *J Bone Joint Surg* 1977; 59B:166–172.
39. Penny JN, Welsh RP: Shoulder impingement syndromes in athletes and their surgical management. *Am J Sports Med* 1981; 9:11–15.
40. Ellman H: Diagnosis and treatment of incomplete rotator cuff tears. *Clin Orthop* 1990;254:64–74.
41. Snyder SJ: Evaluation and treatment of the rotator cuff. *Orthop Clin North Am* 1993;24:173–192.
42. Coonrad RW: Tennis elbow, in Anderson LD (ed): American Academy of Orthopaedic Surgeons *Instructional Course Lectures XXXV*. St. Louis, MO, CV Mosby, 1986, pp 94–101.
43. Runge F: Zur Genese und Behandlung des Schreibekrampfes. *Berl klin Wochenschr* 1873;10:245–248.
44. Nirschl RP: Defining and treating "tennis elbow." *Contemp Surg* 1977;10:13–17.
45. Nirschl RP, Pettrone FA: Tennis elbow: The surgical treatment of lateral epicondylitis. *J Bone Joint Surg* 1979;61A:832–839.
46. Gardner RC: Tennis elbow: Diagnosis, pathology and treatment. Nine severe cases treated by a new reconstructive operation. *Clin Orthop* 1970;72:248–253.
47. Nirschl RP: Muscle and tendon trauma: Tennis elbow, in Morrey BF (ed): *The Elbow and Its Disorders*. Philadelphia, PA, WB Saunders, 1985, pp 481–496.
48. Kleinkort JA, Wood F: Phonophoresis with 1 percent versus 10 percent hydrocortisone. *Phys Ther* 1975;55:1320–1324.
49. Groppel JL, Nirschl RP: A mechanical and electromyographical analysis of the effects of various joint counterforce braces on the tennis player. *Am J Sports Med* 1986;14:195–200.
50. Stanish WD, Rubinovich RM, Curwin S: Eccentric exercise in chronic tendinitis. *Clin Orthop* 1986;208:65–68.
51. Nirschl RP: Prevention and treatment of elbow and shoulder injuries in the tennis player. *Clin Sports Med* 1988;7:289–308.
52. Kurvers H, Verhaar J: The results of operative treatment of medial epicondylitis. *J Bone Joint Surg* 1995;77A:1374–1379.
53. Schaberg JE, Harper MC, Allen WC: The snapping hip syndrome. *Am J Sports Med* 1984;12:361–365.
54. Allen WC, Cope R: Coxa saltans: The snapping hip revisited. *J Am Acad Orthop Surg* 1995;3:303–308.
55. Brignall CG, Stinnsby GD: The snapping hip: Treatment by Z-plasty. *J Bone Joint Surg* 1991;73B:253–254.
56. Clement DB, Taunton JE, Smart GW, et al: A survey of overuse running injuries. *Phys Sportsmed* 1981;9:47–58.
57. Firer P: Results of surgical management of the iliotibial band friction syndrome. *Clin J Sports Med* 1992;2:247–250.
58. Roels J, Martens M, Mulier JC, et al: Patellar tendinitis (jumper's knee). *Am J Sports Med* 1978;6:362–368.
59. Deland JT, Otis JC, Lee KT, et al: Lateral column lengthening with calcaneocuboid fusion: Range of motion in the triple joint complex. *Foot Ankle Int* 1995;16:729–733.
60. Cavanagh PR: *The Running Shoe Book*. Mountain View, CA, Anderson World, 1980, p 270.
61. Clanton TO, Schon LC: Athletic injuries to the soft tissues of the foot and ankle, in Mann RA, Coughlin MJ (eds): *Surgery of the Foot and Ankle*, ed 6. St. Louis, MO, Mosby-Year Book, 1993, vol 2, pp 1095–1224.
62. Woods L, Leach RE: Posterior tibial tendon rupture in athletic people. *Am J Sports Med* 1991;19:495–498.
63. Mann RA, Thompson FM: Rupture of the posterior tibial tendon causing flat foot: Surgical treatment. *J Bone Joint Surg* 1985; 67A:556–561.
64. Inman VT (ed): *Applications to Orthopaedics and Areas for Further Clinical Research in Joints of the Ankle*. Baltimore, MD, Williams & Wilkins, 1976, pp 75–80.
65. Inglis AE, Scott WN, Sculco TP, et al: Ruptures of the tendoachillis: An objective assessment of surgical and non-surgical treatment. *J Bone Joint Surg* 1976;58A:990–993.
66. Lagergren C, Lindholm A: Vascular distribution in the Achilles tendon: An angiographic and microangiographic study. *Acta Chir Scand* 1959;116:491–495.
67. Mann RA, Holmes GB Jr, Seale KS, et al: Chronic rupture of the Achilles tendon: A new technique of repair. *J Bone Joint Surg* 1991;73A:214–219.
68. Wapner KL, Pavlock GS, Hecht PJ, et al: Repair of chronic Achilles tendon rupture with flexor hallucis longus tendon transfer. *Foot Ankle* 1993;14:443–449.
69. James SL, Bates BT, Osternig LR: Injuries to runners. *Am J Sports Med* 1978;6:40–50.
70. Rovere GD, Webb LX, Gristina AG, et al: Musculoskeletal injuries in theatrical dance students. *Am J Sports Med* 1983;11: 195–198.
71. Caine D, Cochrane B, Caine C, et al: An epidemiologic investigation of injuries affecting young competitive female gymnasts. *Am J Sports Med* 1989;17:811–820.
72. Winge S, Jorgensen U, Lassen Nielsen A: Epidemiology of injuries in Danish championship tennis. *Int J Sports Med* 1989; 10:368–371.
73. Zemper ED: Injury rates in a national sample of college football teams: A 2-year prospective study. *Phys Sports Med* 1989;17: 100–113.
74. Arner O, Lindholm A: Subcutaneous rupture of the Achilles tendon: A study of 92 cases. *Acta Chir Scand Suppl* 1959;239.
75. Clancy WG Jr, Neidhart D, Brand RL: Achilles tendinitis in runners: A report of 5 cases. *Am J Sports Med* 1976;4:46–57.
76. Schepsis AA, Leach RE: Surgical management of Achilles tendinitis. *Am J Sports Med* 1987;15:308–315

CHAPTER 56

Clinicians Teaching Orthopaedics: Effective Strategies

Roy A. Meals, MD
Hugh G. Watts, MD

Overview

Doctor means teacher. It is ironic, therefore, that the fully trained surgeon spends 9 or 10 years after college learning to practice orthopaedics, perhaps several additional years learning research methods, but hardly a minute learning to teach.[1] Yet it is teaching that perpetuates and enhances our specialty. In academic environments, promotion committees accentuate this imbalance by rewarding excellence in research and clinical innovation while basically ignoring performance in teaching.

From our own experiences we can recall both effective and ineffective teachers, although we may not be able to readily identify or articulate the differences in their methods. Some teaching methods are obviously better than others, but we tend to teach the way we were taught, and when these methods are suboptimal, learning may be absent.[2,3] For example, a surgeon told his colleague that he had taught his infant daughter how to suture. When asked to have the girl demonstrate this skill, the surgeon replied, "Well, I taught her how to suture. I didn't say she learned."

Worse than ineffective instructional methods are dysfunctional ones, including the classic ABCs of surgical teaching to which we have all at one time or another been exposed: Abuse, Blame, Criticism. Without corrective guidance, an abused learner unconsciously becomes an abusing teacher. This chapter attempts to sensitize the reader to differences in teaching methods available to surgeons and to encourage techniques that optimize surgical learning experiences. Many points to be discussed are intuitive, but surgeons have traditionally lacked a framework, the necessary nontechnical terminology, and a forum for discussing these issues. The strategies discussed are focused on resident-level education, but certainly the same principles can easily be applied to medical students, nurses, and paramedical personnel as well as to continuing medical education. In this era of health care finance reform, leaner full-time faculties and more dependence on volunteer part-time faculty make the imperatives for effective teaching even stronger.

Preadult Versus Adult Learning

As students, we arrive at medical school having been bombarded for two decades with preadult learning experiences. Preadult learning is classroom-oriented and teacher-focused. Here relevance of the presented material is unnecessary or deferred, and the reward to learn is external and artificial—grades. The punishments also are external and artificial—grades. Children have the resilience to memorize and retain the names of the state capitals, the value of pi to 20 decimal places, and similar potentially useful information. In fact, adults can learn such information with equal facility, we just forget it if it is not immediately useful. Remember the Krebs cycle?

By contrast, adult learning is the process of remembering what interests us, and, ideally, only material of immediate relevance to the learner is offered. Thus, in adult learning, the focus is on the learner rather than on the teacher. The student can and wants to use the new information to solve real problems. The student prefers concepts and principles over acquisition of isolated facts. Adult learners also need feedback to monitor their proficiency.[4]

Laboratory opportunities offer excellent adult learning experiences, and the closer the laboratory simulates real-life problems and the more immediate the feedback, the more indelible the message. Hence, the operating room is a good learning laboratory, particularly for surgical skills. In a teaching hospital, there is probably no better adult learning opportunity than the intensive care unit. Here the problems are real and urgent, learner motivation is maximum, and feedback from monitoring the patient's condition is immediate.

Adult learning works best when the students can set their own goals and then become intensely and personally involved. This is easy in surgery. The goal of becoming a doctor is an internal one, and that motivation vastly supersedes the external hurdles of formal examinations. Once a medical student has chosen a specialty, the self-motivation and need for personal involvement become compelling and lifelong. The sense of responsibility for subject mastery becomes personalized, and the drives and rewards are internal and real.

Learner Acquisition of Knowledge, Skills, and Attitude

Teacher goals in adult learning environments are entirely different from those found in preadult environments. The adult teacher presents useful, core material in a memorable way, while gradually making the learner self-responsible and simultaneously rendering himself superfluous. This makes sense and sounds easy, but in the heat of a busy clinic or a stressful operation, old, bad habits can easily take control. As with any new skill, however, practice makes perfect. In this light the following suggestions are offered to help adult teachers perfect their skills.

Knowledge Even having emphasized that adult learning is nonclassroom, real-world problem solving, the adult teacher need not apologize for lecturing. Core information is best imparted in a classroom environment where the pace is leisurely, the presentation sequence is logical and thorough, and questions are encouraged. Lectures should not substitute for reading, but rather embellish it with a synthesis of information and ideas too new, complex, or diffusely distributed to be readily obtained by the student.

Both for lectures and for on-job conversations, the effective teacher selects only the most important material for presentation and offers it in a way that excites the student about the proximity of its relevance.[5] Hence, an effective teacher must be both useful and stimulating (Fig. 1). Entertaining teachers who are not useful are just entertainers. Useful teachers who are not stimulating are bores, merely announcers; and it is a misnomer to call one who is neither creative nor useful a teacher at all.

A useful teacher is easy to describe. Such a teacher, in an orderly fashion, focuses his or her current perspective on the learner. Effective teachers have highly individualized methods of being novel, creative, and stimulating, but they basically capitalize on strong personality traits. Think back on effective teachers in your own experience. Teachers who tend to be mildly obnoxious can make lessons memorable by being real jerks. Good story tellers spin yarns. Self-deprecators painfully relive the agony of personally experienced medical disasters. Artists do chalk talks. Builders use models and cross sections. Whatever it takes, the effective teacher makes the message indelible.

Questions are inevitable and should be encouraged and savored for the attendant, beautiful adult-learning opportunity. After the question, the effective teacher waits silently for 5 seconds and remembers that adult learning is learner focused. To merely answer the question focuses on the teacher. This is a fault of many, including Sherlock Holmes, who additionally belittled his learner by prefacing the answer, "Elementary, my dear Watson." In medical circles, "pimping" is the epitome of self-service and dysfunction, puffing up the teacher's ego at the expense of the student's over a minor and esoteric point.[6] The effective teacher casts ego aside, reflects the question back to the learner, and then guides the student's knowledge and logic until the learner can answer the question. The adult teacher's rewards come not from parading his or her own understanding but from seeing the students achieve their own potential.

Not only does the 5-second pause give the teacher added strength not to blurt an answer, but it warns the learner of the likelihood of some critical thinking ahead. Then reflecting the question back on the learner for a preliminary answer ascertains the learner's level of understanding and initiates the guided inquiry necessary to allow the learner to reason out the answer.

For example, Learner: "How long would you keep this metacarpal fracture casted?" Teacher (after waiting 5 seconds): "How long would you keep it casted?" The ensuing dialogue will be entirely different depending on whether the learner responds, "I keep all fractures casted until I see remodeling of the callus," or "I think most metacarpal fractures are sticky in 3 to 4 weeks and immobilizing them longer risks soft-tissue problems."

Closed-ended questions (eg, "Do most fractures heal?") can move the guided inquiry along quickly, although rather rigidly, and do not probe the depth of the learner's understanding. Open-ended questions (eg, "How do fractures heal?") have the exact opposite results. The effective adult teacher intermixes open-ended and closed-ended questions to keep the discussion generally focused and pertinent to the learner's immediate needs. A string of closed-ended questions becomes nothing more than "What am I thinking?" Continuous open-ended questions remove all limits from the conversation's boundaries and will greatly annoy those who have a tight work schedule.

In situations in which there are multiple learners at the same level of experience, the effective teacher asks a question and then waits 5 seconds before identifying a respondent. All learners are thereby challenged. Conversely, when there are learners at different levels of experience, first asking the most junior person for the answer and then moving up the hierarchy, if necessary, avoids public embarrassment if the medical student knows an answer the chief resident does not. Everyone knows, however, that he or she may be next,

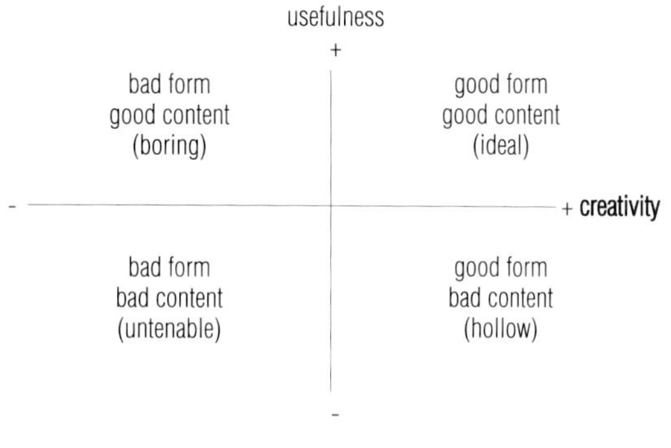

Fig. 1 Teaching styles.

and all become personally aware of any deficits in their own understanding.

Teachers should encourage learners to ask themselves and others meaningful questions forever. Role modeling here is a powerful tool, so is the power of suggestion. "You know, I was wondering last night if there might be a better way to do that. What do you think?"

Skills For imparting technical skills, the educator needs to know where the learner is on a scale of competence and consciousness (Fig. 2). We start out unconsciously incompetent for acquiring a new skill: "That's easy, anybody can put on a cast." We move to conscious incompetence: "This is a lot harder than it looks." Then conscious competence: "I can do it if I concentrate." Finally, unconscious competence: "This is natural, I've never given it a thought."

To effectively teach technical skills, seasoned surgeons have to draw themselves back to the level of conscious competence to guide the learner through the necessary, methodical technical steps. Someone who has recently achieved competence is ideally stationed to lead learners from their consciously incompetent state. This is an example of a near-peer encounter, to be discussed momentarily.

Use of a skills laboratory allows leisurely concentration on a particular technique, and the learner can quickly become consciously competent in a nonstressful setting. Skills laboratories and courses have been particularly successful in the hands-on teaching of internal fixation of fractures, small vessel anastomosis, and arthroscopic techniques.

Attitude The third component of surgical learning is attitude—ethics and behavior, and these traits are irreversibly formulated by a very early age. Although adults with affective problems tend to behave well when closely scrutinized by authority figures, they usually revert to their lifelong dysfunctional patterns once on their own. Therefore, surgical educators can only pick the best people possible, consistently demonstrate the desired behavior and attitudes, and observe the learners early and closely.[7] The mentor's evaluation should include input from less authoritative observers, such as operating room, ward, and clinic nurses. Even the page operators know who is responsible and polite.

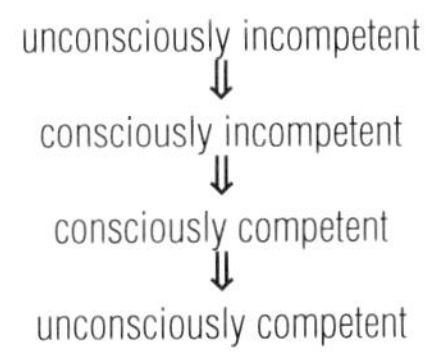

Fig. 2 Maturation of surgical skills.

In the evaluation of attitude, it is important to differentiate between internal and external motivation (Fig. 3). The learner who exhibits desirable values plus desirable behavior will be no problem. The one who demonstrates desirable values but undesirable behavior has solvable problems. The learner who lacks desirable values but demonstrates desirable behavior is dangerous when left unobserved, and the instance where the learner lacks both desirable values and behavior is not remediable, at least by the average orthopaedic teacher. Although transiently painful, everyone benefits when career changes are suggested or enforced on those with documented, unsuitable ethics and behavior.[4]

Catalyzing Acquisition of Knowledge, Skills, and Attitude

Four catalysts facilitate the acquisition of surgical knowledge, skills, and attitude. The first is practice. Few lifelong habits are going to be perfected after one iteration, and practice is inherent in a surgical residency extending over years, if the teacher stresses learner development.[8]

The second is near-peer encounters. We probably can all recall situations in which our best surgical teacher was one who had only recently acquired the knowledge, judgment, technique, or emotional response with which we were then struggling. Where the difference in age and experience of the learners and the teacher is small, the learning environment is nonthreatening and nonjudgmental.[5] The learner can talk, query, and self-test himself to a clearheaded state without fear of reprisal or embarrassment. As an added benefit, the teacher can become confident in the mastery of his or her recently acquired art. In many near-peer encounters, the roles of teacher and student are freely interchangeable. Everyone benefits.

The third facilitator is stress. A moderate level of student stress is good.[9,10] Like lifting weights, too little stress produces no improvement, and too much causes

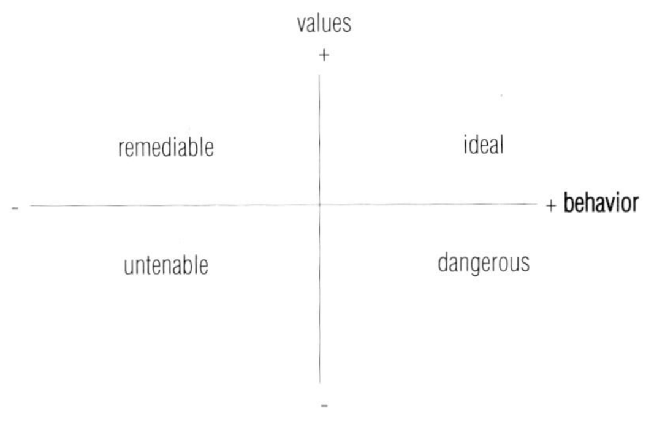

Fig. 3 Attitudes.

Table 1
Differences between feedback and evaluation

Feedback (useful to learner)	Evaluation (not useful to learner)
Facts	Judgments
Absolutes	Comparisons
Nouns and verbs	Adjectives and adverbs
Contemporaneous	Terminal

injury. Here, "war stories" and grilling the more senior residents at conferences are useful techniques. Both methods allow for important maturation of the less experienced learners in an environment that is not immediately and personally hostile.[11]

The fourth catalyst is feedback. This term comes from telemetered rocketry, where feedback is in-flight information used to adjust the course of the rocket so it will strike its target. Similarly, in education feedback is information useful for adjusting the course toward the goal: independent, renewing competence. Feedback is different from evaluation in several important respects.[12,13] Feedback is contemporaneous, in flight; evaluation is after the fact, terminal. Feedback is information, relies on nouns and verbs, and is nonjudgmental. Evaluation is judgmental, comparative, and gets by on adjectives and adverbs (Table 1). Which comments are more likely to help the learner acquire knowledge, skills, and appropriate attitude? (1) Knowledge: "You need to read the article in the most recent issue of the Journal." or "You don't read enough, not nearly as much as your peers." (2) Skills: "Place your sutures closer together to distribute the tension." or "Give me the needle holder, aren't you ever going to learn how to suture?" (3) Attitude: "Some patients think chewing gum in their presence demonstrates a lack of respect." or "You're lousy."?

Anticipating that offering negative feedback is inevitable, the wise teacher offers positive direction as early as possible in an encounter with a learner, such that any subsequent necessary negative feedback is offered and accepted in an atmosphere of trust and cooperation.

Feedback regarding technical skills is nearly intuitive for surgical teachers. "Cut here, retract there." Feedback regarding knowledge, judgment, and behavior, however, is considerably more difficult. If any observations are made at all, judgment, possibly negative, is often substituted: "You klutz!"

Evaluating Performance

Feedback is useful to the learner for making immediate goal-directed changes. Evaluation of the learner's performance at the completion is necessary to document success or failure for continuance in the program, graduation, credentialing, hospital privileges, and so forth.[14] The evaluator should candidly and in detail document observed behaviors and record if they exceed or fall below the norm.[15] Any interpretation of the behavior should be recorded separately from the observations. A good evaluation will begin to distinguish if a problem is one of knowledge, skills, or attitude and starts the counseling process.[16] The residency director's timely review of the evaluations with the resident provides useful feedback—not for the rotation just completed but for subsequent efforts.

Helping Learners Cope With Failure and Mistakes

"Next to being shot at and missed, nothing is really as satisfactory professionally as a good surgical outcome recognized by both the patient and the surgeon."[17] Orthopaedic residents do and will make mistakes. The surgical educator should be prepared to help put a positive spin on the experience so that the trainee can use appropriate coping mechanisms, maintain a psychologically healthy attitude, and improve practice skills.[18] To season the learner before a mistake happens, the teacher should discuss the inevitability of mistakes and relate examples of mistakes made personally, how the mistakes were managed, and what steps were taken to prevent their recurrence.

House officers experience considerable emotional turmoil resulting from their mistakes, and they use a variety of coping mechanisms.[19] Residents who cope by accepting responsibility experience more emotional distress but are more likely to make constructive changes in their habits. Residents who rely on escape-avoidance are more likely to adopt defensive changes in practice. Medical educators should give specific advice about preventing recurrence of the mistake, provide emotional support, and help the resident understand that distress is necessarily associated with learning from the experience.

A morbidity and mortality conference may be a starting point for case review and analyzing how a mistake can be avoided in the future. Possibilities to explore include deficiencies in knowledge, faulty interpretation of information, lapses in routine, and inadequate backup or back-up not consulted. All the residents benefit from such public discussion.

The educator's emotional support and assistance in interpreting the resident's distress is best done in private. Although surgeons may not be particularly adroit in psychological counseling, an awareness of the potential benefits from residents using healthy coping skills, and seeking specialized help when necessary, is certainly a step in the right direction.

Substance Abuse

Surgical learners are not immune to substance abuse, nor are their teachers.[20-22] Several studies indicate a prevalence of alcoholism among faculty and house staff of at least 4% and possibly as high as 14%.

No gender or specialty-specific trends have been noted. The effects of substance abuse among residents on performance and patient care are unknown as is the natural history of substance abuse among this relatively young physician population. Program directors grossly underestimate the prevalence of alcoholism among their trainees.[21] The identification and management of these impaired learners exceed the scope of this paper, but an awareness of the problem and its magnitude is a necessary prelude to any solution.

Summary

The ideal teacher has not yet been invented. Because of differences in personality, effective teachers will have diverse techniques for reaching students, and all students will not be equally affected by any teacher. In adult learning, the focus is on the learner, not on the teacher. The teacher's role is mainly one of setting up an appropriately stressful, close-to-real-life environment and offering near-peer problem-solving opportunities. After that, the teacher observes, offers feedback, and fades away. The student, with perhaps only a vague awareness of the teacher's role in this success, achieves subject mastery along with responsibility for life-long renewal. To complete the cycle, the inspired learner ideally now becomes the inspirational teacher—the truly complete surgeon.

Teaching in the Operating Room

Few things are as important as passing on to our residents the craft of orthopaedic surgery. Who usually does this teaching? In large part it is the clinical surgeon "in the trenches." We are asked to teach these manual skills, yet no one teaches *us* how to teach them.

There have been studies in industry and in the military on how to teach manual skills more effectively, but there have been few objective studies focused on how best to teach *our* orthopaedic skills to those who will follow us. There have been attempts to improve the teaching of surgery by the use of laboratory sessions to "dry run" surgical techniques,[23] as well as attempts to quantify the effectiveness of teaching surgery tried by several surgical specialties,[24,25] and more recently, the use of video camera replays for self-directed learning sessions.[26] But our concern, here, is the search for methods we, who already have the resident in our operating rooms, can use to enhance our own teaching effectiveness. The setting of our teaching is different from that in industry or the military. Realistically, we cannot do an operation several times over, nor can we use up anesthesia time unnecessarily while we labor over an explanation of what needs to be done. It is also difficult to overcome our own urge to have things done perfectly in spite of the fact that our patient's well-being is primary and has been entrusted to us, personally.

The more skilled we become as surgeons, the more we do things unconsciously. This makes teaching more difficult because we often are not aware of many of the things we do. It is hard to remember back to those early days when we learned our surgical skills. Do you remember your very first hip pinning—the nervousness, the desire to please and "look good" to all of the others watching you in the operating room? Should a resident's performance in the operating room require criticism, it can be felt as a severe blow, and it really hurts. If a resident does not know the answer to some question, say about the incidence of a disease, it may be the source of embarrassment, but is not felt anywhere nearly as much as the implication that the resident has poor surgical skills. Take ourselves—most of us would accept (without a huge blow to our pride) that we are not the academic equal of a Nobel Laureate in theoretical physics, but few would be willing to accept being branded as "a poor technical surgeon."

How then can we become better teachers of our surgical craft? We all remember surgeons we have worked with, some of whom were great teachers and others who were little short of rotten. Are there techniques that we can share among those of us "in the trenches" to make each of us more effective teachers of our craft? The following suggestions have been gathered from many individuals, fully experienced orthopaedic surgeons as well as residents at different levels of training. (If any readers of this chapter have suggestions that you would like to pass along, the authors would be grateful to hear about them so that they could be shared in the future.)

Planning on your part is critical to a successful teaching outcome. The teaching session at the operating room should be planned just like any lesson anywhere, although it need not require a formal outline. What needs to be planned? First of all, a goal needs to be established. Stand mentally aside and ask yourself, what is the focus of teaching this resident during today's operation? For example, is the goal to teach the resident how you do this particular operation? Or is it to teach the resident to think ahead to help the scrub technician to be one step ahead, so that the operation flows smoothly. Or perhaps the goal is to encourage the resident's self-reliance. These are different goals and may or may not be appropriate for the given operation today, or for the skills of the particular resident assigned to today's operation. But there should be some thought given to what it is you are trying to teach.

Secondly, your planning needs to prepare the resident. This preparation needs to be done twice before the operation. In the first instance, as soon as it is possible to know the operating room schedule, the resident needs to know who exactly is going to do the surgery. Will it be the attending surgeon, the fellow, the senior resident, or the junior resident? While it is appropriate that all of the assistants should be prepared ahead, there is still a benefit to the resident to feel the stress of knowing that he or she will be the person who really has to know. It allows the resident to mentally do the operation ahead of time, the same way that we all do when we anticipate having to do a new or particularly difficult procedure. At that time there should be a discussion about the procedure so that the resident's reading can be more directed. For example, if you are planning to do a posterior approach to the hip and the resident has read the details of an anterior approach to the hip, it will not be a happy day in the operating room.

A second planning session is needed before the case begins (perhaps in the coffee room or at the scrub sink) to review the reading that the resident has done. There are very likely to be differences between what was read in the text and what you do. (Maybe we should read what the resident plans to read?) The reasons for the differences need to be discussed. It is very confusing for the resident to be proceeding with one operative plan in mind (as prescribed by the reading) only to find in mid-course that you want something done differently. Are these differences a matter of personal preference or a matter of substance? We often do not even recognize when some of our choices are based on personal preference. Residents have a very real problem dealing with personal preferences. Remember that they operate with a number of different surgeons and have to accommodate to each one. (When did you last operate with the other orthopaedists in your hospital to know what their individual preferences were?) It is important to differentiate between a purely personal preference (using a # 2 suture rather than a # 1, which you use primarily because that has always been your habit over the years) versus what you consider a fundamentally important difference for what you see as some significant physiologic or mechanical reason (eg, a nonabsorbable suture rather than an absorbable one). Some surgeons have found it a useful tool to dictate a surgical report *before* the case as a guide for residents. Most surgeons would feel this as a burdensome excess, but if the array of procedures you do is usually limited (eg, total hip and total knee replacements) then such a task is simple. Others are offended by the idea because they feel this makes things too much like a cookbook.

The search to accommodate to personal preferences can lead a resident far astray. A resident may have scouted out from a more senior resident what you like to do. It is easy to get the wrong information: "Dr. ______ *always* does it this way..." (for some particular reason, you did happen to do it that unusual way the time you operated with that senior resident). These planning sessions, and indeed the entire surgical process, can be seen as an opportunity for you to teach the resident about the disease being treated, and the nuances of the decision to operate.

Now that the resident is prepared and the operation has begun, watch out for some common resident difficulties. Major difficulties can be created by the presence of "too many cerebella" in one operating room or by the differences, due to parallax, between what you see from your side of the table and what the resident sees. Much of this can be reduced by optimal positioning of the patient to take advantage of the exquisitely accurate ability of the human eye to perceive verticality and right angles. For example, suppose you are doing a varus osteotomy of the femoral neck, which you are going to fix with a right-angled blade-plate. You want the resident to drive a chisel across the base of the neck of the femur to bring the neck-shaft angle from 150° down to 110°. If the leg is left in the anatomic position, the resident has to align the chisel at what everyone agrees is a 130° angle from the shaft. In addition, the resident has to angle the chisel (from below upward) the amount of femoral anteversion (Fig. 4). Now that is a situation begging for argument and frustration. By contrast, if *you* abduct the patient's leg by the amount you want to change the neck-shaft angle (in this example by 40°) and internally rotate the femur by the amount of the patient's femoral anteversion, the chisel now needs to be driven in at right angles to the long axis of the operating table and parallel with the floor. The osteotomy is made parallel with the chisel. The leg is now aligned with the edge of the table and the fragments fixed. All of the instruments, saw cuts, and leg positioning are aligned parallel, or at

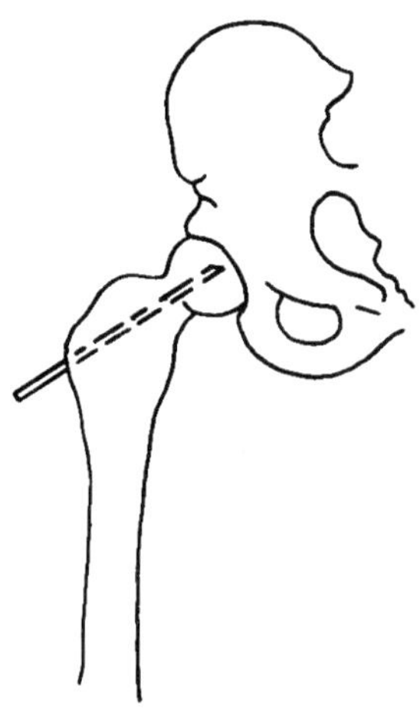

Fig. 4 When planning a varus osteotomy to bring the neck-shaft angle from 150° to 110° (to be fixed with a right-angled blade-plate), you want the resident to line up the chisel at 130° to the shaft of the femur. An angle of 130° is not an intuitive one to the brain, and the exact position of the chisel can be a source of debate between you and the resident.

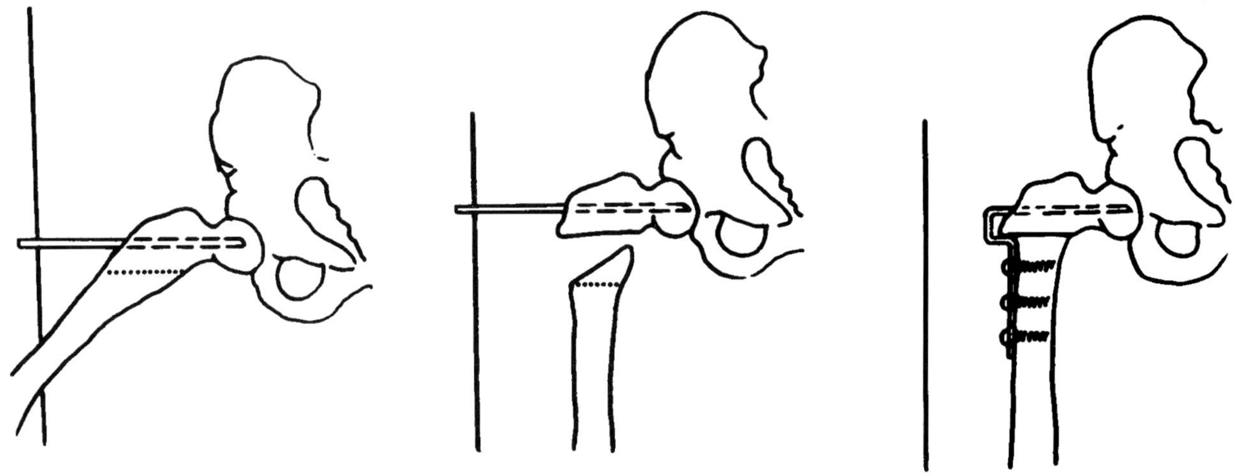

Fig. 5 The brain is highly attuned to perceive right angles and parallels. Use the edge of the operating table as a visual cue easily shared by you and the resident. **Left,** If you abduct the leg so that its proximal part is in the relationship with the acetabulum that you want it to be, the chisel is now driven in at right angles to the near edge of the operating table. The osteotomy is made parallel with the chisel. **Center,** With the proximal fragment held still, the leg is brought parallel with the edge of the operating table and the upper end of the distal fragment cut at right angles to the edge of the table. **Right,** The fragments are fixed as planned.

right angles to the shared reference lines of the table edge and the floor (Fig. 5). This configuration will lead to much less discussion. The same can be done with other osteotomies.

Giving verbal directions to supervise a manual task can be confusing under the best of circumstances. Anxiety on the part of the resident may compound the problem. When you say, "Move your hand up a bit," the poor resident is left to decipher, "Does the surgeon mean move my hand toward the ceiling, or toward the patient's head?" It is worthwhile training yourself to use accurate anatomic directions, for example, "Move your hand cephalad." It may sound stilted at first and will probably require that you constantly remind yourself, but it is worth the effort.

Some residents have a problem with mirror imaging what they have learned. That is, they have watched from the assistant's side of the operating table and find things confusing when they have to mirror image the process as they must do when they move to the surgeon's side. If you suspect this is happening, or if the resident comments to that effect, it may help for you to move across to the resident's side of the operating room table to supervise.

A similar problem can arise if you and the resident do not share the same handedness. Surgical instruments are designed for right-handed use. It is more difficult for a left-handed trainee to learn from a right-handed teacher. Pickleman and Schuenerman[25] found that left-handed residents were consistently rated lower than right-handed residents on their Operative Rating Scale. "We feel the explanation for this lay with the attending surgeons, all of whom were right-handed, and who typically found assisting a left-handed resident to be an annoying experience."[25] Trying to force a left-hander into a right-handed mode may decrease their technical abilities.[27] So what should a right-handed surgeon do when working with a left-handed resident? The most important thing is to recognize the difference, talk about the problems of handedness, and try to explore ways to help the resident achieve the same result, rather than to imitate your exact moves.

Some adult learners are very offended by a teacher who grabs hold of their hand to demonstrate an error in positioning of an instrument, perhaps bringing back bad memories of subjugation to a teaching ogre of the past. Yet sometimes it may be necessary and helpful to position a resident's hand. The offense may be obviated by using another instrument or a Steinmann pin laid on top of the skin to demonstrate the reason for the need to change alignment.

What about the use of teaching aids in the operating room? A number of surgeons have found it useful to have a skeleton in the operating room, while others have atlases of anatomy available that are opened up to the appropriate pages. Some surgeons have outlined the planned operation and written up a set of step-by-step instructions, which they paste on the operating room wall.

Teaching a resident to become independent and to become accustomed to being in charge in the operating room is an important facet of teaching surgery.

Sometimes it may require asking the resident whether the height of the operating table needs to be adjusted or whether the direction of the lights could be improved. This reminds them that they should be thinking about the set-up of the entire operating room. At some point in every resident's training, it is necessary for you to leave the operating room to allow the resident to assume the role of leader. This is usually done in increments where initially the more junior residents are left to close the skin incision. The idea of leaving a resident to do most, if not all, of a case independently can be as terrifying, yet as necessary, as that of leaving your teenage child the keys to the family car.

After the case, review what was done. This is an excellent occasion to provide feedback. "If you were doing the operation again, right now, what would you do differently?" This can be an important opportunity for the resident to make an honest assessment of how well the operation went and for you to make suggestions away from the intensity of the operating room.

If possible, review any surgical notes that the resident has dictated. Residents, particularly the more junior ones, have a tendency to emphasize the minutiae of the procedure ("the fascial layer was then closed with interrupted 2-0 absorbable sutures, and the fat was closed in layers with..."etc.) while overlooking the important issues such as the indications for the specific choice of operation, and the unusual pathologic features found. Such a review of the surgical notes will encourage the resident to be more aware of the "big picture" in subsequent operations.

What happens when things go wrong in the operating room because of a resident's error? First of all, it is vital to pick up the pieces from the patient's perspective. It may be as important, or even more important, to teach the resident the "fall back maneuvers" that you have learned over the years. It is equally important for the surgeon to demonstrate how complications are discussed with the patient or relatives. After the patient's situation has been amended, it is important to pick up the pieces from the resident's perspective. Most residents are stunned when they make a serious blunder. A quiet discussion after the case is over, and away from the operating room, may help to make the event a constructive experience without it being psychologically devastating.

Each of us has his or her own approach to teaching in the operating room. Whatever the approach is, the effectiveness will be enhanced if we take time to think about the processes of teaching that we use.

Teaching by Lecture

As a clinical orthopaedic surgeon, sooner or later you will probably be asked to give a lecture to the residents or your colleagues on some topic for which you are the local expert. You know your stuff or you would not be asked to speak in the first place. The problem is knowing how best to get your message across. Perhaps you consider yourself a poor lecturer, or conversely, a good one. As pointed out by Whitman,[28] there is no gene for good teaching. Can you do better? Probably all of us can do better given some suggestions and, more importantly, an interest in becoming a better lecturer. The following comments are not directed to the academicians who lecture often, but to those who are less frequently asked to teach in the hope that the suggestions offered will enhance effectiveness and reduce anxiety.

Planning

Undoubtedly, the most important part of improving one's teaching has to do with planning. One of the first questions to ask yourself is, "Who is the audience?" If the audience is composed of residents all at one level, the problem is straightforward. What happens if you have some fellows, four levels of residents, and two more of medical students? At what level will you focus your talk? It is difficult to cover all levels and keep all levels awake. It becomes necessary to make a decision as to whom you are directing your talk, which sometimes means that the material will go over the heads of some of the audience (but hopefully will lead them to stretch their horizons).

The second most important question to ask yourself is, "What is the purpose of your talk, that is, what do you want to get across?" Possibilities include facts, ideas, or perhaps a system of how facts and ideas can be organized. If it is facts you are purveying, list on a piece of paper just which facts you think are most important. The same can be done with ideas. The more organized you are with your plan beforehand, the better the teaching session will go. Organization and planning can be a particular lack in the more informal teaching sessions with residents, sessions in which you have been asked to cover a topic that you know like the back of your hand. Although it is easy to feel that little or no planning is needed, lack of planning is often the beginning of a disorganized wander through your experience.

Illustrations

Orthopaedic surgery is such a concrete body of information that it is natural to use illustrations with any lecture. These are usually very helpful, but they can also present problems for the unwary. Because 35-mm slides are the dominant medium used in orthopaedic teaching, they will be the focus of these comments. Depending on the size of the audience and the degree of effort and cost you are able to put into the teaching session, other useful media are overheads and the use of hand drawing.

Slides Slides are a wonderful convenience, but it is important to give thought to the quality and quantity of slides and how you organize them. The quality of your slides depends on the amount of information you try to put on an individual slide and your choice of colors, magnification, and orientation.

How much written information should be on a slide? One wag suggests "Never put more on a slide than you would a T-shirt." A more useful guide is to hold your slide up to the light and see if you can read the writing with your unaided eye. If you cannot, there is too much on the slide.

How many slides should you try to show in a half hour talk? A common guide has been, "no more than four pairs of slides per minute," but there are a number of qualifiers. The number of slides used will vary with the type of material being presented. For example, if you are showing pairs of radiographs or clinical photographs, for example, anteroposterior (AP) views with comparable laterals, more slides can be used. If each slide requires intricate explanation, the number should be reduced.

Slides of differing magnification used to illustrate a single lecture can be distracting. If you are showing clinical photographs of patients and one that shows the patient's body part filling the slide is followed by one that is half or a quarter of the magnification, have one of the slides enlarged so that they match. Also, give some thought to the orientation of your slides. If, for example, you are comparing two postoperative outcomes on radiographs, and one has had the right side done and the other had the left done, it takes a few seconds for the viewer to mentally invert the images to make a quick comparison. Help your viewer by flipping one of the slides over so both are either right or left. In fact, you will do well to decide to give your whole lecture as right or left sided if possible. Some surgeons feel that this is somehow dishonest. But the purpose of the talk is to get over an idea, not to represent a specific patient.

You can help your audience to orient themselves in other ways. Too often slides are projected that show little more than flesh and blood. It can be difficult for the viewer to know which way the patient's head is pointing. Help your viewers. Where possible, first project an overview slide that shows the whole patient, or a schematic of the surgical approach, and then show the detailed view. If you do not have an overview slide, at least take a moment to tell the audience where the patient's head is, or whether the patient is prone or supine.

Some thought must be given to choice of colors, because many colors do not project on a large screen the way they look on a slide sorter or on a computer monitor. For lettering, blues, greens, and reds are especially poor choices for slides that will be used in a large auditorium. Yellow, orange, and white work much better for lettering. The choice of colors for the letters has to be coordinated with that of the background. Very light backgrounds, especially white, can hurt your viewers' eyes. Also, keep in mind that color-blind people may not see red. Once a color scheme has been chosen, use the same scheme throughout the lecture, or the transitions become jarring. If you give many lectures, using the same combination consistently will allow you to make last minute substitutions from one talk to another.

A word about computer-generated slides: The ability to make slides from computer screen images is a wonderful feature of current technology, and it has given us an almost endless array of ways to improve our slides. Unfortunately, this advantage is accompanied by an equally endless array of ways to foul things up, because it is so tempting to use a large palate of colors and a dizzying choice of fonts (styles of type). It is essential to keep in mind that the point of the lecture is the transfer of information or ideas, not a kaleidoscope show. If you do not care to make your own slides, be wary of the graphic artist who may be doing the work for you, because artists are likely to be less interested in the information transferred than they are in showing how beautiful the slides can be. If you make your own slides, there are some useful tips to follow. Limit the number of fonts you use in a lecture series of slides. Fancy fonts may look attractive, but they cannot be read quickly. Slides that use all capital letters are also difficult to read quickly. Omit all border designs. Not only are they distracting, but they take away from the total area of the slide available to you for print. Omit, or at least limit, the fancy effects that make the listener concentrate more on the slides as art objects than on the information you are trying to convey. This does not mean that your slides need to be dull or unattractive. Learn a bit about typesetting and graphics from Robin Williams' *The Mac Is Not A Typewriter*[29] (or *The PC Is Not A Typewriter*[30] if DOS or Windows is your persuasion).

The use of double projectors has considerable merit for illustrating orthopaedic talks, because it allows you to show AP and lateral views of a problem at the same time, or to compare pre- versus postoperative results. However, confusion is bound to occur if you try to advance one tray independently from the other, besides which, many podiums are only equipped with a single slide-advance button, as noted below. Problems come when you do not have matching slides for the two slide trays. If you do not have a slide to project on the right projector to match the one on the left, do not use your favorite flower pictures or those sunset scenes from your recent boat trip to Fiji. Your audience will undoubtedly focus on the nonrelevant slide either dreaming about the beautiful scene and wishing they were there or else critically evaluating your skills as an outdoor photographer, rather than paying full attention to the message that you are trying to get over. In its place, use a blank slide, one that is genuinely opaque. These can be purchased in photo specialty shops. Do not use a blank exposure from the end of a roll. Under the intense light of a projector, the ghostly image is still visible and distracting.

Multimedia Use of video is a great leap forward in teaching, and video projection is increasingly available for teaching sessions, but bear in mind that the potential for chaos increases exponentially with the addition of each medium. Be prepared for the video not to work.

Overheads The use of overheads has not been popular in orthopaedic teaching. They do not project radiographs well, and clinical photos do not work. Furthermore, the bright white background is an eyesore. However, the system can be used effectively for presentation of material where there is not enough time to prepare slides, because overhead transparencies can be produced in ordinary copying machines and in standard laser printers directly from your desktop computer.

Drawing by Hand There is a mesmerizing quality to watching someone illustrate their teaching by drawing. Those in the audience sit with anticipation as the illustration grows in front of them. While the talent to do this varies enormously, those who are interested can enhance their skills by taking drawing lessons. If there is a blackboard or an easel with a large drawing pad at hand, drawing can be the sole technique of illustration or it can be reserved as a backup when all of the modern technology fails (as it will inevitably do at some point...see below).

Speaking Skills

A variety of techniques, such as interactive questioning and role playing, can be used to convey lecture material. These techniques have been discussed above. Regardless of the teaching techniques used, here are some strategies that can help the speaker reduce the likelihood of problems.

Check Out the Podium Technology Beforehand If you use your slides as cue cards, make sure that you can see your slides from the oblique view of the podium. If this is a problem, and you have arrived a few minutes early, you will have time to move the podium forward or angle it for better vision. Also, find out if the auditorium you are about to speak in is equipped with a reverse projection screen. If it is, all your slides will be backwards. Again, arriving early will allow you enough time to sort out the problem.

Check out the slide-advance. Does one button advance both projectors? If there are two infrared remote-advance clickers, pushing the advance on both simultaneously will not result in the desired effect. You need to push first one, then the other. It is not a good idea to become complacent about the workings of the podium, because each year seems to bring some new technology that must be learned. It is a good idea to have a usable pointer of your own just in case the one provided does not work. Pointers are readily available now and relatively cheap. A large-numbered timer is another valuable tool. Bad timing is a great discourtesy to those who follow you and should be avoided, if possible.

Use of the Pointer Keep your finger off the trigger except when you are specifically pointing to an item that needs your audience's attention. Any nervous shakes you are having are hugely magnified and very obvious to the audience when they see the red laser dot dancing all over the front wall of the auditorium or the slide screen.

Humor Do not read your talk. You will bore yourself as well as the audience. Use of humor is a great way to reach your audience as long as it does not become an end in itself. You do not want to have your audience saying to themselves "what a funny lecture," yet not remember anything you said.

Anticipate Disaster What if the slide projector jams, the bulb burns out, or the projectionist slips and all of your slides fall out? Always have a backup plan. You should know your material well enough that you can continue without your slides as prompters. If not, having an outline of the planned talk sitting in your pocket could get you out of trouble. If there is a blackboard, or an easel and paper, even a crude ability to draw may prove to be a lifesaver.

Signify That Your Talk Has Ended Your audience deserves the privilege of showing you their thanks by clapping at the end of your lecture. Think of the times you have been to a lecture and the speaker paused near the end of the talk. The audience nervously tries to decide if the end has arrived and they should clap. Your responsibility is to help them. Make it very clear that you have reached the end. A simple "Thank you" or "Thank you for your attention" will give them the signal and relieve them of embarrassment.

Teaching in Clinic and Conference

Teaching in clinic poses challenges and opportunities different from those encountered when teaching by lecturing or operating. In clinic, the patients' problems cannot be anticipated, so the teaching is extemporaneous. Here, the teacher's role is to extract salient highlights from whatever clinical material is available and capture teachable moments.[31,32] With patients waiting, however, there is a fine line between teaching too much and too little. When the clinic load is light, the teacher may lapse into a stream-of-consciousness ramble that has little relevance to the learners' immediate needs. Conversely, when the clinic is busy, there is a tendency to relapse into a pre-adult teaching mode and disgorge answers rather than guide the learner's inquiry.

These same extemporaneous teaching skills are necessary in the emergency room, for telephone consultations, in morbidity and mortality conference, in weekly service conference, and even on ward rounds, although outpatient surgery has rendered this monument of medical teaching nearly obsolete.[33] Whatever the venue, the teaching will be most effective if it is just at the edge of the learner's current understanding and feeds on an urgent need to know. This edge has to be individualized to the knowledge and experience of the individual learners.[34,35] Artful management of questions, as discussed above, helps define and maintain that edge.

Journal club is a particularly fertile venue for effective adult education. In a relaxed setting and with fewer time demands than clinical settings, residents develop critical reading and thinking skills catalyzed by practice, near-peer interaction, and feedback.[36] Effective management of questions keeps the process focused and relevant. Opportunities abound for the teacher to expand on the article under discussion by recounting relevant personal experiences, both good and bad. Storytelling such as this can enrich not only the learners' knowledge and judgment but also their values and attitudes.[37,38]

The clinic is fertile ground not only for imparting knowledge and reasoning, but also for teaching such clinical skills as physical diagnosis, injections, and casting. "See one, do one, teach one" holds true, and generally, the skills and tools are simpler than those used in the operating room. In the clinic, however, the learner is under the additional scrutiny of an awake patient and any attendant relatives.

It is important to incorporate the patient as an ally in this learning experience. This is easy for painless procedures. The step-by-step technical discussion between teacher and learner should include the patient, so all are being educated and can appreciate the benefits derived by the others. Patients are less willing to accept painful procedures from inexperienced hands. Removing relatives temporarily to the waiting room reduces the call for showmanship on the parts of teacher, learner, and patient. Likewise, planning the procedure—discussing its steps and equipment—away from the patient minimizes confidence-eroding comments during its performance. Finally, let the patient know both before and during the procedure that by words, and by hands if necessary, the teacher's experience is being brought to bear on the problem.

As learners become more experienced with a technique, they need more independence to perfect their skills. The teacher can look in midway through a joint aspiration, for instance; or the teacher can leave during a casting, but instill confidence in the patient and maintain quality control by asking to see the final product.

References

1. Troupin RH: The mini-fellowship in teaching: A senior resident elective. *Invest Radiol* 1990;25:751–753.
2. Meals RA: Teaching clinical judgement: Teaching the choice of surgical procedure in the treatment of arthritis of the hip. *Br J Med Ed* 1973;7:100–102.
3. White JA, Anderson P: Learning by internal medicine residents: Differences and similarities of perceptions by residents and faculty. *J Gen Intern Med* 1995;10:126–132.
4. King TC: Teaching surgeons to teach. *Bull Am Coll Surg* 1987;72:5–9.
5. Schwenk TL, Whitman NA (eds): *Residents as Teachers: A Guide to Educational Practice.* Salt Lake City, UT, University of Utah School of Medicine, 1984, pp 41–43.
6. Brancati FL: The art of pimping. *JAMA* 1989;262:89–90.
7. Lippert FG III, Farmer J, Schafer MF: Professional behavior in the orthopedic resident: A method for evaluation and development. *Clin Orthop* 1983;174:188–192.
8. Whitman N, Lawrence P (eds): *Surgical Teaching: Practice Makes Perfect.* Salt Lake City, UT, University of Utah School of Medicine, 1991, pp 1–14.
9. Barton LL, Friedman AD: Stress and the residency program director. *Arch Pediatr Adolesc Med* 1994;148:101–103.
10. Bunch WH, Dvonch VM, Storr CL, et al: The stresses of the surgical residency. *J Surg Res* 1992;53:268–271.
11. Meals R: Surgical teaching vs. surgical learning. *Loyola Univ Chic Orthop J* 1993;2:35–38.
12. Ende J: Feedback in clinical medical education. *JAMA* 1983;250:777–781.
13. Sprafka S: Suggestions for clinicians providing—and residents seeking—feedback. *J Am Osteopath Assoc* 1992;92:1041–1046.
14. Scheuneman AL, Carley JP, Baker WH: Residency evaluations: Are they worth the effort? *Arch Surg* 1994;129:1067–1073.
15. Opipari M, Baker HH: Procedures to follow when dismissing an intern or resident. *J Am Osteopath Assoc* 1993;93:369–372.
16. Steinert Y, Levitt C: Working with the "problem" resident: Guidelines for definition and intervention. *Fam Med* 1993; 25:627–632.
17. Chase RA: Ruminations of a teaching surgeon. *West J Med* 1992;156:314–315.
18. Bosk CL (ed): *Forgive and Remember: Managing Medical Failure.* Chicago, IL, University of Chicago Press, 1979, pp 1–70.
19. Wu AW, Folkman S, McPhee SJ, et al: How house officers cope with their mistakes. *West J Med* 1993;159:565–569.
20. Lewy R: Alcoholism in house staff physicians: An occupational hazard. *J Occup Med* 1986;28:79–81.
21. McNamara RM, Margulies JL: Chemical dependency in emergency medicine residency programs: Perspective of the program directors. *Ann Emerg Med* 1994;23:1072–1076.
22. Siegel BJ, Fitzgerald FT: A survey on the prevalence of alcoholism among the faculty and house staff of an academic teaching hospital. *West J Med* 1988;148:593–595.
23. Lippert FG III, Spolek GA, Kirkpatrick GS, et al: A psychomotor skills course for orthopaedic residents. *J Med Educ* 1975;50: 982–983.
24. Kopta JA: An approach to the evaluation of operative skills. *Surgery* 1971;70:297–303.
25. Pickleman J, Schuenerman AL: Teaching and evaluating operative technique, in Bartlett R, Selenock G, Strodel W, et al (eds): *Medical Education: A Surgical Perspective.* Chelsea, MI, Lewis Publishers, 1986, pp 55–66.

26. Beckmann CR, Lipscomb GH, Ling FW, et al: Computer-assisted video evaluation of surgical skills. *Obstet Gynecol* 1995; 785:1039–1041.
27. Schuenerman AL, Pickleman J, Freeark RJ: Age, gender, lateral dominance, and prediction of operative skill among general surgery residents. *Surgery* 1985;98:506–515.
28. Whitman NA: *There Is No Gene for Good Teaching: A Handbook on Lecturing for Medical Teachers.* Salt Lake City, UT, University of Utah School of Medicine, 1982.
29. Williams R (ed): *The Mac Is Not a Typewriter: A Style Manual for Creating Professional-Level Type on Your Macintosh.* Berkeley, CA, Peachpit Press, 1990.
30. Williams R (ed): *The PC Is Not a Typewriter: A Style Manual for Creating Professional-Level Type on Your Personal Computer.* Berkeley, CA, Peachpit Press, 1992.
31. Bowling J: Clinical teaching in the ambulatory care setting: How to capture the teachable moment. *JAMA* 1993;93:235–239.
32. Lesky L, Borkan S: Strategies to improve teaching in the ambulatory medicine setting. *Arch Intern Med* 1990;1590:2133–2137.
33. Bartlett R: Teaching from patients, in Bartlett R, Selenock G, Strodel W, et al (eds): *Medical Education: A Surgical Perspective.* Chelsea, MI, Lewis Publishers, 1986, pp 7–22.
34. Ullian J, Bland C, Simpson D: An alternative top defining the role of the clinical teacher. *Acad Med* 1994;69:832–838.
35. Xakelis G, Gjerde C: Ambulatory medical education: Teachers' activities, teaching cost, and residents' satisfaction. *Acad Med* 1995;70:702–707.
36. Moberg-Wolff E, Kosasih J: Journal clubs: Prevalence, format and efficacy in PM&R. *Am J Phys Med Rehabil* 1995;74:224–229.
37. Whitman N: *Creative Medical Teaching.* Salt Lake City, UT, University of Utah School of Medicine, 1990, pp 12–13.
38. Hensel W, Rasco T: Storytelling as a method for teaching values and attitudes. *Acad Med* 1992;67:500–504.

CHAPTER 57

The Use of Computer Technology to Improve the Effectiveness of Orthopaedic Presentations

Jeffrey A. Russell, MS, ATC
A. Louise Fincher, EdD, ATC
G. William Woods, MD

Introduction

Presentations are fundamental to the transfer of orthopaedic knowledge. The effectiveness of any presentation, whether of the stalwart 35-mm slide sort, a static poster exhibit, or a cutting edge multimedia production, depends primarily on how it is perceived by an audience. Many a presenter has stepped into a forum with the intention of educating the audience, only to have those in attendance nod off, riffle through their meeting programs to preview upcoming offerings, or leave shaking their heads. The main objective of any presentation is to impart learning. However, many presentations never even get close to the target, let alone into its bull's-eye, because they are designed, produced, and delivered with nary a modicum of understanding about how to drive a message home.

You, the presenter, can be a quality presenter if you are willing to reassess your abilities and alter those that are problematic. In short, you must become a student of presentation techniques. The caliber of a presenter is not at all proportional to the number of presentations he or she gives. This concept is similar to specificity of exercise training. A marathoner's training cannot focus on sprints, because there is little relationship between the physiology of running 100 meters and that of running 42,000 meters. Running several hundred 100-meter sprints will not do much for the runner's marathon ability; proper long-distance techniques must be part of his or her regimen. Likewise, a presenter must incorporate methods of good presentations, not just do lots of presentations.

Why should this interest a busy orthopaedic professional? You must have something important to say or you would not spend the time and effort necessary to say it. Hendricks[1] describes a "passion to communicate" as the basis for exemplary teaching. A good presenter exudes such a passion. The audience must perceive the presenter's interest in the subject matter and in dispensing information about it. The presentation's recipients must be carried along by the presenter's river of enthusiasm about the topic. Kroenke[2] understands the audience's perspective when he instructs us to remember that those watching a presentation must consume and digest in one sitting what the presenter prepares, rewrites, and rehearses several times.

The objective of this paper is to produce improved orthopaedic presentations by educating orthopaedic presenters. Today's computer technology provides unparalleled capabilities for achieving this goal. Few clinicians today are unacquainted with personal computers. Equipment is decreasing in price, software applications are becoming more powerful, and user interfaces are becoming less obtrusive and more friendly. We have elected to commandeer these resources and desire that you do the same.

Six Basic Steps for Good Presentations

Know Your Audience Widen your understanding of what constitutes an audience. It may be a single viewer of a poster exhibit or it could be a standing-room-only group of 5,000 for a keynote address. Unless you know to whom you are displaying a poster exhibit, presenting a paper or lecture, or showing a multimedia program, you will have great difficulty making the project maximally effective. Although you may not know the recipients personally, usually you will know their professional background (including their associational affiliations), level of training, technical expertise, and, often, the part of the country or world in which they work. Armed with this information, reflect on what the audience wants to hear and direct your presentation toward their desires and needs.

Resolve to Do Excellent Work "The difference between something good and something great is attention to detail."[3] You are responsible for the quality of your work. Do not underestimate the power of your presentation manner. The audience's impression of you as a professional depends chiefly on the image you present while in front of them. Decide before beginning to produce your project that only the best will be acceptable. Then, hold to this decision with diligence and tenacity. Do not allow yourself to slide into complacency. Generally, excellence requires complete conversance not only with the message, but with the means of imparting it. That is, you must understand how to apply the technologies you will use. Computers are supposed to make our lives easier; make yours work for you, not vice versa.

Avoid Misspellings and Poor Grammar Misspellings and poor grammar often are the nemesis of many orthopaedic professionals. Unfortunately, it is much easier to say,

"Oh, I'm a terrible speller," or, "I never could get that grammar right," than it is to proofread, use a dictionary, thesaurus, and writing manual, or run a word processed document through a computerized spell checker or grammar checker. Spelling and grammar are learned skills, just like orthopaedic surgery. Anyone can learn to be better. Determine to put forth the effort required to drive misspelled words and grammatical blunders from your work. This is a very effective means of bringing immediate improvement to presentations. Several excellent resources will assist this process.[4-9]

Heed a word of caution about computerized spell checkers and grammar checkers. Computers cannot substitute for the human brain. You still must proofread your work, as a very effective poetic example from the *Journal of Irreproducible Results*,[10] "Candidate for a Pullet Surprise," underscores. Its title makes enough of a point: you might expect it to read "Candidate for a Pulitzer Prize." Nonetheless, in the article's real title, "Pullet Surprise" will be found correct by any computer spelling software! (A rewrite of this last sentence also will pass the computer's scrutiny: Nun the less, in the art a culls reel tie dull, "Pullet Surprise" will bee found core wrecked bye any come pewter spell in soft where!) In the text of his piece, Zar[10] counts 127 wrong words out of 225; yet, no word is spelled incorrectly. The point is, you yourself must expend some energy to prevent misspellings and grammar problems, because a computer cannot, and will not, do it all for you.

Plan Incessantly The saying goes, "Failure to plan is a plan for failure." It would be unusual to drive from Prescott, Arizona, to Simsbury, Connecticut, without first looking at a map and deciding which roads you should take. There might be several ways to make the trip, but you would have to plan your travel over one of them. This discussion is particularly germane to computer applications in orthopaedic communication.

Basically, the more time you spend planning your poster, presentation, or multimedia program, the less time you will spend in its production. Normally this is not a one-to-one ratio, either. A large amount of wasted production time can be saved by a relatively small investment in planning. Always think with a pencil in your hand. Use an "idea pad" to cultivate the project visually. Planning is an art, not a science, and a good planner is a true craftsman.

Be Intimately Involved in the Production Process We already established that the quality of a project is your responsibility because you are its generator and author. Thus, be very careful how much control you relinquish to your service providers (eg, slidemaking bureaus, desktop publishers, medical school communications departments, etc). Do as much of the work as possible yourself. Where computers are concerned, you probably will enjoy using some of the fantastic graphics applications available in today's market.

Still, it is unreasonable to expect a busy orthopaedic professional to become skilled at the many computer techniques necessary to produce final output in a graphically and visually effective form. There are a number of ways to stay involved in the process, while still maintaining your orthopaedic practice. First, proofread all your service providers' work before they produce your final output. You can word process the text of your poster or slides and export it to whomever will design and produce your final media. This provides you firsthand input to what eventually you will tack to a display board or show on a screen. Get ideas for designs, shapes, colors, typefaces, and layouts from magazines, ads, and other presentations you attend. This is a rich, and limitless, source of creative ammunition.

Visit your graphics service bureau or medical graphics department and ask the employees to explain the technology they apply to your output and show you how it works. Most of them are very willing to showcase their talents and high-end devices. Watching the computers, film recorders, plotters, and other equipment interact to produce your output can be a fascinating experience. However, you must be cautious to use service providers' expertise intelligently, not blindly. Do not fall prey to an unscrupulous or careless vendor who takes advantage of your relative lack of knowledge by impressing you with talk and "glitz" to gain your confidence.

Always Have a Backup Plan The application of computer technology to presentations pushes the limits of that technology because of the inherent pressure of a presentation forum. A presenter, already somewhat apprehensive, an audience, no matter what the size, and a conference, often in unfamiliar out-of-town surroundings, are like a stick of dynamite. The computer system, then, is the fuse. If the technology falters, the whole presentation explodes...unless, of course, the presenter is prepared for the worst. The chances of such unfortunate circumstances are well summarized by Russell's Technology Coefficient: Incidence of Disaster = (Murphy's Law)^n; where $n \rightarrow \infty$.

What would you do if: (1) your medical graphics department called to say its computerized slide recorder's camera malfunctioned and your slides would not be ready in time? (2) the LCD panel provided for your multimedia presentation by a symposium's host organization did not have an input jack that would accept the plug on the cable from your laptop computer? (3) the hard drive on your laptop computer crashed as you were starting it up for your multimedia presentation?

Hypothetical questions 2 and 3 refer to lectures accompanied by computerized projection of audiovisual aids. In most cases, using computer technology (which really means depending on computers) for presentations means pushing the envelope of the computer's function. Because of the variety of factors that must mesh flawlessly, presenting with this methodology is not recommended for the faint of heart. However, if you welcome pressure, excitement, and challenge (and what orthopaedic surgeon does not?) and if you enjoy being distinctive and impactful, computerized presentations will suit you just fine. Yet, with the thrill comes the fine line that separates it from disaster. Hence the caveat to have a backup plan.

Basic Hardware Guidelines

Many factors must be considered when assembling a computer system capable of executing the tasks described in this article. Improvements in computer performance are made so quickly, it is difficult to provide guidance that resists swift obsolescence. Although a sophisticated discussion of the computer is beyond our scope here, we can offer some suggestions about characteristics of useful presentation preparation and delivery systems.

Perhaps the question most frequently asked about computers for graphic applications is which platform is most appropriate, Apple Macintosh or IBM-compatible? We do not intend to settle this argument. While the vast majority of graphic designers and graphic artists and a large percentage of desktop publishers use Macintosh computers, the majority of business laptop computer presenters use IBM-compatibles. The Macintosh has some very compelling features that make it particularly suitable to the creation of graphics. IBM-compatible loyalists have their own passionate reasons for their hardware selections. In our opinion, the PowerPC™ chip developed jointly by Apple, IBM, and Motorola renders the contention about which platform is "best" relatively nondivisive, based on its showcase in Apple Power Macintosh computers. Macintosh may have an edge, though, because Apple has gone out of its way to accommodate the IBM-compatible world by developing a floppy disk "superdrive," which accepts diskettes of either format, and advanced translation software to allow easy file exchanges between the platforms. The most popular professional level software packages usually allow file exchanging between platforms, too. We expect tomorrow's computers to bear an increasing resemblance to one another. Parenthetically, our preference, because of its suitability to high-end graphics and multimedia, is the Power Macintosh.

Much more germane to a discussion of orthopaedic presentation computing are chip speed, memory, and hard disk space. The speed at which a computer chip processes information is, obviously, meaningful to the user's perception of how quickly the computer operates. Where large sets of instructions are present in graphic applications, instruction processing time greatly affects productivity. The significantly reduced cost of very fast chips (eg, Intel Pentium™ chips and Motorola PowerPC™ chips) has brought excellent performance within the grasp of most orthopaedic professionals. Purchase the computer with the highest megahertz of chip speed you can afford. In the PowerPC realm, do not neglect software's contribution to the speed equation. Software written to take advantage of the PowerPC chip's abilities will offer the best performance on a PowerPC computer.

Adequate random access memory, or RAM, is one of the most important parameters of a system. As with chip speed, the usual rule is to equip your computer with as much RAM as you can afford. RAM is expandable (to a maximum allowed by a given computer model) as applications warrant and funds allow. There must be enough RAM to open and use the application software and to manipulate the files. RAM-hungry operating systems (eg, Microsoft Windows 95™) and many of the latest graphics applications need at least 8 megabytes (MB) of RAM, but 16 MB are preferable. Sixteen MB is a minimum for basic multimedia applications. Digital editing and advanced multimedia will work best with even more. Our office desktop computers have 72 MB of RAM.

Adequate hard disk space has become very consequential because of the large size of color graphics and video files. Not very long ago, laptop computers with 80 to 100-MB hard drives were commonplace. Many single graphic files today would consume most of one of these, so manufacturers have developed hard drives that are larger in capacity and smaller in size. The newest AV (audiovisual, or multimedia) laptop computers have one gigabyte hard drives. (A gigabyte is 10^9 bytes, or 1,000 MB.) Hard disk space for desktop computers is less of an issue because these machines do not require portability and can have external storage devices attached. There are many good, relatively inexpensive storage alternatives for such models. We have 700-MB hard disks on our office computers and use removable cartridge drives to augment our storage. We also use compact disc (CD) drives to import files from CD collections of graphics, sounds, or video clips.

General Design Guidelines

Slides, a poster exhibit, or a multimedia program are, effectively, advertisements for you, your institution, and your work. It is critically important that your media are not only visually appealing, but exquisite in their message communication. That is to say, a picture is worth a thousand words only when it speaks a thousand words. There are several tenets of good design mechanics to help you make your point as effectively as possible. One worthwhile evaluation to perform on

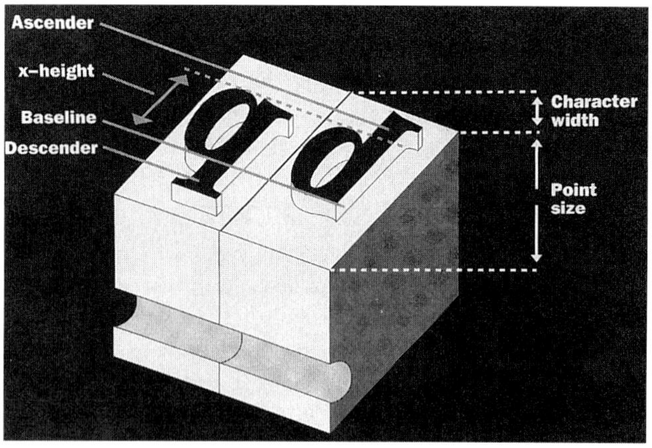

Fig. 1 The anatomy of type (Reproduced with permission from Rabb MY (ed): *The Presentation Design Book: Tips, Techniques and Advice for Creating Effective, Attractive Slides, Overheads, Multimedia Presentations, Screen Shows and More*, ed 2. Chapel Hill, NC, Ventana Press, 1993.)

This is Helvetica, a sans serif typeface that is always a winner.

Futura is another excellent sans serif typeface.

Times, or Times Roman, is a very common serif typeface.

Palatino is a stylish, yet simple, serif typeface.

Optima is attractive, simple, and easy to read.

Tekton is another good choice with a little flair.

Script typefaces, like Brush Script, are not suitable for medical media.

DESIGNER TYPEFACES, SUCH AS ANNA AND *Boulevard, are too complex for medical communications.*

TOTALLY UPPERCASE LETTERING, LIKE TRAJAN, MAKES THE EYES WORK TOO HARD.

Fig. 2 Certain typefaces are much more suitable for scholarly communication than others. In general, the simpler a typeface, the easier it is to read and, thus, the more effective it will be at delivering a message.

your slides is the Nelson Slide Test.[11,12] This "test" simply asks, "Has the information to be presented been prepared specifically for a slide?" The logical corollaries to this propose the same question to the creator of a poster exhibit or multimedia program.

Typography

Typography may be more important to good communication than any other factor. Rabb[13] calls the printed word "a staple of information graphics." How the lettering of your presentation looks will either garner or deflect a viewer's attention. An overall evaluation of the text on a slide is the "Arm's Length Rule."[14] If you cannot read uppercase letters on a slide held at arm's length, redo the slide. Apply similar rules to poster exhibits and multimedia programs. If the text on a poster is not readable from 6 to 10 feet away, make it larger. If someone viewing a multimedia program has to lean forward to read the text on a computer screen, increase the text's size. Exaggerate the increase when the program will be shown on a large screen to an audience; design it for the person in the back row.

The anatomy of type is shown in Figure 1. The following definitions and associated advice will help you design the textual portion of any project.

Typeface A typeface is a set of letters of a single design. For example, Helvetica, Garamond, Garamond Condensed, Times, and Avant Garde are typefaces. A typeface can be considered a family of fonts. Figure 2 shows examples of several typefaces.

Font A font is a series of letters of a single typeface set in a specific point size, stroke weight, and style. For example, 12 point Garamond Semibold Italic is a font. (A technical point: the pulldown menu labeled "Font" in most software more properly should be labeled "Typeface.")

Point Size Point size, which indicates the relative height of a letter, is one of the most confusing parameters in typography. A font's point size is the size of an invisible box that contains the distance from just below the bottom of the lowest descender on a letter in an alphabet to just above the top of the highest ascender (Fig. 1). Seventy-two points equal one inch. In writing (eg, in an abstract), 10 points usually is the smallest acceptable size for good readability. On a poster exhibit the title should be at least 150 points, and any narrative text should be at least 30. Text for slides produced in slidemaking software should be no less than 30 points, although 36 is an even better minimum. Note that letters in different typefaces are not necessarily equal in size when set to the same point size.

Stroke Weight Stroke weight is the width of the lines making up a letter. Typical stroke weights, in order of increasing width, are light, book or regular, medium, semibold or demi, bold, and ultra or extra bold. For maximum readability in presentations, bold stroke is best.

Type Style The style of a letter is any alteration to its standard typeface format. Italic (or oblique), outline, and shadow are some commonly used letter styles. Simple upright type (ie, without an applied style) is most easily read. Italics can be used for emphasis, but they are difficult to read in long phrases and narratives.

Serifs Serifs are the small decorative "tails" and "bulbs," or sculpted ends, on the tops and bottoms of letters in certain typefaces. One purpose of serifs is to transfer the eyes from one letter to the next in reading. See Figure 3 for some samples of serifs.

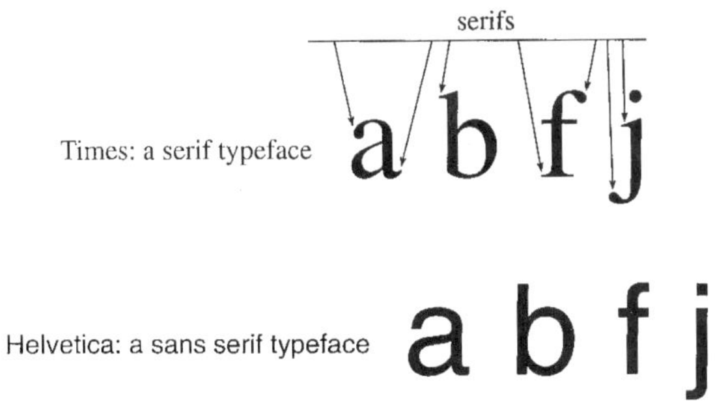

Fig. 3 Serifs are the sculpted ends of a letter's ascenders and descenders.

Sans Serif Sans serif typefaces do not have serifs on their letters (Fig. 3). The ends of their strokes usually are flat and the stroke width is constant across an entire letter. Some experts recommend using primarily sans serif typefaces in research communication because they provide a clean, consistent, easily read look. However, other authorities prefer serif typefaces The strengths of both can be used in your media, if you wish: sans serif type for titles and short phrases, serif type for sections of narrative text.

Leading Leading (pronounced "led–ing") is the amount of space between two lines of type. For practicality, set the leading in your projects according to what pleases your eye. A common leading is 120% of the type size. Simply, be sure you do not squeeze too much text into a given vertical height of space.

Use uppercase and lowercase combination lettering (which is being used in this article) in most instances. If you use a totally uppercase format at all, reserve it for very short titles. THE MAIN REASON FOR THIS GUIDELINE IS THAT UPPERCASE LETTERING IS RATHER DIFFICULT TO READ OVER LONG PHRASES AND SENTENCES. There are no "peaks and valleys" to the letters to assist the eyes in tracking along the line of text. And, some people will not respond favorably to reading entirely uppercase lettering because, as in the world of electronic mail, text exclusively in capitals is the written equivalent of shouting and, thus, is poor etiquette.

Color and Graphics

Computer software and hardware are so advanced that constructing effective presentations is a challenge. Although user interfaces are much improved over a few years ago, the plethora of typefaces, graphic elements, and colors available to even a novice computer user often compel one toward poor judgment in their applications.

Where color choices are concerned, the increasingly popular and accessible 24 bit color, which can display about 16.7 million different colors, is overwhelming. This capability in your computer system is important when incorporating photos to text slides and using still pictures and video in multimedia. However, for text and simple graphic slides and poster exhibits, it only complicates the production process. You must stay focused on good color design for several reasons: (1) presentation colors should be pleasing, (2) using more than a few colors in key elements is distracting, and (3) color guidelines appropriate for poster exhibits and slides vary slightly from those for multimedia presentations.

Select dark colors for the background and light colors for text and graphics, no matter what the medium. Three or four colors should be a maximum; otherwise, you will produce the "rainbow effect,"[15] or what we call "salad bar slides."[14] (Salad bar slides have so many colors they resemble the vividness of the vegetable array on a fresh salad bar. This is terrific at a restaurant when you are hungry, but distracting when you are an audience member in a lecture hall.) Black, navy blue, dark teal, or dark violet make excellent backgrounds and provide a cool, pleasing image. Avoid light backgrounds with dark letters (especially white backgrounds on slides, because the effect on a viewer is similar to reading the wattage on the top of a light bulb when it is turned on). Gradient backgrounds, fading from, for example, black at the bottom of the medium to another dark color at the top, are both effective and common. The most visible colors for text and graphic elements are the tried and true white, golden yellow, ivory, and light blue. It is fine to be creative with your color selection, as long as you preserve good design sense. The overly worn royal blue background with lemon yellow and white lettering is, as Rabb puts it, "the visual correlative of elevator music."[13] The poster exhibit is one medium that could generally benefit from thoughtfully applied accentuating color. Many exhibitors are now using more color as output technologies have progressed.

Modern digital technology has brought us many patterned backgrounds resembling marble, granite, wood grain, cloud formations, and the like. Advanced artistic typography applications let us create very unusual text effects and distortions. Caution is advised when selecting such "new and improved" alternatives, because the graphic effects can distract viewers from your message. Multimedia is probably the only medium where a departure from traditional presentation graphics concepts is beneficial and does not cloud the message being delivered. In short, your overriding concerns should be the attractiveness of the color combinations and the contrast between the background and the text or graphics.

Simplicity is the key to effective diagrams and pictures. "One of the biggest mistakes that can be made is to think that legibility in one form means legibility in another."[16] A photograph that conveys an excellent message in a book or article might serve a presentation much better if converted to a line drawing. Tables and graphs provide another example of this. While a table of data often is appropriate for a journal article where a reader can spend as much time as necessary absorbing it, the same table projected on a slide during a research presentation will not be in front of the audience long enough to allow this luxury. Additionally, most projected tables have a type that is much too small. The preferred mode of information conveyance, then, is a subset of the table's data, a well-designed graph or other schematic representation of the data.[11,12]

Digital Graphic Images

The creation and manipulation of digital images is revolutionizing presentation graphics. In 1989, the Eastman Kodak Company published a book entitled *Slides: Planning and Producing Slide Programs.*[17] In 1993, in an effort to pursue evolving digital production and presentation capabilities, the company wrote an excellent companion book, *More Slides: Planning, Producing, and Presenting Digital Images,*[18] which deals exclusively with the computerization of the slide production process. Much of this information applies equally well to laptop computer-driven multimedia presentations, which only recently have become a truly viable, readily available, and affordable presentation mode. As is typical in the computer world, authoritarianism is difficult because of the continual rapid and substantial developments in the field. However, we offer some basic principles that will allow you to improve both the efficiency of your production process and the effectiveness of your presentations.

Poster exhibits, slides, and multimedia presentations all will smoothly receive digital graphics if you create the projects with the proper application software. We have found the easiest and most cost-effective means of image importation to be Photo CD technology. Your photographic processing facility likely can install your images from slides or negatives on a Photo CD or can refer you to a lab that offers this service. This transfer is done with a transparency scanner and the process installs each image on the CD in five resolutions. Although you can purchase your own transparency scanner to place images directly on your computer's hard drive, we do not recommend this for the busy orthopaedic professional because of the high equipment cost and, with some scanner models, the significant time required to scan the images properly (finding the appropriate brightness, contrast, and color correction settings for each image is time-consuming).

Do not overlook the abundance of clip-art CDs available. The market for these products and, thus, their availability has increased dramatically in the past few years. For a reasonable price you can obtain thousands of images. Several companies offer anatomic and other medical graphics. Virtually anything you can imagine is available in CD clip-art.

Another common and financially accessible technique of obtaining digital images is simple flatbed scanning of photographs and drawings. Today, scanners are available in many offices. Contrast, brightness, and color settings still must be set, but the relative preponderance of scanners heightens the probability that you or someone you know is familiar with flatbed scanning methods. Scanned images are imported into your presentations in the same way you import a Photo CD image.

The most recent development in digital still image capture is the digital camera. There are a number of cameras available at prices from $700 to well into the tens of thousands of dollars. The higher priced models often are 35-mm camera bodies modified for digital photography. In general, the higher a camera's cost, the higher the quality of the images it produces. They work like light-based cameras, except that a digital disk replaces the film. Digitally encoded images in the camera are downloaded to a computer, where they can be manipulated and incorporated into presentations.

Generally, the higher the resolution of an image the better the quality of its final output, but the larger the image's file size. The intended use of the image dictates which of its resolutions to use. If you import a digital image into a text slide, the high quality of that medium and the capability of most film recorders suggest you import a high-resolution (eg, 1,000 dots per inch or greater) file of the image. If you need an image for a multimedia presentation to be viewed on a computer monitor or on a projection screen via an LCD panel, a high-resolution image is of no greater value than a low resolution (eg, 72 dots per inch) image, because the monitor or panel is unable to reproduce high resolutions. Images in the 300 to 600 dots per inch range (typical of popular and affordable desktop scanners) normally are not acceptable for high-quality slide applications.[18] Keep in mind that color images have much larger file sizes than halftone black and white (photographic) images, which, in turn, are much larger than black and white line art files. Particularly for multimedia presentations, the size of the hard disk on which you install your presentation may limit the number of images you use, especially color images.

Much larger file sizes are required for digital video and sound. This technology has developed very quickly in the last few years. Capturing full motion video or

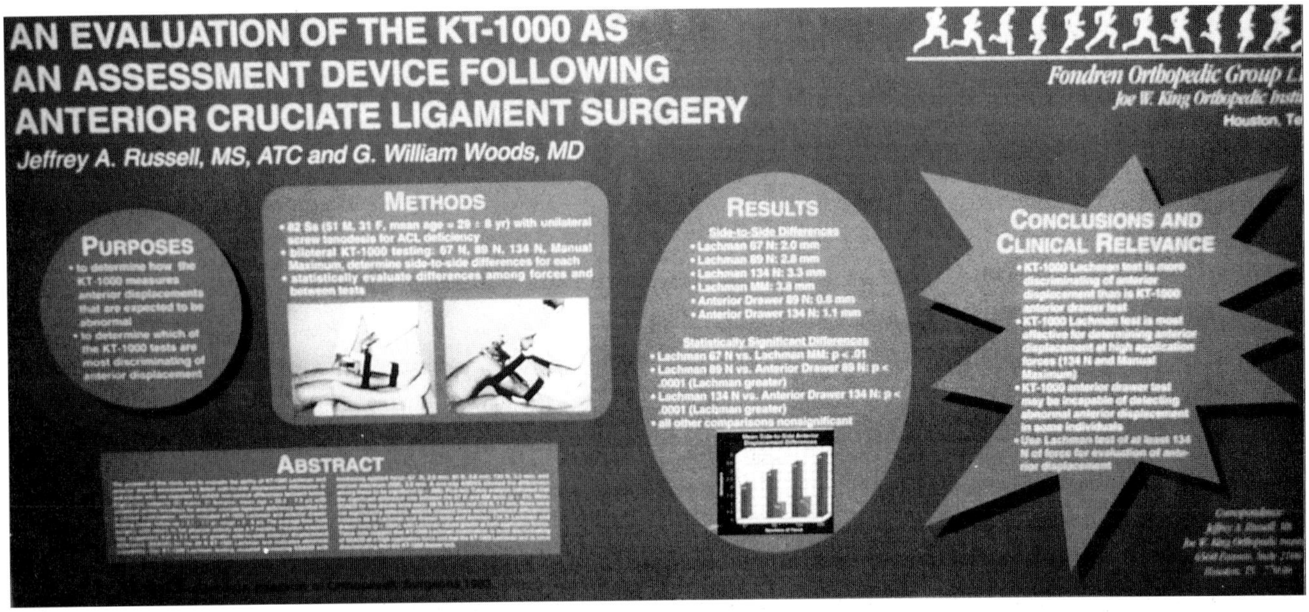

Fig. 4 An example of a poster created with desktop publishing software and output on an electrostatic plotter.

sound and importing it into a multimedia presentation is not only possible, but relatively easy. We caution, however, that if you intend to produce a high-quality project of this type your investment of time and money will be substantial.

One of the most advanced capabilities of high-end digital image systems is image alteration. Digital images exist only on a computer disk, and they can be modified extensively with editing software. Unwanted items in an image can be removed, portions of one image can be added to another, portions of an image can be enhanced or highlighted, colors can be changed, a color image can be changed to black and white, black and white images can be colorized, and much more. This fascinating process requires a significant commitment of time to learn its nuances; it is very much an art. But, the artistic nature of digital image editing notwithstanding, the computer is very forgiving, allowing the user chance after chance to obtain the right results, because, again, there is no "real" image.

Poster Exhibits

Computer technology has greatly expanded the possibilities for producing vibrantly colored, visually emphatic scientific poster exhibits. A wide variety of software products and output devices are available that can generate large format (eg, 3.5 feet high by 8 feet wide, approximately the size of poster exhibit space at the American Academy of Orthopaedic Surgeons [AAOS] Annual Meeting) single pieces of paper (Fig. 4). The entire content of one of these posters is laid out on a computer. The computer operator has complete control over text size, color assignment, and graphic elements. These posters contrast greatly with a multiple piece poster exhibit, which is a collection of small panels on a display tackboard, often with typewritten text. Traveling with a computer-produced, large-format poster is as simple as rolling it up, placing it in a four foot mailing, art, or fishing pole tube, and carrying it under your arm.

A desktop publishing program is well-suited to create large format posters. Computer graphics programs work well, too. We have had success at designing 1:7 scale models of our posters on a popular desktop publishing application (Fig. 5). That is, the computer model, in order to fit within the software's page size requirements, is 1/7 the size of the desired finished product. So, a document 6 inches high by 12.86 inches wide yields an output poster 42 inches high by 90 inches wide, which fits perfectly into the AAOS 4- × 8-ft tackboard format. Similarly, a 24-point title in the computer document is output at 168 points (24 × 7), an easily read size for a poster's title. We prefer not to use text sizes smaller than 6 points on a model (42 points on the final output), except for 4 point type (28 points on output) in an extended narrative, as in an abstract. The effectiveness of a poster exhibit is, we believe, not as much a function of the topic or quality of the research being presented as it is the interest generated by a visually appealing design and an easily understood message. Take great care to adhere to the suggestions presented in the previous general design section.

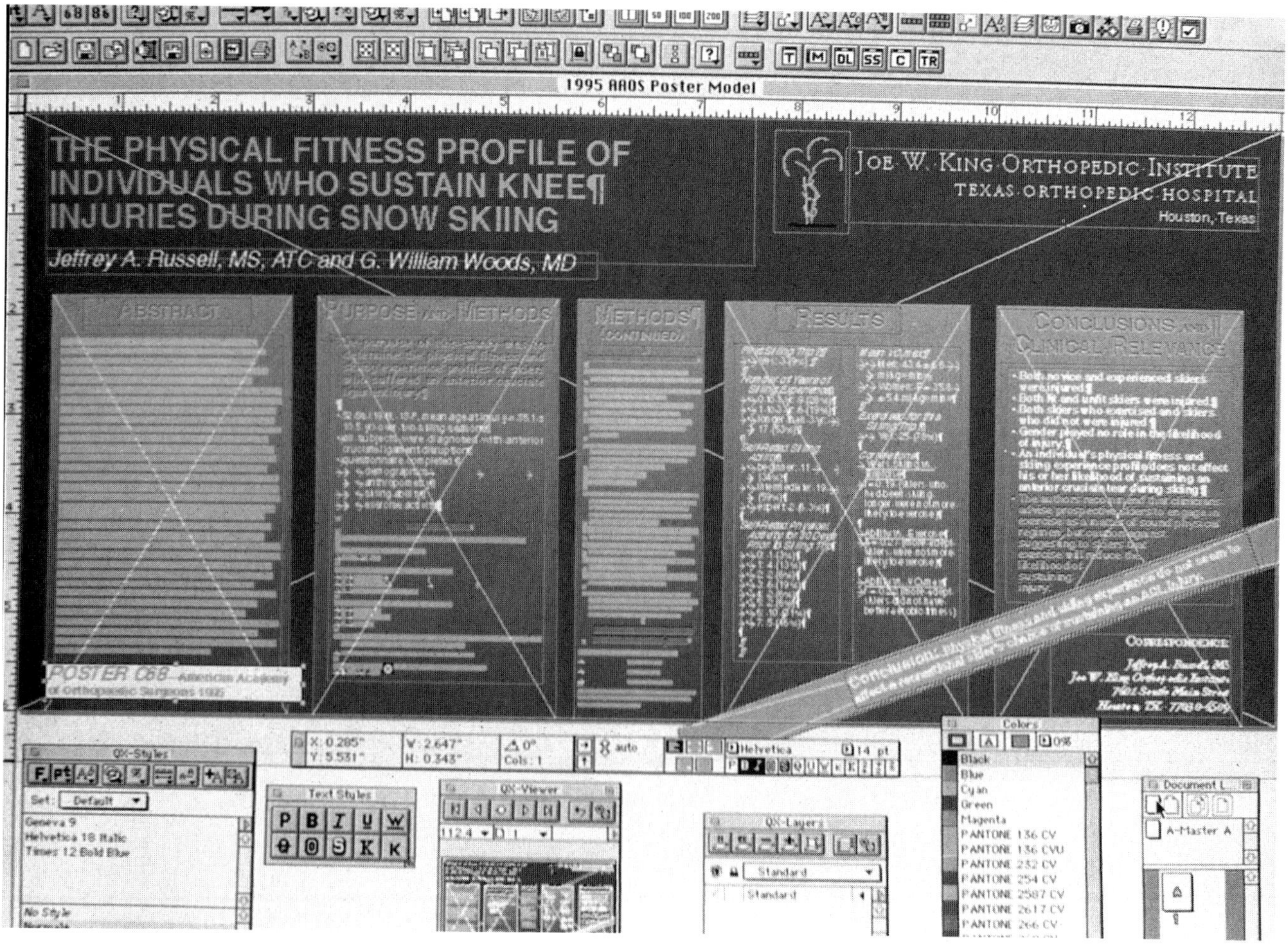

Fig. 5 This computer screen shows a sample of a poster exhibit being composed in a desktop publishing software program called QuarkXPress™ (Courtesy of Quark Inc, Denver, CO).

Computer-designed, large-format posters usually are output on either an electrostatic plotter or an inkjet plotter. Because of the high cost of these devices, most orthopaedic professionals use a service bureau to output their work. Paper and vinyl are the two most common and suitable output media. Posters 36 to 42 inches high by an unlimited length can be output this way, but a 48-inch-high capability undoubtedly will be the next step of this technology. We recommend that paper posters be laminated to protect them when they are being transported and displayed. Lamination also enriches colors and, if matte lamination is used, it will minimize glare from lighting in the exhibit hall.

Inkjet output is much richer in color, and the color coverage is smoother than that of electrostatic output. The Pantone Matching System™, or PMS, (Pantone, Inc, Moonachie, NJ) is a common way of assigning colors to the various parts of a poster. But, neither inkjet nor electrostatic technologies truly reproduce PMS colors. Always obtain color "swatch" samples from your output bureau and use the colors that are richest and not mottled. Dark colors in backgrounds tend to show better coverage and purity than most light colors, because their darkness hides imperfections. Light colors that are exceptions to this are pure yellow, pure cyan, and pure magenta. These are Pantone process colors, meaning all other colors are made from combinations of these three plus black. Medium colors like green, red, and teal also yield acceptable results. The best colors to use for text are white, yellow, and, occasionally, red. Red, cyan, and magenta are good colors for graphic accents.

Graphs, charts, tables, and photographs can be applied to a poster in one of three ways: import and plot, affix within lamination, or affix outside of lamination. Using digital image importation, place a graphic in its desired location on your poster layout model. When the poster is plotted, the graphic will be plotted as part of it. This is the best technique for providing a poster with a consistent look. However, do not expect

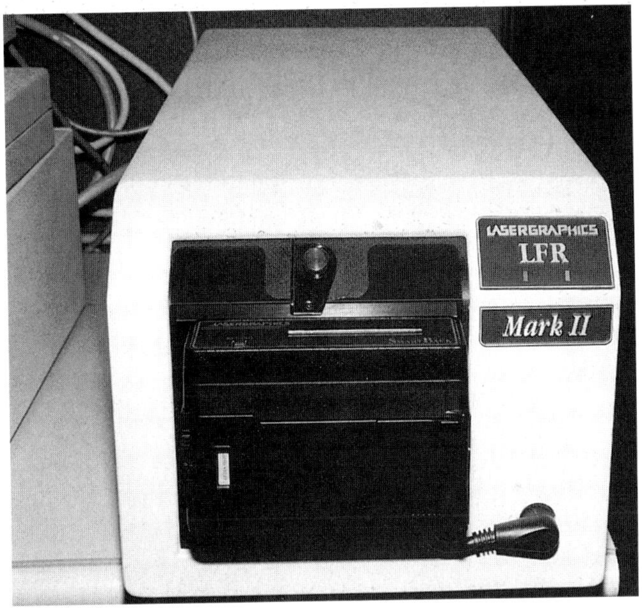

Fig. 6 A typical film recorder for making 35-mm slides from computer files. The camera is the black box in the foreground. The larger, light colored box contains a light source and red, green, and blue filters. The light passes through the filters and exposes the film in the camera, thus producing a colored slide. All colors on a slide are combinations of red, green, and blue light.

plotted photographs to be of finely detailed photographic quality, especially those done on electrostatic plotters.

Photographs or graphics printed on paper can be fastened to a poster in their desired locations and laminated with the poster for protection. The difficulty presented by this technique is potential irregularities in the poster's contour when the poster is rolled up for travel and unrolled for display. Once photographic paper is rolled, it will not behave the same as the bond paper on which the poster is printed.

The third method of including presentation pictures, graphs, and tables in a poster is the simplest: mount the items on heavy cardboard or foam core board. Then, use hook and loop tape to fasten them to their proper locations on the laminated poster. The inconvenience of this method relates, again, to traveling. The graphics must be kept flat and carried separately from the poster, which is rolled up in a tube.

Be forewarned that there will be some anxious moments during production of your first poster exhibit using the procedures described here. Without actually plotting it, there is no way to accurately simulate how the poster will look. Large format output is somewhat costly, and lamination increases the charges even more. Waiting for delivery from the service bureau, to see whether the resulting poster is worth the expense, can be fairly tense. Exquisite attention to planning, design, spelling, and grammar during the production phase will avert disappointment and will greatly enhance your poster presentation.

Slides

Computers are basic to effective slides in most scientific and business disciplines. Advancing technology and software applications have somewhat improved the quality of slides at medical symposia. However, too many presenters have yet to implement the good design concepts previously outlined. We generally oppose using the supposed "presentation ready" slide templates furnished in presentation graphics software packages, having found them rarely accommodating to effective presentations. Specifically, the preset text sizes are much smaller than we recommend for excellent visibility, an issue which is foundational to slide design. Orthopaedic presenters would do well to create their own templates, a rather straightforward process in most reputable software applications. Or, retain a preset template's background and graphic accents while you increase the point size of any type in the template.

Do not be misled about computers and slidemaking. "Writing and visualization are tough mental tasks, demanding an almost paradoxical mix of concentration and free-flowing creativity. Computers and software don't change that."[19] Even the process of scrawling text for your slides on a notepad requires thoughtful effort. Your presentation will be well served if you write the slides' contents on lecture storyboards[14] before you enter any text into a computer. A storyboard is a piece of paper printed with a box containing lines on which to write (1) each slide's number in the presentation sequence; (2) the slide's title, subtitle, and text; and (3) any special notes about what you plan to say when the slide is projected.

There are two typical methods of proceeding from handwritten notes to slides in a software package. Either enter the text of the slides into an outline in the software or import the text into the presentation program from a word-processing program. Personal preference is as significant here as anything. Once in the outline, the text for each slide is combined with a template. Templates have placeholders for each portion of a slide. That is to say, text typed in a title position on an outline is placed where the title placeholder is located on the slide when the template and outline are combined. Similarly, whatever is typed into the subtitle and bullet list positions is dropped into the respective spots on each slide, as well. There are additional placeholders for tables, graphs, etc.

Background colors and shapes, lines that separate the titles from bullet lists, and any other embellishments that are consistent throughout a set of slides usually are applied on the template, too. Colors on a computer monitor differ from the actual colors on a slide. It is wise not to venture too far from standard colors, especially for backgrounds, text, and large graphics, because, if you do, you may find that the final output is rather unattractive when projected.

Slide files on a computer disk are converted to 35-mm slides by a film recorder (Fig. 6). Several recorders are available, ranging in price from approximately $4,000 to $100,000. Production of very high quality slides is possible with desktop film recorders priced up to $15,000. Increasing price typically brings faster operation, but the quality of a text slide imaged by a $50,000 film recorder is not appreciably better than that of a text slide recorded by a $10,000 device. However, the more expensive film recorders are better suited for imaging slides with large file sizes or imported graphics, especially color pictures. An alternative to purchasing your own film recorder is using a service bureau to record your slides. Based on the average per slide cost of $10 to $30 for such service, an investment in a film recorder will be paid back fairly quickly for individuals who do a lot of speaking.

The primary factor that dictates the quality of film recorder output is resolution lines per inch. There is a great difference between 2,000 and 4,000 lines per inch (lpi) when projecting a slide on a screen. Parts of letters and figures that are not horizontal or vertical often show "stairstepping" or "jaggies," images may not be crisp, and color blends may show "banding," or unsmooth transitions, as one color fades to another. The differences in image quality of slides for medical meetings are not nearly as great when the resolution jumps from 4,000 to 8,000 lpi, except, again, when there are imported graphics in a slide. Thus, for those who wish to purchase one, we recommend a film recorder capable of 4,000 lpi imaging.

Photo CD and flatbed scanning technologies, discussed in the digital images section of this article, are ideal for enhancing 35-mm text slides. For instance, heretofore there were two ways of showing a picture and an explanatory text slide simultaneously. You either had to use two projectors, one holding the text slide and the other holding the picture slide, or have a service bureau make a text slide with the accompanying picture inset, or "burned in," often at a cost of $50 to several hundred dollars per slide, depending on its complexity. Now, you can create your text slide on a desktop computer and import to it a digital image. A good quality film recorder will output this file as a beautiful combination slide. There are some caveats, however. Working with digital pictures requires a large amount of computer random access memory (RAM). Also, the film recorder should be high quality, particularly if you import radiographic or 24-bit color images.

Multimedia

The remainder of this article is devoted to multimedia. We have included more information on this topic than on poster exhibits or slides because it is much newer and more complex. Our goal is to describe some of multimedia's characteristics and uses, to instruct you how to get started in multimedia, and to motivate you to apply more advanced methods, if you wish to do so.

Multimedia integrates text, graphics, audio, animation, and motion video in order to present information to an audience via computer. This is not to say, however, that, in order to be classified as multimedia, a presentation must include all of these elements. Multimedia presentations range from simple electronic slide presentations to highly interactive computer programs in kiosks. Orthopaedic professionals can harness the power of multimedia to prepare and deliver dynamic presentations.

Characteristics of Multimedia

Multimedia programs can be categorized in two ways, by their mode of delivery (speaker-driven versus stand-alone) and by their level of interactivity (linear versus interactive).

Speaker-Driven Speaker-driven presentations are given in the typical "live" environment, in which the presenter stands in front of an audience to deliver his or her presentation.

Stand-Alone Stand-alone multimedia presentations, as the name suggests, are designed to run without a presenter. Stand-alone multimedia presentations typically are viewed by an audience of one (or possibly a small group) on a computer monitor.

Linear Linear presentations are structured so that each slide or screen is designed to follow the one just previous to it, with no deviation in the prearranged order. A standard slide presentation is an example of a linear presentation.

Interactive Interactive presentations provide alternate pathways through their instructional content. They allow the presenter or audience to choose direction and pace with navigational buttons or "trigger fields." Interactivity is the main strength of multimedia. Building interactivity into a live presentation makes it possible to change direction during the presentation. Imagine, for example, that during your multimedia presentation you notice that your audience seems extremely interested in a particular aspect of your presentation and asks many questions related to the topic. Imagine further that you had foreseen this possibility and had developed an additional segment describing the topic more thoroughly. Now, as a result of your planning, you can use the power of multimedia to branch to the expanded segment of the program. In a real situation, this application of interactivity would allow you to better meet the needs and interests of

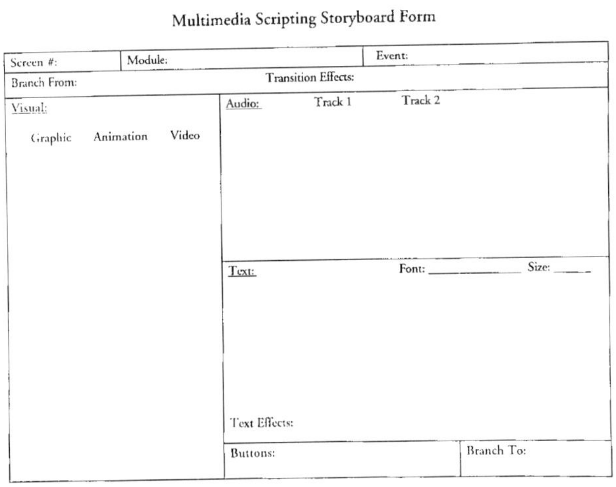

Fig. 7 A storyboard is a beneficial way of scripting a multimedia presentation.

your audience and to display your talents as a highly-effective presenter.

Design Considerations

The dynamic nature of multimedia presentations poses unique design considerations. The complexity of the design process depends largely on the type of multimedia program to be developed (eg, live or stand-alone presentation, linear or interactive). The type and number of media elements to be used also add to the complexity of the design.

Many novice multimedia developers overuse the media elements or use them inappropriately. Each element, whether it is text, a graphic, a sound, or a video clip, should serve one of two distinct purposes: to convey information clearly or to reinforce a point. Value is added not by the number of different effects created, but rather, by how well the effects reinforce your message.

A formal organizational strategy is recommended when planning and integrating the various media elements and multimedia characteristics. Flowcharts and storyboards are two tools commonly used for organizing multimedia presentations. A flowchart is used to frame your program. Once the framework is constructed, storyboards are used to design, in detail, each screen, and to lay out and blend the various media elements (Fig. 7). Detailed storyboards ensure that graphics are matched to the appropriate wording and that the audio is synchronized with the flow of on-screen text. In making storyboards for an interactive presentation, it is necessary to visualize all the navigational pathways and anticipate user choices.

Design Team Few orthopaedic professionals have the time to plan and produce a multimedia program in its entirety. For this reason, successful multimedia projects require a team approach. Professional multimedia design teams usually include a content specialist, an instructional design specialist, a graphic artist, a sound specialist, and a videographer. Your multimedia presentation, depending on its complexity, may not require all of these. Obviously, you are the content specialist. Based on the media elements you plan to use, you can enlist the services of others who possess the necessary skills and experience. In many instances, the multimedia team is made up of one or two individuals who wear a variety of hats. You can create an electronic slide presentation with little, if any, assistance using a presentation program like Adobe Persuasion™.

Background Color and Design The computer screen essentially forms the stage for your multimedia program. For this reason, the visual design and organization of on-screen information directly influence the effectiveness of your presentation.[20]

The background color is the foundation color on which all other colors (text, graphics, interactive buttons, etc) are applied. As discussed earlier, subdued colors like black, navy blue, dark purple, etc, are effective for backgrounds. Most traditional presentation and multimedia development programs include background templates and/or paint programs that allow you to create your own backgrounds. Metaphoric themes within the background design, such as file folder tabs or a spiral notebook layout, can help organize the content of your presentation and provide visual interest. Textured backgrounds, such as those that simulate marble, wood, or paper, can add depth to your screens; however, they should not clash with or distract from the text and graphics that will appear on the screen. Textured backgrounds also can drastically increase the hard disk requirements of your multimedia presentation. If hard disk space is limited, you may want to avoid them.

Text and Graphics Display Computer typefaces must be installed in each computer on which they are used. If you plan to present your multimedia program on a computer other than the one used for its development, be sure the typefaces in the program are installed on the presentation computer. If a presentation has been prepared using a few special typefaces and the computer used to deliver the presentation does not contain them, an impressive presentation will be reduced to mediocrity (or worse) when the computer replaces the special typefaces with ordinary ones. One way to prevent this is to use common typefaces such as Helvetica or Times, which are found on most computers. Another solution is to install copies of your presentation's typefaces on the same disk as your presentation.

Tway[20] recommends that text and graphics be arranged on the screen in a balanced way. This does not imply that the screens should be completely symmetrical. Symmetrical screens can create a dull, uniform look. Slight variations in the layout of your text and graphics will create balance and provide appeal, but these variations must be used in moderation. In overall appearance, the screens should remain somewhat constant in design and color throughout a single presentation. One exception to this rule is the use of a different background color for different modules within the presentation.

Text and graphics should not overcrowd or clutter the screen. Larson[21] recommends the general rule of "less is best." Comparing the computer screen to a sheet of paper, instructional design experts recommend you optimize the "white space." You also should limit the amount of information, presenting only one major point per screen. If a large quantity of information must appear on the screen at one time, consider building the screen for sequential revelation. This technique prevents the audience from being overwhelmed. When building a screen sequentially, graphics should appear first, followed by explanatory text, because graphics that follow text divert attention from the text. When used properly, the combination of text and graphics can guide the audience through a complex process.

Interactivity The quality of interaction ultimately determines its contribution to the overall program. Interactive multimedia presentations require navigational buttons. A stand-alone presentation requires navigational buttons that are easily recognized and consistently placed. In other words, if a button labeled "NEXT SCREEN" appears in the lower right hand corner initially, it should remain there throughout the program. Other essential user control options include: (1) the ability to exit the program from any screen, (2) the freedom to review certain sections, (3) the ability to access "help" from any screen, and (4) the freedom to choose the direction and pace of instruction.[22]

Effects and Transitions Most multimedia development programs provide a variety of special effects for introducing text and graphics and for moving between subsequent frames of a presentation. These effects range from simple dissolves and wipes to intricately designed flying and rolling effects. In most cases, flying text effects are more appropriate for opening segments, when your goal is to grab the attention of your audience. During the main portion of your presentation, simpler text effects are more effective. Too many elaborate effects in the body of a presentation can desensitize the audience to the effects and distract the viewers from your message.

Transition effects signal the audience they are leaving one screen and entering another. Fades, dissolves, and wipes are effective transitions. Transition effects should be consistent throughout your presentation. Using a different transition effect for every screen change will distract your audience.

Sound Digital sound is used in multimedia for sound effects, mood setting (eg, through music), or narration. The three types of digital sound files commonly used in multimedia programs are CD audio stored in CD-ROM format (compact discs), wave audio stored in WAV files, and MIDI (Musical Instrument Digital Interface) synthesizer audio stored in MID files.[23] As with clip art, libraries of digital sound effects and music are available on CD-ROM. Although most library sound files can be used royalty-free, always read the licensing agreement before including a sound in your multimedia presentation.

Narration is very effective for stand-alone multimedia programs. Some multimedia development programs include sound recording and editing features. You also can record sound using a sound editing program like Macromedia's SoundEdit 16™. The process of recording sound for use in a multimedia program, however, is quite technical and requires an understanding of the principles of digital sound.

The quality and file size of digital sound is determined by two factors: the sampling resolution and the sampling rate.[24] Resolution, measured in bits, is the difference between the softest and loudest portions of the sound. Eight-bit digital sound is comparable to the quality of a cassette recording, 12-bit sound is comparable to an LP phonograph record, and 16-bit sound is comparable to CD sound. Sampling rate, measured in kilohertz (kHz), indicates the amount of data stored in one second of sound. Higher sampling rates produce better sound fidelity; however, they also produce larger files. The number of channels used for recording also affects the size of the sound files. Stereo sound (two channels) requires twice as much storage space as monaural sound (one channel). For example, CD quality 16-bit, 44.1 kHz stereo sound requires 10 MB per minute while 8-bit, 22 kHz monaural sound requires only 1.25 MB per minute.

Fortunately, the lower settings (8-bit, 22 kHz) usually are more than adequate for narration. If you can spare the hard disk space, most sound experts recommend recording sound with 16-bit, 44.1 kHz settings and converting it to 8-bit, 22 kHz settings. This technique produces better quality sound than if it was recorded at the lower levels initially.

Digital Video Video, as we typically think of it, exists in an analog format and plays at 30 frames per second (fps). For computers to recognize and store video, the analog video and audio signals must be digitized, or converted to a digital format. Because digital video files are very large (one second of video uses 27 MB of storage space), they require compression for storage

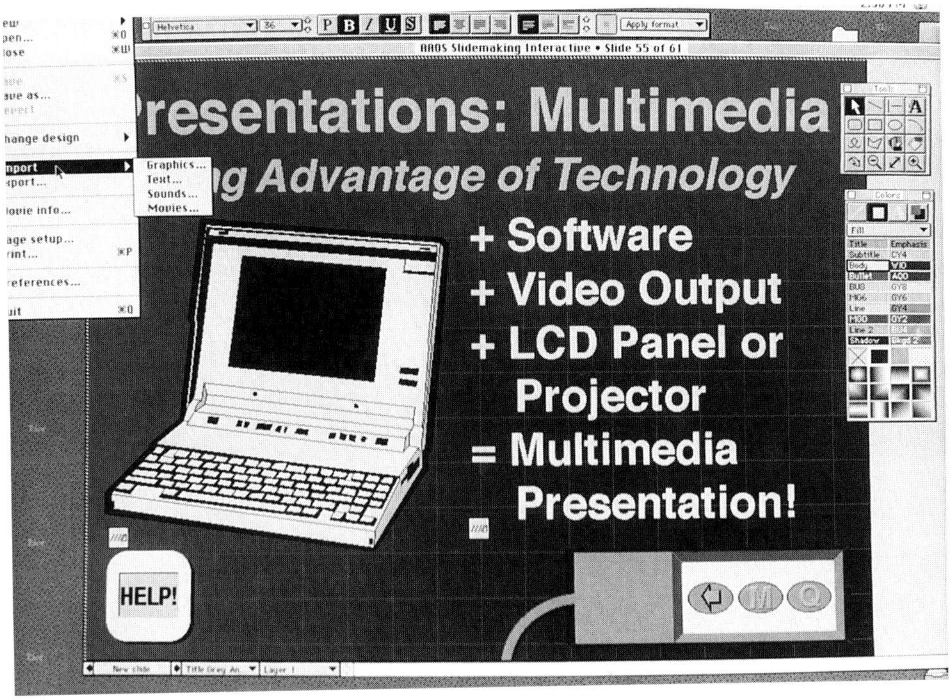

Fig. 8 This computer screen shows a sample of a multimedia presentation being composed in a presentation graphics software program called Adobe Persuasion™ (Courtesy of Adobe Systems, Inc, Mountain View, CA).

on a computer's hard disk. When used in multimedia programs, digital video is decompressed. This process of compressing and decompressing video files is performed by devices called codecs (short for compressor/decompressor).

Until recently, hardware-based codecs like Motion Picture Experts Group (MPEG) provided the only method for digitizing video. This technology produced high quality video (capable of playing video on an entire monitor screen at 30 fps) for a very high price. Software-only codecs, such as Apple's QuickTime™ and Microsoft's Video for Windows™, are more affordable; however, they impose certain limitations. The typical software codec playback window is only 320 by 240 pixels, roughly one quarter the size of the average computer screen. Unless you absolutely need full screen video, this limitation poses no real problem. The most problematic constraint of software-only video is poor image quality and playback rates ranging from 15 to 30 fps. Playback rates less than 30 fps often are choppy or jerky. The development of faster computer chips (Intel's 80486™ and Pentium™ and Motorola's PowerPC™) has greatly improved the playback performance of software codec video, providing rates closer to 30 fps.

Video segments are most effectively used in multimedia to demonstrate a process or emphasize a point. Typically, video segments are displayed in video windows and accompanied by text and graphics. Because of the large size of video files, keep each video segment short, preferably one minute or less. If you plan to produce and digitize your own video, it is extremely important that the original video source be of the highest quality. Ozer[25] has described the video production and capture process as "garbage-in, garbage-out," which means that if the original video is of low quality, the captured video also will be of low quality. A basic knowledge of video formats can improve the quality of your digitized video.

The video formats available, ranged in order from lowest to highest quality, are as follows. VHS and 8-mm formats produce the lowest quality video image. S-VHS, Hi-8, or 3/4-inch video formats produce a higher resolution and fidelity than VHS or 8 mm. They are the bare minimum quality at which digital video should be produced. Betacam SP or 1-inch formats compose the high end of the scale and, therefore, provide the highest quality video image. The equipment necessary to produce this video format is very expensive and is commonly found only in broadcast studios and professional video companies.

Computer Requirements for Multimedia Development

In order to develop multimedia programs, you will need specific computer hardware components.

Random Access Memory (RAM) The average, off-the-shelf multimedia computer has 8 MB of RAM; however, serious multimedia development can require between 16 MB and 128 MB of RAM, depending on the type of multimedia being done and the size of the files being used. Purchase as much RAM as you can afford and be ready to upgrade the RAM once you notice performance deficits.

Hard Disk The newer, faster CPUs (Pentium™ with Windows™ and Power Macintosh™) provide improved playback of video and sound files, increasing the likelihood that the user will use large digital files. Because the files required for multimedia presentations can be enormous, we recommend that you purchase the highest capacity hard disk you can afford. A one gigabyte drive is not unreasonable.

Monitor Computer monitors capable of displaying 24-bit color (16.7 million colors) are the gold standard for developing and displaying high-quality graphic images. Thirteen- and 14-inch monitors (with a resolution of 640 pixels horizontally and 480 lines vertically) are standard for displaying multimedia programs. A larger monitor (17-inch or greater) usually is preferred for developing multimedia. In addition to the monitor, video memory, or VRAM, is important. The more VRAM in your computer, the bigger the monitor and the greater the number of colors your system can support.

CD-ROM A CD-ROM drive (either built-in or external) is essential for serious multimedia development. Two features of CD-ROM drives are extremely important: access time and transfer rate. Access time is the amount of time it takes for the CD-ROM drive to locate information. Transfer rate (measured in kilobytes per second, or kbps) is the rate at which the CD-ROM drive transfers information to the computer. In general, purchase a CD-ROM drive with low access time (400 milliseconds or less) and a high transfer rate (150 kbps or greater).

Multimedia Development Software

Multimedia development software is divided into four categories: traditional presentation, multimedia presentation, multimedia authoring, and high-end authoring systems.[26] Authoring systems, although they offer more features (special effects and range of media elements), are usually more complex and require a greater learning curve.

Consider the following questions when selecting a multimedia development program: (1) What type of multimedia presentations do you plan to develop (both now and in the future)? (2) What is your experience with multimedia? (3) How much money are you willing to spend? (4) What computer platform will you use? If you have not answered these questions, you may find your software selection is not able to perform the tasks you require or is too technical or labor intensive for you and your staff to work with.

If your goal is to develop electronic slide presentations, a traditional presentation program, like Adobe Persuasion™, will be sufficient (Fig. 8). If you intend to use more advanced media elements in combination with advanced level branching, consider a more advanced multimedia authoring package like Macromedia's Director™ (Fig. 9). Director, like many other programs, provides tools for developing graphics, animation, sound, and text internally. This kind of software also serves as an integrator, because it allows developers to create graphics, sound, animation, and video in other software applications and import them.

Presentation Hardware Systems

Laptop Computer The laptop computer, a common companion of many traveling professionals, provides an ideal platform for presenting your multimedia program. Evaluate a potential laptop computer purchase in light of the discussions about RAM and hard disk specifications presented previously in this article.

Liquid Crystal Display (LCD) Panels and Overhead Projectors LCD panels are designed to project a computer monitor's image onto a larger screen with the aid of an overhead projector. There are two types of LCD displays: active matrix and passive matrix. Active matrix panels are critical for the successful delivery of dynamic presentations that include transitions, animation, and video. However, not all of these panels are capable of properly displaying full-motion video. Passive matrix panels definitely are too slow to use for displaying dynamic presentations.

The quality of image displayed by an LCD panel depends principally on the quality of the overhead projector used. There are two types of overhead projectors: transmissive and reflective. A transmissive projector's light comes from below; a reflective projector's light comes from above. LCD panels will work only with transmissive projectors. Because the LCD panel is constructed of multiple layers of glass that can filter much of the light projected by the projector's bulb, brighter projectors produce better images. Panel manufacturers recommend projectors that emit 3,000 to 5,000 lumens for optimal brightness, contrast, and color.[27]

If you plan to use an LCD panel, make certain it is capable of displaying the same range of colors as your computer's monitor. For example, if you create a presentation using 24-bit color (16.7 million colors), but the LCD panel you use to deliver your presentation can display only 256 colors, the appearance of your screens will be noticeably different and of poorer quality.

LCD Projector Portable LCD projectors usually provide more predictable results than LCD panels; however, they also are more expensive. The typical LCD projector consists of three small LCD panels, one for each of the basic color frequencies—red, green, and blue. An internal light source eliminates the need for an overhead projector. LCD projectors employ an active matrix display, which makes them ideal for projecting video images.

Cathode Ray Tube (CRT) Projector The CRT projector, which has three separate phosphor-coated tubes (one each for red, green, and blue), provides greater resolution than the LCD projectors. This type of projector, often seen mounted on the ceiling of an auditorium or meeting room, is characterized by its wide housing.

Remote Control Although you use a computer to deliver your presentation, it is desirable to not be tied to the computer. A remote control, or air mouse, can free you from your computer, yet enable you to control your multimedia presentation. The air mouse is a handheld device that allows you to control the computer's pointer by moving your hand and pressing the remote control's button(s).

The Challenge of Traveling

Lack of familiarity with the computer equipment provided and its compatibility with your multimedia presentation poses the greatest challenge (or, worst nightmare) to successful presentation delivery on the road. Careful planning can prevent disasters. Nevertheless, we refer you again to Russell's Technology Coefficient, presented earlier. A 35-mm slide version of your multimedia presentation is better than no presentation at all. We recommend always creating this backup. When you produce a multimedia project on a presentation software package, normally you will find the capacity to do this.

If you have not requested the right equipment, you have no one to blame but yourself. A prepared checklist of equipment can help guarantee that all equipment needs are met. The following list of questions will help in planning your equipment requirements: (1) What type of computer platform do you need? (Macintosh or Windows) (2) How large a hard disk is required? (3) How much RAM is needed to run your program properly? (4) Do you need to play sound? (5) What type of color monitor do you need, one that is capable of displaying millions of colors (24-bit), thousands of colors (16-bit), or only 256 colors (8-bit)? (6) How will you project the computer screen's image? (LCD panel, LCD projector, CRT projector, computer

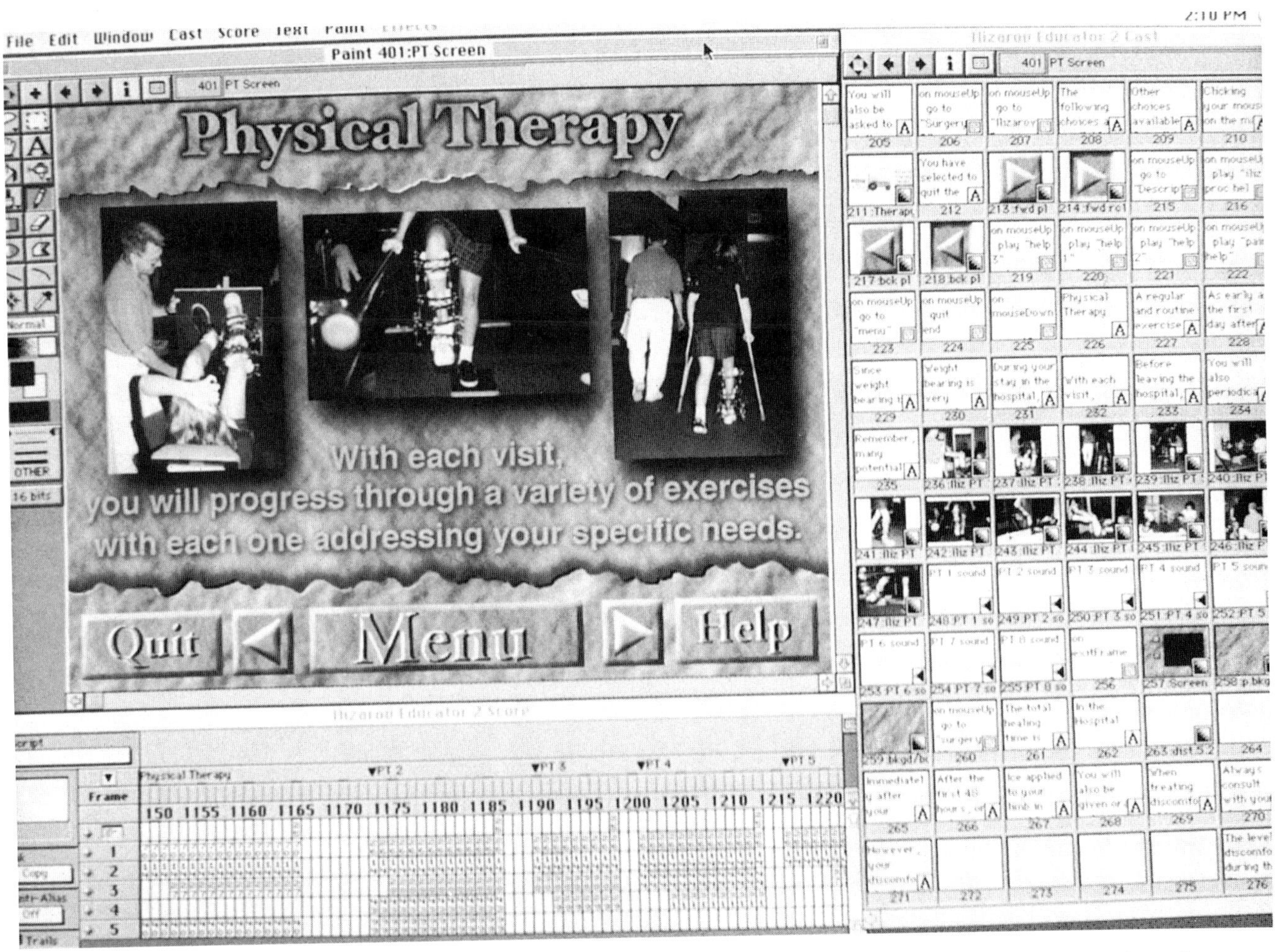

Fig. 9 This computer screen shows a sample of an interactive multimedia program being composed in a multimedia authoring software program called Macromedia Director™ (Courtesy of Macromedia, Inc, San Francisco, CA).

monitor?) (7) Do you need a remote control mouse?

When discussing and requesting equipment, talk directly to the technical person who is in charge of audiovisual equipment for the conference. (Do not be surprised if you find that you are more knowledgeable about computerized presentations than the designated audiovisual technician at any given meeting.) Depending on who is sponsoring the meeting, a computer may or may not be provided at the sponsor's expense. Many presenters prefer to use their own laptop computers. By doing so, usually you can rest assured that your presentation will run. However, you will not know until you arrive at the meeting room how well your computer will interface with the projection system.

Arrive early on the day of your presentation, or seek out your meeting room the day before, to test the room's equipment and practice your presentation. At busy conferences, lunchtime or immediately after the symposium is over for the day are good times to do this.

Always take two copies of your presentation (either on two separate disks or one copy on a removable storage medium and one copy on the hard drive of your laptop) when traveling. Granted, this does become more difficult as the size of your presentation file increases. Most multimedia programs will not fit on a floppy disk. Creating a self-extracting compressed file of the presentation is helpful in many instances. When using a computer provided by the meeting facility, copy your presentation onto the internal hard drive of the computer. Most multimedia programs run more efficiently from the hard drive because their files' information is processed faster than it would be if the files were on a floppy disk or an external storage device.

Conclusion

Clearly, computers have brought new excitement to the world of orthopaedic presentations. This thrilling technology is accompanied by many challenges, however. We recommend that each presenter, even the most experienced, first study and subscribe to the introductory six points made in this article. Once this preparatory work is woven into your presenting, embark on your own experimentation with computer technology. Always adhere to basic design principles. After that, simply try different approaches until you find one that is agreeable to you and that is successful with your audiences. Undoubtedly, in a very short time even greater advances in computer technology will propel our ability to instruct to new heights. Orthopaedic education will never be the same.

Acknowledgment

The authors gratefully acknowledge Charles C. Canton of Houston, Texas, for his technical contributions about IBM-compatible computer technology.

References

1. Hendricks HG (ed): *Teaching to Change Lives.* Portland, OR, Multnomah Press, 1987.
2. Kroenke K: The 10-minute talk. *Am J Med* 1987;83:329–330.
3. Swindoll CR (ed): *Growing Strong in the Seasons of Life.* Grand Rapids, MI, Zondervan, 1983.
4. Bernstein TM (ed): *The Careful Writer: A Modern Guide to English Usage.* New York, NY, Atheneum, 1977.
5. Blauvelt CT, Nelson FRT (eds): *A Manual of Orthopaedic Terminology*, ed 4. St. Louis, MO, CV Mosby, 1990.
6. Day RA (ed): *How to Write and Publish a Scientific Paper*, ed 4. Phoenix, AZ, Oryx Press, 1994.
7. Hoppenfeld S, Zeide MS (eds): *Orthopaedic Dictionary.* Philadelphia, PA, JB Lippincott, 1994.
8. Kilcoyne RF, Farrar E (eds): *Handbook of Orthopedic Terminology.* Boca Raton, FL, CRC Press, 1991.
9. Strunk W, White EB (eds): *The Elements of Style*, ed 3. New York, NY, Macmillan, 1979.
10. Zar JH: Candidate for a pullet surprise. *J Irreproducible Results* 1994;39:13.
11. Nelson RC: Are your presentations sliding away? *Sports Med Bull* 1978;13:8–9.
12. Nelson RC: Are your presentations still sliding away? *Sports Med Bull* 1990;25:14.
13. Rabb MY (ed): *The Presentation Design Book: Tips, Techniques and Advice for Creating Effective, Attractive Slides, Overheads, Multimedia Presentations, Screen Shows and More*, ed 2. Chapel Hill, NC, Ventana Press, 1993.
14. Russell JA, Woods GW: Research communication media: Creating an outstanding impression with abstracts, poster exhibits, and slides, in Schafer M (ed): *Instructional Course Lectures 43.* Rosemont, IL, American Academy of Orthopaedic Surgeons, 1994, pp 625–637.
15. Mandel S (ed): *Technical Presentation Skills.* Menlo Park, CA, Crisp Publications, 1994.
16. Eastman Kodak Company: *Effective Presentation Images.* Rochester, NY, Eastman Kodak, 1993, (Pub No S-101).
17. Bishop A (ed): *Slides: Planning and Producing Slide Programs.* Rochester, NY, Eastman Kodak, 1989, (Pub No S-30).
18. Eastman Kodak Company: *More Slides: Planning, Producing, and Presenting Digital Images.* Rochester, NY, Eastman Kodak, 1993, (Pub No S-30A).
19. Kenny MF (ed): *Presenting Yourself.* Rochester, NY, Eastman Kodak, 1994, (Pub No S-60).
20. Tway LE (ed): *Welcome to Multimedia.* New York, NY, MIS Press, 1992.
21. Larson DE: Effective screen designs for nursing CAI. *Comput Nurs* 1984;2:224–228.
22. Cohen VB: Interactive features in the design of videodisc material. *Educational Technology* 1984;24:16–20.
23. Sirota W: Audio: A sound foundation. *Multimedia World* 1994; 1:92–93.
24. Desmarais N (ed): *Multimedia on the PC: A Guide for Information Professionals.* New York, NY, McGraw-Hill, 1994.
25. Ozer J: Capture their hearts and minds with video. *Presentations* 1995;9:32–38.
26. Martinez CD: All that jazz. *Presentations* 1994;9:44–50.
27. Tuck L: Improving your image with LCD panels. *Presentations* 1994;8:32–34.

Index